Allergens and Allergen Immunotherapy

CLINICAL ALLERGY AND IMMUNOLOGY

Series Editors

MICHAEL A. KALINER, M.D.

Medical Director
Institute for Asthma and Allergy
Washington, D.C.

RICHARD F. LOCKEY, M.D.

Professor of Medicine, Pediatrics, and Public Health
Joy McCann Culverhouse Professor of Allergy and Immunology
Director, Division of Allergy and Immunology
University of South Florida College of Medicine
and James A. Haley Veterans Hospital
Tampa, Florida

ADDITIONAL VOLUMES IN PREPARATION

Allergens and Allergen Immunotherapy

Third Edition, Revised and Expanded

edited by

Richard F. Lockey
Samuel C. Bukantz

University of South Florida College of Medicine and
James A. Haley Veterans' Hospital
Tampa, Florida, U.S.A.

Jean Bousquet

Montpellier University
Montpellier, France

MARCEL DEKKER, INC.   NEW YORK · BASEL

The second edition of this book was edited by Richard F. Lockey and Samuel C. Bukantz.

Library of Congress Cataloging-in-Publication Data
A catalog record for this book is available from the Library of Congress.

ISBN: 0-8247-5650-9

This book is printed on acid-free paper.

Headquarters
Marcel Dekker, Inc., 270 Madison Avenue, New York, NY 10016, U.S.A.
tel: 212-696-9000; fax: 212-685-4540

Distribution and Customer Service
Marcel Dekker, Inc., Cimarron Road, Monticello, New York 12701, U.S.A.
tel: 800-228-1160; fax: 845-796-1772

Eastern Hemisphere Distribution
Marcel Dekker AG, Hutgasse 4, Postfach 812, CH-4001 Basel, Switzerland
tel: 41-61-260-6300; fax: 41-61-260-6333

World Wide Web
http://www.dekker.com

The publisher offers discounts on this book when ordered in bulk quantities. For more information, write to Special Sales/Professional Marketing at the headquarters address above.

PRINTED IN THE UNITED STATES OF AMERICA

To our coeditor,
Samuel C. Bukantz—the compleat teacher,
author, editor, researcher, and clinician

R.F.L
J.B.

Series Introduction

As I look at my library, the most obviously well-read book is the first edition of *Allergen Immunotherapy*. That book helped me establish plans for private practice and served me very well. The second edition, *Allergens and Allergen Immunotherapy,* provided many useful additions to my treatment plans for immunotherapy. Now, there is a third edition, extending the knowledge and applications of the first two books. I might suggest that this book be required reading for all practitioners who prescribe allergy immunotherapy. Where else is theory and practice in such an important subject so well combined and in such useful detail? This book takes the principles of allergens, immunotherapy, and the treatment of allergic disease to a very practical but evidence-based level.

The background for immunotherapy is provided in historical and immunological terms, as well as in aerobiological principles. These chapters provide a solid basis for understanding why we give immunotherapy. Unless one understands the allergens, their importance, and how to decide which is causing patient-related disease, then proper decision-making regarding immunotherapy cannot be applied. Chapters on specific allergens are essential to practitioners prescribing immunotherapy.

As part of my practice, I see patients who have had unsuccessful treatments with allergen immunotherapy. Many of the patients were poor candidates for allergy immunotherapy from the beginning and others were given improper mixes of allergens, administered incorrectly. This book addresses these issues using a very practical approach, detailing how and when to give immunotherapy, for how long, and to which patients. Potential problems encountered in the course of immunotherapy are described and solutions presented.

One of the major advances in prescribing immunotherapy has been the recognition that the constitution of the mixtures and preserving allergenicity are essential to efficacy, and that using sufficient allergen concentration is a minimal prerequisite for long-term benefit. Chapters detailing allergen preparation and administration offer information that is essential to the decision-making process, and these concepts have changed over the past 10 years. Experienced allergists will benefit from re-reading these chapters.

The range of clinical problems for which immunotherapy is an option is described in detail. The usefulness of immunotherapy in allergic rhinoconjunctivitis and asthma, as well as in hymenoptera sensitivity, is presented. Other desensitizations, including drug allergy, are outlined, as are novel treatments such as the newly introduced monoclonal anti-IgE therapy. This is not a clinical allergy text, but it raises and answers the questions of who should get immunotherapy and what to expect. Other forms of treatment besides immunotherapy and their use along with immunotherapy are covered, as are potential future extensions of this treatment. There is limited use of sublingual-swollen immunotherapy in the United States; however, this is a popular form of treatment for mild allergic disease in Europe and the data are presented here.

I find this text to be compelling in its comprehensive approach to the most important disease-modifying treatment available for allergic rhinitis and allergic asthma. It should be read by allergists who want to know where we are with proper immunotherapy and where we are going with this treatment modality. It should be read by those clinicians who use alternative approaches to immunotherapy in order to recognize why allergen immunotherapy is effective and what goes into proper preparation and administration of effective immunotherapy. And, it should be read by clinicians whose patients are receiving immunotherapy to be certain that the immunotherapy prescribed has been ordered appropriately and is being administered correctly.

I am pleased to add this volume to our series of venerable books.

Michael A. Kaliner

Preface

The first edition of *Allergen Immunotherapy*, published in 1991, contains 13 chapters. The second edition, *Allergens and Allergen Immunotherapy* published eight years later, expanded to 33 chapters in order to more precisely define the biochemical and molecular characteristics of the allergen groups, the methods of their manufacture and standardization, and the techniques of their administration in the treatment of allergic diseases.

Global contributions to the understanding of the basic mechanism of the allergic reaction has improved the efficacy of immunotherapy of allergic disease. Many of the scientific contributions have come from around the world, and this prompted the addition of Dr. Jean Bousquet of Marseilles as co-editor. Dr. Bousquet, well-known for his studies of the immunotherapy of allergic diseases and asthma, has been influential in the selection of additional investigators, whose contributions are included in this third edition, and the book has been expanded to 41 chapters.

The chapters have been grouped into five parts.

Part I, Basics   Details the mechanisms of IgE-mediated disease and how immunotherapy affects that mechanism and alters the course of the disease.

Part II, Allergens   Describes inhalational, ingested, and injected allergens as well as those, like latex and drugs, that may have multiple sites of introduction.

Part III, Immunotherapy Techniques   Describes the manufacture and standardization of the allergens for injection and their labeling as allergen vaccines as recommended in 1998 by the World Health Organization.

Part IV, Other Types of Immunotherapy   Describes inhalational and oral routes of administration, the value of DNA vaccines, anti-IgE therapy, and novel approaches to immunotherapy with inhalant allergens.

Part V, Prevention and Management of Adverse Effects   Details how to avoid and treat adverse effects as well as how to prevent and treat anaphylaxis.

All chapters have been updated and organized in a manner that will facilitate use of this volume as a reference source for the use of allergens in immunotherapy.

Particularly interesting, in Part IV, is the chapter by Li and Sampson on the possibility of immunotherapeutic management of food allergy. In their opinion, "Establishment of animal models of food hypersensitivity, including sensitization by the oral route and anaphylaxis by oral challenge, has facilitated the investigation of therapies of food allergy".

Clemens Von Pirquet coined the word "allergy," hoping it would "facilitate new research workers to study the interesting phenomena in the field." With the advent of molecular biology, this has since been realized. While there have been many contributions to the cellular and biological understanding of these "phenomena," basic concepts remain. This, despite the fact that great advances in science have been converting biochemistry to anatomy, when function becomes reduced to structure. Immunotherapy profits by these revelations.

The editors thank Geeta Gehi, whose dedication was absolutely essential to completing this third edition.

Richard F. Lockey
Samuel C. Bukantz
Jean Bousquet

Contents

Contributors

Jonathan A. Bernstein, M.D.   Division of Immunology/ Allergy Section, Department of Internal Medicine, University of Cincinnati College of Medicine, Cincinnati, Ohio, U.S.A.

Jacques de Blic, M.D.   Service de Pneumologie et d'Allergologie Pédiatriques, Hôpital Necker-Enfants Malades, Paris, France

R. Matthew Bloebaum, M.D.   Department of Internal Medicine, University of Texas Medical Branch, Galveston, Texas, U.S.A.

Malcolm N. Blumenthal, M.D.   Departments of Medicine, Pediatrics, and Laboratory Medicine and Pathology, University of Minnesota, Minneapolis, Minnesota, U.S.A.

Jean Bousquet, M.D., Ph.D.   Department of Respiratory Medicine and Allergology, Montpellier University, Montpellier, France

Samuel C. Bukantz, M.D.   Department of Internal Medicine, University of South Florida College of Medicine and James A. Haley Veterans' Administration Hospital, Tampa, Florida, U.S.A.

Wesley Burks, M.D.   Department of Pediatric Allergy and Immunology, Duke University Medical Center, Durham, North Carolina, U.S.A.

Walter G. Canonica, M.D.   Allergy and Respiratory Diseases, Department of Internal Medicine, University of Genoa, Genoa, Italy

Luis Caraballo, M.D., Ph.D.   Department of Immunological Research, University of Cartagena, Cartagena, Colombia

Martin D. Chapman, Ph.D.   Department of Internal Medicine, University of Virginia, and INDOOR Biotechnologies Inc., Charlottesville, Virginia, U.S.A.

Badrul A. Chowdhury, M.D., Ph.D.   Division of Pulmonary and Allergy Drug Products, U.S. Food and Drug Administration, Rockville, Maryland, U.S.A.

Sheldon G. Cohen, M.D.   National Institute of Allergy and Infectious Diseases, National Institutes of Health, Bethesda, Maryland, U.S.A.

Linda Cox, M.D.   Department of Medicine, Nova Southeastern University College of Osteopathic Medicine, Fort Lauderdale, Florida, U.S.A.

Patrick J. DeMarco, M.D.   Department of Internal Medicine, University of South Florida College of Medicine and James A. Haley Veterans' Administration Hospital, Tampa, Florida, U.S.A.

Richard D. deShazo, M.D.   Departments of Medicine and Pediatrics, University of Mississippi Medical Center, Jackson, Mississippi, U.S.A.

Nilesh Dharajiya, M.D.   Department of Internal Medicine, University of Texas Medical Branch, Galveston, Texas, U.S.A.

Stephen R. Durham, M.D., F.R.C.P.   Department of Upper Respiratory Medicine, Imperial College, London, England

Robert E. Esch, Ph.D.   Research and Development, Greer Laboratories, Inc., Lenoir, North Carolina, U.S.A.

Richard Evans III, M.D.   (Retired) Northwestern University Medical School and Children's Memorial Hospital, Chicago, Illinois, U.S.A.

Enrique Fernández-Caldas, Ph.D.   Research and Development, C.B.F. LETI, S.A., Tres Cantos, Madrid, Spain

Fatima Ferreira, Ph.D.   Institute of Genetics, University of Salzburg, Salzburg, Austria

Anthony J. Frew, M.D., F.R.C.P.   Infection, Inflammation and Repair Division, University of Southampton School of Medicine, Southampton, England

David B.K. Golden, M.D.   Division of Allergy-Immunology, Johns Hopkins University, Baltimore, Maryland, U.S.A.

Leslie C. Grammer, M.D.   Department of Medicine, Northwestern University Medical School, Chicago, Illinois, U.S.A.

J. Andrew Grant, M.D., F.A.C.P., F.A.A.A.I.   Departments of Internal Medicine and Microbiology/Immunology, University of Texas Medical Branch, Galveston, Texas, U.S.A.

Priyanka Gupta, M.D.   Division of Allergy-Immunology, Department of Medicine, Northwestern University Medical School, Chicago, Illinois, U.S.A.

Miles Guralnick   Vespa Laboratories, Inc., Spring Mills, Pennsylvania, U.S.A.

Eckard Hamelmann   Department of Pediatric Pneumology and Immunology, University Hospital Charité-Virchow, Berlin, Germany

Ricki M. Helm, Ph.D. Department of Microbiology/Immunology, University of Arkansas for Medical Sciences, Little Rock, Arkansas, U.S.A.

Vivian P. Hernandez-Trujillo, M.D. Department of Allergy/Immunology, University of Tennessee College of Medicine, Memphis, Tennessee, U.S.A.

Donald R. Hoffman, Ph.D. Department of Pathology and Laboratory Medicine, Brody School of Medicine at East Carolina University, Greenville, North Carolina, U.S.A.

W. Elliott Horner, Ph.D. Microbiology, Air Quality Sciences, Inc., Marietta, Georgia

Christian Gauguin Houghton, M.Sc. Department of Formulation and Process Development, ALK-Abelló, Hørsholm, Denmark

Lars Jacobsen, Ph.D. Department of Research and Development, ALK-Abelló, Hørsholm, Denmark

Stephen F. Kemp, M.D. Division of Allergy and Immunology, Department of Medicine, University of Mississippi Medical Center, Jackson, Mississippi, U.S.A.

Te Piao King, Ph.D. Department of Biochemistry, Rockefeller University, New York, New York, U.S.A.

Viswanath P. Kurup, Ph.D. Department of Pediatrics and Medicine, Medical College of Wisconsin, Milwaukee, Wisconsin, U.S.A.

Mark Larché, Ph.D. Department of Allergy and Clinical Immunology, Imperial College London Faculty of Medicine, London, England

Jørgen Nedergaard Larsen, Ph.D. Department of Research and Development, ALK-Abelló, Hørsholm, Denmark

Samuel B. Lehrer, Ph.D. Clinical Immunology, Department of Medicine, Tulane University Health Sciences Center, New Orleans, Louisiana, U.S.A.

Estelle Levetin, Ph.D. Department of Biological Science, University of Tulsa, Tulsa, Oklahoma, U.S.A.

Xiu-Min Li, M.D. Department of Pediatrics, Mount Sinai School of Medicine, New York, New York, U.S.A.

Phillip L. Lieberman, M.D. Department of Medicine and Pediatrics, University of Tennessee College of Medicine, Memphis, Tennessee, U.S.A.

Richard F. Lockey, M.D. Department of Internal Medicine, University of South Florida College of Medicine and James A. Haley Veterans' Administration Hospital, Tampa, Florida, U.S.A.

Manuel Lombardero, Ph.D.   Department of Research and Development, ALK-Abelló, Madrid, Spain

Henning Løwenstein, Ph.D., D.Sc.   Department of Scientific Affairs, ALK-Abelló, Hørsholm, Denmark

Hans-Jørgen Malling, M.D.   Allergy Clinic, National University Hospital, Copenhagen, Denmark

Rauno Mäntyjärvi, M.D.   Department of Clinical Microbiology, University of Kuopio, Kuopio, Finland

François-Bernard Michel, M.D., Ph.D.   Department of Respiratory Diseases, Montpellier University, Montpellier, France

Shyam S. Mohapatra, Ph.D.   Department of Internal Medicine, University of South Florida College of Medicine and James A. Haley Veterans' Administration Hospital, Tampa, Florida, U.S.A.

Nadine Mothes, M.D.   Department of Pathophysiology, University of Vienna, Vienna Medical School, Vienna, Austria

Ulrich R. Müller, M.D.   Medinische Klinik, Spital Bern Ziegler, Bern, Switzerland

Harold S. Nelson, M.D.   Department of Medicine, National Jewish Medical and Research Center, and the University of Colorado Health Sciences Center, Denver, Colorado, U.S.A.

Giovanni Passalacqua, M.D.   Allergy and Respiratory Diseases, Department of Internal Medicine, University of Genoa, Genoa, Italy

Marshall Plaut, M.D.   Division of Allergy, Immunology and Transplantation, National Institute of Allergy and Infectious Diseases, National Institutes of Health, Bethesda, Maryland, U.S.A.

Florentino Polo, Ph.D.   Department of Research and Development, ALK-Abelló, S.A., Madrid, Spain

Anna Pomés, Ph.D.   INDOOR Biotechnologies, Inc., Charlottesville, Virginia, U.S.A.

Claude Ponvert, M.D.   Service de Pneumologie et d'Allergologie Pédiatriques, Hôpital Necker-Enfants Malades, Paris, France

Leonardo Puerta, Ph.D.   Institute of Immunological Research, University of Cartagena, Cartagena, Colombia

Andreas Rosenberg, Ph.D.   Department of Laboratory Medicine and Pathology, University of Minnesota, Minneapolis, Minnesota, U.S.A.

Daniel Rotrosen, M.D. Division of Allergy, Immunology and Transplantation, National Institute of Allergy and Infectious Diseases, National Institutes of Health, Bethesda, Maryland, U.S.A.

Patrick Rufin, M.D. Service de Pneumologie et d'Allergologie Pédiatriques, Hôpital Necker-Enfants Malades, Paris, France

Hugh A. Sampson, M.D. Departments of Pediatrics and Immunobiology, Mount Sinai School of Medicine, New York, New York, U.S.A.

Pierre Scheinmann, M.D. Service de Pneumologie et d'Allergologie Pédiatriques, Hôpital Necker-Enfants Malades, Paris, France

Jay E. Slater, M.D. U.S. Food and Drug Administration, Bethesda, Maryland, U.S.A.

Roland Solensky, M.D. Department of Allergy and Immunology, The Corvallis Clinic, Corvallis, Oregon, U.S.A.

Abba I. Terr, M.D. Department of Medicine, University of California, San Francisco, School of Medicine, San Francisco, California, U.S.A.

Stephen J. Till, M.D., Ph.D. Department of Upper Respiratory Medicine, Imperial College, London, England

Rudolf Valenta, M.D. Department of Pathophysiology, University of Vienna, Vienna Medical School, Vienna, Austria

Erkka Valovirta, M.D., Ph.D. Turku Allergy Center, Turku, Finland

Antonio M. Vignola, M.D., Ph.D. Department of Respiratory Diseases, Palermo University, Palermo, Italy

Hari M. Vijay, Ph.D. Environmental Health Directorate, Health Canada, Ottawa, Ontario, Canada

Tuomas Virtanen, M.D. Department of Clinical Microbiology, University of Kuopio, Kuopio, Finland

Ulrich Wahn, M.D. Department of Pediatric Pneumology and Immunology, University Hospital Charité-Virchow, Berlin, Germany

Kerstin Westritschnig, M.D. Department of Pathophysiology, University of Vienna, Vienna Medical School, Vienna, Austria

John W. Yunginger, M.D. Departments of Pediatrics and Internal Medicine, Mayo Medical School, Rochester, Minnesota, U.S.A.

Allergen Immunotherapy in Historical Perspective

SHELDON G. COHEN

National Institute of Allergy and Infectious Diseases, National Institutes of Health, Bethesda, Maryland, U.S.A.

RICHARD EVANS III

Northwestern University Medical School and Children's Memorial Hospital, Chicago, Illinois, U.S.A.

I. IMMUNITAS

Latin; immunis (adj.), immunitas (n.): exemp(tion) free(dom) from cost, burden, tax, obligation.

Original usage of term pertained to the inferior Roman class of plebeians, artisans, and foreign traders who—deprived of religious, civil, and political rights and advantages of

---

A lengthier account and more detailed coverage of subject material presented in this review can be found in Cohen SG, Evans R. Asthma, allergy and immunotherapy: A historical review. Allergy Proc 1992; Part I, 13:47; Part II, 13:407.

the patrician gentes—were immune to taxation, compulsory military service, and civic obligations and functions. After 294 B.C., with the transition of the monarchy to the Roman Republic, immunitas defined special privileges (e.g., exemptions from compulsory military service and taxation granted by the Roman Senate to sophists, philosophers, teachers, and public physicians). In later years, common use of the Anglicized descriptor immunity continued to have legal relevance. Into the Middle Ages, Church property and clergy were granted immunity from civil taxes. In 1689, the English Bill of Rights formalized Parliamentary immunity protecting members of the British Parliament from liability for statements made during debates on the floor. In France, a century later, a 1790 law prevented arrests of a member of the legislature during periods of legislative sessions without specific authorization of the accused member's chamber.

The first medically relevant usage of the term appears to be that of the Roman poet Lucan [Marcus Annaeus Lucanus (39–65 A.D.)] in "Pharsolia" on referring to the "immunes" of members of the North African Psylli tribe to snakebite. In the scientific literature with definitive medical usage, the term appeared in an 1879 issue of London's *St. George's Hospital Reports (IX:715)*: "In one of the five instances . . . the apparent immunity must have lasted for at least two years, that being the interval between the two diphtheritic visitation." The following year the descriptor found a place in medical terminology with Pasteur's (Fig. 1) report of his seminal work on attenuation of the causal agent of fowl cholera, noting the "(induction) of a benign illness that immunizes (Fr. immunise) against a fatal illness" (1).

II. IMMUNITY THROUGH INTERVENTION

Anthropological records reveal that from the earliest times that humans sought to understand the factors that made for well-being, there were attempts to intervene to prevent deviations from health and well-being. Healers of antiquity, priest-doctors, secular sorcerers, medicine men, practitioners of folk medicine all played influential roles. In the ancient cradles of civilization—Mesopotamia, Babylonia, Assyria, Egypt—magic and mystic methods were created to ward off divine and cosmic-directed afflictions mediated through spirits and demons with tools of intervention such as incantations, rituals, sacrifices, amulets, and talismans. In the biblical era of the Old Testament, freedom from disease and affliction (which were believed to be divine punishment for sin) was sought through the power of prayer and left in the hands of rabbis who took on the dual role of healer. In sixth-century B.C. India, preventive practice became synonymous with following the enlightened morality teachings of Buddha [Gautama (566?–c. 480 B.C.)]. To herbs and dietary manipulations critical for maintaining health and disease promoting balances between internal Yang and Yin forces, ancient China added physical methods. To drain off Yang or Yin excesses, procedures employed insertion of needles (acupuncture) and heat-induced blistering (moxibustion at organ-related skin points along channels of vital flow). According to the tenets originating in classical Greece—with the writings of Hippocrates (460–370 B.C.)—and extended in Roman medicine by Claudius Galen (130–200 A.D.), it was the four internal humors (blood, phlegm, yellow bile, and black bile) that were determinants of health and disease. Their pathogenetic imbalances could be corrected by preventively draining off excesses of the humors through the interventions of bleeding, blistering (by cupping), sweating (by steam baths), purging, and inducing expectoration and emesis.

Regarding pestilence, the observation that survivors of an epidemic were spared from being stricken during return waves of the same illness was described by the ancient

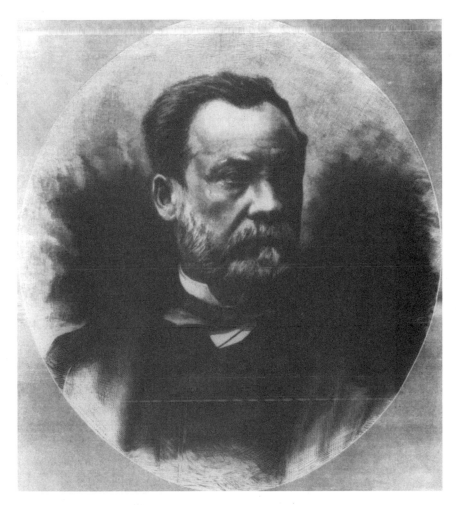

Figure 1   Louis Pasteur, Sc.D. (1822–1895). Founding Director of the Institut Pasteur, Paris. (Courtesy of the National Library of Medicine.)

historians (2) Thucydides (c. 460–400 B.C.) (Fig. 2), who described the plague of Athens, and Procopicus of Byzantine (c. 490–562 A.D.), who wrote about the plague of Justinian that struck Mediterranean ports and coastal towns. First attempts to duplicate this natural phenomenon appeared in the eleventh century, when Chinese itinerant healers developed a method to prevent contracting potentially fatal smallpox. These healers were able to deliberately induce a milder transient pox illness through the medium of dried powder prepared from material recovered from a patient's healing skin pustules and blown into a recipient's nostrils. The practice disseminated along China-Persia-Turkey trade routes ultimately reached Europe and the American colonies following communications with England in 1714–1716 by Timoni, a Constantinople physician (3), and Pylorini, the Venetian counsel in Smyrna (Izmir) (4). Although effective in reducing susceptibility and incidence in epidemic attack, variolation presented difficulties; inoculations sometimes resulted in severe, even fatal, primary illness and recipients could serve as sources of trans- mittable infection until all active lesions healed. A solution to the problem was found in

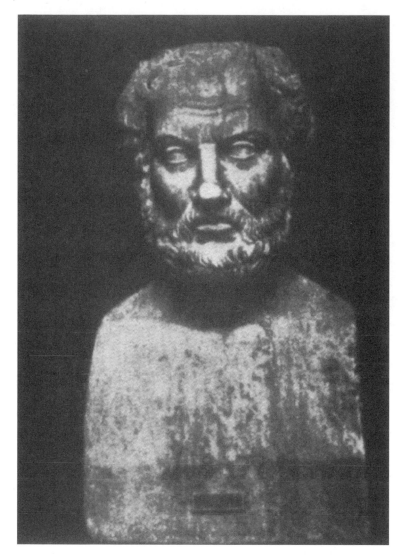

Figure 2 Thucydides (c. 460–400 B.C.). Greek historian. (From Gordon BL. Medicine Throughout Antiquity, 1949. Courtesy of F. A. Davis Company, Philadelphia.)

the investigations of Jenner (Fig. 3), the English rural physician who in 1795 reported a new benign method to prevent smallpox by inducing a single pustule of a related, but different, skin disease, cowpox (vaccinia, from *vaccinus*, Latin, pertaining to a cow)—a lesion resembling smallpox only in appearance. From its name, the procedure became known as vaccination (5).

Jenner's carefully designed protocols carried out in 1796 stimulated experimental leads and raised a number of pertinent questions for future investigators: (1) Were disease-producing and protective (antigenic) qualities interdependent and equivalent? (Jenner had noted that some stored, presumably deteriorated, pox material did not evoke a vaccination lesion; however, he was unable to ascertain whether it still was capable of providing a

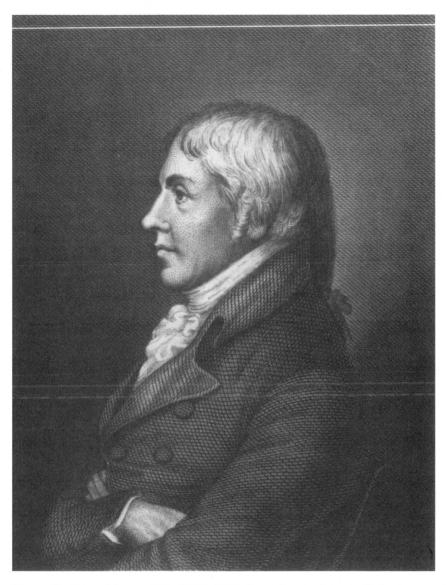

Figure 3   Edward Jenner, M.D. (1749–1823). Practicing physician in Cheltenham, rural England. (Courtesy of the National Library of Medicine.)

protective effect.) (2) Could two different agents share the ability to induce identical protective responses? (Jenner believed vaccination succeeded because smallpox and cowpox were different manifestations of the same disease.) (3) Could the same agent induce both protection against disease and tissue injury? (Jenner's description of the appearance of a local inflammatory lesion after revaccination provided the earliest documentation of hypersensitivity phenomena as a function of the immune response.)

Koch's and Pasteur's early endeavors to develop preventive vaccines were innovative giant steps in establishing immunization as an efficacious measure in disease prevention; they also served as models for later developments of allergen immunotherapy.

Pasteur's use of attenuated microorganisms as vaccines (1) in fowl cholera and sheep anthrax demonstrated that specific antigenic immunizing potential was not impaired by decreasing virulence of a bacterium (5a). Later studies by Salmon and Smith (6) with heat-killed vaccines indicated that immunogenicity also did not require antigen viability.

Some unfortunate outcomes of early immunotherapeutic ventures temporarily hindered the future of immunotherapy with allergens. Koch was premature in introducing injectable preparations of glycerol extracts of tubercle bacilli cultures for the treatment of tuberculosis. His error revealed that violent systemic reactions could result from injection of antigens that acted as specific challenges in delayed hypersensitivity states (7). Pasteur's rabies vaccine met with enthusiastic success, but antigens of the rabbit spinal cords, used as culture medium for the aging rabies virus, also induced simultaneous production of antinervous tissue antibodies and adverse autoimmune neurological reactions (8).

Practical approaches to immunization in the Western world might have had an earlier beginning had cognizance been taken of a centuries-old practice in Egypt. Dating back to antiquity, snake charmers in the temples—and later religious snake dancers among native Southwest American Indians—had found the key to protection from the danger of their craft. Beginning with self-inflicted bites from young snakes as sources of small amounts of venom, and progressing to repetition by large snakes led to tolerant outcomes of otherwise potentially fatal challenges. However, it was not until 1887 that Sewall's (Fig. 4) experimental inoculation of rattlesnake venom in an animal model introduced appreciation and development of antitoxins (9).

The discovery of diphtheria exotoxin (10) spurred the practice of inducing antitoxins in laboratory animals and their therapeutic use by passive immunization (11). The fact that the resultant antitoxins evolved into therapeutically effective agents was due to Ehrlich's (Fig. 5) studies on the chemical nature of antigen-antibody reactions and applications to biological standardization (12). Further, the methods by which antitoxins were obtained enabled early stages of development of allergen immunotherapy (13). Subsequently, development of severe life-threatening hypersensitivity reactions following injection of the antibodies in serum proteins of the actively immunized horse (14) created a virtually insurmountable obstacle in later attempts to initiate therapy of hay fever by passive immunization (13).

III. GENESIS OF ALLERGEN IMMUNOTHERAPY

Discoveries in immunity gave rise to another pioneering area of study within the newly established discipline, and the introduction of immunologically based therapies for infectious diseases soon followed. The impact of widening applications of immunotherapy was largely responsible, in the first half of the nineteenth century, for the evolution of allergy as a separate segment of medical practice. The forerunner of this relationship occurred in 1819, when Bostock, a London physician, precisely described his own personal experience and classical case history of hay fever (15). This landmark account of allergic disease was recorded only 23 years after Jenner's controlled demonstration of the ability of inoculation with cowpox to prevent smallpox (2).

Some 70-odd years after Bostock's report, Wyman identified pollen as the cause of autumnal catarrh in the United States (16). A year later, Blackley published confirmative descriptions based on self-experimentation which established that grass pollen was the cause of his seasonal catarrh, which was noninfective (17). He also made the first investigational reference to allergen immunotherapy when he repeatedly applied grass pollen to

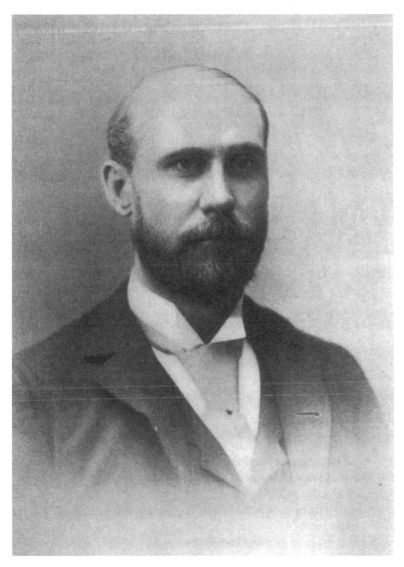

Figure 4 Henry Sewall, M.D., Ph.D. (1855–1936). Professor and Chairman, Department of Physiology, University of Michigan. (From Webb GB, Powell D. Henry Sewall, Physiologist and Physician. 1946. Johns Hopkins; Courtesy of Johns Hopkins University Press, Baltimore.)

his abraded skin areas, but without resultant diminution of local cutaneous reactions or lessened susceptibility.

In 1900, Curtis reported that immunizing injections of watery extracts of certain pollens appeared to benefit patients with coryza and/or asthma caused by these pollens (18). Dunbar (Fig. 6) then attempted to apply the principle of passive immunization developed with diphtheria and tetanus antitoxin to the preventive treatment of human hay fever. He tried using "pollatin," a horse and rabbit antipollen antibody preparation. As a powder or ointment, it was developed for instillation in and absorption from the eyes, nose, and mouth and as pastille inhalational material for asthma (12). Subsequent attempts to

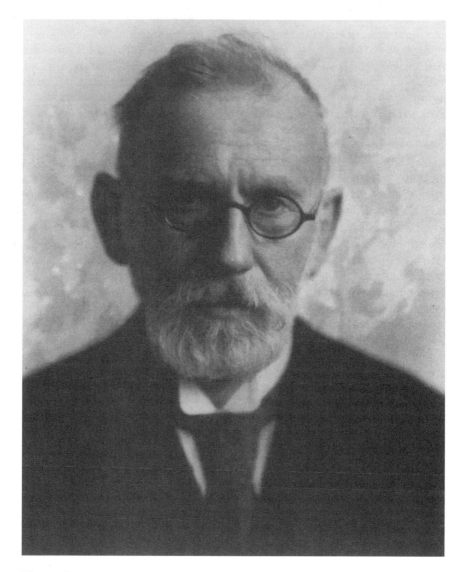

Figure 5   Paul Ehrlich, M.D. (1854–1915). Founding Director of the Institute for Experimental Therapy, Frankfurt. (Courtesy of the National Library of Medicine.)

immunize with grass pollen extract were abandoned because of severe systemic symptoms induced by excessive doses. Dunbar's associate, Prausnitz, had failed to diminish either the mucous membrane reactions or symptom manifestations of hay fever after "thousands" of ocular installations of pollen "toxin" (13). Dunbar then attempted immunization with pollen toxin-antitoxin (T-AT) neutralized mixtures—a technique that had been used with bacterial exotoxins (e.g., tetanus and diphtheria) (19).

While Dunbar's anecdotal reports of success could not be duplicated, the discovery of anaphylaxis formed a new concept of immunity and its relevance to immunotherapy. In 1902, Portier and Richet described anaphylactic shock and death in dogs under immunization

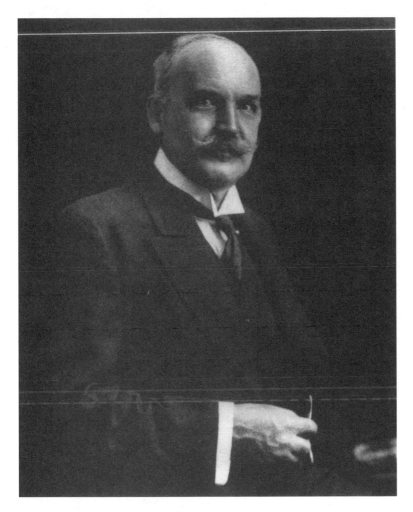

Figure 6   William Dunbar, M.D. (1863–1922). Director of the State Hygienic Institute, Hamburg. (Courtesy of the Hygienisches Institut, Hamburg, Germany.)

with toxins from sea anemones (20). Four years later, these exciting and provocative animal experiments were followed by reports of sudden death in humans after the injection of horse serum antitoxins, and of exhaustive protocols with experimental animals that implicated anaphylactic shock as the likely mechanism (21). Smith made similar observations while standardizing antitoxins, which prompted Otto to refer to the findings as "the Theobald Smith Phenomenon" (22).

Wolff-Eisner applied the concept of hypersensitivity to a conceptual understanding of hay fever (23). Further anaphylactically shocked guinea pigs were discovered to have suffered respiratory obstruction due to contraction and stenosis of bronchiolar smooth muscle that resulted in air trapping and distension of the lungs (24), similar to the characteristic pulmonary changes in human asthma. This finding led Meltzer to conclude that asthma was a manifestation of anaphylaxis (25). The role of the anaphylactic guinea pig as a suitable experimental model for the study of asthma was further enhanced by Otto's

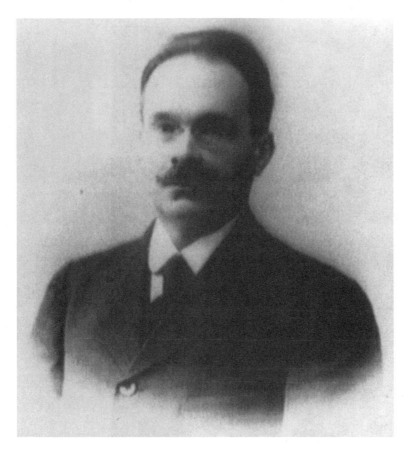

Figure 7   Alexandre Besredka, M.D. (1870–1940). Pasteur Institute, Paris. (Courtesy of the National Library of Medicine.)

demonstration that animals that recovered from induced anaphylactic shock became temporarily refractory to a second shock-inducing dose (26). Additionally, Besredka (Fig. 7) and Steinhardt discovered that repeated injections of progressively larger, but tolerable, doses of antigen eventually protected sensitized guinea pigs from anaphylactic challenge (27). These results suggested that a similar injection technique might success-fully desensitize the presumed human counterpart disorders of asthma and hay fever.

Investigational pursuit of active immunization for hay fever was soon begun in the laboratories of the Inoculation Department at St. Mary's Hospital in London. There Wright had provided the setting for interaction with visiting European masters of microbiology and immunology, giving his students the opportunity to learn about the "new immunother-apy." Wright's enthusiasm was reflected in his frequent prediction that "the physician of the future may yet become an immunisator" (28).

Noon (Fig. 8), Wright's assistant, following Dunbar's concept, also believed that hay fever was caused by a pollen "toxin." To accomplish active immunization, he initiated clinical trials in 1910 with a series of subcutaneous injections of dosages of pollen extracts calculated on a pollen-derived weight basis (Noon unit), and thus introduced preseasonal immunotherapy. Noon's observations provided the following (still pertinent) guidelines:

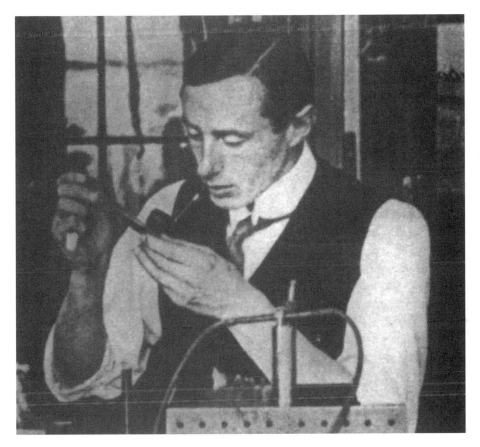

Figure 8 Leonard Noon (1877–1913). Immunologist on staff, Inoculation Department, St. Mary's Hospital, London. (Courtesy of the College of Physicians of Philadelphia.)

(1) a negative phase of decreased resistance develops after initiation of injection treatment; (2) increased resistance to allergen challenge, measured by quantitative ophthalmic tests, is dose dependent; (3) the optimal interval between injections is 1 to 2 weeks; (4) sensitivity may increase if injections are excessive or too frequent; and (5) overdoses may induce systemic reactions (29). Noon's work was continued by his colleague, Freeman, who in 1914 reported results of the first immunotherapeutic trial of 84 patients treated with grass pollen extracts during a 3-year period. The protocols lacked adequate controls, but successful outcomes were recorded with acquired immunity lasting at least 1 year after treatment was discontinued (30). A cluster of related reports indicated that other clinical studies of immunization of hay fever patients by others had been underway, concurrently and independently (31–34).

With the growing appreciation of pollens as allergens, the concept of pollen "toxin" faded and the objective of immunotherapy took on new meaning. Cooke (Fig. 9), at a 1915 meeting at the New York Academy of Medicine, added his summary of favorable result—in a majority of 140 patients treated with pollen extracts (35)—to the series of 45 patients reported from Chicago by Koessler (33). Developments during the next 10 to 15 years were

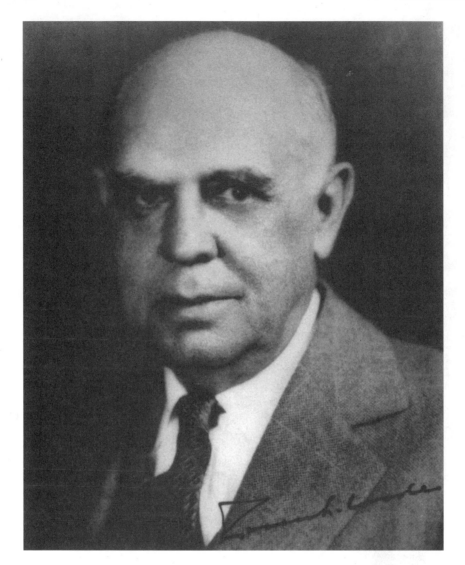

Figure 9 Robert A. Cooke, M.D. (1880–1960). Founding Director of the Institute of Allergy, Roosevelt Hospital, New York. (Courtesy of the National Library of Medicine.)

characterized by an eagerness to accept a continuing stream of favorable reports and adopt an arbitrary and relatively unquestioned technique of immunization therapy. A number of factors influenced the widespread use of this therapeutic method.

1. The scratch test introduced by Schloss in 1912 (36) was popularized by Walker (37) and by Cooke (35) who introduced the intracutaneous skin test technique in 1915. These new diagnostic techniques obviated the need for the more limited ocular test site and permitted practical identification of a wide variety of allergenic substances that might be useful in treatment.

2. Development of methods of extracting allergenic fractions from foods and airborne and environmental materials was extensively pursued by Wodehouse

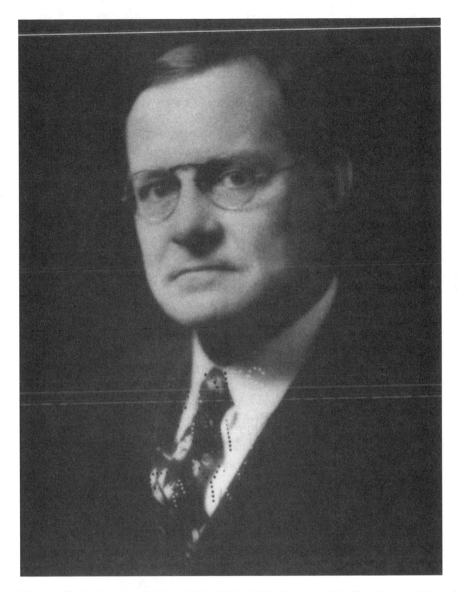

Figure 10   I. Chandler Walker, M.D. (1883–1950). Founder of the first allergy clinic in the United States, at Peter Bent Brigham Hospital, Boston; Department of Medicine, Harvard Medical School. (Courtesy of Frederick E. Walker.)

and Walker (Fig. 10) at the Peter Bent Brigham Hospital in Boston (38,39) and by Coca at a newly established Division of Immunology of New York Hospital (40). A variety of injectable materials became available for the treatment of allergic patients whose problems were not exclusively seasonal.
3. Botanists identified and collected pollens of regional indigenous trees, grasses, and weeds, and developed methods for aerobiological sampling to provide the information and technology essential for specific diagnosis (41–45).

4. Hospital and clinic sections devoted to diagnosis and treatment of allergic disorders (46) were established.
5. Immunization procedures were extended and applied to the treatment of asthma. With favorable results recorded in the treatment of seasonal asthmatic manifestations by pollen immunization, similar benefit was sought for chronic asthma by injections of extracts of perennial allergens and bacterial vaccines (37,47,48).
6. Medications capable of relieving allergic and asthmatic manifestations were relatively unavailable. During those early years, only epinephrine and atropine were mentioned as primary therapeutic agents and iodide, acetyl salicylate, anesthetic ether, morphine, and cocaine and their derivatives (with cautious qualifications) as secondary medications (49). The pharmacological action of ephedrine, with its limited value, was not defined until 1924 by Chen and Schmidt (50).
7. The strong leadership of Cooke and the dedication of Coca provided opportunities for training, experience, and structured courses on preparation and use of allergenic vaccines (51). From these endeavors, an increasing number of clinics were seeded in U.S. cities (52).

Rapid dissemination and application of the newly developed methods for identification of specific agents of hypersensitivity and desensitization therapy for hay fever and asthma patients engendered a new set of problems and questions complicating logical approaches well into the 1940s (52). The era of grant-supported full-time institutional-based academic and research positions in allergy and clinical immunology was then still some three to four decades away. Meanwhile, awaiting definition through research-generated data, there developed wide variability in ideas, criteria for indications, usage of materials, and methods and design of injection treatment plans. Adding to the complexity, a role for airborne mold spores as allergens was introduced by Storm van Leeuwen in 1924 (53). After a searching comprehensive study of the seasonal pollen problem, Thommen (Fig. 11) formulated a set of postulates that offered rational guidelines for the assessment of specific tree, grass, and weed species in the etiology of hay fever and as a source of immunotherapeutic agents (54):

(1) The pollen must contain an excitant of hay fever. (2) The pollen must be anemophilous or wind borne, as regards its mode of pollination. (3) The pollen must be produced in sufficiently large quantities. It is characteristic of wind-pollinated flowers in general that they produce pollen in far greater quantities than do flowers which are insect-pollinated. (4) The pollen must be sufficiently buoyant to be carried considerable distances. (5) The plant producing the pollen must be widely and abundantly distributed.

Principles of preseasonal pollen desensitization were then applied to treatment of patients troubled the year round with vaccines of a variety of perennial allergens that had given positive skin reactions. Of these, house dust as an agent was described by Kern in 1921 (55) and its role became increasingly recognized as an important environmental allergen in respiratory disease. The high prevalence of positive skin tests to dust vaccines initiated widespread use of stock and autogenous house dust vaccines for injection treatment of perennial rhinitis and asthma. Although there often was insufficient evidence to define the allergenic activity of house dust, a positive skin test alone—without differentiation of irritant properties of test materials—was frequently accepted as indication for its use. Some confusion in differentiating house dust–sensitive disease from nonallergic

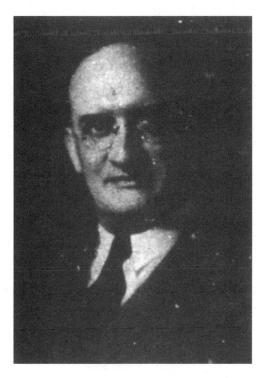

Figure 11   August A. Thommen, M.D. (1892–1943). Director of Allergy Clinic, New York University College of Medicine. (Courtesy of New York Public Library.)

chronic respiratory disease led Boatner and Efron to develop a "purified" house dust vaccine with the objective of increasing the diagnostic significance of a positive skin test to house dust (56).

There was an obvious need to develop suitable guidelines for efficacious injection treatment methods with a minimum of untoward constitutional reactions. Progress depended on the availability of vaccines of uniform strength and stability. Cooke attempted to bypass the problems of variations in allergenic activity of different pollen batches (due to seasonal plant growth factors and/or inadequate storage of collected pollen) by using an assay of total nitrogen content in standardization, although he did note that total nitrogen and allergenic activity were not identical (57,58). Subsequently, with a collaborating chemist, Stull (Fig. 12), he developed and championed a unit based on measurement of the content of protein nitrogen as a more accurate representation of residual stable activity of allergenic fractions (58).

Early treatment programs were developed by trial and error, and efficacy varied accordingly. In general, skin-test reactivity was used for determination of starting dosages, their increments, and frequency of administration. Perennial rhinitis and asthma mandated uninterrupted treatment schedules, but the superiority of perennial versus preseasonal plans for treatment of hay fever could not be settled by impressions and anecdotal reports. Modifications of schedule were devised for applying the principle of desensitization within compressed time frames. Pollen extract injections were given in small daily doses when initiated after seasonal symptoms had already begun (59). An intensive schedule of daily injections was required if initiated within 2 weeks of the anticipated seasonal onset

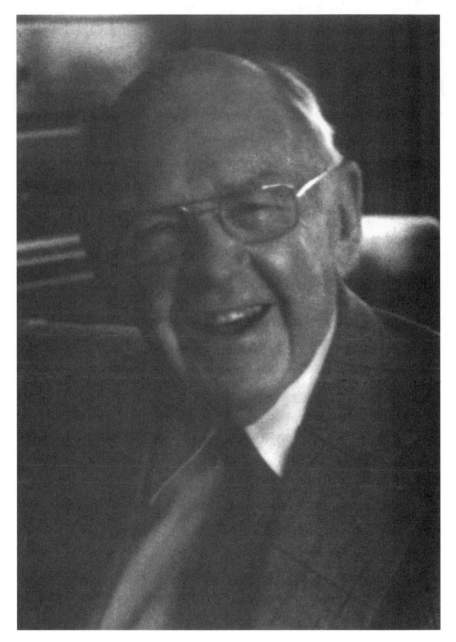

Figure 12 Arthur Stull, Ph.D. (1898–1991). Research Chemist and Director of Allergy Laboratory, Roosevelt Hospital, New York. (Courtesy of Mary Jo Rines.)

(60,61). Other modes and variations for pollen desensitization were described in 1921–1922 (62–66): (1) daily nasal and throat sprays with atomized vaccines (62); (2) pollen-containing ointments applied to the nasal mucosa (63); (3) oral administration (64); (4) intracutaneous injections (65); and (5) a full cycle return to Blackley's attempt 50 years earlier by contact at needle-puncture or skin abraded sites (66).

IV. THE EARLY DEVELOPMENTAL YEARS

In 1931 the (Western) Association for the Study of Allergy and the (Eastern) Society for the Study of Asthma and Allied Conditions established a Joint Committee of Survey and Standardization that achieved one objective by the mid-1930s: approval of medical school and hospital allergy clinics to meet guidelines for allergy training developed by the committee (67). However, the committee was unable to define standards for methods and materials. A lack of correlation between skin-test results and allergic manifestations had been noted in too many patients. Also, the committee believed that proper standardization must await the isolation and purification of etiologically responsible components of allergen vaccine such as Heidelberger and Avery had accomplished by isolating and purifying the specific soluble substances (capular polysaccharide) of the pneumococcus (68).

In 1992, Cooke reported that cutaneous reactivity was not eliminated in patients receiving injection treatments for asthma or allergic conditions due to horse and rabbit danders and sera. This contrasted with desensitization that accomplished complete inactivation of antibody action in animal models of anaphylaxis. Cooke, perceiving that the differences were functions of different mechanisms, referred to the beneficial effects of allergen injections as due to hyposensitization rather than neutralization or desensitization (69). This concept was confirmed in 1926 by Levine and Coca (70) and Jadassohn (71), both of whom found clinical improvement and allergen activity to be independent of effect, if any, on skin-sensitizing ("reaginic") antibody. Levine and Coca's study also demonstrated that a rapid (two- to fourfold) increase in serum reaginic antibody sometimes followed allergen injections. This finding helped to explain some paradoxical observations in treatment programs that had been designed to lessen specific hypersensitivities. For example, (1) severe constitutional reactions followed small increments or even repeated previously well-tolerated dosages, especially in early stages of injection schedules (72); (2) local tolerance diminished even with reduced vaccine dosages; and (3) symptoms of the treated allergic disorder might increase rather than decrease.

Freeman, in 1930, introduced "rush desensitization" in which injections of pollen vaccines were given at 1.5- to 2-hour intervals over a daily 14-hour period, under close observation and in a hospital setting (73). Since the benefits to be derived were generally believed to be outweighed by the danger of severe reactions, rush desensitization found little receptivity in the United States.

In 1935, Cooke's group, relocated in a new Department of Allergy at New York's Roosevelt Hospital, presented evidence in favor of a protective serum factor induced by injection treatments (74). Further, the transferable nature of the factor was indicated by Loveless's report that blood transfusions from ragweed-sensitive donors treated with pollen vaccine injections conferred equivalent beneficial effects on untreated ragweed-sensitive recipients during the hay fever season (75). This finding provided the lead for extended investigation centered at the target tissue cell level.

The ability of posttreatment serum to inhibit reactions between serum containing reaginic antibody and corresponding pollen allergen at passively sensitized cutaneous test sites by the technique of Prausnitz and Kustner (P-K test reaction) (75) was attributed to the effects of "blocking antibody" induced by injection treatment (76). Demonstration, in specifically treated patients, of coexistent, characteristically different—sensitizing and blocking—antibodies provided both the technique and stimulus for continuing study of hyposensitization phenomena. Additionally, relevant contributions by Cooke and associates included demonstrations of: (1) production of the inhibiting factor ("blocking antibody") by nonallergic individuals as a function of normal immune responsiveness (74); (2) specificity of blocking antibody activity and its relationship to the pseudoglobulin serum factor (76); and (3) decreases in serum reagin titers after long-term allergen immunotherapy (77).

Fortuitously, the impetus to search for alternative explanations coincident with the emergence, in 1955, of the National Institute of Allergy and Infectious Diseases (NIAID), a body within the National Institutes of Health, spurred the establishment of the requisite resources to support relevant research endeavors. In an early project, Vannier and Campbell undertook pertinent immunochemical studies on the allergenic fraction of house dust (78). A lead project based on a large multicenter collaborative study later focused on the characterization of other allergens, and a working group was organized under Campbell's chairmanship. Ragweed was the selected prototype for initial investigation by subcommittees for chemistry, animal testing, and clinical trials. The subsequent isolation of the major allergenic fraction of ragweed pollen, designated as antigen E, provided the first quantifiable reagent for standardization of skin test and treatment extracts (79).

V. BACTERIAL VACCINES

A belief that nasopharyngeal bacterial flora were involved in the pathogenesis of the common cold led to a study in London in which Allen developed a respiratory bacterial vaccine (80). The possibility that the immunizing effect of such an autogenous preparation might be of value in the treatment of respiratory illnesses other than the common cold led to its application to hay fever. The introduction, in 1912–1913, of bacterial vaccines for the management of seasonal rhinitis was integrated with an attempt to ameliorate nasopharyngeal and paranasal sinus infection as presumed factors in hay fever (81). Morrey reasoned that a nasal mucosa strengthened by bacterial vaccination would be resistant to the effects of whatever irritants were responsible for hay fever (82). Lowder-milk, in 1914, followed up both reports and utilized both Noon's pollen toxin and Allen's bacterial vaccine formulations in his introduction of immunotherapy (34).

Goodale's report of skin-test reactions to bacterial preparations in vasomotor rhinitis (83) was followed by great interest in putative relationships between bacteria and asthma (84,85). Walker, in popularizing the scratch test, extended the technique to a number of bacterial species along with pollens, perennial inhalants, and foods, and introduced autogenous vaccines into the treatment of asthma (85,86). The groundwork for adopting the concept of bacterial allergy was already in place. It centered around demonstrations of: (1) induced sensitization to bacteria in guinea pig models of anaphylaxis (87); and (2) skin-test and systemic reactivity to bacterial products associated with active infection (e.g., tuberculin) (88).

Further clinical relevance was provided by Rackemann's classic study, which defined intrinsic asthma (89) as a subset in patients with infective asthma, eosinophilia, and family backgrounds of extrinsic allergic diseases—a disorder later characterized by Cooke as presumptively immunologically mediated (90). Subsequent studies of treatment programs demonstrated lack of specificity of positive scratch, intracutaneous, and subcutaneous test reactions to bacterial preparations (91), as well as lack of specific or enhanced efficacy of autogenous over stock bacterial vaccines (92). Although the concept of desensitization or hyposensitization mechanisms as responsible for beneficial effects in infective asthma was put aside, respiratory bacterial vaccines continued to occupy a prominent place in clinical practice. Cooke related respiratory tract infection—especially chronic sinusitis—to asthma, and exacerbations of asthmatic symptoms to incremental overdosages of bacterial vaccine. Based on his experiences, he was a strong proponent of immunotherapy with autogenous vaccines as adjuvants for prevention of recurrences after removal of focal infection, partic ularly from the paranasal sinuses and upper respiratory tract (93).

Respiratory bacterial vaccines became entrenched immunotherapeutic agents. The first report of controlled trials, however, did not appear until 1955 (94); within the next 4 years, publication of two additional studies followed (95,96). Each failed to find efficacy for bacterial vaccines in attempts to prevent or treat asthma that was demonstrably related to respiratory infection. Following these reports, subsequent critical observations, and the diminishing influence of the earlier investigators whose uncontrolled impressions had influenced the clinical scene, respiratory bacterial vaccines slowly fell out of favor.

VI. CLINICAL TRIALS

A new initiative cut to the heart of the accepted role of allergen immunotherapy when Lowell—whose in-depth experience and analytical probing added credibility to his posi- tion—heralded the need for sound investigation to meet the requirements of statistical significance (97). A valid and unbiased evaluation of results of allergen immunotherapy, especially of pollenosis, was not available because controls for the many variables of peri- odic disease were found lacking in published trials. Sample sizes were too limited for tests of significance, and inconsistent seasonal, climatic, environmental, and biologically fluc- tuating factors had not been subjected to adequately controlled study.

"Controlled" studies presented during the preceding 10 years (98–100) were all found to be flawed. Reliance on historical features had not been replaced by placebo controls; double blinding of both subject and evaluator had not been followed; a single test group often consisted of pretreatment and newly entered patients; and comparable groups had not always been balanced for equivalent sensitivities (e.g., by skin-test titrations). Lowell and Franklin then performed a double-blind trial of treatment of allergic rhinitis due to ragweed sensitivity. They reported that patients receiving injections of ragweed pollen vaccine had fewer symptoms and lower medication scores than a control group. The beneficial effect was specific for ragweed, and the effect diminished in varying degrees within 5 months after discontinuing treatments (101). The following year, Fontana et al. reported that any beneficial effect of hyposensitization therapy in ragweed hay fever in children was indistinguishable from differences likely to occur in untreated controls (102). Their study, however, looked only for the presence or disappearance of symptoms, rather than at comparable degrees of severity (103).

Immunotherapy gained credibility with the introduction of new evaluatory measure- ments [i.e., symptom index score and the in vitro measure of leukocyte histamine release (104)], especially in children (105).

VII. ANTIGEN DEPOTS

During the late 1930s, allergen vaccines were modified in an effort to decrease the frequency of injections. Depotlike immunogenic materials were prepared to provide a slow, continuous release of allergen from injection sites. The first attempt used ground raw pollen suspended in olive oil (106). Because particulate bacterial vaccines and modified toxoid proved to be effective immunogens, soluble pollen allergen vaccines next were converted to particulate suspensions by alum precipitation and alum adsorption (107,108). Other modifications included acetylation, heat, and formalin treatment (108), precipitation by tannic (109) and hydrochloric acids (110), and mixture with gelatin (111). Of these, only alum-adsorbed pollen extracts gained any popularity. Treatment of hay fever with an emulsified allergen vaccine was introduced by Naterman, who, in 1937, emulsified a pollen extract with lanolin and olive oil (112). Thirteen years later, he suspended grass and ragweed pollen tannates in peanut oil with aluminum monostearate (113). Malkiel and Feinberg, encouraged by evidence of slow absorption from new penicillin-in-oil depot formulations, prepared extracts of ragweed in sesame oil–aluminum monostearate. With these, however, they were unable to avoid constitutional reactions, while failing to reduce severity of symptoms (114). Furthermore, other investigators detected increased titers of neutralizing antibody in treated patients without clinical benefit, thus casting doubt on the clinical relevance of "blocking" antibody (115,116).

Clinical trials with repository therapy, initiated by Loveless in 1947 (117), gave highly favorable results as reported 10 years later (118). This stimulated the first major departure from conventional injection treatment schedules. Loveless, firmly believing that successful treatment was a function of induced "blocking" antibody, aimed her protocols at maintaining the highest possible humoral levels of blocking antibody. She was convinced that the threshold of conjunctival responses to graded local challenges was a valid measure of systemic sensitivity and that suppression of both depended on the generation of neutralizing factor. Although there were no data to equate desired results with those reported for influenza vaccine (119), she used the depot medium that Freund and McDermott had developed (120) as an immunogen adjuvant in experimental animal models. A large dose of pollen vaccine, calculated as the cumulative total that would be given in the course of a conventional preseason schedule, was emulsified in oil with an emulsion stabilizer, and administered as a single intramuscular injection (117,118). A number of anecdotal reports by Brown spoke of "thousands" of uniformly successful results of treatment with emulsified vaccines of pollen and other airborne allergens (121). However, adverse reactions consisting of late formation and persistence of nodules, sterile abscesses and granulomata, and a potential for induction of delayed hypersensitivity to injected antigens were found inherent in emulsion therapy. Furthermore, subsequent controlled studies failed to confirm significant therapeutic effectiveness (122–124). Finally, emulsion therapy was discontinued after a report that mineral oil and mineral oil adjuvants induced plasma cell myelomas in a certain strain of mice (125) and the U.S. Food and Drug Administration did not approve the repository emulsion for therapy.

VIII.   ORAL ROUTE TO TOLERANCE AND DESENSITIZATION

Possibilities for inducing protection by feeding on causative agents date back to stories of poisons in antiquity. In the first century B.C., Mithradates VI (131–63 B.C.) (Fig. 13), King of Pontus in Asia Minor, noted that ducks who fed on plants known to be poisonous to humans did not manifest any apparent ill effects. Applying this observation, he incorporated ducks' blood in an antidote he attempted to develop against poisons—an early concept of passive immunization. Further, in preparing himself for the ever-present possibility of a palace revolt, Mithradates sought to gain immunity from poisoning by swallowing small amounts of poisons—particularly toadstool toxins—in gradually increasing dosages (126). So successful was the outcome of his experiments that he later failed to achieve attempted suicide by ingesting large doses of the same poisons (127). For many subsequent centuries, the technique of gaining tolerance or active immunity through incremental dosage schedules continued to be known as mithradatising.

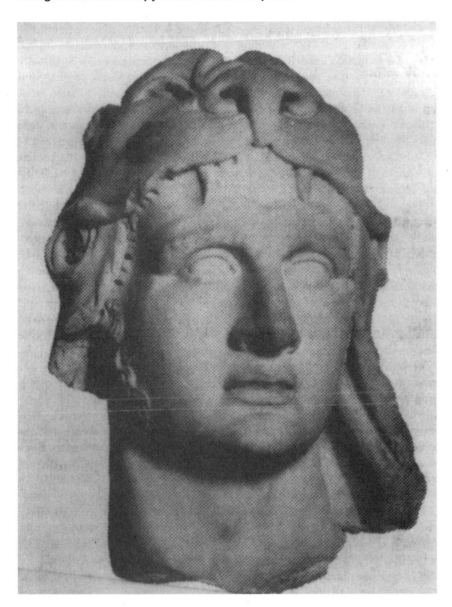

Figure 13 Mithradates VI Eupator (c. 131–63 B.C.). King of Pontus; Asia Minor. (Courtesy of the Musee de Louvre, Paris.)

The renowned Greek physician who practiced in Rome, Claudius Galen (130–200 A.D.), had noted that snake venoms taken by mouth were devoid of the systemic toxic actions effected by snake bites (128). According to folklore, this knowledge allowed snake charmers of the classic Greco-Roman era to acquire protection against potentially fatal bites by drinking from serpent-infested waters that contained traces of their venoms (129)—a less traumatic method than seeking protection through self-inflicted bites.

Moving to a more recent era and the beginning of the scientific study of immunity, in 1891 Ehrlich provided experimental evidence of orally achieved toxin tolerance in mice by feeding them the toxins ricin and abrin (130). Then germane to delayed hypersensitivity, in 1946 Chase demonstrated an inhibiting effect of prior feeding (131). The earliest recorded journal item of clinical relevance was noted in a description of plant-induced allergic contact dermatitis in 1829 (132). In his discussion, Dakin reported that chewing poison ivy leaves, both as a prevention and a cure, was recommended by some "good meaning, marvelous, mystical physicians," despite adverse side effects—eruption, swelling, redness, and intolerable itching around the verge of the anus. It was also a practice seen among native North Americans (Indians), who chewed and swallowed the juice of early shoots as a preventive against the development of poison ivy dermatitis during ensuing summer months (133). Apparently, this method had been found to be of some value since it was used in rural areas and by park workers, and considered an example of effective homeopathic autotherapy (134). A novel modification reported partial immunity after drinking milk from cows deliberately fed poison ivy in grass mixtures (135).

The first move to explain the procedure that originated in folk medicine in terms of immune phenomena began with the approach of Strickler in 1918. Although unable to demonstrate circulating blood antibodies in patients affected by poison ivy and poison oak dermatitis, Strickler postulated the likely pathogenesis to be a form of "tissue immunity" to the plant toxins. Believing the mechanism to be similar to that of hay fever, he introduced an adaptation of desensitization for treatment and prevention of the plant-related contact dermatitis with extracts of the alcohol-soluble leaf fraction given by intramuscular injection (136). The following year, Schamberg introduced an oral approach to prophylactic desensitization utilizing incremental drop dosages of a tincture of *Rhus toxicodendron* (137). Strickler's follow-up report 3 years later indicated favorable acceptance of intramuscular injection, oral methods, and a combination of both (133). Although trials during subsequent years supported this early usage (138), there were differing reports varying from only short-term immunizing effects (139) to lack of either clinical benefit (140) or increased tolerance (141).

Despite divergence of opinion, the oral method of preventive therapy remained popular for 50-some years. Alcohol and acetone extracts in vegetable oils were prepared from a variety of plant source polyhydric phenols (e.g., the Rhus ivy-oak-sumac group, primula, geranium, tulip, and chrysanthemum). In 1940, Shellmire expanded the spectrum of plant sources of delayed hypersensitivity by identifying ether-soluble fractions of pollens responsible for producing allergic contact dermatitis through airborne exposure. These were distinct from water-soluble pollen albumins implicated in the immediate hypersensitivity phenomenon of hay fever. Through Shellmire's work, preparations of specific pollen oleoresins were then made available for oral desensitization (142).

Proponents in the 1940s and 1950s based their belief in the validity of desensitization methods for plant contact dermatitis on the concept of cell-associated "antibody" to chemical haptens in the pathogenesis of delayed cutaneous hypersensitivity. However, there were complicating problems in the nature of induced dermatitis at locally injected or previously involved distal sites, exacerbations of existing lesions, stomatitis, gastroenteritis, anal pruritis, and dermatitis from mucous membrane contact with oral preparations. Additionally, in the face of lack of convincing evidence of efficacy, the practice gradually faded from popular usage.

On a parallel track, similar thought was being given to treatment of another group of allergic disorders that Coca in 1923 characterized as atopic—hay fever, asthma, and eczema. The first case record of desensitization to an allergenic food came from England, in 1908, with Schoffield's report of successful reversal of severe egg in-induced asthma, urticaria, and angioedema in a 13-year old boy by the daily feedings of egg in homeopathic doses (143). Three years later, Finzio, in Italy, reported similar success with cow's milk in infants (144). Shortly thereafter, favorable results of trials of desensitization to foods in children were reported in the United States by Schloss—in a study that coincidentally established practicability of the scratch test in hypersensitivity (145)—and in work by Talbot (146). Because of possible anaphylactic reactions to only a minute amount of an allergenic food in an exquisitely sensitive individual, Pagniez and Vallery-Radot, in 1916, prefed patients with food digests consisting predominantly of peptones. Theoretically, these foods were reduced in allergenicity by the treatment process but retained immunogenic specificity (147,148). Acceptance of oral food desensitization plans declined with later negative experiences (149,150).

The first use of an orally administered pollen-related preparation appeared in the homeopathic literature of 1890 with the description of "ambrose," a tincture of fresh flower heads and young shoots, recommended for the treatment of hay fever (151). Impressed by an experience in which asthma caused by inhalation of ipecac was prevented with drop doses of syrup or tincture of ipecac, Curtis explored a like possibility in hay fever. In 1900—in conjunction with introduction of flower and pollen vaccines—he noted preliminary efficacious results with tincture and fluid extracts of ragweed flowers and pollen taken by mouth (152). Touart later reported varying responses in six patients given enteric-coated tablet triturates of grass and ragweed pollen (64). In 1927, Black demonstrated that large doses of orally administered ragweed extract effectively lowered nasal threshold responses to inhalational challenges (153), but later reported a large series of patients with results less favorable than could be expected after injection treatments (154). Urbach attempted to bypass distressing gastrointestinal symptoms following ingestion of pollen vaccines by advocating oral administration of specific pollen digest peptones ("propetan") (155). Since collection of pollen supplies was difficult, Urbach prepared peptone derivatives of blossoms of trees, grasses, and grass seeds for use as orally administered allergens (156). Passive transfer experiments by Bernstein and Feinberg calculated that more than a pound of raw pollen would be required orally to reach a circulating antigen concentration obtained by injection of maximally tolerated doses of pollen vaccine (157). Additionally convincing lack of efficacy confirmed by a later multicenter, collaborative, placebo-controlled study followed (158).

IX. DRUGS AND BIOLOGICAL PRODUCTS

The purported effectiveness of oral desensitization to foods was soon applied to drug hypersensitivity, and a report of successful oral desensitization of a malaria patient with anaphylactic hypersensitivity to quinine appeared in the French literature (159). When the allergenic character of pharmaceutical and biological products derived from plant and animal sources became increasingly evident, attempts were made to desensitize reactive patients who otherwise would be deprived of essential specific therapy. An early problem was treatment of the horse-sensitive patient with horse antidiphtheria or antitetanus antiserum (160). The cautious injections of horse dander vaccine offered some measure of protection after long-term treatment (161). However, the potential for anaphylaxis resulting from the large volumes of therapeutic antisera required was too great. Even a minute dose could cause a fatal reaction (162), and early trials had failed to accomplish desensitization (163,164).

Success was achieved in use of dried and pulverized ipecacuanha plant root for treatment of ipecac-sensitive asthmatic pharmacists and physicians and of beef or pork insulin for desensitization injection of sensitive diabetics who required insulin replacement therapy (165,166).

Freeman's method of "rush inoculation" with pollen vaccines (73) was not generally accepted. However, the principle was effectively applied in treating drug hypersensitivities requiring prompt resumption of therapy, such as with insulin to control diabetes (167) and penicillin when required as the essential antibiotic to control a specific and severe infection (168). This procedure probably induced transient anaphylactic desensitization, as first demonstrated in the guinea pig (27), or by mechanism of hapten inhibition (169). Over 40 to 50 years, a number of publications affirmed effective desensitization to pharmaceutical products responsible for hypersensitivity reactions (170–172).

X. INSECT ANTIGENS

In classical Greece of the fourth century B.C., the philosopher-biologist Aristotle, who had written extensively on the life history, types, and behavior patterns of bees, in his *Historia Animalia* noted their ability to sting large animals to death—even one as large as a horse. Yet it was recognized that beekeepers in the course of their work could be repeatedly or periodically stung without ill effect. No attempt was made to duplicate this observed natural phenomenon until the early years of the twentieth century, when the possibility of ameliorating insect hypersensitivity was provided by the description of favorable responses to injection treatments with extracts of gnats (173) and bees (174). Hyposensitization to other species was also explored using mosquito (175) and flea (176) extracts. Some failed attempts were not understood until the acquisition of knowledge that delayed (cell-mediated) hypersensitivity and biochemistry of inflammation were responsible mechanisms.

Whether hypersensitivity-induced states owed their reduction to the raising of blocking antibodies or to later defined mechanisms of regulatory control of IgE production, elements of cell-mediated immunity did not lend themselves to comparable diminishing effects sought in allergen immunotherapy for immediate hypersensitivity disorders.

Fine hairs and epithelial scales shed by swarming insects were also identified as airborne allergens responsible for conjunctivitis, rhinitis, and asthma which could be managed by hyposensitization (177,178). Benson reported extensive studies of Hymenoptera allergy and hyposensitization with whole-body vaccine. Efficacy of treatment was demonstrated for anaphylactic sensitivity to the venom of stings and for inhalant allergy to body parts and emanations incurred by exposed beekeepers (179). Hyposensitization therapy employed whole-body vaccines until Loveless—based on her discovery and definition of neutralizing ("blocking") factor as therapeutically responsible for the efficacy of pollen hyposensitization in hay fever—sought the same objective for the Hymenoptera–anaphylactically sensitive patient. She then introduced several variations: (1) use of isolated contents of dissected venom sacs in conventional hyposensitization schedules; (2) single repository immunization with venom emulsified in oil adjuvant; (3) "rush" desensitization; and (4) deliberate controlled stinging with captured wasps to ascertain establishment and maintenance of a protective state (180,181). Later studies confirmed the far greater efficacy of venom allergens (Chapter 18).

XI. NONSPECIFIC IMMUNOTHERAPY

Attempts were made to duplicate the benefits of specific hyposensitization by altering, initiating, or regulating immune system function through injections with a variety of nonspecific antigens (e.g., typhoid and mixed coliform vaccines, cow's milk, snake venom, soybean, and creation of a sterile fixation abscess with injection of turpentine) (182,183). It was thought that repeated injections of small doses of protein-digested peptones might evoke subclinical anaphylactic mechanisms with resultant desensitization to a multiplicity of allergens (184).

Another global approach employing the administration of autogenous blood visualized that injected (autohemato- and autoserotherapeutic) samples contained absorbed causative allergens in quantities too small to produce an attack, yet sufficiently minutely antigenic to induce tolerance (185).

Another indirect approach considered possible benefits that might be derived from attempted hyposensitization responses to antigens to which specific sensitization resulted from past infection but were concurrently inactive and unrelated to the etiology of asthma. Two such agents—tuberculin (186) and the highly reaginic and anaphylactic antibody-inducing extract of *Ascaris lumbricoides* (187)—were given to correspondingly positive skin test reactors according to conventional hyposensitization schedules.

If unable to accomplish specific hyposensitization, therapy attempted to neutralize the alleged mediator of allergic reactions (i.e., histamine). Histamine "desensitization" was first introduced in 1932 for treatment of cold urticaria in the expectation that daily incremental injections would achieve correspondingly increased degrees of tolerance to histamine and thereby diminish allergic symptoms (188). Enzymatic destruction of released histamine in urticaria and atopic dermatitis was then attempted with parenteral or oral administration of histaminase (189). An immune-mediated blocking of histamine was postulated through injections of a histamine-linked antigen [(histamine-azo-depreciated horse serum) "hapamine"] to induce antihistamine antibodies (190). While some of these modalities were initially encouraging, later studies failed to confirm their benefit. Favorable symptomatic improvements of empirical but nonspecific, treatment designed to modulate immune functions could not be determined without controlled clinical trials. The use of these agents fell by the wayside as new scientific knowledge of mechanisms of allergy were acquired (191).

XII. CONCLUDING COMMENTS

In this review of the evolution of allergen immunotherapy (Table 1) as a method introduced into clinical medicine almost a century ago, two retrospective considerations are particularly noteworthy. The first relates to the several decades of trial and error, recorded observations, and the transition from loosely conducted trials to controlled clinical investigative protocols. Relevant knowledge of the value of allergen immunotherapy was not advanced much beyond appreciation that varied approaches helped some treated patients, some of the time, to variable degrees. Establishing a requisite informational base still looks to: (1) epidemiological studies of a scope and design to provide in-depth understanding of the natural history of asthma and allergic disease; and (2) large-scale clinical trials from which to construct critical criteria for exact indications, and use of materials and methods by which immunotherapeutic regimens can be properly evaluated.

Second is awareness of the enormous impact and influence that allergen immunotherapy had on the launching, development, and continuation of allergy as a medical specialty. For 40 to 50 years following the original description of skin test and hyposensitization techniques, these modalities served as the mainstays of allergy when there was little else to offer in the way of adequate and feasible management. So firmly

Table 1   Pioneering Highlights Along the Pathway to the Development and Understanding of Allergen Immunotherapy

Time	Observation/finding	Credit
430 B.C.	First recorded perception of immunity; recovery from plague endowed protection from repeated attack.	Thucydides
63 B.C.	Oral tolerance: method derived from repetitious ingestion of incremental, minute, subtoxic doses of plant poisons (126).	Mithradates VI
1712–1776	Variolation: ancient oriental method, introduction of induced active immunity (2,3).	Emanuel Timoni, Giacomo Pilorini
1798	Vaccination: immunity induced through biologically related inoculum (4).	Edward Jenner
1880–1884	Immune responses not dependent on pathogenicity (1) or viability (6) of inocula.	Louis Pasteur, Daniel Salmon, and Theobold Smith
1880	Conceptual method for exhausting susceptibility to hay fever by repetitious application of pollen to abraded skin (17).	Charles Blackley
1897	Immunizing method derived from inoculation series of minute sublethal doses of rattlesnake venom (9).	Henry Sewall
1890	Passive immunization with tetanus and diphtheria antitoxins; introduction of therapeutic antisera (11).	Shibasaburo Kitasato and Emil von Behring
1891–1907	Adverse outcomes: hypersensitivity disorders mediated by immunizing agents.	
	Severe nonantibody reactions to biological product of disease agent tuberculin (88); systemic cell-mediated delayed hypersensitivity.	Robert Koch
	Anaphylaxis; immediate hypersensitivity mechanism (20).	Paul Portier and Charles Richet
	Systemic foreign serum sickness (13) and local tissue reaction (Arthus phenomenon) (193); antigen-antibody complex mechanism.	Clemens von Pirquet and Béla Schick; Maurice Arthus
1897	Standardization of diphtheria antitoxin; introduction of concept of biological standardization with application to immunogens and antisera (12).	Paul Ehrlich
1903	Conceptual immunization for hay fever with grass pollen "toxin" (proteid isolate) and foreign species antisera (12).	William Dunbar
1907–1913	Protection against anaphylactic challenges: animal models.	
	"Antianaphylaxis"; transient desensitization following recovery from anaphylactic shock due to temporary depletion of anaphylactic antibody (126).	Richard Otto
	Temporary protection (desensitization) induced by repeated subanaphylactic doses of antigen through neutralization or exhaustion of anaphylactic antibody (27).	Alexandre Besredka
	"Masked anaphylaxis," partial refractory state: antigen prevented from reaching shock tissue by excess of circulating anaphylactic antibody (194).	Richard Weil
1911–1914	First reported successful immunization against grass pollen "toxin" for hay fever (29,30).	Leonard Noon and John Freeman
1917–1919	"Injection treatments" for desensitization expanded to allergens beyond pollens (37).	I. Chandler Walker

(Continued)

Table 1   Continued

Time	Observation/finding	Credit
1917	Development of techniques for extraction of allergens: availability of expanded testing and treatment reagents made available (38,39).	Roger Wodehouse
1919	Oral tolerance to plant oil-soluble fraction agent of contact dermatitis: derivitive modification of Native American preventive practice of chewing "poison ivy" shoots (133,136).	Jay Schamberg
1921	Differentiation between antibodies (Ab) involved in states of hypersensitiveness and desensitization: anaphylactic Ab, precipitin, and atopic reagin (192).	Arthur Coca and Ellen Grove
1922	"Desensitization" by procedure of Besredka in an anaphylactic animal model not attainable in human hypersensitiveness objective of hyposensitization" (69).	Robert Cooke
1922	Constitutional reactions from hyposensitization injection treatments: cause, nature, and prevention (72).	Robert Cooke
1922	Identification of house dust as a ubiquitous allergen: expanded scope of hyposensitization programs for the treatment of perennial rhinitis and asthma (195).	Robert Cooke
1926	Increase in serum reaginic antibodies following hyposensitization injection treatments explaining nature of reactions to injections of pollen vaccines (196).	Philip Levine and Arthur Coca
1932	Arbitrary incorporation of bacterial vaccines in hyposensitization treatments influenced by concept of immunological mechanism in infective asthma (90).	Robert Cooke
1933	Laboratory technique of assay of allergenic vaccines: protein nitrogen unit standardization for guide to hyposensitization schedule (197).	Arthur Stull and Robert Cooke
1935	Identification of blocking antibody as a product of hyposensitization treatment: its chemical and immunological differentiation and inhibiting action on atopic reagin + allergen (74).	Robert Cooke and Arthur Stull
1937	Guideline for prevention of precipitin-mediated serum disease by desensitization: contraindication in coexisting presence of atopic reagins to foreign species antisera (198).	Louis Tuft
1940	Depot allergenic vaccines for delayed absorption: alum adsorption (108).	Arthur Stull, Robert Cooke, and William Sherman
1947–1957	Repository adjuvant therapy with single injection of water-in-oil emulsified vaccine (117,118).	Mary Loveless
1956	Desensitization to anaphylactic challenge of stinging insect venom (180).	Mary Loveless
1962	Densitization to anaphylactic drug hypersensitivity in penicillin model explained by hapten-inhibition mechanism.	Charles Parker and Herman Eisen
1967–1987	Identification and assay of immunoglobulin E as the reaginic antibody (199) and function of a cytokine, IL-4, in its synthesis (200); presenting new vistas for exploring applications of cellular and molecular immunological phenomena to allergen immunotherapy through regulatory control of IgE.	Kimishiga and Teruko Ishizaka; William Paul

had arbitrary patterns of allergen immunotherapy been implanted in clinical practice, that only recently was an internationally representative effort made to sort out bias and unproven impressions from verifiable fact, and an attempt made to reach consensus (191).

This review, then, leaves allergen immunotherapy with a major question: With the advent of newer, effective symptom-relieving pharmacological agents and new relevant knowledge on chemical mediators of inflammation, were the empirical aspects of allergen immunotherapy perpetuated beyond justification? At the same time, this consideration leaves the history of allergen immunotherapy in the midstream of new technologies in molecular biology, informational advances, and research opportunities. Current interests and activities in the design of modified antigens of enhanced efficacy, immunochemical characterization and standardization of allergen vaccines, and definition of responsible immune mechanisms and targeted responses ultimately may provide answers to questions pursued by a century of pioneering research in biomedical science—particularly immuno-chemistry and cellular immunology—and clinical investigation. Later chapters deal with many of these relevant advances.

XIII. SALIENT POINTS

Although "injection treatments" with pollen vaccines were introduced into clinical practice in the early 1900s, development of the method is rooted in the genesis and evolution of immune function dating back to antiquity. An appreciation of allergen immunotherapy viewed in this historical context follows.

1. Immunity, as a naturally occurring phenomenon, was recognized as early as the fifth century B.C., with the observation that those who recovered from epidemic illness during the plague of Athens were not similarly stricken a second time (2).
2. By applications of the principles of nature, prototype methods introduced the phenomenon of induced immunity as a result of deliberate exposure to causative agents: (a) tolerance to plant poisons by ingestion of subtoxic doses (Mithradates VI, 63 B.C.); and (b) protection from smallpox by contact with material recovered from disease lesions (variolation; eleventh-century Chinese healers).
3. Modification of variolation introduced methods for inducing immunity with reduced risk by inoculations of: (a) biologically related agent of mild disease [vaccination (4)]; (b) nonpathogenic attenuated microorganisms (1); and (c) killed bacteria (6). Although relatively harmless procedures, inocula demonstrated potential for producing inflammatory effects concurrent with immunity (later defined as sensitization mechanisms).
4. Demonstration of protection of an animal model from lethal snake venom by inoculation series of sublethal doses (9) provided the introductory approach to the development of methods for immunization against microbial toxins and identification of the antibody product, antitoxin, in blood serum (11).
5. Systemic shock reaction of anaphylaxis—discovered as an adverse effect of immunization (20)—provided animal models for the study of hypersensitivity as an aberrant immune phenomenon (21); particularly relevant was the challenged-sensitized guinea pig whose respiratory manifestations suggested a counterpart expression of human hay fever and asthma. Discovery of refrac

tory state following recovery from shock—attributed to temporary depletion of anaphylactic antibody (22)—led to development of the method of "desensitization" by repeated injections of incremental tolerated doses of antigens (27).

6. In the erroneous belief that seasonal hay fever was caused by grass pollen toxin, serial injections of pollen solutions—designed to induce immunity by production of serum antitoxin—introduced the concept of allergen immunotherapy (29,30). This method was subsequently defined as an approach to reverse sensitization to pollen proteins and expanded in scope by employing vaccines derived from a variety of airborne seasonal and perennial allergens (38,39).

7. Serum factors associated with hypersensitivity and desensitization treatments were differentiated as skin-sensitizing antibody (ssa) and precipitating antibody (pa), respectively (192). Detection of concurrent induction of pa and increase in levels of ssa—identical with naturally occurring atopic disease reagins—following injections of allergen extracts accounted for local and constitutional reactions associated with therapy (70).

8. Desensitization, as effected in animal anaphylactic models, when recognized as not attainable in allergen immunotherapy, aimed at the objective of inducing diminished (hypo) sensitization (69). Studies of antibody raised by allergen-hyposensitizing injections demonstrated its chemical properties and its "blocking" of reactions of skin sensitizing (reaginic) antibodies with allergens to explain putative responsible immune mechanisms (74).

9. Demonstrated adjuvant effect of allergen vaccine incorporated in oil-in-water emulsion (75) had the inherent potential for inducing plasma cell neoplastic proliferation as a function of hyperimmunization (125), and was thus contraindicated in allergen immunotherapy.

10. Desensitization of anaphylactic drug reactivity (e.g., penicillin and insulin) was accomplished by a special rush protocol of immunotherapeutic injections designed to effect the mechanism of hapten inhibition (169).

ACKNOWLEDGMENTS

In the search and collection of original source material, we drew heavily upon the resources of the National Library of Medicine (NLM) and the archival and special collections of the NLM History of Medicine Division (HMD). For valued interactions and expert assistance graciously extended by information specialists of the Library Reference Section and HMD staff, our many thanks and special appreciation. We also gratefully acknowledge and thank Patricia E. Richardson, NIAID editorial assistant, for dedicated technical skills and assistance in the assembly and organization of materials from which this chapter was constructed.

REFERENCES

1. Pasteur L. De l'attenuation du virus du cholra des poules. CRend Acad Sci 1880; 91:673.
2. Thucydides. The Peloponesian War (Smith C F, transl). Cambridge, MA: Harvard University Press, 1958: v2, Bk 2, Ch 47:54.
3. Timoni E. A Letter Containing the Method of Inoculating the Small Pox; Practiced With Success at Constantinople. Phil Trans R Soc London 1714; 339:72.

4.   Pylarinum J. Nova et tuta Variolas per Transplantatonem Methodus, nuper inventa et in ufum tracta. Phil Trans R Soc London 1716; 347:393.

5.   Jenner E. An Inquiry Into the Causes and Effects of the Variolae. Sampson Low, Soho, London, 1798.

5a. Pasteur L, Chamberland C, Roux E. Compte Rendu Sommaire des experiences faites a' Pouilly-le-Fort, pres' Melun, sur la vaccination charboneusse. CR Acad Sci 1881; 92:1378.

6.   Salmon DE, Smith T. On a new method of producing immunity from contagious diseases. Proc Biol Soc Wash 1884/86; 3:29.

7.   Koch R. Forsetzung der Muttheilungen "uber ein Hermittel gegen Tuberculose. Dtsch Med Wschr 1891; 9:101.

8.   Pasteur L. Method pour prevenir la rage apres' morsure. CRend Acad Sci 1885; 101:765.

9.   Sewall H. Experiments on the preventive inoculation of rattlesnake venom. J Physiol 1887; 8:205.

10. Roux PPE, Yersin AEJ. Contribution a' l'etude de la diphterie. Ann Inst Pasteur 1889; 2:629.

11. Behring EA von, Kitasato S. Ueber das zustandekommen der diphtherie-immunitat und der tetanus-immunitat bei thieren. Dtsch Med Wschr 1890; 16:1113.

12. Ehrlich P. Die Wertbestimmunung des Diphtherieheislserums. Klin Jb 1897; 6:299.

13. Dunbar WP. The present state of our knowledge of hay-fever, J Hygiene 1902; 13:105.

14. Pirquet von Cesenatico C P, Schick B. Die Serumkrankheit, Vienna: F. Deutch, 1905.

15. Bostock J. Case of periodical affection of the eyes and chest. Med Chir Trans 1819; 10:161.

16. Wyman M. Autumnal Catarrh. Cambridge, MA: Hurd and Houghton, 1872.

17. Blackley CH. Hay Fever; Its Causes, Treatment, and Effective Prevention. London: Balliere, 1880.

18. Curtis HH. The immunizing cure of hay fever. Med News 1900; 77:16.

19. Park WH. Toxin-antitoxin immunization against diphtheria. J Am Med Assoc 1922; 79:1584.

20. Portier P, Richet C. De l'action anaphylactique de certains venins. CR Soc Biol 1902; 54:170.

21. Rosenau MJ, Anderson JF. A study of the cause of sudden death following the injection of horse serum. In: Hygienic Laboratory Bulletin 29. Washington, DC: Government Printing Office, 1906.

22. Otto R. Das Theobald Smithsche Phanomenon der Serum-Veberfindlichkeit. In: Gendenkschr. f.d. verstorb Generalstabsarzt. Berlin: von Leuthold, 1906: vol. 1, 153.

23. Wolff-Eisner A. Das Heufieber. Munchen: J. F. Lehman, 1906.

24. Auer J, Lewis PA. The physiology of the immediate reaction of anaphylaxis in the guinea pig. J Exp Med 1910; 12:151.

25. Meltzer SJ. Bronchial asthma as a phenomenon of anaphylaxis. J Am Med Assoc 1910; 55:1021.

26. Otto R. Zur frage der serum-ueberempfindlichkeit. Munch Med Wschr 1907; 54:1664.

27. Besredka A, Steinhardt E. De l'anaphylaxie et de l'antianaphylaxie vis-a-vis due serum de cheval. Ann Inst Pasteur 1907; 21:117, 384.

28. Colebrook L. Almoth Wright. Provocative Doctor and Thinker. London: William Heinemann Medical Books Ltd., 1954:61.

29. Noon L. Prophylactic inoculation against hay fever. Lancet 1911; 1:1572.

30. Freeman J. Vaccination against hay fever; report of results during the last three years. Lancet 1914; 1:1178.

31. Clowes GHA. A preliminary communication on certain specific reactions exhibited in hay fever cases. Proc Soc Exp Biol Med 1913; 10:70.

32. Lowdermilk RC. Personal Communication to Duke WW. Cited in Duke WW. Allergy. Asthma, Hay Fever, Urticaria and Allied Manifestations of Reaction. St Louis: Mosby, 1925:222.

33. Koessler KK. The specific treatment of hayfever by active immunization. Ill Med J 1914; 24:120.

34. Lowdermilk RC. Hay-fever. J Am Med Assoc 1914; 63:141.

35. Cooke RA. The treatment of hay fever by active immunization. Laryngoscope 1915; 25:108.

36. Schloss O. A case of allergy to common foods. Am J Dis Child 1912; 3:341.

37. Walker IC. Studies on the sensitization of patients with bronchial asthma (Study series III–XXXVI). J Med Res 1917:35–37.

38. Wodehouse RP. Immunochemical study and immunochemistry of protein series. J Immunol 1917; 11:VI. cat hair, 227; VII. horse dander, 237; VIII. dog hair, 243.

39. Wodehouse RP. IX. Immunochemical studies of the plant proteins: Wheat seed and other cereals. Am J Botany 1917; 4:417.

40. Coca AF. Studies in specific hypersensitiveness. XV. The preparation of fluid extracts and solutions for use in the diagnosis and treatment of the allergies, with notes on the collection of pollens. J Immunol 1922; 7:163.

41. Goodale JL. Preliminary notes on the anaphylactic skin reactions exacted in hay fever subjects by the pollen of various species of plants. Boston Med Surg J 1914; 171:695.

42. Goodale JL. Pollen therapy in hay fever. Boston Med Surg J 1915; 173:42.

43. Wodehouse RP. Hay Fever Plants. Waltham, MA: Chronica Botanica Co., 1945.

44. Durham OC. The contribution of air analysis to the study of allergy. J Lab Clin Med 1925; 13:967.

45. Unger L, Harris MC. Stepping Stones in Allergy. Minneapolis, MN: Craftsman Press, 1975:75.

46. Cohen SG. Firsts in allergy. N Engl Reg Allergy Proc 1983; 4:309; 1984; 5:48; 5:247.

47. Cooke RA. Protein sensitization in the human with special reference to bronchial asthma and hay fever. Med Clin North Am 1917; 1:721.

48. Cooke RA. Studies in specific hypersensitiveness. New etiologic factors in bronchial asthma. J Immunol 1922; 7:147.

49. Duke WW. Allergy, Asthma, Hay Fever, Urticaria and Allied Manifestations of Reaction. St. Louis: C. V. Mosby, 1925; 237–241.

50. Chen KK, Schmidt CF. The action of ephedrine, the active principle of the Chinese drug MaHuang. J Pharmacol Exp Ther 1924; 24: 192.

51. Cohen SG. Firsts in allergy: IV. The contributions of Arthur F. Coca, M. D. (18751959). N Engl Reg Allergy Proc 1985; 6:285.

52. Cohen SG. The American Academy of Allergy, An historical review. J Allergy Clin Immunol 1976; 64:III. Soc Study Allergy Allied Cond 342; VI. Stand Cert 375:VII. Res 390.

53. Storm van Leeuwen W. Bronchial asthma in relation to climate. Proc R Soc Med 1924; 17:19.

54. Thommen AA. Etiology of hay fever: Studies in hay fever. NY State J Med 1930; 30:437.

55. Kern RA. Dust sensitization in bronchial asthma. Med Clin North Am 1921; 5:751.

56. Boatner CH, Efron BG. Studies with antigens. XII. Preparation and properties of concentrates of house dust allergen. J Invest Dermatol 1942; 5:7.

57. Cooke RA. Human sensitization. J Immunol 1916; 1:201.

58. Stull A, Cooke RA, Tenant J. The allergen content of protein extracts; its determination and deterioration. J Allergy 1933; 4:455.

59. Thommen AA. The specific treatment of hay fever. In: Asthma and Hay Fever in Theory and Practice (Coca AF, Walzer M, Thommen AA, eds.). London: Balliere, Tindall, & Cox, London, 1931; 757–774.

60. Bernton HS. Plantain hay fever and asthma. J Am Med Assoc 1925; 84:944.

61. Kahn IS, Grothaus EM. Studies in pollen sensitivities. Med J Rec 1925; 121:664.

62. MacKenzie GM. Desensitization of hay fever patients by specific local application. J Am Med Assoc 1922; 78:787.

63. Caulfield AHW. Desensitization of hay fever patients by injection and local application. J Am Med Assoc 1922; 79:125.

64. Touart MD. Hay fever; desensitization by ingestion of pollen protein. NY Med J 1922; 116:199.

65. Phillips EW. Relief of hay fever in intradermal injections of pollen extracts. J Am Med Assoc 1922; 79:125.

66. Le Noir P, Richet C Jr, Renard. Skin test for anaphylaxis. Bull Soc Med Hop 1921; 45:1283 (abstr); J Am Med Assoc 77:1770.

67. Report of the Joint Committee on Standards. J Allergy 1935; 6:408.

68. Heidelberger M, Avery OT. The soluble specific substance of pneumococcus. J Exp Med 1924; 40:301.

69. Cooke RA. Studies in specific hypersensitiveness, IX. On the phenomenon of hyposensitization (the clinically lessened sensitiveness of allergy). J Immunol 1922; 7:219.

70. Levine P, Coca A. Studies in hypersensitiveness. 1926; J Immunol, XX. A quantitative study of the interaction of atopic reagins and atopen. 11:411; XXII. On the nature of alleviating effect of the specific treatment of atopic conditions. 11:449.

71. Jadassohn W. Beitrage zun idosynkrasie problem. Klin Wschnschr 1926; 5(2):1957.

72. Cooke RA. Studies in specific hypersensitiveness. III. On constitutional reactions: The dangers of the diagnostic cutaneous test and therapeutic injection of allergens. J Immunol 1922; 7:119.

73. Freeman J. Rush inoculation with special reference to hay fever treatment. Lancet 1930; 1:744.

74. Cooke RA, Barnard JH, Hebald S, Stull A. Serological evidence of immunity with coexisting sensitization in a type of human allergy (hay fever). J Exp Med 1935; 62:733.

75. Loveless MH. Application of immunologic principles to the management of hay fever, including a preliminary report on the use of Freund's adjuvant. Am J Med Sci 1947; 214:559.

76. Cooke RA, Loveless M, Stull A. Studies on immunity in a type of human allergy (hay fever): serologic response of non-sensitive individuals to pollen injections. J Exp Med 1937; 66:689.

77. Sherman WB, Stull A, Cooke RA. Serologic changes in hay fever cases treated over a period of years. J Allergy 1940; 11:225.

78. Vannier WE, Campbell DH. The isolation and purification of purified house dust allergen fraction. J Allergy 1959; 30:198.

79. King TP, Norman PS. Isolation studies of allergens from ragweed pollen. Biochemistry 1962; 1:709.

80. Allen RW. The common cold: Its pathology and treatment. Lancet 1908; 2(1): 1589; (2) 1689.

81. Farrington PM. Hay fever. Memphis Med J 1912; 32:381.

82. Morrey CB. Vaccination with mixed cultures from the nose in hay fever. J Am Med Assoc 1913; 61:1806.

83. Goodale JL. Preliminary notes on skin reactions excited by various bacterial proteins in certain vasomotor disturbances of the upper air passages. Boston Med Surg J 1916; 174:223.

84. Walker IC. Studies on the sensitization of patients with bronchial asthma to bacterial proteins as demonstrated by the skin reaction and the methods employed in the preparation of those proteins. J Med Res 1917; 35:487.

85. Walker IC. The treatment with bacterial vaccines of bronchial asthmatics who are not sensitive to proteins. J Med Res 1917; 37:51.

86. Walker JW, Adkinson J. Studies on staphylococcus pyogenes aureus, albus and citreus and on Micrococcus tetragenous and M. catarrhalis. J Med Res 1917; 35:373; subsequent articles in this series appeared in 35:391, 36:293.

87. Kraus R, Doerr R. Uber bacterienanaphylaxie. Wien Klin Wschr 1908; 21:1008.

88. Koch R. Fortsetzung der muttheilungen uber ein Heilmittel gegen Tuberculose. Dtsch Med Wschr 1891; 9:101.

89. Rackemann FM. A clinical study of one hundred and fifty cases of bronchial asthma. Arch Intern Med 1918; 22:552.

90. Cooke RA. Infective asthma: indication of its allergic nature. Am J Med Sci 1932; 183, 309.

91. Walzer M. Asthma. In: Asthma and Hay Fever in Theory and Practice (Coca AF, Walzer M, Thomen AA, eds). Springfield, IL: Charles C. Thomas, 1931:260 261.

92. Hooker SB, Anderson LM. Heterogeneity of streptococci isolated from sputum with active critique on serological classification of streptococci. J Immunol 1929; 16:291.

93. Cooke RA. Infective asthma with pharmacopeia. In: Allergy in Theory and Practice (Cooke RA, ed). Philadelphia: W. B. Saunders Co., 1947:151–152.

94. Frankland AW, Hughes WH, Garrill RH. Autogenous bacterial vaccines in the treatment of asthma. Br Med J 1955; 2:941.

95. Johnstone DE. Study of the value of bacterial vaccines in the treatment of bronchial asthma associated with respiratory infections. Am J Dis Child 1957; 94:1.

96. Helander E. Bacterial vaccines in the treatment of bronchial asthma. Acta Allergy 1959; 13:47.

97. Lowell FC. American Academy of Allergy Presidential Address. J Allergy 1960; 31:185.

98. Brun E. Control examination of specificity of specific desensitization in asthma. Acta Allergol 1949; 2:122.

99. Frankland AW, Augustin R. Prophylaxis of summer hay-fever and asthma: Controlled trial comparing crude grass-pollen extracts with isolated main protein component. Lancet 1954; 1:1055.

100. Johnstone DE. Study of the role of antigen dosage in treatment of pollenosis and pollen-asthma. Am J Dis Child 1957; 94:1.

101. Lowell FC, Franklin W. A double blind study of the effectiveness and specificity of injection therapy in ragweed hay fever. N Engl J Med 1965; 273:675.

102. Fontana VC, Holt LE Jr, Mainland D. Effectiveness of hyposensitization therapy in ragweed hay-fever in children. J Am Med Assoc 1967; 195:109.

103. Lowell FC, Franklin W, Fontana VJ, Holt LE, Jr, Mainland D. Hyposensitization therapy in ragweed hay fever. J Am Med Assoc 1966; 195:1071 (lett).

104. Norman PS, Winkenwerder WL, Lichtenstein LM. Immunotherapy of hay fever with ragweed antigen E: Comparisons with whole pollen extracts and placeboes. J Allergy 1968; 42:93.

105. Sadan N, Rhyne MB, Mellits ED et al. Immunotherapy of pollenosis in children. Investigation of the immunologic basis of clinical improvement. N Engl J Med 1969; 280:623.

106. Sutton C. Hay fever. Med Clin North Am 1923; 7:605.

107. Zoss AR, Koch CA, Hirose RS. Alum-ragweed precipitate: Preparation and clinical investigation; preliminary report. J Allergy 1937; 8:829.

108. Stull A, Cooke RA, Sherman WB et al. Experimental and clinical studies of fresh and modified pollen extracts. J Allergy 1940; 11:439.

109. Naterman H. The treatment of hay fever by injections of suspended pollen tannate. J Allergy 1941; 12:378.

110. Rockwell G. Preparation of a slowly absorbed pollen antigen. Ohio State Med J 1941; 37:651.

111. Spain W, Fuchs A, Strauss M. A slowly absorbed gelatin-pollen extract for the treatment of hay fever. J Allergy 1941; 12:365.

112. Naterman HL. The treatment of hay fever by injections of pollen extract emulsified in lanolin and olive oil. N Engl J Med 1937; 218:797.

113. Naterman HL. Pollen tannate suspended in peanut oil with aluminum monostearate in the treatment of hay fever. J Allergy 1950; 22:175.

114. Malkiel S, Feinberg SM. Effect of slowly absorbing antigen (ragweed) on neutralizing antibody titer. J Allergy 1950; 21:525.

115. Gelfand HH, Frank DE. Studies on the blocking antibody in serum of ragweed treated patients. II. Its relation to clinical results. J Allergy 1944; 15:332.

116. Alexander HL, Johnson MC, Bukantz SC. Studies on correlation of symptoms of ragweed hay fever and titer of thermostable antibody. J Allergy 1948; 19:1.

117. Loveless MH. Application of immunologic principles to the management of hay fever, including a preliminary report on the use of Freund's adjuvant. Am J Med Sci 1947; 214:559.

118. Loveless MH. Repository immunization in pollen allergy. J Immunol 1957; 79:68.

119. Henle W, Henle G. Effect of adjuvants of vaccination of human beings against influenza. Proc Soc Exp Biol Med 1945; 59:179.

120. Freund J, McDermott K. Sensitization to horse serum by means of adjuvants. Proc Soc Exp Biol Med 1942; 49:548.

121. Brown EA. II. The treatment of ragweed pollenosis with a single annual emulsified extract injection. Ann Allergy 1958; 16:28, thru XI. Tree pollenosis effects of single annual injections of emulsified extracts in 560 multiply allergic patients. Ann Allergy 1960; 18:1200.

122. Feinberg SM, Rabinowitz HI, Pruzanski JJ et al. Repository antigen injections. J Allergy 1960; 31:421.

123. Sherman WB, Brown EB, Karol ES et al. Respository emulsion treatment of ragweed pollenosis. J Allergy 1962; 33:473.

124. Arbesman CE, Reisman RE. Hyposensitization therapy including repository: A double blind study. J Allergy 1964; 35:12.

125. Potter M, Boyce ER. Induction of plasma cell neoplasms in strain BALB/c mice with mineral oil and mineral oil adjuvants. Nature 1962; 193:1086.

126. Pliny Natural History. Jones WHS trans. Cambridge, MA: Harvard University Press, 1956: v7, Bk 15 139.

127. White H, transl. Appian's Roman History. Cambridge, MA: Harvard University Press, 1962: Bk 12, Chap 16 453.

128. Galen. De Temperamentis. Coxe JR. Writing of Hippocrates a)Id Galen (epitomized from the original Latin translation). Philadelphia: Lindsay and Blakiston, 1846:493.

129. Pliny. Cited by Urbach E, Gottlieb PM. Allergy. New York: Grune & Stratton, 1943:252.

130. Ehrlich P. Experimentelle intersuchungen uber immunitat. Dsch Med Wochenschr I. Uber ricin, 1891; 17:976, II. Uber abrin. 1891; 17:1218.

131. Chase MW. Inhibition of experimental drug allergy by prior feeding of the sensitizing agent. Proc Soc Exp Biol Med 1946; 61:257.

132. Dakin R. Remarks on a cutaneous affliction produced by certain poisonous vegetables. Am J Med Sci 1829; 1:98.

133. Strickler A. The toxin treatment of dermatitis venenata. J Am Med Assoc 1921; 77:910.

134. Duncan CH. Autotherapy in ivy poisoning. J Am Med Assoc 1916; 104:901.

135. Diffenbach WW. Treatment of ivy poisoning. South Cal Pract 1917; 32:91.

136. Strickler A. The treatment of dermatitis venenata by vegetable toxins. J Cutan Dis 1918; 36:327.

137. Schamberg JF. Desensitization against ivy poisoning. J Am Med Assoc 1919; 73:1213.

138. Blank JM, Coca AF. Study of the prophylactic action of an extract of poison ivy in the control of Rhus dermatitis. J Allergy 1936; 7:552.

139. Molitch M, Poliakoff S. Prevention of dermatitis venenata due to poison ivy in children. Arch Derm Syph 1936; 33:725.

140. Bachman LC. Prophylaxis of poison ivy: Use of an almond oil extract in children. J Pediatr 1938; 12:31.

141. Sompayrac LM. Negative results of rhus antigen treatment of experimental ivy poisoning. Am J Med Sci 1938; 195:361.

142. Shelmire B. Contact dermatitis from vegetation. Patch testing and treatment with plant oleoresins. South Med 1940; 38:337.

143. Schoffield AT. A case of egg poisoning. Lancet 1908; 1:716.

144. Finzio G (1911). Anaf. familiare per il latte di mucca. Tentativie di terapia antianaf. Pediatria 1911; 19:641.

145. Schloss OM. A case of allergy to common foods. Am J Dis Child 1912; 3:341.

146. Talbot FB. Asthma in children, III. Its treatment. Long Island Med J 1917; 11:245.

147. Pagniez P, Vallery-Radot P. Etude physiologique et therapeutique d'un cas d'urticaire geante. Anaphylaxie et anti-anaphylaxie alimentaires. Nouv Presse Med 1916, 24.529.

148. Luithlen F. Ueberempfindlichkeit und ernahrungstherapie. Wien Med Wschnschr 1926; 76:907.

149. Rowe AH. Desensitization to foods with reference to propeptanes. J Allergy 1931; 3:68.

150. Rowe AH. Food Allergy. Its Manifestation and Control and the Elimination Diets, A Compendium. Springfield, IL: Charles C Thomas, 1972:71.

151. Wrightman HB, discussion of Iliff EH, Gay LN. Treatment with oral ragweed pollen. J Allergy 1941; 12:601.

152. Curtis HH. The immunizing cure of hay fever. Med News 1900; 77:16.

153. Black JH. The oral administration of pollen. J Lab Clin Med 1927; 12:1156.

154. Black JH. The oral administration of ragweed pollen. J Allergy 1939; 10:156.

155. Urbach E. Desensibilisiering pollen ullergischer individuen auforalem wege mittels art-spezitischer pollenpeptone. Klin Wchnshr 1931; 10:534.

156. Urbach E. Die biologiche behandlung des henfiebers. Munchen Med Wchnschr 1937; 84:488.

157. Bernstein TB, Feinberg SM. Oral ragweed pollen therapy Clinical results and experiments in gastrointestinal absorption. Arch Intern Med 1938; 62:297.

158. Feinberg SM, Foran FL, Lichtenstein ML. Oral pollen therapy in ragweed pollinosis. J Am Med Assoc 1940; 115:231.

159. Heran J, Saint-Girans F. Un cas d'anaphylaxie a la quinine chez un paludeen intolerance absolus et urticaria. Antianaphylaxie par voie gastrique. Paris Med 1917; 7:161.

160. Goodale JL. Anaphylactic reactions occurring in horse asthma after the administration of diphtheria antitoxin. Boston Med Surg J 1914; 170:837.

161. Feinberg SM. Allergy in Practice. Chicago: Year Book Publishers, 1946; 536.

162. Boughton TH. Anaphylactic deaths in asthmatics. J Am Med Assoc 1912; 73:1912.

163. Kerley CG. Accidents in foreign protein administration. Arch Pediatr 1917; 34:457.

164. Tuft L. Fatalities following injection of foreign serum; report of unusual case. Am J Med Sci 1928; 175:325.

165. Widal F, Abrami P, Joltrain E. Anaphylaxie a l'ipeca. Presse Med 1922; 32:341.

166. Jeanneret R. Desensitization in insulin urticaria. Rev Med Suisse Rom 1929; 49:99; Abstr J Am Med Assoc 1929; 92:2197.

167. Corcoran AC. Note in rapid desensitization in a case of hypersensitiveness to insulin. Am J Med Sci 1938; 196:357.

168. Reisman RE, Rose NR, Witebsky E et al. Penicillin allergy and desensitization. J Allergy 1962; 33:178.

169. Parker CW, Shapiro J, Kern M, Eisen HN. Hypersensitivity to penicillenic acid derivatives in human beings with penicillin allergy. J Exp Med 1962; 115, 821.

170. O'Donovan WJ, Klorfajn I. Sensitivity to penicillin: Anaphylaxis and desensitization. Lancet 1946; 2:444.

171. Peck SM, Siegel S, Bergamini R. Successful desensitization in penicillin sensitivity. J Am Med Assoc 1947; 134:1546.

172. Crofton J. Desensitization to streptomycin and P. A. S. Br Med J 1953; 2:1014.

173. Clewes, cited by Freeman J. Toxic idiopathies; the relationship between hay and other pollen fevers, animal asthmas, food idiosyncracies, bronchial and spasmotic asthma, etc. Proc R Soc Med 1919–1920; 13:129.

174. Braun LIB. Notes on desensitization of a patient hypersensitive to bee stings. South Afr Med Rec 1925; 23:408.

175. Benson RL. Diagnosis and treatment of sensitization to mosquitoes. J Allergy 1936; 8:47.

176. Mclvor BC, Cherney LS. Studies in insect bite desensitization. Am J Trop Med 1941; 21:493.

177. Parlato SJ. A case of coryza and asthma due to sand flies. J Allergy 1929; 1:35.

178. Figley KD. Asthma due to May fly. Am J Med Sci 1929; 178:338.

179. Benson RL, Semenov H. Allergy in its relation to bee sting. J Allergy 1930; 1:105.

180. Loveless MH, Fackler WR. Wasp venom allergy and immunity. Ann Allergy 1956; 14:347.

181. Loveless MH. Immunization in wasp-sting allergy through venom-repositories and periodic insect stings. J Immunol 1962; 89:204.

182. Walzer M. Asthma. In: Asthma and Hay Fever in Theory and Practice (Coca AF, Walzer M, Thommen AA, eds). London: Balliere, Tindall & Cox, 1931:297–304.

183. Feinberg SM. Allergy in Practice. Chicago: Year Book Publishers, 1946; 544–553.

184. Auld AG. Further remarks on the treatment of asthma by peptone. Br Med J 1918; 2:49.

185. Kahn MH, Emsheimer HW. Autogenous defibrinated blood in the treatment of bronchial asthma. Arch Intern Med 1916; 18:445.

186. Storm Van Leewuen W, Varekamp H. On the tuberculin treatment of bronchial asthma and hay fever. Lancet 1921; 2:1366.

187. Brunner M. In: Asthma and Hay Fever in Theory and Practice (Coca AF, Walzer M, Thommen AA, eds.). London: Balliere, Tindall & Cox, 1931:301–302.

188. Bray GW. A case of physical allergy: A localized and generalized allergic type of reaction to cold. J Allergy 1932; 3:367.

189. Laymon CW, Cumming H. Histaminase in the treatment of urticaria and atopic dermatitis. J Invest Dermatol 1939; 2:301.

190. Sheldon JM, Fell N, Johnson JH et al. A clinical study of histamine azoprotein in allergic disease: A preliminary report. J Allergy 1941; 13:18.

191. Thompson RA, Bousquet J, Cohen SG et al. Current status of allergen immunotherapy. Shortened version of World Health Organization/International Union of Immunological Societies Working Group Report. Lancet 1989; 1:259.

192. Coca AF, Grove EF. Studies in hypersensitiveness XII. A study of the atopic reagins. J Immunol 1925; 10:445.

193. Arthus M. Injections répétées de sérum de cheval chez le lapin. CR Soc Biol (Paris) 1903; 55:817.

194. Weil R. The nature of anaphylaxis and the relations between anaphylaxis and immunity. J Med Res 1913; 27:497.

195. Cooke RA. Studies in specific hypersensitiveness; new etiologic factors in bronchial asthma. J Immunol 1922; 7:147.

196. Levine P, Coca AF. Studies in hypersensitiveness XXII. On the nature of the alleviating effect by the specific treatment of atopic conditions. J Immunol 1926; 11:449.

197. Stull A, Cooke RA, Tenant J. The allergen content of pollen extracts: Its determination and deterioration. J Allergy 1933; 4:455.

198. Tuft L. Clinical Allergy. Philadelphia: Saunders, 1937;739.

199. Ishizaka K, Ishizaka T. Identification of gamma-E antibodies as a carrier of reaginic antibody. J Immunol 1967; 99:1187.

200. Paul W, Ohara J. B-cell stimulatory factor-I/interleukin 4. Ann Rev Immunol 1987; 5:429.

2

Definition of an Allergen (Immunobiology)

MALCOLM N. BLUMENTHAL and ANDREAS ROSENBERG

University of Minnesota, Minneapolis, Minnesota, U.S.A.

I. INTRODUCTION

A variety of terms have been used to define the substance that stimulates an atopic reaction. Which words are used depends upon the terms chosen to denote the sensitivity. In the context of a general immunological reaction, the triggering substance is called an antigen. An antigen in modern usage is any substance that, as a result of coming into contact with appropriate tissues of an animal body, induces a state of sensitivity and/or resistance to infection or other substances after a latent period. In addition, the stimulating substances react specifically and in a demonstrable way with the responding tissues and/or antibody of the sensitized subject in vivo or in vitro. When allergy, defined as an adverse immune reaction, is used to express the state of sensitivity, von Pirquet called the exciting substances (or "antigen") that causes the sensitivity an "allergen." He stated that "the allergens comprise, besides the antigen proper, the many protein substances which lead to non-production of antibodies but to supersensitivity." The antibody that is produced by the

37

allergen was given the name "allergin," a term rarely used today. Coca coined the word "atopy" as a type of sensitized state and called the exciting substance an "atopen" and the reacting antibody a "reagin" or skin-sensitizing antibody. For experimental anaphylaxis in animals, the antigen is called an anaphylactogen, and the antibody an anaphylactin or anaphylactic antibody (1,2).

Through the years, the term "atopy" has been defined as an adverse immune reaction involving immunoglobulin E (IgE). The term "allergen" has been used to define the substance that is involved in atopy and induces reaginic or specific IgE antibodies. Allergens are defined in terms of the body's response to them. The immune response in atopy results from the interaction of the host with an allergen and other modulating environmental factors. It appears that only certain members of the general population are allergenically predisposed. Atopic conditions were originally identified by Cooke and Vander Veer as a genetically defined condition (1). Exposure to the allergen can be by inhalation, contact, ingestion, or injection. Typically, the dose-stimulated IgE production by an allergen is low. The resulting antibodies have high affinity. Not all individuals have a demonstrable IgE response to "known" allergens. The response to an allergen is determined by its properties, environmental factors, and host factors, including genetic susceptibility (3).

Although an allergen at present is defined as an antigen that will induce and interact specifically with IgE, the differences between allergens and antigens are blurred. The question arises of whether all antigens can be allergens under proper conditions.

II. PROPERTIES OF AN ALLERGEN/ANTIGEN/IMMUNOGEN

An operationally defined antigen (1) shows immunogenicity (i.e., a capacity to stimulate the formation of corresponding antibody and/or establish a state of sensitivity) and (2) reacts specifically with those antibodies and/or the responding tissue. The two properties are not always associated or are both known to be present. If only immunogenicity is observed, we define the molecules responsible more broadly as immunogens. Haptens (low-molecular-weight compounds such as drugs) are not immunogens but react specifically with the corresponding antibody that has been formed against hapten-protein complexes. Immunogenicity is not an inherent property of a molecule, as its molecular weight is. A molecule acts as an antigen if an organism recognizes it as foreign and its immune system responds to it. Thus, a molecule might function as an antigen in one organism but not in another. This chapter is concerned with molecules recognized as antigens by the humoral system of humans.

Any molecule able to elicit a humoral response in an organism is called an antigen. The specific antibody response is directed toward a unique surface region of the antigen. Such contiguous regions are called B-cell epitopes and generally have a surface area of 500 Å^2 (4). The surface of the antigen-binding region of the antibodies (the variable regions of light and heavy chains) is called the paratope and forms a tightly fitting complementary surface. The complementary juxtapositioning of charges and hydrophobic mountains or valleys produces the free energy for the binding reaction. The precise fit of the two surfaces excludes most of the hydration water, tightening the complex (5). Therefore, the elicitation of a response to an antigen indicates the appearance of antibodies specific to one or more epitopes on the antigen surface. Because the antibody is directed toward an epitope, that antibody will recognize another antigen if it carries the same or a very similar epitope. This is the basis for observed cross-reactivity between antigens and antisera. The surface of an antigen represents a quilt of putative epitopes (6). How many of those putative epitopes dominate the antibody response varies from case to case. The structure and position of dominating epitopes has been described only for a few protein antigens (5).

One of the major problems concerning allergenic response has been the identification of inherent structural features of a subclass of antigens that would make them uniquely suitable for acting as allergens. The number of identified allergens among the multitude of antigens surrounding us has been increasing rapidly. Whereas in the year 1995 we had about 250–300 plant and animal allergens identified, the number has been increasing since. Each aqueous extract of a plant and tissue reveals in electrophoresis 10 to 50 bands able to react with sera of people reporting sensitivity to the source. This Western blotting tells us about antibody binding in presence of an excess of antigen in vitro. Whether the reported antigens are able to act as allergens and produce a response in vivo is not always known. In some patients up to 50% of IgE is directed toward a single plant or animal while in others a single response represents only a fraction of IgE present (7). As a rule, there is enough unidentified IgE present, often called bystander antibody, to account for undetected sensitivity to many plants and animals. The total response load to allergens in an individual is as yet undetermined. Testing with 10 to 20 of the most common allergens reveals a distribution of responses from a few to many of the allergens presented. It is now known that the limit of skin-test sensitivity is related to the affinity of the antibody (8), and lower-affinity antibodies present in concentrations capable of causing symptoms may remain undetected by skin test unless titration of the response is carried out. This is most obvious in the case of children whose antibodies generally show lower affinity (9).

The sea of molecules acting as allergens is organized according to a schema proposed by WHO/IUIS. The molecules are labeled by the three or four first letters of the genus they are isolated from and by an arabic numeral indicating the sequence of isolation (3). *Der p* 1 is the first isolate from *Dermatophagoides petronyssinus*, house dust mite. Efforts to classify allergens by grouping molecules with homologies in sequence and defining allergens in a group as iso-allergens has not yielded very useful insights. The definition of major and minor allergens is a local functional classification because no special structural features associated with allergenicity have been found.

The question of whether all antigens can act as allergens given the right circumstances or whether allergens represent a structurally restricted class of antigens is of great importance for clinical considerations. To answer this question we must first consider if antigens themselves represent a restricted population of substances that have the unique property of being able to initiate a humoral response. Antigens/allergens are generally proteins, polysaccharides, glycoproteins, and lipoproteins of animal and vegetable origin. They can also be haptens or other small molecules complexed to proteins of the responding organism. Antigen response to tissue from different individuals involves all the types of molecules listed above. It does not appear at this point that these molecule types can be distinguished as allergic or nonallergic on an a priori structural basis (10).

To explore the possible positioning of allergens within the antigen family, features of an antigen in its function as an initiator of humoral response has to be considered. First, antigens, regardless of their allergenic properties, can be divided into two classes: those eliciting a thymus dependent response and those initiating a thymus-independent response. More precisely, thymus-dependence means that to act as antigen and trigger a humoral, antibody-based response, the molecule has to be able to first interact and activate antigen-specific T-cells. This activation proceeds by an initial proteolytic digestion of the peptide chain of the putative antigen. This is carried out as a first step of interaction with a number

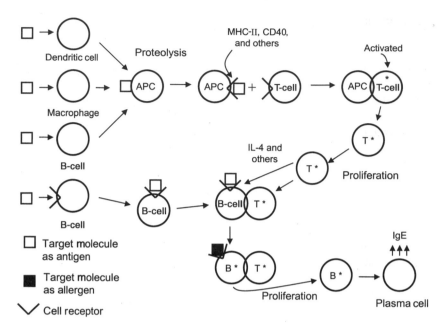

Figure 1 Conversion of antigen to allergen.

of antigen presenting cell (APC) types, the most prominent among them dendritic cells, macrophages, and even B-cells. The 13-amino-acid–long proteolytic fraction of the chain, called the T-cell epitope, is then bound to the MHC-II complex on the APC and presented to the T-cell receptor complex on the specific T-cell to be activated. The interaction involves additional binding of receptor pairs on the two cells. This complex interaction leads to activated T-cells that, both by exogenous effector molecules and by cognate inter-action, activate the B-cell clones chosen by antigen binding to their B-cell receptor (BCR). The activated clones proliferate and differentiate into antibody-producing plasma cells. The rough outline of this essential process leading to production of all subclasses of anti-bodies is roughly sketched in Fig. 1. Most protein antigens activate this T-cell–linked path of activation. The thymus-independent pathway allows direct activation of the specific B-cell clones, eliminating the need for the T-cell epitope. Most bacterial sugar-based antigens belong to this class. Hundreds of aeroallergens and other kind of allergens isolated contain protein and trigger the T-cell–dependent pathway. In addition to these two classes of anti-gens, a third, superantigen class exists, where antigens are able to trigger a general nonspe-cific activation of T-cell response leading to wide antibody response. There has been some speculation about the superantigenic nature of some allergic response (11).

Thus, all antigens can be divided into two classes. The first class is T-cell depend-ent and the second T-cell independent. Allergens seem to belong to the first class. There are two reasons for this. First, despite the prevalence and efficiency of the sugar- and lipid-dominated antigens of the second class, we know that the interaction between the sugar and lipid epitopes and the corresponding para-types is thermodynamically quite different from the interactions shown by the protein epitopes. The free energy of interaction is lower, as a rule, than that seen for protein epitopes (12). For allergens presented at a very low level this might constitute a major obstacle. Individual sugar groups linked to proteins can and often do participate in the topographic features of protein epitopes. Because the

T-cell epitopes represent a 13-residue sequence, a length allowing good binding to the MHC II complex, an antigen must have a peptide backbone of sufficient length. Most allergens encountered have sufficiently long peptide chains. Despite this and the well-known promiscuity of the MHC II complex for allergens of low molecular weight (4000 or less), this might still present a problem. The postulated requirement explains the preference of allergens for T-cell–dependent activation from an observational point of view. The mechanistic explanation most likely lies in the necessity for the presence of activated T-cells during the switch of heavy-chain synthesis to the ε chain. In this context one could argue that the limitation for allergenic nature of some antigens may lie in the specific motifs of T-cell sequence present. However, the promiscuity of the human leukocyte antigen (HLA) complex combined with the large number of T-cell epitopes of different sequences possible has produced what appears as a plethora of universal motifs present in all T-cell epitopes sequenced so far (13).

The T-cell–dependent class of antigens can be further subdivided into those prone to become allergens and those that are not; consideration must be given to the function of antibodies in general and those specifically involved with interaction with allergens. The most important feature for an antibody is its ability to recognize an antigen and to form a complex with its target epitope. It can, and under suitable conditions does, form networks with an antigen; however, this is not its exclusive property. The function of an antibody to allergen is to arm an antibody receptor situated on effector cells, such as mast cells, and wait for the antigen/allergen to come and cross-link the receptors. It is the cross-linking reaction that an allergen, in general, must accomplish. For that purpose an allergen must carry at least two suitably separated epitopes allowing the molecule to form a bridge. One epitope might be enough for the functioning of an antigen, but it is certainly not enough for an allergen. It appears for some purified allergens that the IgE response is predominantly toward three or four dominant epitopes (14). The IgG and IgE responses in the same sensitized individual (15) recognize the same epitopes. The spatial distribution of the epitopes is known in a very few cases (16). It stands to reason, from a receptor aggregation point of view, that a favorable topography of epitopes would contribute greatly to the potency of an allergen. One might argue that the necessary high affinity of an antibody would limit the inherited libraries capable of producing such antibodies and thus restrict some antigens to become allergens. This probably is not true, because although IgE affinities toward allergens are exceptionally high, nonallergic individuals are able to mount an equally high affinity response of IgG to the same allergens, acting in this case as antigens (14). Thus, high affinity by itself is not a necessary step toward atopy. In addition, in skin test–negative clinically allergic people, lower-affinity antibodies can act in allergic reactions. It has been shown that affinity is correlated with the ability to cross-link receptors (17). Thus, high affinity is correlated with the strength of atopic reactions, but achieving that affinity seems not to be the limiting factor in characterizing allergens among antigens.

The necessity of link formation of two separated epitopes might also induce a lower limit in molecular weight where crowding on small surfaces could limit a cross-linking activity. Studies of *Amb a* 5 reveal that at least three epitopes are present on that 2500 MW protein (15). How much smaller it can go without the necessity of dimerization or polymerization of the putative allergen is not known; it is likely, however, that the probability of finding an antigen with allergenic properties is lessened at the lower molecular weight.

There has been lot of speculation that the presence of enzymes among recognized allergens relates to the necessary role of proteolytic activity for disruption of the cohesion of epithelial barriers hindering the movement of allergens in tissue (18). However, despite the preponderance of proteolytic enzyme activity in mite droppings, many of the allergens reported are not proteolytic enzymes. Some of the most efficient allergens known, such as peanut, are storage proteins. Tropomyosin of shrimp appears as *Pen a* 1, and cockroach, *Bla g*, belongs to the calycin family. Furthermore, allergens such as lactoglobulin do not have proteolytic activity. Among the major sets of proteins, enzymes are often more water soluble than structural or membrane proteins. In corn extracts, only a fraction of water-soluble allergens are found in the extracts based on isopropanol (19). It is therefore unlikely that proteolytic activity is necessary for allergens. However, unanswered is the more broadly formulated question of whether proteolytic activity correlates with the allergenic potential of an antigen. This cannot be answered until the preponderance of proteolytic enzymes among allergens is known and compared with that among proteins in general.

For antigens to act as allergens, they must elicit T-cell–dependent responses and be able to form at least two, and preferably three or four, spatially separated epitopes. This establishes some lower molecular weight limit and raises the question of whether the majority of T-cell–dependent antigens become allergens. They certainly have the ability, but whether they become an antigen depends on the circumstances. A series of investigations of allergy-prone families found that, although the tendency to be sensitive to allergens is inherited, the choice of allergens among antigens seems to be totally random. There was no correlation between the selectivity allergen of the mother and father and of the children. Thus, all antigens encountered that fulfill the two criteria above can become allergens by a purely random process (20).

Another observation supporting this model is the fact that most people, both atopic and nonallergic, mount a vigorous response to antigens, utilizing all subclasses of immunoglobulins except IgE. The atopic people mount the same response, but in addition they have an IgE response (21). The major difference in immune antibody response to antigen and allergen is consequently quite narrowly localized. The additional production of high-affinity IgE is directed to the dominant epitopes of the antigen. The epitopes seem to be the same ones recognized by other antibody classes. There is no evidence up to now of tolerance in nonatopic individuals. Unusual patterns of response by other subclasses of antibodies has been frequently mentioned, especially the appearance of enhanced IgG4 response. This may appear in individual circumstances, but studies of large populations of immune-response profiles to allergens have not revealed any systematic differences.

There is intrinsically very little in the structure of the T-cell–dependent subclass of antigens that determines whether they will become allergens or not. There is, to our knowledge, no reliable report of a common structural feature in allergens. Allergens are created by the selective response to them as they are presented as normal antigens; consequently, antigen-allergen switch for a molecule ultimately rests in the circumstances under which the presentation takes place.

III. ALLERGEN: ROUTE OF EXPOSURE

Exposure to the allergen appears necessary to the development of an IgE immune response. Typically, the mucosal surfaces and skin are the body's barriers to encounters with allergens and other environmental factors. The presence of these barriers safeguards the internal milieu by keeping foreign items out. The relative importance of these barriers, as well as of the parenteral routes in the development of the immune response, especially with regard to an allergen, is not clear. It is thought that the mucosal surfaces, present in the upper and lower respiratory tract, GI tract, genital tract, and mammary glands, are most important. Both the innate and adaptive immune systems are involved. The physical barriers of the skin, gastrointestinal tract, and respiratory tract may prevent penetration of high-molecular-weight allergens. Schneeberger reported that the molecular weight cutoff above which nasal and alveolar membranes are impermeable is between 40,000 and 60,000 (22). IgE sensitivity has also been found following injection of allergens, such as penicillin or enzymes delivered by stinging insects (3). The innate mucosal immune factors consist of many components including complement, secretory leukocytes, protease inhibitors, surfactant protein, defensin, mucins, slatherin, lactoferrin, cystatins, lysozyme, manose-binding lectin, thrombospondins, and collectin, as well as secretory agglutins. The adaptive mucosal immune system involves two main systems: (1) the tonsils, Peyers patches, and isolated lymphoid follicles; and (2) the diffuse mucosal immune system, consisting of intra-epithelial lymphocytes and the lamina propria. The organized mucosal tissues play an important role in the inductive stage of an immune response. The experimental literature suggests that a response leading to primary allergen sensitization to both inhalants and ingestants is provided principally via the production of a population of cytokines (23). The importance of the resulting immunoglobulin production regarding the response to allergens has not been well studied. IgA is the main mucosal antibody. Its response is quantitatively among the highest, but the affinities associated are low, though they still provide quite high capacity.

The duration and amount of exposure, as well as the presence of other modulating pollutants are a few of the many environmental factors that influence the type of response to an antigen/allergen. Marsh has estimated that the mean adult annual dosage of individual allergenic components is probably in the nanogram range (3). Allergens appear to induce IgE production at relatively low doses. The ambient level of mite allergen $Der\ p$ that a normal individual is exposed to has been measured to fluctuate around 100 pg/m^3. As a result of many studies, a consensus has been reached that mite content of house dust > 2 $\mu g/g$ dust is associated with sensitization in children (23). Clinical studies suggest that days of exposure for parasitic allergens and months for some constant allergen exposure to years of exposure for seasonal allergens such as pollen are needed to develop reaginic/IgE antibodies. Tada and Ishizaka suggest that the routes of entry used by the allergen that are most likely to induce IgE antibody formation are the respiratory and gastrointestinal tracts, because the IgE-producing microenvironments are found predominantly in these locations (24).

IV. ENVIRONMENTAL FACTORS MODULATING THE IMMUNE RESPONSE TO ALLERGENS

There has been, in the Western world, a substantial increase in atopy prevalence over the last few decades (25). Changes in diagnostic procedures and genetic composition appear to be insufficient to explain most of this increase. The environment must be of major importance in the development and increased prevalence of atopy. Western living conditions, allergens, air pollution from sources such as smoke and diesel fumes, and infections all may influence the immune system and determine the ability of the individual to develop or not develop atopy. Atopy is thought to involve the persistent presence of the T helper cell 2 (TH2) profile. One of the major hypotheses regarding this increase in atopic reactions is the hygiene hypothesis (26). The basis of the hygiene theory is that newborns have a TH2 profile, and after birth the majority change to a T helper cell 1 (TH1) profile associated with an increase in interferon-gamma (IFN-γ), resulting in decreased susceptibility to atopy. Those having a persisting TH2 profile with a decrease in the production of INF-γ and increased production of interleukin-4 (IL-4) appear to have a susceptibility to asthma and allergies. Bacterial infections and endotoxin trigger changes toward a TH1 profile. Investigations suggest that an increase in INF-γ production is associated with protection against asthma and atopy. A possible explanation for the protective effects of exposure to bacteria or their products during the period when sensitization occurs in early life is its stimulation to increased IFN-γ production. The lack of microbial stimulation of sufficient intensity in early life may, paradoxically, influence the maturation of the immune system, causing a predominance of the TH2 subtype in genetically susceptible individuals. This was stressed in several early studies involving mycobacteria. Changes in infant diet, early use of antibiotics, and reduced exposure to bacterial infections predisposes individuals to the persistence of TH2 response in childhood. It also has been suggested that only those infections that are able to prompt a strong cell-mediated immune response and long-memory immunity play a positive role here in a shift toward the TH1-type response and prevention of asthma and atopy.

Exposure to allergens from domestic pets, such as dogs and cats, as well as mite exposure have shown a relationship to atopic sensitization (27). Community studies in Europe indicate that early exposure to farm animals has a protective effect against sensitization and asthma. A protective effect may have resulted from exposure to bacterial endotoxins. The presence of cats in a home has been associated with a decrease in the incidence and prevalence of asthma. It has been suggested that domestic animals can be a source of endotoxin, which is a stimulant of IL-12, and may bias the overall immune response away from an atopic or TH2 response. The results seen in some studies may be due to selection and environmental bias. There are many problems with accepting the hygiene hypothesis. These include the finding that asthma and atopy are more prevalent in the core city compared with the suburbs and the observation that autoimmune processes, which are thought to involve TH1, are increasing. Other environmental factors such as diesel fumes, occupational inhalants, and allergen exposure have been noted to affect the immune response to allergens and the resulting clinical picture. It appears at this point that environmental factors may enhance either sensitization or normalization (26).

V. GENETIC FACTORS MODULATING THE IMMUNE RESPONSE TO ALLERGENS

The atopic immune response, by definition, is a complex condition involving genetic as well as environmental factors (Fig. 2). The evidence for genetic factors being involved in the different phenotypes of atopy has consisted of their aggregation in families, increased prevalence in first-degree relatives, and increased concordance in monozygotic twins compared with dizygotic twins. Genetic investigations to determine where the genes are located have used many approaches, including forward genetics, candidate genes, genome screens, fine mapping, and functional genomics using statistical linkage and association analysis. These methods considered genetic heterogeneity, gene-gene interac-

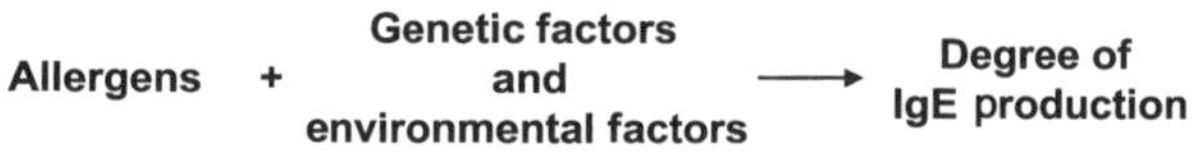

Allergens + Genetic factors and environmental factors ⟶ Degree of IgE production

Figure 2 Environmental and genetic factors involved in IgE response to allergen.

tion, and gene-environment interaction. Atopy, defined as an adverse specific IgE immune reaction, has been studied using a variety of phenotypes, including serum IgE levels, skin test reactivity, specific skin test reactivity, and specific serum IgE levels. Candidate gene approaches using these phenotypes have stressed the importance of several areas, including the cytokine cluster on chromosome 5q, TNF on chromosome 6p, FcεRIb on chromosome 11q, and the IL-4 receptor on chromosome 16q. Several groups have used the positional genetic approach to study atopy phenotypes. Using serum IgE as well as allergen skin test reactivity as a phenotype, a variety of loci have been identified, especially those on chromosomes 5q, 11q, and 12q (28). Evidence of gene-gene interaction was noted by the Collaborative Study of the Genetics of Asthma (CSGA) in a subset analysis (29). Specific IgE responses as measured by skin test reactivity or specific serum IgE levels have also been investigated. Early association studies have demonstrated that several purified allergens, such as ragweed *Amb a* 5 and 6, Olive *Ole e* I, and *Lillilum perenne* 1, 2, and 3, have been associated with the HLA system (30). Genome screens using specific skin test reactivity to mites, cockroaches, and mold have detected a few other potential chromosomal areas with no replication reported (31). The HLA system is one of the necessary components for the development of a T-cell–dependent specific immune response; however, additional factors are needed for the development of such a T-cell response. On the basis of the proposed atopic model, another point of restriction involves the binding of the complex formed by the HLA system and the critical peptide of the allergen with the specific T-cell receptor (TCR) complex. A critical relationship may exist between the structure determined by the HLA class II region genes and the availability of selected TCR variable region genes that affect the binding of foreign peptides. The arrangement of TCR elements on the alpha and beta chains appears to determine the antigen specificity of the T-cell. Studies of genomic polymorphism in humans at the TCR alpha and beta region suggest that there may be restriction of the IgE response to a particular allergen.

The current understanding of the immune system suggests that the upregulation of IgE synthesis in atopy is due to the induction of IgE isotype utilization at the DNA level in B-cells. The start of IgE synthesis appears to involve a number of signals followed by direct T- and B-cell interaction. They require prior engagement of the TCR with antigenic fragments (peptides) that are recognized on MHC class II molecules on antigen presentation cells (APCs). Interferon-α appears to be a major downregulator of IgE synthesis. There are at least two major genetic controls of atopy. One, which is non–epitope specific, is noted using the phenotypes of total serum IgE levels and skin test reactivity in general. The genes may reside on a variety of different loci and chromosomes, i.e., IL-4 on chromosome 5q, IgE receptor on chromosome 11q, and INF-γ on chromosome 12q. Another is epitope specific and appears to be associated with the HLA system. Therefore, there appear to be several levels involved in selectivity: (1) the epitope-specific level, which is related to the HLA system; (2) the purified allergen level (molecular selection), which is only partially HLA associated and is dependent on size; and (3) the complex or natural allergen level, involving many epitopes selective for organisms. There are probably too many surface epitopes to demonstrate any specific HLA association.

VI. ALLERGIC SENSITIZATION

The development of an atopic condition is dependent on sensitization involving the primary encounter with the allergen that leads to immune recognition. The involved immune system's primary function is protection of the organism from infectious microbes as well as from other foreign substances that may possess a diverse collection of pathogenic mechanisms. The responding system has been divided into the innate immune system and the adaptive immune system. The innate immune system is the host defense mechanism that is encoded in the germline genes of the host. It involves barrier mechanisms such as the epithelial cell layers, secreted mucus layers and epithelial cilia, soluble proteins and bioactive small molecules in biological fluids (i.e., complement and defensin) released from cells (cytokines, chemokines, and bioactive amines and enzymes), as well as cell surface receptors that use binding molecular patterns expressed on the surfaces of invading microbes and other foreign substances for identification. The adaptive system exhibits specificity for its target antigens. It is based primarily on the antigen-specific receptors on the surfaces of the T and B lymphocytes. The antigen-specific receptors of the adaptive response are assembled by somatic rearrangement of germline gene elements to form both intact T-cell receptors and B-cell antigen-specific receptors (Ig).

The innate and adaptive immune systems work together. The innate system is the first line of host defense. The adaptive response becomes prominent as antigen-specific T- and B-cells undergo clonal expansion. The antigen-specific cells amplify their response by recruiting innate effector mechanisms to bring about the complete control of invading microbes and other foreign antigens. The innate and adaptive immune responses are different in their mechanisms of action. Synergy between them is essential for an intact, fully effective immune response involving exposure to the allergen. The immune response to an allergen involves a variety of cells. The process of the immune response to an allergen most likely begins with involvement of the innate immune system, which sets the stage for the development of an adaptive response to the allergen, resulting in the production of allergen-specific IgE. Once formed, the resultant allergen-specific IgE attaches via high-affinity IgE receptors (FcεRI, such as on mast cells and basophils) and low-affinity IgE receptors (FcεRII, such as on a variety of other cells including eosinophils and platelets). This primary sensitization occurs in predisposed naive individuals on their initial encounter with the allergen. The pathway for sensitization is quite similar to the future recognition reaction in sensitized people; however, the cellular participants are probably different. The cells recruited for response cannot come from the memory cell compartment, but only from the naive cell population. Furthermore, the absence of traces of high-affinity antibody favors cells that do not use the Ig as receptor in the antigen-presenting function. This may push the concentration limits for recognition higher than those that develop in sensitized individuals. There is persistence of the robustness of the IgE immune response into old age (32).

VII. ALLERGIC ATOPIC REACTIONS AND INFLAMMATION (INCLUDING PATHOLOGY)

The resulting clinical allergic reactions may vary from symptoms of sneezing, nasal discharge, and nasal congestion associated with allergic rhinitis; to coughing, wheezing, and shortness of breath with evidence of reversible airway obstruction; to urticaria, angioedema, and anaphylaxis. Inflammation is an important feature of these conditions. It consists of a dynamic complex of cytological and histological reactions that occur in tissues in response to an injury or abnormal stimulation caused by a physical, chemical, or biological agent.

Once the individual begins to develop sensitization to the allergen, inflammation is initiated. Upon reexposure to the allergen, the immune system is further activated, resulting in more inflammation, ultimately determining the clinical picture of allergy/atopy. One of the steps following reexposure to the allergen involves the interaction with its specific IgE, attached by way of FcεRI and FcεRII to cells containing mediating substances. The ultimate allergic reaction results from the involvement of a variety of cells ranging from T-cells involved in the development of the specific immune reaction as well as monocytes and macrophages and cells of the myeloid series, including granulocytes (i.e., mast cells, eosinophils, neutrophils, and platelets). The interactions between these cells are of importance in the inflammatory response, which is involved in atopy. Mediators released by some cells regulate the function of the others. The acute symptoms of allergies, such as sneezing, wheezing, and urticaria, may be due to the release of mediators from the mast cells, such as histamine, whereas the chronic symptoms such as bronchial hyperreactivity may be explained on the basis of eosinophil-mediated tissue damage. The T-cells, which are of major importance in atopy, are of the TH2 type and produce IL-4 and IL-5, which potentiate the terminal differentiation and activation of the eosinophils. Basic proteins, together with the platelet-activating factor and leukotrienes secreted by eosinophils, probably also contribute to these chronic symptoms. Cellular communication and control through the release of mediators is important in the regulation of the inflammatory response. Important mediators are thought to include histamine, cytokines, and leukotrienes. Cell adhesion molecules are also important in inflammation. A series of cell adhesion molecules mediate interaction between vascular endothelium and leukocyte cell surfaces. The three major families of adhesion molecules that have been identified and contribute to this process are integrins, selectins, and immunoglobulin-like receptors. Other mediators of the inflammatory response that may be important are the complement system and heat shock proteins. Therefore, as a result of the introduction of the allergen in a sensitized individual, a variety of cells and humoral components are activated, resulting in inflammation and determining the clinical picture. The end result for exposure to an allergen is transient and/or chronic inflammation. The molecular and tissue changes found are common to all inflammatory processes. The difference between atopic allergy and all other inflammatory processes lies in causation. Atopic allergy is linked to aberrant humoral response to foreign molecules, whether these responses are IgE, IgG, or direct cellular reactions, as in the case of some late-phase reactions (33,34).

The nature of the immune reaction to an allergen and the resulting clinical picture is dependent upon many steps influenced by host and environmental factors, such as properties of the allergen, route of exposure, and genetic controls.

VIII. SALIENT POINTS

1. Allergens/antigens have two properties: (1) immunogenicity (i.e., the capacity to stimulate the formation of the corresponding antibody and/or a state of sensitivity) and (2) the ability to react specifically with those antibodies and/or the responding tissue. The two properties are not always associated.
2. Allergens are antigens that induce the production of an IgE-specific antibody that will interact with the inducing antigen.
3. From a chemical standpoint, there seems to be little to differentiate allergens from other antigens.
4. There appear to be four conditions for a molecule to become an allergen: (1) It must possess a surface to which the antibody can form a complementary surface; (2) it must have an amino acid sequence in its backbone able to bind the

Table 1 Definitions

Allergens are a subclass of antigens that stimulate the production of and combine with the IgE
subclass of antibodies.

Antigens are substances that have immunogenicity, leading to the production of antibodies with
which the antigens will react.

B-cell epitopes are specific surface areas on antigens toward which the specificity of a single
antibody is directed.

Haptens are substances that are not immunogenic (cannot stimulate humoral response without the
help of carrier substances) but combine specifically with the formed antibody.

Immunogens are substances that stimulate specific immune response, such as the production of an
antibody.

T-cell epitopes are approximately 13-amino-acids–long proteolytic fragments of the antigen
backbone and are necessary to activate the antigen-specific T-cells.

T helper cell 1 (TH1) profile is a specific pattern of effector molecules, where INF-γ is dominant,
derived from activated T-cells.

T helper cell 2 (TH2) profile is a specific pattern of effector molecules, of which IL-4 and IL-5
are dominant, derived from activated T-cells.

MHC-II alleles of the responding individual; (3) the free energy of interaction
of the allergen with the antibody should be adequate to ensure binding at low
concentrations; and (4) it must form at least two epitopes able to act as a bridge.

5. The nature of the immune reaction to an allergen is dependent upon many steps
    influenced by host and environmental factors.

6. Genetic factors include multiple genes regulating non–epitope-specific factors,
    such as those on chromosome 5q, as well as those that are allergen epitope
    specific, including genes in the MHC on chromosome 6.

7. The duration, route, and amount of exposure, as well as the presence of other
    modulating pollutants, are a few of the environmental factors that influence the
    type of response to an allergen.

8. Atopy, clinically defined, is an inflammatory condition resulting from an aller-
    gen producing an adverse immune reaction.

ACKNOWLEDGMENTS

This work was supported in part by NIH grants 5U01HL49609 and M01-RR00400 from
the National Center for Research Resources, National Institutes of Health.

REFERENCES

1. Blumenthal MN. Historical perspectives. In: Bjorksten B, Blumenthal MN, eds. Genetics of
    Allergy and Asthma: Methods for Investigative Studies. New York: Marcel Dekker, 1996:1–8.
2. Gell PGH, Coombs RRA. Clinical Aspects of Immunology. Philadelphia: FA Davis, 1963.
3. Marsh D, Blumenthal MN. Genetic and Environmental Factors in Clinical Allergy.
    Minneapolis: University of Minnesota, 1990.
4. Wilson IA, Stanfield RL. Antibody-antigen interactions: New structures and new
    conformational changes. Curr Opin Struct Biol 1994; 4:857–867.
5. Davies DR, Padlan EA, Sheriff S. Antibody-antigen complexes. Ann Rev Biochem 1990;
    59:439–473.

6. Jemmerson R. Epitope mapping by proteolysis of antigen-antibody complexes: Protein footprinting. Methods Mol Biol 1996; 66:97–108.

7. Hamra MA, Rosenberg A, Blumenthal MN. Comparison of specific and total IgE levels in monoresponders and polyresponders. J Allergy Clin Immunol 1995; 95:1(2):336.

8. Pierson-Mullany LK, Jackola DR, Blumenthal MN, Rosenberg A. Evidence of an affinity threshold for IgE-allergen binding in the percutaneous skin test reaction. Clin Exp Allergy 2002; 32(1):107–116.

9. Jackola D, Liebeler C, Blumenthal MN, Rosenberg A. Allergen skin test reaction patterns in children (≤ 10 y.o.) from atopic families suggest age-dependent changes in allergen-IgE binding in early life. Int Arch Allergy Immunol 2003; in press.

10. Kraft D, Sehon AH. Molecular Biology and Immunology of Allergens. Boca Raton, FL: CRC Press, 1993.

11. Snow RE, Chapman LJ, Frew AJ, Holgate ST, Stevenson FK. Is the IgE response driven by a B cell super antigen? J Allergy Clin Immunol 1997; 99:1(2):S437.

12. Bundle DR, Bauman H, Brisson JR, Gagne SM, Zdanov A, Cygler M. Solution structure of a trisaccharide-antibody complex: Comparison of NMR measurements with a crystal structure. Biochemistry 1994; 33:5183–5192.

13. Van Neerven RJ, Ebner C, Yssel H, Kapsenberg ML, Lamb JR. T cell response to allergens: Epitope specificity and clinical relevance. Immunol Today 1996; 17:526–532.

14. Pierson-Mullany LK, Jackola DR, Blumenthal MN, Rosenberg A. Characterization of polyclonal allergen-specific IgE responses by affinity distributions. Mol Immunol 2000; 37(10):613–620.

15. Kim KE, Rosenberg A, Roberts S, Blumenthal MN. The affinity of allergen specific IgE and the competition between IgE and IgG for the allergen in *Amb a V* sensitive individuals. Mol Immunol 1996; 33(10):873–880.

16. Topham CM, Srinivasin N, Thorpe CY, Overington JP, Kalsheker NA. Comparative modeling of major house dust mite allergen *Der p 1*: Structure validation using an extended environmental amino-acid propensity table. Protein Eng 1994; 7:869–894.

17. Mita H, Yasueda H, Akiyama K. Affinity of IgE antibody to antigen influences allergen-induced histamine release. Clin Exp Allergy 2000; 30:1582–1589.

18. Robinson C, Kalsheker NA, Srinivasan N, King CM, Garrod DR, Thompson RJ, Stewart GA. On the potential significance of the enzymatic activity of mite allergens to immunogenicity: Clues to structure and function revealed by molecular characterization. Clin Exp Allergy 1997; 27:10–21.

19. Lehrer SB, Reese G, Ortega H, El-Dhar JM, Goldby B, Malo JL. IgE antibody reactivity to aqueous-soluble, alcohol-soluble and transgenic core proteins. J Allergy Clin Immunol 1997; 99:1(2):S147.

20. Jackola DR, Liebeler CL, Blumenthal MN, Rosenberg A. Absence of inherited selectivity restrictions in humoral responses to allergens. 2003; personal communication.

21. Jackola DR, Pierson-Mullany LK, Liebeler CL, Blumenthal MN, Rosenberg A. Variable binding affinities for allergen suggest a "selective competition" among immunoglobulins in atopic and non-atopic humans. Mol Immunol 2002; 39(5–6):367–377.

22. Schneeberger EE. The permeability of the alveolar-capillary membrane to ultrastructural protein tracers. Ann NY Acad Sci 1974; 221:238–243.

23. Kuehr J, Frischer T, Meinert R, Barth R, Forster J, Schraub S, Urbanek R, Kazmaus W. Mite allergen exposure is a risk for the incidence of specific sensitization. J Allergy Clin Immunol 1994; 94:44–52.

24. Tada T, Ishizaka K. Distribution of gamma E forming cells in lymphoid tissues of the human and monkey. J Immunol 1970; 104(2):377–387.

25. Blumenthal MN. Epidemiology and Genetics of Asthma and Allergy. In: Allergy, 2nd ed. (Kaplan AP, ed.) Philadelphia: Saunders, 1997:407–420.

26. Liu AH, Murphy JR. Hygiene hypothesis: Fact or fiction? J Allergy Clin Immunol 2003; 111:471–478.
27. Ownby DR, Johnson CC, Peterson EL. Exposure to dogs and cats in the first year of life and risk of allergic sensitization at 6 to 7 years of age. J Am Mmed Assoc 2002; 288(8):963–72.
28. Blumenthal JB, Blumenthal MN. Genetics of asthma. Med Clin North Am 2002; 86(5):937–50.
29. Xu JF, Meyers DA, Ober C, Blumenthal MN, Mellen B, Barnes K, King RA, Lester LA, Howard TD, Solway J, Langefeld C, Beaty TH, Rich SS, Bleecker ER, Cox NJ, CSGA. Genome wide screen and identifying gene-gene interactions for asthma susceptibility loci in three U.S. populations: Collaborative Study on the Genetics of Asthma (CSGA). Am J Hum Genet 2001; 68:1437–1446.
30. Blumenthal MN. Genetics of Asthma, Allergy and Related Conditions. In: Genetics of Allergy and Asthma: Methods for Investigative Studies (Bjorksten B, Blumenthal MN, eds.) New York: Marcel Dekker, 1996:327–356.
31. Blumenthal MN, Ober C, Bleecker E, Beaty T, Banks-Schlegel S, Florance AM, Langefeld CD, Rich SS, CSGA. Linkage analysis of a genome scan for skin test reactivity to allergens. Am J Res Crit Care Med 2001; 163(5,2):A960.
32. Jackola DR, Pierson-Mullany LK, Daniels LR, Corazalla E, Rosenberg A, Blumenthal MN. Robustness into advanced age of atopy-specific mechanisms in atopy-prone families. Gerontol A Biol Sci Med Sci 2003; 58(2):99–107.
33. Lympany PA, Lee T. Inflammation. In: Genetics of Allergy and Asthma: Methods for Investigative Studies (Bjorksten B, Blumenthal MN, eds.). New York: Marcel Dekker, 1996:241–280.
34. Barnes P. Inflammation. In: Bronchial Asthma: Mechanisms and Therapeutics (Weiss EB, Stein M, eds.). Boston: Little, Brown 1993:80–94

3

Allergen Nomenclature

MARTIN D. CHAPMAN

INDOOR Biotechnologies, Inc., and University of Virginia, Charlottesville, Virginia, U.S.A.

I. HISTORICAL INTRODUCTION

As with most biochemical disciplines, the history of allergen nomenclature dates back to the time when allergens were fractionated using a variety of "classical" biochemical separation techniques and the active (most allergenic) fraction was usually named according to the whim of the investigator. For allergens, this dates to the 1940s through the late 1950s, when early attempts were made to purify pollen and house dust allergens using phenol extraction, salt precipitation, and electrophoretic techniques. In the early 1960s, ion exchange and gel filtration media were introduced and ragweed "antigen E" was the first allergen to be purified. This allergen, named by King and Norman, was one of five precipitin lines (labeled A–E) that reacted with rabbit polyclonal antibodies to ragweed in Ouchterlony immunodiffusion tests. Following purification, precipitin line E, or "antigen E" was shown to be a potent allergen (1). Later, Marsh, working in Cambridge, England, isolated an important allergen from rye grass pollen (*Lolium perenne*) and used the name "Rye 1" to indicate that this was the first allergen purified from this species (2). In the 1970s, the field advanced apace and many allergens were purified from ragweed, rye grass, insect venoms, and other sources. The field was led by the laboratory of the late Dr. David Marsh, who had moved to Johns Hopkins University in Baltimore, Maryland. There ragweed allergens Ra3, Ra4, Ra5, and Ra6 and rye grass allergens Rye 2 and Rye 3 were isolated and used for immunological and genetic studies of hay fever. At the same time, Ohman identified a major cat allergen (Cat-1) (3) and Elsayed purified allergen M from codfish (4).

The state of the art in the early 1970s was reviewed in a seminal chapter by Marsh in *The Antigens* (ed. Michael Sela), which described the molecular properties of allergens, the factors that influenced allergenicity, the immune response to allergens, and immunogenetic studies of IgE responses to purified pollen allergens (5). This chapter provided the first clear definition of a "major" allergen, which Marsh defined as a highly purified allergen that induced immediate skin test responses in >90% of allergic individuals—this in contrast to a "minor" allergen, to which <20% of patients had skin test responses. A less stringent standard was subsequently adopted, and today a major allergen is defined as one to which >50% of allergic patients react.

With the introduction of crossed immunoelectrophoresis (CIE) and crossed radioimmunoelectrophoresis (CRIE) for allergen identification by Lowenstein and colleagues in Scandinavia, there was a tremendous proliferation of the number of antigenic proteins and CIE/CRIE peaks identified as allergens (6). Typically, 10 to 50 peaks could be detected in a given allergen based on reactivity with rabbit polyclonal antibodies or IgE antibodies. These peaks were given a plethora of names such as Dp5, Dp42, Ag12, etc. Inevitably, this led to the same allergens being referred to by different names in different laboratories. Thus, mite antigen P_1 was also known as Dp42 or Ag12. It was clear that a unified nomenclature was urgently needed.

A. Three Men in a Boat

The origins of the systematic allergen nomenclature can be traced to a meeting among Drs. David Marsh (at that time at Johns Hopkins University, Baltimore), Henning Lowenstein (at that time at the University of Copenhagen, Denmark) and Thomas Platts-Mills (at that time at Clinical Research Centre, Harrow, UK) on a boat ride on Lake Boedensee, Konstanz, Germany, during the 13th Symposium of the Collegicum Internationale Allergologicum in July 1980 (7). The idea was simply to develop a systematic nomenclature based on the Linnean system, with numerals used to indicate different allergens. It was decided to adopt a system whereby the allergen was described based on the first three letters of the genus and the first letter of the species (in italics) and then by a Roman numeral to indicate the allergen in the chronological order of purification. Thus, ragweed antigen E became *Ambrosia artemisifolia* allergen I or *Amb a* I, and Rye 1 became *Lolium perenne* allergen I or *Lol p* I.

An allergen nomenclature subcommittee was formed under the auspices of the World Health Organization (WHO) and the International Union of Immunological Societies (IUIS), and criteria for including allergens in the systematic nomenclature were established. These included strict criteria for biochemical purity, as well as criteria for determining the allergenic activity of the purified protein. A committee chaired by Marsh and including Lowenstein, Platts-Mills, Dr. Te Piao King (Rockefeller University, New York), and Dr. Larry Goodfriend (McGill University, Canada) prepared a list of allergens that fulfilled the inclusion criteria and established a process for investigators to submit names of newly identified allergens. The original list, published in the *Bulletin of the*

World Health Organization in 1986, included 27 highly purified allergens from grass, weed and tree pollens, and house dust mites (8).

The systematic allergen nomenclature was quickly adopted by allergy researchers and proved to be a great success. It was logical, easily understood, and readily assimilated by allergists and other clinicians who were not directly involved with the nitty-gritty of allergen immunochemistry. The nomenclature *Der p* I, *Fel d* I, *Lol p* I, *Amb a* I was used at scientific meetings and in the literature, and expanded rapidly to include newly isolated allergens.

II. THE REVISED ALLERGEN NOMENCLATURE

A. Allergens

The widespread use of molecular cloning techniques to identify allergens in the late 1980s and 1990s led to an exponential increase in the number of allergens described. A large number of allergen nucleotide sequences were generated from cDNA- or PCR-based sequencing, and it soon became apparent that the use of Roman numerals (e.g., *Lol p* I through *Lol p* XI) was unwieldy (9–11). The use of italics to denote a purified protein was inconsistent with nomenclature used in bacterial genetics and the HLA system, where italicized names denote a gene product and roman typeface indicates an expressed protein. In 1994 the allergen nomenclature was revised so that the allergen phenotype was shown in roman type and arabic numerals were adopted. Thus *Amb a* I, *Lol p* I, and *Der p* I in the original 1986 nomenclature are referred to as Amb a 1, Lol p 1, and Der p 1 in the current nomenclature, which has been published in several scientific journals (12–14).

1. Inclusion Criteria

A key part of the systematic WHO/IUIS nomenclature is that the allergen should satisfy biochemical criteria, which define the molecular structure of the protein, and immunological criteria, which define its importance as an allergen. Originally, the biochemical criteria were based on establishing protein purity (e.g., by SDS-PAGE, IEF, or HPLC and physicochemical properties including MW, pI, and N-terminal amino acid sequence) (8). Nowadays, the full nucleotide or amino acid sequence is generally required. An outline of the inclusion criteria is shown in Table 1. An important aspect of these criteria is that

Table 1 Allergens: Criteria for Inclusion in the WHO/IUIS Nomenclature

1. The molecular and structural properties should be clearly and unambiguously defined, including:
   - Purification of the allergen protein to homogeneity.
   - Determination of molecular weight, pI, and carbohydrate composition.
   - Determination of nucleotide and/or amino acid sequence.
   - Production of monospecific or monoclonal antibodies to the allergen.
2. The importance of the allergen in causing IgE responses should be defined by:
   - Comparing the prevalence of serum IgE antibodies in large population(s) of allergic patients. Ideally, at least 50 or more patients should be tested.
   - Demonstrating biological activity, e.g., by skin testing or histamine release assay.
   - Investigating whether depletion of the allergen from an allergic extract (e.g., by immunoabsorption) reduces IgE binding activity.
   - Demonstrating, where possible, that recombinant allergens have comparable IgE antibody binding activity to the natural allergen.

they should provide a "handle" whereby other investigators can identify the same allergen and make comparative studies. Originally, this was achieved by purifying the protein, developing monospecific or monoclonal antibodies to it, and providing either the allergen or antibodies to other researchers for verification. Nucleotide and amino acid sequencing unambiguously identifies the allergen and enables sequence variation between cDNA clones of the same allergen to be defined (15,16). Allergen preparations, sequences, and antibodies submitted for inclusion in the systematic nomenclature are expected to be made available to other investigators for research studies.

A second set of inclusion criteria is based on demonstrating the allergenic activity of the purified allergen, both in vitro and in vivo. Researchers use a variety of techniques for measuring IgE antibodies in vitro, including radioallergosorbent (RAST)-based techniques, CIE/CRIE, radioimmunoassays using labeled allergens, enzyme immunoassay (ELISA), and immunoblotting. These techniques differ in sensitivity, and their efficacy may be affected by a variety of factors. For example, CIE/CRIE is dependent on the quality of polyclonal rabbit antisera. Immunoblotting, which has largely replaced CIE techniques, relies on the allergen being resistant to heating in detergents used for electrophoresis. Whatever technique is used, it is important to screen a large number of sera from an unselected allergic population to establish the prevalence of reactivity. Ideally, 50 or more sera should be screened, although allergens can be included in the nomenclature if the prevalence of IgE reactivity is >5% and they elicit IgE responses in as few as five patients (Table 1,12). "Chimeric" ELISA systems are now available that allow a large number of sera to be screened for IgE antibodies to specific allergens. The assays use a captured monoclonal antibody to bind allergen. Serum IgE antibodies that bind to the allergen complex are detected by biotinylated anti-IgE (Fig. 1). The assay is quantitated using a chimeric mouse anti–Der p 2 and human IgE epsilon antibody and provides results in nanograms per milliliter of allergen-specific IgE. Chimeric ELISA for measuring IgE antibody to Der p 1, Der p 2, and Fel d 1 correlate with Pharmacia CAP measurements and provide useful tools for comparing the prevalence of IgE to specific allergens (17,18).

It is often easier to isolate sequences from cDNA libraries and screen them against panels of sera than it is to work with patients themselves! However, demonstrating that the allergen has biological activity in vivo is critical, especially since many allergens are now produced as recombinant molecules before the natural allergen is purified (if ever). Several mite, cockroach, and fungal allergens (e.g., *Aspergillus, Alternaria, Cladosporium*) have been defined solely using recombinant proteins, and it is unlikely, in most cases, that much effort will be directed toward isolating the natural allergens (9–11,15,16). In these cases, the allergenic activity of the bacterial or yeast expressed recombinant protein should be confirmed in vivo by quantitative skin testing or in vitro by histamine release assays. Skin testing studies have been carried out using a number of recombinant allergens, including Bet v 1, Asp f 1, Bla g 4, Bla g 5, Der p 2, Der p 5, and Blo t 5. These allergens have shown very good biological activity using picogram amounts of proteins.

2. Resolving Ambiguities in Nomenclature

Every system has its faults, and allergen nomenclature is no exception. Early on it was recognized that because the system had Linnaean roots, some unrelated allergens would have the same name: *Candida* allergens could be confused with dog allergen (*Canis domesticus*), there are multiple related species of *Vespula* (Vespid) allergens, and *Periplaneta americana* (American cockroach) allergen needs to be distinguished from *Persea americana* (avocado)! These ambiguities have been overcome by adding an additional letter to either the genus or

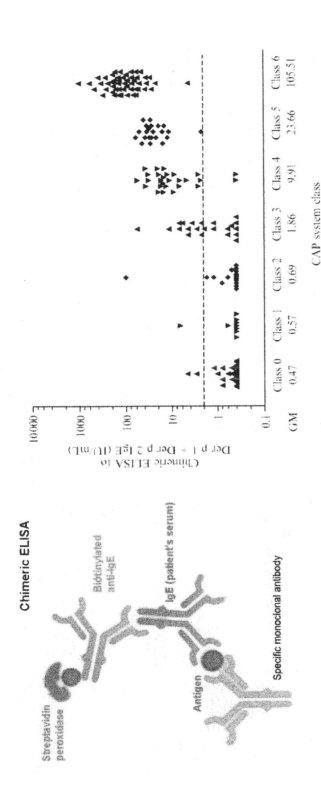

Figure 1 Chimeric ELISA for measuring allergen-specific IgE. *A*: Schematic graphic of the ELISA. Microtiter plates are coated with monoclonal antibodyfollowed by the relevant allergen and incubated with patient's serum. IgE antibodies that bind to the allergen complex are detected using biotinylated anti-IgE and streptavidin peroxidase. A chimeric IgE anti–Der p 2 is used to generate a control curve, and IgE values for patient's serum are interpolated from this curve. *B*: Correlation between the chimeric ELISA for IgE antibody to Der p 1 and Der p 2 and the Pharmacia CAP system for measuring IgE to house dust mite. Chimeric ELISA values for IgE anti–Der p 1 and IgE anti–Der p 2 were summed and compared with the CAP system. Sera were obtained from 212 patients with asthma, wheezing, and/or rhinitis. There was an excellent quantitative correlation between the chimeric ELISA and CAP ($r = 0.86$, $p < 0.001$). (Reproduced from Trombone et al., Clin Exp Allergy 32:1323–1328, 2002, with permission.)

species name. The preceding examples thus become Cand a 1 (*C. albicans* allergen 1); Ves v 1 or Ves vi 1, to indicate *V. vulgaris* and *V. vidua* allergens, respectively; and Per a 1 and Pers a 1 for the cockroach and avocado allergens. Dog allergen is referred to as Can f 1, from *Canis familiaris*.

Many allergens have biochemical names that describe their biological function and may precede the allergen nomenclature. Examples include egg allergens (ovomucoid and ovalbumin), insect allergens (phospholipase As and hyaluronidases), and tropomyosins from shrimp, mite, and cockroach. In fact, it is common to be able to designate allergens to particular protein families based on sequence homology searches, which have provided important clues to their biological function. Allergens may be enzymes, e.g., proteases (Der p 1, Der p 3, Der p 9) or glutathione transferases (Der p 8, Bla g 5); ligand binding proteins (Bla g 4, Rat n 1, Can f 1, Bos d 2); storage proteins (peanut, Ara h 1); hemoglobins (midge, Chi t 1); plant pathogenesis–related proteins (Bet v 1); or have as yet undetermined functions (mite Group 5 and Group 7 allergens, Group 1 and Group 5 grass pollen allergens). Although several mite and fungal allergens are proteolytic enzymes, the dog allergen Can f 1 has 60% homology to human Van Ebner's gland protein (VEGH), which is a cysteine protease inhibitor. A cystatin allergen (Fel d 3) has also been cloned from a cat skin cDNA library. Fel d 3 has a conserved cysteine protease inhibitor motif that is partially preserved in Can f 1, a lipocalin (Fig. 2) (19). In the allergy literature, it is preferable to use the systematic allergen nomenclature. However, in other contexts, such as comparisons of biochemical activities or protein structure, it may be appropriate or more useful to use the biochemical names. A selected list of the allergen nomenclature and biochemical names of inhalant, food, and venom allergens is shown in Table 2.

The use of molecular cloning has led to the rapid identification of allergen sequences, and multiple allergens have been cloned from several sources. Six or more allergens have been defined from each of the following sources: mite (*Dermatophagoides*), grass and ragweed pollen, cockroach, *Aspergillus, Alternaria*, and latex (Table 2). Homologous allergens have also been cloned from related species, and this can create problems for naming the homologues or unrelated allergens from other species. Mite is a good example. Structural homologues of *Dermatophagoides* allergens have been cloned from *Euroglyphus maynei* (Eur m 1), *Lepidoglyphus destructor* (Lep d 2), and *Blomia tropicalis*

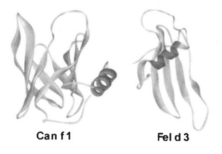

Can f 1   Fel d 3

Figure 2 Molecular modeling of the three-dimensional structures of Can f 1 and Fel d 3, which are thought to function as cysteine protease inhibitors. Fel d 3 has a cysteine protease inhibitor motif (QVVAG) that is located at the tip of the central loop at the bottom of the figure. Similar residues are located in the flattened loop region at the base of the Can f 1 structure. These loop regions are thought to bind to cysteine proteases and inhibit their activity. (Fel d 3 structure reproduced with permission from Clin Exp Allergy 31:1279–1286, 2001.)

Table 2 Molecular Properties of Common Allergens

Source	Allergen	MW(kDA)	Homology/function
Inhalants			
Indoor			
House dust mite (*Dermatophagoides pteronyssinus*)	Der p 1	25	Cysteine protease[b]
	Der p 2	14	Epididymal protein?[b]
	Der p 3	30	Serine protease
	Der p 5	14	Unknown
Cat (*Felis domesticus*)	Fel d 1	36	(Uteroglobin)[b]
Dog (*Canis familiariss*)	Can f 1	25	Cysteine protease inhibitor?[b]
Mouse (*Mus muscularis*)	Mus m 1		Lipocalin (territory marking protein
Rat (*Rattus norvegicus*)	Rat n 1	21	Pheromone-binding lipocalin[b]
Cockroach (*Blattella germanica*)	Bla g 2	36	Inactive aspartic protease
Outdoor			
Pollen—grasses			
Rye (*Lolium perenne*)	Lol p 1	28	Unknown
Timothy (*Phleum pratense*)	Phl p 5	32	Unknown
Bermuda (*Cynodon dactylon*)	Cyn d 1	32	Unknown
Weeds			
Ragweed (*Artemisia artemisifolia*)	Amb a 1	38[a]	Pectate lyase[b]
	Amb a 5	5	Neurophysins[b]
Trees			
Birch (*Betula verucosa*)	Bet v 1	17	Pathogenesis-related protein[b]
Foods			
Milk	β-Lactolobulin	36	Retinol-binding[a,b] protein (calycin)[b]
Egg	Ovomucoid	29	Trypsin inhibitor
Codfish (*Gadus callarias*)	Gad c 1	12	Ca-binding protein (muscle parvalbumin)
Peanut (*Arachis hypogea*)	Ara h 1	63	Vicilin (seed-storage protein)[b]
Venoms			
Bee (*Apis melifera*)	Api m 1	19.5	Phospholipase A_2[b]
Wasp (*Polestes annularis*)	Pol a 5	23	Mammalian testis proteins
Hornet (*Vespa crabro*)	Ves c 5	23	Mammalian testis proteins
Fire ant (*Solenopsis invicta*)	Sol i 2	13	Unknown
Fungi			
Aspergillus fumigatus	Asp f 1	18	Cytotoxin (mitogillin)
Alternaria alternata	Alt a 1	29	Unknown
Latex			
Hevea brasiliensis	Hev b 1	58	Elongation factor
	Hev b 5	16	Unknown—homologous to kiwi fruit protein of unknown function

[a] Most allergens have a single polypeptide chain; dimers are indicated.
[b] Allergens of known three-dimensional structure are also indicated.

(Blo t 5), which show >40% homology to the *Dermatophagoides* allergens (11). The problem comes in numbering other allergens cloned from *Lepidoglyphus* or *Blomia* cDNA libraries that may be unrelated to *Dermatophagoides* allergens. Calling the allergen, for example, Blo t 3, in the absence of evidence that *Blomia* produces a homologous allergen to Der p 3, would cause complications if such a homologue were identified at a later date. In these cases, it may be better to use Blo t 11, for example, for the *Blomia* allergen, reserving numbers 1–10 for any allergens related to *Dermatophagoides* that may subsequently be identified.

B.   Isoallergens, Isoforms and Variants

Originally, isoallergens were broadly defined by Marsh and others as multiple molecular forms of the same allergen, sharing extensive antigenic (IgE) cross-reactivity. The revised nomenclature defines isoallergens as allergens from a single species, with similar molecular size, identical biological function, and ≥67% amino acid sequence identity (8). Some allergens that were previously "grandfathered" into the nomenclature as separate entities share extensive sequence homology and some antigenic cross-reactivity, but are named independently and are not considered to be isoallergens. Examples include Lol p 2 and Lol p 3 (65% homology), and Amb a 1 and Amb a 2 (65% homology). The word "group" is now being used more often to describe structurally related allergens from different species within the same genus, or from closely related genera. In these cases, the levels of amino acid sequence identity can range from as little as 40% to ~90%. Similarities in tertiary structure and biological function are also taken into account in describing allergen groups. Examples include the Group 2 mite allergens (Der p 2, Der f 2 and Lep d 2, Gly d 2 and Tyr p 2), showing 40% to 88% homology, and the Group 5 ragweed allergens (Amb a 5, Amb t 5, and Amb p 5), showing ~45% homology. The *Dermatophagoides* Group 2 allergen structures have been determined by X-ray crystallography and nuclear magnetic resonance spectroscopy (NMR). The structures of the Group 2 allergens from other species were modeled on the *Dermatophagoides* structures (Fig. 3). This enabled the structural basis for antigenic relationships between members of the group to be defined (20–22).

The term "variant" or "isoform" is used to indicate allergen sequences that show a limited number of amino acid substitutions (i.e., polymorphic variants of the same allergen). Typically, variants may be identified by sequencing several cDNA clones of a given allergen. Variants have been reported for Der p 1, Der p 2, Amb a 1, Cry j 1, and for the most prolific Bet v 1, for which 42 sequences have been deposited in the GenBank database. Isoallergens and variants are denoted by the addition of four numeral suffixes to the allergen name. The first two numerals distinguish isoallergens and the last two distinguish variants. Thus, for ragweed Amb a 1, which occurs as four isoallergens, showing 12% to 24% difference in amino acid sequence, the nomenclature is as follows:

> *Allergen*: Amb a 1
> *Isoallergens*: Amb a 1.01, Amb a 1.02, Amb a 1.03, Amb a 1.04

Three variants of each isoallergen occur, showing >97% sequence homology:

> *Isoforms*: Amb a 1.0101, Amb a 1.0102, Amb a 1.0103
> Amb a 1.0201, Amb a 1.0202, Amb a 1.0203, etc.

Examples showing precisely how the nomenclature for isoforms of mite Group 2 allergens and for the Group 1 allergens of cockroach have been published (20,23). The

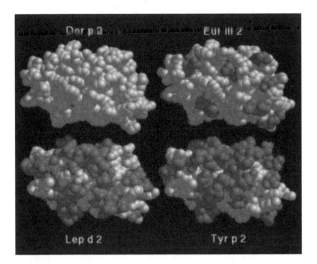

Figure 3 Space-filling models of Group 2 allergens from house dust mite. Amino acid substitutions are shown in gray scale. The space-filling model of Der p 2 was generated from nuclear magnetic resonance spectroscopy studies and has subsequently been confirmed by X-ray crystallography (22). Eur m 2 shows 85% sequence identity with Der p 2, and seven of the substituted amino acids are shown in gray on the surface structure. There is extensive cross-reactivity between Der p 2 and Eur m 2. In contrast, Lep d 2 and Tyr p 2 show only 40% amino acid identity with the other Group 2 allergens. They show many substitutions on the antigenic surface of the molecules and show limited antigenic cross-reactivity for mAb and human IgE. (Reproduced from Smith et al., J Allergy Clin Immunol 107:977–984, 2001, with permission.)

Group 1 allergens from tree pollen have an unusually high number of isoallergens and variants. The 42 Bet v 1 sequences are derived from 31 isoallergens, which show from 73% to 98% sequence homology and are named Bet v 1.0101 through Bet v 1.3101. The Group 1 allergen from hornbeam (*Carpinus betulus*), Car b 1, has three isoallergens that show 74% to 88% homology (Car b 1.01, 1.02, and 1.03), and the nomenclature committee's most recent records show 15 sequences of Car b 1. Ten variants of hazel pollen allergen, Cor a 1, have also been recorded. The reasons the Group 1 tree pollen allergens have so many variants are unclear. Latex provides another example of distinctions in nomenclature. Hevein is an important latex allergen, designated Hev b 6, which occurs as a 20-kDa precursor with two fragments derived from the same transcript. These moieties are all variants of Hev b 6 and are distinguished as Hev b 6.01 (prohevein, 20-kDa precursor), Hev b 6.02 (5-kDa hevein), and Hev b 6.03 (a 14-kDa C-terminal fragment).

III. NOMENCLATURE FOR ALLERGEN GENES AND RECOMBINANT OR SYNTHETIC PEPTIDES

In the revised nomenclature, italicized letters are reserved to designate allergen genes. Two genomic allergen sequences have been determined from animal dander allergens: cat allergen, Fel d 1, and mouse urinary allergen, Mus m 1. Fel d 1 has two separate genes encoding chain 1 and chain 2 of the molecule, which are designed Fel d 1A and Fel d 1B, respectively (24). Genomic sequences of Bet v 1, Cor a 1, and apple allergen, Mal d 1, have also been determined.

When recombinant allergens were introduced, researchers often used the term "native allergen" to distinguish the natural protein from the recombinant allergen. However, because "native" has implications for protein structure (i.e., native conformation), it was decided that the term "natural allergen" should be used to indicate any allergen purified from natural source material. Natural allergens may be denoted by the prefix "n" to distinguish them from recombinant allergens, which are identified by the prefix "r" before the allergen name (e.g., nBet v 1 and rBet v 1). There is no distinction between recombinant allergens produced in bacterial, yeast, or mammalian expression systems. Synthetic peptides are identified by the prefix "s", with the particular peptide residues indicated in parentheses after the allergen name. Thus, a synthetic peptide encompassing residues 100–120 of Bet v 1.0101 would be denoted as sBet v 1.0101 (100–120). At this point, the nomenclature, while technically sound, begins to become cumbersome and rather long-winded for most purposes. Additional refinements to the nomenclature cover substitutions of different amino acid residues within synthetic peptides. This aspect of the nomenclature (which is based on that used for synthetic peptides of immunoglobulin sequences) is detailed in the revised nomenclature document, to which aficionados are referred for full details (8).

IV. THE IUIS SUBCOMMITTEE ON ALLERGEN NOMENCLATURE

Allergens to be considered for inclusion in the nomenclature are reviewed by an IUIS subcommittee, which is currently chaired by Dr. Wayne Thomas, Institute for Child Health, Western Australia, and has eight members (Table 3). The committee meets annually at an international allergy/immunology meeting and discusses new proposals it has received during the year, together with any proposed changes or additions to the nomenclature. There is also a committee-at-large, which is open to any scientist with an interest in allergens, to whom decisions made by the subcommittee are circulated. The procedure for submitting candidate names for allergens to the subcommittee is straightforward. Having purified the allergen and demonstrated its allergenicity, investigators should download the "new allergen name" form from the nomenclature subcommittee Web site (www.allergen.org) and send the completed form to the subcommittee prior to publishing articles describing the allergen. The subcommittee will provisionally accept the author's

Table 3 The IUIS Subcommittee on Allergen Nomenclature, 2003–2005

Name	Institution	Country
Wayne R. Thomas, Ph.D. (chairman)	Western Australia Institute for Child Health	Perth, Australia
Jorgen N. Larsson, Ph.D. (secretary)	ALK-ABELLO	Horsholm, Denmark
Robert C. Aalberse, Ph.D.	University of Amsterdam	Amsterdam, The Netherlands
Donald Hoffman, Ph.D.	East Carolina University	Greenville, NC, U.S.A.
Thomas A.E. Platts-Mills, M.D. Ph.D.	University of Virginia	Charlottesville, VA, U.S.A.
Otto Scheiner, Ph.D.	University of Vienna	Vienna, Austria
Martin D. Chapman, Ph.D.	INDOOR Biotechnologies, Inc.	Charlottesville, VA, U.S.A.
Viswanath P. Kurup, Ph.D.	Medical College of Wisconsin	Milwaukee, WI, U.S.A.

Table 4 Online Allergen Databases

Database	Locator
WHO/IUIS Allergen Nomenclature	www.allergen.org[a]
Structural Database of Allergenic Proteins (SDAP)	http://fermi.utmb.edu/SDAP
Food Allergy Research and Resource Program (Farrp)	www.allergenonline.com
Protall	www.ifr.bbsrc.ac.uk/protall
ALLERbase	www.dadamo.com/allerbase
Allergome	www.allergome.org
Central Science Laboratory (York, UK)	http://www.csl.gov.uk/allergen/

[a] Official Web site of the WHO/IUIS Subcommittee on Allergen Nomenclature.

suggested allergen name, or assign the allergen a name, provided that the inclusion criteria are satisfied. The name will later be confirmed at a full meeting of the subcommittee. Occasionally, the subcommittee has to resolve differences between investigators who may be using different names for the same allergen, or disputes concerning the chronological order of allergen identification. These issues can normally be resolved by objective evaluation of each case.

A. Allergen Databases

The official Web site for the WHO/IUIS Sub-committee on Allergen Nomenclature, www.allergen.org, lists all allergens and isoforms that are recognized by the subcommittee and is updated on a regular basis. Over the past 5 years, several other allergen databases have been generated by academic institutions, research organizations, and industry-sponsored groups (Table 4). These sites differ in their focus and emphasis, but are useful sources of information about allergens. The Structural Database of Allergenic Proteins (SDAP) was developed at the Sealy Center for Structural Biology, University of Texas Medical Branch, and provides detailed structural data on allergens in the WHO/IUIS nomenclature, including sequence information, PDB files, and programs to analyze IgE epitopes. Amino acid and nucleotide sequence information is also compiled in the SWISS-PROT and NCBI databases. The Farrp and Protall databases focus on food allergens and provide sequence similarity searches (Farrp) and clinical data (skin tests, provocation tests) (Protall). The Allergome database provides regular updates on allergens from publications in the scientific literature. The reader is referred to Table 4 to ascertain which of these sites may be of interest.

V. CONCLUDING REMARKS

The three men in a boat did a remarkably good job! The use of the systematic allergen nomenclature has been extremely successful and has significantly enhanced research in the area. The current list comprises 353 allergens and 190 isoallergens. The nomenclature continues to be revised. One topic under discussion is whether it is valid to include an allergen in the system if it has been demonstrated to cause IgE-mediated reactions in only five patients (the present policy) or represents <5% of a particular patient population. The problem with including allergens according to these criteria is that the number of allergens becomes very large and, unless the allergens are used in research or clinical studies, an element of redundancy is built into the system. Conversely, it has been argued that the nomenclature is only a standardized name that permits precise communication about a particular allergen and that relative allergenic influence is not necessarily significant, provided that allergenic activity is clearly documented.

Another topic that continues to evoke discussion is the use of the generic terms "major" and "minor" in reference to an allergen. Relatively few allergens fulfill the criteria originally used by Marsh to define a major allergen (i.e., one that causes IgE response in ≥90% of allergic patients, such as Bet v 1, Fel d 1, Der p 2, or Lol p 1). However, there are a large number of allergens that cause sensitization in >50% of patients, and Lowenstein used this figure (50%) to define major allergens in the early 1980s (6). Scientists like to describe their allergens as "major" because this is effective in promoting their research and carries some weight in securing research funding. The question continues to be, "What defines a major allergen?" Demonstrating a high prevalence of IgE-mediated sensitization and that the protein has allergenic activity in vivo is a minimal requirement, given the increasing sensitivity of assays to detect IgE antibodies. The contribution of the allergen to the total potency of the vaccine should be considered (e.g., by absorption studies), as well as the amount of IgE antibody directed against the allergen, compared with other allergens purified or cloned from the same source. Other criteria include whether the allergen induces strong T-cell response and, for indoor allergens, whether it is a suitable marker of exposure in house dust and air samples. All of these criteria need to be taken into account, and ultimately, the onus is on researchers to establish the importance of their allergens by designing more creative and objective experiments.

For most purposes, allergists need only be familiar with the nomenclature for allergens (Lol p 1, Amb a 1, etc.), rather than isoallergens and peptides, for example. As measurements of allergens in extracts/vaccines or for environmental exposure become a routine part of the care of allergic patients, allergists will need to know what the allergens are and how to distinguish them. Having a systematic nomenclature will help this process. However, the nomenclature of isoallergens and variants will largely be used by researchers, allergen manufacturers, and biotechnology companies that need to identify minor differences between allergens. The systematic nomenclature is a proven success and is versatile enough to evolve with advances in molecular biology and protein science that will occur over the next decade.

VI. SALIENT POINTS

1. A systematic nomenclature for all allergens that cause disease in humans has been formulated by a subcommittee of the World Health Organization and the International Union of Immunological Societies.

2. Allergens are described using the first three letters of the genus, followed by a single letter for the species and an arabic numeral to indicate the chronological order of allergen purification (for example, *Dermatophagoides pteronyssinus* allergen 1 = Der p 1).

3. To be included in the systematic nomenclature, allergens have to satisfy criteria of biochemical purity and criteria to establish their allergenic importance. It is important that the molecular structure of an allergen is defined without ambiguity and that allergenic activity is demonstrated in a large, unselected population of allergic patients.

4. Modifications of the nomenclature are used to identify isoallergens, isoforms, allergen genes, recombinant allergens, and synthetic peptides. For example, Bet v 1.10 is an isoallergen of Bet v 1, and Bet v 1.0101 is an isoform or variant of the Bet v 1.10 isoallergen. The prefixes "r" and "s" denote recombinant and synthetic peptides of allergens, respectively. Allergen genes are denoted by italics; e.g., *Fel d* 1A and *Fel d* 1B are the genes encoding chain 1 and chain 2 of Fel d 1, respectively.

This chapter has reviewed the systematic IUIS allergen nomenclature as revised in 1994. Other views expressed in the chapter are personal opinions and do not necessarily reflect the views of the IUIS Subcommittee on Allergen Nomenclature. The nomenclature is being updated, and a third revision is expected to be published by 2004. The author is grateful to Drs. Anna Pomés and Jorgen Larsen for assistance in preparing this chapter.

REFERENCES

1. King TP, Norman PS. Isolation of allergens from ragweed pollen. Biochemistry 1962; 1:709–720.
2. Johnson P, Marsh DG. The isolation and characterization of allergens from the pollen of rye grass (*Lolium perenne*). Eur Polymer J 1965; 1:63–77.
3. Ohman JL, Lowell F, Bloch KJ. Allergens of mammalian origin: III. Properties of major feline allergen. J Immunol 1974; 113:1668–1677.
4. Elsayed S, Aas K. Characterization of a major allergen (cod): Chemical composition and immunological properties. Int Arch Allergy Appl Immunol 1970; 38:536–548.
5. Marsh DG. Allergens and the genetics of allergy. In: The Antigens, vol III. (Sela M, ed.) New York: Academic Press, 1975: 271–350.
6. Lowenstein H. Quantitative immunoelectrophoretic methods as a tool for the identification and analysis of allergens. Prog Allergy 1978; 25:1–62.
7. DeWeck A, Ring J. Collegicum Internationale Allergologicum: History and Aims of a Special International Community Devoted to Allergy Research, 1954–1996. Munich: MMV Medizin Verlag.
8. Marsh DG, Goodfriend L, King TP, Lowenstein H, Platts-Mills TAE. Allergen nomenclature. Bull World Health Organ 1986; 64:767–770.
9. Scheiner O, Kraft DG. Basic and practical aspects of recombinant allergens. Allergy 1995; 50:384–391.
10. Thomas WR. Molecular analysis of house dust mite allergens. In: Allergic Mechanisms and Immunotherapaeutic Strategies (Roberts AM, Walker MR, eds.). Chichester: John Wiley & Sons, 1997; 77–98.
11. Platts–Mills TAE, Vervloet D, Thomas WR, Aalberse RC, Chapman MD. Indoor allergens and asthma: Report of the third international workshop. J Allergy Clin Immunol 1997; 101:S1–S24.
12. King TP, Hoffman, Lowenstein H, Marsh DG, Platts-Mills TAE, Thomas WR. Allergen nomenclature. Bull World Health Organ 1994; 72:797–80.
13. King TP, Hoffman D, Lowenstein H, Marsh DG, Platts–Mills TAE, Thomas WR. Allergen nomenclature. Int Arch Allergy Appl Immunol 1994; 105:224–233.
14. King TP, Hoffman D, Lowenstein H, Marsh DG, Platts–Mills TAE, Thomas W. Allergen nomenclature. Allergy 1995, 50(9):765–774.
15. Chapmpan MD, Smith AM, Vailes LD, Arruda K, Dhanaraj V. Recombinant allergens for diagnosis and therapy of allergic diseases. J Allergy Clin Immunol 2000;106:409–418.
16. Pomés A, Smith AM, Grégoire C, Vailes LD, Arruda LK, Chapman MD. Functional properties

of cloned allergens from dust mite, cockroach, and cat—Are they relevant to allergenicity? ACI Int 2001; 13:162–169.

17. Ichikawa K, Iwasaki E, Baba M, Chapman MD. High prevalence of sensitization to cat allergen among Japanese children with asthma, living without cats. Clin Exp Allergy 1998; 29:754–761.

18. Trombone APF, Tobias KRC, Ferriani VPL, Schuurman J, Aalberse RC, Smith AM, Chapman MD, Arruda LK. Use of chimeric ELISA to investigate immunoglobulin E antibody responses to Der p 1 and Der p 2 in mite-allergic patients with asthma, wheezing and/or rhinitis. Clin Exp Allergy 2002; 32:1323–1328.

19. Vailes LD, Sun AW, Ichikawa K, Wu Z, Sulahian TH, Chapman MD, Guyre PM. High-level expression of immunoreactive recombinant cat allergen (Fel d 1): Targeting to antigen-presenting cells. J Allergy Clin Immunol 2002; 110:757–762.

20. Smith AM, Benjamin DC, Hozic N, Derewenda U, Smith WA, Thomas WR, Gafvelin G, van Hage-Hamsten M, Chapman MD. The molecular basis of antigenic cross-reactivity between the group 2 mite allergens. J Allergy Clin Immunol 2001; 107:977–984.

21. Gafvelin G, Johansson E, Lundin A, Smith AM, Chapman MD, Benjamin DC, Derewenda U, van Hage-Hamsten M. Cross-reactivity studies of a new group 2 allergen from the dust mite *Glycyphagus domesticus*, Gly d 2, and group 2 allergens from *Dermatophagoides pteronyssinus, Lepidoglyphus destructor*, and *Tyrophagus putrescentiae* with recombinant allergens. J Allergy Clin Immunol 2001; 107(3):511–518.

22. Derewenda U, Li J, Derewenda Z, Dauter Z, Mueller GA, Rule GS, Benjamin DC. The crystal structure of a major dust mite allergen Der p 2 and its biological implications. J Mol Biol 2002; 318:189–197.

23. Melen E, Pomes A, Vailes LD, Arruda KL, Chapman MD. Molecular cloning of Per a 1 and definition of the cross-reactive Group 1 cockroach allergens. J Allergy Clin Immunol 1999; 103:859–864.

24. Griffith IJ, Craig S, Pollock J, Yu XB, Morganstern JP, Rogers BL. Expression and genomic structure of the genes encoding Fd 1, the major allergen from the domestic cat. Gene 1992; 113:263–268.

4

Mechanisms of IgE-Mediated Allergic Reactions

**R. MATTHEW BLOEBAUM, NILESH DHARAJIYA, and
J. ANDREW GRANT**

University of Texas Medical Branch, Galveston, Texas, U.S.A.

I. INTRODUCTION

Immunoglobulin E (IgE), a key player in allergic inflammatory processes in allergic rhinitis, asthma, anaphylaxis, allergic gastroenteritis, and perhaps atopic dermatitis, is one of five immunoglobulin classes making up the humoral immune system. The IgE immune system, very recent in phylogenetic development, is found only in mammals (1). Though originally intended to ward off parasites, it has proved to be a double-edged sword, with harmful effects imparted on the host as well. Binding of multivalent antigens to IgE antibodies on their cell membranes initiates a chain reaction that releases pro-inflammatory mediators and cytokines from mast cells and basophils. There is strong organ specificity in this response due to homing of mast cells to mucosal tissues exposed to the external environment, local synthesis of IgE, upregulation of the receptor FcεRI on mast cells by IgE, consequent downregulation of FcγR, and slow dissociation of IgE from FcεRI.

Though the concentration of IgE is very low in the circulation, local synthesis of IgE easily compensates for the loss of IgE from the surface of mast cells, resulting in a prolonged inflammatory potential. This chapter provides an overview of the basic immunobiology of IgE and specific cells that participate in pathophysiologic mechanisms of the allergic response.

Von Pirquet coined the term "allergy" for the first time in 1906, in describing the role of antigens in protective immune responses as well as hypersensitivity reactions. Allergy, as so defined, was an "uncommitted" biological response, that may lead to immunity (favorable effect) or allergic diseases (harmful effect). The term "atopy" (from the Greek *atopos*, which means "out of place") was initially used to define a predilection for the production of IgE in immune responses to environmental antigens. However, current literature uses "allergy" and "atopy" as synonyms. Prausnitz and Kustner, in 1921, first demonstrated the presence of a factor in the blood of allergic subjects that, when transferred to the skin of nonallergic individuals, rendered them sensitive to allergens (2). In 1966 Ishizaka identified this substance as IgE, which was termed "reaginic" antibodies (3). IgE derived its name from the erythema that the allergens provoke in allergic skin. A major hurdle to the development of this field was the very low concentration of IgE in the serum, well below the threshold for detection by protein assays at that time. The discovery of a rare IgE-secreting myeloma by Johansson revolutionized the field (4). The protein from this cell line and a few other IgE myelomas has been used as a standard for the measurement of IgE concentrations in the blood and was the source of material for structural analyses. Messenger RNA from this cell line was utilized for cloning ε-chain cDNA, which propelled the growth of structural data for IgE. In 1982 Capron demonstrated for the first time that IgE plays an important role in defense against parasites in elegant studies showing IgE-mediated killing of schistosomes in vitro (5). Epidemiological studies done in areas of endemic schistosomiasis and other parasitic diseases strengthened the role of IgE in conferring protection against parasites. IgE-secreting cells are observed in abundance in the respiratory mucosa, gastrointestinal tract, and skin, which are sites of entry of parasites.

A typical allergic response is characterized by the overproduction of IgE in response to common environmental antigens, such as those present in pollen, foods, drugs, house dust mites, animal danders, fungal spores, and insect venoms. These antigens are called allergens, the majority of which are proteins or glycoproteins. Allergens cross-link IgE molecules bound to the high-affinity receptor FcεRI on the surface of mast cells and basophils, leading to aggregation of FcεRI receptors and subsequent activation of these cells. The outcome of this signaling and activation process includes (1) mast cell degranulation with secretion of preformed mediators that are stored in cytoplasmic granules, (2) de novo synthesis of pro-inflammatory lipid mediators, and (3) the synthesis and secretion of cytokines and chemokines. The immune system takes only a few minutes to respond to an allergen, resulting in the term "immediate hypersensitivity," also classified as "type I hypersensitivity" in the Gel and Coombs classification. The characteristic feature of type I hypersensitivity that separates it from other immunological reactions is the rapid appearance of symptoms typical of allergic diseases. A late-phase response ensues after several hours, with influx of T-cells, monocytes, eosinophils, and basophils. This allergic response is initiated by activation and secretion of mast cells and is the fundamental pathophysiological mechanism of allergic rhinitis, asthma, food allergy, atopic dermatitis, and anaphylaxis.

Though unfavorable for the host at first sight, IgE-mediated reactions help to exclude harmful agents from the body and thus impart a survival benefit to the host. Shortly after an insect sting, a local allergic reaction with itching and swelling is a strong stimulus to flee, with reduced potential for disease transmission. In addition, the quick initiation of gastrointestinal symptoms after onset of a parasitic infection may improve host defense and purging of the infection.

II. STRUCTURE OF IgE

IgE, like all other immunoglobulins, is a heterotetramer of two heavy (H) and two light (L) chains with variable (V) and constant (C) regions. The basic structure of all components involves immunoglobulin (Ig) domains having about 110 amino acids in β-sheet configuration (Fig. 1). The heavy chain of IgE is called the ϵ chain. Like IgM, the IgE heavy chain consists of four C_H (present in the C region of the heavy chain) domains. In contrast, IgG, IgD, and IgA possess three C_H domains; and because of the missing Ig domain, C_H2 and C_H3 domains of IgG, IgD, and IgA are homologous to C_H3 and C_H4 in IgE and IgM. This observation suggests that the extra domains in IgE and IgM are $C_\epsilon2$ and $C_\mu2$, respectively. The V regions of the L and H chains form a pair of antigen-binding sites. The antigen-binding fragment (Fab) consists of these antigen-binding sites together with the adjacent $C_\epsilon1$ domain pair. The remaining Ig domains form the Fc (constant) fragment of the antibody, which can bind to cellular receptors. Like all other immunoglobulins, IgE is also glycosylated, and differential glycosylation may affect interaction of IgE with its receptor.

Baird and colleagues first provided experimental evidence that the IgE molecule is highly bent based on fluorescence energy transfer experiments (6). Later it was confirmed that there is a smooth curve in the linker regions between $C_\epsilon1$ and $C_\epsilon4$. More precise X-ray crystallographic structures and neutron-scattering profiles identified that the $C_\epsilon3$-$C_\epsilon4$ domains are perpendicular to the $C_\epsilon2$ domains (7). The bend between $C_\epsilon2$ and $C_\epsilon3$ is more acute, providing more flexibility to the $C_\epsilon2$-$C_\epsilon3$ linker region. Thus, the extra $C_\epsilon2$ domain in IgE imparts distinctive physicochemical properties and isotype-specific functions to IgE. It is interesting to note that the only other antibody containing an extra C_H2 domain, IgM, forms a table-like structure when bound to multivalent antigen, with the $C_\mu3$-$C_\mu4$ region forming the top and $C_\mu2$-Fab elements attached to the multivalent antigen forming the legs. Thus, there is a 90° angle between $C_\mu2$ and $C_\mu3$ regions, recapitulating the orien-

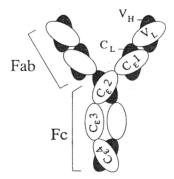

Figure 1 The human IgE molecule consists of two identical light (L) chains (κ or λ) and two identical heavy (H) chains, folded into domains. Each chain has a variable (V) region in which the amino acid sequence is variable and a constant (C) region with no variation in structure. The IgE H chain is called an ϵ chain. Indicated are the two antigen-binding fragments (Fab) and the C region fragment (Fc) in which the receptor binding sites are located. In each Fab, a disulphide bridge links C_L to $C_\epsilon1$. In the Fc fragment, two bridges link the $C_\epsilon2$ domains of the ϵ chains. (Adapted from Ref. 1.)

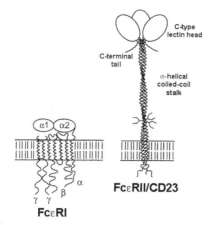

Figure 2   Schematic representations of the IgE receptors FcεRI and FcεRII/CD23. (Adapted from Ref. 1.)

tation of the corresponding domains of IgE. IgE binds to its receptors at sites on the $C_\varepsilon 3$ domain.

III. IgE RECEPTORS

The biological activity of IgE is mediated through the action of two types of receptors, the high-affinity receptor FcεRI and the low-affinity receptor FcεRII.

A. FcεRI

FcεRI, the high-affinity receptor for IgE, belongs to an immunoglobulin superfamily of proteins. This receptor was first identified on a rat basophilic leukemia (RBL) cell line. It is highly abundant (~200,000 molecules/cell) on mast cell and basophil membranes and lower in numbers on other cells. In humans, FcεRI is present as a αβγ2 heterotetramer on mast cells and basophils (Fig. 2) and as a αγ2 heterotrimer in monocytes, Langerhans cells, and blood dendritic cells (Table 1). In contrast, rodent FcεRI has an obligatory αβγ2

Table 1   An Overview of the FcεR1 Subtypes Expressed by Different Human Cells with Known Cell Functions

Cell type	Subunit composition	Associated cell function
Mast cells, basophils	Tetrameric	Cell activation and degranulation in allergic diseases
Monocytes, blood dendritic cells, Langerhans cells	Trimeric	Antigen presentation and modulation of cell differentiation
Neutrophils	Unknown	Allergic diseases
Eosinophils	Unknown, possibly trimeric	Defense against parasitic infections
Platelet	Unknown	Unknown

Source: Adapted from Ref. 40.

heterotetrameric structure on all cells. The α chain of the receptor forms the binding site for the Fc region of IgE, whereas β and γ chains are the functional signal transduction units of FcεRI receptors.

The FcεRIα chain, like the α chains of other immunoglobulin receptors, is a type I integral membrane protein having the Fc binding sites in their extracellular (N-terminal) region. The extracellular part of FcεRIα contains two immunoglobulin-like domains designated as α1 and α2 (Fig. 2). Structural analyses of α1 and α2 reveal that the domains are positioned at an acute angle with formation of a convex surface on the top of the molecule and a marked cleft directed toward the membrane. Present on this convex surface is a hydrophobic patch formed by α1, α2 and the interface region that is a putative contact site for binding to IgE Fc. The α chain has a single spanning transmembrane region followed by cytoplasmic tail of varying length. FcεRIα is heavily *N*-glycosylated, but the carbohydrate component is not required for IgE binding. The glycosylation sites prevent aggregation of FcεRIα chains in the absence of antigen. However, binding of a multivalent antigen overcomes the intrinsic resistance of α chains to interaction, allowing receptor aggregation. Intracellular assembly of the α and γ chains of FcεRI is necessary for surface expression; this interaction masks a retention signal present on the α chain, and it helps in export of the receptor complex from the endoplasmic reticulum to the cell surface and to the Golgi body where terminal glycosylation takes place. FcεRIα is not a conventional signal-transducing molecule. The short cytoplasmic tail (~17 amino acids) does not interact with any signaling target. Indeed, deletion of FcεRIα does not compromise FcεRI signaling (8).

FcεRI β and γ chains contain immunoreceptor tyrosine-based activation motifs (ITAMs) in their cytoplasmic tails. ITAMs act as acceptors of high-energy phosphates and provide docking sites for other signaling proteins. However, there is subtle difference in the ITAM motifs of β and γ chains, which forms the basis for their distinct functional properties. This is reflected in differential binding affinities of protein tyrosine kinases (PTKs) to these ITAMs. Two species of PTKs are associated with FcεRI, the src kinases Lyn and Syk. Lyn preferentially binds to the β chain ITAM, whereas Syk can bind to both β and γ chains but has higher affinity for the latter. FcεRIβ also enhances FcεRI maturation and the assembly process, leading to an increase in surface expression and an amplification of signal transduction capacity within the cells (9).

B. IgE and FcεRI Interaction

The IgE–FcεRI complex has a ratio of 1:1. That is, one IgE molecule binds with one FcεRIα chain (Fig. 3A). This interaction is characterized by an association constant K_a of 10^{10} M^{-1}. This exceptionally high affinity of IgE for FcεRIα is the reason for the very slow dissociation rate and longer half-life of about 20 h for IgE on the receptor. The longevity of this interaction is extended to ~14 days by restricted diffusion of IgE and rebinding to cell receptors. Crystallization studies have revealed that the two $C_\varepsilon 3$ domains of IgE Fc bind to distinct sites on FcεRIα (10). Binding of IgE to FcεRIα leads to conformational changes in IgE with substantial movement of $C_\varepsilon 2$, as shown in Fig. 3B. The biological significance of the univalency of IgE is to provide a safeguard against possible receptor cross-linking by a single Ig molecule with consequent activation of cells in the absence of antigen; this property prevents the catastrophic events that might follow such activation. Other measures that prevent nonspecific signaling are a fundamental requirement of the adaptive immune system, considering the pro-inflammatory and potentially harmful nature of the signal transduced by IgE ligation.

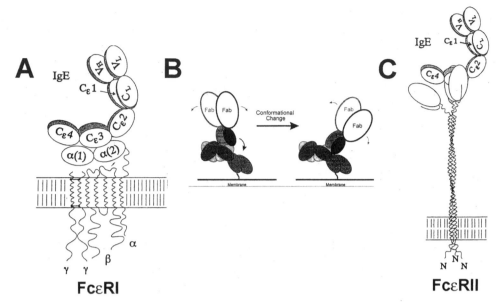

Figure 3 *A*: Schematic of an IgE molecule bound to FcεRI. IgE adopts a bent conformation so that the N-terminal region of the $C_\varepsilon 3$ domain of IgE contacts the second domain of the FcεRI α chain. *B*: There is substantial conformational change of $C_\varepsilon 2$ upon receptor binding to the IgE molecule. *C*: The interaction between human FcεRII and IgE. Two lectin-like regions of membrane-bound FcεRII combine with the two $C_\varepsilon 3$ domains of IgE. (*A* and *C* are adapted from Ref. 1, and *B* from Ref. 30 with permission from the *Annual Review of Immunology*, Volume 21 ©2003 by Annual Reviews www.annualreviews.org.)

C. FcεRII (CD23)

Ishizaka first demonstrated the presence of IgE-binding factors in the culture supernatants of antigen- or mitogen-stimulated lymphocytes and their involvement in regulation of the IgE antibody response (11). Subsequently, Spiegelberg showed the presence of low-affinity receptors for IgE on lymphocytes that differed from FcεRI expressed on mast cells and basophils (12). This receptor was designated FcεRII, and later Yukawa identified it as CD23 (13). CD23 is found on B and T lymphocytes, monocytes, macrophages, NK cells, Langerhans cells, eosinophils, and platelets. It is a single-chain transmembrane glycoprotein. In humans, two receptor isoforms are generated due to different mRNA transcription initiation sites and splicing patterns, resulting in a difference of six to seven amino acids. FcεRIIα is a developmentally regulated gene expressed only on B-cells before their differentiation into immunoglobulin-secreting plasma cells, while FcεRIIb is inducible by IL-4 on all of the cells mentioned above. The difference in biological activities of these two isoforms is still unknown. There is one distinguishing feature of FcεRII: It is the only antibody receptor that is not a member of the immunoglobulin superfamily. The presence of a C-type (calcium-dependent) lectin domain on FcεRII places it in the family of proteins that includes the asialoglycoprotein receptor, the adhesion molecules, and carbohydrate pattern recognition receptors. It has been classified as a type II integral membrane protein with the N-terminal on the cytoplasmic side. The association constant K_a for IgE and CD23 interaction is $2–7 \times 10^6$ M^{-1}; thus, FcεRII (CD23) is also known as a low-affinity receptor for IgE.

The lectin domains of FcεRII are separated from the cell membrane by a three-stranded coiled-coil stalk (also known as a "leucine zipper") (Fig. 2). The lectin domains provide binding sites for CD23 ligands such as IgE; complement receptors CR2, CR3, and CR4; and vitronectin. The presence of calcium ions is obligatory to maintain the proper fold of the lectin domain and binding to carbohydrate substitutes in complement receptors. CD23 exists on the cell membrane as an equilibrium mixture of a 45-kDa monomer and a trimer; the latter has a 10-fold higher affinity for IgE (14). A possible mode of interaction between CD23 and IgE is shown in Fig. 3C, with two lectin heads binding to the two sites on the IgE molecule.

D. Functions of CD23

There is evidence that CD23 is important for antigen presentation by human B lymphocytes. CD23 is bound to the B-cell membrane along with the HLA-DR complex, and together they undergo endocytosis and recycling. This association may form a mechanism by which the peptides are transported by the HLA-DR into the peptide-loading compartments of the cell. CD23 also may have a role in regulation of IgE synthesis by providing negative feedback. CD23 knockout mice overexpress IgE, whereas transgenic mice overexpressing CD23 are deficient in IgE (15). In the mouse, IgE can bind with low affinity to FcγRII and propagate a negative signaling event when the IgE concentration increases beyond certain limits. CD23 expressed on enterocytes helps in transmigration of IgE-antigen complexes found in the intestinal lumen to the underlying tissue where local reaction can be elicited.

IV. SIGNAL TRANSDUCTION

The IgE–FcεRI signaling cascade follows three basic principles: (1) signaling molecules are recruited to the receptor, (2) posttranslational modification activates the catalytic activity of the signaling proteins, and (3) pluripotent adapter proteins affect the activity of the effector proteins toward a particular intracellular target. After IgE–FcεRI complexes are brought together by allergen bound to two or more IgE antibodies, internal signaling is essential for the cell to make a response (Fig. 4). The first event is activation of Lyn, a src-family PTK associated with the single β subunit of FcεRI; this provides the mechanism whereby the β chain can amplify the activation signal. Then Lyn phosphorylates tyrosine residues on the ITAMs of the β and γ chains; this event leads to recruitment of more Lyn molecules to the β chain. It also initiates recruitment and activation of a second kinase Syk to the two γ chains. Active Syk then phosphorylates many substrates, including adapter proteins LAT (linker for activation of T-cells), SLP76 (a SH2-domain-containing leukocyte protein of 76 kDa), and Vav. Syk is essential for completion of the signaling events.

Another event following antigen-receptor interaction is activation of phospholipase Cγ1 (PLCγ1); this enzyme then catalyzes the breakdown of membrane phospholipids to generate two second messengers: inositol-1,4,5-triphosphate (PIP3) and diacylglycerol (DAG). These signaling molecules in turn release calcium from the intracellular stores and activate protein kinase C (PKC) isoforms. Recruitment of PLCγ1 to the membrane is accomplished by LAT adapter protein in T-cells and probably in mast cells. After recruitment to the membrane, PLCγ1 is tyrosine phosphorylated by Syk and by Bruton tyrosine kinase (the defective protein in X-linked agammaglobulinemia) (16). Other important molecules participating in signaling following IgE–FcεRI activation include adapter

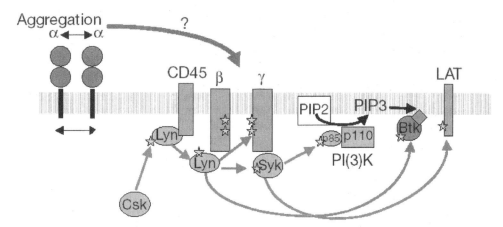

Figure 4 Early event of signaling though the FcεRI. FcεRIα chains are aggregated by cross-linking. Information concerning aggregation is passed, by an unknown mechanism, to the β and γ chain signaling subunits. Lyn activation occurs, which subsequently phosphorylates the β and γ ITAMS. The phosphorylated ITAMS of the γ chain are then able to recruit Syk, which is then phosphorylated/activated by Lyn. Targets of Lyn and Syk include the activation of PI3 kinase to produce the activation of downstream kinases and adapter proteins. Stars represent phosphorylation sites. (Adapted from Ref. 42.)

proteins such as Grb-2, a guanine nucleotide exchange factor Sos, kinases such as those in the Ras/Raf/MEK/ERK cascade, and transcription factors such as Elk-1 and NFAT. A detailed description of this cascade of events can be found elsewhere (17). The completion of these signaling pathways is required for the functional response of basophils and mast cells to IgE linkage by allergens: degranulation, the synthesis and release of lipid mediators, and the production and secretion of cytokines chemokines, and growth factors.

V. SYNTHESIS AND REGULATION OF IgE AND FcεRI

IgE-producing plasma cells are most abundant in skin and in the lymphoid tissue associated with the gastrointestinal and respiratory tracts; the highest numbers are in the tonsils and adenoids. IgE produced by these cells can be found in the mucosal secretions of these tissues, attached to tissue mast cells, and in the systemic circulation. In humans, production of IgE is first evident as early as the eleventh week of gestational life; however, it is modest due to limited fetal antigenic exposure. It steadily rises in childhood and reaches maximum levels by the early teenage years, and then IgE levels decline throughout adulthood. Several studies have shown that basal IgE production is under genetic control, and racial factors are also very important in control of IgE levels (18). Levels of IgE are higher in children with a genetic predisposition to be atopic, and levels rise more quickly.

IgE has the lowest concentration of all immunoglobulin classes in human serum. The normal adult level is 50–300 ng/ml versus 10 mg/ml of IgG. The half-life of IgE in serum is 1–5 days, in contrast to 20 days for IgG. About half of total IgE is found in circulation, with the rest sequestered into the tissues. The comparatively lower level of IgE in serum clearly indicates that it is not meant to neutralize the antigens accumulating in blood or tissues. Logically, there should be amplification after contact of allergens with IgE on the surface of reactive cells. In this way, even small amounts of IgE molecules can provoke an appropriate immune response to commonly encountered antigens. Thus, the immune system has elegantly designed immune surveillance in circulation by IgG and IgM, in secretions by IgA, and in tissues by IgE.

VI. IMMUNOGLOBULIN CLASS SWITCHING

Class switching is the basis for a B-cell changing from synthesis of IgM, the first immunoglobulin expressed, to IgE. Class switching occurs in three distinct stages: (1) germline gene transcription, (2) class switch recombination, and (3) B-cell differentiation into Ig-secreting plasma cells (19). Details of the mechanism and factors involved in the regulation of class switching are beyond the scope of this chapter; however, an outline of the entire process is presented in Fig. 5. The phenomenon of class switching is linked to cell division; the IgE switch requires more cycles than IgG. Cells may leave this process at any time by terminal differentiation of B-cells into Ig-secreting plasma cells or by apoptosis. In the mucosal microenvironment, synthesis of IgE is favored at the expense of IgG. The local concentration of IgE is directly linked to the expression of FcεRI on mast cells and basophils. This mechanism couples the expression of receptors to that of IgE; thus, local synthesis and secretion of IgE leads to upregulation of FcεRI on neighboring mast cells and on circulating basophils.

Differentiation of B-cells into IgE-secreting plasma cells is a complex cascade of events in which cytokines play a crucial role. IL-4, the prototypic TH2 cytokine, is the most important stimulus for IgE synthesis. Recent studies have emphasized that both IL-4 and IL-13 can induce transcription of germline ε mRNA and class switching in B-cells. These cytokines activate transcription at a specific immunoglobulin locus. This event is dependent on the signaling molecule STAT-6. Gene knockout studies in mice have revealed that mice deficient in either IL-4 or STAT-6 are incapable of IgE synthesis in response to antigen challenge (20). On the contrary, individuals with mutations in IL-4 that cause a gain of function show enhanced IgE responses and predisposition to atopic diseases. CD40–CD154 (CD40 ligand) interaction provides the second signal essential for IgE class switching and B-cell growth; complete deficiency of CD40 abrogates IgE responses. CD40 is present on B-cells; CD154 is on T-cells, which also secrete the first signal, IL-4 and IL-13 (Fig. 6).

IgE–FcεRI signaling forms an autoregulatory loop in mast cells and basophils by which surface expression of FcεRI is modulated by the surrounding IgE concentration. This conclusion is supported by the observation that mice deficient in IgE synthesis have mast cells that do not express FcεRI. Another observation supporting the linkage between the local concentration of IgE and the cellular expression of FcεRI receptors was made during trials of monoclonal anti-IgE. This antibody quickly reduced the serum concentration of free IgE and was associated with a profound reduction in the expression of FcεRI on blood basophils (21).

The upregulation of FcεRI is biphasic; the first phase involves stabilization of the receptor complex on the cell surface, leading to decreased degradation and increased accumulation from the intracellular pool without the need for de novo synthesis. Stabilization occurs when the receptor is occupied by IgE. The FcεRIβ chain plays a pivotal role in stabilization of the entire receptor complex. The gene for the FcεRIβ chain is on the long arm (q) of chromosome 11; Adra et al. have reported a potential linkage in this region with allergic disorders (22). In the second phase, when all intracellular FcεRI is at the surface, there is synthesis of new complexes from preexisting transcripts. Overall, the total number

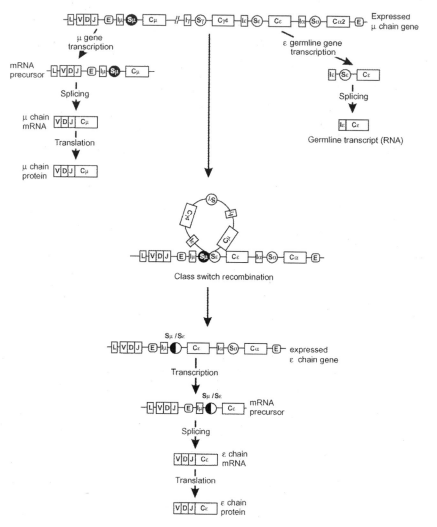

Figure 5 Mechanism of IgE class switch recombination. This schematic diagram shows the major events in this complex process. Part of chromosome 14q32 where immunoglobulin heavy chain genes are located is depicted at the very top of the figure. Genes for the variable (V), diversity (D), and joining (J) regions are located on the left side. Genes for the constant region of the heavy chain are located downstream from the V, D, and J regions in the following order, corresponding to the respective class and subclass of the antibody: Cμ (constant region for IgM), Cδ(IgD), Cγ3 (IgG3), Cγ1 (IgG1), Cα1 (IgA1), Cγ2 (IgG2), Cγ4, Cε (IgE), and Cα2 (IgA2) (shown in part here). Initially, B-cells have transcription from left to right through the Cμ region with ultimate synthesis of the μ heavy chain for IgM (shown in the upper left portion of the figure). As the cell differentiates, it may generate any of the other classes and subclasses of heavy chains. Class switch recombination is responsible for this change in cell function, and it occurs by somatic recombination between Cμ and one of the seven constant region genes downstream of it. Recombination signal sequences (shown as Sγ, Sε, etc.) are the sites where actual switch recombination occurs, and the intervening DNA is looped out (shown in the middle part of the figure). Recombined DNA is then transcribed, spliced, and translated into the ε chain of IgE, as shown in the bottom part of the figure. (Adapted from Ref. 30 with permission from the *Annual Review of Immunology*, Volume 21 ©2003 by Annual Reviews www.annualreviews.org.)

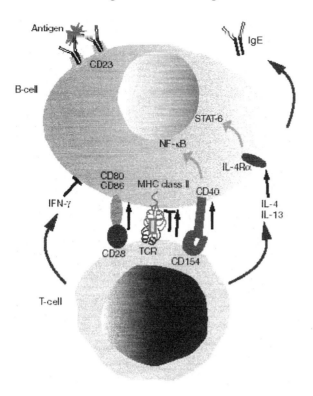

Figure 6 Molecular control of the IgE response. The T-cell provides the pivotal stimulus that drives maturation and differentiation of B-cells into IgE-secreting plasma cells. In this figure, the stimulatory effects of T-cells are indicated by the arrows; an inhibitory effect is indicated by a blocked line. Antigen presented through the MHC class II receptor can be either stimulatory or inhibitory. Both CD86/80–CD28 and CD40–CD154 interactions promote IgE production through direct effects on T-cells and B-cells, respectively. IL-4 and IL-13, both ligands of the IL-4Rα receptor, are the most potent inducers of B-cell activation and differentiation, whereas interferon-gamma (IFN-γ) is major negative regulator. Signal transduction through the IL-4Rα receptor ultimately results in activation of the signaling molecule STAT-6, and the CD40–CD154 interaction signals through the NF-κB pathway. These cumulative effects result in increased IgE production by initiating ε transcript synthesis and class switching as shown in Fig. 5. (Adapted from Ref. 41.)

of FcεRI receptors on the cell surface is linked more to stabilization of the surface complex with reduced loss of the receptor from the surface than to regulation of receptor synthesis.

The potent effects of IgE–FcεRI signaling lasts only while the receptor is engaged and phosphorylated. Negative feedback regulatory mechanisms are in place to stop induction of the signaling pathway in the absence of antigen or when sufficient IgE concentrations are reached. One of these mechanisms is binding of IgE to the low-affinity IgG receptor FcγRII, which exists in two isotypes, activating and inhibitory. FcγRIIb is an inhibitory receptor containing an ITIM motif on the intracellular aspect that can transmit negative signals when the receptor is ligated. This receptor may thus regulate mast cell function independent of FcεRI. Further evidence of this model is provided by studies in FcγRIIb knockout mice that can have markedly enhanced IgE-associated anaphylaxis (23). CD23 also provides negative regulatory effects on IgE production. In vitro experiments using B cells have shown that cross-linking of IgE and CD23 results in downregulation of

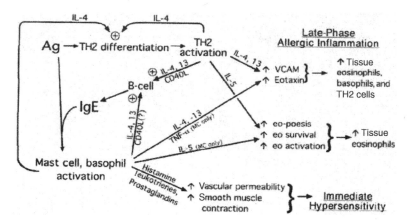

Figure 7 Cellular and molecular mechanisms of an allergic response. (Adapted from Ref. 27.)

IgE synthesis when the IgE concentration is of the same order as K_d, around 10^{-4} M. This clearly denotes that much higher concentrations of IgE than are required for sensitization of mast cells and basophils ($K_d \sim 10^{-10}$ M) cause activation of a negative feedback loop.

VII. CELLS INVOLVED IN IgE-MEDIATED ALLERGIC REACTIONS

An overview of the allergic reaction is presented in Fig. 7. Within 5 minutes of the initiation of an allergic reaction, release of preformed mediators causes slight vascular engorgement and the beginning of edema. Smooth muscle contraction may occur. Fifteen to 20 minutes into the reaction, many cells are recruited into the vessel wall, especially eosinophils, with a slight increase in perivascular lymphocytes. Three hours after antigen exposure, a leukocytosis is seen with neutrophils predominating, and a day after allergen exposure there is an increase in the number of tissue mononuclear cells (24). This section will focus on the function of several cells, their relation to the allergic reaction, and the propagation of the allergic response through IgE mechanisms.

Mast cells and basophils have been grouped together based on their roles in the allergic response and staining properties; the granules of both cells are stained by basophilic dyes. Both cell types contain high concentrations of FcεRI on their cell surface and have similar outcomes when cross-linking of these receptors occurs. The common consequences of cellular activation include degranulation with release of preformed mediators (especially histamine), de novo synthesis of pro-inflammatory lipid mediators, and synthesis and secretion of cytokines and chemokines (25). However, fundamental differences between these cell types include their nuclear morphology, location in vivo, factors controlling differentiation, mediator content, cell surface adhesion molecules, and response to chemical activating agents (26).

A. Mast Cells

Mast cells are derived from CD34+ hematopoetic progenitor cells originating in the bone marrow but migrating to peripheral tissues to complete the maturation process (25,27). Typically, these cells are recovered in the skin, conjunctiva, gut, and respiratory mucosa, all tissues that have contact with the outside environment. These cells are in loose connective tissue and near vessels, nerves, glandular ducts, and beneath cutaneous tissues and mucosal and serosal surfaces. This implies that the original evolution of mast cells was for protection against foreign invaders (28). Mast cells hamper invasion of microbes as part of the innate immune response until the more specific acquired immune response develops.

After an immature mast cell reaches its resident tissue, stem cell factor (SCF) is the crucial survival and proliferation factor needed to complete maturation. SCF is synthesized by fibroblasts and endothelial cells. Another means of identifying mast cells is the surface receptor for SCF, called Kit. IL-3 will work to enhance its development (25). Other cytokines that may influence the proliferation, maturation, survival, and activation of mast cells include IL-4, IL-5, and IFN-γ. IL-4 upregulates the expression of enzymes synthesizing leukotrienes and other inflammation-associated genes (28). In the tissue, the mast cell will reside for a few days, depending on the techniques used to study the mast cell, and some may survive up to 14 days. There are two major subtypes of mast cells based upon their secretory protease content. In humans, these subtypes are (1) MC_T, which is identified by tryptase alone and is located mainly in the mucosa of the lung and small intestine, and (2) MC_{TC}, which has tryptase plus chymase and is the predominant type found in skin, blood vessels, and the gastrointestinal submucosa (26,27). The best means of identifying mast cells is by staining tryptase.

It is reasonable to consider the mast cell as the orchestrator of the allergic response (29). Because of its proximity to the world outside the body, it usually is the initial response cell to an allergen. The mast cell propagates this response though IgE antibodies linked to FcϵRI. The density of FcϵRI ranges from 10^4 to 10^6 on each mast cell. Amazingly, aggregation of only 1% to 15% of these receptors is required for degranulation (26,30). The importance of both IgE and FcϵRI in the allergic response is undisputed: If FcϵRI is not expressed, then IgE-mediated allergic reactions cannot occur, and no other mechanism has been shown to compensate, even partially, for its absence (31). This is not to discount the other methods by which mast cells can be activated, including the complement fragments C3a and C5a, nerve growth factor, and IgG. However, the response is strongest in the mast cell through allergen bridging the IgE–FcϵRI complex (27).

When mast cell activation occurs, particularly by cross-linking of IgE–FcϵRI, many of the signs, symptoms, and pathological changes of the immediate allergic response can be attributed to the release of mediators through degranulation. In the asthmatic patient, this includes enhancement of airway hyperreactivity, bronchial mucosal edema, mucus secretion, smooth muscle contraction, increased eosinophil infiltration, and an overall increase in the number of proliferating cells in the airway epithelium (25,32). This response parallels reactions of the skin, gut mucosa, and nasal mucosa in other allergic reactions. Many of these responses result from enhanced vascular permeability, increased blood flow secondary to vasodilatation, increased loss of intravascular fluid from postcapillary venules, as well as stimulation of cutaneous nerves (30). Mast cell activation also has the effect of increasing mast cell numbers in the affected tissue, which causes continued sensitivity and difficulty. Additionally, mast cells appear to be integral to the late-phase response since inhibition of mast cell mediators or interference with mast cell activation not only blocks the onset of the acute-phase response in asthmatics, but also inhibits the development of the late-phase response (33).

As mentioned previously, mast cells release preformed mediators, manufacture lipid mediators, and produce and secrete cytokines (Table 2). Two of the preformed mediators include histamine and tryptase. Histamine induces vasodilation, increases glandular secretion, and affects smooth muscle cells, endothelial cells, and nerve cells (27,29). It is

Table 2 Selected Products of Human Basophils and Mast Cells

Feature	Mast cells	Basophils
Preformed mediators	Histamine, tryptase and/or chymase, major basic protein, many acid hydrolases, cathepsin, heparin and/or chondroitin sulphates, peroxidase, carboxypeptidases, TNF-α	Histamine, neutral protease with bradykinin-generating activity, major basic protein, Charcot-Leyden crystal, chondroitin sulphates, peroxidase, carboxypeptidase, A, IL-4
Lipid mediators	Prostaglandin D2, leukotriene C4, platelet-activating factor	Leukotriene C4
Cytokines and chemokines	TNF-α, MIP-1α, IL-3, IL-4, IL-5, IL-6, IL-8, IL-10, IL-13, IL-16, GM-CSF, MCP-1	IL-4, IL-13, MIP-1α

GM-CSF, granulocyte-macrophage colony–stimulating factor; IL, interleukin; MCP-1, monocyte chemotactic protein 1; MIP-1α, macrophage inflammatory protein 1α.

responsible for the barrage of symptoms that allergy patients exhibit and therefore makes an excellent target for pharmacotherapy. Tryptase breaks down kininogens found in the blood, leading to the generation of kinins, potent mediators that can act on blood vessels to cause plasma extravasation and sensory nerves to stimulate reflexes (34). Again, this is an attractive target for therapy. Both of these mediators can upregulate the production of RANTES and GM-CSF, important chemotactic factors for the recruitment of inflammatory cells (29). Mast cells also store significant amounts of certain cytokines, the most important being tumor necrosis factor α (TNF-α).

Lipid mediators produced upon IgE cross-linking include prostaglandin D2 and leukotriene (LT) C4. Both are bronchoconstrictors and may enhance vascular permeability. Prostaglandin D2 plays a role in the recruitment of neutrophils (27).

The late-phase allergic response is characterized by structural changes seen in mucosa or skin. Mast cells serve as managers of the allergic response, and possibly the most important action of mast cells is the production of cytokines. One cytokine produced is IL-4. This cytokine is responsible for upregulation of adhesion molecules, including very late antigen-4 (VLA-4) on the local epithelium. VLA-4 binds to cells expressing vascular cell adhesion molecule-1 (VCAM-1), including T lymphocytes, basophils, eosinophils, and monocytes. This interaction is essential for recruitment of inflammatory cells (30,34). IL-4 is critical for the differentiation of CD4+ lymphocytes into T helper type 2 (TH2) cells, furthermore, this cytokine may influence the strength and/or persistence of the associated immune responses. As discussed earlier, IL-4 sets up the environment for IgE synthesis in B lymphocytes (29). Other cytokines produced by mast cells include TNF-α, IL-3, GM-CSF, IL-5, IL-6, IL-8, IL-16, and the chemokine macrophage inflammatory protein 1α (MIP-1α).

B. Basophils

Like mast cells, basophils develop from CD34+ pluripotent stem cells (26). However, these cells remain in the bone marrow until fully differentiated and mature; then they escape into the circulation. IL-3 is the dominant cytokine in this maturation process and is sufficient to differentiate stem cells into basophils in culture (27). Once in circulation, the half-life of basophils is hours to days. Unlike eosinophils and mast cells, the majority of basophils are found within the circulation. Atopic individuals tend to have modest basophilia.

Basophils possess a large number of the FcεRI receptors, ranging from 5000 to 1 million on each cell. These cells are of equal sensitivity to mast cells to activation induced when allergens cross-link IgE–FcεRI complexes. Cross-linking of as few as 15% of FcεRI receptors is required for degranulation. It is worth noting that FcεRII has not been identified on basophils (26). Several other mechanisms for activating basophils have been identified. The complement fragments C3a and C5a can induce release of histamine. Chemokines such as eotaxin 1 and 2 and monocytes chemotactic peptide 1, 3, and 4 can attract basophils to sites of allergic inflammation and induce degranulation. Other cytokines such IL-3 can prime basophils to respond more effectively to other triggers.

Another similarity between mast cells and basophils is that upon activation, they release preformed mediators, manufacture lipid mediators, and produce cytokines and chemokines. Although basophils do not reside in the peripheral tissues, they may be recruited after mast cell activation. Histamine is the only preformed mediator of basophils with direct potent vasoactive effects, and there is evidence that the edema seen during the late-phase reaction originates from basophils, suggesting that a continuing late-phase reaction is due in part to the many mediators released and produced by stimulation of basophils. Other mediators released from basophils include proteoglycans and major basic protein (in small amounts) (Table 2). Only minute amounts of tryptase are released during basophil degranulation. Finally, basophils have small amounts of stored IL-4. LTC4 and its metabolites are the most important newly generated lipid mediators released from basophils. Basophils can produce some platelet activating factor and free oxygen radicals, but do not produce LTB4 or prostaglandin D2. Through the production of cytokines such as IL-4 and IL-13, basophils have a role in driving T-cell differentiation into TH2 cells. Furthermore, since basophils express CD40 ligand (CD154), these cells may contribute to both IgE class switching and local IgE production.

C. Eosinophils

Blood and tissue eosinophilia are hallmarks of allergy and asthma (27). Eosinophils are closely related to basophils; both cells differentiate and mature in the bone marrow from CD34+ pluripotent stem cells, with release of mature cells into the bloodstream. IL-5 is the major differentiation/maturation factor for eosinophils. Immature CD34+ cells may also be recruited to sites of allergic inflammation where differentiation into eosinophils is induced by the local production of cytokines, especially IL-5 (35). An abundance of eosinophils and precursor cells are released from the bone marrow following allergen challenge. Most of the eosinophils are resident in tissues, especially the digestive tract and the lungs. An important event in the recruitment of eosinophils includes upregulation of endothelial VCAM-1. Eotaxin 1, 2, and 3 are members of the chemokine family of cytokines and potent chemotactic factors for eosinophils. Platelet activating factor and LTB4 also promote attraction of eosinophils into local tissues.

Eosinophils express the FcεRI receptor. However, unlike basophils and mast cells, the fundamental structure on normal eosinophils is thought to be αγ2, but this remains controversial (Table 1). Cross-linking of IgE bound to FcεRI with anti-IgE causes degranulation of eosinophils in subjects that have hypereosinophilic disease. However, the applicability of this finding to allergic diseases is unknown. Smith et al. have recently shown that intracellular amounts of the α subunit of FcεRI are considerably less in eosinophils than in basophils. Further, direct cross-linking using an antibody directed against the α subunit of FcεRI did not cause degranulation of eosinophils (36). This data suggests that FcεRI is unlikely to be important for degranulation of eosinophils in atopic disease. However, stimulation by complement fragments, leukotrienes, platelet activating factor, and chemokines can lead to degranulation of eosinophils. In addition, IgG and IgA may induce eosinophil activation. Many of these triggers are present in the microenvironment of allergic inflammation. Activation imparts prolonged survival benefit to eosinophils.

The two known roles of eosinophils are in fighting helminth infections and causing allergic inflammation. Perhaps the most important phenomenon of eosinophil activation is the release of preformed basic mediators that are stored in granules. The granules include major basic protein, eosinophil-derived neurotoxin, eosinophilic cationic protein, and eosinophilic peroxidase, all of which are toxic to respiratory epithelial cells and to parasites. Like mast cells and basophils, eosinophils can also synthesize eicosanoids and cytokines. For example, eosinophils are a major source of LTC4 during allergic inflammation. Specific cytokines synthesized by eosinophils include TGF-β, IL-1, IL-3, IL-4, IL-5, IL-8, and TNF-α. The actual role of these cytokines in allergic reactions has not been completely determined (27,30).

D. Antigen-Presenting Cells

Antigen-presenting cells (APCs), including monocytes, macrophages, Langerhans cells, and dendritic cells, also play an important role in IgE-mediated allergic disease. These cells possess both FcεRI and FcεRII on the cell surface; the FcεRI present on APCs is most commonly the trimeric complex (Table 1). Expression of the FcεRI receptor on some cells (mast cells and basophils) is constitutive, but on the APC this expression seems variable. For example, in nonatopic individuals, Langerhans cells express low amounts of FcεRI. When these cells are examined in the lesional skin of atopic dermatitis, there is a high density of FcεRI. Interestingly, there is also high density of the high-affinity receptor in the normal oral mucosa (37).

APCs have a variety of roles in propagating allergic disease, participating in both the sensitization phase and the elicitation phase of an allergic response (38). During the sensitization phase, an immature APC may recognize and internalize a specific allergen via IgE–FcεRI receptor recognition (39). It is important to note that this mode of endocytosis can capture and internalize large allergens that are not normally engulfed by the usual pathway, pinocytosis (40). Endocytosis of this complex results in direct transport of allergens to endosomes, which are distinctive MHC class II–rich compartments, where processing and assembly occur (37).

Once the allergen has been captured, the immature APCs—specifically dendritic cells and Langerhans cells—travel to lymphatic tissues. Here the APCs have an important role in priming T lymphocytes that subsequently develop into effector cells and memory T lymphocytes. B-cell maturation and differentiation into cells synthesizing allergen-specific IgE is also facilitated by APC and TH2 cells (30). It is important to note that while maturing dendritic cells are in the lymphoid tissues, there is a profound change of their receptor expression. There is both upregulation of certain chemokine receptors (CXCR4, CCR4, and CCR7) and downregulation of cognate receptors (37). Subsequently, APCs may be recruited back to sites of allergic inflammation.

Upon arrival back in the effector tissues, the mature APC is quite capable of participation in the allergic response. Each cell may have a greatly enhanced number of FcεRI receptors on its surface, which can bind to IgE molecules with various specificities. This allows a significant enhancement of cross-linking by a defined allergen at the cell surface (40). As with mast cells, this cross-linking may trigger the synthesis and release of mediators that initiate a local inflammatory reaction. Most investigators believe that APCs crucially contribute to the development of chronic allergic disease in the skin and respiratory tract (37,40).

E. Lymphocytes

If mast cells are the orchestrators of the allergic response, then lymphocytes should be considered the backbone. B lymphocytes differentiate into plasma cells that serve as the factories for IgE production. Binding of IgE to FcεRII has two different effects: inhibition or amplification of IgE antibody production (41). Further, as stated above, FcεRII facilitates antigen presentation to T lymphocytes.

CD4+ T lymphocytes differentiate into either pro-inflammatory TH1 cells or proallergic TH2 cells depending on the regulatory cytokine stimulation present. In the absence of IL-12, these cells will produce IL-4, downregulating the release of IFN-γ (30). This may explain the observation that when antigen is presented in the absence of ongoing infections (where TH1 cells release abundant amounts of IL-12), T-cell differentiation is likely to be to TH2 cells by default.

In addition, TH2 cells play a supporting role in the production of IgE by B lymphocytes. The cytokine products of TH2 cells provide many signals in the pathogenesis of allergic inflammation, such as promotion of eosinophil development and recruitment, mucus production, IgE receptor expression, and adhesion molecules (Fig. 7). In a sense, the TH2 lymphocyte sets up the milieu for the allergic reaction to occur. Chronic allergic inflammation may be driven primarily by allergen-specific T lymphocytes (33).

VIII. SALIENT POINTS

1. IgE is the principal antibody class responsible for inducing allergic reactions. Although it is present in the lowest concentration of the five antibody classes in serum, about half of IgE is bound to cells in the tissues, where it plays a fundamental role of immunosurveillance.

2. IgE can bind to mast cells and basophils via a high-affinity FcεRI receptor. On these cells, the receptor is a heterotetramer αβγ2. Cross-linking of the IgE–FcεRI by allergens initiates a complex array of signals in these cells that leads to degranulation with release of preformed mediators including histamine and subsequent synthesis of pro-inflammatory lipid mediators and cytokines. FcεRI is also found on antigen-presenting cells (APCs), including monocytes, Langerhans cells, and dendritic cells; its structure is a heterotrimer αγ2. The purpose of IgE on these cells includes facilitation of antigen presentation.

3. IgE can also bind to a low-affinity FcεRII receptor on lymphocytes, APCs, and eosinophils. This complex may function in antigen presentation and in regulation of IgE synthesis.

4. Most mast cells reside in loose connective tissues so that they are in close contact with the external environment. There are two phenotypes of mast cells:

(1) MC_T cells have granular tryptase alone and are found in the mucosa of the lung and small intestine, and (2) MC_{TC} cells have both tryptase and chymase in their granules and are located in skin, blood vessels, and the gastrointestinal submucosa. The maturation of mast cells is principally under the direction of stem cell factor, but other cytokines are also important, especially IL-4.

5. The mast cell initiates the immediate reaction to allergens occurring within minutes of exposure. Histamine, tryptase, chymase, and tumor necrosis factor α are principal mediators released from granules. The principal lipid mediators synthesized after cell stimulation are LTC4 and prostaglandin D2. A number of newly synthesized cytokines have been recovered from activated mast cells; these are critical to driving the remainder of the allergic response.

6. Basophils, eosinophils, TH2 lymphocytes, and monocytes are recruited to the local environment and release additional mediators that lead to the late-phase allergic response. Basophils mature in the bone marrow under the influence of cytokines, principally IL-3. Basophils are activated by allergens cross-linking the IgE–FcεRI complex and/or complement fragments C3a and C5a causing release of histamine, LTC4, and cytokines including IL-4 and IL-13. These cells also express CD40 ligand (CD154) and can interact with B lymphocytes to drive maturation to IgE-forming plasma cells.

7. Eosinophils mature in the bone marrow principally under the influence of IL-5. They circulate in large numbers in allergic individuals, especially following allergen challenge, and are attracted to inflammatory sites by chemokines and other factors. When activated, these cells release cationic granules that may be toxic for parasites as well as host respiratory cells. Also, their survival is prolonged.

8. Antigen-presenting cells (APCs) include monocytes, macrophages, Langerhans cells, and dendritic cells. These cells may have surface FcεRI and FcεRII receptors for IgE. These cells may use IgE for antigen recognition and internalization. The cells circulate to regional lymphatic tissues. There APCs function to activate T-cells and participate in B-cell differentiation into IgE-secreting plasma cells. APCs may return to sites of allergic inflammation to become significant effector cells.

9. T lymphocytes differentiate into TH2 helper cells under stimulation by IL-4. This process is antagonized by IL-12 synthesized by TH1 cells. TH2 cells release critical cytokines that drive much of the allergic response.

10. B lymphocytes differentiate into IgE-forming plasma cells under the influence of IL-4 and IL-13. A second signal for the differentiation of B lymphocytes is the coupling of CD40 ligand (CD154) on T-cells to CD40 expressed on B-cells.

REFERENCES

1. Sutton BJ, Gould HJ. The human IgE network. Nature 1993; 366(6454):421–428.
2. Prausnitz C, Kustner H. Zentralblat fur bacteriologie, Infectionskrankheiten und Hygiene Abt 1 1921; 86:160–169.
3. Ishizaka K, Ishizaka T. Physicochemical properties of reaginic antibody: 1. Association of reaginic activity with an immunoglobulin other than gammaA- or gammaG-globulin. J Allergy 1966; 37(3):169–185.

4. Johansson SG, Bennich H, Wide L. A new class of immunoglobulin in human serum. Immunology 1968; 14(2):265–272.

5. Capron A, Dessaint JP, Capron M, Joseph M, Torpier G. Effector mechanisms of immunity to schistosomes and their regulation. Immunol Rev 1982; 61:41–66.

6. Zheng Y, Shopes B, Holowka D, Baird B. Conformations of IgE bound to its receptor Fc epsilon RI and in solution. Biochemistry 1991; 30(38):9125–9132.

7. Beavil AJ, Young RJ, Sutton BJ, Perkins SJ. Bent domain structure of recombinant human IgE-Fc in solution by X-ray and neutron scattering in conjunction with an automated curve fitting procedure. Biochemistry 1995; 34(44):14449–14461.

8. Alber G, Miller L, Jelsema CL, Varin-Blank N, Metzger H. Structure-function relationships in the mast cell high affinity receptor for IgE: Role of the cytoplasmic domains and of the beta subunit. J Biol Chem 1991; 266(33):22613–22620.

9. Donnadieu E, Jouvin MH, Kinet JP. A second amplifier function for the allergy-associated Fc(epsilon)RI-beta subunit. Immunity 2000; 12(5):515–523.

10. Garman SC, Wurzburg BA, Tarchevskaya SS, Kinet JP, Jardetzky TS. Structure of the Fc fragment of human IgE bound to its high-affinity receptor Fc epsilonRI alpha. Nature 2000; 406(6793):259–266.

11. Ishizaka K. Regulation of IgE synthesis. Annu Rev Immunol 1984; 2:159–182.

12. Spiegelberg HL. Structure and function of Fc receptors for IgE on lymphocytes, monocytes, and macrophages. Adv Immunol 1984; 35:61–88.

13. Yukawa K, Kikutani H, Owaki H, Yamasaki K, Yokota A, Nakamura H, Barsumian El, Hardy RR, Suemura M, Kishimoto T. A B cell-specific differentiation antigen, CD23, is a receptor for IgE (Fc epsilon R) on lymphocytes. J Immunol 1987; 138(8):2576–2580.

14. Kilmon MA, Ghirlando R, Strub MP, Beavil RL, Gould HJ, Conrad DH. Regulation of IgE production requires oligomerization of CD23. J Immunol 2001; 167(6):3139–3145.

15. Payet M, Conrad DH. IgE regulation in CD23 knockout and transgenic mice. Allergy 1999; 54(11):1125–1129.

16. Scharenberg AM, El-Hillal O, Fruman DA, Beitz LO, Li Z, Lin S, Gout I, Cantley LS, Rawlings DJ, Kihet JP. Phosphatidylinositol-3,4,5-trisphosphate (PtdIns-3,4,5-P3)/Tec kinase-dependent calcium signaling pathway: A target for SHIP-mediated inhibitory signals. EMBO J 1998; 17(7):1961–1972.

17. Rivera J. Molecular adapters in Fc(epsilon)RI signaling and the allergic response. Curr Opin Immunol 2002; 14(6):688–693.

18. Orgel HA, Lenoir MA, Bazaral M. Serum IgG, IgA, IgM, and IgE levels and allergy in Filipino children in the United States. J Allergy Clin Immunol 1974; 53(4):213–222.

19. Gould HJ, Beavil RL, Vercelli D. IgE isotype determination: Epsilon-germline gene transcription, DNA recombination and B-cell differentiation. Br Med Bull 2000; 56(4):908–924.

20. Shimoda K, van Deursen J, Sangster MY, Sarawar SR, Carson RT, Tripp RA, Chu C, Quelle FW, Nosaka T, Vignali DA, Doherty PC, Grojueld G, Paul WE, Ihle JN. Lack of IL-4-induced Th2 response and IgE class switching in mice with disrupted Stat6 gene. Nature 1996; 380(6575):630–633.

21. MacGlashan D Jr, Xia HZ, Schwartz LB, Gong J. IgE-regulated loss, not IgE-regulated synthesis, controls expression of Fc(epsilon)RI in human basophils. J Leukoc Biol 2001; 70(2):207–218.

22. Adra CN, Mao XQ, Kawada H, Gao PS, Korzycka B, Donate JL, Shaldon SR, Coull P, Dubowitz M, Enomoto T, Ozawa A, Syed SA, Horiuchi T, Khaeraja R, Khan R, Lin SR, Flinter F, Beales P, Hagihara A, Inoko H, Shirakawa T, Hopkin JM. Chromosome 11q13 and atopic asthma. Clin Genet 1999; 55(6):431–437.

23. Ravetch JV, Lanier LL. Immune inhibitory receptors. Science 2000; 290(5489):84–89.

24. Peters S, Zangrilli J, Fish J. Late phase allergic reactions. In: Allergy: Principles and Practice (Adkinson N, Busse W, Ellis E, Middleton E, Reed C, Yunginger J, eds.). St. Louis: Mosby-YearBook, 1998: 342–352.

25. Kawakami T, Galli SJ. Regulation of mast-cell and basophil function and survival by IgE. Nat Rev Immunol 2002; 2(10):773–786.

26. Grant JA, Li H. Biology of basophils. In: Allergy: Principles and Practice (Adkinson N, Busse W, Ellis E, Middleton E, Reed C, Yunginger J, eds.). St. Louis: Mosby-YearBook, 1998: 277–284.

27. Prussin C, Metcalfe DD. IgE, mast cells, basophils, and eosinophils. J Allergy Clin Immunol 2003; 111(suppl 2):S486–S494.

28. Boyce JA. Mast cells: Beyond IgE. J Allergy Clin Immunol 2003; 111(1):24–32.

29. Pawankar R. Mast cells as orchestrators of the allergic reaction: The IgE-IgE receptor mast cell network. Curr Opin Allergy Clin Immunol 2001; 1(1):3–6.

30. Gould HJ, Sutton BJ, Beavil AJ, Beavil RL, McCloskey N, Coker HA, Fear D, Smurthwaite L. The biology of IgE and the basis of allergic disease. Annu Rev Immunol 2003; 21:579–628.

31. Kinet JP. The high-affinity IgE receptor (Fc epsilon RI): From physiology to pathology. Annu Rev Immunol 1999; 17:931–972.

32. Broide DH. Molecular and cellular mechanisms of allergic disease. J Allergy Clin Immunol 2001; 108(suppl 2):S65–S71.

33. Oettgen HC, Geha RS. IgE regulation and roles in asthma pathogenesis. J Allergy Clin Immunol 2001; 107(3):429–440.

34. Togias A. Unique mechanistic features of allergic rhinitis. J Allergy Clin Immunol 2000; 105(6 pt 2):S599–S604.

35. Denburg JA, Sehmi R, Saito H, Pil-Seob J, Inman MD, O'Byrne PM. Systemic aspects of allergic disease: bone marrow responses. J Allergy Clin Immunol 2000; 106(suppl 5):S242–S246.

36. Smith SJ, Ying S, Meng Q, Sullivan MH, Barkans J, Kon OM, Sihra B, Larche M, Levi-Schaffer. Blood eosinophils from atopic donors express messenger RNA for the alpha, beta, and gamma subunits of the high-affinity IgE receptor (Fc epsilon RI) and intracellular, but not cell surface, alpha subunit protein. J Allergy Clin Immunol 2000; 105(2 pt 1):309–317.

37. von Bubnoff D, Geiger E, Bieber T. Antigen-presenting cells in allergy. J Allergy Clin Immunol 2001; 108(3):329–339.

38. Novak N, Kraft S, Bieber T. Unraveling the mission of Fc epsilon RI on antigen-presenting cells. J Allergy Clin Immunol 2003; 111(1):38–44.

39. Saini SS, MacGlashan D. How IgE upregulates the allergic response. Curr Opin Immunol 2002; 14(6):694–697.

40. Novak N, Kraft S, Bieber T. IgE receptors. Curr Opin Immunol 2001; 13(6):721–726.

41. Corry DB, Kheradmand F. Induction and regulation of the IgE response. Nature 1999; 402(suppl 6760):B18–B23.

42. Turner H, Kinet JP. Signalling through the high-affinity IgE receptor Fc epsilon RI. Nature 1999; 402(suppl 6760):B24–B30.

5

Immunological Responses to Allergen Immunotherapy

STEPHEN J. TILL and STEPHEN R. DURHAM

Imperial College, London, England

I. INTRODUCTION

Allergen injection immunotherapy is highly effective in carefully selected patients with IgE-mediated disease (1–4). Patient selection is important, and the risk/benefit ratio must be assessed in the individual patient. The underlying mechanisms of immunotherapy are important since they may provide insight into the mechanism of allergic (and immunological) disorders in general. For example, allergen injection immunotherapy is allergen specific. This enables one to observe the effects of specific modulation of the immune response in a patient in whom the provoking factor(s) (common aeroallergen or venom) is known. The effects of the allergen exposure may be observed either during experimental provocation in a clinical laboratory or during natural environmental conditions. Similarly, the influence of immunotherapy on clinical, immunological, and pathological changes may be observed under controlled conditions. This is in contrast to other immunological diseases where the antigen is unknown and no specific treatment is available.

In this chapter the known causes and immunopathological mechanisms during early and late-phase responses after allergen provocation and/or during natural exposure are

85

considered. Allergic inflammation is characterized by IgE-dependent reactions and tissue eosinophilia. These are largely under the regulation of T-cells and the balance of TH1/TH2 (T helper 1 or T helper 2 cells) cytokines. A review of the effects of immunotherapy on serum antibody measurements and effector cells is followed by a section on how immunotherapy may alter T-cell responses to allergens by inducing immune deviation, IL-10–producing regulatory T-cells, or both. The final section addresses whether immunotherapy may induce long-lived responses and thereby modify the natural course of allergic disease and how new knowledge of mechanisms has led to more specific, targeted immunotherapeutic strategies that are still under evaluation.

II. ALLERGIC RESPONSE

The nature of the allergic response depends on the type of allergen, the allergen dose, and the route of exposure. Respiratory allergy frequently involves the upper and lower airways, resulting in rhinitis and/or asthma. Systemic penetration, either by venoms following insect stings or intravenous administration of drugs (e.g., penicillin), results in immediate systemic reactions, including anaphylaxis. In contrast, ingested food allergens may provoke immediate oral symptoms followed by upper airway obstruction, nausea, vomiting, and diarrhea, with or without systemic reactions. Such allergic responses occur in atopic, genetically predisposed individuals characterized immunologically by a heightened tendency to develop IgE antibody responses and clinically by a positive skin-prick test to one or more common inhaled aeroallergens. A proportion of such individuals may have no clinical manifestations. Allergy (the clinical manifestation of atopic disorders) may result in rhinoconjunctivitis, asthma, eczema, anaphylaxis, or food allergy as indicated above. The cardinal feature of these immediate-type responses is the IgE-dependent activation of mast cells and/or basophils, either at mucosal surfaces or in the systemic circulation.

A. Provocation Tests

Following local allergen installation in the nose or eyes or inhalation into the bronchi, immediate symptoms develop of sneeze, itch, and watery discharge, or wheezing/chest tightness, respectively, which are maximal at 15 to 30 min and resolve within 1 to 3 h. A proportion of subjects develop a late-allergic response, manifest in the nose (if at all) largely as nasal obstruction, and in the bronchi as a second fall in 1 s forced expiratory volume (FEV1), which is maximal at 6 to 12 h and resolves within 24 h.

The immediate response of an IgE-dependent activation is the release of a plethora of mediators, including histamine, tryptase, TAME-esterase, bradykinin, leukotrienes (including LTC_4, LTD_4, and LTE_4), prostaglandins [including $PGF_{2\alpha}$ and PGD_2 (specific for mast cells)], and platelet activating factor. These mediators collectively induce vasodilatation, increased vascular permeability, mucosal edema, increased mucus production from submucosal glands and goblet cells within the respiratory/gastric epithelium, and smooth muscle contraction (particularly in the lower respiratory tract). The late-phase response, by contrast, is characterized by the recruitment, activation, and persistence of inflammatory cells at the sites of allergic inflammation. For example, when ragweed hay fever patients were challenged with increasing concentrations of allergen, using aqueous ragweed extract or increasing numbers of ragweed pollen grains, the early response was accompanied by an increase in histamine, TAME-esterase, bradykinin, and PGD_2 (5).

After several hours, the late phase of mediator release included histamine, TAME-esterase, and bradykinin, but not PGD_2. The mast cell is the most likely source of these mediators during the early response, and the lack of a second rise in PGD_2 suggests that the late increase in histamine results from a secondary influx of basophils.

One problem with nasal lavage is that T-cells tend to compartmentalize in tissue rather than transmigrate into nasal fluid (6). Immunohistochemical studies of nasal biopsies following allergen challenge demonstrated, however, that late nasal responses were accompanied not only by recruitment of neutrophils and eosinophils, but also by an increase in CD4+ T-cells and CD25+ T-cells [interleukin-2 (IL-2) receptor–positive, presumed activated].

In situ hybridization studies demonstrated that the dominant cytokines expressed at the mRNA level were interleukin-4 (IL-4), IL-5, and IL-13—so-called TH2-type cytokines—which are known to characterize human allergic disorders (7,8). In contrast, few mRNA-positive cells for interferon-gamma (IFN-γ) and IL-2 so-called TH1-type cytokines were observed, with no changes in the number of these cells during the late phase following allergen provocation. IL-4 and IL-13 promote "step 1" in B-cell switching to IgE production. Both cytokines induce the production of a sterile RNA transcript (Iϵ), a necessary precursor to "step 2," which involves genetic recombination between the variable region of the immunoglobulin gene and the IgE heavy chain under the regulation of CD40/CD40-ligand interaction between T- and B-cells (9).

Increases in cells positive for IL-3, IL-5, and granulocyte-macrophage colony stimulating factor (GM-CSF) were also observed. These cytokines are important in eosinophil differentiation from CD34+ bone marrow stem cell precursors and the recruitment, priming, and activation of eosinophils for release of inflammatory mediators at sites of allergic inflammation. IL-5, in particular, is specific for eosinophils and promotes the terminal differentiation of the cell from committed precursors. Eosinophil recruitment is also dependent on specific adhesion pathways and the influence of specific chemokines. VCAM-1, which is expressed on vascular endothelium following allergen provocation, results in specific eosinophil adhesion via interaction with VLA-4 on the surface of these cells (10). VCAM-1 is upregulated by both IL-4 and IL-13 (11). Eotaxin is a potent eosinophil chemoattractant produced at sites of allergic inflammation and that acts via the CCR3 receptor to recruit eosinophils (12,13). The persistence of eosinophils in tissue is also dependent on suppression of programmed cell death (apoptosis), which occurs under the influence of IL-3, IL-5, and GM-CSF (14). Studies have confirmed that there is upregulation of these various eosinophil-specific (and nonspecific) pathways during late-phase responses in the nose, and downregulation—for example, by topical corticosteroids—during inhibition of allergen-induced late responses (15).

B. Natural Allergen Exposure

These events, including recruitment and activation of inflammatory cells, mediator release, T-cell activation, TH2-type cytokine production, and activation of specific chemokine and adhesion pathways, have also been documented within the nasal mucosa during natural seasonal pollen exposure (16,17) and in patients with perennial allergic rhinitis and sensitivity to indoor allergens, particularly house dust mite (18). Thus, eosinophils and eosinophil granule proteins are detectable in nasal lavage or filter papers (or plastic imprints) applied directly to the nasal mucosa during the pollen season (19). A characteristic feature of natural allergen exposure, not evident following provocation of the nasal mucosa in the laboratory, is the transepithelial migration of basophils, eosinophils, and, particularly, mast cells during the pollen season (20–22). Similarly, patients with current symptomatic asthma have increased numbers of mast cells detectable in brushings of the bronchial epithelium, again reflecting this migratory process (23).

C. T-Cells and the Allergic Response

T-cells and the cytokines they produce are thought to play a major role in orchestrating allergic inflammation. Initial studies in mice revealed two distinct CD4+ T-cell subsets based on their profiles of cytokine production (24). TH1 cells produce IFN-γ and IL-2, but not IL-4 or IL-5, following activation. TH2 cells produce mainly IL-4, IL-13, and IL-5, but not IL-2 or IFN-γ. This functional dichotomy of CD4+ T helper cells was subsequently demonstrated in humans by analysis of T-cell clones obtained from atopic donors, healthy subjects, and patients with infectious diseases. Factors that determine the evolution of either TH1 or TH2 responses include the nature and dose of antigen. For example, high doses of allergen may preferentially favor the induction of TH1-type responses (25). A second factor is the nature of the antigen presenting cells, with macrophages favoring TH1 responses, possibly via production of IL-12, and with antigen presentation by B-cells, particularly at low antigen concentrations, favoring the development of TH2 cells (25). Different dendritic cell subsets, DC1 and DC2 cells, have also been implicated in the development of TH1 and TH2 responses (reviewed in Ref. 26). DC2-type cells have been identified in atopic subjects (27), and their ability to drive TH2 responses appears to relate to low levels of IL-12 expression.

Both IL-12 and IFN-γ promote or sustain TH1 responses (28,29); whereas IL-4 is the major growth factor promoting the differentiation of TH2 cells (29). A third factor is the nature of the costimulatory signals. After processing by antigen-presenting cells, specific peptides are presented in the context of class II molecules to the antigen-specific T-cell receptor. Activation requires the interaction of other molecules on antigen-presenting cells and T-cells, respectively, including HLA-DR with CD4, B7-1/B7-2 with CD28/CTLA-4, and CD40 with CD40-ligand. It has been suggested that preferential costimulation via the B7-2 molecule may favor TH2 responses (30). Lack of costimulation may result in a state of T-cell unresponsiveness or anergy (31).

III. INFLUENCE OF IMMUNOTHERAPY

Studies have provided insight into how immunotherapy may influence the inflammatory processes that characterize the allergic response. Whereas early work focused on circulating antibodies, more recent studies highlight the potential influence of immunotherapy on T-cell responses. Most work has examined the effect of subcutaneous immunotherapy rather than immunotherapy by alternative routes. Mechanisms are likely to be heterogeneous, depending on the nature of the allergen; the site of allergy; the route, dose, and duration of immunotherapy; the use of different adjuvants; and the genetic status of the host.

A. Provocation Tests

A characteristic feature of immunotherapy is its ability to inhibit late responses in the skin (32), nose (33), and lung (34), but it is not clear whether suppression of the late response is predictive of clinical improvement following immunotherapy. The effects of immunotherapy on the early response after antigen exposure have been variable; some studies confirm inhibition of the early response in the skin, whereas others have shown only temporary inhibition of the early response in the skin (35) and no inhibition in the lung (34). The interesting discovery, within a group of house dust mite–sensitive children, that suppression of the early skin response was predictive of a prolonged suppression following discontinuation of immunotherapy, requires confirmation in a prospective study (36).

B. Serum Antibody Concentrations

In conventional grass pollen immunotherapy, serum IgE concentrations show little or no change in response to treatment (37), though seasonal increases in IgE may be blunted following prolonged therapy (38). A possible unwanted effect of immunotherapy is the development of new IgE responses to allergenic components of the pollen vaccine used for treatment (39), although the clinical significance of this phenomenon has not been determined.

Immunotherapy with aeroallergens is associated with rises in serum concentrations of allergen-specific IgG and IgG4 within the first year of treatment (37,40). Increased venom-specific IgG4 can also be detected within 60 days of starting bee venom immunotherapy (41). The rise in IgG antibodies has led to the proposal that antibodies have "blocking" activity by competing with IgE for allergen binding, thereby inhibiting the IgE-dependent activation of mast cells, basophils, or other IgE receptor–expressing cells. In accordance with this model, allergen-specific IgG4 induced by immunotherapy can block allergen-induced IgE-dependent histamine release by basophils (42,43). These IgG antibodies are also able to suppress allergen-specific T-cell responses in vitro by inhibiting IgE-mediated allergen presentation by B-cells (44,45). However, a major objection to the hypothesis that IgG underlies the efficacy of immunotherapy is the observation that IgG concentrations are unrelated to the clinical response to treatment (40,46,47). For example, immunotherapy in "rush" protocols is effective long before any changes in antibody synthesis can be detected. Nevertheless, to refute a role for allergen-specific IgG on the basis of a lack of correlation between clinical response and quantity of antibody is probably too simplistic. Michils and colleagues investigated the IgG antibody response to venom immunotherapy and observed the usual increase in IgG titers, but reported for the first time that this was preceded by a change in the fine specificity of IgG antibodies (48). Allergen-specific IgG isolated from patients allergic to bee venom displayed a fine specificity spectrum to the major bee venom allergen that was distinct from that of allergen-specific IgG derived from individuals protected either naturally or by successful immunotherapy (49). These observations stress the importance of studying the *activity* of allergen-specific IgG, as a blocking antibody or otherwise, as opposed to measuring crude levels in sera.

Finally, the role of other antibody classes, particularly IgA, in tissues or mucosal secretions (as opposed to measurements performed in peripheral blood) requires further study.

C. Effector Cells

Immunotherapy has a profound effect on the production of inflammatory mediators during both early and late-phase responses. In a study of ragweed-sensitive patients, Creticos and colleagues measured concentrations of histamine, TAME-esterase, and PGD_2 following ragweed pollen provocation (50). In untreated subjects, there was a dose-dependent increase in the concentrations of these mediators in lavage fluid and inhibition of the early nasal response, and there was a significant reduction in concentrations of mediators in nasal fluid of patients who had received immunotherapy.

A characteristic feature of symptomatic seasonal or perennial allergic rhinitis is transepithelial migration of mast cells (20,21). This was demonstrated originally by metachromatic staining of mast cells and, more recently, with immunohistochemical techniques confirming that this seasonal migration of mast cells involves mucosal-type (tryptase-only positive cells) and not connective tissue–type (tryptase$^+$/chymase$^+$) mast cells, which remain confined to the lamina propria and connective tissue (20). Nasal scrapings obtained before and after house dust mite immunotherapy of children demonstrated a significant reduction in metachromatic cells, which were presumed to be mast cells (51). Nevertheless, this observation has not been reproduced in grass pollen immunotherapy, since similar seasonal increases in epithelial mast cell numbers were seen in both actively treated and placebo groups (22).

Successful immunotherapy has been associated with a decrease in eosinophils in the skin and nose following allergen provocation. In grass-sensitive patients, a trend for decreased eosinophil recruitment accompanied inhibition of the late cutaneous response (52,53). Furin and colleagues measured the percentages of eosinophils in nasal lavage fluid before and 24 h after nasal allergen provocation in untreated patients and those receiving ragweed allergen immunotherapy (54). A dose-dependent reduction in nasal eosinophilia was observed in relation to the dose used for maintenance immunotherapy. The effect of grass pollen immunotherapy on eosinophil numbers in nasal mucosal biopsies has also been examined under conditions of allergen challenge and natural seasonal exposure. In the allergen challenge model, nasal biopsies were collected from placebo and actively treated patients before and 24 h after allergen provocation (55). Inhibition of the late nasal response was associated with a decrease in the numbers of eosinophils but not neutrophils recruited in response to the challenge. Similarly, the seasonal increases in numbers of eosinophils within nasal epithelium and lamina propria were reduced in patients who had received 2 years of grass pollen immunotherapy compared with placebo-treated subjects (22) (Fig. 1). Moreover, in immunotherapy patients significant correlations were observed between eosinophil numbers and overall symptoms, suggesting that inhibition of eosinophilia during natural grass pollen exposure may contribute to the clinical efficacy.

Rak and colleagues studied patients with birch pollen asthma before and during the pollen season compared with a group of untreated control subjects (56). Nonspecific airway responsiveness was measured before and several times during the pollen season. Fiber-optic bronchoscopy and bronchoalveolar lavage were used to quantify local bronchial eosinophil counts and local concentrations of eosinophil cationic protein (ECP). Untreated subjects developed a time-dependent increased airway hyperreactivity (i.e., decrease in histamine PC20) during the pollen season, accompanied by a significant increase in ECP, while patients who had received immunotherapy developed comparatively fewer symptoms and less bronchial hyperactivity toward the end of the pollen season. Prevention of seasonal increases in airway responsiveness was accompanied by a decrease in local bronchial eosinophil counts and ECP concentrations.

Although basophils have been detected in nasal fluid and in skin (using the skin window technique) following local allergen provocation, a specific monoclonal antibody that allows basophils to be quantified in nasal mucosal tissue has only recently emerged (57). Using this as a marker, the effect of grass pollen immunotherapy on basophils in the

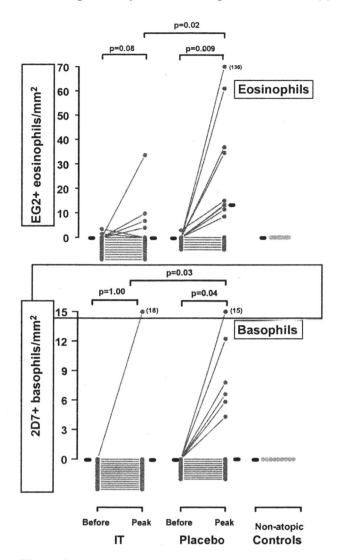

Figure 1 Eosinophil and basophil cell numbers within the nasal epithelium of immunotherapy- and placebo-treated hay fever patients. During a randomized, placebo-controlled trial of grass pollen immunotherapy, nasal biopsies were taken at baseline, out of the pollen season ("before"), and at the peak of the pollen season following 2 years of treatment ("peak"). Biopsies were processed for immunohistochemistry for basophils (2D7+) and eosinophils (EG2+). Significant seasonal increases in intra-epithelial basophils were seen only in placebo-treated patients. Basophils and eosinophils were absent in the epithelium of nonatopic control subjects (during the pollen season).

nose during natural seasonal exposure was examined. Immunotherapy did not appear to reduce seasonal increases in basophils in the nasal mucosal lamina propria. On the other hand, when the epithelium was examined for basophils, cells could be observed in only 1 of 20 immunotherapy patients, whereas they were present in 6 of 17 placebo subjects (22) (Fig. 1). This suggests that immunotherapy may act to reduce the seasonal recruitment of both basophils and eosinophils into the nasal epithelium.

D.   T-Cell Responses in Peripheral Blood

The importance of T-cells in directing allergic responses has created particular interest in the modification of T-cell responses to allergen following immunotherapy. By altering the T-cell response to subsequent allergen exposure, particularly by modifying the pattern of cytokines produced, immunotherapy may suppress late responses and improve clinical symptoms. For example, a reduction in expression of IL-5 and IL-4 might suppress allergen-induced eosinophil and IgE responses in tissues. Alternatively, immunotherapy might increase expression of "protective" cytokines acting to dampen the allergic inflammatory response. Collectively, these outcomes could be achieved by immune deviation of CD4+ T helper cells away from a TH2 phenotype and toward a TH1 phenotype, or through the induction of T-cell populations with "regulatory" or "suppressor" type activity.

The majority of studies addressing these issues have employed readouts based on isolating and culturing T-cells from peripheral venous blood and testing their reactivity to allergen extracts in vitro. A number of early studies of patients treated with venom or pollen immunotherapy reported a reduction in the global reactivity (i.e., proliferation) of peripheral blood T-cells to allergen (58–61). Superimposed on this reduced reactivity was a shift away from TH2 toward TH1 responses following treatment (50,60,62–64).

IL-10 is expressed by a variety of human immune cells, including both TH1 and TH2 cells, B-cells, monocytes/macrophages, dendritic cells, mast cells, and eosinophils. In mouse models, IL-10 has been associated with suppression of colitis (65), delayed-type hypersensitivity (66), graft rejection (67), arthritis (68), experimental autoimmune encephalomyelitis (69), and allergic inflammation (70–72). IL-10 has a number of documented anti-allergic properties that may be important to immunotherapy (Fig. 2) (reviewed in 73). These include modulation of IL-4–induced B-cell IgE production in favor of IgG4 (74), inhibition of IgE-dependent mast cell activation (75), and inhibition of human eosinophil cytokine production and survival (76). In human T-cells, IL-10 suppresses production of pro-allergic cytokines such as IL-5 (77) and is able to induce a state of antigen-specific hyporesponsiveness ("anergy") (78).

The presence of peripheral blood T-cells that produce IL-10 in response to allergen stimulation after immunotherapy has emerged as a consistent finding from numerous studies. Bellinghausen and colleagues (79) were the first to describe IL-10 production after venom immunotherapy. Akdis and colleagues (80) similarly described an increase in IL-10 production in response to venom immunotherapy, and this was superimposed on a global suppression of T-cell cytokine and proliferative responses to stimulation with venom allergen in vitro. The same investigators observed a similar IL-10 response to venom allergen in vitro in beekeepers who developed natural tolerance to venom by repetitive stings. When IL-10 was neutralized with anti–IL-10 antibodies, proliferation and cytokine production were restored. In contrast, the addition of IL-2—a fundamental and ubiquitous growth factor for activated T-cells—restored proliferation but led to a preferential restoration of TH1 cytokine production with production of IL-4 remaining suppressed. These observations raise the possibility that after immunotherapy IL-10 production may globally inhibit T-cell responses to allergen, but in the context of appropriate microenvironmental cytokines it may also effect a concomitant shift away from TH2 to TH1 cytokine production. Induction of IL-10–producing T-cells has now also been identified following conventional immunotherapy with grass pollen (Fig. 3) (81).

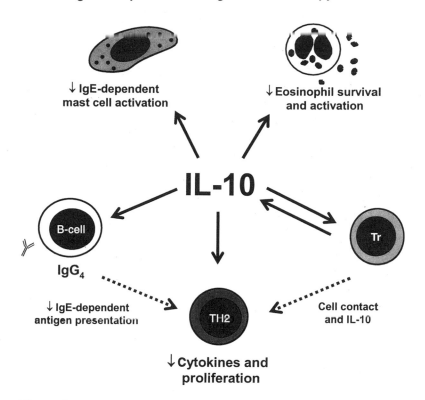

Figure 2 Summary of potential anti-allergic properties of IL-10. "Tr" represents IL-10–producing regulatory T-cells.

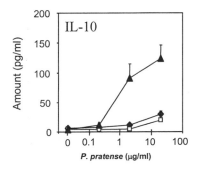

Figure 3 Effect of grass pollen immunotherapy on IL-10 production by peripheral blood T-cells. Peripheral blood mononuclear cells were isolated from 10 hay fever patients (closed triangle) who had received at least 18 months of conventional grass pollen immunotherapy, 11 untreated hay fever patients (closed diamond), and 12 nonatopic controls (open squares). Peripheral blood mononuclear cells were stimulated for 6 days with *P. pretense* (Timothy grass) extract. Values show mean IL-10 production as measured by ELISA in culture supernatants ($p < 0.05$ for immunotherapy patients vs. atopic or nonatopic controls).

E.   T-Cell Responses in Tissue

Studies performed by our group have examined T-cell responses after grass pollen immunotherapy in nasal mucosal and skin tissue following grass pollen immunotherapy. The experimental basis for this approach has been to collect nasal or cutaneous biopsy specimens after allergen challenge or natural seasonal exposure and to examine cytokine production in vivo using antisense RNA probes that identify specific cytokine mRNAs. While treatment appears to be associated with reduced accumulation of T-cells in skin and nose following allergen challenge, there was no attenuation of the T-cell response in the nasal mucosa during natural exposure to grass pollen exposure, suggesting that factors other than T-cell numbers probably account for clinical efficacy.

The first study to describe modulation of T-cell cytokine responses, with a shift in favor of allergen-induced TH1 cytokines, was published by Varney and colleagues in 1993 (52). After one year of grass pollen immunotherapy as part of a controlled trial, intradermal challenge with grass pollen extract was associated with a reduction in the cutaneous late-phase response in actively treated subjects. When this site was biopsied at 24 h, contrary to expectation, a reduction in numbers of IL-4 or IL-5 mRNA–expressing cells was not observed. However, modest but significant increases in IFN-γ and IL-2 mRNA–expressing cells suggested local immune deviation. Subsequently, skin biopsies collected after 2 years of immunotherapy were examined for expression of mRNA encoding one of the subunits of IL-12—a potent regulator of TH1 responses, including at sites of active allergic inflammation (82). IL-12 mRNA expression did indeed increase after immunotherapy and correlated positively with IFN-γ mRNA expression (83). While the majority of IL-12 mRNA–expressing cells were demonstrated to be CD68+ macrophages, a primary mechanism by which immunotherapy is able to induce this response in macrophages has yet to be proposed. When patients were subsequently followed up after 7 years of grass pollen immunotherapy, IL-4 mRNA expression in response to intradermal allergen challenge was decreased (84), suggesting that changes to cytokine responses after immunotherapy may evolve during prolonged treatment.

It is studies of immunological changes within the respiratory mucosa in response to inhaled allergens—i.e., the site of the disease—that are arguably of greatest relevance. With this in mind, nasal mucosal biopsies were collected from a cohort of immunotherapy- and placebo-treated patients 1 year into a double-blind trial 24 h after intranasal allergen provocation. Consistent with the skin model, immunotherapy increased allergen-dependent IFN-γ mRNA expression within the nasal mucosal lamina propria, with no reductions in IL-4 and IL-5 mRNA. Subsequently, cytokine mRNA expression was examined in nasal biopsies of grass pollen immunotherapy patients following natural pollen exposure during the summer pollen season (85). Seasonal increases in IL-5–producing cells were observed in placebo- but not immunotherapy-treated patients. Conversely, significant increases in interferon-gamma–expressing cells were observed during the pollen season only in immunotherapy-treated patients. Furthermore, an increase in the ratio of interferon-gamma/IL-5–producing cells was significant in the immunotherapy-versus to the placebo-treated group (Fig. 4) (86). Few other investigators have addressed the impact of immunotherapy on cytokine responses at mucosal surfaces. However, one study did examine the effect of immunotherapy with modified birch pollen allergens on cytokine concentrations in nasal lavage fluid during the pollen season (87). While IFN-γ and IL-5 were increased and decreased, respectively, in the actively treated group, these investigators could not identify any modulation of peripheral blood T-cell cytokine

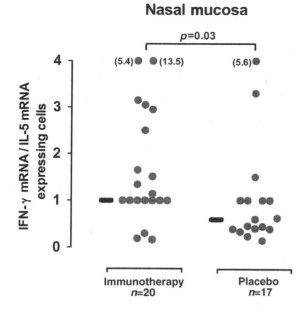

Figure 4 Ratio of IL-5 to IFN-γ mRNA–expressing cells in the nasal mucosa of immunotherapy patients. In a double-blind trial of grass pollen immunotherapy, nasal biopsies were obtained during the peak pollen season following 2 years of immunotherapy. IL-5 and IFN-γ mRNA–expressing cells were examined by in situ hybridization. Clinical improvement in the immunotherapy-treated group was associated with an increased ratio of IFN-γ to IL-5 mRNA–expressing cells in the nasal mucosa ($p = 0.03$).

responses in the same subjects. These findings further support the concept that local rather than peripheral immune modulation is necessary for clinically successful immunotherapy.

Expression of IL-10 mRNA has been described in skin biopsies taken from wasp venom immunotherapy patients following cutaneous allergen challenge (88). Additionally, a rise in IL-10 concentrations within nasal lavage fluid during the pollen season was reported in patients who received intranasal immunotherapy with weed vaccine (89). Taken together, these studies suggest that immunotherapy may act either by immune deviation of TH2 lymphocyte responses in favor of TH1 responses or by IL-10–induced allergen-specific T-cell nonresponsiveness (Fig. 5).

IV. DURATION OF EFFECT OF IMMUNOTHERAPY

Long-lived changes in memory T-cell function may induce prolonged clinical remission and/or prevent the progress of allergic disease. Although not conclusive, several studies support this view. Johnstone demonstrated in a controlled trial in children that immunotherapy for patients with rhinitis reduced the prevalence of asthma in subsequent years (90). Tree pollen immunotherapy for 3 years was associated with persistently reduced seasonal symptoms for up to 6 years following discontinuation, although no control group was followed in this study (91). One study in mite-sensitive children demonstrated that specific immunotherapy for one year did not result in maintained clinical improvement the following year (92). However, a retrospective study showed that mite-sensitive children treated

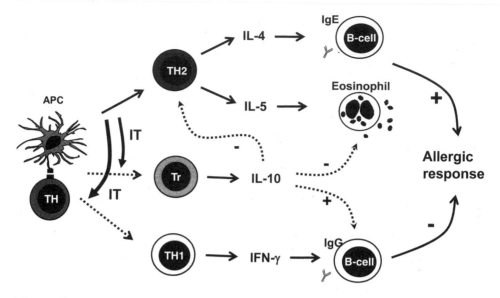

Figure 5 Summary of the effects of immunotherapy on T-cell responses. Immunotherapy read-dresses the balance between TH2/TH1 responses, in favor of TH1 responses. An increase in IL-10–producing T-cells, possibly regulatory T-cells (Tr), is also seen. The relationship between these events remains controversial.

for greater than 3 years as opposed to less than 3 years showed prolonged remission (36). A double-blind withdrawal of grass pollen immunotherapy following 4 years of treatment accomplished prolonged remission for at least 3 years after discontinuation (84). These studies indicate that immunotherapy can have a long-term benefit. Prolonged remission is accompanied by diminished immunological responses as shown by persistent suppression of the late skin response and a decrease of CD3+ and IL-4 mRNA+ cells in skin biopsies taken 24 h following intradermal allergen challenge (84).

V. NOVEL STRATEGIES FOR IMMUNOTHERAPY

The reasons for studying the mechanism of immunotherapy include the possibility of developing more advanced and targeted manipulations of the allergic response to improve both the efficacy and the safety profile of immunotherapy.

Although immunotherapy, using standardized vaccines in a specialist setting, is a safe form of treatment, administration of native allergen has occasionally been associated with IgE-mediated systemic reactions and, rarely, anaphylaxis. This has stimulated inter-est in the development of vaccines that reproduce the modulation of T-cell responses obtained with conventional immunotherapy without cross-linking IgE on mast cells. One ingenious approach has been to develop recombinant, genetically modified allergen proteins that have reduced binding to IgE while still containing the tolerance-producing T-cell epitopes. For example, Valenta and colleagues have developed both hypoallergenic recombinant fragments and a hypoallergenic trimer of the major birch pollen allergen *Bet v* 1 (93). These derivatives induced smaller inflammatory responses when tested in skin (94) and nose (95), though their efficacy in immunotherapy has yet to be evaluated. An additional advantage of using recombinant allergen proteins for immunotherapy is avoidance of the development of new IgE responses to allergenic components of the pollen vaccine used for treatment (39). Based on the same rationale, other investigators have proposed using allergen-derived peptides that do not bind IgE due to the absence of tertiary structure but that stimulate T-cells. Muller and colleagues administered bee venom–derived peptides to a few patients, though in the absence of placebo control claims of efficacy can only be regarded as anecdotal (41). Others have sought to evaluate allergen-derived peptides for the treatment of aeroallergy. The results of a trial of 27 amino acid peptides derived from the cat allergen *Fel d* 1 and given subcutaneously showed only weak efficacy (96). Others have extended this work to look at smaller peptide vaccines given by the intradermal route. In a small trial of cat allergen peptides, inhibition of peripheral blood T-cell responses in vitro was accompanied by modest reductions in early and late cutaneous responses to allergen (97). Nevertheless, peptide treatment did not result in a statistically significant improvement in symptoms over placebo treatment.

Alternative strategies for immunotherapy include the use of novel adjuvants to potentiate the ability of allergen vaccines to induce TH2 to TH1 immune deviation. These include monophosphoryl lipid A (MPL) derived from the lipid A region of lipopolysaccharide (LPS). MPL is a promoter of TH1 responses, perhaps through induction of IL-12 production by APCs (98,99). In a double-blind placebo-controlled trial, a tyrosine-absorbed glutaraldehyde-modified grass pollen vaccine containing MPL reduced hay fever symptoms and medication requirements and increased allergen-specific IgG (100). Similarly, immunostimulatory sequences (ISS) of DNA containing CpG motifs stimulate TH1 responses by a mechanism that probably involves induction of macrophage and/or dendritic cell IL-12 production (101,102), and inhibit airway inflammation in murine models of asthma (103). ISS may be more effective as an adjuvant when directly conjugated to allergen (104,105). An ISS–ragweed allergen (*Amb a* 1) conjugate given intradermally suppressed murine allergic responses (106), and clinical studies in human ragweed hay fever are in progress.

VI. SALIENT POINTS

1. Allergen injection immunotherapy is effective in selected patients with IgE-mediated disease and sensitivity to one or limited numbers of allergens.
2. Allergic disorders in humans are characterized by TH2 T-cell responses with preferential production of IL-4 and IL-5.
3. Immunotherapy inhibits allergen-induced late responses in the nose, skin, and lung.
4. The most significant effect of immunotherapy on serum antibodies is an increase in allergen-specific IgG, especially IgG4. These antibodies block some of the effects of IgE in vitro, but the clinical importance of these antibodies remains controversial.
5. Immunotherapy inhibits recruitment of eosinophils to the nose and lung.
6. Basophils that are observed within the nasal epithelial cell layer in some subjects during the pollen season are not present after immunotherapy.
7. Immunotherapy alters the TH2/TH1 balance in favor of TH1 responses, as detected in some peripheral blood T-cell studies and in the skin and nose following allergen exposure.

8. Local rather than peripheral immune modulation appears to be necessary for clinically successful immunotherapy.
9. IL-10–producing T-cells can be detected in blood after immunotherapy. IL-10 has numerous potential anti-allergic properties and promotes IgG_4 production by B-cells.
10. Immunotherapy studies in venom-, mite-, and grass-sensitive patients suggest that 3–5 years of immunotherapy has a prolonged effect (3 years minimum) following discontinuation, representing the only treatment with the potential to modify the course of allergic disease.
11. Novel approaches that directly target the T-cell response are being studied. These include non–IgE-binding recombinant allergens, allergen-derived peptides, and novel TH1-promoting adjuvants derived from bacteria such as MPL and ISS.

ACKNOWLEDGMENTS

This work was supported by the Medical Research Council, UK; the National Asthma Campaign, UK; and ALK Abello, Horsholm, Denmark.

REFERENCES

1. Malling H, Weeke B. Immunotherapy. Position paper of the European Academy of Allergy and Clinical Immunology. Allergy 1993; 48(suppl):9–35.
2. Frew AJ. British Society for Allergy and Clinical Immunology Working Party. Injection immunotherapy. Br Med J 1993; 307:919–923.
3. Bousquet J, Lockey R, Malling HJ (eds.). Allergen immunotherapy: Therapeutic vaccines for allergic diseases. A WHO position paper. J Allergy Clin Immunol 1998; 102:558–562.
4. Lockey RF. ARIA: Global guidelines and new forms of allergen immunotherapy. J Allergy Clin Immunol 2001; 108:497–499.
5. Naclerio RM, Proud D, Togias AG, Adkinson NF Jr, Meyers DA, Kagey-Sobotka A, Plaut M, Norman PS, Lichtenstein LM. Inflammatory mediators in late antigen-induced rhinitis. N Engl J Med 1985; 313:65–70.
6. Varney VA, Jacobson MR, Sudderick RM, Robinson DS, Irani AM, Schwartz LB, Mackay IS, Kay AB, Durham SR. Immunohistology of the nasal mucosa following allergen-induced rhinitis: Identification of activated T-cells, eosinophils and neutrophils. Am Rev Respir Dis 1992; 145:170–176.
7. Durham SR, Ying S, Varney VA, Jacobson MR, Sudderick RM, Mackay IS, Kay AB, Hamid QA. Cytokine messenger RNA expression for IL-3, IL-4, IL-5 and GM-CSF in the nasal mucosa after local allergen provocation: Relationship to tissue eosinophilia. J Immunol 1992; 148:2390–2394.
8. Ghaffar O, Laberge S, Jacobson MR, Lowhagen O, Rak S, Durham SR, Hamid Q. IL-13 mRNA and immunoreactivity in allergen induced rhinitis: Comparison with IL-4 expression and modulation by topical glucocorticoid therapy. Am J Respir Cell Mol Biol 1997; 17:17–24.
9. Sutton BI, Gould HI. Human IgE synthesis. Nature 1993; 366:421–428.
10. Schleimer RP, Sterbinsky SA, Kaiser J, Bickel CA, Klunk DA, Tomioka K, Newman W, Luscinskas FW, Gimbrone MA Jr, McIntyre BW. IL-4 induces adherence of human eosinophils and basophils but not neutrophils to endothelium: Association with expression of VCAM-l. J Immunol 1992, 148.1086 1092.

11. Ying S, Meng Qiu, Taborda-Barata L, Robinson DS, Durham SR, Kay AB. Associations between IL-13 and IL-4 (mRNA and protein), VCAM-1 expression and the infiltration of eosinophils, macrophages and T-cells in the allergen-induced late-phase cutaneous response in atopic subjects. J Immunol 1997; 158:5050–5057.

12. Heath H, Qin S, Rao P, Wu L, LaRosa G, Kassam N, Ponath PD, Mackay CR. Chemokine receptor usage by human eosinophils: The importance of CCR3 demonstrated using an antagonistic monoclonal antibody. J Clin Invest 1997; 99:178–184.

13. Ying S, Robinson DS, Meng Q, Rottman J, Kennedy R, Ringler DJ, Mackay CR, Daugherty BL, Springer MS, Durham SR, Williams TJ, Kay AB. Enhanced expression of eotaxin and CCR3 mRNA and protein in atopic asthma: Association with airway hyperresponsiveness and predominant co-localization of eotaxin mRNA to bronchial epithelial and endothelial cells. Eur J Immunol 1997; 27:3507–3516.

14. Her E, Frazer I, Austen KF, Owen WF. Eosinophil hematopoietins antagonize the programmed cell death of eosinophils: Cytokine and glucocorticoid effects on eosinophils maintained by endothelial cell–conditioned medium. J Clin Invest 1991; 88:1982–1987.

15. Rak S, Jacobson MR, Sudderick RM, Masuyama K, Juliusson S, Kay AB, Hamid Q, Lowhagen O, Durham SR. Influence of prolonged treatment with topical corticosteroid (fluticasone propionate) on early and late phase nasal responses and cellular infiltration in the nasal mucosa after allergen challenge. Clin Exp Allergy 1994; 24:930–939.

16. Masuyama K, Till SJ, Jacobson MR, Kamil A, Cameron L, Juliusson S, Lowhagen O, Kay AB, Hamid Q, Durham SR. Nasal eosinophilia and IL-5 mRNA expression in seasonal allergic rhinitis: Effect of topical corticosteroids. J Allergy Clin Immunol 1998; 102:610–617.

17. Cameron LA, Durham SR, Jacobson MR, Masuyama K, Juliusson S, Gould HJ, Lowhagen O, Minshall EM, Hamid QA. Expression of IL-4, C epsilon RNA, and I epsilon RNA in the nasal mucosa of patients with seasonal rhinitis: Effect of topical corticosteroids. J Allergy Clin Immunol 1998; 101:330–336.

18. Bradding P, Feather IH, Wilson S, Bardin PG, Heusser CH, Holgate ST, Howarth PH. Immunolocalization of cytokines in the nasal mucosa of normal and perennial rhinitic subjects: The mast cell as a source of IL-4, IL-5, and IL-6 in human allergic mucosal inflammation. J Immunol 1993; 151:3853–3865.

19. Pipkorn U, Karlsson G, Enerback L. The cellular response of the human allergic mucosa to natural allergen exposure. J Allergy Clin Immunol 1988; 81:1046–1054.

20. Gomez E, Clague JE, Gatland D, Davies RJ. Effect of topical corticosteroids on seasonally induced increases in nasal mast cells. Br Med J 1988; 296:1572–1573.

21. Bentley AM, Jacobson MR, Cumberworth V, Barkans JR, Moqbel R, Schwartz LB, Irani AM, Kay AB, Durham SR. Immunohistology of the nasal mucosa in seasonal allergic rhinitis: Increases in activated eosinophils and epithelial mast cells. J Allergy Clin Immunol 1992; 89:821–829.

22. Wilson DR, Irani AM, Walker SM, Jacobson MR, Mackay IS, Schwartz LB, Durham SR. Grass pollen immunotherapy inhibits seasonal increases in basophils and eosinophils in the nasal epithelium. Clin Exp Allergy 2001; 31:1705–1713.

23. Gibson PG, Allen CJ, Yang JP, Wong BJ, Dolovich J, Denburg J, Hargreave FE. Intraepithelial mast cells in allergic and nonallergic asthma: Assessment using bronchial brushings. Am Rev Respir Dis 1993; 148:80–86.

24. Mosmann TR, Cherwinski H, Bond MW, Giedlin MA, Coffman RL. Two types of murine helper T-cell clone: I. Definition according to profiles of lymphokine activities and secreted proteins. J Immunol 1986; 136:2348–2357.

25. Secrist H, DeKruyff RH, Umetsu DT. Interleukin-4 production by CD4+ T-cells from allergic individuals is modulated by antigen concentration and antigen-presenting cell type. J Exp Med 1995; 181:1081–1089.

26. Kapsenberg ML, Hilkens CM, Wierenga EA, Kalinski P. The paradigm of type 1 and type 2

antigen-presenting cells. Implications for atopic allergy. Clin Exp Allergy 1999; 29(suppl):33–36.

27.   Reider N, Reider D, Ebner S, Holzmann S, Herold M, Fritsch P, Romani N. Dendritic cells contribute to the development of atopy by an insufficiency in IL-12 production. J Allergy Clin Immunol 2002; 109:89–95.

28.   Manetti R, Parronchi P, Giudizi MG, Piccinni MP, Maggi E, Trinchieri G, Romagnani S. Natural killer cell stimulatory factor (interleukin 12 [IL-12]) induces T helper type 1 (Th1)–specific immune responses and inhibits the development of IL-4 producing Th cells. J Exp Med 1993; 177:1199–1204.

29.   Maggi E, Parronchi P, Manetti R, et al. Reciprocal regulatory effects of IFN-gamma and IL-4 on the in vitro development of human Th1 and Th2 clones. J lmmunol 1992; 148:2142–2147.

30.   Freeman GJ, Boussiotis VA, Anumanthan A, Bernstein GM, Ke XY, Rennert PD, Gray GS, Gribben JG, Nadler LM. B7-1 and B7-2 do not deliver identical costimulatory signals since B7-2 but not B7-1 preferentially costimulates the initial production of IL-4. Immunity 1995; 2:523–532.

31.   Harding FA, McArthur JG, Gross JA, Raulet DH, Allison JP. CD28-mediated signalling costimulates murine T-cells and prevents induction of anergy in T-cell clones. Nature 1992; 356:607–609.

32.   Pienkowski MM, Norman PS, Lichtenstein LM. Suppression of late phase skin reactions by immunotherapy with ragweed extract. J Allergy Clin lmmunol 1985; 76:729–734.

33.   Iliopoulos O, Proud D, Adkinson NF Jr, Creticos PS, Norman PS, Kagey-Sobotka A, Lichtenstein LM, Naclerio RM. Effects of immunotherapy on the early, late and rechallenge nasal reaction to provocation with allergen: Changes in inflammatory mediators and cells. J Allergy Clin Immunol 1991; 87:855–866.

34.   Warner JO, Price JF, Soothill JF, Hey EN. Controlled trial of hyposensitisation to *Dermatophagoides pteronyssinus* in children with asthma. Lancet 1978; 2:912–915.

35.   Walker S, Varney V, Jacobson MR, Durham SR. Grass pollen immunotherapy: Efficacy and safety during a four year follow-up study. Allergy 1995; 50:405–413.

36.   Des Roches A, Paradis L, Knani J, Hejjaoui A, Dhivert H, Chanez P, Bousquet J. Immunotherapy with a standardized *Dermatophagoides pteronyssinus* extract: V. Duration of efficacy of immunotherapy after its cessation. Allergy 1996; 51:430–433.

37.   Gehlhar K, Schlaak M, Becker W, Bufe A. Monitoring allergen immunotherapy of pollen-allergic patients: The ratio of allergen-specific IgG4 to IgG1 correlates with clinical outcome. Clin Exp Allergy 1999; 29:497–506.

38.   Lichtenstein L, Ishizaka K, Norman P, Sobotka A, Hill B. IgE antibody measurements in ragweed hayfever: Relationship to clinical severity and the results of immunotherapy. J Clin Invest 1973; 52:472–82

39.   Moverare R, Elfman L, Vesterinen E, Metso T, Haahtela T. Development of new IgE specificities to allergenic components in birch pollen extract during specific immunotherapy studied with immunoblotting and Pharmacia CAP System. Allergy 2002; 57:423–430.

40.   McHugh SM, Lavelle B, Kemeny DM, Patel S, Ewan PW. A placebo-controlled trial of immunotherapy with two extracts of *Dermatophagoides pteronyssinus* in allergic rhinitis, comparing clinical outcome with changes in antigen-specific IgE, IgG, and IgG subclasses. J Allergy Clin Immunol 1990; 86:521–531.

41.   Muller U, Akdis CA, Fricker M, Akdis M, Blesken T, Bettens F, Blaser K. Successful immunotherapy with T-cell epitope peptides of bee venom phospholipase A2 induces specific T-cell anergy in patients allergic to bee venom. J Allergy Clin Immunol 1998; 101:747–54.

42.   Garcia BE, Sanz ML, Gato JJ, Fernandez J, Oehling A. IgG4 blocking effect on the release of antigen-specific histamine. J Investig Allergol Clin Immunol 1993; 3:26–33.

43.   Lambin P, Bouzoumou A, Murrieta M, Debbia M, Rouger P, Leynadier F, Levy DA.

Purification of human IgG4 subclass with allergen-specific blocking activity. J Immunol Methods 1993; 165:99–111,

44. van Neerven RJ, Wikborg T, Lund G, Jacobsen B, Brinch-Nielsen A, Arnved J, Ipsen H. Blocking antibodies induced by specific allergy vaccination prevent the activation of CD4+ T-cells by inhibiting serum-IgE–facilitated allergen presentation. J Immunol 1999; 163:2944–2952.

45. Wachholz PA, Kristensen N, Till SJ, Durham SR. Inhibition of allergen-IgE binding to B-cells by IgG antibodies following grass pollen immunotherapy. (Submitted.)

46. Djurup R, Malling HJ. High IgG4 antibody level is associated with failure of immunotherapy with inhalant allergens. Clin Allergy 1987; 17:459–468.

47. Ewan PW, Deighton J, Wilson AB, Lachmann PJ. (1993) Venom-specific IgG antibodies in bee and wasp allergy: Lack of correlation with protection from stings. Clin Exp Allergy 1993; 23:647–660.

48. Michils A, Ledent C, Mairesse M, Gossart B, Duchateau J. Wasp venom immunotherapy changes IgG antibody specificity. Clin Exp Allergy 1997; 27:1036–1042.

49. Michils A, Mairesse M, Ledent C, Gossart B, Baldassarre S, Duchateau J. Modified antigenic reactivity of anti-phospholipase A2 IgG antibodies in patients allergic to bee venom: Conversion with immunotherapy and relation to subclass expression. J Allergy Clin Immunol 1998; 102:118–126.

50. Creticos PS, Adkinson NF Jr, Kagey-Sobotka A, Proud D, Meier HL, Naclerio RM, Lichtenstein LM, Norman PS. Nasal challenge with ragweed in hayfever patients: Effect of immunotherapy. J Clin Invest 1985; 76:2247–2253.

51. Otsuka H, Mezawa A, Ohnishi M, Okubo K, Sehi H, Okuda M. Changes in nasal metachromatic cells during allergen immunotherapy. Clin Exp Allergy 1991; 21:115–120.

52. Varney VA, Hamid QA, Gaga M, Ying S, Jacobson M, Frew AJ, Kay AB, Durham SR. Influence of grass pollen immunotherapy on cellular infiltration and cytokine mRNA expression during allergen-induced late-phase cutaneous responses. J Clin Invest 1993; 92:644–651.

53. Nish WA, Charlesworth EN, Davis TL, Whisman BA, Valtier S, Charlesworth MG, Leiferman KM. The effect of immunotherapy on the cutaneous late phase response to antigen. J Allergy Clin Immunol 1994; 93:484–493.

54. Furin MJ, Norman PS, Creticos PS, Proud D, Kagey-Sobotka A, Lichtenstein LM, Naclerio RM. Immunotherapy decreases antigen-induced eosinophil migration into the nasal cavity. J Allergy Clin Immunol 1991; 88:27–32.

55. Durham SR, Ying S, Varney VA, Jacobson MR, Sudderick RM, Mackay IS, Kay AB, Hamid QA. Grass pollen immunotherapy inhibits allergen-induced infiltration of CD4+ T-cells and eosinophils in the nasal mucosa and increases the number of cells expressing messenger RNA for interferon-gamma. J Allergy Clin Immunol 1996; 97:1356–1365.

56. Rak S, Lowhagen O, Venge P. The effect of immunotherapy on bronchial hyperresponsiveness and eosinophil cationic protein in pollen-allergic patients. J Allergy Clin Immunol 1988; 82:470–480.

57. Kepley CL, Craig SS, Schwartz LB. Identification and partial characterization of a unique marker for human basophils. J Immunol 1995; 154:6548–6555.

58. Jutel M, Pichler WJ, Skrbic D, Urwyler A, Dahinden C, Muller UR. Bee venom immunotherapy results in decrease of IL-4 and IL-5 and increase of IFN-gamma secretion in specific allergen-stimulated T-cell cultures. J Immunol 1995; 154:4187–4194.

59. Akdis CA, Akdis M, Blesken T, Wymann D, Alkan SS, Muller U, Blaser K. Epitope-specific T-cell tolerance to phospholipase A2 in bee venom immunotherapy and recovery by IL-2 and IL-15 in vitro. J Clin Invest 1996; 98:1676–1683.

60. Ebner C, Siemann U, Bohle B, Willheim M, Wiedermann U, Schenk S, Klotz F, Ebner H, Kraft Dh, Scheiner O. Immunological changes during specific immunotherapy of grass pollen allergy: Reduced lymphoproliferative responses to allergen and shift from TH2 to TH1 in T-

cell clones specific for Phl p 1, a major grass pollen allergen. Clin Exp Allergy 1997; 27:1007–1015.

61. Eusebius NP, Papalia L, Suphioglu C, McLellan SC, Varney M, Rolland JM, O'Hehir RE. Oligoclonal analysis of the atopic T-cell response to the group 1 allergen of *Cynodon dactylon* (bermuda grass) pollen: Pre- and post- allergen-specific immunotherapy. Int Arch Allergy Immunol 2002; 127:234–244.

62. Secrist J, Chelen CJ, Wen Y, Marshall JD, Umetsu DT. Allergen immunotherapy decreases interleukin-4 production in CD4+ T-cells from allergic individuals. J Exp Med 1993; 178:2123–2130.

63. McHugh SM, Deighton J, Stewart AG, Lachmann PJ, Ewan PW. Bee venom immunotherapy induces a shift in cytokine responses from a Th2 to a Th1 dominant pattern: Comparison of rush and conventional immunotherapy. Clin Exp Allergy 1995; 25:828–838.

64. Akoum H, Tsicopoulos A, Vorng H, Wallaert B, Dessaint JP, Joseph M, Hamid Q, Tonnel AB. Venom immunotherapy modulates interleukin-4 and interferon-gamma messenger RNA expression of peripheral T-cells. Immunology 1996; 87:593–598.

65. Kuhn R, Lohler J, Rennick D, Rajewsky K, Muller W. Interleukin-10–deficient mice develop chronic enterocolitis. Cell 1993; 75:263–274.

66. Flores-Villanueva PO, Zheng XX, Strom TB, Stadecker MJ. Recombinant IL-10 and IL-10/Fc treatment down-regulate egg antigen-specific delayed hypersensitivity reactions and egg granuloma formation in schistosomiasis. J Immunol 1996; 156:3315–3320.

67. Kingsley CI, Karim M, Bushell AR, Wood KJ. CD25+CD4+ regulatory T-cells prevent graft rejection: CTLA-4–and IL-10–dependent immunoregulation of alloresponses. J Immunol 2002; 168:1080–1086.

68. Quattrocchi E, Dallman MJ, Dhillon AP, Quaglia A, Bagnato G, Feldmann M. Murine IL-10 gene transfer inhibits established collagen-induced arthritis and reduces adenovirus-mediated inflammatory responses in mouse liver. J Immunol 2001; 166:5970–5978.

69. Cua DJ, Hutchins B, LaFace DM, Stohlman SA, Coffman RL. Central nervous system expression of IL-10 inhibits autoimmune encephalomyelitis. J Immunol 2001; 166:602–608.

70. Tournoy KG, Kips JC, Pauwels RA. Endogenous interleukin-10 suppresses allergen-induced airway inflammation and nonspecific airway responsiveness. Clin Exp Allergy 2000; 30:775–783.

71. Oh JW, Seroogy CM, Meyer EH, Akbari O, Berry G, Fathman CG, Dekruyff RH, Umetsu DT. CD4 T-helper cells engineered to produce IL-10 prevent allergen-induced airway hyperreactivity and inflammation. J Allergy Clin Immunol 2002; 110:460–468.

72. Akbari O, DeKruyff RH, Umetsu DT. Pulmonary dendritic cells producing IL-10 mediate tolerance induced by respiratory exposure to antigen. Nat Immunol 2001; 2:725–731.

73. Bellinghausen I, Knop J, Saloga J. The role of interleukin 10 in the regulation of allergic immune responses. Int Arch Allergy Immunol 2001; 126:97–101.

74. Jeannin P, Lecoanet S, Delneste Y, Gauchat JF, Bonnefoy JY. IgE versus IgG4 production can be differentially regulated by IL-10. J Immunol 1998; 160:3555–3561.

75. Royer B, Varadaradjalou S, Saas P, Guillosson JJ, Kantelip JP, Arock M. Inhibition of IgE-induced activation of human mast cells by IL-10. Clin Exp Allergy 2001; 31:694–704.

76. Takanaski S, Nonaka R, Xing Z, O'Byrne P, Dolovich J, Jordana M. Interleukin 10 inhibits lipopolysaccharide-induced survival and cytokine production by human peripheral blood eosinophils. J Exp Med 1994; 180:711–715.

77. Schandene L, Alonso-Vega C, Willems F, Gerard C, Delvaux A, Velu T, Devos R, de Boer M, Goldman M. B7/CD28-dependent IL-5 production by human resting T-cells is inhibited by IL-10. J Immunol 1994; 152:4368–4374.

78. Groux H, Bigler M, de Vries JE, Roncarolo MG. Interleukin-10 induces a long-term antigen-specific anergic state in human CD4+ T-cells. J Exp Med 1996; 184:19–29.

79. Bellinghausen I, Metz G, Enk AH, Christmann S, Knop J, Saloga J. Insect venom

immunotherapy induces interleukin-10 production and a Th2- to-Th1 shift, and changes surface marker expression in venom-allergic subjects. Eur J Immunol 1997; 27:1131–1139.

80. Akdis CA, Blesken T, Akdis M, Wuthrich B, Blaser K. Role of interleukin 10 in specific immunotherapy. J Clin Invest 1998; 102:98–106.

81. Francis JN, Till SJ, Durham SR. Induction of IL-10+CD4+CD25+ T-cells by grass pollen immunotherapy. J Allergy Clin Immunol 2003; 111(6):1255–1261

82. Varga EM, Wachholz P, Nouri-Aria KT, Verhoef A, Corrigan CJ, Till SJ, Durham SR. T-cells from human allergen-induced late asthmatic responses express IL-12 receptor β2 subunit mRNA and respond to IL-12 in vitro. J Immunol 2000; 165:2877–2885.

83. Hamid Q, Schotman E, Jacobson MR, Walker SM, Durham SR. Increases in interleukin-12 (IL-12) messenger RNA+ (mRNA+) cells accompany inhibition of allergen induced late skin responses following successful grass pollen immunotherapy. J Allergy Clin Immunol 1997; 99:254–260.

84. Durham SR, Walker SM, Varga EM, Jacobson MR, O'Brien F, Noble W, Till SJ, Hamid QA, Nouri-Aria KT. Long-term clinical efficacy of grass-pollen immunotherapy. N Engl J Med 1999; 341:468–475.

85. Wilson DR, Nouri-Aria KT, Walker SM, Pajno GB, O'Brien F, Jacobson MR, Mackay IS, Durham SR. Grass pollen immunotherapy: Symptomatic improvement correlates with reductions in eosinophils and IL-5 mRNA expression in the nasal mucosa during the pollen season. J Allergy Clin Immunol 2001; 107:971–976.

86. Wachholz P, Nouri-Aria KT, Verhoef A, Walker SM, Till SJ, Durham SR. Grass pollen immunotherapy for hayfever is associated with increases in local nasal mucosal but not peripheral Th1/Th2 ratios. Immunology 2002; 105:56–62.

87. Klimek L, Dormann D, Jarman ER, Cromwell O, Riechelmann H, Reske-Kunz AB. Short-term preseasonal birch pollen allergoid immunotherapy influences symptoms, specific nasal provocation and cytokine levels in nasal secretions, but not peripheral T-cell responses, in patients with allergic rhinitis. Clin Exp Allergy 1999; 29:1326–1335.

88. Nasser SM, Ying S, Meng Q, Kay AB, Ewan PW. Interleukin-10 levels increase in cutaneous biopsies of patients undergoing wasp venom immunotherapy. Eur J Immunol 2001; 31:3704–3713.

89. Gaglani B, Borish L, Bartelson BL, Buchmeier A, Keller L, Nelson HS. Nasal immunotherapy in weed-induced allergic rhinitis. Ann Allergy Asthma Immunol 1997; 79:259–265.

90. Johnstone DE. Some aspects of the natural history of asthma. Ann Allergy 1982; 49:793–802.

91. Jacobsen L, Nuchel Petersen B, Wihl JA, Lowenstein H, Ipsen H. Immunotherapy with partially purified and standardized tree pollen extracts: IV. Results from long-term (6-year) follow-up. Allergy 1997; 52:914–920.

92. Price IF, Warner JO, Hey EN, Turner MW, Soothill IF. A controlled trial of hyposensitisation with absorbed tyrosine *Dermatophagoides pteronyssinus* antigen in childhood asthma: In vivo aspects. Clin Allergy 1984; 14:209–219.

93. Valenta R, Vrtala S, Focke-Tejkl M, Twardosz A, Swoboda I, Bugajska-Schretter A, Spitzauer S, Kraft D. Synthetic and genetically engineered allergen derivatives for specific immunotherapy of type I allergy. Clin Allergy Immunol 2002; 16:495–517.

94. Nopp A, Hallden G, Lundahl J, Johansson E, Vrtala S, Valenta R, Gronneberg R, Van Hage-Hamsten M. Comparison of inflammatory responses to genetically engineered hypoallergenic derivatives of the major birch pollen allergen bet v 1 and to recombinant bet v 1 wild type in skin chamber fluids collected from birch pollen-allergic patients. J Allergy Clin Immunol 2000; 106:101–109.

95. van Hage-Hamsten M, Johansson E, Roquet A, Peterson C, Andersson M, Greiff L, Vrtala S, Valenta R, Gronneberg R. Nasal challenges with recombinant derivatives of the major birch pollen allergen Bet v 1 induce fewer symptoms and lower mediator release than rBet v 1 wild-type in patients with allergic rhinitis. Clin Exp Allergy 2002; 32:1448–1453.

96. Norman PS, Ohman JL Jr, Long AA, Creticos PS, Gefter MA, Shaked Z, Wood RA, Eggleston PA, Hafner KB, Rao P, Lichtenstein LM, Jones NH, Nicodemus CF. Treatment of cat allergy with T-cell reactive peptides. Am J Respir Crit Care Med 1996; 154:1623–1628.

97. Oldfield WL, Larche M, Kay AB. Effect of T-cell peptides derived from Fel d 1 on allergic reactions and cytokine production in patients sensitive to cats: A randomised controlled trial. Lancet 2002; 360:47–53.

98. Salkowski CA, Detore GR, Vogel SN. Lipopolysaccharide and monophosphoryl lipid A differentially regulate interleukin-12, gamma interferon, and interleukin-10 mRNA production in murine macrophages. Infect Immun 1997; 65:3239–3247.

99. Ismaili J, Rennesson J, Aksoy E, Vekemans J, Vincart B, Amraoui Z, Van Laethem F, Goldman M, Dubois PM. Monophosphoryl lipid A activates both human dendritic cells and T cells. J Immunol 2002; 168:926–932.

100. Drachenberg KJ, Wheeler AW, Stuebner P, Horak F. A well-tolerated grass pollen–specific allergy vaccine containing a novel adjuvant, monophosphoryl lipid A, reduces allergic symptoms after only four preseasonal injections. Allergy 2001; 56:498–505.

101. Chu RS, Targoni OS, Krieg AM, Lehmann PV, Harding CV. CpG oligodeoxynucleotides act as adjuvants that switch on T helper 1 (Th1) immunity. J Exp Med 1997; 186:1623–1631.

102. Jakob T, Walker PS, Krieg AM, von Stebut E, Udey MC, Vogel JC. Bacterial DNA and CpG-containing oligodeoxynucleotides activate cutaneous dendritic cells and induce IL-12 production: Implications for the augmentation of Th1 responses. Int Arch Allergy Immunol 1999; 118:457–461.

103. Kline JN, Waldschmidt TJ, Businga TR, Lemish JE, Weinstock JV, Thorne PS, Krieg AM. Modulation of airway inflammation by CpG oligodeoxynucleotides in a murine model of asthma. J Immunol 1998; 160:2555–2559.

104. Tighe H, Takabayashi K, Schwartz D, Van Nest G, Tuck S, Eiden JJ, Kagey-Sobotka A, Creticos PS, Lichtenstein LM, Spiegelberg HL, Raz E. Conjugation of immunostimulatory DNA to the short ragweed allergen amb a 1 enhances its immunogenicity and reduces its allergenicity. J Allergy Clin Immunol 2000; 106:124–134.

105. Marshall JD, Abtahi S, Eiden JJ, Tuck S, Milley R, Haycock F, Reid MJ, Kagey-Sobotka A, Creticos PS, Lichtenstein LM, Van Nest G. Immunostimulatory sequence DNA linked to the Amb a 1 allergen promotes T(H)1 cytokine expression while downregulating T(H)2 cytokine expression in PBMCs from human patients with ragweed allergy. J Allergy Clin Immunol 2001; 108:191–197.

106. Santeliz JV, Van Nest G, Traquina P, Larsen E, Wills-Karp M. Amb a 1–linked CpG oligodeoxynucleotides reverse established airway hyperresponsiveness in a murine model of asthma. J Allergy Clin Immunol 2002; 109:455–462.

6

Primary and Secondary Prevention of Allergy and Asthma by Allergen Therapeutic Vaccines

JEAN BOUSQUET

Montpellier University, Montpellier, France

I. INTRODUCTION

Although pharmacological intervention to treat established asthma is highly effective in controlling symptoms and improving the quality of life, no strategies have been devised to cure the condition and few are available to modify the natural course of the disease. This inevitably focuses attention on prevention as the optimal approach to avoid having to treat a chronic life-long and incurable disease.

Three levels of prevention can be considered (1).

Primary prevention should be introduced before any evidence arises of sensitization to allergens capable of inducing allergic respiratory disease. Because there is evidence that allergic sensitization, the most common precursor to development of asthma, can occur antenatally (2), much of the focus of primary prevention will be on perinatal interventions. However, there is very little information concerning allergen vaccination of either the mother or the neonate.

Secondary prevention is employed after primary sensitization to an allergen has occurred, but before there is any evidence of disease. Often this will focus specifically on the first years of life. Although this is not specifically stated in the WHO document, the secondary prevention of allergy may also refer to the prevention of new sensitizations in a patient already sensitized to certain allergens. Secondary prevention of asthma can also be attempted in occupational rhinitis and in patients with allergic rhinitis or children with nonasthmatic allergic conditions, using, as appropriate, allergen immunotherapy, anti-IgE therapy, and/or pharmacotherapy (3,4).

Tertiary prevention involves the avoidance of allergens and nonspecific triggers once asthma or other allergic disease is already established. It is accepted that tertiary prevention should be started when the first signs of asthma occur. However, increasing evidence suggests that the histopathology of the disease is fully established by this time.

II. PRIMARY PREVENTION OF ALLERGY USING ALLERGEN VACCINATION

The immune status and allergen exposure of the mother may influence the immune response of the offspring after birth and may contribute to the primary prevention of allergy. This has been demonstrated in animal studies.

The progeny of rats immunized with egg albumin display prolonged suppression of IgE responsiveness to egg-specific albumin (5). An identical effect was produced by injecting the progeny of nonimmunized rats with small amounts anti–egg-albumin–specific IgG during the first few days of life. Both manipulations also elevated the primary IgG response to a subsequent immunization (6). Feeding antigen to the progeny of (IgG-transmitting) immune mothers showed that passive and active immunity in the young rat both suppressed the IgE responsiveness (7).

Preconception maternal immunization with dust mite vaccines inhibits the type I hypersensitivity response of offspring, as shown by female A/Sn mice immunized or not with *Dermatophagoides pteronyssinus* and mated with unimmunized male C57BL/6 mice (8). Allergen immunization of NIH/OlaHsd female mice during pregnancy and postpartum significantly reduced the IgE response in their progeny, whereas the IgG2a response to the same allergen was increased. Allergen immunization of the female mice 3 days into pregnancy resulted in a significantly lower IgE response in progeny compared with the response by progeny of nonimmunized female mice and progeny of female mice immunized 17 days into pregnancy (9). IgE suppression is detectable in the progeny of immunized female mice during the first 4 months of life, but not thereafter (10). However, when the initial immunization at age 3 or 4 months was followed by further application of both allergens, IgE suppression persisted up to an age of more than 1 year.

In ovalbumin-sensitized BALB/c mice TH2/TH0 immunity present during pregnancy has a decisive impact on shaping the TH1/TH2 T-cell profile in response to postnatal allergen exposure (11). In a mouse model of TH2 immunity, BALB/c mice were sensitized to ovalbumin (OVA) before mating followed by allergen aerosol exposure during pregnancy. At the end of pregnancy, the mice developed allergen-specific TH2/TH0 immunity and immediate-type hypersensitivity responses to OVA. To assess whether prenatal allergen exposure favors postnatal onset of a TH2-type immune response, the progeny were immunized to a novel antigen by a single injection of β-lactoglobulin (BLG). In contrast to offspring from nonsensitized mothers, offspring from OVA-sensitized mice showed both higher anti BLG immunoglobulin titers and higher frequencies of immediate type skin test responses.

If applicable to man, these findings may allow the development of new strategies to prevent allergy and asthma by maternally transferred or neonatally injected allergen-specific monoclonal IgG antibodies.

The effect of maternal allergen vaccination on immediate skin test reactivity, specific Lol p 1 IgG and IgE antibodies, and total IgE was studied in 14 children allergic to grass pollen (12). Fourteen additional children from the same allergic mothers, to whom vaccination had not been given during the pregnancy, served as controls. Levels of Lol p 1 IgG and total IgE were lower in the sera of children born to mothers who received allergen vaccine (not statistically significant) compared with their control cohorts. Paired cord blood and maternal blood samples drawn at delivery showed similar levels of Lol p 1 IgG, indicating that blocking antibody readily crosses the placenta. This study suggests that allergen vaccination during pregnancy may have an inhibitory effect on immediate skin reactivity to grass allergens in some offspring. Whether tolerance to other allergens can be induced in children by maternal vaccination remains to be determined.

III. SECONDARY PREVENTION OF ASTHMA USING ALLERGEN VACCINATION

Although drugs are highly effective and usually without important side effects, they result in only symptomatic treatment; allergen vaccination is the only treatment that may alter the natural course of the disease (13–15).

Long-term efficacy of allergen vaccination following discontinuation of allergen immunotherapy has been demonstrated for subcutaneous vaccination (16–20). However, in a study by Naclerio et al. (19), 1 year following discontinuation of ragweed immunotherapy, nasal challenges showed partial recrudescence of mediator responses even though patient reports during the season indicated continued suppression of symptoms. Long-term efficacy remains to be documented for local allergen vaccination (21).

Allergen vaccination is primarily used to control allergic diseases, but data suggests that allergen vaccination may be preventive. Allergic sensitization usually begins early in life, and symptoms often start within the first decade. Allergen vaccination is less effective in older asthmatic patients than in children, and inflammation and remodeling of the airways in asthma are a poor prognosticator of effective allergen vaccination. Moreover, if allergen vaccination is used as a preventive treatment, it should be started as soon as allergy has been diagnosed (22).

Allergen vaccination of patients with only allergic rhinoconjunctivitis may prevent the onset of asthma. An early study by Johnstone (23), using several different allergens, showed that 28% of children receiving allergen vaccination developed asthma compared with 78% of placebo-treated children. To answer the question "Does specific allergen vaccination stop the development and onset of asthma?" the Preventive Allergy Treatment (PAT) study was started in children ages 7 to 13 (24). This study, performed as a multicenter study in Austria, Denmark, Finland, Germany, and Sweden, involved 205 children age 6–14 years. After 3 years of allergen vaccination, a significantly greater number of children in the control group developed asthma compared with the active group (Fig. 1). Before the start of vaccination, 20% of the children had symptoms of mild asthma during the pollen season(s). Among those without asthma and only with allergic rhinitis, the actively treated children had significantly fewer cases of new-onset asthma than the control group after 3 years on allergen immunotherapy (for clinical diagnosis of asthma,

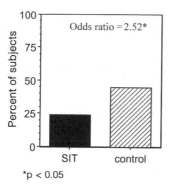

Figure 1 Percentage of children after 3 years of immunoptherapy with asthma among the 152 children without asthma before treatment. (From Ref. 24.)

odds ratio = 2.52; $p < 0.05$). Methacholine bronchial provocation test results improved significantly in the actively treated group only ($p < 0.05$).

The long-lasting effects of sublingual-swallow immunotherapy (SLIT) in 60 children with asthma due to house dust mite were examined in a 10-year prospective parallel group controlled study (25). Thirty-five children received a 4- to 5-year course of SLIT with standardized extracts, and 25 received only drug therapy. The children were evaluated at three time points (baseline, end of SLIT, and 4 to 5 years after SLIT discontinuation) for the presence of asthma, use of anti-asthma drugs, response to skin prick tests, and concentrations of specific IgE (Fig. 2). After 3 years of SLIT, there was a significant difference versus baseline for the presence of asthma ($p < 0.001$) and the use of asthma medications ($p < 0.01$), whereas no differences were observed in the control groups. The mean peak expiratory flow rate, at completion of the study (10 years), was significantly higher in the active group than in the control group. Sublingual-swallow immunotherapy was effective in children and maintained clinical efficacy for 4 to 5 years after discontinuation.

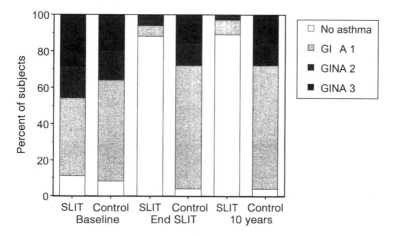

Figure 2 Percentage of patients with different asthma severity or without asthma before treatment, 3 years after the begining of SLIT swallow with mites (end SLIT), and 7 years after its cessation (10 years). (From Ref. 25.)

IV. SECONDARY PREVENTION OF NEW SENSITIZATIONS USING ALLERGEN VACCINATION

A. Clinical Studies

Several longitudinal studies report that allergic sensitization increases with age from childhood to adulthood. One study (26) found that monosensitized children may become polysensitized. House dust mite (HDM) sensitization and, to a lesser degree, pollen sensitization seem to play a "triggering" role in the development of polysensitization, since a high proportion of children originally monosensitized to HDM or to pollen became polysensitized.

A study was designed to determine whether allergen vaccination with standardized allergen vaccines prevented the development of new sensitizations over a 3-year period (27). Twenty-two children, monosensitized to HDM, who received allergen immunotherapy with standardized allergen vaccines were compared with 22 other age-matched control subjects who were monosensitized to HDM. The initial investigation included a full clinical history, skin tests with a panel of standardized allergens, and the measurement of allergen-specific IgE, depending on the results of skin tests. Children were followed on an annual basis for 3 years, and the development of new sensitizations in each group was recorded. Ten of 22 (45.5%) children who were receiving allergen vaccination did not have new sensitivities, compared with zero of 22 (0%) in the control group ($p = 0.001$, chi-square test). This study suggests that allergen vaccination in children monosensitized to HDM alters the natural course of allergy by preventing the development of new sensitizations (Fig. 3).

A second study was carried out to increase knowledge of the ability of allergen vaccination to affect the onset of new sensitizations in monosensitized subjects (28). One hundred and thirty-four children (age range 5–8 years) with intermittent asthma, with or without rhinitis, and with single sensitization to HDM (skin prick test and serum-specific IgE), were enrolled. Subcutaneous allergen vaccination was offered to the parents of all the children, but was accepted by only 75 (SIT group). The remaining 63 children were

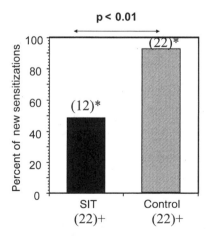

Figure 3 Percentage of children monosensitized to mites who developed new sensitizations after treatment for 3 years by SIT compared with an untreated control group. * = number with new sensitivities; + = number in each group. (From Ref. 27.)

treated with medication only and were considered the control group. Vaccination with mite mix was administered to the treated group during the first 3 years, and all patients were followed for a total of 6 years. All patients were checked for allergic sensitization(s) by skin prick tests and serum-specific IgE every year until the end of the follow-up period. Both groups were comparable in terms of age, sex, and disease characteristics. One hundred and twenty-three children completed the follow-up study. At the end of the study, 52 out of 69 children (75.4%) in the SIT group showed no new sensitization, compared with 18 out of 54 children (33.3%) in the control group ($p < 0.0002$). *Parietaria*, grass, and olive pollen were the most common allergens responsible for the new sensitization(s). The investigators concluded that allergen vaccination may prevent the onset of new sensitizations in children with respiratory symptoms monosensitized to HDM.

A third, retrospective study was conducted to compare the prevention of new sensitizations in monosensitized subjects treated with allergen vaccination or anti-allergic medications (29). A very large number of patients were studied: 8396 monosensitized patients with respiratory symptoms were selected according to an open, retrospective design (28). Group A, 7182 patients, were given allergen vaccination (and anti-allergic drugs as needed) for 4 years and then treated only with medications for at least 3 years. Group B, 1214 patients, were treated only with medications for at least 7 years. All patients underwent prick testing with a standard panel of allergens, and total and specific IgE concentrations were obtained before and after 4 years of treatment and again 3 years later. Group demographics were very similar. In group A 23.75% of patients and in group B 68.03% were polysensitized after 4 years ($p < 0.0001$) and 26.95% and 76.77%, respectively, after 7 years ($p < 0.0001$). Asthmatic subjects were more prone to develop polysensitization compared with subjects with only rhinitis (32.14% vs. 27.29% after 4 years, 36.5% vs. 31.33% after 7 years; $p < 0.0001$). Specific IgE decreased by 24.11% in group A and increased by 23.87% in group B ($p < 0.0001$). Total IgE decreased by 17.53% in group A and increased by 13.71% in group B ($p < 0.0001$).

In a fourth study, preseasonal grass pollen vaccination was administered for 3 years to children who were examined 6 years after discontinuing treatment (30). Thirteen patients with previous allergen vaccination and 10 patients in the control group were prospectively followed. During the observation time, scores for overall hay fever symptoms ($p < 0.004$) and individual symptoms for eyes ($p < 0.02$), nose ($p < 0.04$), and chest ($p < 0.01$) as well as combined symptom and medication scores ($p < 0.002$) remained lower in the group with previous allergen vaccination. Only 23% of patients with previous pollen asthma who had received allergen vaccination experienced pollen-associated lower respiratory tract symptoms, compared with 70% in the control group ($p < 0.05$). Eight years after commencement of allergen immunotherapy, 61% of the initially pollen-monosensitized children had developed new sensitization to perennial allergens compared with 100% in the control group ($p < 0.05$). This study confirmed that allergen vaccination in children with pollen allergy reduces the onset of new sensitization and therefore has the potential to modify the natural course of allergic disease.

B. Putative Mechanisms

There is now sufficient evidence to support the effect of allergen vaccination in the prevention of new sensitizations in children with mono- or paucisensitizations. However, it appears that the prevention of new sensitizations by allergen vaccination is inconsistent in patients with multiple sensitivities, suggesting that mono- and polysensitized patients present a different ability to synthetize IgE when exposed to new allergens. The mechanisms of these findings are still unclear but may be related to the effect of immunotherapy in the TH1/TH2 balance (31,32) and the immune reactivity of mono- and polysensitized patients.

Nonallergic healthy individuals develop an immune response toward allergens. T-cell clones (TCCs) with specificity for Bet v 1, the major birch pollen allergen, can be established from their blood and analyzed for epitope specificity (33,34). All TCCs revealed the TH phenotype, and the majority of them produced IL-4 and IFN-γ; however, most TCCs revealed a low IL-4/IFN-γ ratio. Immunoblot revealed Bet v 1–specific IgG in nonallergic individuals, whereas no IgE could be detected (34). These results indicate that T-cells from allergic (35) and nonallergic (33) individuals recognize the same epitopes on allergenic molecules, leading to activation, which then results in differential production of cytokines and consequently to differential isotype switching in allergen-specific B-cells.

Allergen immunotherapy induces reduced lymphoproliferative responses to allergen and a shift from TH2 to TH1 in T-cell clones specific for the allergen administered (36). It also appears that there is a global reduction of the TH2 response after immunotherapy (37).

The IL-4/IFN-γ balance differs between mono- and polysensitized patients. Peripheral blood mononuclear cells (PBMCs) stimulated by polyclonal activators have a lower IL-4/IFN-γ ratio in monosensitized patients compared with polysensitized ones (38). It is therefore possible that new allergens will lead to an IgG immune response rather than an IgE one in monosensitized individuals. However, during the pollen season, PBMCs of monosensitized patients allergic to grass pollen have an increased IL-4 response (39).

The reduction of the allergen-specific TH2 response by immunotherapy may be involved in the lack of induction of new TH2 cells in mono- or paucisensitized patients and prevent the onset of new sensitizations. On the other hand, monosensitized children who do not receive immunotherapy will have a gradual increase in TH2 responses and thereby may become sensitized to new allergens. Polysensitized individuals already have a high TH2 response, and there is no prevention for the development of new sensitizations by immunotherapy.

V. CONCLUSION

In the future, allergen vaccination may be effective in the secondary prevention of asthma (40) (Fig. 4). Allergen vaccination is the only treatment that may alter the natural course of allergic diseases (20). Allergen vaccination in children with rhinitis prevents the onset of persistent asthma (24). Moreover, allergen vaccination in monosensitized young children has been found to reduce the onset of new sensitizations. However, more studies are needed to determine how SIT may modify the allergic disease or impair progression to asthma. It is therefore proposed that allergen vaccination should be started early in the disease process in order to modify the spontaneous long-term progress of the allergic inflammation and disease (13,41,42).

VI. SALIENT POINTS

1. Primary prevention of allergy and asthma cannot be achieved with current methods of immunotherapy.

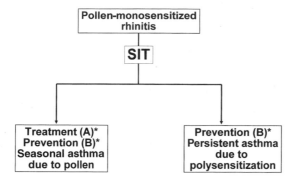

Figure 4 Level of evidence (37) for the treatment and secondary prevention of asthma in children sensitized to pollen receiving SIT (see Chapter 27).

2. Secondary prevention of asthma may be achieved using injectable immunotherapy and possibly using sublingual-swallow immunotherapy.
3. Specific immunotherapy appears to prevent the onset of new sensitizations in monosensitized patients.

REFERENCES

1. Johansson SGO, Haahtela T, Asher I, Boner A, Chuchalin A, Custovic A, et al. Prevention of allergy and asthma: Interim report. Allergy 2000; 55(11):1069–1088.
2. Jones CA, Holloway JA, Warner JO. Does atopic disease start in foetal life? Allergy 2000; 55(1):2–10.
3. Iikura Y, Naspitz CK, Mikawa H, Talaricoficho S, Baba M, Sole D, et al. Prevention of asthma by ketotifen in infants with atopic dermatitis. Ann Allergy 1992; 68(3):233–236.
4. Warner JO. A double-blinded, randomized, placebo-controlled trial of cetirizine in preventing the onset of asthma in children with atopic dermatitis: 18 months' treatment and 18 months' posttreatment follow-up. J Allergy Clin Immunol 2001; 108(6):929–937.
5. Jarrett E, Hall E. Selective suppression of IgE antibody responsiveness by maternal influence. Nature 1979; 280(5718):145–147.
6. Jarrett EE, Hall E. IgE suppression by maternal IgG. Immunology 1983; 48(1):49–58.
7. Jarrett EE, Hall E. The development of IgE-suppressive immunocompetence in young animals: Influence of exposure to antigen in the presence or absence of maternal immunity. Immunology 1984; 53(2):365–373.
8. Victor JR Jr, Fusaro AE, Duarte AJ, Sato MN. Preconception maternal immunization to dust mite inhibits the type I hypersensitivity response of offspring. J Allergy Clin Immunol 2003; 111(2):269–277.
9. Melkild I, Groeng EC, Leikvold RB, Granum B, Lovik M. Maternal allergen immunization during pregnancy in a mouse model reduces adult allergy-related antibody responses in the offspring. Clin Exp Allergy 2002; 32(9):1370–1376.
10. Lange H, Kiesch B, Linden I, Otto M, Thierse HJ, Shaw L, et al. Reversal of the adult IgE high responder phenotype in mice by maternally transferred allergen-specific monoclonal IgG antibodies during a sensitive period in early ontogeny. Eur J Immunol 2002; 32(11):3133–3141.
11. Herz U, Ahrens B, Scheffold A, Joachim R, Radbruch A, Renz H. Impact of in utero Th2 immunity on T cell deviation and subsequent immediate-type hypersensitivity in the neonate. Eur J Immunol 2000; 30(2):714–718.

12. Glovsky MM, Ghekiere L, Rejzek E. Effect of maternal immunotherapy on immediate skin test reactivity, specific rye I IgG and IgE antibody, and total IgE of the children. Ann Allergy 1991; 67(1):21–24.

13. Bousquet J, Lockey R, Malling H. WHO Position Paper. Allergen immunotherapy: Therapeutic vaccines for allergic diseases. Allergy 1998; 53(suppl):54.

14. Bousquet J, Van Cauwenberge P, Khaltaev N. Allergic rhinitis and its impact on asthma. J Allergy Clin Immunol 2001; 108(suppl 5):S147–S334.

15. Passalacqua G, Canonica GW. Long-lasting clinical efficacy of allergen specific immunotherapy. Allergy 2002; 57(4):275–276.

16. Grammer LC, Shaughnessy MA, Suszko IM, Shaughnessy JJ, Patterson R. Persistence of efficacy after a brief course of polymerized ragweed allergen: A controlled study. J Allergy Clin Immunol 1984; 73(4):484–489.

17. Mosbech H, Osterballe O. Does the effect of immunotherapy last after termination of treatment? Follow-up study in patients with grass pollen rhinitis. Allergy 1988; 43(7):523–529.

18. Des-Roches A, Paradis L, Knani J, Hejjaoui A, Dhivert H, Chanez P, et al. Immunotherapy with a standardized *Dermatophagoides pteronyssinus* extract: V. Duration of efficacy of immunotherapy after its cessation. Allergy 1996; 51:430–433.

19. Naclerio RM, Proud D, Moylan B, Balcer S, Freidhoff L, Kagey-Sobotka A, et al. A double-blind study of the discontinuation of ragweed immunotherapy. J Allergy Clin Immunol 1997; 100(3):293–300.

20. Durham SR, Walker SM, Varga EM, Jacobson MR, O'Brien F, Noble W, et al. Long-term clinical efficacy of grass-pollen immunotherapy [see comments]. N Engl J Med 1999; 341(7):468–475.

21. Filiaci F, Zambetti G, Romeo R, Ciofalo A, Luce M, Germano F. Non-specific hyperreactivity before and after nasal specific immunotherapy. Allergol Immunopathol 1999; 27(1):24–28.

22. Demoly P, Bousquet J, Michel FB. Immunotherapy in allergic rhinitis: A prevention for asthma? Curr Probl Dermatol 1999; 28:119–123.

23. Johnstone DE. Immunotherapy in children: Past, present, and future (part I). Ann Allergy 1981; 46(1):1–7.

24. Moller C, Dreborg S, Ferdousi HA, Halken S, Host A, Jacobsen L, et al. Pollen immunotherapy reduces the development of asthma in children with seasonal rhinoconjunctivitis (the PAT-study). J Allergy Clin Immunol 2002; 109(2):251–256.

25. Di Rienzo V, Marcucci F, Puccinelli P, Parmiani S, Frati F, Sensi L, et al. Long-lasting effect of sublingual immunotherapy in children with asthma due to house dust mite: A 10-year prospective study. Clin Exp Allergy 2003; 33(2):206–210.

26. Silvestri M, Rossi GA, Cozzani S, Pulvirenti G, Fasce L. Age-dependent tendency to become sensitized to other classes of aeroallergens in atopic asthmatic children. Ann Allergy Asthma Immunol 1999; 83(4):335–340.

27. Des-Roches A, Paradis L, Ménardo J-L, Bouges S, Daurès J-P, Bousquet J. Immunotherapy with a standardized *Dermatophagoides pteronyssinus* extract: VI. Specific immunotherapy prevents the onset of new sensitizations in children. J Allergy Clin Immunol 1997; 99:450–453.

28. Pajno GB, Barberio G, De Luca F, Morabito L, Parmiani S. Prevention of new sensitizations in asthmatic children monosensitized to house dust mite by specific immunotherapy: A six-year follow-up study. Clin Exp Allergy 2001; 31(9):1392–1397.

29. Purello-D'Ambrosio F, Gangemi S, Merendino RA, Isola S, Puccinelli P, Parmiani S, et al. Prevention of new sensitizations in monosensitized subjects submitted to specific immunotherapy or not: A retrospective study. Clin Exp Allergy 2001; 31(8):1295–1302.

30. Eng PA, Reinhold M, Gnehm HP. Long-term efficacy of preseasonal grass pollen immunotherapy in children. Allergy 2002; 57(4):306–312.

31. Durham SR, Till SJ. Immunologic changes associated with allergen immunotherapy. J Allergy Clin Immunol 1998; 102(2):157–164.

32. Wachholz PA, Nouri-Aria KT, Wilson DR, Walker SM, Verhoef A, Till SJ, et al. Grass pollen immunotherapy for hayfever is associated with increases in local nasal but not peripheral Th1:Th2 cytokine ratios. Immunology 2002; 105(1):56–62.

33. Ebner C, Schenk S, Najafian N, Siemann U, Steiner R, Fischer GW, et al. Nonallergic individuals recognize the same T cell epitopes of Bet v 1, the major birch pollen allergen, as atopic patients. J Immunol 1995; 154(4):1932–1940.

34. Ebner C, Siemann U, Najafian N, Scheiner O, Kraft D. Characterization of allergen (Bet v 1)-specific T cell lines and clones from non-allergic individuals. Int Arch Allergy Immunol 1995; 107(1–3):183–185.

35. Ebner C, Szepfalusi Z, Ferreira F, Jilek A, Valenta R, Parronchi P, et al. Identification of multiple T cell epitopes on Bet v I, the major birch pollen allergen, using specific T cell clones and overlapping peptides. J Immunol 1993; 150(3):1047–1054.

36. Ebner C, Siemann U, Bohle B, Willheim M, Wiedermann U, Schenk S, et al. Immunological changes during specific immunotherapy of grass pollen allergy: Reduced lymphoproliferative responses to allergen and shift from TH2 to TH1 in T-cell clones specific for Phl p 1, a major grass pollen allergen [see comments]. Clin Exp Allergy 1997; 27(9):1007–1015.

37. Varney VA, Hamid QA, Gaga M, Ying S, Jacobson M, Frew AJ, et al. Influence of grass pollen immunotherapy on cellular infiltration and cytokine mRNA expression during allergen-induced late-phase cutaneous responses. J Clin Invest 1993; 92(2):644–651.

38. Pene J, Rivier A, Lagier B, Becker WM, Michel FB, Bousquet J. Differences in IL-4 release by PBMC are related with heterogeneity of atopy. Immunology 1994; 81(1):58–64.

39. Lagier B, Pons N, Rivier A, Chanal I, Chanez P, Bousquet J, et al. Seasonal variations of interleukin-4 and interferon-gamma release by peripheral blood mononuclear cells from atopic subjects stimulated by polyclonal activators. J Allergy Clin Immunol 1995; 96(6 pt 1):932–940.

40. Ebner C, Szepfalusi Z, Ferreira F, Jilek A, Valenta R, Parronchi P, et al. Identification of multiple T cell epitopes on Bet v I, the major birch pollen allergen, using specific T cell clones and overlapping peptides. J Immunol 1993; 150(3):1047–1054.

41. Bousquet J. Pro: Immunotherapy is clinically indicated in the management of allergic asthma. Am J Respir Crit Care Med 2001; 164(12):2139–2140; discussion 2141–2142.

42. Malling H, Weeke B. Immunotherapy. Position Paper of the European Academy of Allergy and Clinical Immunology. Allergy 1993; 48(suppl 14):9–35.

43. Ownby DR, Adinoff AD. The appropriate use of skin testing and allergen immunotherapy in young children. J Allergy Clin Immunol 1994; 94(4):662–665.

7

In Vitro Tests to Monitor Efficacy of Immunotherapy

JOHN W. YUNGINGER

Mayo Medical School, Rochester, Minnesota, U.S.A.

I. In Vitro Studies
II. Salient Points
    References

Although allergen immunotherapy has been utilized for nearly 100 years, its exact mechanism of action is not known. Allergen immunotherapy induces a wide variety of humoral and cellular immune changes (Table 1), but it has been difficult to correlate individual immune changes with the clinical response to immunotherapy. This chapter reviews several immunological tests that have been used to monitor the immune changes induced by allergen immunotherapy.

I. IN VITRO STUDIES

A. Humoral Immune Assays

1. Allergen-Specific IgG

The first discovered immunological effect of immunotherapy was the production in the sera of treated patients of heat-stable blocking antibody (1), subsequently identified as IgG (2). The concentration of IgG antibody correlated with the quantity of allergen administered (3), but in most published studies of inhalant immunotherapy, the IgG antibody levels could not be correlated with the degree of symptom relief.

Following the 1980 introduction of Hymenoptera venoms for immunotherapy of Hymenoptera sting–sensitive individuals in the United States, it was proposed that

Table 1   Immunological Changes Associated with Allergen Immunotherapy

Redirection of T-cell responses:
   Decreased TH2 cytokine production (IL-4, IL-5, IL-13)
   Increased TH1 cytokine production (IL-2, IFN-γ)
Generation of allergen-specific suppressor T lymphocytes
Suppression of allergen-specific IgE antibody response
Generation of allergen-specific IgG antibody response

venom-specific IgG antibodies might be of even greater clinical importance in parenteral allergic disorders than in inhalant allergic diseases. An IgG antibody level of 3 μg/ml or greater had been found to correlate with protection from sting reaction, as assessed by deliberate sting challenges (4). In a subsequent report involving 211 sting-sensitive persons, only 2 of 126 venom-immunized persons with IgG antibody levels above 3 μg/ml exhibited symptoms when stung; however, only 14 of 85 persons with IgG antibody levels less than 3 μg/ml experienced sting anaphylaxis (Table 2) (5). Thus, the predictive value of a venom-specific IgG antibody level of 3 μg/ml or lower was quite poor as a predictor of either reaction or nonreaction to a sting. A similar lack of correlation between venom-specific IgG antibody levels and severity of field sting reactions was noted in a study of 54 sting-sensitive persons in the UK. (6).

Of the four human IgG subclasses, IgG4 antibodies have been of particular interest because they are disproportionately stimulated by allergen immunotherapy (7). Postimmunotherapy increases in specific IgG4 antibodies may be stimulated by IL-10 (see below) (8). However, the utility of allergen-specific IgG4 measurements in clinical practice remains limited. Elevated IgG4 antibodies cannot always be correlated with the success of immunotherapy (9), and nonimmunized asthmatic children and adults have both total and specific IgG4 antibody levels comparable to those in nonallergic children and adults (10).

2. Allergen-Specific IgE

Peak levels of serum IgE antibodies to seasonal pollen from trees, grasses (11), and weeds (12) occur about 4 to 6 weeks following the pollination season, then slowly decline to a nadir just prior to the next pollination season. Immunotherapy to inhalant allergens initially produces an increase in allergen-specific IgE serum antibodies (13), followed by a progressive decline in specific IgE levels and a blunting of the seasonal rise in specific IgE that occurs in sensitized individuals who do not receive immunotherapy (14). However, this decline in specific IgE antibodies does not correlate well with the degree of clinical improvement induced by immunotherapy; improvement in symptoms often predates the decline in allergen-specific IgE antibody.

Table 2   Venom-Specific IgG Antibody Levels and Responses to Deliberate Insect Sting Challenges in 211 Venom-Immunized Patients

Patient group	IgG antibody < 3 μg/ml	IgG antibody > 3 μg/ml	Total
Reactors	14	2	16
Nonreactors	71	124	195
Total	85	126	211

Source: Ref. 5.

3. Secretory IgA and IgG Antibodies

Nasal washings from ragweed- and grass-sensitive individuals contain measurable levels of allergen-specific IgA and IgG antibodies (15,16), and antibodies in both classes increase following allergen immunotherapy. However, the quantities of these IgG antibodies cannot be correlated with the degree of symptom relief produced by treatment (15). In addition, frequent intranasal nebulization of blocking antibody to ragweed during the pollination season does not produce significant relief of symptoms (17).

B. Cellular Immune Assays

1. Basophil Sensitivity to Allergen

Peripheral blood leukocytes from persons with allergic rhinitis release histamine when challenged in vitro with allergen. Following allergen immunotherapy, leukocytes from some, but not all, treated persons become less reactive to in vitro challenge (18,19).

2. Antigen-Specific T Suppressor Cells

Peripheral blood mononuclear cells (PBMCs) from allergic individuals can proliferate and produce lymphokines when stimulated in vitro by the addition of allergen (20). Immunotherapy induces the formation of circulating suppressor T-cells that inhibit antigen-induced proliferation of these autologous lymphocytes (21).

3. Histamine-Releasing Factors

PBMCs from allergic individuals can generate histamine-releasing factors (HRFs) that are capable of inducing histamine release from mast cells and basophils by either IgE-independent (22) or IgE-dependent (23) mechanisms. In a double-blind, placebo-controlled immunotherapy study, Kuna and colleagues (24) obtained PBMCs from 24 grass-sensitive asthmatic individuals prior to and after 2 years of immunotherapy treatment. Placebo-treated persons experienced increased symptoms during the pollen season, and their PBMCs exhibited increased HRF production. Conversely, persons receiving active immunotherapy exhibited fewer seasonal symptoms, and their PBMCs showed a significant decline in spontaneous HRF production in vitro that paralleled declines in the individuals' nonspecific bronchial reactivity to nebulized histamine.

C. Cytokine Assays

The development of allergic disease is marked by enhanced IgE synthesis, enhanced T-cell production of TH2 cytokines (IL-4, IL-5, IL-13), and reduced T-cell production of TH1 cytokines, such as interferon-gamma (IFN-γ) (25). The ability to quantitate in vitro cytokine production by cultured peripheral blood leukocytes has permitted more precise study of T-cell changes induced by allergen immunotherapy. There is increasing experimental evidence suggesting that allergen immunotherapy redirects T-cell responses away from TH2 cytokine production and toward TH1 cytokine production.

Insect sting allergy is the prototypical example of a parenteral hypersensitivity disorder, and several investigators have studied PBMCs from honeybee sting–allergic patients undergoing venom immunotherapy. McHugh and colleagues (26) compared in vitro proliferation and cytokine production by PBMCs from patients undergoing rush (one-day) or conventional (weekly) immunotherapy regimens. One day after rush immunotherapy, IL-4 production decreased markedly, while in the conventional immunotherapy group

IL-4 production fell more gradually, becoming undetectable by 6 months. Swiss investigators (27,28) noted that after 2 months of rush immunotherapy with whole bee venom, the secretion of both TH2 cytokines (IL-4, IL-5, and/or IL-13) and TH1 cytokines (IL-2 and/or IFN-γ) from bee venom phospholipase A (PLA)–stimulated PBMCs was abolished. By culturing the PBMCs with PLA in the presence of IL-2 or IL-15, the specific TH1 cytokine suppression could be overcome, whereas culturing the PBMCs with PLA in the presence of IL-4 only partially restored TH2 cytokine production (28). Venom immunotherapy had no effect on cytokine secretion when PBMCs were stimulated in vitro with tetanus toxoid, a control antigen (27). Belgian investigators (29) extended these observations to yellow jacket sting–sensitive patients, documenting postimmunotherapy increases in IFN-γ–producing stimulated CD4+ and CD8+ T-cells and decreases in the percentage of IL-4–producing CD4+ and CD8+ T-cells.

Subsequent studies showed that rush venom immunotherapy evoked IL-10 production, initially by CD4+CD25+ allergen-specific T-cells, and later by B-cells and monocytes (Fig. 1) (8). IL-10 acts to induce peripheral T-cell anergy to honeybee venom PLA by blocking CD28 tyrosine phosphorylation and binding to phosphatidylinositol 3-kinase (PI3-K) (30). Anergic T-cells cultured with PLA in the presence of IL-2 or IL-15 restored proliferation and stimulated production of IFN-γ and IgG4 antibodies, whereas anergic T-cells cultured with PLA in the presence of IL-4 reactivated T-cell IL-4, IL-5, and IL-13 production and stimulated IgE antibody production (31).

Cytokine assays have also been used to study patients receiving inhalant immunotherapy. Compared with nonallergic individuals, persons with perennial allergic rhinitis have elevated serum levels of IL-4 (32). Dust mite immunotherapy (*n* = 39 patients), but not pharmacological therapy (*n* = 10 patients), was associated with a decline in both serum IL-4 levels and allergen-specific IgE antibody levels. The percentage decline in IL-4 levels, but not the decline in specific IgE, was correlated with improvement in clinical symptoms.

Using *Dermatophagoides pteronyssinus* vaccine administered by rush immunotherapy, Lack et al. (33) treated 10 mite-sensitive persons, all of whom were also allergic to

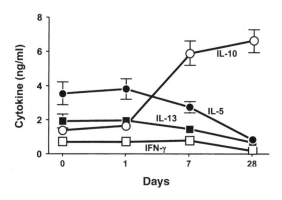

Figure 1 Changes in cytokine production in PBMC cultures during honeybee venom–specific immunotherapy. PBMCs from one patient were stimulated with PLA before and after 1, 7, and 28 days of immunotherapy. Cytokines were determined in supernatants taken after 5 days of culture. IL-5, IL-13, and IFN-γ decreased continuously, while simultaneously IL-10 increased. Results shown are mean ± SD of triplicate cultures. Similar results were obtained in eight other immunized patients. (From Ref. 8.)

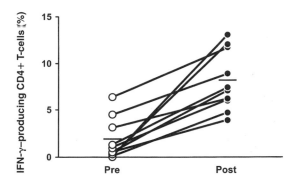

Figure 2 Rush immunotherapy with house dust mite vaccine induced a selective increase in IFN-γ production by the CD4+ T-cell population. Shown is the percentage of IFN-γ–producing CD4+ T-cells before and after maintenance dose of immunotherapy was reached. Group mean values are shown by horizontal bars. $p < 0.01$ compared with pretreatment value. (From Ref. 33.)

cat dander. In blood samples obtained when the volunteers had reached maintenance doses, the numbers of peripheral blood CD8+ T-cells increased, and T-cell proliferative response to mite antigen was suppressed. In vitro stimulation by mite vaccine induced a marked increase in IFN-γ production by CD4+ cells (Fig. 2). There was a strong correlation between the increases in IFN-γ and the suppression of cutaneous reactivity to mite allergen. However, no changes were noted in IFN-γ production or T-cell proliferative responses to in vitro stimulation with cat allergen, documenting that the cytokine response to immunotherapy was allergen specific. In another mite immunotherapy study, O'Brien et al. (34) found that immunotherapy in 15 mite-sensitive persons was associated with decreased expression of IL-4 and IFN-γ in isolated PBMCs following in vitro stimulation with purified Der p 2 allergen. The two patients who still expressed IL-4 postimmunotherapy also exhibited little clinical benefit from the immunotherapy. Ebner and colleagues (35) studied eight timothy grass pollen–sensitive patients, from whom sera and PBMCs were obtained prior to conventional immunotherapy, after reaching maintenance dose at 3 months and after 1 year of treatment. In vitro lymphocyte proliferation to timothy grass extract and to recombinant Phl p 1 decreased after 3 months. Specific IgG, IgG1, and IgG4 antibodies rose progressively, while specific IgE antibodies remained elevated. Peripheral blood Phl p 1–specific T-cell clones isolated during treatment showed a progressive decline in IL-4 production, while IFN-γ production was variable. Although seven of the eight patients improved clinically following immunotherapy, the lack of an untreated control group and the small number of patients precluded study of correlations between symptoms and immunological changes.

In a randomized, double-blind, placebo-controlled, parallel group study involving 37 grass pollen–sensitive adults, Wilson and colleagues (36) obtained out-of-season and peak-season nasal biopsies to investigate local immune changes induced by 2 years of grass pollen immunotherapy. Placebo-treated patients exhibited significant seasonal increases in nasal mucosal eosinophils, CD25+ cells, CD3+ cells, and IL-15 mRNA–expressing cells. However, these increases were not seen in the immunized patients, who showed significant seasonal increases in nasal mucosal IFN-γ mRNA+ cells (37). Symptom scores were significantly correlated with mucosal eosinophils (Fig. 3) and IL-5 mRNA–expressing cells. Immunotherapy also reduced the seasonal rise in nasal epithelial basophils, but

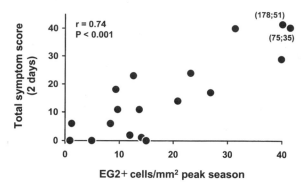

Figure 3 Correlation between symptom scores at the time of nasal biopsy and numbers of eosinophils stained with specific monoclonal antibody EG2 in the nasal mucosa at the peak of the pollen season after 2 years of immunotherapy. Correlation was performed using the Spearman rank correlation method. (From Ref. 36.)

epithelial and submucosal neutrophils remained constant (38). Interestingly, these cytokine changes occurred only in the nasal mucosa; peripheral blood T-cells showed no alterations in allergen-induced proliferative responses or cytokine production post-therapy (37).

IL-12 is a cytokine produced by tissue macrophages and B lymphocytes that stimulates proliferation of TH1-type T lymphocytes. To determine if immunotherapy stimulates IL-12 production, Hamid et al. (39) employed in situ hybridization to examine biopsies from grass pollen–induced late-phase skin tests in 20 grass-sensitive persons, including 10 who had completed 4 years of grass immunotherapy and 10 who were not immunized. Only biopsies from the immunized persons showed IL-12 mRNA+ cells, and the number of IL-12+ cells correlated positively with the number of IFN-γ+ cells and inversely with the number of IL-4+ cells. Compared with the nonimmunized group, immunized persons showed a marked reduction in the size of the late skin response to grass pollen vaccine. The same investigator group has shown that grass pollen immunotherapy inhibits the infiltration of IL-4+ T-cells and activated eosinophils into the nasal mucosa following nasal provocation challenges with grass pollen (40). In addition, immunotherapy was associated with an increase in nasal biopsy cells expressing mRNA for IFN-γ; this increased expression could be correlated with decreased allergy symptom scores and decreased medication requirements during the grass pollination season.

II. SALIENT POINTS

1. Allergen immunotherapy induces an initial rise and then a gradual fall in allergen-specific IgE antibodies, while induced allergen-specific IgG1 and IgG4 antibodies increase gradually over time. The magnitude of the IgG antibody response varies directly with the delivered dose of allergen.
2. Allergen immunotherapy also induces allergen-specific IgG and IgA antibodies in respiratory secretions.
3. Allergen immunotherapy reduces the in vitro reactivity of PBMCs to added allergen, in part due to the generation of allergen-specific suppressor T lymphocytes.

4. Successful allergen immunotherapy redirects T-cell responses away from TH2 (IL-4, IL-5, IL-13) cytokine production and toward TH1 (IL-2, IFN-γ) cytokine production

5. No single immunological test perfectly correlates with the clinical response to immunotherapy.

REFERENCES

1. Cooke RA, Barnard JH, Hebald S, Stull A. Serologic evidence of immunity with coexisting sensitization in a type of human allergy (hay fever). J Exp Med 1935; 62:733–750.

2. Lichtenstein LM, Holtzman NA, Burnett LS. A quantitative in vitro study of the chromatographic distribution and immunoglobulin characteristics of human blocking antibody. J Immunol 1968; 101:317–324.

3. Lichtenstein LM, Norman PS, Winkenwerder WL. Clinical and in vitro studies on the role of immunotherapy in ragweed hay fever. Am J Med 1968; 44:514–524.

4. Golden DBK, Meyers DA, Kagey-Sobotka A, Valentine MD, Lichtenstein LM. Clinical relevance of the venom-specific immunoglobulin G antibody level during immunotherapy. J Allergy Clin Immunol 1982; 69:489–493.

5. Golden DBK, Lawrence ID, Hamilton RG, Kagey-Sobotka A, Valentine MD, Lichtenstein LM. Clinical correlation of the venom-specific IgG antibody level during maintenance venom immunotherapy. J Allergy Clin Immunol 1992; 90:386–393.

6. Ewan PW, Deighton J, Wilson AB, Lachmann PJ. Venom-specific IgG antibodies in bee and wasp allergy: Lack of correlation with protection from stings. Clin Exp Allergy 1993; 23:647–660.

7. Aalberse RC, Van Milligan F, Tan KY, Stapel SO. Allergen-specific IgG4 in atopic disease. Allergy 1993; 48:559–569.

8. Akdis CA, Blesken T, Akdis M, Wüthrich B, Blaser K. Role of interleukin 10 in specific immunotherapy. J Clin Invest 1998; 102:98–106.

9. Djurup R, Malling HJ. High IgG4 antibody level is associated with failure of immunotherapy with inhalant allergens. Clin Allergy 1987; 17:459–468.

10. Homburger HA, Maurer K, Sachs MI, O'Connell EJ, Jacob GL, Caron J. Serum IgG4 concentrations and allergen-specific IgG4 antibodies compared in adults and children with asthma and nonallergic subjects. J Allergy Clin Immunol 1986; 77:427–434.

11. Berg T, Johansson SGO. In vitro diagnosis of atopic allergy. IV. Seasonal variations of IgE antibody in children allergic to pollens: A study of nontreated children and of children treated with inhalation of disodium cromoglycate. Int Arch Allergy Appl Immunol 1971; 41:452–462.

12. Yunginger JW, Gleich GJ. Seasonal changes in IgE antibodies and their relationship to IgG antibodies during immunotherapy for ragweed hay fever. J Clin Invest 1973; 52:1268–1275.

13. Lichtenstein LM, Ishizaka K, Norman PS, Sobotka AK, Hill BM. IgE antibody measurements in ragweed hay fever: Relationship to clinical severity and the results of immunotherapy. J Clin Invest 1973; 52:472–482.

14. Gleich GJ, Zimmermann EM, Henderson LL, Yunginger JW. Effect of immunotherapy on immunoglobulin E and immunoglobulin G antibodies to ragweed antigens: A six-year prospective study. J Allergy Clin Immunol 1982; 70:261–271.

15. Platts-Mills TAE, von Maur RK, Ishizaka K, Norman PS, Lichtenstein LM. IgA and IgG anti-ragweed antibodies in nasal secretions; Quantitative measurements of antibodies and correlation with inhibition of histamine release. J Clin Invest 1976; 57:1041–1050.

16. Platts-Mills TAE. Local production of IgG, IgA, and IgE antibodies in grass pollen hay fever. J Immunol 1979; 122:2218–2225.

17. Gleich GJ, Yunginger JW. Ragweed hay fever: Treatment by local passive administration of IgG antibody. Clin Allergy 1975; 5:79–87.

18. Lichtenstein LM, Norman PS, Winkenwerder WL, Osler AG. In vitro studies of human ragweed allergy: Changes in cellular and humoral activity associated with specific desensitization. J Clin Invest 1966; 45:1126–1136.

19. Pruzansky JJ, Patterson R. Histamine release from leukocytes of hypersensitive individuals. II. Reduced sensitivity of leukocytes after injection therapy. J Allergy 1967; 39:44–50.

20. Rocklin RE, Pence H, Kaplan H, Evans R. Cell-mediated immune response of ragweed-sensitive patients to ragweed antigen E: In vitro lymphocyte transformation and elaboration of lymphocyte mediators. J Clin Invest 1974; 53:735–744.

21. Rocklin RE, Sheffer AL, Greineder DK, Melmon KL. Generation of antigen-specific suppressor cells during allergy desensitization. N Engl J Med 1980; 302:1213–1219.

22. Alam R, Kuna P, Rozniecki J, Kuzminska B. The magnitude of the spontaneous production of histamine-releasing factor (HRF) by lymphocytes in vitro correlates with the state of bronchial hyperreactivity in patients with asthma. J Allergy Clin Immunol 1987; 79:103–108.

23. MacDonald SM, Rafnar T, Langdon J, Lichtenstein LM. Molecular identification of an IgE-dependent histamine-releasing factor. Science 1995; 269:688–690.

24. Kuna P, Alam R, Kuzminska B, Rozniecki J. The effect of preseasonal immunotherapy on the production of histamine releasing factor (HRF) by mononuclear cells from patients with seasonal asthma: Results of a double-blind, placebo-controlled, randomized study. J Allergy Clin Immunol 1989; 83:816–824.

25. Durham SR, Ying S, Varney VA, Jacobson MR, Sudderick RM, Mackay IS, Kay AB, Hamid QA. Cytokine messenger RNA expression for IL-3, IL-4, IL-5, and granulocyte/macrophage colony-stimulating factor in the nasal mucosa after local allergen provocation: Relationship to tissue eosinophilia. J Immunol 1992; 148:2390–2394.

26. McHugh SM, Deighton J, Stewart AG, Lachmann PJ, Ewan PW. Bee venom immunotherapy induces a shift in cytokine responses from a TH-2 to a TH-1 dominant pattern: Comparison of rush and conventional immunotherapy. Clin Exp Allergy 1995; 25:828–838.

27. Jutel M, Pichler WJ, Skrbic D, Urwyler A, Dahinden C, Muller UR. Bee venom immunotherapy results in decrease of IL-4 and IL-5 and increase of IFN-gamma secretion in specific allergen-stimulated T cell cultures. J Immunol 1995; 154:4187–4194.

28. Akdis CA, Akdis M, Blesken T, Wymann D, Alkan SS, Muller U, Blaser K. Epitope-specific T cell tolerance to phospholipase A2 in bee venom immunotherapy and recovery by IL-2 and IL-15 in vitro. J Clin Invest 1996; 98:1676–1683.

29. Schuerwegh AJ, De Clerck LS, Bridts CH, Stevens WJ. Wasp venom immunotherapy induces a shift from IL-4-producing towards interferon-gamma–producing CD4+ and CD8+ T lymphocytes. Clin Exp Allergy 2001; 31:740–746.

30. Joss A, Akdis M, Faith A, Blaser K, Akdis CA. IL-10 directly acts on T cells by specifically altering the CD-28 costimulation pathway. Eur J Immunol 2000; 30:1683–1690.

31. Akdis CA, Blaser K. IL-10–induced anergy in peripheral T cell and reactivation by microenvironmental cytokines: Two key steps in specific immunotherapy. FASEB J 1999; 13:603–609.

32. Ohashi Y, Nakai Y, Okamoto H, Ohno Y, Sakamoto H, Sugiura Y, Kakinoki Y, Tanaka A, Kishimoto K, Washio Y, Hayashi M. Serum level of interleukin-4 in patients with perennial allergic rhinitis during allergen-specific immunotherapy. Scand J Immunol 1996; 43:680–686.

33. Lack G, Nelson HS, Amran D, Oshiba A, Jung T, Bradley KL, Giclas PC, Gelfand EW. Rush immunotherapy results in allergen-specific alterations in lymphocyte function and interferon-gamma production in CD4(+) T cells. J Allergy Clin Immunol 1997; 99:530–538.

34. O'Brien RM, Byron KA, Varigos GA, Thomas WR. House dust mite immunotherapy results in a decrease in Der p 2–specific IFN-gamma and IL-4 expression by circulating T lymphocytes. Clin Exp Allergy 1997; 27:46–51.

35. Ebner C, Siemann U, Bohle B, Willheim M, Wiedermann U, Schenk S, Klotz F, Ebner H, Kraft D, Scheiner O. Immunological changes during specific immunotherapy of grass pollen allergy: Reduced lymphoproliferative responses to allergen and shift from TH2 to TH1 in

T-cell clones specific for Phl p 1, a major grass pollen allergen. Clin Exp Allergy 1997; 27:1007–1015.

36. Wilson DR, Nouri-Aria KT, Walker SM, Pajno GB, O'Brien F, Jacobson MR, Mackay IS, Durham SR. Grass pollen immunotherapy: Symptomatic improvement correlates with reductions in eosinophils and IL-5 mRNA expression in the nasal mucosa during the pollen season. J Allergy Clin Immunol 2001; 107:971–976.

37. Wachholz PA, Nouri-Aria KT, Wilson DR, Walker SM, Verhoef A, Till SJ, Durham SR. Grass pollen immunotherapy for hayfever is associated with increases in local nasal but not peripheral Th1:Th2 cytokine ratios. Immunology 2002; 105:56–62.

38. Wilson DR, Irani A-MA, Walker SM, Jacobson MR, Mackay IS, Schwartz LB, Durham SR. Grass pollen immunotherapy inhibits seasonal increases in basophils and eosinophils in the nasal epithelium. Clin Exp Allergy 2001; 31:1705–1713.

39. Hamid QA, Schotman E, Jacobson MR, Walker SM, Durham SR. Increases in IL-2 messenger RNA+ cells accompany inhibition of allergen-induced late skin responses after successful grass pollen immunotherapy. J Allergy Clin Immunol 1997; 99:254–260.

40. Durham SR, Ying S, Varney VA, Jacobson MR, Sudderick RM, Mackay IS, Kay AB, Hamid QA. Grass pollen immunotherapy inhibits allergen-induced infiltration of CD4+ T lymphocytes and eosinophils in the nasal mucosa and increases the number of cells expressing messenger RNA for interferon-gamma. J Allergy Clin Immunol 1996; 97:1356–1365.

8

Aerobiology

W. ELLIOTT HORNER

Air Quality Sciences, Inc., Marietta, Georgia, U.S.A.

ESTELLE LEVETIN

University of Tulsa, Tulsa, Oklahoma, U.S.A.

SAMUEL B. LEHRER

Tulane University Heath Sciences Center, New Orleans, Louisiana, U.S.A.

I. INTRODUCTION

Awareness of the health effects of airborne agents is almost as old as written history. In Western civilization, suggestion of unhealthy "air" is mentioned in the early books of the Bible (Leviticus 14:35–48) and among ancient Roman writings. Blackley (1) provided perhaps the first modern treatise on aerobiology when he presumed that "bronchial catarrh" was due to emanations from freshly cut hay. Pasteur's classic experiments on germ theory compared microbial growths in sterile broths that were either exposed to or protected from air. Although it was not directed toward aerobiology, airborne spores made the experiment work. Airborne material was considered a disease agent long before it was possible to sample the air for biological particles. Gregory's treatise (2) is an excellent additional source on, and indeed a salient part of, aerobiology history.

II. OUTDOOR ALLERGENS

A. Sampling

Plant pollen and fungal spores are the two major groups of outdoor allergenic particles. Plants and fungi are sufficiently distinct to represent different kingdoms, but many species of each group rely on airborne dispersal of propagules. Airborne pollen of plants moves male genetic material to other plants. In fungi, airborne spores colonize new and often remote substrates. To be effective, these particles must remain aloft, and hence entrained, in the flow of air. Airborne pollen and spores have adaptations of size and shape that make them more buoyant in air and more easily carried by air currents. The same properties that keep particles aloft, though, hinder the collection of particles onto a sampling surface. Thus, the central problem of aeroallergen sampling is that the particles are designed to be effectively dispersed, which makes them hard to capture.

Airborne particles may be collected either by passive or by active sampling (3). Passive sampling collects particles that are permitted to settle from air by the force of gravity; these sampling techniques are called settle or gravity slides, plates, and traps. Active sampling removes particles from the air by some mechanical, physical, or electrical device. It is important to note that particles carried in an airstream tend to stay with the airstream until some force pulls—or accelerates—the particles free of the airstream.

Settle traps collect particles by gravity; this exerts a very small force on spores and pollen. Hence, the recovery of aeroallergen particles by gravity is heavily biased toward larger particles, since smaller particles are more likely to be relifted by very slight air currents. This significant qualitative bias is particularly important with spores, but also affects smaller pollen. Settle traps are also not quantitative. That is, the particle count from settle plates is derived from an unknown quantity of air and cannot be expressed as a concentration. These limitations preclude the widespread use of settle plates. Historically, in spite of these limitations, remarkable progress has been made with settle traps in describing the common pollen and molds and their patterns of abundance. It is also important from an allergological point of view that most of the molds currently available as commercial allergen extracts are fungi that are readily recovered on settle plates. Thus, to a degree, the selection of fungi for allergen vaccination is based on spore size and relative numbers, rather than allergological importance.

A number of active samplers are available commercially for sampling airborne particulates (4). The common types are impactors, impingers, and filters (Table 1). Filters act as particle sieves, retaining particles from an airstream as the air passes through the filter. Impingers collect the particles from an airstream by passing (bubbling) the air through a volume of fluid and trapping the particles in the fluid. Impingers and filters are used for research purposes to collect allergen samples over a long time period or allergen that is associated with particles of unknown size. Virtually all aeroallergen sampling for pollen and fungal spores is conducted with impactor-type samplers.

The common aeroallergen impactor samplers work by accelerating an airstream onto a sampling surface or accelerating a surface through an airstream. This forces the airstream to turn sharply around the surface. The momentum of particles entrained in the airstream prevents the particles from turning so sharply and forces them to break free of the airstream and impact the sampling surface. Hence, smaller particles (generally those of less mass) have to be accelerated to a greater velocity than larger particles to break free of the airstream. This, in general, is why pollen grains are easier to sample than spores.

Two impactor-type samplers that are widely used in outdoor aeroallergen studies are the Rotorod (Multidata, St. Louis Park, MN) rotating-rod sampler and the Burkard (Burkard Manufacturing, Rickmansworth, United Kingdom) suction-type spore trap (Fig. 1). The Rotorod is more widely used in the United State, but the Burkard has a greater acceleration velocity and hence is more efficient for collecting fungal spores (5). The Kramer-Collins (G-R Electric Manufacturing Co., Manhattan, KS), Allergenco (Environmental Monitoring

Table 1 Comparison of Active Samplers Used for Aerobiology

Sampler type	Example(s)	Advantage	Limitation
Impactor: non-culture	Burkard,[a] Rotorod[b]	Detects particles regardless of viability or culturability	Spore counts assignable only to categories, some rather broad
Impactor: non-culture	Air-o-Cell[c]	As above, inexpensive, very clear visual background	As above, not well characterized
Impactor: culture	Andersen,[d] SAS[e]	Many fungi in culture may be identified with certainty	Only culturable propagules detected, only sporulating types identifiable
Impinger	AGI[f]	Sample may be split for different types of analyses; longer-duration samples	Low sample volume, delicate instrument
Filter cassette	Mixed cellulose ester, or polycarbonate	Inexpensive; sample may be split for different types of analyses; longer-duration samples	Some propagules may be damaged by desiccation
Filter membrane	Air-Sentinel[g] PTFE membrane	Higher volume sampled than with impinger; sample may be split for different analyses; longer sample times possible	High volume restricts indoor use; expensive; antibody required for immunoassay

[a] Burkard Manufacturing, Rickmansworth, UK
[b] Multidata, St. Louis Park, MN
[c] Zefon International, St. Petersburg, FL
[d] Thermo Andersen, Franklin, MA
[e] Bioscience International, Rockville, MD
[f] Ace Glass, Vineland, NJ
[g] Quan-Tec Air, Rochester, MN

Systems, Charleston, SC) (Fig. 2), and Lanzoni (Lanzoli S.R.L., Bologna, Italy) samplers are other suction-type impactor samplers that are used for pollen and spore collection (Table 2). The first widely used active—and hence volumetric—sampler for airborne pollen and spores was the Hirst spore trap. Almost immediately, the Hirst sampler was used to study allergenic spores and pollen as well as the airborne plant pathogens it was designed to study. Indeed, one of the first papers that included spore trap data suggested that basidiomycete (mushrooms and allies) spores might be important allergens (6). This idea is now gaining wider acceptance over 35 years later (7–9). The Burkard, Lanzoni, and Kramer-Collins samplers are based on the Hirst spore trap, as are, in part, the Allergenco, Air-Ø-Cell (Zefon International, St. Peterbug, FL), and others. Subsequently, other types of less expensive, rotating impactor samplers—rotoslide, rotobar, and rotorod—were developed and became widely used in the allergy field to track pollen and spore counts. These samplers accelerate the sampling surface through the airstream but attain the same result of forcing particles out of the airstream and onto the sampling surface (3).

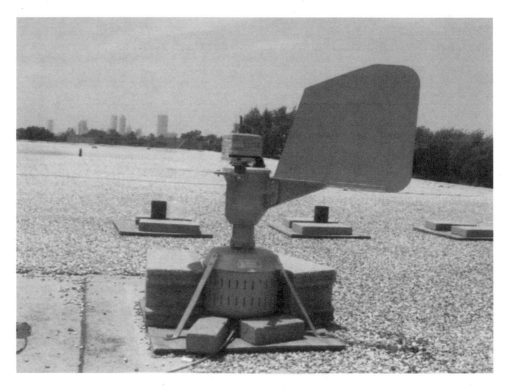

Figure 1 Recording Burkard spore trap (suction-type impactor) installed on a rooftop. This sampler can be configured to record for 7 days or for 24 hours.

Regardless of design, these active samplers make up the technology that permits quantitative aerobiology. Thus, aerobiology can now provide reliable approximations of airborne pollen and spore levels. The major remaining limitation, however, is that the data as reported by the news media always pertain to yesterday, and allergy patients need to know the counts for tomorrow or even for the upcoming season. In addition, pollen forecasts can aid physicians in developing treatment plans for patients and in planning clinical trials. Such forecasting requires prediction models based on a large database of observations. Fortunately, such databases are being acquired, and pollen forecasting models are being developed in various parts of the world (10).

B. Analysis

Three general types of analysis, each with its own strengths and limitations, are used for airborne allergen detection: direct microscopy, culture analysis, and immunoassays (5,11). Molecular techniques are also now beginning to be applied to aerobiology. Microscopy can be performed immediately. Although irrelevant for pollen and immunochemical analysis of allergens, direct microscopy for fungal spores does not need the 3- to 10-day incubation necessary for culture analyses. This is very important since many spores and all pollen cannot grow on agar. Microscopy requires extensive training, though, and the accuracy is very dependent on the skill level of the practitioner. Also, many different fungi produce similar spores that, once released, cannot be clearly identified, except as to the general group. This presents a limit to the specificity of these fungal spore counts, since

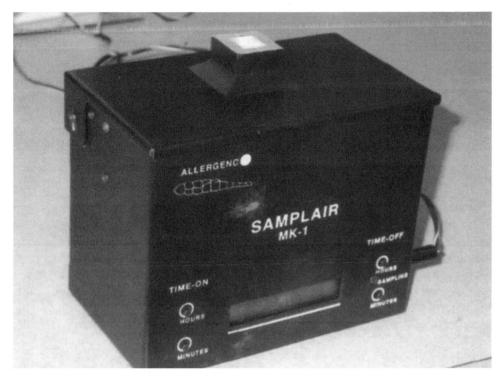

Figure 2 Allergenco suction-type spore trap. This sampler collects multiple, discrete samples at predetermined intervals and can be used to monitor outdoor trends or for indoor investigations.

Table 2 Comparison of Selected Features of Commonly Used Outdoor Aeroallergen Impactor Samplers (Non-culture)

Sampler	Salient feature	Advantage	Limitation
Burkard[a]	Continuous recording sample	Well characterized, wind oriented, small particle efficiency	Somewhat more expensive, although price difference now less
Rotorod[b]	Intermittent, overlaid samples	Wind oriented, operational simplicity	Less efficient for small particles (spores)
Allergenco[c]	Intermittent, discrete samples	Small particle efficiency	Not wind oriented
Kramer-Collins[d]	Continuous recording sample	Wind oriented, small particle efficiency	Relatively few in use

[a] Burkard Manufacturing, Rickmansworth, UK
[b] Multidata, St. Louis Park, MN
[c] Environmental Monitoring Systems, Charleston, SC
[d] G-R Electric Manufacturing Co. Manhattan, KS

even experienced counters must "lump" spores into rather broad categories on the basis of similar spore shape, size, and coloration. This is like viewing a landscape through a wide-angle lens, but one that may be slightly out of focus.

Culture analysis is useful only for fungal spores as opposed to pollen and only for those spores that can germinate and grow on the nutrient medium used (12,13). This can be a significant limitation. Culture analysis can be used for impactor samples or for samples from impingers or filter samplers. The greatest strength of this method is that the fungi recovered are in culture and hence can be identified precisely by technicians that are familiar with a particular group of fungi. The major problem is that dead spores will not grow, although they may still be allergenic. Moreover, if the spores are alive but the agar medium selected is unsuitable for growth of a particular species, that species will likely not be detected. This is like viewing a landscape through a sharply focused lens, but one with a narrow field of view.

Specific allergen molecules can also be measured immunochemically either in impinger fluid or in filter washings, provided that a specific assay is available for the target allergen (5,11). This very important technology requires widely available skills (conducting ELISAs), rather than the highly specialized skills necessary for identifying spores or colonies microscopically. A drawback of the technique is the equipment expense. The major constraint, however, is that the antigen (allergen) of interest must be isolated and specific antibodies must be prepared against it. This approach requires a significant research effort to obtain the antibody but has been applied successively to, and is now commercially available for, dust mite, cockroach, cat, and dog allergens.

In principle, immunoassay measures of fungal and pollen allergens should be a cost-effective and rapid means to monitor airborne levels. The great strength of immunoassays relative to DNA-based assays (discussed later) is that the allergen is directly detected. Even though immunoassays may directly measure the molecule of interest, unfortunately, no practical applications of immunoassays have been established for ongoing monitoring. The attempts to use immunoassays for environmental monitoring to date have focused on fungi occurring indoors, commonly referred to as molds. Molds are fungi that, unlike mushrooms, produce microscopic reproductive structures. When fungi grow indoors, the terms "fungus" and "mold" are often used interchangeably.

The power of molecular detection and quantification techniques has only begun to be applied to monitoring airborne molds. Molecular detection systems for clinically relevant molds have been available for some time, but these are not designed to exclude effects from environmental interferences. From the perspective of measuring allergens, though, pollen (and likely mold) allergens can be carried on particles other than intact pollen grains (or spores) (14). So these allergens may occur in the absence of DNA, or the amounts of allergen and DNA target may not correlate. The correlation of DNA target and allergen can be evaluated with other allergens with established techniques for measuring environmental levels, such as mite, pet, rodent, and roach. The application of DNA-based techniques just in the last few years indicates that detection, routine monitoring, and even reliable forecasting of mold spores (and perhaps pollen) may soon be possible. One method of outdoor monitoring is discussed next. Other methods chiefly applied to indoor measures are discussed later.

One method uses polymerase chain reaction (PCR) assays to detect spores of specific molds collected on spore trap samplers (15). Although developed for a specific agricultural application, it was designed to complement an ongoing air monitoring program, such as is used in aeroallergen monitoring. Additionally, the samplers used are the same type used in aeroallergen monitoring, and the data generated are used for a forecasting model, such as a model for forecasting aeroallergen levels (16). This system may be readily adaptable to aeroallergen monitoring and even forecasting if suitable primers for molds and even pollens of interest to physicians and patients are included.

Microscopy remains the standard analytical mode for outdoor aerobiology monitoring. Results can be obtained within the day and pollen are readily detected. Indoor aerobiology has become more important as fungal growth in buildings becomes more widely recognized as a potential health problem. This controversial topic is discussed in Section III. Relative to outdoor monitoring programs, indoor aerobiology sampling more often focuses on locating a suspected source in a building. Here pollens are typically not of interest since indoor plants are not usually wind pollinated. Furthermore, speciation of fungi indoors is crucial since some fungi that grow indoors have known health effects, yet related and less harmful species of the same genus may be growing and producing abundant spores outdoors. Without identifying these as different species, it might appear that the fungus indoors is merely a contaminant from outdoors (17,18).

1. Pollen

Anthesis (pollen release) leads to pollen spread through the air and, in turn, to deposition either on another flower (pollination) or onto mucosa (19). During the flowering period of wind-pollinated (anemophilous) plants, the local concentration of a pollen type can reach hundreds or even thousands of grains per cubic meter of air. The onset, duration, and peak of pollen concentrations depend on several factors (20–22). These include the type of plant and the region of growth (e.g., north/south, mountain/lowland). Seasonal weather trends are also important, including parameters such as "degree-days," which is a measure of how many days in a season are warm and how warm those days are. Finally, regional day-to-day weather patterns are crucial. Periods of cold weather suppress anthesis and rain washes pollen grains from the air, whereas warm, breezy weather promotes anthesis and also keeps pollen aloft.

Most temperature zone airborne pollen grains are between 12 and 40 µm in size (23). Impactor-type samplers are efficient enough to accurately sample most pollens. For practical purposes, pollens are generally divided into three seasonal types. These are trees in the spring, grasses in the summer, and weeds through the summer and fall. Although these seasonal ranges are typical for these pollen groups, there are substantial year-to-year differences regarding the beginning date, the peak pollen concentration, and the length of the season for each pollen.

Examples of the possible variation for oak, grass, and ragweed are presented in Table 3. These data are from the Aeroallergen Monitoring Network, 1996 Pollen and Spore Report, American Academy of Allergy, Asthma, and Immunology (24). Data are submitted to this network from stations at sites across North America. Current locations are mapped on their Web site (www.aaaai.org/nab).

Note that the environmental cues for anthesis of these plant types differ. The beginning of oak anthesis—or onset of the season—is governed by seasonal development (i.e., the number of warm days that have occurred so far in the spring). However, the amount of pollen production—or the "severity" of the pollen season—is affected by the soil moisture levels earlier in the season, since this affects the number of flower buds that develop. In comparison, some trees form flower buds in the autumn, and hence the previous (autumn) moisture levels affect the amount of pollen or severity of the pollen season for these trees. Some trees, such as birches, actually initiate bud formation the previous spring. So the weather in one spring determines the potential pollen load the following spring (25).

Table 3 Beginning Date, Duration, and Peak Concentrations for Oak, Grass, and Ragweed Pollen

Pollen type	Station[a]	Start (date)[b]	Duration (days)[c]	Peak (date, concentration)
Oak	LA	2/22	82	3/26 (2321)
	KY	4/4	56	4/29 (1358)
	MN	5/16	30	5/21 (999)
Grass	LA	1/2	>330	4/2 (56)
	KY	4/19	195	5/17 (75)
	MN	6/5	96	6/25 (37)
Ragweed	LA	7/30	>120	10/4 (358)
	KY	8/6	120	8/30 (201)
	MN	8/5	>80	9/3 (228)

[a] Reported from three American Academy of Allergy, Asthma, and Immunol network stations in 1996: Lafayette, LA (30° N latitude); Lexington, KY (38° N); and Mankato, MN (44° N).
[b] Start date is when pollen was recorded on at least 3 of 5 consecutive days.
[c] End dates for the season are when that pollen was recorded on 2 or fewer of 5 consecutive days.

Present weather conditions, temperature, humidity, and wind also are very important factors determining day-to-day fluctuations of pollen counts.

Many temperate grasses grow from seed each year, so the time of onset and the amount of pollen released depend on current growing season and daily weather patterns. Most weeds, including ragweed, also grow from seed each year and so, like grasses, the abundance of pollen depends on current growing season conditions and daily weather patterns. The beginning of grass season varies somewhat between years with an early or late spring. Ragweed, in particular, is a "short day" plant, and flowering is initiated by lengthening nights rather than by current or accumulated temperature. So ragweed season starts predictably near the beginning of August each year in the northern United State. The end of the season varies, though, with the first hard frost in a region. In most southern states, pollen release begins in late August and continues through October.

2. Fungi

Fungi are more difficult than pollen to assess from an allergy standpoint. There are several reasons for this, including the greater number of fungal species, the variety of spore shapes and sizes, the difficulty of sampling for fungal spores, and the greater skill needed to identify fungal spores. Airborne spore concentrations also respond at least as quickly as pollen to short-term environmental changes (26,27). Fungal spore release is also less seasonally limited than pollen. Indeed, many fungal spores can be released at almost any time of the year, when suitable temperature and moisture conditions exist, and often are released within hours or even minutes of events such as rainfall.

High-quality fungal allergen extracts are very difficult to produce compared with pollen extracts (9). Regarding management of allergic disease, fungal allergens are not as well characterized as pollen, and apparently many cross-react extensively (28). Thus, there are no standardized fungal extracts, and sensitized patients may respond to a number of fungi other than the one to which they were originally sensitized (29). Finally, although season does moderate the abundance of fungal spores, spore "seasons" are much less defined in nature than pollen seasons (27). This means that there often is no clear season for mold spores, and avoiding exposure is thus far more difficult.

Fungi can be grouped by taxonomy or by their ecology (i.e., their role in nature). Textbooks typically discuss fungi by taxonomic groups, but mention of their ecology is also useful since it relates to their life cycles and why and when they produce spores.

The major taxonomic groups of true fungi that are currently recognized are the ascomycetes, basidiomycetes, and zygomycetes (30). Many textbooks still discuss the "fungi imperfecti" as a separate group. Almost all of these are forms of ascomycetes that produce asexual spores called conidia; perhaps 10% are asexual states of basidiomycetes. These are treated as conidial forms of ascomycetes (or basidiomycetes) rather than as a separate taxonomic group. Most of the familiar fungal allergens are conidial forms of ascomycetes, including *Cladosporium*, *Alternaria*, *Penicillium*, *Fusarium*, *Epicoccum*, *Drechslera*, *Curvularia*, and *Aspergillus*.

The ecological groupings of fungi are relevant to allergy since fungi of similar ecological types may sporulate in response to similar environmental conditions. Hence, high spore counts of a number of these fungi may occur at the same time. The great majority of airborne spores are produced by one of three general ecological types of fungi. These are the phylloplane fungi, basidiomycetes, and the soil and litter fungi.

Phylloplane (leaf surface) fungi live on the surfaces of leaves. Most of these are microfungi that are asexual states of ascomycetes. Some familiar examples are *Alternaria*, *Cladosporium*, *Epicoccum*, and *Curvularia*. Leaf surfaces are exposed to periodic drying and ultraviolet radiation and accumulate exudates from the leaves and organic detritus from the air. Thus, phylloplane fungi are adapted to continual wetting/drying cycles, tolerate harmful exposures (cleansers), and use organic debris (skin scales/soap residues) as a nutrient source. Hence, the shower wall of a domestic bathroom remarkably mimics a leaf surface. Since plant leaves abound in almost every habitable region of the earth, these fungi are usually prevalent and frequently dominant in the outdoor air spora and are readily available to colonize suitable indoor surfaces.

Basidiomycetes include mushrooms, puffballs, conks, and related fungi. *Pleurotus*, *Ganoderma*, *Psilocybe*, *Calvatia*, and *Coprinus* are among the basidiomycetes known to produce allergens. Surveys with noncommercial allergen extracts indicate that the prevalence of reactivity to basidiomycetes is comparable to the prevalence of reactivity to conidial fungi (7). Very few commercial extracts of basidiomycetes are available, and these are not well characterized. Hence, the true prevalence of basidiomycete sensitization among broader clinical populations remains unknown.

Basidiomycetes typically live in association with plant roots or as decomposers of plant litter and/or wood. In fact, the most efficient wood decomposers are basidiomycetes, and these occur wherever there are shade trees, lawns, or parks or wherever wood becomes sufficiently wet to permit decay.

Two additional groups of basidiomycetes are the rust fungi and the smut fungi; these are important plant pathogens that attack a wide range of both native and cultivated plants. There are approximately 6000 species of rust fungi and 1200 species of smut fungi. Unlike other basidiomycetes, these fungi lack macroscopic reproductive structures and are identified only by the lesions or spore masses produced on the host plant. Both groups produce airborne spores, which are frequently abundant in the atmosphere and recognized as allergenic (31–34). A variety of smut spore allergen extracts are available for testing and allergen immunotherapy, but only one rust extract—from stem rust of wheat, the commercial label of which is "stem rust"—is currently FDA approved.

Most soil and litter fungi are asexual states of ascomycetes. Among these are the allergenic fungi *Penicillium*, *Aspergillus*, and *Fusarium*. Some species of these genera are also capable of producing mycotoxins, which are secondary metabolites produced by some species of fungi during their growth in organic materials (30). The most common route of exposure is by ingestion of food contaminated with toxigenic fungi. The toxins can cause acute or chronic disease in animals, with effects ranging from neurotoxic to carcinogenic to immune-suppressive. For these reasons the amounts of mycotoxins permissible in grains, seeds, and nuts is tightly regulated by governments throughout the world. These fungi are also common in the outdoor airspora. Spores, especially of *Penicillium* and *Aspergillus*, are recovered in almost all air samples, although they are not usually the dominant species; some species of *Penicillium* are claimed to be the most common forms of eukaryotic life on the planet. Although some of these are specialized fungi, many degrade various organic detritus and are widespread.

Many soil and litter fungi can also tolerate indoor conditions. Just as the wall of a residential shower is reasonably similar to a leaf surface, so indoor dust can mimic soil. Likewise, cellulosic building materials—wallpaper, paper coating on wallboard, acoustic ceiling tile—if they become wet, are serviceable substitutes for moldering leaves. Thus, soil and litter fungi are abundant in outdoor air on almost all days without snow cover, and even their indoor presence can be high in buildings with moisture problems.

In order to become airborne, spores must be either propelled into the air or positioned so that air currents can pick them up. This can be a formidable task for particles only a few microns in diameter, since there is a boundary layer of very still air up to 1 mm around most surfaces (6). Spores must penetrate this boundary layer to become airborne. With few exceptions, the spores of leaf surface fungi are passively released. As the spores are produced, they are fragmented from the fungus body, but no motion is imparted (i.e., there is no "kick"). This is true of essentially all conidial (imperfect) fungi, including the common allergenic fungi.

Most soil and litter fungi, such as the phylloplane fungi, produce spores that are passively liberated. Spores of these fungi require some external physical disturbance in order to become airborne. With leaf surface fungi, shaking by the wind is often sufficient (35). When the spores are shaken loose, they fall free of the leaf and are picked up by air currents. These spores are like dust, though, and are held by wet surfaces. Thus, spores of phylloplane fungi become airborne in greater quantities during dry conditions. For soil or litter—or other moldy organic material—any disturbance is usually sufficient to dislodge quantities of spores. The same disturbance will also generate air currents, which can lift and disperse the spores.

Conversely, many perfect-state (or sexual) spores of ascomycetes and basidiomycetes are actively discharged. Ascospores are often impelled through the boundary layer and gain sufficient height to become entrained in air currents. With many cup fungi, the explosive discharge can easily be seen as a puff or cloud of spores. Mushroom spores are flung away from the spore-producing tissues so that the spores can fall free of the mushroom cap and be picked up by air currents.

Avoidance measures are most successful when the factors affecting spore concentrations can be conveyed to the patient. Dry, windy days during the growing season tend to have high spore concentrations from phylloplane fungi (Fig. 3). Patients with strong allergies to *Cladosporium* might avoid walking in parks or woods on those days. Disturbing or handling mulch or decaying organic matter will likely release plumes of spores from soil and litter fungi on any day (36). Patients allergic to *Aspergillus* or *Penicillium* should probably avoid handling yard or garden wastes and especially refrain from any composting activities. Actively discharged ascospores and basidiospores also reach high concentrations under particular conditions. Ascospore concentrations

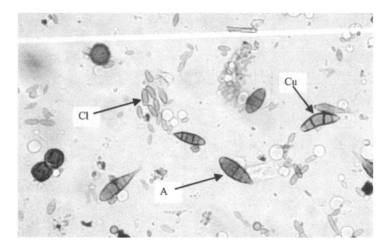

Figure 3 Spore trap sample typical of "dry" airspora. Numerous *Cladosporium* spores (Cl) are present, as well as multiseptate *Alternaria* spores (A) and one *Curvularia* spore (Cu). (Original magnification 400x.)

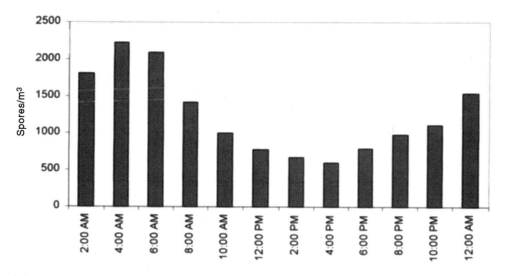

Figure 4 Diurnal rhythm of airborne basidiospores in Tulsa, Oklahoma, during May 1998; values are monthly averages for the hours indicated.

frequently peak following rain. Except during drought conditions, basidiospore concentrations are especially high during spring and fall, and peak during the early morning hours, roughly from midnight to 8 A.M. (Fig. 4).

C. Variability

1. Temporal

Pollen and spore concentrations in the air can vary dramatically from year to year, day to day, or even within a few hours (2,20–22,26,27,36,37). General differences in weather from year to year affect plant growth and hence pollen levels. Table 4 shows the variation

Table 4   Seasonal Characteristics for Mulberry Pollen in Tulsa, Oklahoma

Year	Start date	Peak concentration (grains/m³)	Peak date	End date	Season duration (days)	Seasonal total
1991	3/24	881	4/2	4/21	28	7876
1992	4/7	175	4/12	4/25	18	764
1993	4/11	1197	4/16	5/2	21	5888
1994	3/29	1236	4/6	4/22	25	7611
1995	3/23	565	3/31	4/15	23	2459
1996	4/17	244	4/20	5/11	24	1922
1997	3/29	782	4/2	5/16	49	5791
1998	4/3	439	4/22	5/6	32	3541
1999	4/1	853	4/7	4/27	27	6751
2000	3/24	717	4/5	4/12	20	6290

of the *Morus* (mulberry) pollen season over a 10-year period in Tulsa, Oklahoma. The season start date varied by 25 days and the seasonal total varied by an order of magnitude. Directly and indirectly, such yearly variations also affect fungal spore levels. Patterns of pollen and spore concentration also vary within seasons on a daily basis and even very predictably on a diurnal pattern.

All pollen are notably seasonal, occurring only during the flowering season of the plant. Some fungi, including many mushrooms, also fruit and release spores in definite seasons each year. Conversely, there will probably be some species of basidiomycetes (mushrooms and wood decay fungi) fruiting during any part of the year, other than months when the temperature is below freezing. There is a definite fall mushroom peak that is reflected in gradually increasing basidiospore counts in late summer and fall for many sampling stations (see current reports at www.aaaai.org/nab). Other fungi, particularly the leaf-surface fungi that are widely used for allergen testing, can release spores throughout the year when temperature and moisture levels are favorable. The highest levels tend to be in the fall, however, coinciding with senescence of the vegetation for the year.

Within any of these pollen or spore seasons there are diurnal patterns that are clinically important. Note that the observed peak time at any sampling station is modified by distance to the source. A sampler adjacent to an oak-filled park will record the peak when anthesis is truly peaking. A sampler in an urban center, however (where many are located), may show the peak several hours later due to the time required for atmospheric mixing and transport of pollen clouds. The time delay is affected both by the pollen cloud traveling from the source and by the need for vertical mixing to raise a portion of the cloud high enough to reach most aeroallergen stations located atop buildings rather than at "nose level." Hence, a few hours may pass before transport and vertical air mixing can bring pollen to urban rooftops (21). Since grass pollen tends to be released in the morning, local airborne peaks will be before noon; however, pollen from distant sources leads to afternoon peaks. Almost all ragweed pollen is released between 6:30 and 8:30 A.M. However, at this time the pollen is wet and clumped together, ending up on the surface of adjacent ragweed leaves. The pollen slowly dries as the morning humidity decreases and becomes airborne later in the morning (38). Thus, ragweed pollen peaks may occur at midday at urban rooftop sampling stations.

There is also evidence of a smaller, postmidnight peak in pollen concentrations (39,40). After sunset, atmospheric convection and vertical mixing slows and particles begin settling (41,42). In calm air, settling rates range from approximately 1.5 (ragweed) to 8.8 (rye grass) cm/s for angiosperm pollen grains (some gymnosperm pollens such as pine pollen settle faster). This permits the pollen dispersed from 160 up to 950 m to settle back to near ground level in 3 hours of calm air.

The release of many fungal spores also follows circadian patterns. These peaks generally coincide with the time of day when conditions are favorable for the spores to land on favorable substrates (2). The near-ground concentrations of basidiospores are frequently highest between midnight and dawn (Fig. 4). Remember that these spores are forcibly liberated and fall from the fruit body to be picked up by air currents. Hence, very light air currents are sufficient and the high humidities of predawn protect the spore from desiccation. Spore concentrations of the potato late blight fungus, *Phytophthora infestans*, peak in a postdawn pattern, between 6 A.M. and noon. These spores are passively liberated, so they will not become airborne until morning breezes begin, but infection of new leaves is unsuccessful after leaves dry out by late morning. Rust and smut spores and powdery mildews do not require as much moisture as *Phytophthora* to infect leaves. Hence, spore release later in the day is not as detrimental and is actually advantageous because convective wind has increased and spore clouds are better mixed through the foliage. There is a midday peak of these fungi between 10 A.M. and 3 P.M. There are other patterns as well; for example, *Cladosporium* and other phylloplane fungi tend to peak between midday and early afternoon.

2. Spatial

The clinical interest in pollen and spore counts is based on knowledge of the exposure of the individual patient. Although the local spore and pollen count is typically the variable used to estimate exposure, this is unfortunately only a rough estimate of the exposure for any individual. Because the bioaerosol concentration differs over short spaces, the reported pollen or spore counts may be either higher or lower than those to which an individual patient is exposed. Three common sources of spatial variation affect pollen and spore concentrations in a particular location: long-distance transport, local (neighborhood) sources, and height.

There are only a few reported studies of long-distance transport of pollen and spores (43,44). Notable among these is the trans-Atlantic "jump" that coffee rust made from Africa to South America. Every year, clouds of birch pollen from central Europe move across Scandinavia, inducing symptoms in the spring before birch releases pollen in Scandinavia. Each winter, mountain cedar pollen (*Juniperus ashei*) is carried from central Texas to Oklahoma, Missouri, and other states by southerly winds (45–49). In fact, trajectory analysis shows that the source of *Juniperus* pollen trapped in London, Ontario, on 27 January 1999 was released from the Texas population of *J. ashei* on the previous day. Likewise, wheat in the central and northern plains of the United State is infected with stem rust from spores that are blown northward from overwintering crops along the U.S.-Mexico border (44). These spores, as well as pollen transported long distances, are very well mixed and contribute to the overall background levels of airborne spores and pollen.

Clinicians and patients should be aware of the factors that modify local pollen and spore count reports. The spatial variation of local pollen loads is known from studies where arrays of samplers were positioned around metropolitan areas. These indicate that substantial differences can occur in pollen loads only a few kilometers apart (50); spore concentrations drop very quickly with height above ground (51). Hence, pollen or spore concentrations may differ markedly within a few thousand meters along the ground or a few dozen meters above the ground. However, the typical aeroallergen sampling station for a city is a single sampler on a rooftop (often urban), far above "nose level." A rooftop or other elevated location does not reflect what most patients are exposed to since atmospheric mixing is required to raise pollen and spores to the height of most samplers. Atmospheric mixing also homogenizes the spatial variation seen near ground level, which value is judiciously considered as a regional count.

Although counting a regionally "homogenized" sample saves considerable labor, the spore/pollen counts obtained are less relevant to the exposure of any single individual. The clinician should recognize this inherent conflict between a regional estimate and the local exposure of the individual patient. It is also crucial for allergy patients to understand and account for this, as pollen and spore counts become available and are reported daily from more localities. Hence, the birch pollen count may always be low if the reporting station in town has very few birches nearby. However, if a patient lives in a suburb filled with birches, his or her exposure in the early spring will be far greater than the pollen report indicates.

3. Pollen/Spore Reports: Clinical Aspects

Pollen and spore counts are now routinely reported in many cities in North America and in Europe. This is valuable for both the clinician and the allergy patient. Aeroallergen counts are a useful additional piece of diagnostic information since these counts can also provide guidance to the patient on avoidance and on scheduling medication. Several points need to be considered as these counts are used more frequently. These involve timing issues as well as "local effects," which were discussed earlier. A significant problem with all current pollen and spore reports is that they report the levels that were in the air yesterday. Generally, the samplers run for 24 h and are then counted and reported. Clinicians should emphasize to their patients the need to track pollen and spore counts but to associate yesterday's symptoms with today's counts. This will hopefully become an obsolete precaution when prediction models become sufficiently reliable to give advance notice of high peaks of pollen or spores.

The current status of pollen forecasting has been reviewed (10). Progress is being made in day-to-day as well as seasonal forecasting. Once pollen release for a particular species begins, airborne pollen concentrations typically show a Gaussian distribution; however, meteorological factors influence day-to-day pollen release. Forecasting models utilize various meteorological parameters combined with day of the season to predict daily pollen levels. For example, Norris-Hill (52) used accumulated average temperature combined with maximum temperature, relative humidity, and rainfall to predict daily grass pollen concentrations in London. This forecasting model was 71% accurate in predicting grass pollen levels. Levetin and Van de Water (48,49) used an empirical model based on sunshine, temperature, relative humidity, and wind speed to predict pollen release for mountain cedar. The release forecast is combined with regional meteorological conditions and wind trajectories generated using HYSPLIT-4 (Hybrid Single-Particle Lagrangian Integrated Trajectory), an atmospheric dispersion model available online from the NOAA (National Oceanic and Atmospheric Administration) Air Resources Laboratory (http://www.arl.noaa.gov), to predict the downwind dispersal of mountain cedar (48).

III. INDOOR ALLERGENS

In the last quarter century, major allergenic components of "house dust" have been identified, including allergens from dust mites, cats, dogs, mice, cockroaches, and certain molds. This is arguably the most significant advancement during that time in understanding the "ecology" of allergic respiratory diseases. The immunochemical characterization of these major indoor allergens was determined with quantitative assays that reliably measured the levels of these allergens in settled dust. This, in turn, has allowed exposure to be more reliably assessed and related to disease. A thorough discussion of these aspects has been compiled (53), other chapters in this volume address these individual indoor allergens in greater detail.

A. Sampling

As with outdoor allergens, air is the most relevant medium to measure for allergen content, since it is the major exposure route for respiratory allergens. However, indoor air sampling has important limitations (Fig. 4). Several of the important indoor allergens occur on particles of fairly large aerodynamic diameter (e.g., 10–40 μm for mite fecal pellets, and nearly as large for cockroach allergens). Particles of this size settle rather quickly. Hence, the allergen-bearing particles are airborne only transiently, which makes airborne exposure technically difficult to measure.

Another technical problem is the volume of air that must be sampled in order to obtain a quantifiable amount of the allergen. Allergens are often present at low concentrations, and thus several cubic meters may need to be sampled to recover enough allergen to assay reliably. In outdoor air, this is not a problem, since the pool of available air is very large. In indoor air, however, the pool of air is limited by the room size. If the sampler is very efficient, then the air passing through the sampler will be depleted, or "cleaned," of the allergen. If a significant portion of the room air is thus passed through the sampler, then the sampler is effectively cleaning the room air and reducing the allergen level that is being measured.

ELISA assays can measure the allergen content of sample material recovered from various samplers. The size of the particles on which allergens are distributed can be assessed by determining the allergen content of cascade impinger fluids or other air samplers that are selective for particle size. Allergens eluted from the membrane filters of personal exposure "cassette" samplers can also be measured by ELISA assays. These have been used successfully in various settings. Settled dust can also be eluted and the allergen content of the eluate can be measured. Since air sampling is relatively difficult and expensive to do accurately, dust samples are widely used to obtain estimates of allergen exposure.

Although measuring allergens in dust rather than air is not obvious as an exposure index, this is generally regarded as the best available index. Numerous quantitative analyses of indoor environments have now been conducted and show that allergen content in dust does reflect allergen exposure indoors. Dust is usually processed through a 50-mesh (250-μm) sieve to obtain the fine dust fraction. This fine dust contains essentially all of the allergenic material and is more homogeneous (and reproducible) than unsieved dust. Since results are expressed as allergen units per gram of dust, the sieved material is also less likely to be biased by the presence of large (heavy) particles.

B. Assessment

ELISA assays, using monoclonal antibodies directed against specific allergens, have been available since the early 1990s (53). These are objective, are reproducible, are cost-effective, have been widely used, and have produced a sufficiently large database to permit evaluation of what is high or low in the sampled environment. For some allergens, the clinically relevant concentrations have also been estimated. Furthermore, the distribution of allergens within houses and the efficacy of allergen reduction strategies can be assessed. The development of DNA-based techniques (discussed in Section II) to quantify indoor mold may significantly impact the way that indoor mold is measured, if those techniques gain commercial acceptance. A current limitation is the novel aspect of the data, which, as with any new technique, limits the interpretation since there is no previous experience.

C. Mites

Dust mites, distributed in almost all spaces that are occupied by humans, concentrate in upholstered furniture, mattresses, and carpeting, which tend to accumulate human skin scales. There are several major allergens of dust mites. Environmental assessments are most frequently conducted on the group 1 mite allergens, Der p 1 and Der f 1, from *Dermatophagoides pteronyssinus* and *D. farinae*, respectively. These allergens are present on rather large particles (fecal pellets) that settle out of the air quickly. Since these allergens are only transiently airborne, most assessments are conducted from settled dust samples rather than from air. The clinical relevance of this has been challenged, although the consensus of mite allergen researchers is that dust sampling is a practical approach to assessing exposure. Environmental assessment of these allergens in the fine dust fraction requires eluting the dust and measuring the allergen content of the eluate by ELISA. Surfaces to be sampled should be slowly vacuumed, covering 1 m^2 in 2 min. Residential or hand-held (mains-powered) vacuums may be used, with dust collection bags fitted into the vacuum inlet.

Mite exposure can be assessed by directly counting mites in dust, by measuring guanine levels in dust, or by directly measuring the allergen content. Mite counts demand a high level of expertise and require more time than ELISA. Guanine estimates are fast and inexpensive, but may be affected by other components of dust. Guanine estimates may ultimately prove most useful as an initial screening tool to identify samples that are very low or very high. The ELISA assays are relatively fast and require less specialized training than the traditional method of counting and identifying mites. The ELISA assays are also quantitative over the concentration range of interest. Consequently, these ELISAs have been applied and the results have confirmed and extended what was known about mite ecology. Mite allergen levels correlate with mite counts and hence are concentrated in portions of the house with high mite counts. Mite levels, however, vary dramatically from house to house, for reasons that remain unknown. It is clear, though, that further assessments are likely to help elucidate why some houses are more heavily infested than other houses and that the ability to conduct these assessments is now widely available.

Studies have corroborated that building characteristics can influence levels of mite allergen exposure and that young children may be especially affected by elevated mite allergen exposure (54,55). In particular, in New Zealand it was shown that although mite allergens are detectable in many public buildings, the levels are far below those in houses (54). The type of construction of houses and cleaning regimes both significantly affected dust mite allergen levels. Hence, environmental factors can affect the level of exposure. This is of particular concern since exposure relates to allergic asthma development (53,55).

Based on cross-sectional and at least one longitudinal survey, levels of Group 1 allergens below 2 µg/g fine dust are regarded as unlikely to cause allergic disease (53). Levels above 2 µg/g, however, increase the risk of sensitization among atopic individuals. An extensive longitudinal study in Germany substantiated the premise that reduced allergen exposure in early childhood decreases the risk of developing childhood asthma (55). This premise is supported by several studies summarized earlier (53), but in this particular study, the risk of developing allergic asthma was increased at exposure levels as low as 0.8 µ/g. The importance of environmental control—especially in the home—needs to be further emphasized to allergy patients.

D. Mammalian Allergens

The most common aeroallergen exposure from mammals is probably from pets (dogs, cats, rabbits, guinea pigs, etc.). Occupational exposure (for laboratory and farm workers) to mammal allergens is also common; there is also exposure to allergens from pest mammals (domestic mice, rats, etc.). Exposure assessment to these allergens has become possible through the development of ELISA assays directed against the major allergens of these species. The most is known about levels of the major cat allergen, Fel d 1, in houses (53). As with mite allergen exposure, the risk of sensitization is greatly increased with exposure to higher levels of cat allergen in house dust during early childhood (55).

Unlike the insect and mite allergens, however, cat allergen is borne on very small particles (<5 µm diameter) that remain airborne for long periods of time. Thus, airborne measurements are feasible and have shown that significant amounts of allergen remain aloft for long periods of time after disturbance. Although feasible, airborne sampling remains primarily a research tool. In most cases, cat allergen levels are assessed in settled dust, as with mite and cockroach allergens. Levels of cat allergen Fel d 1 above 8 µg/g dust have been associated with symptom development in sensitized individuals. ELISA assays have also been developed for mouse allergen and other specialized allergens.

E. Insect Allergens

A number of insects are either known to or suspected to be able to cause sensitization. Exposure to most of these is outdoors and is seasonal, such as with caddis fly. Except for caddis fly, however, few experimental data are available for these outdoor insect exposures. The most common inhalant allergy to insects is to cockroach, and the exposure is predominantly or exclusively indoors.

Cockroach infestation is generally considered a problem of substandard or crowded housing or a problem of semitropical and tropical regions. The development of ELISA assays for cockroach allergens, however, has provided an objective measure of cockroach allergens in settled dust. Assays are available for the two major allergens from the German cockroach, Bla g 1 and Bla g 2. Bla g 1 cross-reacts with Per a 1, the major allergen from the American cockroach, but Bla g 2 is the more clinically relevant of the German cockroach allergens. Exposure to Bla g 2 levels above 1 unit/g dust are provisionally considered to be a risk factor for sensitization (53). With results of these assessments becoming available, evidence is mounting that cockroach exposure is relatively widespread, at least in the warmer parts of North America and Europe.

Many of the environmental assessment considerations that apply to dust mites also apply to cockroach allergens. The allergens are typically sampled in settled dust rather

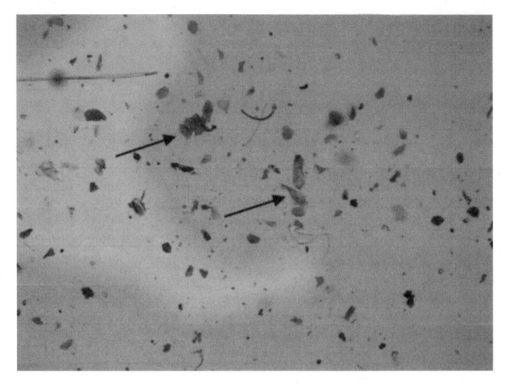

Figure 5 Spore trap sample taken from a clean indoor environment. The predominant particle type is skin scales (arrows). (Original magnification 100x.)

than air. The allergen apparently is on rather large particles and settles quickly; therefore, air monitoring is seldom successful.

F. Fungi

Exposure to fungi occurs indoors as well as outdoors (56). Although all indoor spaces will have some spores that are brought in with outside air, it is generally agreed that indoor spaces should not support active growth of fungi, both for the general health of the occupants and because fungal growth rots the building materials (Fig. 5). Indoor fungal exposures are likely or even unavoidable if there is adequate moisture in the building. Excess moisture in buildings is not desirable. When present, it is usually due to design flaws, inappropriate operating conditions, accidents, or natural disasters. Hence, indoor exposures to fungi occurs. Studies have shown an association between respiratory complaints, including asthma, and moisture or mold in buildings (57–60).

Although the exposure levels that are important for allergic sensitization are not known, active fungal growth often raises spore counts and, theoretically, the risk of allergic sensitization. Active fungal growth—depending on species—may also produce various metabolites, including mycotoxins, glucans, and microbial volatile organic compounds (MVOCs). All of these have been implicated as causing complaints in moldy buildings, although there are no precise, thoroughly documented risk assessments for these exposures. As with any other pollutant, when mold contamination is present, it should be rectified.

Fungi have benefited little from the advances in assessment that have been derived from immunochemical assays for allergens. This is due largely to the complexity of the fungi. Although fungi are often very important indoor allergens, there are usually many species present, rather than only one or two, as with mites, rodents, or pets Each fungus may have numerous allergens—as many as 20 is not unusual—rather than only a few allergens in each species, as for cat, mite, and cockroach. Major fungal allergens have been identified, but only a few have been isolated by traditional methods. Current efforts to produce recombinant fungal allergens may prove to be the most effective way to accumulate sufficient amounts to immunize and to screen for monoclonal antibodies. Assays are available for the major allergens of *Alternaria alternata* and for *Aspergillus fumigatus*.

There have been at least four immunoassays developed for Alt a 1, the major allergen of *A. alternata*. These are based on polyclonal and/or monoclonal antibodies (61–64). The principal application to date has been to aid in the measurement of Alt a 1 in commercial allergen extracts. These assays have also been used to measure the allergen content in dust samples from indoor environments (65). The prevalence of dust samples with detectable levels of Alt a 1 was very low, however; only 6 samples of 1531 tested positive. Although in principle these assays can also be applied to measures of airborne allergen, based on the previous observation, only rather high levels are likely to be detected.

An assay developed with polyclonal and monoclonal antibodies was developed to quantify the major allergen Asp f 1 of *A. fumigatus* (66). The levels of Asp f 1 were greatly increased in actively growing cultures relative to dormant spores. Asp f 1 was detected with this assay in some environm ental samples, but only those samples collected in areas suspected of active mold growth. Asp f 1 levels measured with this assay in dust and in air of office environments failed to detect Asp f 1 in dust and detected low levels of Asp f 1 in less than 5% of air samples (67). Since some samples were from wet building locations where culturable *A. fumigatus* was detected, the presence of Asp f 1 was reasonably expected. The scarcity of samples with detectable Asp f 1 may reflect a very low production of this allergen in indoor environments or interfering environmental substances. However, *A. fumigatus* is not among the molds that most commonly colonize water-damaged materials indoors.

Analysis of fungal aeroallergens is also just beginning to benefit from DNA-based techniques. A system to measure levels of common molds in environmental samples has been developed using quantitative PCR (68). This system has been used to characterize the populations of specific indoor molds (69). The only limitation seems to be in the selection of appropriate target molds. PCR has also been used to reliably quantify total airborne fungi (70). Measures of total airborne fungi may be useful where any mold is undesirable, such as in clinical environments as part of a control program for nosocomial infections. Aeroallergen monitoring needs to distinguish the types of molds, though, which limits the usefulness of this system for that application.

The DNA-based systems measure either all fungi or specific, predetermined fungi. Neither option is optimal for aeroallergen monitoring. Some degree of identification is necessary; counts of total fungi have limited use. However, many fungi are not readily culturable, and many fungal spores are not sufficiently distinctive for identification on spore trap analysis, so there are certainly fungi that are abundant and allergenic but that have never been identified in air samples. Thus, a specific assay that relies on a predetermined "target list" will exclude any previously unrecognized fungal allergens. This will be resolved only by fully characterizing airborne fungal communities. DNA-based techniques such as terminal-RFLP (tRFLP) analysis are used to study both culturable and noncultur-able species in other microbial communities and may be useful in completely determining airborne mold exposure.

Sampling for indoor fungi should be directed toward detecting whether active growth is present or identifying a source (71). In either case, the objective is to eliminate the active growth. If mold growth is visible, then samples of the moldy material may be examined in order to identify the fungus. If mold growth is suspected but not visible, then air sampling may help detect an indoor source. It is important to note that there are no accepted guidelines for safe concentrations of airborne spore levels.

Although other types have been used, the air samplers that are commonly used indoors are impactors, either the culture plate or spore trap type. The same limitations and biases that apply to air samplers apply indoors. The interpretation of indoor spore levels is more complex, though. Spores from outdoors are usually present in indoor air, although at lower levels than outdoors. Hence, spores from indoor fungi must be detected against this background. Since the outdoor spore load also varies, an outdoor sample is always needed in order to determine the expected indoor background. Indoor growth may then be detected by changes in the types of spores in the indoor spore load or by spore concentrations above the current outdoor levels.

There are no stable guidelines for acceptable indoor spore loads. This is due in part to the lack of a well-substantiated relationship between exposure and health effects. Perhaps the best guideline at present is that exposure to active fungal growth indoors should be avoided, as reiterated by several consensus documents (71–73).

Although many fungi, such as *Cladosporium* species, can colonize indoor substrates, *Penicillium* and *Aspergillus* species are often abundant indoors (Fig. 6), especially in problem buildings (72,73). In a study from 1717 buildings across the United States, Shelton et al. (74) found that the most common fungi cultured were *Cladosporium, Penicillium,* nonsporulating fungi, and *Aspergillus.* The conidia of both *Penicillium* and *Aspergillus* are known to be allergenic, and some species of *Aspergillus* are potential human pathogens,

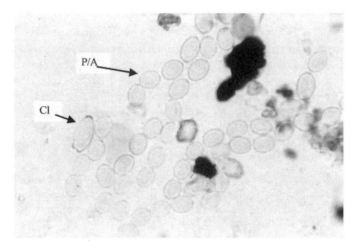

Figure 6   Spore trap sample taken in indoor environment with abundant *Penicillium/Aspergillus*-type spores (P/A). *Penicillium/Aspergillus*-type spores are in chains; *Cladosporium* spore (Cl) is included with three attachment scars. (Original magnification 1000x.)

capable of causing hypersensitivity pneumonitis, sinusitis, and aspergillosis. In addition, some species in both genera are known to produce mycotoxins, the clinical significance of which remains unknown (75). Although these two genera are often the dominant indoor taxa in problem buildings, the attention of the news media has focused primarily on *Stachybotrys chartarum* contamination.

Stachybotrys chartarum is a cellulose-degrading soil fungus in the natural environment. Indoors it is commonly found on water-damaged materials containing cellulose, such as ceiling tiles, the paper facing of gypsum wallboard, cardboard, paper, jute, and straw. Barnes et al. (76) found that 9.4% of patients tested (out of 139) contained IgE antibodies against *S. chartarum*; however, the media frenzy about this fungus relates to its "toxic" properties, not its allergenic properties. Some strains of *S. chartarum* produce numerous mycotoxins, including macrocyclic trichothecenes, which can cause stachybotrytoxicosis in farm animals (77). This condition has a long history and is well accepted in veterinary medicine, and results from the consumption of *Stachybotrys*-colonized wet hay or fodder by horses or other farm animals (78). Also, farm workers handling *Stachybotrys*-contaminated fodder have reported various symptoms, including cough, burning sensation in the mouth, and cutaneous irritation (79). *Stachybotrys* toxins have been suspected as the cause of infant deaths due to pulmonary hemorrhage, although this association is controversial and not proven. The resulting stories in the news media frightened many people and led to the closing of many schools and other public buildings when *Stachybotrys* contamination was discovered. Even more controversial are the claims of neurological effects due to exposure to *Stachybotrys* toxins. Animal studies on rats and mice showing damaging effects of the toxins on pulmonary tissue used very high concentrations of spores instilled intranasally (79,80). Extrapolation of these studies to human respiratory exposure in contaminated buildings is not possible, and in addition, not all strains are toxigenic. Studies (77,78) suggest that isolates identified as *S. chartarum* may actually belong to more than one species, and that these species may have different toxicological properties. Until more data are available, the health effects due to *Stachybotrys chartarum* exposure remain unknown (81,82).

However, the remaining valid questions about mold growth indoors, and *S. chartarum* in particular, will not foster controversy if pragmatic approaches are followed. Barring incidents such as storm damage or plumbing accidents, materials in a building that is well constructed and maintained will not be wet enough for *S. chartarum* or other molds to grow. If mold is growing in a building, repairs are needed and should be made promptly. Further, materials with visible mold growth should be deemed unsanitary, and either cleaned or removed in an appropriate manner. Regardless of the exact mechanism or exposure level involved, pragmatic action to eliminate mold exposure should preclude any health effects and will also prevent the building from rotting.

IV. SALIENT POINTS

1. The science of volumetric aerobiology is about 50 years old.
2. Exposure to pollen and spores varies significantly by season, locale, weather, and even time of day.
3. Pollens have a distinctly seasonal distribution, although some seasons are more confined than others.
4. The mix and concentration of airborne fungal spores are far more variable than those of pollen, both in spatial and temporal patterns.

5. Some pollen and mold allergens are likely associated with fragments or other particles, rather than pollen grains or fungal spores.
6. Available samplers and analysis techniques each have strengths and weaknesses. These should be recognized and considered in designing a sampling or monitoring strategy.
7. Pollen and spore counts reported from a regional station are affected by height of the sampler and proximity to significant sources and regional background levels.
8. Patients should be educated about the variation between regional counts, local exposure, and the time lag inherent in pollen and spore reporting.
9. Exposure to fungal allergens in indoor air may exceed outdoor exposure due to longer periods of time spent indoors and growth of fungi indoors.
10. Epidemiological evidence indicates that exposure to sustained fungal growth indoors may be associated with respiratory complaints. Plausible mechanism(s) include exposure to fungal allergens and/or other metabolites, or a combination of these.

REFERENCES

1. Blackley CH. Experimental Researches on the Causes and Nature of Catarrhus Aestivus (hay fever, asthma). London: Balliere, Tindall & Cox, 1873.
2. Gregory PH. The Microbiology of the Atmosphere. London: London Hill Books, 1961.
3. Lacey J, Venette J. Outdoor air sampling techniques. In: Bioaerosols Handbook (Cox CS, Wathes CM, eds.). Boca Raton, FL: CRC Press, 1995: 407–471.
4. Buttner MP, Willeke K, Grinsphun SA. Sampling and analysis of airborne microorganisms. In: Manual of Environmental Microbiology (Hurst CJ, ed.). Washington, DC: ASM Press, 1997: 629–640.
5. Madelin TM, Madelin MF. Biological analysis of fungi and associated molds. In: Bioaerosols Handbook (Cox CS, Wathes CM, eds.). Boca Raton, FL: CRC Press, 1995: 361–386.
6. Gregory PH, Hirst JM. Possible role of basidiospores as air-borne allergens. Nature (London) 1952; 170:414.
7. Lehrer SB, Hughes JM, Altman LC, Bousquet J, Davies RJ, Gell L, Li J, Lopez M, Malling HJ, Mathison DA, Sastre J, Schultze-Werninghaus G, Schwartz HJ. Prevalence of basidiomycete allergy in the USA and Europe and its relationship to allergic respiratory symptoms. Allergy 1994; 49:460–465.
8. Lopez M, Voigtlander JR, Lehrer SB, Salvaggio JE. Bronchoprovocation studies in basidiospore-sensitive allergic subjects with asthma. J Allergy Clin Immunol 1989; 84:242–246.
9. Horner WE, O'Neil CE, Lehrer SB. Basidiospore aeroallergens. Clin Rev Allergy 1992; 10:191–211.
10. Levetin E, Van de Water P. Pollen count forecasting. Immunol Allergy Clin North Am 2003 (in press).
11. Chapman MD. Analytical methods: Immunoassays. In: Bioaerosols (Burge HA, ed.). Boca Raton, FL: CRC Press, 1995: 235–248.
12. Burge HP, Solomon WR, Boise JR. Comparative merits of eight popular media in aerometric studies of fungi. J Allergy Clin Immunol 1977; 60:199–203.
13. Morring KL, Sorenson WG, Attfield MD. Sampling for airborne fungi: A statistical comparison of media. Am Ind Hyg Assoc J 1983; 44:662–664.
14. Spieksma FTM, Kramps JA, van der Linden AC, Nikkels BH, Plomp A, Koerten HK, Dijkman JH. Evidence of grass-pollen allergenic activity in the smaller micronic atmospheric aerosol fraction. Clin Exp Allergy 1990; 20:273–280.

15. Calderon C, Ward E, Freeman J, Foster SJ, McCartney HA. Detection of airborne inoculum of *Pyrenopeziza brassicae* in oilseed rape crops by polymerase chain reaction (PCR) assays. Plant Pathol 2002; 51:303–310.

16. Calderon C, Ward E, Freeman J, and McCartney HA. Detection of airborne fungal spores sampled by rotating-arm and Hirst-type spore traps using polymerase chain reaction assays. J Aerosol Sci 2001; 33:283–296.

17. Burge HA. Toxigenic potential of indoor microbial aerosols. In: Short-Term Bioassays in the Analysis of Complex Environmental Mixtures, vol. V (Sandhu SS, DeMarini DM, et al., eds.). New York: Plenum, 1987.

18. Miller JD. Fungi as contaminants in indoor air. Atmos Environ 1992; 26:2163–2172.

19. Rantio-Lehtimaki A. Aerobiology of pollen and pollen antigens. In: Bioaerosols Handbook (Cox CS, Wathes CM, eds.). Boca Raton, FL: CRC Press, 1995: 387–406.

20. Ogden EC, Hayes JV, Raynor GS. Diurnal patterns of pollen emissions in Ambrosia, Phleum, zea, and Ricinus. Am J Botany 1969; 56:16–21.

21. Rantio-Lehtimaki A, Helander ML, Pessi A-M. Circadian periodicity of airborne pollen and spores: Significance of sampling height. Aerobiologia 1991; 7:129–135.

22. Trigo MdM, Cabezuda B, Recio M, Toro FJ. Annual, daily and diurnal variations of Urticaceae airborne pollen in Malaga (Spain). Aerobiologia 1996; 12:85–90.

23. Smith EG. Sampling and Identifying Allergenic Pollen and Molds, 1st ed. San Antonio, TX: Blewstone Press, 1984.

24. Anon. The 1996 pollen and spore report. Am Acad Allergy Asthma Immunol 1997.

25. Dahl A, Strandhede S-O. Predicting the intensity of the birch pollen season. Aerobiologia 1996; 12:97–106.

26. Calderon C, Lacey J, McCartney HA, Rosas I. Seasonal and diurnal variation of airborne basidiomycete spore concentrations in Mexico City. Grana 1995; 34:260–268.

27. Kramer CL. Seasonality of airborne fungi. In: Phenology and Seasonality Modeling (Lieth H, ed.) New York: Springer-Verlag, 1974.

28. Horner WE, Helbling A, Salvaggio JE, Lehrer SB. Fungal allergens. Clin Microbiol Rev 1995; 8:161–179.

29. O'Neil CE, Hughes JM, Butcher BT, Salvaggio JE, Lehrer SB. Basidiospore extracts: Evidence of common antigenic/allergenic epitopes. Int Arch Allergy Appl Immunol 1988; 85:161–166.

30. Kendrick B. The Fifth Kingdom 3rd ed. Waterloo, Ontario: Mycologue, 2000.

31. Hamilton ED. Studies on the air spora. Acta Allergol 1959; 13:143–175.

32. McDevitt TJ, Mallea M, Dominick T, Holte KE. Allergic evaluation of cereal smuts Ann Allergy 1977; 38:12–15.

33. Halwagy M. Seasonal airspora at three sites in Kuwait 1977–1982. Mycol Res 1989; 93:208–213.

34. Crotzer V, Levetin E. The aerobiological significance of smut spores in Tulsa, Oklahoma. Aerobiologia 1996; 12:177–184.

35. Aylor DE. The role of intermittent wind in the dispersal of fungal pathogens. Ann Rev Phytopathol 1990; 28:73–92.

36. Burch M, Levetin E. Effect of meteorological conditions on spore plumes. Int J Biometeorol 2002; 46(3):107–117.

37. Haselwandter K, Ebner MR, Frank A. Seasonal fluctuations of airborne fungal allergens. Mycol Res 1989; 92:170–176.

38. Bianchi DE, Scwemmin DJ, Wagner WH. Pollen release in the common ragweed (*Ambrosia artemiiifolia*). Bot Gazette 1959; 4:235–243.

39. Smart IJ, Knox RB. Aerobiology of grass pollen in the city atmosphere of Melbourne: Quantitative analysis of seasonal and diurnal changes. Aust J Bot 1979; 27:317–331.

40. Kapyla M. Diurnal fluctuation of non-arboreal pollen in the air in Finland. Grana 1981; 20:55–59.

41. Rosas I, Escamilla B, Calderon C, Mosino P. The daily variations of airborne fungal spores in Mexico City. Aerobiologia 1990; 6:153–158.

42. Spieksma FTM, Tonkelar JF. Four-hourly fluctuations in grass-pollen concentrations in relation to wet versus dry weather, and to short versus long over-land advection. Int J Biometeorol 1986; 30:351–358.

43. Aylor DE. A framework for examining inter-regional aerial transport of fungal spores. Agricult Meteorol 1986; 38:263–288.

44. Levetin E. Aerobiology of agricultural pathogens. In: Manual of Environmental Microbiology, 2nd ed. (Hurst CJ, Crawford RL, Knudsen GR, McInerney MJ, Stetzenbach LD, eds.). Washington DC: American Society of Microbiology Press, 2002: 884–897.

45. Levetin E, Buck P. Evidence of mountain cedar pollen in Tulsa. Ann Allergy 1986; 56:295–299.

46. Levetin E. A long-term study of winter and early spring pollen in Tulsa, Oklahoma. Aerobiologia 1998; 14:21–28.

47. Rogers C, Levetin E. Evidence of long-distance transport of mountain cedar pollen into Tulsa, Oklahoma. Int J Biometeorol 1998; 42:65–72.

48. Van de Water P, Levetin E. An assessment of predictive forecasting of *Juniperus ashei* pollen movement in the southern Great Plains. Int J Biometeorol 2003 (in press).

49. Van de Water P, Levetin E. The contribution of upwind pollen sources to the characterization of *Juniperus ashei* phenology. Grana 2001; 40:133–141.

50. Norris-Hill J, Emberlin J. Diurnal variation of pollen concentration in the air of north-central London. Grana 1991; 30:229–234.

51. Lyon FL, Kramer CL, Eversmeyer MG. Vertical variation of airspora concentrations in the atmosphere. Grana 1984; 23:123–125.

52. Norris-Hill J. The modelling of daily Poaceae pollen concentrations. Grana 1995; 34:182–188.

53. Johnston RB, et al. Clearing the Air: Asthma and Indoor Air Exposures. Washington, DC: National Academy Press, 2000.

54. Wickens K, Martin I, Pearce N, Fitzharris P, Kent R, Holbrook N, Siebers R, Smith S, Trethowen H, Lewis S, Town I, Crane J. House dust mite allergen levels in public places in New Zealand. J Allergy Clin Immunol 1997; 99:587–593.

55. Wahn U, Lau S, Bergmann R, et al. Indoor allergen exposure is a risk factor for sensitization during the first three years of life. J Allergy Clin Immunol. 1997; 99:763–769.

56. Horner WE, Lehrer SB, Salvaggio JE. Fungi. Immunol Allergy Clin North Am 1994; 14:551–566.

57. Verhoeff AP, Burge HA. Health risk assessment of fungi in home environments. Ann Allergy Asthma Immunol 1997; 78:544–554.

58. Peat JK, Dickerson J, Li J. Effects of damp and mould in home on respiratory health: A review of the literature. Allergy 1998; 53:120–128.

59. Bornehag CG, Blomquist G, Gyntelberg F, Järvholm B, Malmberg P, Nordvall L, Nielsen A, Pershagen G, Sundell J. Dampness in buildings and health. Indoor Air 2001; 11:72–86.

60. Zock J-P, Jarvis D, Luczynska C, Sunyer J, Burney P. Housing characteristics, reported mold exposure, and asthma in the European Community Respiratory Health Survey. J Allergy Clin Immunol 2002; 110:285–292.

61. Portnoy J, Brothers D, Pacheco F, Landuyt J, Barnes C. Monoclonal antibody–based assay for Alt a 1, a major *Alternaria* allergen. Ann Allergy Asthma Immunol 1998; 81:59–64.

62. Aden E, Weber B, Bossert J, Teppke M, Frank E, Wahl R, Fiebig H, Cromwell O. Standardization of *Alternaria alternata*: Extraction and quantification of Alt a 1 by using a mAb-based 2-site binding assay. J Allergy Clin Immunol 1999; 104:128–135.

63. Asturias JA, Arilla MC, Ibarrola I, Eraso E, Gonzalez-Rioja R, Martinez A. A sensitive two-site enzyme-linked immunosorbent assay for measurement of the major *Alternaria alternata* allergen Alt a 1. Ann Allergy Asthma Immunol 2003; 90:529–535.

64. Duffort O, Barber D, Polo F. Quantification assay for the major allergen in *Alternaria alternata*, Alt a 1. Alergol Inmunol Clin 2002; 17:162–168.

65. Vailes L, Shridhara S, Cromwell O, Weber B, Breitenbach M, Chapman M. Quantitation of the major fungal allergens, Alt a 1 and Asp f 1, in commercial allergenic products. J Allergy Clin Immunol 2001; 107:641–666.

66. Arruda LK, Mann BJ, Chapman MD. Slective expression of a major allergen and cytotoxin, Asp f 1, in Aspergillus fumigatus: Implications for the immuno-pathogenesis of Aspergillus-related diseases. J Immunol 1992; 149:3354–3359.

67. Ryan TJ, Whitehead LW, Connor TH, Burau KD. Survey of the Asp f 1 allergen in office environments. Appl Occup Environ Hyg 2001; 16:679–684.

68. Haugland RA, Vesper SJ, Wymer LJ. Quantitative measurement of *Stachybotrys chartarum* conidia using real time detection of PCR products with the TaqMan (TM) fluorogenic probe system. Mol Cell Probes 1999; 13:329–340.

69. Roe JD, Haugland RA, Vesper SJ, Wymer LJ. Quantification of *Stachybotrys chartarum* conidia in indoor dust using real time, fluorescent probe–based detection of PCR products. J Expo Anal Environ Epidemiol 2001; 11:12–20.

70. Zhou G, Whong W-Z, Ong T, Chen B. Development of a fungus-specific PCR assay for detecting low-level fungi in an indoor environment. Mol Cell Probes 2000; 14:339–348.

71. Flannigan B, Miller JD. Overview. In: Health Effects of Fungi in Indoor Environments (Samson RA, Flannigan B, Flannigan ME, Verhoeff AP, Adan OCG, Hoekstra ES, eds.). Amsterdam: Elsevier, 1994.

72. Gravesen A, Nielsen PA, Iversen R, Nielsen KF. Microfungal contamination of damp buildings: Examples of risk constructions and risk materials. Environ Health Perspect 1999; 107(suppl 3):505–508.

73. Flannigan B. Microorganisms in indoor air. In: Microorganisms in Home and Indoor Work Environments (Flannigan B, Samson RA, Miller JD, eds.). New York: Taylor and Francis, 2001: 17–31.

74. Shelton BG, Kirkland KH, Flanders WD, Morris, GK. Profiles of airborne fungi in buildings and outdoor environments in the United States. Appl Environ Microbiol 2002; 68:1743–1753.

75. Yang CS, Johanning E. Airborne fungi and mycotoxins. In: Manual of Environmental Microbiology, 2nd ed. (Hurst CJ, Crawford RL, Knudsen GR, McInerney MJ, Stetzenbach LD, eds.). Washington DC: American Society of Microbiology Press, 2002: 839–852.

76. Barnes C, Buckley S, Pacheco F, Portnoy J. IgE reactive proteins from *Stachybotrys chartarum*. Ann Allergy Asthma Immunol 2002; 89:29–33.

77. Cruse M, Telerant R, Gallagher T, Lee T, Taylor JW. Cryptic species in *Stachybotrys chartarum*. Mycologia 2002; 94:814–822.

78. Andersen B, Nielsen K, Jarvis BB. Characterization of *Stachybotrys* from water-damaged buildings based on morphology, growth, and metabolite production. Mycologia 2002; 94:392–403.

79. Nikulin M, Reijula K, Jarvis BB, Hintikka E-L. Experimental lung mycotoxicosis in mice induced by *Stachybotrys atra*. Int J Exp Pathol 1996; 77:213–218.

80. Rao CY, Brain JD, Burge HA. Reduction of pulmonary toxicity of *Stachybotrys chartarum* spores by methanol extraction of mycotoxins. Appl Environ Microbiol 2000; 66:2817–2821.

81. Burge HA. Fungi: Toxic killers or unavoidable nuisances. Ann Allergy Asthma Immunol 2001; 87(suppl):52–56.

82. Kuhn DM, Ghannoum MA. Indoor mold, toxigenic fungi, and *Stachybotrys chartarum:* Infectious disease perspective. Clin Microbiol Rev 2003; 16:144–172.

9

Pharmacoeconomic Considerations for Allergen Immunotherapy

JONATHAN A. BERNSTEIN

University of Cincinnati College of Medicine, Cincinnati, Ohio, U.S.A.

I. INTRODUCTION

Since the beginning of the 1990s, medical health care reimbursements in the United States have evolved from a loosely controlled fee-for-service system into highly regulated managed-care organizations. Physicians, patients, employers, insurance companies, and local and federal government health agencies have a heightened awareness of increased health care costs and the driving forces behind them. This has resulted in the reexamination of recognized standard approaches for the diagnosis and management of many common medical disorders.

Pharmacoeconomics has emerged as an important means for assessing the cost versus benefit of medical diagnostic procedures and therapeutic interventions. Studies have been conducted for potential new therapeutic agents, educational programs, and diagnostic or screening procedures in almost every medical and surgical specialty. The demonstration that a drug, educational program, or diagnostic/screening procedure improves short- and long-term medical outcomes and improves quality of life in a cost-effective manner, is influential in modifying standard health care approaches.

Pharmacoeconomics has already had a significant impact on the specialty of allergy and clinical immunology. For example, most new investigational drug protocols for the treatment of allergic rhinitis, asthma, and other allergic/immuonological diseases now include quality-of-life questionnaires (1). They also often monitor for changes in such parameters as lost days from school and work, which correlate with indirect costs associated with specific disease management (2). Another example is the advent of asthma self-management programs, which reduce asthma morbidity cost-effectively and are now considered an essential part of the overall care of asthma patients (3,4).

As yet there are no controlled pharmacoeconomic studies assessing the benefits of allergen immunotherapy in the treatment of allergic rhinitis and allergic asthma. One uncontrolled study compared 166 children with asthma receiving immunotherapy with 248 children with asthma on no immunotherapy. After 10 years there was no difference in the number of hospital admissions or quality of life. However, the children receiving immunotherapy experienced fewer acute exacerbations and required fewer drugs (5). No information was provided regarding improvement in lung function. There are reports of high patient satisfaction after immunotherapy, but none of these studies formally address quality of life or cost-effectiveness (6,7).

Because allergen immunotherapy is commonly used to treat allergic diseases, it constitutes a significant cost. Therefore, the benefits of allergen immunotherapy should be scrutinized to determine if it is cost-effective. Since there is a paucity of information on pharmacoeconomics for allergen immunotherapy, a logical analysis must be based on existing experimental data and the current understanding of such treatment.

This chapter focuses on six key factors that must be addressed in order to arrive at proper conclusions regarding the pharmacoeconomics of allergen immunotherapy: (1) prevalence of allergic rhinitis and allergic asthma in the United States; (2) economic impact (direct and indirect costs) associated with the treatment of allergic rhinitis and allergic asthma; (3) efficacy in reducing allergic rhinitis and allergic asthma, preventing the onset of allergic asthma in patients with allergic rhinitis, and limiting the complications associated with allergic rhinitis; (4) proper diagnosis of allergic rhinitis/allergic asthma and selection of patients who will benefit optimally; (5) appropriate initiation; and (6) cost analyses comparing immunotherapy with avoidance measures and the continuous use of medication.

II. PREVALENCE OF ALLERGIC DISEASES

Allergic rhinitis is the most prevalent chronic disease diagnosed in patients 18 years of age or younger (8). It is the fifth most prevalent chronic disease diagnosed by physicians in the United States (8). The National Health Interview Survey distributed by the Centers for Disease Control and Prevention in 1994 indicated that the incidence of allergic rhinitis is 10% (26 million) in the United States and its prevalence is increasing (9). A 23-year follow-up study of college students revealed that the frequency of allergic rhinitis increases with age (10).

A self-administered questionnaire distributed to 15,000 households representative of the U.S. population with respect to gender, age, geographic locale, population density, and household income was used to evaluate the prevalence of allergic rhintis (11). Table 1

Table 1 Prevalence of Self-Diagnosed Allergic Rhinitis[a]

Variable	Percentage
Total	14.2
Gender	
Male	13.7
Female	14.3
Age (years)	
≤17	9.1
18–34	18.4
35–49	17.6
50–64	14.2
≥65	7.8
Region	
Northeast	
New England	13.2
Middle Atlantic	13.8
Midwest	
East North Central	11.7
West North Central	13.7
South	
South Atlantic	13.7
East South Central	12.7
West South Central	15.5
Pacific	
Mountain	20.2
Pacific	16.4
Population density	
Rural (<100,000)	12.4
Urban	
100,000–499,999	12.6
500,000–1,999,999	14.4
≥2 million	15.1
Household income ($)	
<12,500	9.4
12,500–24,999	12.8
25,000–39,999	13.4
40,000–59,999	15.8
≥60,000	15.9

[a] Extrapolated to the total base population of 22,285 responders.
Used with permission from Ref. 11.

summarizes the prevalence of self-diagnosed allergic rhinitis with respect to each of these demographic variables. Extrapolation of this survey's results from 1993 census data indicates that 14.2% of the U.S. population, or at least 35.9 million persons, have allergic rhinitis, and 31.5% of the population, or approximately 79.5 million persons, experience ≥7 days of nasal/ocular symptoms each year (Fig. 1) (11). The results can be critiqued on several points. First, the investigators did not utilize a validated questionnaire; second, they did not confirm with objective testing self-reported symptoms or diagnosis of allergic

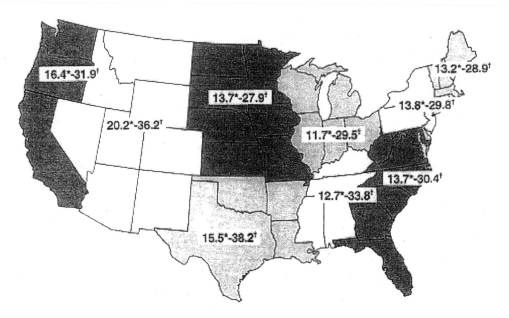

Figure 1 Prevalence by geographic area of patients with allergic rhinitis (*) or ≥7 days of nasal/ocular symptoms in the previous 12 months (†) (11).

rhinitis; third, there was no attempt to distinguish perennial allergic rhinitis from nonallergic rhinitis; and fourth, there was a high nonresponder rate (33.7%). The latter may reflect the likelihood that the majority of individuals who completed and returned the questionnaires might have been symptomatic (11).

The prevalence of allergic diseases is increasing not only in the United States, but in other countries in the world as well (12–14).

III. ECONOMIC IMPACT OF ALLERGIC DISEASES

Cost-analysis study of allergic rhinitis using data from the 1996 Medical Expenditure Panel Survey estimates that 7.7% of the population have allergic rhinitis and that the total direct costs for this disease are $4.6 billion per year. The majority of these costs are attributed to prescription medications (46.6%) and outpatient medical visits (51.9%) (15). The majority of prescription medication costs are for second-generation antihistamines. In addition, 58% of the population surveyed were on more than one medication, with individual medication expenditures ranging from $70 (no insurance) to $213 (comprehensive insurance) per year (15). This same study estimated that the annual direct costs to manage allergic rhinitis patients who are on versus not on allergen immunotherapy were 5.8-fold higher ($661 vs. $114). Costs for outpatient doctor visits for patients on such therapy were $524 versus $42 per year. Finally, annual medication costs were higher for those receiving immunotherapy ($135 vs. $70), and patients with private insurance were more likely to receive immunotherapy (81% vs. 63%).

Cost-analysis studies can be criticized in that they are often associated with underreporting of disease or recall bias, and there is no assessment of disease severity (15). In the preceding case, there was also no attempt to assess morbidity, such as reduction of sinusitis

Table 2   Direct Costs Associated with Self-Reported Allergic Rhinitis in 1993

Item	Millions of dollars/year
Medications	
Prescription	907
Nonprescription	1389
Total	2296
Physician visits[a]	1130
Total overall	3426

[a] Does not include diagnostic tests or allergen immunotherapy.
Used with permission from Ref. 16.

or new-onset asthma—important considerations in evaluating the cost-effectiveness of disease management.

The economic impact of allergic rhinitis is better appreciated when one considers that such patients have a threefold increased risk of developing asthma (14). Therefore, a significant percentage of the approximately 4.5% of the U.S. population who have asthma (nearly 10 million individuals) experience exacerbations in response to allergens and excitants. Collectively, allergic rhinitis and asthma affect approximately 15%, or 40 million people, in the United States. The prevalence of other comorbid features of allergic rhinitis, such as sinusitis and otitis media with effusion, further magnifies the health and economic impact (10,16).

Direct costs for disease management include physician office and emergency room visits, hospitalizations, and pharmacological and avoidance intervention measures. Indirect costs refer to lost income from impairment of an individual's quality of life and missed days from work and school. Table 2 presents the estimated direct costs of treating allergic rhinitis in the United States, which exceed $4.6 billion each year (15,16). This figure does not count indirect costs, which are estimated to approximate or equal direct costs. Conservative estimates of direct costs to treat patients with allergic rhinitis with acute and chronic sinusitis and otitis media with effusion amount to an additional $2.4 billion each year (17). Finally, a portion of the total annual (direct and indirect) costs to treat asthma, now estimated to exceed $13 billion a year, must also be considered since many individuals with allergic rhinitis also have allergic asthma (18). Together, total health care spending in the United States to treat allergic rhinitis and associated conditions approximates $18 billion yearly, almost 3% of total annual health care costs.

IV.   EFFICACY OF ALLERGEN IMMUNOTHERAPY

Both the prevalence of allergic diseases and the magnitude of the associated health care costs require that the advantages and disadvantages of the available therapeutic interventions be carefully examined. Allergen immunotherapy is defined as "the repeated administration of specific allergens to patients with IgE-mediated conditions, for the purpose of providing protection against the allergic symptoms and inflammatory reactions associated with natural exposure to these allergens" (19).

The initial and successful use of allergen immunotherapy was reported by Noon in 1911, and evidence now indicates that such therapy effectively downregulates the

IgE-mediated immune response (19,20). Thus, allergen immunotherapy attenuates the inflammatory responses associated with allergic rhinitis and allergic asthma.

The inability to achieve a better understanding and to truly measure the cost-effectiveness of allergen immunotherapy is magnified by the absence of objective biomarkers with which patients who respond optimally to this treatment can be selected. Similarly, there are no objective tests to determine when the optimal benefits of allergen immunotherapy have been achieved. Allergen skin testing and in vitro assays of specific IgE are useful to confirm potential triggers but are seldom useful for determining whether the duration of allergen immunotherapy is sufficient to induce long-term tolerance (19). This requires the clinician to decide on initiating, continuing, and ultimately discontinuing such therapy based solely on the presence or absence of a patient's symptoms. Helpful criteria to determine clinical improvement include (1) reduction of symptom scores, (2) increased time interval between injections associated with continual improvement in symptoms, (3) improved spirometric outcome for patients with asthma, and (4) reduction of medication requirements.

Allergen immunotherapy is effective in treating allergic rhinitis, allergic conjunctivitis, allergic asthma, and stinging insect hypersensitivity (19,21,22). Double-blind, placebo-controlled studies demonstrate that allergen-specific immunotherapy is effective for seasonal allergies to tree, grass, and ragweed pollen and cat, dust mite, *Alternaria*, and *Cladosporium* induced allergic rhinitis (23–36). Likewise, there are three meta-analyses all indicating that allergen immunotherapy is effective in treating asthma (37–39). Finally, immunotherapy in individuals with Hymenoptera stinging insect–induced anaphylaxis experience almost complete protection from subsequent laboratory or field stings (40). Durham et al. have also demonstrated that effective grass pollen immunotherapy has a long-lasting effect on patients with allergic rhinitis that obviates the need for medical management for several years after discontinuation, a further tribute to its cost-effectiveness (41). More significantly, a prospective specific pollen immunotherapy trial has demonstrated that this treatment can decrease the progression to asthma in children with seasonal rhinoconjunctivitis (42,43).

V. PROPER DIAGNOSIS AND PATIENT SELECTION FOR IMMUNOTHERAPY

The effectiveness of allergen immunotherapy does not necessarily indicate that it offers distinct advantages over other forms of therapy. The decision to initiate such therapy must consider other factors. A primary consideration for initiating allergen immunotherapy requires an accurate diagnosis of allergic rhinitis, allergic asthma, or Hymenoptera hypersensitivity. To ensure that patients selected for immunotherapy will benefit, it is essential that a detailed history be obtained to differentiate allergic from nonallergic rhinitis and/or asthma with confirmation by allergy skin testing or by specific IgE in vitro assays using standard methods of application and interpretation (44). The Joint Task Force on Practice Parameters for Allergy Diagnostic Testing has published consensual guidelines for allergen skin testing (45). These highlight the fact that proper training and expertise are required for the application and interpretation of allergy skin tests and in vitro specific IgE tests. The Food and Drug Administration has developed a standardized method to ensure proficiency of skin testing for assessing the potency of allergen extracts (46). Close attention to optimal skin testing methods will prevent the incorrect interpretation of skin test results and inappropriate use of allergen immunotherapy.

Studies confirm that management of patients with allergic rhinitis and/or allergic asthma by allergists provides more effective and cost-efficient clinical outcomes (47). This is attributed to more accurate recognition of allergic disease and minimization of inappropriate treatment and ultimately complications. Pharmacoeconomic studies assessing the cost-effectiveness of allergen immunotherapy must account for the savings in health care costs that allergists/immunologists achieve by adhering to standard recommendations to diagnose allergic diseases and appropriately administer allergen immunotherapy.

VI. APPROPRIATE INITIATION OF ALLERGEN IMMUNOTHERAPY

The guidelines for initiating allergen immunotherapy require sound decision analysis based on clinical experience and knowledge of immunopathogenic allergic mechanisms (21). The consensus recommendations by the Joint Task Force on Practice Parameters for initiating allergen immunotherapy are (1) correlation of symptoms and clinical course with evidence of specific IgE to relevant allergens, (2) inability to adequately control symptoms with avoidance measures and appropriate medications, (3) patient concerns and apprehensions about pharmacotherapy versus allergen immunotherapy, and (4) the absence of significant risk for systemic allergic reactions (19,21).

The first criterion for initiating immunotherapy—correlating symptoms with appropriate evidence of specific IgE sensitization—was covered in Section V. Second, patients, when appropriate, should be educated on practical avoidance measures for indoor and outdoor allergens in the home and work environments (19,48,49). Compliance with such recommendations is often poor. Patients often perceive environmental avoidance measures as impractical and impacting negatively on their quality of life. For example, patients allergic to their pets often have strong emotional attachments to them and are not willing to remove them from their homes. Most dust mite–sensitive patients, even when requested to do so, do not implement dust mite avoidance measures. Patients allergic to outdoor aeroallergens often have to restrict their outdoor activity during the peak pollen seasons (50).

Allergists/immunologists should be more knowledgeable about the cost-effectiveness of scientifically based avoidance measures to be more effective in educating their patients about their benefits. For example, it is not always necessary to remove pets from the home of an allergic patient. Removing the animal from the bedroom, applying bedding encasements, and using a free-standing HEPA filter and a HEPA vacuum cleaner significantly reduce animal allergen levels (51).

To maximize compliance, physicians should question patients during each office visit about the measures they have taken in their home or workplace to reduce indoor allergen exposure. Continuous reinforcement about the long-term benefits of allergen avoidance is essential to maximize patient compliance (52). Avoidance measures should improve patient response to medication and/or allergen immunotherapy.

Third, the initial treatment of allergic rhinitis should include a medication regimen tailored to the severity of the patient's symptoms and tolerance of medications (44). However, even though medications are often effective for symptomatic control, many patients do not want to use them chronically or experience side effects from them, which limits their use (44). Patients' wishes and/or apprehensions about any form of therapy are an integral part of their individualized care.

The fourth criterion for initiating immunotherapy is to be sure that the patient has no contraindications and is at no significant risk for systemic allergic reactions. Contraindications include a high risk factor for a systemic reaction, poorly controlled asthma, significant immunodeficient disease, heart disease, autoimmune disease, and the need for medication such as a beta-blocker (19,21,22).

VII. COST ANALYSIS: MEDICATION VERSUS ALLERGEN IMMUNOTHERAPY

Pharmacological treatment of allergic rhinitis often includes the combined use of a topical intranasal corticosteroid spray (~$69 per prescription) and a nonsedating antihistamine with or without a decongestant (~$70–100 for a 30-day supply), costing a maximum of approximately $170/month or $2040 per year and $10,200 for 5 years. This treatment does not include the cost of physician office visits, antibiotics for secondary sinus or otitis media infections, and the indirect costs that result from missed days at school and work. The costs for treating asthma are even more substantial, especially when one considers that many patients with asthma have concomitant allergic rhinitis (15). Treatment of asthma each month commonly includes, at the very least, a short- and/or long-acting β_2-agonist bronchodilator (~$30 per canister for a short-acting β_2-agonist and ~$100 per 30-day supply for a long-acting β_2-agonist) and an inhalational glucocorticosteroid (~$65 for low dose, $93 for moderate dose, $137 for high dose), the combined cost of which is approximately $1930–2910 each year if all of these medications are required. This cost for drugs does not include other direct and indirect expenses.

The average cost of appropriately prescribed allergen immunotherapy over a 5-year period is less than the cost of treatment with medication alone, and favorable results lead to reduced requirements for and discontinuation of the use of medications. Table 3 illustrates the costs to provide immunotherapy to a patient for 5 years in three different medical facilities in the United States (53). The average 5-year cost to administer immunotherapy is approximately $2000 compared with over $10,000 for medication alone. Assuming a most conservative estimate of 50% efficacy for immunotherapy and a 50% reduction of medication, the combined total cost of allergen immunotherapy and medication compared with medication alone is still less expensive ($5000 vs. $10,000). However, after 5 years, medication alone would have been effective only in controlling symptoms and not in

Table 3   Cost Comparison of Immunotherapy at Three Separate Institutions with Daily Medication Use over 5 Years in the United States

	Year 1	Year 2	Year 3	Year 4	Year 5	Total 5 years[a]
Site 1[b]	$1774	$750	$750	$750	$750	$4773
Site 2[b]	$1690	$755	$755	$755	$755	$4710
Site 3[b]	$1974	$646	$646	$646	$646	$4560
Medications[c]	$2040	$2040	$2040	$2040	$2040	$10,200

[a] Total costs do not include the cost of a yearly office visit to assess the patient's progress on immunotherapy. Reimbursement for allergy injections will vary regionally across the United States and between insurance carriers. Costs are based on receiving two injections each visit; if maintenance injections are given more frequently than once a month, costs will be higher.
[b] Estimated costs from a center in each of three different parts of the United States.
[c] Estimated annual medication costs if an antihistamine/decongestant and intranasal corticosteroid spray are used on a daily basis; prices will vary geographically and between pharmacies.
Source: Ref. 53.

modifying the underlying allergic immune response, the major advantage of allergen immunotherapy. The disappearance of symptoms or absence of progression of disease to asthma after long-term immunotherapy implies a further economic advantage (41).

These estimated economic benefits of allergen immunotherapy are not supported by the cost analysis survey previously cited (15). This may reflect a lack of a standardized approach to diagnose allergic disease and initiate immunotherapy. A discussion of the economic advantages of allergen immunotherapy, however, is incomplete without taking into consideration quality-of-life issues, which are included in this cost analysis. The Rhinoconjunctivitis Quality of Life Questionnaire (RQLQ) is an example of a disease-specific instrument used to assess patients with allergic rhinitis (1,2). Table 4 summarizes the quality-of-life parameters that are measured by this questionnaire (54), and Fig. 2 illustrates an example of RQLQ profiles of subjects experiencing nasal/ocular symptoms (54). Individuals exhibit consistently higher scores, directly corresponding to a poorer quality of life, compared with normal healthy controls. Therefore, disease-specific quality-of-life questionnaires, such as the RQLQ questionnaire, provide a quantitative method for approximating indirect costs associated with poorly controlled diseases such as allergic rhinitis and allergic asthma.

VIII. CONCLUSIONS

Given the preponderance of evidence demonstrating the effectiveness of allergen immunotherapy, the question that needs to be addressed is not whether immunotherapy

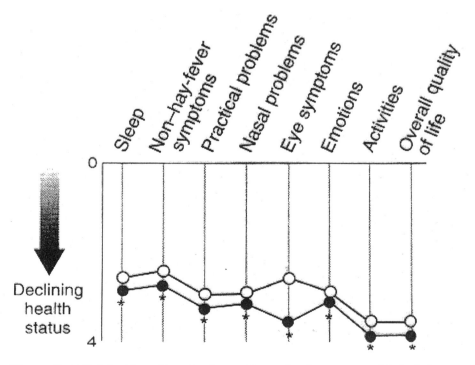

Figure 2 RQLQ health profiles of patients with nasal/ocular symptoms (black circles; $n = 312$) versus healthy controls (white circles; $n = 96$). Higher score indicates poorer health status. *$p < 0.01$ versus control. (From Ref. 54.)

Table 4 Quality-of-Life Parameters Measured by the Rhinoconjunctivitis Quality of Life Questionnaire

Dimension (items)

Sleep
   Lack of a good night's sleep
   Wake during the night
   Difficulty getting to sleep
Non–hay fever symptoms
   Tiredness
   Fatigue
   Worn out
   Reduced productivity
   Poor concentration
   Thirst
   Headache
Practical problems
   Need to blow nose repeatedly
   Need to rub nose/eyes
   Inconvenience of having to carry
   tissues or handkerchief
Nasal symptoms
   Stuffy/blocked
   Sneezing
   Runny
   Itchy
Eye symptoms
   Itchy
   Watery
   Swollen
   Sore
Emotions
   Irritable
   Frustrated
   Impatient or restless
   Embarrassed by nose/eye symptoms

Activities[a]
   Bicycling
   Cooking
   Dancing
   Doing home maintenance
   Doing housework
   Gardening
   Eating
   Jogging, exercising, or running
   Attending public events
   Driving a car
   Watching TV or a movie
   Singing
   Mowing the lawn
   Playing with pets
   Doing regular social activities
   Talking (public speaking)
   Studying or doing homework
   Taking a test or quiz
   Visiting friends or relatives
   Going for a walk
   Having sexual intercourse
   Carrying out activities at work
   Reading
   Playing sports

[a] Examples listed in the questionnaire. Subjects may provide additional activities.
Borrowed with permission from Ref. 54.

should be implemented to treat allergic rhinitis, allergic asthma, and Hymenoptera sensitivity, but rather at what point during the course of disease it should be implemented. A study published in 1968 indicates that children with allergic rhinitis treated with immunotherapy have significantly reduced chances of later developing asthma (55). A European study confirms this observation (43). Early treatment intervention with allergen immunotherapy in patients with allergic rhinitis or mild allergic asthma downmodulates inflammatory responses and lessens the severity of future disease (43,55). Another investigation found that early intervention, including immunotherapy, in the management of allergic rhinitis and asthma by an allergist/immunologist is more effective in improving clinical outcomes while reducing overall resource utilization and net costs than care provided by a general internist (47). Expert care encompasses specialized clinical, pharmaceutical, and immunological skills, including allergen immunotherapy. Although the optimal time to implement such therapy has not been determined, it should be administered early in the course of the disease, based on the same rationale used to recommend early introduction of inhaled glucocorticoids to treat asthma to reduce disease severity and improve clinical outcomes (56,57).

Further outcome studies are necessary to determine more precisely the cost-effectiveness of allergen immunotherapy compared with the chronic use of medications and avoidance measures. Such studies should take into account indirect costs and quality-of-life issues. Since the course of allergic rhinitis or allergic asthma is variable among individuals, such studies are difficult to do. Cost-effectiveness analysis studies using "construction and analysis of reference case" methods may prove useful to better demonstrate the beneficial pharmacoeconomic impact of allergen immunotherapy to treat allergic diseases (58–60).

IX. SALIENT POINTS

1. Allergic diseases, which include allergic rhinitis and allergic asthma, are prevalent in the United States. Hymenoptera hypersensitivity affects up to 0.4% of the population.
2. The direct and indirect costs of allergic rhinitis, allergic asthma, and their complications (i.e., sinusitis and otitis media) in the United States approach $18 billion each year.
3. The average cost of allergen immunotherapy over a 5-year period is less expensive than treatment with medication alone.
4. Early intervention with allergen immunotherapy in appropriately selected patients with allergic rhinitis reduces the likelihood that the patient will develop allergic asthma.
5. Controlled pharmacoeconomic cost-effective studies are needed to compare allergen immunotherapy, pharmacological therapy, and avoidance measures for the management of allergic rhinitis and allergic asthma.
6. Future outcome studies should incorporate quality-of-life evaluations to compare direct and indirect costs of allergen immunotherapy with the costs of medications and avoidance measures.

REFERENCES

1. Juniper EF, Guyatt GH. Development and testing of a new measure of health status for clinical trials in rhinoconjunctivitis. Clin Exp Allergy 1991; 21:77–83.
2. Juniper EF, Guyatt GH, Dolovich J. Assessment of quality of life in adolescents with allergic rhinoconjunctivitis: Development and testing a questionnaire for clinical trials. J Allergy Clin Immunol 1994; 93:413–423.
3. Kotses H, Bernstein IL, Bernstein DI, et al. A self-management program for adult asthma. Part I: Development and evaluation. J Allergy Clin Immunol 1995; 95:529–540.
4. Taitel MS, Kotses H, Bernstein IL, et al. A self-management program for adult asthma. Part II: Cost-benefit analysis. J Allergy Clin Immunol 1995; 95:672–676.
5. Calvo M, Marin F, Grob K, Sanhaera M, Kylling L, Alborniz C, Stickler A. Ten-year follow-up in pediatric patients with allergic bronchial asthma: Evaluation of specific immunotherapy. J Investig Allergol Clin Immunol 1994; 4:126–131.

6.   Gozalo-Reques F, Estrada-Rodriquez JL, Martin Hurtado S, Alvarez Cuesto E. Patient satisfaction and allergen immunotherapy. J Investig Allergol Clin Immunol 1999; 9:101–105.

7.   Yilmaz M, Bingol G, Altintas D, Kendirli SG. Effect of SIT on quality of life. Allergy 2000; 55:302.

8.   Naclerio RM. Allergic rhinitis. N Eng J Med 1991; 325:860–869.

9.   Adams PF, Marano MA. Current estimates from the National Health Interview Survey, 1994. In: Vital and Health Statistics. U.S. Dept. of Health and Human Services Publication (PHS) 96–1521. Series 10, no. 193. Hyattsville, MD: National Center for Health Statistics, 1995.

10. Settipane RJ, Hagy GW, Settipane GA. Long-term risk factors for developing asthma and allergic rhinitis: A 23-year follow-up of college students. Allergy Proc 1984; 15:21–25.

11. Nathan RA, Meltzer EO, Selner JC, Storms W. Prevalence of allergic rhinitis in the United States. J Allergy Clin Immunol 1997; 99:S808–S814.

12. Wright AL, Holberg CJ, Marinez FD, et al. Epidemiology of physician-diagnosed allergic rhinitis in childhood. Pediatrics 1994; 94:895–901.

13. Royal College of General Practitioners, Office of Population Censuses and Surveys, Department of Health and Social Security. Morbidity Statistics from General Practice 1981–82: Third National Study. Series MB5, no 1. London: Her Majesty's Stationery Office, 1986.

14. Aberg N. Asthma and allergic in Swedish conscripts. Clin Exp Allergy 1989; 19:59–63.

15. Law AW, Reed SD, Sundy JS, Schulman KA. Direct costs of allergic rhinitis in the United States: Estimates from the 1996 Medical Expenditure Panel Survey. J Allergy Clin Immunol 2003; 111:296–300.

16. Storms W, Meltzer EO, Nathan RA, Selner JC. The economic impact of allergic rhinitis. J Allergy Clin Immunol 1997; 99:S820–S824.

17. Kaliner MA, Osguthorpe JD, Fireman P, et al. Sinusitis: Bench to bedside. J Allergy Clin Immunol 1997; 99:S829–S848.

18. Weiss KB, Gergen PJ, Hodgson TA. An economic evaluation of asthma in the United States. N Engl J Med 1992; 326:862–866.

19. Nicklas RA, Bernstein IL, Blessing-Moore J, et al. Practice parameters for allergen immunotherapy. J Allergy Clin Immunol 1996; 98:1001–1011.

20. Noon L. Prophylactic inoculation against hay fever. Lancet 1911; 1:1572–1573.

21. Li JT, Lockey RF, Bernstein IL, et al., eds. Allergen immunotherapy: A practice parameter. Ann Allergy Asthma Immunol 2003; 90:1–40.

22. Bousquet J, Lockey RF, Malling H-J, eds. WHO Position Paper: Allergen immunotherapy: Therapeutic vaccines for allergic diseases. Eur J Allergy Clin Immunol 1998; 53:1–42.

23. Frankland AW, Augustin R. Prophylaxis of summer hay fever and asthma: A controlled trial comparing crude grass-pollen extracts with the isolated main protein component. Lancet 1954; 1:1055–1057.

24. Lowell FC, Franklin W. A double-blind study of the effectiveness and specificity of injection therapy in ragweed hay fever. N Engl J Med 1965; 273:675–679.

25. Pence HL, Mitchell DQ, Greely RL, Updegraff BR, Selfridge HA. Immunotherapy for mountain cedar pollinosis: A double-blind controlled study. J Allergy Clin Immunol 1976; 58:39–50.

26. Ahlstedt S, Eriksson NE. Immunotherapy in atopic allergy-antibody titres and avidities during hyposensitization with birch and timothy pollen allergens. Int Arch Allergy 1977; 55:400–411.

27. Ohman JL Jr, Marsh DG, Goldman M. Antibody responses following immunotherapy with cat pelt extract. J Allergy Clin Immunol 1982; 69:319–326.

28. Ohman JL, Findlay SR, Leitermann KM. Immunotherapy in cat-induced asthma: Double-blind trial with evaluation of *in vivo* and *in vitro* responses. J Allergy Clin Immunol 1984; 74:230–239.

29. Taylor WW, Ohman JL, Lowell FC. Immunotherapy in cat-induced asthma: Double-blind trial with evaluation of bronchial responses to at allergen and histamine. J Allergy Clin Immunol 1978; 61:283–287.

30. Chapman MD, Platts-Mills TAE, Gabriel M, Ng HK, Allan WG, Hill LE, Nunn AJ. Antibody response following prolonged hyposensitization with *Dermatophagoides pteronyssinus* extract. Int Arch Allergy 1980; 61:431–440.

31. D'Souza MF, Pepys J, Wells ID, Tai E, Palmer F, Overell BG, McGrath IT, Megson M. Hyposensitization with *Dermatophagoides pteronyssinus* in house dust allergy: A controlled study of clinical and immunologic effects. Clin Allergy 1973; 3:177–193.

32. Metzger WJ, Donnelly BA, Richerson HB. Modification of late asthmatic responses (LAR) during immunotherapy for *Alternaria*-induced asthma. J Allergy Clin Immunol 1983; 71:119.

33. Horst M, Hejjaoui A, Horst V, et al. Double-blind, placebo-controlled rush immunotherapy with a standardized *Alternaria* extract. J Allergy Clin Immunol 1990; 85:460–472.

34. Dreborg S, Agrell B, Foucard T, Kjellman NI, Koivikko A, Nilsson S. A double-blind multi-center immunotherapy trial in children using a purified and standardized *Cladosporium herbarum* preparation: I. Clinical results. Allergy Clin Immunol 1986; 131:140.

35. Malling H-J. Diagnosis and immunotherapy of mold allergy: V. Clinical efficacy and side effects immunotherapy with *Cladosporium herbarum*. Allergy 1986; 41:505–519.

36. Adkinson NF, Eggleston PA, Eney D, et al. A controlled trial of immunotherapy for asthma in allergic children. N Eng J Med 1997; 336:324–331.

37. Abramson MJ, Puy RM, Weiner JM. Allergen immunotherapy effective in asthma? A meta-analysis of randomized controlled trials. Am J Respir Crit Care Med 1995; 151:969–974.

38. Bousquet J, Michel FB, Malling HJ. Is allergen immunotherapy effective in asthma? A meta-analysis of randomized clinical trials. Am J Respir Crit Care Med 1995; 152:1737–1738.

39. Klimek L, Malling HJ. Specific immunotherapy (hyposensitization) in allergic rhinoconjuctivitis: Meta-analysis of effectiveness and side effects. HNO 1999; 47:602–610.

40. Hunt KJ, Valentine MD, Sobotka AK, et al. A controlled trial of immunotherapy in insect hypersensitivity. N Engl J Med 1978; 299:157–161.

41. Durham SR, Walker SM, Varga EM, Jacobson MR, O'Brien F, Noble W, Till SJ, Hamid QA, Novri-Aria KT. Long-term clinical efficacy of grass-pollen immunotherapy. N Engl J Med 1999; 341:468–475.

42. Moller C, Dreborg S, Ferdousi HA, et al. Pollen immunotherapy reduces the development of asthma in children with seasonal rhinoconjunctivitis (the PAT-study). J Allergy Clin Immunol 2002; 109:251–256.

43. Jacobsen L, Moller C, Dreborg S, et al. Five-year follow-up on the PAT study: A 3-year course of specific immunotherapy (SIT) results in long-term prevention of asthma in children. Paper presented at the EAACI in Paris, 6/03.

44. Bernstein JA. Allergic rhinitis: Helping patients lead an unrestricted life. Postgrad Med 1993; 93:124–132.

45. Bernstein IL, Storms WW. Practice parameters for allergy diagnostic testing. Ann Allergy 1995; 75:543–625.

46. Turkeltaub PC. Proficiency Test Method. Rockville MD: U.S. Food and Drug Administration, Center for Biologics Evaluation and Research, Office of Vaccines Research and Review, Division of Allergenic Products and Parasitology.

47. Vollmer WM, O'Hollaren M, Ettinger KM, Stibolt T, Wilkins J, Buist AS, Linton KL, Osborne ML. Specialty differences in the management of asthma. Arch Intern Med 1997; 157:1201–1208.

48. Duff AL, Platts-Mills TA. Allergens and asthma. Pediatr Clin North Am 1992; 39(6):1277–1291.

49. Ehnert B, Lau-Schadendorf S, Weber A, et al. Reducing domestic exposure to dust mite allergen reduces bronchial hyperreactivity in sensitive children with asthma. J Allergy Clin Immunol 1992; 90:135–138.

50. Huss K, Squire EN Jr, Carpenter GB, et al. Effective education of adults with asthma who are allergic to dust mites. J Allergy Clin Immunol 1992; 89:836–843.

51. van der Heide S, Kauffman HF, Bubois AE, de Monchy JG. Allergen reduction measures in houses of allergic asthmatic patients: Effects of air-cleaners and allergen impermeable mattress covers. Eur Respir J 1997; 10:1217–1223.

52. Callahan KA, Eggleston PA, Rand CS, et al. Knowledge and practice of dust mite control by specialty care. Ann Allegy Asthma Immunol 2003; 90:302–307.

53. Sullivan TJ, Selner JC, Patterson R, et al. Expert care and immunotherapy for asthma. Am Coll Allergy Asthma Immunol 1996; 1–25.

54. Meltzer EO, Nathan RA, Selner JC, Storms W. Quality of life and rhinitic symptoms: Results of a nationwide survey with the SF-36 and RQLQ questionnaires. J Allergy Clin Immunol 1997; 99:S815–S819.

55. Johnstone DE, Dutton A. The value of hyposensitization therapy for bronchial asthma in children: A 14-year study. Pediatrics 1968; 42(5):793–802.

56. Konig P, Shaffer J. The effect of drug therapy on long-term outcome of childhood asthma: A possible preview of the international guidelines. J Allergy Clin Immunol 1996; 98:1103–1111.

57. Agertoft L, Pedersen S. Effects of long-term treatment with an inhaled corticosteroid on growth and pulmonary function in asthmatic children. Respir Med 1994; 88:84–87.

58. Weinstein MC, Siegel JE, Gold MR, Kamlet MS, Russell LB. Recommendations of the Panel on Cost-Effectiveness in Health and Medicine. J Am Med Assoc 1996; 276:1253–1258.

59. Russell LB, Gold MR, Siegel JE, Daniels N, Weinstein MC. The role of cost-effectiveness analysis in health and medicine. J Am Med Assoc 1996; 276:1172–1777.

60. Smith JM. Effectively costing out options. J Am Med Assoc 1996; 276:1180.

10

Tree Pollen Allergens

NADINE MOTHES, KERSTIN WESTRITSCHNIG, and RUDOLF VALENTA

University of Vienna, Vienna Medical School, Vienna, Austria

I. INTRODUCTION

IgE-mediated allergy affects more than 25% of the population (1). Besides mites and grass pollen, trees are the most important allergen sources (2). Pollen, fruits, and seeds are the major allergen-containing elements in trees. Wind-pollinated trees with heavy pollen production are the major sources of respiratory allergens. Other trees bear fruits and seeds that may cause different forms of food allergy. In the northern and middle parts of Europe and North America and in certain parts of Australia, birch (*Betula verrucosa*), belonging to the order Fagales, represents the most important elicitor of respiratory manifestations of allergy (e.g., rhinitis, conjunctivitis, and asthma) (3). Other trees belonging to the same botanical order (hazel, alder, hornbeam, oak, and chestnut) contain cross-reactive allergens and also represent major triggers of allergic symptoms (4). Botanically distinct tree species (e.g., Rosaceae) may contain allergens in their seeds (fruits), which cross-react with pollen allergens and therefore elicit food allergy in pollen-allergic individuals (5,6).

The order Fagales represents the predominant allergen source in the northern parts of Europe and America, as well as in certain areas of Australia. Pollen from olive trees and cypress are abundant in the Mediterranean area. Japanese cedar is prominent in Japan. Plantain is found in the Mediterranean area as well as in America. Maple trees, found in America, may also represent a relevant allergen source (7–10). Plants that are wind pollinated are the most potent allergen sources, in contrast to insect-pollinated plants, which rarely elicit allergic symptoms. The allergens of these sources are mostly known and have been identified and characterized using cDNA cloning techniques (reviewed in 11). The tree pollen allergens characterized to date represent low-molecular-weight intracellular proteins or glycoproteins that are rapidly released after contact with aqueous solutions (12,13). Mucosal contact with the allergen molecules leads to allergic sensitization, a process characterized by the production of allergen-specific IgE antibodies (reviewed in 14).

An exciting development was the discovery that cross-reactivity observed among certain species (e.g., trees belonging to the order Fagales) can be attributed to the structural and immunological similarity of relevant cross-reactive allergens (summarized in 4). This finding implies that diagnosis and immunotherapy may be performed with a few cross-reactive marker allergens that harbor a large proportion of the cross-reactive epitopes (11,15–17).

II. TAXONOMY

Among the 250,000 well-described pollen-producing plant species existing, fewer than 100 represent potent sources in terms of pollen allergy (7,8,18,19). Pollens of closely related trees contain cross-reactive allergen molecules (e.g., order Fagales—major birch pollen allergen, Bet v 1) that are absent in pollen from unrelated trees (subclass: Rosidae, genus *Prunus)* but present in their fruits (apple, cherry) (20). Table 1 displays the taxonomy of the most relevant allergenic plants with emphasis on trees and highlights the most common allergenic sources with asterisks. While the subclass Rosidae (e.g., apple, cherry) mainly represents a source of allergenic fruits, Coniferophytina (e.g., cypress, pine), Hamamelididae (e.g., birch, alder, hazel, oak, beech) and Asteridae (e.g., olive, plantain) represent trees that are potent sources of pollen allergens. In general, trees that are wind pollinated tend to represent more relevant allergen sources than trees that are insect-pollinated. Among the Coniferophytina, the genera *Cupressus* (e.g., cypress), *Pinus* (e.g., pine), and *Cryptomeria* (e.g., cedar) are the most important sources of pollen allergens (Table 1). The Hamamelididae comprise weeds and trees. Among them, the order Fagales contains the most potent elicitors of tree pollen allergy [families Betulaceae (e.g., birch), Fagaceae (e.g., beech), and Corylaceae (e.g., hazel)]. Among the Asteridae, again including trees and weeds, the family Oleaceae—in particular *Olea* (olive)—represents the major tree pollen allergen source. The botanical relationships shown in Table 1 are summarized according to Ref. 3.

III. TREE POLLEN IDENTIFICATION

Pollen grains represent single cells that are enclosed within an inner wall, the intine, and an outer wall, the exine. The walls protect the pollen during distribution and contain

Table 1 Taxonomy of the Most Relevant Allergenic Plants—**Plantae**

Magnoliophyta—Angiosperms				Pinales
Hamamelides	**Rosidae**	**Dillenidae**	**Asteridae**	
Fagales	**Fabales**	**Salicales**	**Scrophulariales**	**Pinales**
Fagaceae*	Fabaceae	Salicaceae	Oleaceae*	Pinaceae
Fagus (beech)	*Acacia* (wattle)	*Salix* (willow)	*Olea* (olive)	*Pinus* (pine)
Quercus (white oak)	*Prosopis* (mesquite)	*Populus* (cottonwood)	*Fraxinus* (ash)	Cupressaceae*
Castanea (chestnut)	**Myrtales**		*Ligustrum* (privet)	*Cupressus* (cypress)
Betulaceae*	Myrtaceae		*Syringa* (lilac)	*Juniperus* (cedar)
Betula (birch)	*Eucalyptus*		Plantaginaceae	Taxodiaceae
Alnus (alder)	*Melaleuca*		*Plantago* (plantain)	*Cryptomeria* (sugi)
Corylaceae*	**Sapindales**			
Corylus (hazel)	Aceraceae			
Carpinus (hornbeam)	*Acer* (maple)			
Ostrya (hop hornbeam)				
Hamamelidales				
Platanaceae				
Platanus (plane tree)				
Urticales				
Ulmaceae				
Ulmus (elm)				
Juglandales				
Juglandaceae				
Juglans (walnut)				
Carya (hickory)				

Plants are listed following taxonomical guidelines. Classifications are printed in bold: kingdom, division, class, subclass, and order. Family names are underlined. The most common trees causing allergic symptoms are highlighted with asterisks.

Taxonomical classification of tree species producing allergenic pollen is according to the Integrated Taxonomic Information System (http://www.itis.usda.gov). For further information see also Watson L, Dallwitz MJ. The Families of Flowering Plants: Descriptions, Illustrations, Identification, and Information Retrieval (1992 onward). Version: 14 December 2000 (http://biodiversity.bio.uno.edu/delta/angio/).

apertures, the number, position, and features of which help to identify the originating species by light microscopy (7). It is important to collect air samples and to identify and analyze pollen and other allergen sources for several reasons. Measurements of pollen loads during certain periods of the year permit prediction of allergen exposure, and such information can be distributed to allergic patients to help them avoid exposure (9). The allergist needs to know which species of allergenic pollen are present in the atmosphere, the number of allergenic pollen grains in a given volume of air, and the time and spatial variations of concentrations of airborne allergenic pollen. Knowledge of pollen loads during certain periods and in certain countries also allows allergic patients to plan their vacations and traveling schedules (21). An interesting correlation between date of birth and sensitization against certain pollen has been described. Children who were born in early spring and summer are more frequently sensitized against birch and grass pollen, respectively (22). There is also compelling evidence that sensitization to certain pollen (e.g., birch) is more common in children with heavy pollen exposure early in life than in children who experienced mild pollen exposure (23).

A number of methods are used to collect and quantitate pollen in the air (24). One of the most widely used techniques is the rotorod system (Stanford Research Institute, California), which consists of a rotating impact sampler and uses the suction trapping technique. The rotorod system measures average concentration during the sampling period but fails to detect variations in concentration within this period. Volumetric traps allow continuous isokinetic sampling and record variations in the concentrations of pollen and spores during the sample period. The collected samples may be counted on the basis of pollen morphology, which, however, does not allow discrimination between closely related pollen species. Alternatively, collected samples can be analyzed with antibodies to allow the quantitative determination of allergens in collected samples. This has the advantage that, in addition to pollen-associated allergens, those allergens that are released from pollen and become adsorbed to other carrier particles (e.g., aerosols) can be measured. In this context it has been reported that pollen from birch and related trees can release allergens by a process of artificial pollen germination that occurs when pollen is exposed to humidity (13). Incidentally, certain carrier molecules (diesel exhaust particles) have been found to act as adjuvants by driving the allergen-specific immune response into a preferential TH2 pathway that is accompanied by increased production of IgE antibodies (25). For these reasons it appears that the actual measurement of allergenic molecules using antibody-based assays can give much more accurate information about true allergen exposure than mere pollen counting. Another argument for true antibody-based measurement of allergen exposure is the observation that pollen may contain greatly varying amounts of allergens depending on the maturation state of the pollen and depending on the cultivar (26,27).

IV. DISTRIBUTION OF TREES

Trees of both the divisions angiosperms (flowering plants) and gymnosperms (nonflowering plants) have a role in eliciting allergic symptoms in patients. The most allergenic trees are birch, olive, and cypress. Of less allergenic importance are alder, hazel, *plane tree*, and chestnut. Trees belonging to the order Fagales grow in Europe, Northwest Africa, East Asia, and North America to the area of the Andes. Olive trees, being a member of the order Scrophulariales, are the dominant tree pollen source in the Mediterranean areas, but also are found in North and South America, South Africa, and Australia. Both Fagales and

Scrophulariales belong to the division of the angiosperms. Of lesser or uncertain importance in the elicitation of allergic symptoms are maple trees, which grow in Middle Europe and North America; plane trees, which grow in Southern and Central Europe, Western Asia, North America, South Africa, Australia, and New Zealand; and *Eucalyptus* trees, which can be found in Australia, South America, Africa, and Eastern Asia. *Melaleuca* is not wind pollinated and thus not allergenic (28). There is little known about the sensitization potency of trees belonging to the families Juglandaceae (e.g., walnut, pecan), Leguminosae (e.g., *Wattle*) and Salicaceae (willow, cottonwood), which also exist in southern parts of the world.

Other important tree families in inducing allergy belong to the nonflowering plants (gymnosperms) and include the Pinaceae (pine) and Cupressaceae (cypress and cedar), which grow in Mediterranean areas, Australia, New Zealand, South America, and parts of Asia (China, India). The Taxodiaceae (sugi), another representative of the gymnosperms, dominates in Japan and grows to a lesser degree in China, Mediterranean areas, and North America (10).

Two papers investigating the sensitization profiles of allergic patients from different parts of the world have revealed interesting differences depending on geographic areas (29,30). Birch pollen–allergic patients from the northern parts of Europe are mainly sensitized against the major birch pollen allergen, Bet v 1, which therefore may be considered a genuine marker for birch sensitization (30). By contrast, patients from the more southern parts of Europe appear positive in a birch pollen extract–based diagnostic test, but when tested with pure recombinant allergens are more frequently positive to cross-reactive allergens (e.g., profilin, calcium-binding allergens). It is therefore likely that these patients are sensitized against other allergen sources and, due to cross-reactivity, appear positive in the birch pollen extract test. Similar results were obtained when an allergic population from Central Africa was tested with recombinant allergens, indicating that the IgE reactivity profile reflects local pollen exposure (29). These studies and another study performed with recombinant *Parietaria* allergens (31) emphasize the importance of diagnostic testing with recombinant allergens for accurate determination of the sensitizing allergen source.

V. CLONING OF TREE POLLEN ALLERGENS

The diagnosis and specific immunotherapy of pollinosis are currently performed with allergen extracts or vaccines obtained by simple extraction procedures in aqueous buffers. Many attempts have been made to improve the quality of the extracts, and it has long been recognized that extracts may lack important allergens, contain nonallergenic materials, and vary greatly in their composition (32). Furthermore, it is technically impossible to purify all of the major and minor allergens of a natural allergen source to obtain adequate materials for diagnostic testing. However, due to application of molecular biology techniques to the field of allergen characterization, most relevant allergens of the common allergen sources have been produced as recombinant molecules (32).

In principle, there are two strategies that can be applied to obtain the allergen-encoding cDNA (17). The first approach uses IgE antibodies of allergic patients to isolate cDNA coding for allergens from expression cDNA libraries that have been constructed from the allergen sources (Fig. 1). The standard procedure for the isolation of allergen-encoding cDNA involves the isolation of mRNA from the allergen source. This mRNA is converted to cDNA by reverse transcription and then inserted into a vector suitable for the

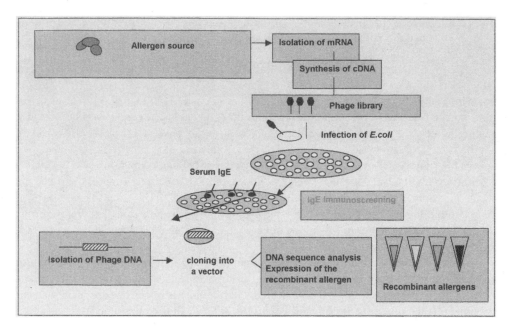

Figure 1 Production of recombinant allergens. Description of the procedure from the isolation of mRNA from the allergen source to the production of recombinant allergens. mRNA is isolated from the allergen source and cDNA is synthesized. Allergen-encoding cDNAs can be isolated directly with IgE antibodies from allergic patients using immunoscreening technology. Next, the allergen-encoding cDNA is inserted in suitable vectors (viral, plasmid DNA) and can be expressed as recombinant protein in various host organisms (e.g., prokaryotic, eukaryotic organisms).

construction of a library or used as a template for polymerase chain reaction (PCR) amplification. Using serum IgE from allergic patients, clones expressing allergens can be isolated by immunoreactivity, purified, and subjected to sequence analysis. After the allergen-encoding cDNA has been inserted into expression vectors, recombinant allergens can be produced according to established protocols in large amounts and of high purity (Fig. 1). The second strategy uses DNA-based screening technologies (e.g., DNA-based screening of libraries, rT-PCR approaches) for the isolation of allergen-encoding cDNA; the procedure for the preparation of recombinant allergens remains the same.

The first isolated tree pollen allergen cDNA coded for Bet v 1, the major birch pollen allergen (33). Bet v 1 was obtained after IgE immunoscreening of a cDNA library that was constructed from mature birch pollen. With the same approach, a cDNA coding for Bet v 2 (profilin), a highly cross-reactive birch pollen allergen and the first known plant-actin binding protein, was isolated (34). Bet v 3 and Bet v 4, both calcium-binding birch pollen allergens (35–37), and Aln g 4, a calcium-binding pollen allergen from alder pollen, were obtained by expression cDNA cloning (38).

Using DNA-based approaches, oligonucleotides constructed according to the amino acid sequences of the allergen molecules can be used for screening of libraries or for PCR amplification. The PCR approach was used to clone Aln g 1, the major alder allergen; Car b 1, the major hornbeam allergen; and Cor a 1, the major hazel allergen (39–41). The PCR approach was also used to clone the major olive pollen allergen, Ole e 1, olive pollen profilin, Ole e 2, and Lig v 1, the major allergen from privet pollen (42–44). The spectrum of olive pollen allergens, including Ole 3–8, is almost complete (45). Cry j 1 and Cry j 2, the major allergens of Japanese cedar, were obtained by DNA-based screening of cDNA libraries (46,47). On the basis of similarity at the protein and nucleic acid level with Bet v 1, the major birch pollen allergen, an rT-PCR approach was used to isolate the cDNA coding for Mal d 1, the major apple allergen, Api g 1, the major celery allergen, Pru av 1, the major cherry allergen, and others relevant for food allergy and documented cross-reactivity (48–50). Table 2 gives an overview of tree allergens, and their biological functions and characteristics. The spectrum of tree pollen allergens and tree nut allergens has been reviewed in several publications (45,79,86). The rapid progress in the field of recombinant allergens holds promise that most of the traditional allergen raw extracts will be soon replaced by recombinant allergens covering the complete epitope repertoire of the extracts (11,87).

VI. BIOLOGICAL FUNCTIONS AND STRUCTURAL CHARACTERISTICS OF TREE POLLEN ALLERGENS

During the past decade the molecular nature of the most common environmental allergens has been revealed through the application of molecular biology techniques for allergen characterization (87). The DNA and deduced amino acid sequences can be obtained by sequencing the allergen-encoding cDNAs and thus allow comparisons with sequences deposited in databases. Using this approach the biological functions of various allergens can be either revealed or projected. For example, it was found that the cDNA and amino acid sequence of the major birch pollen allergen, Bet v 1, showed significant sequence homology with a group of proteins that were found to be upregulated when plants were wounded, infected, or subjected to stressful conditions, and accordingly these proteins were designated pathogenesis-related proteins (i.e., PR proteins) (33). Although to date there are no definitive experimental data to support the conjecture that the family of Bet v 1–related allergens contribute to the plant defense system, it is possible that they have protective functions (88). On the other hand, other functions (e.g., RNAse activity, lipid carrier) have been claimed for the Bet v 1 allergen family on the basis of in vitro experiments and structural data (89–91).

Numerous Bet v 1–homologous allergens have been identified in pollen of trees belonging to the order Fagales (e.g., Aln g 1, alder; Cor a 1, hazel; Car b 1, hornbeam; Que a 1, white oak and Cas s 1, chestnut) (see www.allergen.org/List.htm). Figure 2 demonstrates the relationship among Bet v 1–related plant allergens on the basis of sequence identities. Almost all of the displayed proteins contain cross-reactive IgE epitopes (see Pharmacia home page: http://www.diagnostics.nu/). However, it is also known that even birch pollen contains proteins with high sequence identity to Bet v 1 but without relevant allergenic activity (92). The existence of these hypoallergenic Bet v 1 isoforms and of nonallergenic proteins with high sequence homology to Bet v 1 (93) demonstrates that sequence homology per se cannot predict with certainty whether a protein is allergenic or not.

Table 2 gives an overview of tree pollen allergens grouped according to botanical classification. Each of the different trees contains a spectrum of allergens. However, it turns out that certain allergenic molecules occur in different trees as proteins with significant sequence homology and cross-reactive epitopes. In general, it is possible to identify certain groups of cross-reactive allergens. For example, there are the Bet v 1–related allergens Aln g 1, Cor a 1, Car b 1, and Cas s 1, which can be found in pollen of trees belonging to the

Table 2 Tree Pollen Allergens

Allergen	Source	Scientific name	Allergen description	MW (kDa)	References
Fagales					
Bet v 1	Birch	*Betula verrucosa*	PR10	17	33
Bet v 2			Profilin	15	34
Bet v 3			Ca^{2+}-binding protein	23.7	35
Bet v 4			Ca^{2+}-binding protein	9.3	36,37
Bet v 5			Isoflavone red	35	51
Bet v 6				33.5	AAC05116*
Bet v 7			Cyclophilin	18	52
Bet v 8			Pectin esterase	66	53
Aln g 1	Alder	*Alnus glutinosa*	Homologue: Bet v 1, PR10	17	39
Aln g 4			Ca^{2+}-binding protein		38
Cor a 1	Hazel	*Corylus avellana*	Homologue: Bet v 1, PR10		41
Cor a 2			Profilin	14	**
Cor a 8			Lipid transfer protein	9	**
Cor a 9			11S globulin-like protein	40	54
Cor a 10			Luminal binding protein	70	AJ295617**
Cor a 11			7S vicilin-like protein	48	AF441864**
Car b 1	Hornbeam	*Carpinus betulus*	PR10	17	40
Cas s 1	Chestnut	*Castanea sativa*	PR10	22	55
Cas s 5			Chitinase		CAA64868 *
Cas s 8			Lipid transfer protein	9.7	56
Que a 1	While oak	*Quercus alba*	PR10	17	57
Hamamelidales					
Pla a 1	London plane tree	*Platanus acerifolia*		18	58,59
Pla a 2				43	P82967**
Scrophulariales					
Ole e 1	Olive tree	*Olea europea*		16	42
Ole e 2			Profilin	15–18	60
Ole e 3			Ca^{2+}-binding protein	9.2	61,62
Ole e 4				32	63
Ole e 5			Superoxide dismutase	16	63
Ole e 6				10	64
Ole e 7					65
Olc c 8			Ca^{2+}-binding protein	21	66
Ole e 9				46,4	67,68
Fra e 1	Ash	*Fraxinus excelsior*		20	69,70
Lig v 1	Privet	*Ligustrum vulgare*		20	44
Syr v 1	Lilac	*Syringa vulgaris*		20	71
Syr v 3					***
Pla l 1	English plantain	*Platanus lanceoloata*		18	72
Pinales					
Cry j 1	Sugi	*Cryptomeria japonica*	Pectate lyase	41–45	46,73,74
Cry j 2			Polymethylgalacturunase		47,75,76
Cha o 1	Japonese cypress	*Cupressus japonica*			77
Cha o 2					78
Cup a 1	Cypress	*Cupressus arizonica*		43	79
Cup a 3					***
Cup s 1	Common cypress	*Cupressus sempervirens*		43	AAF72629*
Jun a 1	Mountain cedar	*Juniperus ashei*	Pectate lyase	43	80
Jun a 2					81
Jun a 3			PR5	30	82
Jun o 2	Prickly juniper	*Juniperus oxycedrus*			83
Jun o 4			Ca^{2+}-binding protein	29	AF031471**
Jun s 1	Mountain cedar	*Juniperus ashei*		50	84
Jun v 1	Eastern red cedar	*Juniperus virginiana*		43	85

Allergenic molecules are listed according to their taxonomical orders (underlined). Allergen source, name, function, molecular weight (kDa), and references or accession numbers are shown. The different databases are indicated by asterisks:*http://www.allergenonline.com; ** International Union of Immunological Societies Allergen Nomenclature Subcommittee; http://www.allergen.org/List.htm; *** SDAP—Structural Database of Allergenic Proteins.

	Asparagus	Carrot	Celery	Tomato	Soybean	Pea	Medicago	Pear	Apricot	Cherry	Apple	Beech	Hornbeam	Alder	Hazel	Birch
Birch	39	38	40	47	49	54	55	58	60	59	66	69	79	81	83	100
Hazel	40	41	40	46	53	53	55	59	63	59	67	69	92	82	100	
Alder	41	39	40	40	50	50	52	55	61	57	64	67	79	100		
Hornbeam	39	42	40	46	51	51	56	56	62	58	66	68	100			
Beech	39	41	42	49	57	54	55	70	74	74	71	100				
Apple	39	40	45	47	50	51	54	70	79	76	100					
Cherry	37	40	43	49	55	51	51	84	76	100						
Apricot	37	44	50	50	53	51	52	73	100							
Pear	35	39	40	43	54	50	50	100								
Medicago	33	36	40	42	66	83	100									
Pea	29	33	39	39	70	100										
Soybean	34	37	40	41	100											
Tomato	43	32	40	100												
Celery	32	51	100													
Carrot	33	100														
Asparagus	100															

Figure 2 Sequence identity (%) between Bet v 1–homologous proteins from different sources. The percentage of sequence identity between Bet v 1–related allergens from various sources is displayed. (http://www.diagnostics.nu/)

order Fagales. These allergens are also expressed in fruits and seeds of unrelated trees and, due to cross-reactivity, elicit symptoms of food allergy in pollen-allergic patients (6,94).

A second group of highly cross-reactive allergens is represented by the profilins, which are actin-binding proteins (34,95–98). They include birch profilin, Bet v 2, hazel profilin, Cor a 2, and Ole e 2, from olive, and numerous other profilins. Bet v 2, birch profilin, is probably the most widely distributed and conserved allergen described thus far (34). It belongs to a family of proteins that are structurally conserved low-molecular-weight (12–15 kDa) eukaryotic proteins.

Profilins represent actin-binding proteins, which are expressed in all eukaryotic cells; they regulate actin functions but also bind to phosphoinositides and proline-rich proteins, thus linking signal transduction and reassembly of the cytoskeleton (99).

Bet v 3 and Bet v 4 and also Ole e 3 (61) and Ole e 8 belong to the group of calcium-binding proteins (100). Sequence analysis of allergen-encoding cDNA revealed the presence of typical calcium-binding motifs (i.e., binding sites for calcium), termed EF-hands, within allergens from various sources (100). Bet v 3 represents a three–EF-hand allergen, highly expressed in mature pollen (35), whereas Bet v 4 contains only two EF-hands (36,37). Two–EF-and calcium-binding allergens have been found in a variety of pollens from trees, grasses, and weeds (101). Furthermore, Jun o 2 and Ole e 8 represent four–EF-hand calcium-binding allergens isolated from cypress and olive pollen (66,83). The calcium-binding allergens are mainly expressed in pollen as opposed to other plant tissues and therefore are responsible only for pollen, and not for food cross-reactivity. IgE inhibition experiments indicate that there is extensive IgE cross-reactivity between members of the different EF-hand allergens (101). Furthermore, IgE recognition of the calcium-binding allergens is in most cases stronger when the proteins contain calcium. This indicates that patients were sensitized preferentially against the conformation of the calcium-bound proteins (102). The first three-dimensional structure of a two–EF-hand allergen from timothy grass, Phl p 7, with extensive cross-reactivity to tree pollen allergens has been determined (103).

Another group of pollen allergens is represented by the major olive pollen allergen, Ole e 1, which shares sequence identity and cross-reactive epitopes with allergens from ash (Fra e 1) (69,70), privet (Lig v 1) (44), lilac (Syr v 1) (71), and plantain (Pla l 1) (72). There is a similar degree of sequence homology between the major cedar pollen allergen, Cry j 1, and the major ragweed allergens, Amb a 1 and Amb a 2 (73,74,104). Furthermore, the cedar allergen, Cry j 2, is highly homologous to polygalacturonases of several other plants, but the degree of cross-reactivity seems to be more limited (75). Table 2 gives an overview of the tree pollen allergens and provides information about their sources, scientific names, biological functions, molecular weights (kDa), and references regarding their description.

All of the tree pollen allergens are low-molecular-weight proteins or glycoproteins that rapidly elute from pollen after contact with aqueous solutions (105). The use of immunogold electron microscopy has revealed that these allergens are mainly intracellular proteins that either elute from pollen or, under certain conditions, are expelled from pollen by rupture or abortive germination (12,13,106). The analysis of the three-dimensional structures of important pollen allergens has not revealed structural motifs common among unrelated allergens but show that cross-reactivity is due to structural similarity (107).

VII. CROSS-REACTIVITY BETWEEN TREE POLLEN ALLERGENS

During the last decade the most common allergens have been identified by molecular cloning and produced as recombinant allergens (87). In this context IgE inhibition studies performed with purified recombinant allergens have greatly enhanced our understanding of cross-reactivity at the molecular level (87). Figure 3 illustrates as an example the cross-reactivity within the family of Bet v 1–related allergens. Allergens containing cross-reactive IgE epitopes have been described in pollen, fruits, vegetables, nuts, and seeds (94). Accordingly Bet v 1–sensitized patients frequently suffer from an oral allergy syndrome caused by ingestion of food containing cross-reactive allergens. Due to extensive cross-reactivity among the Bet v 1–related allergens, it is not surprising that immunotherapy with birch pollen vaccine alone had beneficial effects on allergy to pollens of related trees and on food allergy (108).

It turns out that cross-reactivity has in principle two facets that can be applied for diagnosis and therapy. Certain allergens/epitopes are restricted to certain allergen sources and thus can be used as marker molecules to confirm sensitization to these sources (109). For example, Bet v 1 cross-reacts mainly with pollen allergens of trees belonging to the Fagales order, the major grass pollen allergens (e.g., Phl p 1, Phl p 2, Phl p 5 from timothy grass) are only present in grasses, and certain weed allergens (e.g., Par j 2 from *Parietaria*) are markers for sensitization to a certain weed (31). Based on this observation it has been proposed to use such species-specific marker allergens to confirm sensitization to certain allergen sources. These marker allergens can thus be used as diagnostic gatekeepers to confirm the suitability of patients for immunotherapy with a given allergen extract (109). Another argument for using major species-specific marker allergens as an inclusion criterion for immunotherapy is that the currently used allergen extracts are mainly standardized regarding these major allergens.

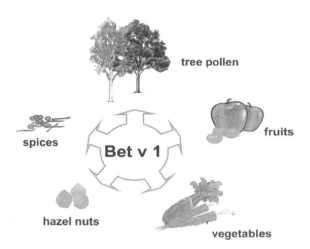

Figure 3 Bet v 1 cross-reactive allergens can be found in pollens of trees belonging to the Fagales, fruits, vegetables, nuts, and spices. (Reprinted with permission from Ref. 109.)

However, allergens have been identified that exhibit very broad cross-reactivity and thus indicate polysensitization. These allergens include the group of profilins and calcium-binding allergens. Patients who are sensitized to profilin (e.g., Bet v 2, Phl p 12) cross-react in most cases with profilins from various unrelated plants and suffer from pollen and plant food polysensitization (109). Patients who are sensitized to calcium-binding allergens (e.g., Bet v 4, Phl p 7) suffer in most cases from multiple pollen sensitization to trees, grasses, and weeds (109). Such patients may benefit less from allergen vaccine–based immunotherapy because the currently used therapeutic vaccines are not standardized regarding these molecules and it is known that patients with polysensitization benefit less from allergen-specific immunotherapy (110). In vitro diagnostic tests equipped with recombinant marker allergens to facilitate the selection of patients for immunotherapy with birch pollen and grass pollen extracts have been made available by diagnostic companies and can be used by clinicians (see Pharmacia home page: http://www.diagnostics.nu/).

VIII. TRANSITION FROM ALLERGEN EXTRACT/VACCINE–BASED DIAGNOSIS AND THERAPY TO RECOMBINANT ALLERGEN-BASED DIAGNOSIS AND THERAPY

The fast progress in the field of allergen characterization through the application of molecular cloning techniques has provided us with recombinant allergens covering most allergen sources, including trees. Recombinant allergens allow the individual sensitization profiles of allergic patients to be dissected out, a process that has been designated component-resolved diagnosis (CRD) (32). The diagnostic information obtained by CRD is much more profound than that obtainable by extract-based diagnosis. Extract-based diagnosis will identify potential allergen sources but does not provide any information regarding the disease-eliciting allergens within the given allergen source. In order to utilize the full spectrum of recombinant allergens for allergy diagnosis, novel forms of multi-allergen tests are currently being developed (111). Some of the new tests combine chip and microarray technology, whereas others simply utilize nitrocellulose-based test systems for the elucidation of the patient's reactivity profile in a single test (111–113). To allow precise quantitative measurements of IgE and IgG levels, recombinant allergens have also been used in established quantitative and automated in vitro allergy test systems. Recombinant allergen–based tests have been used to dissect the sensitization profiles of patients from various populations (29,30,114), to monitor the development of allergies from early childhood on (115), to investigate the development of IgE profiles in the natural course of allergic disease (116), and to study the effects of allergen-specific immunotherapy (116–119). Using the new recombinant allergen–based tests, several interesting results have been obtained regarding the pathomechanisms operative in allergic diseases and the potential mechanisms behind allergen-specific immunotherapy.

The monitoring of IgE and IgG responses during allergen-specific immunotherapy has reemphasized the importance of true blocking antibodies in the success of allergen-specific immunotherapy (116,117,119). The finding that allergen vaccines induce a highly heterogeneous immune response against the individual components in the vaccine has underlined the need for improvement of therapeutic allergen preparations (119). Moreover, it turns out that injection of allergen vaccines may induce IgE reactivity against new allergens in patients (118,120). Although the clinical relevance of these findings has not yet been investigated, these data support the idea that patients would benefit if they were treated according to their individual sensitization profiles. The concept of treating allergic patients according to their sensitization profiles with purified recombinant allergens, termed component-resolved immunotherapy (CRIT), has therefore been proposed (32). During the last few years several candidate molecules have been developed by recombinant DNA technology (14,87). These molecules are characterized by strongly reduced allergenic activity, although T-cell epitopes and immunogenicity (i.e., the capacity to induce protective IgG responses) have been maintained. The recombinant hypoallergenic allergen derivatives have been evaluated in vitro in experimental animal models, and regarding reduced allergenic activity by in vivo provocation testing in patients (14,87). The first immunotherapy study performed with hypoallergenic derivatives of the major birch pollen allergen, Bet v 1, has been performed, and several other immunotherapy studies with recombinant allergens have been initiated.

IX. SALIENT POINTS

1. The most significant tree pollen allergens are derived from wind pollinated trees belonging to the order Fagales (e.g., birch) and from olive, cedar, and cypress.
2. The most common and important tree allergens have been produced as recombinant allergens equivalent to their natural counterparts. Panels of recombinant allergens resembling the epitope complexity of natural allergen extracts have become available.
3. The molecular characterization of tree pollen allergens has revealed that there are families of cross-reactive allergens that are characterized by high sequence homology and immunological cross-reactivity.
4. Recombinant allergen–based diagnostic tests are now available for routine clinical use to determine the sensitization profiles of patients and to improve the selection of the most accurate treatment forms. They have been used successfully for

research to establish patients' sensitization profiles, to reveal pathomechanisms underlying allergic diseases, and to study the effects of allergen-specific immunotherapy.

5. Recombinant allergen derivatives with reduced allergenic activity have been developed and evaluated. Currently, the first immunotherapy trials are being performed with the new molecules to study the mechanisms, efficacy, and safety of component-resolved immunotherapy with recombinant allergen molecules.

REFERENCES

1. Kay AB. Allergy and Allergic Diseases. Oxford, UK: Blackwell Science, 1997.
2. Wuthrich B, Schindler C, Leuenberger P, Ackermann-Liebrich U. Prevalence of atopy and pollinosis in the adult population of Switzerland (SAPALDIA study): Swiss Study on Air Pollution and Lung Diseases in Adults. Int Arch Allergy Immunol 1995; 106:149–156.
3. Integrated Taxonomic Information System (http://www.itis.usda.gov). See also Watson L, Dallwitz MJ. The Families of Flowering Plants: Descriptions, Illustrations, Identification, and Information Retrieval. (1992 onward). Version: 14 December 2000 (http://biodiversity.bio. uno.edu/delta/angio/)).
4. Valenta R, Steinberger P, Duchene M, Kraft D. Immunological and structural similarities among allergens: Prerequisite for a specific and component-based therapy of allergy. Immunol Cell Biol 1996; 74:187–194.
5. Valenta R, Kraft D. Type I allergic reactions to plant-derived food: A consequence of primary sensitization to pollen allergens. J Allergy Clin Immunol 1996; 97:893–895.
6. Kazemi-Shirazi L, Pauli G, Purohit A, Spitzauer S, Fröschl R, Hoffmann-Sommergruber K, Breiteneder H, Scheiner O, Kraft D, Valenta R. Quantitative IgE ingibition experiments with purified recombinant allergens indicate pollen-derived allergens as the sensitizing agents responsible for many forms of plant food allergy. J Allergy Clin Immunol 2000; 105:116–125.
7. Accorsi CA, Bandini-Mazzanti M, Romano B, et al. Allergenic pollen: Morphology and microscopic photographs. In: Allergenic Pollen, and Pollenosis in Europe (D'Amato G, Spieksma FThM, Bonini S, eds.). Oxford, England: Blackwell Scientific, 1991: 24–44.
8. D'Amato G, Spieksma FThM, Liccardi G, Jager S, Russo M, Kontou-Fili K, Nikkels H, Wuthrich B, Bonini S. Pollen Related Allergy in Europe: Position paper of the European Acadamy of Allergology and Clinical Immunology. Allergy 1998; 53:567–578.
9. Rantio-Lehtimäki A. Sampling airborne pollen and pollen antigens. In: Allergenic Pollens and Pollenosis in Europe (D'Amato G, Spieksma FTM, Bonini S, eds.). Oxford, England: Blackwell Scientific, 1991.
10. D'Amato G, Bonini S, Bousquet J, Durham SR, Platts-Mills TAE. Pollenosis 2000 Global Approach. Naples: JGC Editions, 2001.
11. Valenta R, Kraft D. Recombinant allergens for diagnosis and therapy of allergic diseases. Curr Opin Immunol 1995; 7:751–756.
12. Grote M, Vrtala S, Valenta R. Monitoring of two allergens, Bet v 1 and profilin, in dry and rehydrated birch pollen by immunogold electron microscopy and immunoblotting. J Histochem Cytochem 1993; 41:745–750.
13. Grote M, Valenta R, Reichelt R. Abortive pollen germination: A mechanism of allergen release in birch, alder, and hazel revealed by immunogold electron microscopy. J Allergy Clin Immunol 2003; 111:1017–1023.
14. Valenta R. The future of antigen-specific immunotherapy of allergy. Nat Rev Immunol 2002; 2:446–453.
15. Lockey RF, Bukantz SC, eds. Allergen Immunotherapy, 2nd ed. New York: Marcel Dekker, 1998.

16. Valenta R, Ball T, Focke M, Linhart B, Mothes N, Niederberger V, Spitzauer S, Swoboda I, Vrtala S, Westritschnig K, Kraft D. Immunotherapy of allergic disease. Adv Immunol 2003 (in press).

17. Valenta R, Vrtala S, Laffer S, Spitzauer S, Kraft D. Recombinant allergens. Allergy 1998; 53:552–561.

18. Gregory PH. The Microbiology of the Atmosphere. Aylesbury: L. Hill, 1973.

19. Thommen AA. Etiology of hay fever: Studies in hay fever. N Y State J Med 1930; 437–441.

20. Ebner C, Hirschwehr R, Bauer L, Breiteneder H, Valenta R, Ebner H, Kraft D, Scheiner O. Identification of allergens in fruits and vegetables: IgE cross-reactivities with the important birch pollen allergens Bet v 1 and Bet v 2 (birch profilin). J Allergy Clin Immunol 1995; 95:962–969.

21. Jäger S, Emberlin J, Gallop R, Toth J, Marks B, Berger U, Horak F. The European pollen information service center in the internet. Allergy Suppl 1997; 52:32.

22. Aalberse RC, Nieuwenhuys EJ, Hey M, Stapel SO. "Horoscope effect" not only for seasonal but also for non-seasonal allergens. Clin Exp Allergy 1992; 22:1003–1006.

23. Kihlstrom A, Lilja G, Pershagen G, Hedlin G. Exposure to birch pollen in infancy and development of atopic disease in childhood. J Allergy Clin Immunol 2002; 110:78–84.

24. Rantio-Lehtimäki A, Helander ML, Pessi AM. Significance of sampling height of airborne particles for aerobiological information. Allergy 1991; 46:68–76.

25. Diaz-Sanchez D, Tsien A, Fleming J, Saxon A. Combined diesel exhaust particulate and ragweed allergen challenge markedly enhances human in cico nasal ragweed-specific IgE and skews cytokine production to a T helper cell 2 type pattern. J Immunol 1997; 158:2406–2413.

26. Mittermann I, Swoboda I, Pierson E, Eller N, Kraft D, Valenta R, Heberle-Bors E. Molecular cloning and characterization of profilin from tobacco (*Nicotina tabacum*): Increased profilin expression during pollen maturation. Plant Mol Biol 1995; 27:137–146.

27. Castro AJ, de Dios Alche J, Cuevas J, Romero PJ, Alche V, Rodriguez-Garcia MI. Pollen from different olive tree cultivars contains varying amounts of the major allergen Ole e 1. Int Arch Allergy Immunol 2003; 131:164–173.

28. Stablein JJ, Buchholtz GA, Lockey RF. Melaleuca tree and respiratory disease. Ann Allergy Asthma Immunol 2002; 89:523–530.

29. Westritschnig K, Sibanda E, Thomas W, Auer H, Aspock H, Pittner G, Vrtala S, Spitzauer S, Kraft D, Valenta R. Analysis of the sensitization profile towards allergens in central Africa. Clin Exp Allergy 2003; 33:22–27.

30. Moverare R, Westritschnig K, Svensson M, Hayek B, Bende M, Pauli G, Sorva R, Haahtela T, Valenta R, Elfman L. Different IgE reactivity profiles in birch pollen-sensitive patients from six European populations revealed by recombinant allergens: An imprint of local sensitization. Int Arch Allergy Immunol 2002; 128:325–335.

31. Stumvoll S, Westritschnig K, Lidholm J, Spitzauer S, Colombo P, Duro G, Kraft D, Geraci D, Valenta R. Identification of cross-reactive and genuine *Parietaria judaica* pollen allergens. J Allergy Clin Immunol 2003; 111:974–979.

32. Valenta R, Lidholm J, Niederberger V, Hayek B, Kraft D, Gronlund H. The recombinant allergen–based concept of component-resolved diagnostics and immunotherapy (CRD and CRIT). Clin Exp Allergy 1999; 29:896–904.

33. Breiteneder H, Pettenburger K, Bito A, Valenta R, Kraft D, Rumpold H, Scheiner O, Breitenbach M. The gene coding for the major birch pollen allergen, Bet v 1, is highly homologous to a pea disease resistance response gene. EMBO J 1989; 8:1935–1938.

34. Valenta R, Duchene M, Pettenburger K, Sillaber C, Valent P, Bettelheim P, Breitenbach M, Rumpold H, Kraft D, Scheiner O. Identification of profilin as a novel pollen allergen: IgE autoreactivity in sensitized individuals. Science 1991; 253:557–560.

35. Seiberler S, Scheiner O, Kraft D, Lonsdale D, Valenta R. Characterization of a birch pollen allergen, Bet v III, representing a novel class of Ca^{2+} binding proteins: Specific expression in

mature pollen and dependence of patients' IgE binding on protein-bound Ca^{2+}. EMBO J 1994; 13:3481–3486.

36. Twardosz A, Hayek B, Seiberler S, Vangelista L, Elfmann L, Grönlund H, Kraft D, Valenta R. Molecular characterization, expression in *Escherichia coli* and epitope analysis of a two EF-hand calcium-binding birch pollen allergen, Bet v 4. Biochem Biophys Res Commun 1997; 239:197–204.

37. Engel E, Richter K, Obermeyer G, Briza P, Kungl AJ, Simon B, Auer M, Ebner C, Rheinberger HJ, Breitenbach M, Ferreira F. Immunological and biological properties of Bet v 4, a novel birch pollen allergen with two EF-hand calcium-binding domains. J Biol Chem 1997; 272:8630–8637.

38. Hayek B, Vangelista L, Pastore A, Sperr WR, Valent P, Vrtala S, Niederberger V, Twardosz A, Kraft D, Valenta R. Molecular and immunological characterization of a highly cross-reactive two EF-hand calcium-binding alder pollen allergen, Aln g 4: Structural basis for calcium-modulated IgE recognition. J Immunol 1998; 161:7031–7039.

39. Breiteneder H, Ferreira F, Reikerstorfer A, Duchene M, Valenta R, Hoffmann-Sommergruber K, Ebner C, Breitenbach M, Kraft D, Scheiner O. cDNA cloning and expression in *Escherichia coli* of Aln g I, the major allergen in pollen of alder (*Alnus glutinosa*). J Allergy Clin Immunol 1992; 90:909–917.

40. Larson JN, Stroman P, Ipsen H. PCR based cloning and sequencing of isogenes encoding the tree pollen major allergen Car b I from *Carpinus betulus*, hornbeam. Mol Immunol 1992; 29:703–711.

41. Breiteneder H, Ferreira F, Hoffmann-Sommergruber K, Ebner C, Breitenbach M, Kraft D, Scheiner O. Four recombinant isoforms of Cor a I, the major allergen of hazel pollen, show different IgE-binding properties. Eur J Biochem 1993; 212:355–362.

42. Villalba M, Batanero E, Monsalve RI, Delapena MAG, Lahoz C, Rodriguez R. Cloning and expression of Ole e 1, the major allergen from olive tree pollen: Polymorphism analysis and tissue specificity. J Biol Chem 1994; 269:15217–15222.

43. Asturias JA, Arilla MC, Gomez-Bayon N, Martinez A, Martinez J, Palacios R. Cloning, expression and structural analysis of profilins from different plant species. Allergy Suppl 1997; 52:32.

44. Batanero E, Gonzalez de la Pena MA, Villalba M, Monsalve RI, Martin-Esteban M, Rodriguez R. Isolation, cDNA cloning and expression of Lig v 1, the major allergen from privet pollen. Clin Exp Allergy 1996; 26:1401–1410.

45. Rodriguez R, Villalba M, Monsalve RI, Batanero E. The spectrum of olive pollen allergens. Int Arch Allergy Immunol 2001; 125:185–195.

46. Sone T, Komiyama N, Shimizu K, Kusakabe T, Morikubo K, Kino K. Cloning and sequencing of cDNA coding for Cry j I, a major allergen of Japanese cedar pollen. Biochem Biophys Res Commun 1994; 199:619–628.

47. Komiyama N, Sone T, Shimizu K, Morikubo K, Kino K. cDNA cloning and expression of Cry j II, the second major allergen of Japanese cedar pollen. Biochem Biophys Res Commun 1994; 201:1021–1028.

48. Vanek-Krebitz M, Hoffmann-Sommergruber K, Laimer da Camara Machado M, Ebner C, Kraft D, Scheiner O, Breiteneder H. Cloning and sequencing of Mal d 1, the major allergen from apple (*Malus domestica*), and its immunological relationship to Bet v 1, the major birch pollen allergen. Biochem Biophys Res Commun 1995; 214:538–551.

49. Breiteneder H, Hoffmann-Sommergruber K, O'Riordain G, Susani M, Ahorn H, Ebner C, Kraft D, Scheiner O. Molecular characterization of Api g 1, the major allergen of celery (*Apium graveolens*), and its immunological and structural relationships to a group of 17 kDa tree pollen allergens. Eur J Biochem 1995; 233:484–489.

50. Scheurer S, Pastorello EA, Wangorsch A, Kastner M, Haustein D, Vieths S. Recombinant allergens Pru av 1 and Pru av 4 and a newly identified lipid transfer protein in the in vitro diagnosis of cherry allergy. J Allergy Clin Immunol 2001; 107:724–731.

51. Karamloo F, Schmitz N, Scheurer S, Foetisch K, Hoffmann A, Hausstein D, Vieths S. Molecular cloning and characterization of a birch pollen minor allergen, Bet v 5, belonging to a family of isoflavone reductase–related proteins. J Allergy Clin Immunol 1999; 104:991–999.

52. Cadot P, Diaz JF, Proost P, Van Damme J, Engelborghs Y, Stevens EA, Ceuppens JL. Purification and characterization of an 18-kD allergen of birch (*Betula verrucosa*) pollen: Identification as a cyclophilin. J Allergy Clin Immunol 2000; 105:286–291.

53. Mahler V, Fischer S, Heiss S, Duchene M, Kraft D, Valenta R. cDNA cloning and characterization of a cross-reactive birch pollen allergen: Identification as a pectin esterase. Int Arch Allergy Immunol 2001; 124:64–66.

54. Beyer K, Grishina G, Bardina L, Grishin A, Sampson HA. Identification of an 11S globulin as a major hazelnut food allergen in hazelnut-induced systemic reactions. J Allergy Clin Immunol 2002; 110:517–523.

55. Kos T, Hoffmann-Sommergruber K, Ferreira F, Hirschwehr R, Ahorn H, Horak F, Jäger S, Sperr WR, Kraft D, Scheiner O. Purification, characterization and N-terminal amino acid sequence of a new major allergen from European chestnut pollen, Cas s 1. Biochem Biophys Res Commun 1993; 196:1086–1092.

56. Díaz-Perales A, Lombardero M, Sánchez-Monge R, García-Sellés FJ, Pernas M, Fernández-Rivas M, Barber D, Salcedo G. Lipid-transfer proteins as potential plant panallergens: Cross-reactivity among proteins of Artemisia pollen, Castaneae nut and Rosaceae fruits, with different IgE-binding capacities. Clin Exp Allergy 2000; 30:1403–1410.

57. Ipsen H, Hansen OC. The NH2-terminal amino acid sequence of the immunochemically partial identical major allergens of alder (*Alnus glutinosa*) Aln g I, birch (*Betula verrucosa*) Bet v I, hornbeam (*Carpinus betulus*) Car b I and oak (*Quercus alba*) Que a I pollens. Mol Immunol 1991; 28:1279–1288.

58. Asturias JA, Ibarrola I, Eraso E, Arilla MC, Martinez A. The major *Platanus acerifolia* pollen allergen Pla a 1 has sequence homology to invertase inhibitors. Clin Exp Allergy 2003; 33:978–985.

59. Asturias JA, Ibarrola I, Bartolome B, Ojeda I, Malet A, Martinez A. Purification and characterization of Pla a 1, a major allergen from *Platanus acerifolia* pollen. Allergy 2002; 57:221–227.

60. Asturias JA, Arilla MC, Gomez-Bayon N, Martinez J, Martinez A, Palacios R. Cloning and expression of the panallergen profilin and the major allergen (Ole e 1) from olive tree pollen. J Allergy Clin Immunol 1997; 100:365–372.

61. Batanero E, Villalba M, Ledesma A, Puente XSM, Rodriguez R. Ole e 3, an olive-tree allergen, belongs to a widespread family of pollen proteins. Eur J Biochem 1996; 241:772–778.

62. Ledesma A, Villalba M, Rodriguez R. Molecular cloning and expression of active Ole e 3, a major allergen from olive-tree pollen and member of a novel family of calcium-binding proteins (polcalcins) involved in allergy. Eur J Biochem 1998; 258:454–459.

63. Boluda L, Alonso C, Fernandez-Caldas E. Characterization of two new allergens of Olea europea, Ole e 4 and Ole e 5. Allergy Suppl 1997; 52–81.

64. Batanero E, Ledesma A, Villalba M, Rodriguez R. Purification, amino acid sequence and immunological characterization of Ole e 6, a cysteine-enriched allergen from olive tree pollen. FEBS Lett 1997; 410:293–296.

65. Tejera ML, Villalba M, Batanero E, Rodriguez R. Identification, isolation, and characterization of Ole e 7, a new allergen of olive tree pollen. J Allergy Clin Immunol 1999; 104:797–802.

66. Ledesma A, Villalba M, Rodriguez R. Cloning, expression and characterization of a novel four EF-hand Ca(2+)-binding protein from olive pollen with allergenic activity. FEBS Lett 2000; 466:192–196.

67. Huecas S, Villalba M, Rodriguez R. Ole e 9, a major olive pollen allergen is a 1,3-beta-glucanase: Isolation, characterization, amino acid sequence, and tissue specificity. J Biol Chem 2001; 276:27959–27066.

68. Palomares O, Villalba M, Rodriguez R. The C-terminal segment of the 1,3-beta-glucanase Ole e 9 from olive (*Olea europaea*) pollen is an independent domain with allergenic activity: Expression in *Pichia pastoris* and characterization. Biochem J 2003; 369:593–601.

69. Niederberger V, Purohit A, Oster JP, Spitzauer S, Valenta R, Pauli G. The allergen profile of ash (*Fraxinus excelsior*) pollen: Cross-reactivity with allergens from various plant species. Clin Exp Allergy 2002; 32:933–941.

70. Hemmer W, Focke M, Wantke F, Götz M, Jarisch R, Jäger S. Ash (*Fraxinus excelsior*) pollen allergy in Central Europe: Specific role of pollen pan allergens and the major allergen of ash pollen, Fra e 1. Allergy 2000; 55:923–930.

71. Batanero E, Villalba M, Lopez-Otin C, Rodriguez R. Isolation and characterization of an olive allergen–like protein from lilac pollen. Eur J Biochem 1994; 221:187–193.

72. Calabozo B, Barber D, Polo F. Studies on the carbohydrate moiety of Pla l 1 allergen. identification of a major N-glycan and significance for the immunoglobulin E-binding activity. Clin Exp Allergy 2002; 32:1628–1634.

73. Taniai M, Ando S, Usui T, Kurimoto M, Sakaguchi M, Inouye S, Matuhasi T. N-terminal amino acid sequence of a major allergen of Japanese cedar pollen (Cry j I). FEBS Lett 1988; 239:329–332.

74. Griffith IJ, Lussier A, Garman R, Koury R, Yeung H, Pollock J. The cDNA cloning of Cry j I, the major allergen of *Cryptomeria japonica* (Japanese cedar) (abst). J Allergy Clin Immunol 1993; 91:339.

75. Sakaguchi M, Inouye S, Taniai M, Ando S, Usui M, Matuhasi T. Identification of the second major allergen of Japanese cedar pollen. Allergy 1990; 45:309–312.

76. Tamura Y, Kawaguchi J, Serizawa N, Hirahara K, Shiraishi A, Nigi H, Taniguchi Y, Toda M, Inouye S, Takemori T, Sakaguchi M. Analysis of sequential immunoglobulin E-binding epitope of Japanese cedar pollen allergen (Cry j 2) in humans, monkeys and mice. Clin Exp Allergy 2003; 33:211–217.

77. Suzuki M, Komiyama N, Itoh M, Itoh H, Sone T, Kino K, Takagi I, Ohta N. Purification, characterization and molecular cloning of Cha o 1, a major allergen of *Chamaecyparis obtusa* (Japanese cypress) Pollen Mol Immunol 1996; 33:451–460.

78. Mori T, Yokoyama M, Komiyama N, Okano M, Kino K. Purification, identification and cDNA cloning of Cha o 2, the second major allergen of Japanese cypress pollen. Biochem Biophys Res Commun 1999; 263:166–171.

79. Mistrello G, Roncarolo D, Zanoni D, Zanotta S, Amato S, Falagiani P, Ariano R. Allergenic relevance of *Cupressus arizonica* pollen extract and biological characterization of the allergoid. Int Arch Allergy Immunol 2002; 129:296–304.

80. Liu D, Midor-Horiuti T, White MA, Brooks EG, Goldblum RM, Czerwinski EW. Crystallization and preliminary X-ray diffraction analysis of Jun a 1, the major allergen isolated from pollen of the mountain cedar *Juniperus ashei*. Acta Crystallogr D Biol Crystallogr 2003; 59:1052–1054.

81. Yokoyama M, Miyahara M, Shimizu K, Kino K, Tsunoo H. Purification, identification, and cDNA cloning of Jun a 2, the second major allergen of mountain cedar pollen. Biochem Biophys Res Commun 2000; 275:195–202.

82. Midoro-Horiuti T, Goldblum RM, Kurosky A, Wood TG, Brooks EG. Variable expression of pathogenesis-related protein allergen in mountain cedar (*Juniperus ashei*) pollen. J Immunol 2000; 164:2188–2192.

83. Tinghino R, Barletta B, Palumbo S, Afferni C, Iacovacci P, Mari A, Di Felice G, Pini C. Molecular characterization of a cross-reactive Juniperus oxycedrus pollen allergen, Jun o 2: A novel calcium-binding allergen J Allergy Clin Immunol 1998; 101:772–777.

84. Gross GN, Zimburean JM, Capra JD. Isolation and partial characterization of the allergen in mountain cedar pollen. Scand J Immunol 1978; 8:437–441.

85. Midoro-Horiuti T, Goldblum RM, Brooks EG. Identification of mutations in the genes for the pollen allergens of eastern red cedar (*Juniperus virginiana*). Clin Exp Allergy 2001; 31:771–778.

86. Roux KH, Teuber SS, Sathe SK. Tree nut allergens. Int Arch Allergy Immunol 2003; 131:234–244.

87. Valenta R, Kraft D. From allergen structure to new forms of allergen-specific immunotherapy. Curr Opin Immunol 2002; 14:718–727.

88. Hoffmann-Sommergruber K. Plant allergens and pathogenesis-related proteins: What do they have in common? Int Arch Allergy Immunol 2000; 122:155–166.

89. Bufe A, Spangfort MD, Kahlert H, Schlaak M, Becker WM. The major birch pollen allergen, Bet v 1, shows ribonuclease activity. Planta 1996; 199:413–415.

90. Markovic-Housley Z, Degano M, Lamba D, von Roepenack-Lahaye E, Clemens S, Susani M, Ferreira F, Scheiner O, Breiteneder H. Crystal structure of a hypoallergenic isoform of the major birch pollen allergen Bet v 1 and its likely biological function as a plant steroid carrier. J Mol Biol 2003; 325:123–133.

91. Mogensen JE, Wimmer R, Larsen JN, Spangfort MD, Otzen DE. The major birch allergen, Bet v 1, shows affinity for a broad spectrum of physiological ligands. J Biol Chem 2002; 277:23684–23592.

92. Ferreira F, Hirtenlehner K, Jilek A, Godnik-Cvar J, Breiteneder H, Grimm R, Hoffmann-Sommergruber K, Scheiner O, Kraft D, Breitenbach M, Rheinberger HJ, Ebner C. Dissection of immunglobulin E and T lymphocyte reactivity of isoforms of the major birch pollen allergen Bet v 1: Potential use of hypoallergenic isoforms for immunotherapy. J Exp Med 1996; 183:599–609.

93. Laffer S, Hamdi S, Lupinek C, Sperr WR, Valent P, Verdino P, Keller W, Grote M, Hoffmann-Sommergruber K, Scheiner O, Kraft D, Rideau M, Valenta R. Molecular characterization of recombinant T1, a non-allergenic periwinkle (Catharanthus roseus) protein, with sequence similarity to the Bet v 1 plant allergen family. Biochem J 2003; 373:261–269.

94. Hoffmann-Sommergruber K, O'Riordain G, Ahorn H, Ebner C, Laimer-Da-Camara-Machado M, Puhringer H, Scheiner O, Breiteneder H. Molecular characterization of Dau c 1, the Bet v 1 homologous protein from carrot and its cross-reactivity with Bet v 1 and Api g 1. Clin Exp Allergy 1999;29:840–847.

95. Valenta R, Ferreira F, Grote M, Swoboda I, Vrtala S, Duchene M, Deviller P, Meagher RB, McKinney E, Heberle-Bors E, Kraft D, Scheiner O. Identification of profilin as an actin-binding protein in higher plants. J Biol Chem 1993; 268:22777–22781.

96. van Ree R, Voitenko V, van Leeuwen WA, Aalberse RC. Profilin is a cross-reactive allergen in pollen and vegetable foods. Int Arch Allergy Immunol 1992; 98:97–104.

97. Vallier P, DeChamp C, Valenta R, Vial O, Deviller P. Purification and characterization of an allergen from celery immunochemically related to an allergen present in several other plant species: Identification as a profilin. Clin Exp Allergy 1992; 22:774–782.

98. Valenta R, Duchene M, Ebner C, Valent P, Sillaber C, Deviller P, Ferreira F, Teijkl M, Edelmann H, Kraft D, Scheiner O. Profilins constitute a novel family of functional plant pan-allergens. J Exp Med 1992; 175:377–385.

99. Staiger CJ, Gibbon, Kovar DR, Zonie LE. Profilin and actin-depolymerizing factor: Modulators of actin organization in plants. Trends Plant Sci 1997; 2:275–281.

100. Valenta R, Hayek B, Seiberler S, Bugajska-Schretter A, Niederberger V, Twardosz A, Natter S, Vangelista L, Pastore A, Spitzauer S, Kraft D. Calcium-binding allergens: From plants to man. Int Arch Allergy Immunol 1998; 117:160–166.

101. Tinghino R, Twardosz A, Barletta B, Puggioni EM, Iacovacci P, Butteroni C, Afferni C, Mari A, Hayek B, Di Felice G, Focke M, Westritschnig K, Valenta R, Pini C. Molecular, structural, and immunologic relationships between different families of recombinant calcium-binding pollen allergens. J Allergy Clin Immunol 2002; 109:314–320.

102. Valenta R, Twardosz A, Swoboda I, Hayek B, Spitzauer S, Kraft D. Calcium-binding proteins in Type I allergy: Elicitors and vaccines. In: Calcium: The Molecular Basis of calcium Action in Biology and Medicine (Pochet R, Donato R, Haiech J, Heizmann C, Gerke V, eds.). Dordrecht, Netherlands: Kluwer Academic, 2000: 365–377.

103. Verdino P, Westritschnig K, Valenta R, Keller W. The cross-reactive calcium-binding pollen allergen, Phl p 7, reveals a novel dimer assembly. EMBO J 2002; 21:5007–5016.

104. Rafnar T, Friffith IJ, Kuo M, Bond JF, Rogers BL, Klapper DG. Cloning of Amb a I (antigen E), the major allergen family of short ragweed pollen. J Biol Chem 1995; 95:970–978.

105. Vrtala S, Grote M, Duchene M, vanRee R, Kraft D, Scheiner O, Valenta R. Properties of tree and grass pollen allergens: Reinvestigation of the linkage between solubility and allergenicity. Int Arch Allergy Immunol 1993; 102:160–169.

106. Grote M, Vrtala S, Niederberger V, Wiermann R, Valenta R, Reichelt R. Release of allergen-bearing cytoplasm from hydrated pollen: A mechanism common to a variety of grass (Poaceae) species revealed by electron microscopy. J Allergy Clin Immunol 2001; 108:109–115.

107. Valenta R, Kraft D. Recombinant allergen molecules: Tools to study effector cell activation. Immunol Rev 2001; 179:119–127.

108. Asero R. Fennel, cucumber, and melon allergy successfully treated with pollen-specific injection immunotherapy. Ann Allergy Asthma Immunol 2000; 84:460–462.

109. Kazemi-Shirazi L, Niederberger V, Linhart B, Lidholm J, Kraft D, Valenta R. Recombinant marker allergens: Diagnostic gate keepers for therapy of allergy. Int Arch Allergy Immunol 2002; 127:259–268.

110. Bousquet J, Becker WM, Hejjaoui A, Chanal I, Lebel B, Dhivert H, Michel FB. Differences in clinical and immunologic reactivity of patients allergic to grass pollens and to multiple-pollen species: II. Efficacy of a double-blind, placebo-controlled, specific immunotherapy with standardized extracts. J Allergy Clin Immunol 1991; 88:43–53.

111. Hiller R, Laffer S, Harwanegg C, Huber M, Schmidt WM, Twardosz A, Barletta B, Becker WM, Blaser K, Breiteneder H, Chapman M, Crameri R, Duchene M, Ferreira F, Fiebig H, Hoffmann-Sommergruber K, King TP, Kleber-Janke T, Kurup VP, Lehrer SB, Lidholm J, Muller U, Pini C, Reese G, Scheiner O, Scheynius A, Shen HD, Spitzauer S, Suck R, Swoboda I, Thomas W, Tinghino R, Van Hage-Hamsten M, Virtanen T, Kraft D, Muller MW, Valenta R. Microarrayed allergen molecules: diagnostic gatekeepers for allergy treatment. FASEB J 2002; 16:414–416.

112. Suck R, Nandy A, Weber B, Stock M, Fiebig H, Cromwell O. Rapid method for arrayed investigation of IgE-reactivity profiles using natural and recombinant allergens. Allergy 2002; 57:821–824.

113. Harwanegg C, Laffer S, Hiller R, Mueller MW, Kraft D, Spitzauer S, Valenta R. Microarrayed recombinant allergens for diagnosis of allergy. Clin Exp Allergy 2003; 33:7–13.

114. Laffer S, Spitzauer S, Susani M, Pairleitner H, Schweiger C, Gronlund H, Menz G, Pauli G, Ishii T, Nolte H, Ebner C, Sehon AH, Kraft D, Eichler HG, Valenta R. Comparison of recombinant timothy grass pollen allergens with natural extract for diagnosis of grass pollen allergy in different populations. J Allergy Clin Immunol 1996; 98:652–658.

115. Niederberger V, Niggemann B, Kraft D, Spitzauer S, Valenta R. Evolution of IgM, IgE and IgG(1–4) antibody responses in early childhood monitored with recombinant allergen components: Implications for class switch mechanisms. Eur J Immunol 2002; 32:576–584.

116. Ball T, Fuchs T, Sperr WR, Valent P, Vangelista L, Kraft D, Valenta R. B cell epitopes of the major timothy grass pollen allergen, Phl p 1, revealed by gene fragmentation as candidates for immunotherapy. FASEB J 1999; 13:1277–1290.

117. Ball T, Sperr WR, Valent P, Lidholm J, Spitzauer S, Ebner C, Kraft D, Valenta R. Induction of antibody responses to new B cell epitopes indicates vaccination character of allergen immunotherapy. Eur J Immunol 1999; 29:2026–2036.

118. Moverare R, Elfman L, Vesterinen E, Metso T, Haahtela T. Development of new IgE specificities to allergenic components in birch pollen extract during specific immunotherapy studied with immunoblotting and Pharmacia CAP System. Allergy 2002; 57:423–430.

119. Mothes N, Heinzkill M, Drachenberg KJ, Sperr WR, Krauth MT, Majlesi H, Semper P, Valent P, Niederberger V, Kraft D, Valenta R. Allergen-specific Immunotherapy with a

monophosphoryl lipid A–adjuvanted vaccine: Reduced seasonally boosted IgE production and inhibition of basophil histamine release by therapy-induced blocking antibodies. Clin Exp Allergy 2003; 33:1–11.

120. van Hage-Hamsten M, Valenta R. Specific immunotherapy: The induction of new IgE specificities? Allergy 2002; 57:375–358.

11

Grass Pollen Allergens

ROBERT E. ESCH

Greer Laboratories, Inc., Lenoir, North Carolina, U.S.A.

I. INTRODUCTION

Grass pollens represent a major component of the airborne allergen load during the spring and summer months in most parts of the world. They are responsible for the symptoms in the majority of allergic rhinitis patients and can also trigger asthma. The diagnosis and treatment of grass pollen allergy with grass pollen allergen extracts/vaccines is nearly a hundred years old, and their use for immunotherapy is unequaled by any other allergen vaccine. Since Charles Blackley's initial investigations (1) during the 1870s that led to the identification of grass pollen as the cause of his own illness, the study of grass pollen allergens has continued to fascinate botanists, allergists/immunologists, and, more recently, molecular biologists. In this chapter, the grass family (Poaceae), ecology, and pollen allergens are described. Special attention is given to the molecular characteristics of grass pollen allergens with regard to their cross-reactivities.

1861   II.   CLASSIFICATION AND TAXONOMY

1862   The grasses belong to the family Poaceae (Gramineae) and are grouped with the sedges,
1863   rushes, and other monocots belonging to the order Poales. The family Poaceae is the fourth
1864   largest family of flowering plants, with more than 600 genera and 10,000 species. The
1865   family has historically been divided into two major groups, the pooids and the panicoids,
1866   based on the structure of the spikelet, the basic unit of inflorescence (2). The pollen
1867   antigens of the pooids and panicoids are immunochemically distinct, as are other charac-
1868   teristics including leaf anatomy, embryo anatomy, and karyotype. These and additional
1869   morphological, physiological, biochemical, and cytological comparisons have led to
18610 the recognition of up to nine subfamilies and as many as 60 tribes. Most agrostologists
18611 today recognize five or six subfamilies, although the placement of tribes is variable. A
18612 taxonomic grouping of common grass genera is presented in Table 1. The classification
18613 system is based on that of Watson and Dallwitz (3) with minor modifications. Over 95%
18614 of the allergenically important grass species belong to the three subfamilies Pooideae,
18615 Chloridoideae, and Panicoideae.

18616   III.   THE GRASS FLOWER AND POLLEN

18617 Flowers of the allergenic grasses have obvious characteristics for wind pollination:
18618 reduced perianth, small and smooth pollen grains, high pollen-ovule ratio, and feathery
18619 stigmas. The flower head, known as the inflorescence (Fig. 1), is made up of spikelets,
18620 which are highly modified branches consisting of a pair of bracts called glumes that
18621 protect the immature spikelet and a rachilla, on which are borne one to several florets.
18622 There is wide variation in spikelet structure, size, and shape, and this is of great value in
18623 the identification and classification of grasses.
18624   Pollination in grasses is of short duration and regularly occurs at a certain time of
18625 day or night. The breeding systems of the grasses are extremely varied. Some grasses are
18626 cleistogamous (self-fertile) or entomophilous (insect pollinated) and therefore are not
18627 allergenically important. Polyploidy is common among the grasses, and hybridization is
18628 known to contribute to the adaptation and evolution of many grass groups, especially
18629 among the tribe Triticeae, the cereal grasses.
18630   The pollen structure is unique to the family, but is too uniform to be useful taxo-
18631 nomically (Fig. 2). The pollen is more or less spheroidal to ovoid, 20–55 μm in diameter.
18632 The pollen grain wall consists of two layers, the exine (outer wall) and the intine (inner
18633 wall), and a single germination aperture or pore. Pollen antigens are stored in both
18634 the exine and intine walls, most being localized in the intine. A wide range of pollen anti-
18635 gens, including those that are allergenic, undoubtedly play a major role in the recognition
18636 of a suitable reproductive partner and thus may be expected to be species specific. Many
18637 grass pollen antigens also have wide taxonomic spans. Upon moistening, exine- and
18638 intine-associated components are released into the medium (Fig. 3). The kinetics of anti-
18639 gen release from grass pollen suggest minimal structural compartmentalization compared
18640 with pollen derived from other plant families (4).
18641   Variations in a patient's allergic symptoms during the year depend in part on the
18642 pattern of seasonal pollen exposure. The expected seasonal levels of grass pollen for a
18643 given geographic locality in the United States can be obtained from various sources, includ-
18644 ing the American Academy of Allergy, Asthma, and Immunology (AAAAI) Aerobiology
18645 Committee's Annual Pollen and Spore Report (5). Grass pollen are most abundant during

Table 1 Taxonomic Relationships Between Common Grasses

Subfamily	Tribe	Genus and species	Common name
Bambusoideae	Oryzeae	*Oryza sativa*	Cultivated rice
		Zizania aquatica	Wild rice
		Ehrharta erecta	Panic, veldt grass
Arundinoideae	Arundineae	*Phragmites communis*	Common reed
		Cortoderia	Pampas grass
	Aristideae	*Aristida* spp.	Three-awns
	Stipeae	*Stipa* spp.	Needlegrass
Panicoideae	Paniceae	*Digitaria sanguinalis*	Crabgrass
		Paspalum notatum	Bahia grass
		Panicum miliaceum	Common millet
		Panicum virgatum	Switch grass
		Stentaphrum secundatum	Buffalo grass, Saint Augustine grass
	Andropogoneae	*Eremochloa ophiuroides*	Centipede grass
		Saccharum officinarum	Sugar cane
		Sorghum halepense	Johnson grass
		Sorghum sudanense	Sudan grass
		Zea mays	Corn, maize
Chloridoideae	Chlorideae	*Bouteloua* spp.	Grama grass
		Buchloë dactyloides	Buffalo grass
		Choris spp.	Finger grass
		Cynodon dactylon	Bermuda, couch grass
	Aeluropodeae	*Distichlis spicata*	Salt grass
	Eragrosteae	*Eragrostis* spp.	Love grass
		Eleusine indica	Goose grass
		Tridens flavus	Purpletop
Pooideae	Poaceae	*Bromus inermis*	Smooth brome
		Dactylis glomerata	Orchard grass, cocksfoot
		Festuca elatior	Meadow fescue
		Lolium multiforme	Italian rye
		Lolium perenne	Perennial rye
		Poa compressa	Canada bluegrass
		Poa pratensis	Kentucky bluegrass (June grass)
	Avenae (incl. Agrostideae and Phalarideae)	*Agrostis alba*	Redtop, bent grass
		Anthoxanthum odoratum	Sweet vernal
		Avena sativa	Cultivated oat
		Holcus lanatus	Velvet grass
		Koeleria cristata	June grass
		Phalaris arundinacea	Reed canary
		Phalaris canariensis	Canary
		Phleum pratense	Timothy grass
	Triticeae	*Agropyron repens*	Quack, wheat grass
		Elymus spp.	Wild rye
		Hordeum vulgare	Barley
		Secale cereale	Cultivated rye
		Triticum aestivum	Wheat

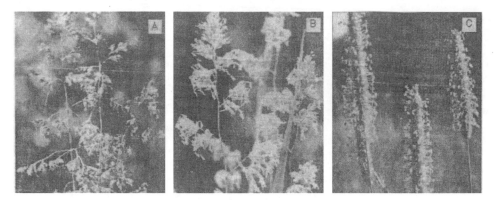

Figure 1 Grass inflorescence, the arrangement of the flowers on the stem, is illustrated by the three pooids (*A*) Kentucky bluegrass with panicles, a compound inflorescence, bearing flowers along slender, spreading branches; (*B*) orchard grass with panicles bearing clusters of flowers near the ends of stout branches; and (*C*) timothy grass with spikes, or cylindrical clusters of flowers with no stalks.

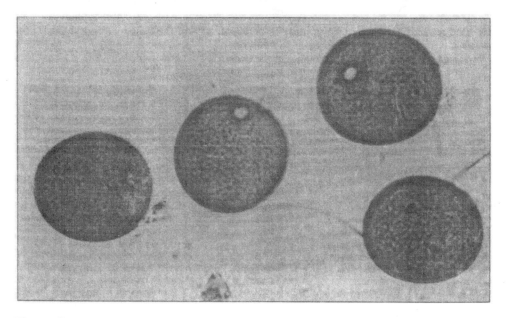

Figure 2 The pollen grains of the grasses are remarkably uniform. They are spheroidal, and in most allergenic species they range from about 20 μm to less than 50 μm in diameter. The exine is thin and has a characteristically granular texture without adornments of any kind. The most distinctive characteristic is the single germ pore, consisting of a small aperture surrounded by a thickened rim of the exine and covered by a transparent membrane.

the spring and summer months and account for a significant portion of the total pollen count during this time. Because whole pollen grains are too large to be respirable, it has been difficult to explain how grass pollen provoke asthmatic symptoms. Several possibilities, including the presence of submicronic particles possessing allergenic activity, have been suggested as the trigger of asthma attacks. The existence of such particles has been confirmed by specialized airborne sampling and immunochemical detection methods (6,7)

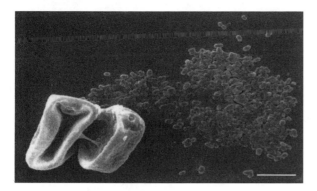

Figure 3 Ryegrass pollen ruptures after slight wetting with sedimenting mist droplets. The cytoplasmic debris from the ruptured pollen forms an aerosol of respirable particles that are loaded with allergens. (From Ref. 9.)

and has been shown to correlate to weather (e.g., thunderstorms) and epidemics of asthma (8). A primary source of such particles has been identified as starch granules (0.6–2.5 μm in diameter) that are released from grass pollen upon contact with moisture. Other sources, including pollen fragments (9), orbicules (10), and allergen-adsorbed aerosols, remain to be investigated

IV. ECOLOGY AND HABITAT

Grasses occur on all continents, from desert to polar regions and in freshwater to marine habitats, and account for about 25–35% of the earth's vegetation. The steppes of Eurasia, the prairies and plains of central and western North America, and the pampa of Argentina represent the most extensive grassland areas of the temperate zone. Less extensive grasslands are found in the velds of South Africa and in Australia and New Zealand. Tropical and subtropical grasslands are located in central Africa and in central South America. In the grasslands, drought, fire, and grazing by animals are the major ecological challenges for a plant's survival. The growth tissue in most plants is located at the tip of the leaf or shoot, and once clipped, it will not grow back. In contrast, the growth tissue in the grasses is located near the base of the leaf or the shoot, and growth continues even after the grass plant is cropped, burned, or grazed. This and other distinctive features—including basal tillering; protection of the flower and fruit within the spikelet; a great diversity of habitats; and alternative photosynthetic pathways, breeding systems, and dispersal mechanisms—allow grasses to survive and dominate in areas where other plants cannot.

The distribution of grass species are delimited by conditions of soil, moisture, temperature, exposure, and altitude. Some species are restricted in habitat, found only in salt marshes or alpine summits. Their geographical range, however, may be extensive. A species found on one mountain range may also be found at the same altitude on another mountain range. Other, more tolerant species, such as *Festuca rubra*, can be found in meadows, bogs, marshes, and hills of North America, Eurasia, and North Africa.

Seventy percent of the world's farmland is planted in crop grasses, with sugar cane (*Saccharum officinarum*), wheat (*Triticum aestivum*), rice (*Oryza sativa*), and maize (*Zea mays*) being the most widely cultivated. Bamboos are a critical part of the economy of many tropical areas because they contribute young shoots for food, fiber for paper, and stems for construction. Grasses are cultivated for livestock feed, for erosion control, and as ornamentals. Many grasses introduced into cultivation escape and become established over wide areas. Their seeds may be carried long distances in cattle cars as impurities in the seed of crop plants and by birds and insects. Often, they become troublesome weeds. The turfgrasses are planted to cover lawns, parks, roadsides, cemeteries, golf courses, and sporting fields. Considerable energy is spent maintaining turfgrasses in areas where they would normally not survive. The lawn industry, which accounts for more than a billion dollars in sales of seed, fertilizers, chemicals, paraphernalia, and services, supports the maintenence of grasses in regions that would otherwise be deciduous forests and deserts. Of the hundreds of genera of grasses recognized, only a few are known to cause allergic disease. The major grass species responsible for inducing allergic symptoms are usually those that are cultivated and, therefore, are prevalent where people live (Table 1).

A. Bambusoideae

The Bambusoideae are the most primitive extant grasses and are associated with forest and aquatic habitats. Bamboos are distributed on the continents of Asia, Africa, and North and South America. They are the least understood in terms of their classification and evolution among the grasses. Bamboos are not allergenically important due to the infrequency of flowering, with up to 120 years elapsing between pollinations in many species. The woody bamboos inhabit the tropical regions as well as temperate regions in Asia. The most primitive grasses are represented among the herbaceous bamboos that inhabit the tropical rain forests. Due to the relative lack of wind in their habitats, they have developed animal pollination. The more advanced climbing and herbacious bamboos have adapted to colder climates of the Himalaya and Andes mountains. The only native bamboos in North America are the two species *Arundinaria tecta* and *A. gigantea* (giant or switch cane), which grow in moist ground from southern Maryland and Ohio to Florida and Texas. The rices, a herbaceous and mainly aquatic group, are in the Bambusoideae subfamily based on their leaf blade anatomy and the presence of six stamens. The Asian species *Oryza sativa* and the wild rice of North America, *Zinania aquatica*, are the best-known species.

B. Arundineae

The Arundineae are thought to represent the direct descendants of the earliest grasses that moved into the open savanna ecosystem. This subfamily is a heterogeneous group of unrelated genera and tribes that do not fit into the other, relatively well-defined subfamilies. As a group, they are distributed mainly in the tropical and temperate regions of the southern hemisphere. Of the some 75 genera represented in the subfamily, only about 5 are native to North America. This group includes giant reed (*Arundo*) and the common reed (*Phragmites communis*), which are frequently planted to control erosion. The female plants of the South American pampasgrass (*Cortaderia*), with their large, plumose panicles, are commonly grown as ornamentals in warmer regions of the world. The some 250 species of *Aristida* (three-awns), having adapted to the semiarid habitats of South Africa and northern Mexico, are one of the more successful genera of this subfamily.

C. Pooideae

The temperate zones are dominated by grasses belonging to the subfamily Pooideae. The major tribes, consisting of about 155 genera, are distributed across the world in relatively well-defined latitudinal belts, with the majority of genera found in the Northern Hemisphere. The center of pooid distribution is the Mediterranean area, and they have adapted to cool and cold climates of the open steppes or meadows. They are virtually absent at low elevations in both humid and dry tropical areas. Species of *Bromus*, *Poa*, *Festuca*, and *Agropyron* can be found only at high altitudes in mountainous regions of tropical latitudes. The pooids account for approximately 70–85% of the grasses in Canada and the northwestern United States, 40–50% in the middle latitudes, and less than 15–25% in the southern United States. The cool-season turfgrasses representing this subfamily include the genera *Poa* (bluegrasses), *Agrostis* (bent grasses), *Festuca* (fescues), and *Lolium* (ryegrasses). These represent the major allergenic grass genera along with *Dactylis glomerata* (orchard grass), *Phleum pratense* (timothy grass), and *Anthoxanthum odoratum* (vernal grass), which are common in meadows, pastures, and waste places. The subfamily also includes the important cultivated cereals *Triticum aestivum* (wheat), *Secale cereale* (rye), and *Hordeum vulgare* (barley).

D. Chloridoideae

The members of the subfamily Chloridoideae are well distributed over North America, Africa, and Australia. The chloridoids have adapted to a wide range of ecotypes, especially the warm and arid habitats, with high winter temperatures and summer or nonseasonal rainfall. Over 50% of the grass species in the southwestern United States are chloridoid, compared with less than 10% of the total in the northwestern United States. The centers of distribution are in the savannas of southern Africa and in the open grasslands of Queensland. Their success in the warm, arid environments is due to the distinct physiological and anatomical features of their C_4 dicarboxylic acid pathway of photosynthesis, referred to as the Kranz syndrome. The popular southern turfgrass *Cynodon dacylon* (Bermuda grass) is widespread throughout the warmer regions of the world and is a major allergenic species. Several species of *Bouteloua* (grama grass) and *Buchloë* (buffalo grass) are the outstanding range forage grasses and occur widely in the central and western United States.

E. Panicoideae

The subfamily Panicoideae dominates the humid, tropical to subtropical environments of the savannas of Indochina and Africa as well as the moist New World tropics, especially northeastern South America. Over 75% of the grasses in the Panama Canal Zone are panicoid, compared with 50% in the southern United States, but only about 5% of the species belong to this subfamily in the northwestern United States. The subfamily includes the largest of the grass genera, *Panicum*, with about 600 species distributed throughout the warmer parts of the world, and the cultivated species *Saccharum officinarum* (sugar cane) and *Sorghum vulgare* (sorghum). Allergenically important species include *Paspalum notatum* (Bahia grass), an important forage and erosion control grass in the Gulf Coast states of the United States, and *Sorghum halepense* (Johnson grass), a forage grass and frequently a troublesome weed in the warmer and tropical regions of both hemispheres.

V. MOLECULAR CHARACTERISTICS AND CROSS-REACTIVITIES OF GRASS POLLEN ALLERGENS

Since the pioneering work of David Marsh and co-workers (11–13) with the perennial ryegrass Group 1, 2, and 3 allergens during the 1960s and 1970s, a number of new allergens have been identified, isolated, and characterized. The techniques of molecular biology and protein chemistry have contributed to the increased knowledge regarding the structure and possible function of grass pollen allergens. Murine monoclonal antibodies raised against specific allergens have been used to define allergenically important and cross-reactive B-cell epitopes. Cloning of cDNA and nucleic acid sequencing has accelerated the availibility of primary structure data. Recombinant allergen fragments and synthetic peptides have been useful in delineating determinants involved in T-cell recognition. High-resolution electrophoretic and immunoblotting techniques have led to the identification of new allergen groups and the detection of microheterogeneity (isoallergens or isoforms) within the grass allergen groups.

The availability of highly purified and well-characterized allergen molecules will undoubtedly continue to lead to further advances and the prospects of better diagnostic and therapeutic approaches.

A. Group 1 Antigens

The grass Group 1 allergens are acidic glycoproteins with molecular weights (MW) in the 27–35 kDa range and exist in at least four isoallergenic forms or isoforms distinguished by their respective pIs. Histochemical examination has localized this glycoprotein in the exine and cytoplasm of the pollen grain (14). The complete Group 1 amino acid sequences from perennial ryegrass (Lol p 1), timothy grass (Phl p 1), velvet grass (Hol l 1), Johnson grass (Sor h 1), and Bermuda grass (Cyn d 1) have been determined and the sequences of internal peptide fragments or N-terminal sequences from several other grass species have been reported (15–17). The degree of glycosylation varies between 2% and 7%, and the monosaccharides fucose, arabinose, xylose, mannose, and N-acetylglucosamine have been detected. The carbohydrate moiety does not appear to play an important role in the allergenicity of the Group 1 allergens, although IgE antibodies toward the carbohydrate structures have been detected in a select group of subjects (18).

The Group 1 allergens belong to a subfamily of structurally related proteins called beta-expansins, which are cell wall–loosening proteins. Their activity shows specificity to grass cell walls, suggesting that they act on the matrix polymers specific to grasses, e.g., glucuronoarabinoxylan or mixed-linked 1,3:1:4-β-glucan (19). The expansin activity of grass Group 1 allergens has been attributed to a papain-like proteinase activity (20,21), but this proposed mechanism of action has been challenged (22). Structural modeling of the presumed cellulose-binding domain of Lol p 1 suggests a close structural relationship between its cellulose-binding and allergenic properties (23).

Allergens homologous to Lol p 1 have been detected in pollen extracts from all grass species examined to date, and in each case greater than 95% of allergic subjects were highly reactive to the respective Group 1 allergens. Patient sensitivity to the Group 1 allergens has been found to correlate with sensitivity to the whole pollen extract as measured by both skin test and histamine release assays. Extensive immunological cross-reactivity among the Group 1 allergens from taxonomically related grasses is also firmly established. For these reasons, a potency assay based on the Group 1 content of grass pollen extracts has been proposed as an approach to grass pollen allergen extract standardization (24).

Two important cross-reactive allergenic determinants or sites have been localized on the pooid grass Group 1 allergen molecule with the aid of murine monoclonal antibodies that were selected for their ability to inhibit human IgE binding to grass Group 1 allergens. One site has been localized on a 28-mer located at the C-terminus (25) (amino acid residues 213–240) of the molecule, and the second site has been localized within amino acid residues 23–35 (26). Continuous B-cell epitopes on Phl p 1 that represent five major IgE-reactive regions of the allergen molecule have been identified by a gene fragmentation approach. The IgE binding fragments, generated from a random fragment expression library of Phl p 1 (27) and Hol l 1 (28) cDNA, represented regions localized at C-terminus, N-terminus, and in the center of the allergen sequence. The allergenic epitopes of the Group 1 allergen of Bermuda grass (Cyn d 1) appear to be different from those defined for the pooid grasses (29) in spite of a 70–75% sequence homology. Nonconservative amino acid substitutions in allergenically important regions may explain the lack of cross-reactivity between Cyn d 1 and the other grass Group 1 allergens (17).

A major human T-cell determinant has been localized within amino acid residues 191–210 utilizing overlapping peptides spanning the entire Lol p 1 molecule (15). Subsequent studies revealed multiple T-cell determinants distributed throughout the molecule, including cross-reactive T-cell epitopes shared with grass Group 2, Group 3, and Group 5 allergens (30–34).

B. Group 2 Antigens

The grass Group 2 allergens are acidic proteins (MW = 11,000) toward which 35–50% of grass-allergic subjects are sensitive. The perennial ryegrass Group 2 antigens exist in at least two immunochemically indistinguishable isoforms, Lol p 2A (pI = 5.0) and Lol p 2B (pI = 5.1–5.3). The complete primary structure of Lol p 2A was determined by peptide sequencing of the purified protein and found to contain 97 amino acids without evidence of glycosylation sites (34). The complete primary structure of an orchard grass Group 2 antigen, Dac g 2, was deduced from the nucleotide sequence of the cDNA encoding the protein and was found to be 97% identical to the Lol p 2 sequence (35). Mapping of IgE-reactive epitopes was attempted using a model based on the solution structure of Phl p 2 and recombinant Phl p 2 fragments spanning the entire molecule (36). Only relatively long fragments representing the N-terminal and C-terminal regions of the molecule showed strong IgE reactivity. No reactivity could be detected when synthetic dodecapeptides spanning the complete Phl p 2 sequence were evaluated. These results indicate that grass Group 2 IgE epitopes are highly conformation dependent.

The amino acid sequences of Group 2 and 3 allergens are also highly homologous. Lol p 2A and Lol p 3 possess 59% identical amino acids, and this percentage increases to 67% when similar amino acids are equated. A similar homology was found for Dac g 2 and Dac g 3, with 66% sequence identity and 79% sequence similarity. This sequence homology translates to a high degree of cross-reactivity at the B- and T-cell levels (30,37).

C. Group 3 Antigens

The grass Group 3 allergens are basic proteins (MW = 11–14 kDa, pI = 9.0–9.4) with a reported frequency of sensitization of 35% to 70% among grass pollen–allergic subjects. The Group 3 allergens from perennial ryegrass and orchard grass pollen have been isolated and characterized at the molecular level (38,39). The complete primary structures of Lol p 3 and Dac g 3 revealed a 92.6% similarity and 84.2% identity, and the mature proteins lack cysteine and show no evidence of glycosylation. In spite of this high degree of homology, computer analyses detected differences in their predicted secondary structure and antigenic sites.

D. Group 4 Antigens

The grass Group 4 allergens are high-molecular-weight basic glycoproteins (MW = 50–60 kDa, pI = 8.6–10.4) of unknown biochemical function. The initial report by Marsh found only a 20% sensitization rate toward Lol p 4 among grass-allergic subjects, but other studies suggest that Group 4 allergens or a similar group of high-molecular-weight basic glycoproteins from timothy grass, orchard grass, and Bermuda grass may be responsible for sensitization rates of 50–75%. The complete primary structure of a Group 4 allergen has not yet been reported, although some information is available from amino acid sequence data of a limited number of tryptic fragments. Using monoclonal antibodies raised against Dac g 4, related proteins from a various pooid and chlorodoid grass species were detected on SDS-PAGE immunoblots. ELISA inhibition experiments, however, revealed cross-reactivity only among the pooid grasses (40). Allergenic determinants have been localized on two Lol p 4 peptide fragments (MW = 17.4 and 11.0 kDa) by CNBr cleavage of the purified protein. Fragmentation of these Lol p 4 fragments with trypsin or chymotrypsin completely destroyed their IgE binding capacity, hampering further resolution and delineation of the allergenic sites (41). A decapeptide sequence of Phl p 4 shows significant sequence similarity to peptides from the major allergen family of ragweed pollen, Amb a 1 and Amb a 2 (42). Phl p 4 specific monoclonal antibody and human IgE antibody binding could be inhibited by preadsorption with Amb a 1. Rabbit and human antibodies directed toward Phl p 4 react with allergens present in various tree and weed pollen as well as vegetables and fruits (43,44). Together, these findings suggest the possibility of common IgE-binding epitopes on grass Group 4 allergens and various unrelated pollen and plant foods. Studies with the Group 4 allergen from Bermuda grass (45) suggest that the carbohydrate moiety, accounting for about 7.5% of the mass, may be an important allergenic determinant of the molecule. Periodate oxidation reduced the IgE binding activity of the allergen by approximately 50%. The predominant N-linked oligosaccharides of the molecule are unique among plant glycoproteins in that they possess α-(1,3)-linked fucose without any xylose (46).

E. Group 5 Antigens (Includes Group 9 Antigens)

The Group 5 allergens are a heterogeneous group of proteins with pIs ranging from 4.2 to 7.0 for Phl p 5 isoforms (47) and from 9.0 to 10.2 for the Lol p 5 (formerly Lol p 9/1b) isoforms and Poa p 5 isoforms (48,49). Comparison of the deduced amino acid sequences of the three Group 5 allergens shows a high degree of homology (80–90%), which is consistent with the high degree of cross-reactivity observed. Their having similar molecular weights to the Group 1 allergens (27–35 kDa for Group 1 and 27–38 kDa for Group 5) may explain why traditional protein fractionation methods based on molecular size failed to establish the identity of the Group 5 allergens. The Group 5 allergens, together with the Group 1 allergens, account for the majority of the IgE binding reactivity of most grass-allergic sera. In contrast to the Group 1 allergens, Group 5 allergens have been identified only among the subfamily Pooideae, and polyclonal antibodies raised against Group 5 allergens failed to detect cross-reactive antigens outside of the subfamily. Furthermore, Northern analysis with Poa p V probes could only identify homologous transcripts among the pooids (50). Thus, it appears that Group 5 allergens are restricted to a single subfamily of grasses, and if similar proteins are produced by the panicoid, chloridoid, and arundinoid grasses, they are immunochemically and genetically unique.

By using recombinant and synthetic allergen fragments, investigators have localized IgE binding determinants in the central and C-terminal regions of the Lol p 5 molecule

(51,52) to both the N-terminal and C-terminal ends of Phl p 5 (53) and predominantly on a C-terminal fragment of Poa p 5 (Poa p 9) (54). At least four continuous and five discontinuous IgE binding sites were localized on the Group 5 allergen from velvet grass pollen (Hol l 5), and each were differentially recognized by individual patient IgE antibodies (55). Taken together, these studies suggest either a extremely heterogeneous human B-cell response to Group 5 allergens or a marked difference in the epitope structures of Group 5 proteins derived from the different grass species.

A remarkable characteristic of the Group 5 allergens is their association with intracellular starch granules within the pollen grain. The cDNA sequence of Lol p 5 revealed the flanking transit peptide sequences typical of chloroplast-targeted proteins, and thus it has been proposed that Lol p 5 is synthesized as a pre-allergen in the cytosol and transported to the amyloplast for posttranslational modification (56). This model may explain the existence of the multiple isoforms and the molecular weight heterogeneity of Group 5 allergens isolated from pollen extracts. The size of the starch granules (0.6–2.5 µm in diameter) and their sudden appearance in air samples following rainfall is suggestive of a role in triggering asthmatic reactions. Phl p 5 has been shown to possess ribonuclease activity, and the homologous Group 5 allergens from the other grass species may be expected to possess this activity as well (57). It is interesting to speculate on the role of ribonuclease activity at the level of pollen–stigma interaction: Its release during hydration and stigma contact might facilitate the reproductive responses of the stigma.

T-cell determinants have been localized on Lol p 5 and Phl p 5 allergens by generating specific T-cell lines or clones and measuring proliferative responses to a series of overlapping Group 5 synthetic peptides spanning the entire sequence of the molecule (32,33,58,59). T-cell determinants were spread throughout the allergen molecule. Regions of high reactivity were found in specific patients but differed among patients. Isoform-specific T-cell epitopes were also detected with Phl p 5a and Phl p 5b fragments. The observed diversity of the human T-cell response and specificity shown by individual patient responses suggest that immunotherapy with allergen peptides is not feasible.

F. Group 6 Antigens

The Group 6 allergens from timothy grass pollen, Phl p 6, are polypeptides (MW = 12–13 kDa, pI = 5.2–5.5) toward which a majority of timothy grass pollen–sensitive subjects react (60,61). The Group 6 allergens have so far been detected only in timothy grass pollen extracts. Phl p 6 is a pollen-specific protein localized on the polysaccharide-containing wall-precursor bodies or P-particles (60). The amino acid sequence deduced from the cDNA sequence revealed no cysteines and one potential glycosylation site, although no carbohydrate structures were detected (61). The N-terminal sequence of Phl p 6 is highly homologous to internal Phl p 5 sequences, and epitope mapping studies with rPhl p 6 fragments indicate that the N-terminus of the molecule is required for IgE recognition. Sequence analysis of cDNA encoding the complete Phl p 6 allergen provides evidence for an independent gene family arising from gene duplication. Comparison of the complete Phl p 6 and Phl p 5 sequences showed only a 55–60% match even though the N- and C-termini of Phl p 6 showed about a 95% similarity to the internal Phl p 5 protein sequence. Both unique and shared epitopes have been identified on Phl p 5 and, 6 allergens using antibodies raised against Phl p 5 and Phl p 6, and allergenic cross-reactivity has been detected by immunoadsorption studies (62). Epitope mapping studies with rPhl p 6 fragments indicate that the N-terminus of the molecule is required for IgE recognition.

G. Group 7 Antigens

The Group 7 allergens (MW = 8–12 kDa) from Bermuda (Cyn d 7) and timothy grass pollen (Phl p 7) were identified and isolated from a cDNA expression library using serum IgE from grass-allergic individuals (63,64). The Group 7 allergens belong to a new family of Ca^{2+}-binding proteins, characterized by the presence of two potential EF-hand calcium-binding domains. Approximately 35% of grass pollen–allergic subjects possessed IgE antibodies toward the recombinant Cyn d 7. In addition, approximately 10% of pollen-allergic patients possessed IgE antibodies toward Group 7–homologous allergens present in the pollen of monocotyledonic and dicotyledonic plants. The deduced amino acid sequence of this protein shows significant sequence similarity with a variety of Ca^{2+}-binding proteins, including the pollen allergens Bet v 4 from birch, Aln g 4 from alder, Ole e 3 from olive, Bra r 1 from oilseed rape, and calmodulin from the fungus *Fusarium oxysporum*. A three-dimensional model of Phl p 7 with two calcium-binding domains (EF-hands) shows a novel dimer assembly adopting a barrel-like structure with an extended hydrophobic cavity providing a ligand-binding site (65). Structural similarities with other pollen allergens with two EF-hands (Bet v 4, Aln g 4, Ole e 3, Cyn d 7, and Bra r 1), three EF-hands (Bet v 3), and four EF-hands (Jun o 4 and Ole e 8) have also been suggested by molecular modeling studies (66). Cross-reactivity with Bet v 4 has been established and a cross-reactive allergenic epitope was localized to the region representing the Ca^{2+}-binding domain II of the molecule, which shows a 83.3% amino acid sequence identity between Bet v 4 and Cyn d 7. The Cyn d 7 clone hybridized to transcripts in 13 other grass pollens using RNA gel blot analysis, suggesting that homologous proteins with similar allergenic activity may be present in other grass pollens. In addition, pollen extracts derived from 16 unrelated genera exhibited cross-reactivity with Aln g 4 and Jun o 4, suggesting that calcium-binding allergens are widely distributed in pollen from various plants.

H. Group 10 Antigens (Cytochrome c)

Cytochrome c (MW = 11 kDa, pI = 10) from timothy grass, perennial ryegrass, and Bermuda grass pollens has been demonstrated to be allergenic in humans having allergies to the respective pollen. Its importance as an allergen based on sensitization rates has not been thoroughly documented. This allergen group has been proposed as a model system for studying the molecular basis of cross-reactivity because a vast knowledge base exists for cytochrome structure and function (67).

I. Group 11 Antigens

The Group 11 allergens are a group of glycoproteins (MW – 16–18 kDa, pI = 5.0 6.0) structurally similar to the Kunitz soybean trypsin inhibitor, but lack the active site and appear not to possess inhibitory activity. Proteins that are homologous to Lol p 11 have been reported in other grass and non-grass pollen, including timothy grass, maize, tomato, and olive (68,69). This allergen may have eluded detection in conventional immunoblotting techniques using SDS-PAGE under reducing conditions, because there are three potential disulfide bridges present that may be required for maintaining the IgE-binding peptide epitopes.

Among individuals with IgE antibodies against grass pollen, approximately 65% possessed IgE antibodies toward Lol p 11, and of these, about 35% possessed IgE antibodies against the carbohydrate moiety. Monosaccharide analysis suggested that *N*-glycan (mannose-type) or arabinoxylan substitutions may represent the IgE-binding carbohydrate group(s). The *N*-glycan structures appear to be involved in IgE binding, as is bee venom phospholipase A_2, an allergen with known *N*-glycan IgE binding epitopes, which is a potent inhibitor of IgE binding to Lol p 11. The recombinant form of Phl p 11, expressed as a soluble fusion protein in *Escherichia coli*, induced histamine release from basophils and skin reactivity in grass pollen–sensitized subjects. The unglycosylated rPhl p 11 showed a reduced prevalence of IgE reactivity among grass pollen–positive sera and little or no cross-reactivity with other members of this allergen family, suggesting its diagnostic utility in identifying the primary sensitizer in allergic individuals.

J. Group 12 Antigens (Profilin)

Profilin, purified from grass pollen, has been suggested as an important allergen because antiprofilin IgE antibodies can be detected in 20–50% of grass-sensititive subjects (70). Because profilin is a highly conserved protein present in all organisms, the potential role of this allergen as a "panallergen" has been proposed (71). The cDNA sequences of timothy grass, Bermuda grass, and birch (*Betula verrucosa*) pollen encoding for the respective profilins are 80% homologous, but profilins from unrelated sources are much more variable and typically are less than 50% homologous (72). Allergic patients with multiple pollen and plant-derived food sensitizations frequently possess IgE antibodies toward profilin. However, the clinical relevance of the cross-reacting IgE antibodies could not be established (73).

K. Group 13 Antigens

The Group 13 allergens (MW = 50–60 kDa, pI = 6.0–7.5) have similar molecular weights to the grass Group 4 allergens and are difficult to distinguish by one-dimensional SDS-PAGE. This and the finding that Group 13 allergens are highly susceptible to proteolytic degradation may explain why they were not identified earlier. Approximately 42–75% of grass-sensitive subjects possess IgE antibodies to the Group 13 allergens, and allergenic proteins homologous to Phl p 13 have been detected in all grass pollen extracts examined to date. The deduced amino acid sequence from the cloned cDNA of Phl p 13, consisting of 394 residues, indicated homology with pollen-specific polygalacturonases (74). The observation that Group 13 allergens show increased susceptibility to proteolytic degradation after removal of low-molecular-weight constituents may be of interest to manufacturers of allergen extracts because dialysis and gel filtration are commonly used for their production.

VI. GRASS POLLEN ALLERGEN CROSS-REACTIVITY

Grass-allergic subjects almost always display multiple grass pollen sensitivities. Because many grass species coexist in the same geographical area, simultaneous sensitization to pollen from multiple grass species is expected. RAST and ELISA inhibition assays have revealed extensive allergenic cross-reactivity among taxonomically related grasses, suggesting that sensitization to one pollen species could lead to multiple grass pollen sensitivities.

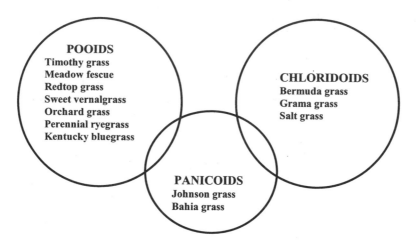

Figure 4 A Venn diagram representing cross-reactivity groupings of major allergenic grasses based on their taxonomic and immunological relationships. The grass species within each subfamily group are highly cross-reactive and are difficult to differentiate immunologically. The two groups pooids and chloridoids are allergenically distinct and require separate diagnoses and immunotherapies. The panicoids, Johnson and Bahia grass, are allergenically cross-reactive with both the pooids and chloridoids.

The pattern of allergenic cross-reactivity among the pollen species closely follows their taxonomic relationships (Fig. 4). All studies found the highest degree of allergenic cross-reactivity among pollen extracts derived from grasses of the same subfamily. Martin et al. (75), using a human serum pool from allergic North American subjects with pollen extracts from the three subfamilies Pooideae (brome, meadow fescue, perennial ryegrass, timothy, sweet vernal, redtop, Kentucky bluegrass, and Western wheatgrass), Chloridoideae (salt grass, Bermuda grass, and grama grass), and Panicoideae (Bahia grass and Johnson grass), detected little or no cross-reactivity between pooid and chloridoid pollen, while the panacoid grasses showed moderate cross-reactivity with both the pooids and chloridoids. González et al. (76), employing sera from European subjects selected for reactivity toward each pollen group, detected little or no allergenic cross-reactivity between the pooids (perennial ryegrass, timothy, and cultivated rye) and Bermuda grass. *P. communis* (common reed), an arundinoid, showed moderate cross-reactivity with both the pooids and chloridoids. In a study involving 209 individual sera with reactivity toward grass pollen, extensive cross-reactivity was detected among 14 different species of pooids, with the highest responses directed toward *P. pratensis, F. rubra, P. pratense*, and *D. glomerata*. Excluding *P. communis*, an arundinoid, *C. dactylon*, a chloridoid, and *Z. mays*, a panicoid, any one grass species was sufficient for in vitro diagnosis of grass pollen allergy (77). No studies have examined possible allergenic cross-reactivities between arundinoid and panicoid pollens.

The availability of purified grass pollen allergens, allergen fragments, and recombinant allergens has allowed for more refined studies that detect cross-reactivity among allergens derived from the same species as well as among homologous allergens from different species. Of particular interest is the strong homology between the C-terminal end of the Group 1 molecule (amino acid residues 145–240) and the entire 97-amino-acid sequence of the grass Group 2 and Group 3 allergens. The human immune response to the three ryegrass allergens is associated with histocompatibility leukocyte antigen (HLA) DR3, and concordant reactivity to all three allergens is common. These observations may be explained by cross-reactivity among Lol p 1, Lol p 2, and Lol p 3, which has been detected at both the B-cell level and the T-cell level. Some human T-cell clones are reactive to the purified protein of the three allergen groups and the Group 5 allergen. Stretches of homologous segments with an amphipathic nature suggest the presence of structural similarities that may account for this cross-reactivity.

The cross-reactive nature of the ubiquitous protein profilin is illustrated by the serological cross-reactivity between grass pollen profilins and profilins from other pollen and vegetable foods. Human antiprofilin IgE antibodies have been shown to cross-react with almost all plant profilins. The presence of highly conserved structures among plant profilins may explain the reports of coincident oral allergies to fruits and vegetables eaten by grass-allergic subjects (70,78,79) as well as allergenic cross-reactivities occasionally detected between unrelated pollens. The Group 4 and Group 7 allergens may also be useful diagnostic markers to identify patients with multiple sensitizations caused by cross-reactivity. For example, grass Group 4–related proteins have been identified in unrelated plant foods including peanut, apple, celery, and carrot root as well as mugwort and birch pollen. Approximately 20% of polysensitized individuals possess IgE antibodies toward calcium-binding pollen proteins. Among the calcium-binding proteins, Phl p 7 contained most of the relevant IgE epitopes in the population studied and may be a useful molecule for detecting sensitization to this group of cross-reactive pollen allergens.

Cross-reactive carbohydrate determinants (CCDs) of grass pollen allergens have also been implicated in serological cross-reactions among a variety of pollen and vegetable foods (80,81). The ß(1-2)-xylose– and α(1-3)-fucose–containing glycans on glycoproteins from several plants, molluscs, and insects have been shown to be highly cross-reactive. The clinical significance of anti-carbohydrate IgE antibodies has not been established, and the role of CCDs in allergic sensitization remains to be explored (82). In this regard, the grass Group 11 allergens and Cyn d 4 (BG60) may present a unique opportunity to investigate the role of both carbohydrate and peptide epitopes in allergenic cross-reactivity among glycoproteins from related and unrelated sources. The presence of conserved amino acids and cysteine positions in the primary structure of Lol p 11 suggests homology with pollen glycoproteins from maize, rice, tomato, olive tree, and privet.

Since grass pollen immunotherapy was pioneered by Freeman and Noon (83) almost a century ago, the specificity of grass immunotherapy has been questioned. Freeman advocated the use of only extracts/vaccines from timothy grass pollen for the diagnosis and treatment of grass allergy in Great Britain, as did Cooke and Vander Veer (84) in the United States Leavengood et al. (85) selected a group of patients showing multiple sensitivities to pooid, panicoid, and chloridoid grasses and treated them with vaccines prepared only from timothy and Bermuda grass pollens. The treatment significantly reduced the skin test responses to all of the grass pollens, suggesting that treatment with the two grass pollen vaccines may be sufficient for effective treatment in these grass-allergic patients. The current practice parameters for allergen immunotherapy established by both the American Academy of Allergy, Asthma, and Immunology and the American College of Allergy, Asthma, and Immunology specifically state that information regarding allergen cross-reactivity should be used in the selection of relevant allergens for immunotherapy because limiting the number of allergens in a treatment vial may be necessary to attain optimal therapeutic doses for the individual patient (86). The molecular and clinical evidence for cross-reactivity among grass pollen allergens supports the notion that effective diagnosis and immunotherapy can be accomplished with a limited number of grass pollen extracts/vaccines. The use of representative extracts/vaccines from the major grass subfamilies appears to be a reliable strategy, and the selection of the species should be based on their prevalence. For example, timothy grass (or any of the pooids), Bermuda grass, and Johnson grass, which represent the three major allergenic grass subfamilies, should be sufficient for clinical practice.

VII. CONCLUSION

Grasses are ubiquitous and their pollens are important aeroallergens in most parts of the world. Only a few grass species have been positively identified as important sources of allergens, but less conspicuous grass species may add to the aeroallergen load due to their cross-reactivity. The degree of allergenic cross-reactivity tends to correlate with taxonomic grouping, and the treatment of grass allergy with vaccines derived from representative species has been shown to be efficacious. Cross-reactivities between homologous proteins from different grass species and their clinical relevance have long been established. There is evidence of cross-reactivities between grass pollen allergens and proteins derived from diverse plant sources, including other pollens, fruits, and vegetables. Clinical investigations to establish the relevance of such cross-reactivities are still needed.

New immunochemical and molecular biological approaches to the study of grass pollen allergens have greatly increased the knowledge about this important group of pollen allergens. Due to their worldwide importance, grass allergens are a subject of great interest among researchers from virtually every continent, and more than 70 grass pollen allergen structures have been identified, purified, and sequenced. Two groups independently sequenced and assembled more than 90% of the rice (*Oryza sativa*) genome (87,88). Because the members of the grass family are closely related and their genomes share extensive synteny, this genetic information will undoubtedly have a great impact on grass pollen allergen research. It is expected that in the next few years the molecular structure of all of the major grass allergen groups will have been established. The human immune responses at both the B-cell and T-cell levels are being studied to define relevant structures on the grass allergen molecules, and novel diagnostic and therapeutic approaches based on their immunological activities are in progress. Together with advances being made with allergens from other environmental sources, the study of grass pollens will contribute to a better understanding of allergic responses to these ubiquitous allergens.

VIII. SALIENT POINTS

1. Grasses are ubiquitous, and grass pollen allergens are of worldwide importance.
2. Of the hundreds of grass genera and thousands of species, only a small number are allergenically important. Most of these species are cultivated.
3. The pooids account for most grass species in Canada and the northwestern United States and are prevalent in the cooler regions of the world; the chloridoids are well established especially in the warm and arid habitats with high winter temperatures, such as the southwestern United States; and the panicoids dominate the humid tropical environments, including the southern United States and northeastern South America.

4. Allergic symptoms depend on pollen exposure. Particles that are significantly smaller than the size of grass pollen grains and capable of entering the lower airway have been implicated as major causes of allergic reactions.

5. Eleven groups of structurally related allergens have been identified and characterized across multiple grass subfamilies.

6. Grass-allergic patients often display multiple sensitivities. Simultaneous sensitization to multiple species are expected based on the numerous grass species pollinating at a given time and place and on the high degree of cross-reactivity among them.

7. Allergenic cross-reactivities have been documented among homologous allergens produced by taxonomically related grasses and between allergens produced in a single grass species.

8. The presence of conserved structures among the proteins and various carbohydrate determinants of pollen and vegetable foods is consistent with coincident allergic reactions to fruits and vegetables as well as unrelated pollens in grass pollen–allergic patients.

9. Diagnosis and immunotherapy with a limited number of grass allergen vaccines representing the subfamilies Pooideae, Chloridoideae, and Panicoideae may be effective in most grass-allergic patients.

10. Advances made with the rice genome project should be leveraged to increase understanding of the structure, expression, and function of grass pollen allergens.

REFERENCES

1. Waite KJ. Blackley and the development of hay fever as a disease of civilization in the nineteenth century. Med Hist 1995; 39:186–196.
2. Hitchcock AS. Manual of the Grasses of the United States, 2nd ed., rev. by A. Chase. Misc. Publ. 200. Washington, DC: USDA, 1951.
3. Watson L, Dallwitz MJ. The Grass Genera of the World, 2nd ed. Wallingford, UK: CAB International, 1994.
4. Barunuik JN, Bolick M, Esch R, Buckely CE. Quantification of pollen solute release using pollen grain column chromatography. Allergy 1992; 47:411–417.
5. Aeroallergen Monitoring Network. 1996 Pollen and Spore Report. Milwaukee: AAAA&I, 1997.
6. Habenicht HA, Burge HA, Muilenburg ML, Solomon WR. Allergen carriage by atmospheric aerosol: II. Ragweed-pollen determinants in submicronic atmospheric fractions. J Allergy Clin Immunol 1984; 74:64–67.
7. Schumacher MJ, Griffith RD, O'Rourke MK. Recognition of pollen and other particulate aeroantigens by immunoblot microscopy. J Allergy Clin Immunol 1988; 82:608–616.
8. Knox RB. Grass pollen, thunderstorms and asthma. Clin Exp Allergy 1993; 23:354–359.
9. Taylor PE, Flagan RC, Valenta R, Glovsky MM. JA. Release of allergens as respirable aerosols: A link between grass pollen and asthma. J Allergy Clin Immunol 2002; 109:51–56.
10. Vinckier S, Smets E. The potential role of orbicules as a vector of allergens. Allergy 2001; 56:1129–1136.
11. Johnson P, Marsh DG. Allergens from common rye grass pollen (*Lolium perenne*): I. Chemical composition and structure. Immunochemistry 1966; 3:91–100.
12. Johnson P, Marsh DG. Isoallergens from rye grass pollen. Nature 1965; 206:935–937.
13. Marsh DG, Haddad ZH, Campbell DH. A new method for determining the distribution of allergenic fractions in biological materials: its application to grass pollen extracts. J Allergy 1970; 46:107–121.

14. Howlett BJ, Vithanage HIMV, Knox RB. Immunofluorescence localization of two water soluble glycoproteins, including the major allergen of rye-grass, *Lolium perenne*. Histochem J 1981; 13:461–480.

15. Perez M, Ishioka GY, Walker LE, Chesnut RW. cDNA cloning and immunological characterization of the rye grass allergen Lol p I. J Biol Chem 1990; 265:16210–16215.

16. Laffer S, Valenta R, Vrtala S, Susani M, van Ree R, Kraft D, Scheiner O, Duchêne M. Complementary DNA cloning of the major allergen Phl p 1 from timothy grass (*Phleum pratense*): Recombinant Phl p 1 inhibits IgE binding to group 1 allergens from eight different grass species. J Allergy Clin Immunol 1994; 94:689–698.

17. Smith PM, Suphioglu C, Griffith IJ, Theriault K, Knox B, Singh MB. Cloning and expression in yeast *Pichia pastoris* of a biologically active form of Cyn d 1, the major allergen of Bermuda grass pollen. J Allergy Clin Immunol 1996; 98:331–343.

18. Petersen A, Becker W-M, Moll H, Blumke M, Schlaak M. Studies on the carbohydrate moieties of the timothy grass pollen allergen Phl p I. Electrophoresis 1995; 16:869–875.

19. Cosgrove DJ. Loosening of plant cell walls by expansins. Nature 2000; 407:321–326.

20. Grobe K, Becker WM, Schlaak M, Petersen A. Grass group 1 allergens (beta-expansins) are novel, papain-related proteinases. Eur J Biochem 1999; 263:33–40.

21. Grobe K, Poppelmann M, Becker WM, Petersen A. Properties of group 1 allergens from grass pollen and their relation to cathepsin B, a member of the C1 family of cysteine proteinases. Eur J Biochem 2002; 269:2083–2092.

22. Li LC, Cosgrove DJ. Grass group 1 pollen allergens (beta-expansins) lack proteinase activity and do not cause wall loosening via proteolysis. Eur J Biochem 2001; 268:4217–4226.

23. Barre A, Rouge P. Homology modeling of the cellulose-binding domain of a pollen allergen from rye grass: Structural basis for the cellulose recognition and associated allergenic properties. Biochem Biophys Res Commun 2002; 296:1346–1351.

24. Baer H, Maloney CJ, Norman P, Marsh DG. The potency and group I antigen content of six commercially prepared grass pollen extracts. J Allergy Clin Immunol 1974; 54:157–164.

25. Esch RE, Klapper DG. Isolation and characterization of a major cross-reactive grass group I allergenic determinant. Mol Immunol 1989; 26:557–561.

26. Hiller KM, Esch RE, Klapper DG. Mapping of an allergenically important determinant of grass group 1 allergens. J Allergy Clin Immunol 1997; 100:335–340.

27. Ball T, Fuchs T, Sperr R, Valent P, Vangelista L, Kraft D, Valenta R. B cell epitopes of the major timothy grass pollen allergen, Phl p 1, revealed by gene fragmentation as candidates for immunotherapy. FASEB J 1999; 13:1277–1290.

28. Shramm G, Bufe A, Petersen A, Haas H, Schlaak M, Becker WM. Mapping of IgE-binding epitopes on the recombinant major group 1 allergen of velvet grass pollen, rHol l 1. J Allergy Clin Immunol 1997; 99:781–787.

29. Han S, Chang Z, Chang H, Chi C, Wang J, Lin C. Identification and characterization of epitopes on Cyn d I, the major allergen of Bermuda grass pollen. J Allergy Clin Immunol 1993; 91:1035–1041.

30. Baskar S, Parronchi P, Mohapatra S, Romagnani S, Ansari AA. Human T cell responses to purified pollen allergens of the grass, *Lolium perenne*: Analysis of relationship between structural homology and T cell recognition. J Immunol 1992; 148:2378–2383.

31. Mohapatra SS, Mohapatra S, Yang M, Ansari AA, Parronchi P, Maggi E, Romagnani S. Molecular basis of cross-reactivity among allergen-specific human T cells: T-cell receptor Vα gene usage and epitope structure. Immunology 1994; 81:15–20.

32. Müller W-D, Karamfilov T, Bufe A, Fahlbush B, Wolf I, Jüger L. Group 5 allergens of timothy grass (Phl p 5) bear cross-reacting T cell epitopes with group 1 allergens of rye grass (Lol p 1). Int Arch Allergy Immunol 1996; 109:352–355.

33. Burton MD, Papalia L, Eusebius NP, O'Hehir RE, Rolland JM. Characterization of the human T cell response to rye grass pollen allergens Lol p 1 and Lol p 5. Allergy 2002; 57:1136–1144.

34. Ansari AA, Shenbagamurthi P, Marsh DG. Complete primary structure of a *Lolium perenne* (perennial rye grass) pollen allergen, Lol p II. J Biol Chem 1989, 263:11181–11185.

35. Roberts AM, Bevan LJ, Flora PS, Jepson I, Walker MR. Nucleotide sequence of cDNA encoding the group II allergen cocksfoot/orchard grass (*Dactylis glomerata*), Dac g II. Allergy 1993; 48:615–623.

36. De Marino S, Castiglione Morelli MA, Fraternali F, Tamborini E, Musco G, Vrtala S, Dolecek C, Arosio P, Valenta R, Pastore A. An immunoglobulin-like fold in a major plant allergen: The solution structure of Phl p 2 from timothy grass pollen. Structure Fold Des 1999; 7:943–952.

37. Ansari AA, Kihara TK, Marsh DG. Immunochemical studies of *Lolium perenne* (rye grass) pollen allergens Lol p I, II, and III. J Immunol 1987; 139:4034–4041.

38. Ansari AA, Shenbagamurthi P, Marsh DG. Complte primary structure of a *Lolium perenne* (perennial rye grass) pollen allergen, Lol p III: Comparison with known Lol p I and II sequences. Biochemistry 1989; 28:8665–8670.

39. Guérin-Marchand C, Sénéchal H, Bouin A-P, Leduc-Brodard V, Taudou G, Weyer A, Peltre G, David B. Cloning, sequencin and immunlogical characterization of Dac g 3, a major allergen from *Dactylis glomerata* pollen. Mol Immunol 1996; 33:797–806.

40. Leduc-Brodard V, Inacio F, Jaquinod M, Forest E, David B, Peltre G. Characterization of Dac g 4, a major basic allergen from *Dactylis glomerata* pollen. J Allergy Clin Immunol 1996; 98:1065–1072.

41. Jaggi KS, Ekramoddoullah AKM, Kisil FT. Allergenic fragments of ryegrass (*Lolium perenne*) pollen allergen Lol p IV. Int Arch Allergy Appl Immunol 1989; 89:342–348.

42. Fischer S, Grote M, Fahlbusch B, Müller WD, Kraft D, Valenta R. Characterization of Phl p 4, a major timothy grass (*Phleum pratense*) pollen allergen. J Allergy Clin Immunol 1996; 98:189–198.

43. Grote M, Stumvoll S, Reichelt R, Lidholm J, Rudolf V. Identification of an allergen related to Phl p 4, a major timothy grass pollen allergen, in pollen, vegatables, and fruits by immunogold electron microscopy. Biol Chem 2002; 383:1441–1445.

44. Stumvoll S, Lidholm J, Thunberg R, DeWitt AM, Eibensteiner P, Swoboda I, Bugajska-Schretter A, Spitzauer S, Vangelista L, Kazemi-Shirazi L, Sperr WR, Valent P, Kraft D, Valenta R. Purification, structural and immunological characterization of a timothy grass (*Phleum pratense*) pollen allergen, Phl p 4, with cross-reactive potential. Biol Chem 2002; 383:1383–1396.

45. Su S-N, Shu P, Gai-Xuong L, Yang S-Y, Huang S-W, Lee Y-C. Immunologic and physico-chemical studies of Bermuda grass pollen antigen BG60. J Allergy Clin Immunol 1996; 98:486–494.

46. Ohsuga H, Su S-N, Takahashi N, Yang S-Y, Nakagawa H, Shimada I, Arata Y, Lee Y-C. The carbohydrate moiety of the Bermuda grass antigen BG60: New oligosaccharides of plant origin. J Biol Chem 1996; 273:26653–26658.

47. Matthiesen F, Lowenstein H. Group V allergens in grass pollen: I. Purification and characterization of group V allergen from *Phleum pratense* pollen, Phl p V. Clin Exp Allergy 1991; 21:297–307.

48. Silvanovich A, Astwood J, Zhang L, Olsen E, Kisil F, Sehon A. Mohapatra S, Hill R. Nucleotide sequence analysis of three cDNAs coding for Poa p IX isoallergens of Kentucky bluegrass pollen. J Biol Chem 1991; 266:1204–1210.

49. Ong EK, Griffith IJ, Knox RB, Singh MB. Cloning of a cDNA encoding a group V (group IX) allergen isoform from rye-grass pollen that demonstrates specific antigenic immunoreactivity. Gene 1993; 134:235–240.

50. Smith PM, Ong EK, Knox RB, Singh MB. Immunological relationships among group I and group V allergens from grass pollen. Mol Immunol 1994; 31:491–498.

51. Ong EK, Knox RB, Singh MB. Mapping of the antigenic and allergenic epitopes of Lol p VB using gene fragmentation. Mol Immunol 1995; 32:295–302.

52. Suphioglu C, Blaher B, Rolland JM, McCluskey J, Schappi G, Kenrick J, Singh MB, Knox RB. Molecular basis of IgE-recognition of Lol p 5, a major allergen of rye-grass pollen. Mol Immunol 1998; 35:293–305.

53. Bufe A, Becker W-M, Schramm G, Petersen A, Mamat U, Schlaak M. Major allergen Phl p Va (timothy grass) bears at least two different IgE-reactive epitopes. J Allergy Clin Immunol 1994; 94:173–181.

54. Zhang L, Olsen E, Kisil FT, Hill RD, Sehon AH, Mohapatra SS. Mapping of antibody binding epitopes of a recombinant Poa p IX allergen. Mol Immunol 1992; 29:1383–1389.

55. Schramm G, Bufe A, Petersen A, Haas H, Merget R, Schlaak M, Becker WM. Discontinuous IgE-binding epitopes contain multiple continuous epitope regions: Results of an epitope mapping on recombinant Hol l 5, a major allergen from velvet grass pollen. Clin Exp Allergy. 2001; 31:331–341.

56. Singh MB, Hough T, Theerakulpisut P, Avjioglu A, Davies S, Smith PM, Taylor P, Simpson RJ, Ward LD, McCluskey J, Puy R, Know B. Isolation of cDNA encoding a newly identified major allergenic protein of rye-grass pollen: Intracellular targeting to the amyloplast. Proc Natl Acad Sci USA 1991; 88:1384–1388.

57. Bufe A. Uhlig U, Scholzen T, Matousek J, Schlaak M, Weber W. A nonspecific, single-stranded nuclease activity with characteristics of a topisomerase found in a major grass pollen allergen: Possible biological significance. Biol Chem 1999; 380:1009–1016.

58. Blaher B, Suphioglu C, Knox RB, Singh MB, McCluskey J, Rolland JM. Identification of T-cell epitopes of Lol p 9, a major allergen of ryegrass (*Lolium perenne*) pollen. J Allergy Clin Immunol 1996; 98:124–132.

59. Wurtzen P, Wissenbach M, Ipsen H, Bufe A, Arnved J, van Neerven RJ. Highly heterogeneous Phl p 5-specific T cells from patients with allergic rhinitis differentially recognize recombinant Phl p 5 isoallergens. J Allergy Clin Immunol 1999; 104:115–122.

60. Vrtala S, Fischer S, Grote M, Vangelista L, Pastore A, Sperr WR, Valent P, Reichelt R, Kraft D, Valenta R. Molecular, immunological and structural characterization of Phl p 6, a major allergen and P-particle–associated protein from Timothy grass (*Phleum pratense*) pollen. J Immunol 1999; 163:5489–5496.

61. Petersen A, Bufe A, Schramm G, Schlaak M, Becker W-M. Characterization of the allergen group VI in timothy grass pollen (Phl p 6): II. cDNA cloning of Phl p 6 and structural comparison to group V. Int Arch Allergy Immunol 1995; 108:55–59.

62. Petersen A, Bufe A, Schlaak M, Becker W-H. Characterization of the allergen group VI in timothy grass pollen (Phl p 6): I. Immunological and biochemical studies. Int Arch Allergy Immunol 1995; 108:49–54.

63. Suphioglu C, Ferreira F, Knox RB. Molecular cloning and immunological characterisation of Cyn d 7, a novel calcium-binding allergen from Bermuda grass pollen. FEBS Lett 1997; 402:167–172.

64. Niederberger V, Hayek B, Vrtala S, Laffer S, Twardosz A, Vangelista L, Sperr WR, Valent P, Rumpold H, Kraft D, Ehrenberger K, Valenta R, Spitzauer S. Calcium-dependent immunoglobulin E recognition of the apo- and calcium-bound form of a cross-reactive two EF-hand timothy grass pollen allergen, Phl p 7. FASEB J 1999; 13:843–856.

65. Verdino P, Westritschnig K, Valenta R, Keller W. The cross-reactive calcium-binding pollen allergen Phl p 7, reveals a novel dimer assembly. EMBO J 2002; 21:5007–5016.

66. Tinghino R, Twardosz A, Barletta B, Puggioni EM, Iacovacci P, Butteroni C, Afferni C, Mari A, Hayek B, Di Felice G, Focke M, Westritschnig K, Valenta R, Pini C. Molecular, structural and immunological relationships between different families of recombinant calcium-binding pollen allergens. J Allergy Clin Immunol 2002; 109:314–320.

67. Ekramoddoullah AKM, Kisil FT, Sehon AH. Allergenic cross-reactivity of cytochromes c of Kentucky bluegrass and perennial ryegrass pollen. Mol Immunol 1982; 19:1527–1534.

68. van Ree R, Hoffman DR, Vandijk W, Brodard V, Mahieu K, Koeleman CAM, Grande M, van Leeuwen A, Aalberse RC. Lol p XI, a new major grass pollen allergen, is a member of

a family of soybean trypsin inhibitor-related proteins. J Allergy Clin Immunol 1995; 970–978.

69. Marknell DeWitt A, Niederberger V, Lehtonen P, Spitzauer S, Sperr WB, Valent P, Valenta R, Lidholm J. Molecular and immunological characterization of a novel timothy grass (*Phleum pratense*) pollen allergen, Phl p 11. Clin Exp Allergy 2002; 32:1329–1340.

70. van Ree R, Voitenko V, van Leeuwen WA, Aalberse RC. Profilin is a cross-reactive allergen in pollen and vegetable foods. Int Arch Allergy Immunol 1992; 98:97–104.

71. Valenta R, Duchene M, Vrtala S, Valent P, Sillaber CV, Ferreira F, Tejkl M, Hirschwehr R, Ebner C, Kraft D, Scheiner O. Profilin, a novel plant pan-allergen. Int Arch Allergy Immunol 1992; 99:271–273.

72. Valenta R, Ball T, Vrtala S, Duchene M, Kraft D, Scheiner O. cDNA cloning and expression of timothy grass (*Phleum pratense*) pollen profilin in *Escherichia coli*: Comparison with birch pollen profilin. Biochem Biophys Res Commun 1994; 199:106–118.

73. Wensing M, Akkerdaas JH, van Leeuwen WA, Stapel SO, Bruijnzeel-Koomen C, Aalberse RC, Bast B, Knulst AC, van Ree R. IgE to Bet v 1 and profilin: Cross-reactivity patterns and clinical relevance. J Allergy Clin Immunol 2002; 11:435–442.

74. Suck R, Petersen A, Hagen S, Cromwell O, Becker WM, Fiebig H. Complementary DNA cloning and expression of a newly recognized high molecular mass allergen Phl p 13 from timothy grass (*Phleum pratense*). Clin Exp Allergy 2000; 30:324–332.

75. Martin BG, Mansfield LE, Nelson HS. Cross-allergenicity among the grasses. Ann Allergy 1985; 54: 99–104.

76. Gonzales RM, Cortés C, Conde J, Negro JM, Rodriguez J, Tursi A, Wüthrich B, Carreira J. Cross-reactivity among five major pollen allergens. Ann Allergy 1987; 59: 149–154.

77. van Ree R, van Leeuwen WA, Aalberse RC. How far can we simplify in vitro diagnostics for grass pollen allergy? A study with 17 whole pollen extracts and purified natural and recombinant major allergens. J Allergy Clin Immunol 1998; 102:184–190.

78. De Martino M, Novembre E, Cozza G, De Marco A, Bonazza P, Vierucci A. Sensitivity to tomato and peanut allergens in children monosensitized to grass pollen. Allergy 1988; 43:206–213.

79. Petersen A, Vieths S, Aulepp H, Schlaak M, Becker W-H. Ubiquitous structures responsible for IgE cross-reactivity between tomato fruit and grass pollen allergens. J Allergy Clin Immunol 1996; 98:805–813.

80. Calkhoven PG, Aalbers M, Koshte VL, Pos O, Oie HD, Aalberse RC. Cross-reactivity among birch pollen, vegetables and fruits as detected by IgE antibodies is due to at least three distinct cross-reactive structures. Allergy 1987; 42:382–390.

81. Mari A. Multiple pollen sensitization: A molecular approach to the diagnosis. Int Arch Allergy Immunol 2001; 125:57–65.

82. Aalberse RC, Akkerdaas JH, van Ree R. Cross-reactivity of IgE antibodies to allergens. Allergy 2001; 56:478–490.

83. Freeman J, Noon L. Further observations on the treatment of hayfever by hypodermic inoculations of pollen vaccine. Lancet 1911; 2:814–817.

84. Cooke RA, Vander Veer A. Human sensitization. J Immunol 1916; 1:201–237.

85. Leavengood DC, Renard RL, Martin BG, Nelson HS. Cross allergenicity among grasses determined by tissue threshold changes. J Allergy Clin Immunol 76:789–794.

86. Joint Task Force on Practice Parameters (AAAAI, ACAAI, JCAAI). Allergen immunotherapy: A practice parameter. Ann Allergy 2003; 90:S1–S40.

87. Yu J, Hu S, Wang J, et al. A draft sequence of the rice genome (*Oryza sativa* L. spp *indica*). Science 2002; 296:79–92.

88. Goff SA, Ricke D, Lan TH, et al. A draft sequence of the rice genome (*Orysa saliva* L. spp *japonica*). Science 2002; 296:92–100.

12

Weed Pollen Allergens

SHYAM S. MOHAPATRA and RICHARD F. LOCKEY

*University of South Florida College of Medicine and James A. Haley
Veterans' Hospital, Tampa, Florida, U.S.A.*

FLORENTINO POLO

ALK-Abello, Madrid, Spain

I. INTRODUCTION

Ragweed pollen is one of the most important sources of allergenic proteins in different parts of the Americas, and it is widespread globally. Although ragweed pollination begins in midsummer and extends to late autumn, its pollinating season varies depending on the geographical location. Immunotherapy with ragweed allergen vaccine has been established as a variably effective therapeutic regimen for ragweed-allergic patients. There are many other allergenic weeds, both related and unrelated to ragweed. Ragweeds, by far, are the most important clinically and hence have been studied thoroughly. Investigators, using molecular biological techniques, have succeeded in advancing the knowledge of the allergenic constituents of ragweed and have provided information on the molecular structure of its allergens and their potential cross-reactivity. Special attention is given in this chapter to the integration of the morphological, taxonomical, and aerobiological aspects, as well as the biochemical and clinically relevant aspects of weed pollen allergens.

Table 1 Botanical Classification of Important Allergenic Weeds

Family	Genus	Common name	Clinical importance
Compositae	*Ambrosia*	Ragweed	+++
	Franseria	False ragweed	−
	Iva	Marsh elder	+
	Xanthicum	Cocklebur	−
	Artemisia	Sage, mugwort	++
	Chrysanthemum	Daisy	+
	Taraxacum	Dandelion	−
	Parthemum	Guayule	+
	Parthenium	American feverfew	++
Amaranthaceae	*Amaranthus*	Pigweed, amaranthus	+
	Atriplex	Orache, scale	+
	Beta	Beet	+
	Chenopodium	Lamb's quarters	+
		Burning bush	
		Russian thistle	
		Pellitory	
	Kochica	Nettle	+
	Salsola	Patterson's curse	+
Urticaceae	*Parietaria*	Ram	++
	Urtica	Plantain	+
Boraginaceae	*Echium*	Sorrel, dock	+
Brassicaceae	*Brassica*	Mustard	+
Plantaginaceae	*Plantago*	English plantain	+
Polygonaceae	*Rumex*	Unknown	+

Relative clinical importance of the weeds is as follows: +++, major; ++, moderate: +, minor; and −, no or little importance. *Source*: Ref. 2.

II. TAXONOMY OF WEEDS

Of the families of weeds that have been identified, some have been implicated in pollen allergy, some have not, and the importance of others as allergens is unknown. Table 1 provides a comprehensive list of the prevalent weeds with their botanical classifications (taxonomic family and genus), common names, and relative clinical importance (1). A botanist or aerobiologist should be consulted for detailed information on the prevalent weeds in one's surrounding geographical area. The exposure records as collected and compiled by the American Academy of Allergy, Asthma, and Immunology can be obtained by calling the Pollen Hotline, 1-800-POLLEN, or by writing to the American Academy of Allergy, Asthma, and Immunology, 611 East Wells Street, Milwaukee, WI 53202-3889.

III. WEED AND POLLEN IDENTIFICATION

Although there are many species of ragweeds, their morphology is strikingly similar (2). Some of the important weeds of the United States are shown in Fig. 1. The characteristic features of short ragweed include a finely divided leaf, each leaf being subdivided into three or more segments, which are further divided, giving a typical fernlike appearance.

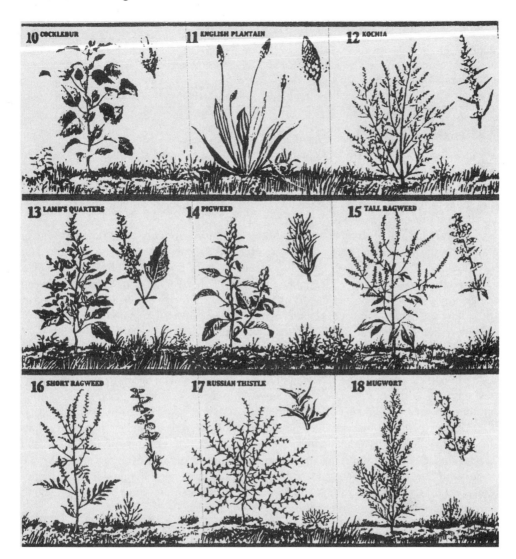

Figure 1 Illustration of some common allergenic weeds in the United States. *Source:* Poster on Center Laboratories Guide to Allergenic Trees, Weeds and Grasses of the United States.

The pyramid-shaped plants grow in the thousands in various parts of the United States, mostly on river banks and on land that has been disturbed. They branch extensively, with a ground spread spanning 3 to 4 feet and a height of 4 to 5 feet, producing greenish-yellow flower spikes. In marked contrast to short ragweed, giant ragweed features broad leaves, which may be three- or five-lobed or undivided, with blades of the leaf carried down the leaf stalk as narrow wings on each side. Giant ragweed branches above the ground as a columnar bush frequently attaining a height between 10 and 15 feet. Western ragweed is similar to short ragweed in size and habitat. However, these weeds typically have inconsistently divided leaves and grow each spring from the roots rather than the seeds. Western giant ragweed differs from its eastern counterpart by its wingless leaves and its tendency

Table 2 The Characteristic Anatomical Features of Ragweed Pollen

Tricolporate: three furrows (boat-shaped portion of grain surface), each enclosing a pore
Subechinate: surface coarsely granular, beset with spines
Small: greatest diameter 18 to 20 μm
Exine: medium size; subechinate; beset with short spines, approximately 1.7 to 3.4 μm apart

Source: Ref. 2.

to branch well above the ground, rising from the root on a central stalk. Southern ragweed has slender, lance-shaped leaves with one or more large teeth near its base and is much smaller than other ragweeds. All of the preceding ragweed species are to be distinguished from clinically less important species that are essentially similar in their general appearance but are distinguished by their spinier seed pods.

Toward the end of summer, most ragweeds produce extremely small flowers borne in immense numbers on small heads, which are arranged in long spikes at the top of the plant and at the ends of side branches. The spikes stand out in the ragweed plant, and these spike-like structures produce pollen. The pollen grains of the large number of different ragweed species vary considerably in size and form, but they are all light and buoyant and are shed in large quantities over prolonged periods. Table 2 summarizes the anatomical features of ragweed pollen (3). Ragweed pollen causes allergic rhinitis, but its relatively large size (~12 μm) suggests that ragweed pollen may be less likely to penetrate past the glottis and cause asthma (4). However, a study by Agarwal et al. revealed that airborne ragweed allergens are present in particles of less than 10 μm in diameter. Ragweed plant debris exists in different-sized particles both before and after the ragweed season. These allergenic particles may contribute to out-of-pollination-season symptoms in many ragweed-sensitive subjects (5).

Other weeds that may produce pollen and cause hay fever include mugwort, plantain, pellitory, sunflower, marsh elder, cocklebur, sagebrush, chenopods, amaranths, and Russian thistle. Each of these has morphological features distinct from ragweed (Fig. 1). Most of these weeds are suspected to cause allergic asthma, allergic rhinitis, and conjunctivitis; however, except for a small number of species, few studies have been conducted to confirm their importance or to characterize their allergens.

Mugwort (*Artemisia vulgaris*), which also belongs to the Compositae family, is an aromatic, perennial weed with stalks 2 to 4 feet long, petiolate leaves, and small, inconspicuous flower heads. It preferably grows on ruderal soils in urban, suburban, and rural areas and pollinates in late summer (6). Pollen grains of mugwort are oblate-spheroidal, 18 to 22 μm in diameter, and normally tricolporate.

The genus *Plantago* belongs to the family Plantaginaceae and comprises about 250 species. One of the most common species is *Plantago lanceolata* (English plantain or ribwort), which has been associated with hay fever since the beginning of last century (7). English plantain is a biennial or perennial herbaceous weed. It has a basal rosette of ribbed lanceolate leaves and leafless stems up to 2 feet long bearing dense spikes of hermaphroditic flowers protected by oval bracts. It grows in moist soils, waste places, fields, and pastures. Spheroidal, multipored (with six to eight pores), pollen grains (24–28 μm) are airborne during the pollination period, which occurs in spring and summer.

The genus *Parietaria* (pellitory), which belongs to he Urticaceae family, is composed of a number of allergenically related species. The most common and best-studied species are *P. judaica* and *P. officinalis*. They are perennial weeds with a barely ramified hairy stem 1 to 3 feet in height. They possess oval or lanceolate leaves and axillary agglomerated flowers. The preferred habitat has been defined for some *Parietaria* species. *P. officinalis* is mainly found in mountainous zones, whereas *P. judaica* grows on walls in urban coastal areas. Nevertheless, there are no clear limits to their distribution, and two or more species may grow simultaneously in most regions. *Parietaria* plants produce large amounts of small (12–18 µm) spheroidal tricolporate pollen grains, which are released through a mechanism of propulsion operated by the elastic filament of the anther, ensuring the success of wind-borne pollination. *Parietaria* has a very long pollen season, which extends over several months. Depending on the climate, the pollination may last nearly the whole year, as happens, for instance, in southern Italy, where it starts in February and persists until December, with two cycles of flowering (8).

IV. DISTRIBUTION OF WEEDS

The important and clinically relevant weeds of the world are listed in Table 3 (4). Ragweed is the most important weed in terms of its allergenic pollen worldwide and in the United

Table 3 Allergenically Relevant Weeds of the World

Country	Weeds
Argentina	Short ragweed
Australia	Capeweed, wattle, plantain, dock, goosefoot family, Paterson's curse, wild mustard
Brazil	Ragweed
Canada	Ragweed, goosefoot family, pigweed, Russian thistle, sage, dock, plantain
Chile	Lamb's quarters, English plantain, cocklebur, dock, sorrell
Colombia	Pigweed family
Cuba	Short ragweed, goosefoot, pigweed family
Ecuador	Goosefoot and pigweed families
Egypt	Goosefoot and pigweed families
France	Ragweed, sagebrush, plantain, pellitory, goosefoot and pigweed families
Russia	Sagebrush, ragweed
Germany	Dock, nettle, plantain, goosefoot family, sagebrush
Great Britain	Sunflower family, plantain, sorrels and docks, nettle, goosefoot, mugwort
Hawaii	Goosefoot and pigweed families
Hungary	Plantain, dock, goosefoot, hemp, ragweed, sagebrush, pigweed, cocklebur
India	Cocklebur, hemp, sagebrush, dock, goosefoot and pigweed families, castor bean, mugwort
Italy	Pellitory, mugwort, sunflower, warnwood, burweed
Japan	Sagebrush, ragweed
Netherlands	Ragweed, sagebrush, sedges, cattails
New Zealand	Plantain, dock, goosefoot family
Portugal	Goosefoot and pigweed families, cocklebur, plantain, sage, pellitory
Romania	Goosefoot, sages, ragweed
Sweden	Dock, sagebrush, goosefoot family, pellitory
United States	Ragweeds (short, giant, western, southern, slender, and false ragweeds), burweed, marsh elder, cocklebur, sages, pigweed, Russian thistle, firebush
Yugoslavia	Hemp, pellitory, dock, goosefoot and pigweed families, ragweed, plantain, castor bean

Source: Ref. 1.

States There are nearly 60 species included in the ragweed family. In the eastern United States, the common or short ragweed and its relative, the giant ragweed, grow in great profusion in roadside ditches and disturbed areas. These two species are the major ragweeds found in the northeastern United States, including parts of Canada, but they are much less abundant in the western states and on the Pacific coast. Western ragweed prevails in the states west of the Rocky Mountains, on the Pacific coast, and in the south and southwestern states from Louisiana to Arizona. Southern ragweed, with typically lance-shaped leaves, is important as a cause of hay fever, but is mainly confined to the central United States. The slender and bur ragweeds are among the false ragweeds, which consist of about 25 species that exist in the United States, and these are common in the Southwest and in Colorado; the latter also ranges northward into Canada, where it is abundant in most arid regions.

Seasonal pollen dispersal is important since it suggests the critical period of avoidance for ragweed-sensitive individuals in various locations. Frenz and associates (9) compared ragweed pollen dispersal in the United States using volumetric techniques and recorded the date of first and final pollen capture and the date of maximum airborne pollen concentration at locations ranging from 30° to 45° north latitude. Sixteen cities located at 38° N have similar peak dates, achieving maximal pollen concentration in late August or early September. Four cities located south of 38° N experience later peak dates, reaching maximum pollen levels in mid-October.

Mugwort is widely spread, especially in the temperate and humid zones of the Northern Hemisphere and along the Mediterranean basin. The pollen of mugwort has been considered the most important cause of pollinosis at the end of summer and beginning of autumn in Europe, with pollination in Central Europe occurring at the end of July and through August, while in the Mediterranean areas it takes place mostly in September and the beginning of October (10).

English plantain is distributed in the temperate zones of both hemispheres. It was introduced from Europe in North America and is now found throughout Canada and the United States. English plantain is also widespread in Asia and Australia. The pollen season begins in April or early May, peaking in May–July, depending on the latitude and climatic conditions, and continuing throughout the remainder of summer and early fall. The clinical importance of pollinosis caused by English plantain has been underestimated for a long time because of the low frequency of monosensitized patients and the overlap of the pollen season with that of grasses. Nevertheless, a high incidence of allergy to English plantain pollen has been reported in the last two decades in different geographic areas, particularly in the Mediterranean basin and Australia (11,12).

Parietaria is the most important allergenic plant in most regions of the Mediterranean-surrounding countries (8). The abundance of this plant, and hence its allergenic relevance, decreases in Europe as the latitude increases, although sensitization to *Parietaria* has been reported to occur as far north as southern England (13). Only one report identifying *Parietaria* as a cause of respiratory allergy in the United States has been published so far, in which 8 out of 100 sequential patients with seasonal respiratory allergy referred to the allergist practice prick-tested positive to *Parietaria* (14). One important characteristic of *Parietaria* is the very long pollination period, resulting in multiseasonal or even almost perennial symptoms shown by allergic patients, ranging from mild rhinoconjunctivitis to severe asthma. The prevalence of asthma is very high (40–60%) in certain regions, such as central and southern Italy (15).

V. MOLECULAR CHARACTERISTICS OF RAGWEED POLLEN ALLERGENS

Although a number of allergens from diverse weeds have been studied, the most extensively studied is short ragweed. The allergens isolated and characterized from various weeds are listed in Table 4 (16–19). Crossed-radioimmunoelectrophoresis of aqueous short ragweed pollen extract detected 22 distinct proteins, which bound to specific human IgE antibodies (16,17). However, not all of these allergens have been fully characterized.

The predominant allergen from short ragweed pollen, Amb a 1 (formerly known as antigen E), first purified and identified in 1964 (16–18), consists of an α- and a β-chain. Amb a 1 constitutes about 6% of the protein content of short ragweed pollen, and about 90% of ragweed-sensitive subjects have antibodies directed to Amb a 1. Using site-specific monoclonal antibodies, a small number of major antigenic determinants were found on the native Amb a 1 molecule (20). The cloning of Amb a 1 polypeptide subunits revealed that short ragweed pollen contained four isoforms of Amb a 1, designated as 1.1, 1.2, 1.3, and 1.4 (21). The IgE binding ability of these isoforms indicated that they differ in their capacity to bind human IgE, with a ranking of 1.1 > 1.3 > 1.4 > 1.2. T-cell responses to these individual isoforms of Amb a 1, measured by the stimulation index (SI), which is an index of T-cell proliferation compared with control cells showing a different ranking: 1.1, SI = 25; 1.2, SI = 4.2; 1.3, SI 9.1, and 1.4, SI-8.3. Together, these studies confirm that Amb a 1 is the dominant allergen of short ragweed pollen (21).

Table 4 Weed Pollen Allergens

Botanical name (common name)	Allergens	Molecular weight (kDa)
Ambrosia artemisiifolia (short ragweed)	Amb a 1 (antigen E)	38
	Amb a 2 (antigen K)	38
	Amb a 3 (Ra 3)	11
	Amb a 5 (Ra 5)	5
	Amb a 6 (Ra 6)	10
	Amb a 7 (Ra 7)	12
	Amb a	11
Ambrosia trifida (giant ragweed)	Amb t 5 (Ra 5G)	4.4
Artemisia vulgaris (mugwort)	Art v 1	27–29
	Art v 2 (Ag 7)	35
	Art v 3 (LTP)	12
	Art v 4 (profilin)	14
	Art v ? (Art v I)	60
Parietaria judaica (pellitory of the wall)	Par j 1	10–15
	Par j 2	11.3
	Par j 3 (profilin)	14
Parietaria officinalis	Par o 1	11–15
Plantago lanceolata (English plantain)	Pla l 1	17–20
Chenopodium album (lamb's quarters)	Che a 1	17
Salsola kali (Russian thistle)	Sal k 1	43
Helianthus annuus (sunflower)	Hel a 1	34
	Hel a 2 (profilin)	15.7
Mercurialis annua	Mer a 1 (profilin)	14–15

The second most important short ragweed allergen, Amb a 2, is closely related to Amb a 1 (65% amino acid identity). Amb a 1 is present in both pollen and flower heads of short ragweed, while Amb a 2 is detectable only in flower heads. Recombinant (*Escherichia coli* produced) and native Amb a 2 differ in their ability to bind human IgG antibodies (22), indicating that the recombinant protein is not as allergenic as the native protein. About 58% of the 7-cell lines were stimulatable with Amb a 2, exhibiting an average SI of 14 (21).

Amb a 3 is a basic glycoprotein, having a single polypeptide chain composed of 101 amino acid residues (23). Clinical testing has shown that Amb a 3 is highly allergenic in about 30–50% of short ragweed–sensitive patients (24) and therefore is a minor allergen. The antibody and T lymphocyte recognition regions on short ragweed allergen Amb a 3 (Ra3) have been characterized (25).

One of the most studied among the minor allergens is Amb a 5. About 10–20% of short ragweed–allergic subjects are sensitized to this allergen (26,27). The Amb 5 allergens have been cloned and sequenced from different species of ragweed and have been characterized with respect to their B- and T-cell epitopes (28). The 3-D structures of Amb t 5 and Amb a 5 were also derived by two-dimensional spectroscopy (29,30). The HLA association study of human allergic immune response demonstrated that all Amb 5 allergens were restricted by the same DR molecule (31).

A few other minor allergens have also been defined in the pollens of short ragweed. Radioallergosorbent test (RAST) analysis has determined that 17–51% of ragweed-allergic patients exhibit IgE antibodies that bind to these minor allergens. Three other allergens, including Amb a 6, have been described in short ragweed pollen (32–34).

In addition to the ragweed pollen allergens, allergens found in other weeds are important in different geographic regions of the world. These include mugwort (35–42), English plantain (43–46), *Parietaria* (47–57), sunflower (58,59), lamb's quarter (60), Russian thistle (61), and parthenium (62).

Mugwort pollens contain approximately 40 extractable proteins, of which 10 appear to be allergens (35). Five allergens from mugwort have been characterized, although one of them is not included yet in the official list of allergens of the International Union of Immunological Societies (IUIS), in spite of having been the first allergen isolated from this pollen, because no sequence information is available. This allergen, which was termed *Art v* I in the article dealing with its purification (36), is a monomeric acidic glycoprotein of 60 kDa in SDS-PAGE that is recognized by the IgE from 73% of mugwort allergic patients.

The allergen named Art v 1 in the official list of allergens is a different glycoprotein, with 108 amino acid residues and high sugar content (30–40%), to which 95% of the individuals allergic to mugwort have specific IgE. Art v 1 is a modular glycoprotein with an N-terminal cysteine-rich domain homologous to plant defensins and a C-terminal domain rich in hydroxyproline residues some of which are Ø-glycosylated (37). The carbohydrate moiety is highly heterogeneous (two major series of peaks centered around 13.4 and 15.6 kDa are observed in mass spectra of the natural allergen), and it greatly influences the electrophoretic mobility of the allergen, since the apparent molecular weight in SDS-PAGE is as high as 27–29 kDa. Besides, it seems that the carbohydrate moiety of Art v 1 plays an important role in the allergenicity (37). A single immunodominant T-cell epitope recognized by 81% of patients has been identified (38).

Art v 2 is also a glycosylated protein (10% carbohydrate content) that consists of two identical polypeptide chains covalently linked by disulfide bridges. It exists in at least six different isoforms. Art v 2 cannot be considered as a major allergen, since it bound IgE from only 33% of sera from patients with pollinosis caused by mugwort (39).

Two plant panallergens, lipid transfer protein (LTP) and profilin, have been identified in mugwort pollen. Art v 3 belongs to the LTP family. The N-terminal amino acid sequence of this allergen, covering more than one-third of its complete sequence, showed a 40–50% sequence identity with LTPs from Rosaceae fruits (40). The rate of positive skin prick tests for Art v 3 is 40% in mugwort-allergic patients (41). The name Art v 4 has been assigned to mugwort profilin. Thirty-six percent of mugwort-sensitive patients have IgE antibodies against this allergen (42).

English plantain pollen contains 5 to 10 allergenic proteins (43–45). The prevalence of specific IgE to the major allergen Pla l 1 in plantain-allergic patients is about 90%. Pla l 1 is a mixture of isoforms that may occur in glycosylated and unglycosylated forms (45,46). Three Pla l 1 variants have been sequenced that display about 40% sequence identity with the major *Olea europaea* pollen, allergen Ole e 1 (46).

Although authors differ on the number of allergens present in *Parietaria* pollen, all agree that a highly heterogeneous glycoprotein with a molecular weight in the range of 10–15 kDa is the main allergen, inducing an IgE response in at least 95% of *Parietaria*-allergic patients (47,48). The major allergens from *P. judaica* and *P. officinalis*, Par j 1 and Par o 1, isolated from their respective pollens exhibit very similar physicochemical and immunochemical properties (49–51). Different Par j 1 isoforms and variants have been isolated both from the natural source and through recombinant expression (52–54). Another allergen, Par j 2, sharing 45% sequence identity and an immunodominant IgE epitope with Par j 1, has been produced as a recombinant protein (55,56). Both Par j 1 and Par j 2 are related to the plant LTP family. The panallergen profilin has also been identified in *P. judaica* pollen and named Par j 3 (57).

VI. WEED POLLEN ALLERGEN CROSS-REACTIVITY

Plants having a close taxonomic relationship will probably have pollen proteins with homologous sequences. Clinical studies have revealed that skin test–positive ragweed-allergic patients are also positive to pollen proteins derived from several distinct plant families (63). The cross-reactivity among weed pollen allergens may be categorized as interspecies and intraspecies cross-reactivity. Table 5 summarizes the Western blotting

Table 5 Cross-reactivity Among Weed Pollen Allergens[a]

Ragweed species	Anti–Amb a 1 pAbs	Anti–Amb a 2 pAbs	Anti–Amb a 2 mAb
False ragweed (*Franseria acanthicarpa*)	Yes	Yes	No
Slender ragweed (*F. envifolia*)	Yes	Yes	No
Wooly ragweed (*F. tormentosa*)	Yes	Yes	No
Short ragweed (*A. artimisiifolia*)	Yes	Yes	Yes
Southern ragweed (*A. bidentata*)	Yes	Yes	No
Western ragweed (*A. psilostachya*)	Yes	Yes	Yes
Western giant ragweed (*A. aptera*)	Yes	Yes	No
Giant ragweed (*A. trifida*)	Yes	Yes	No

Abbreviations: pAb, polyclonal antibodies; mAb, monoclonal antibody.
[a]Western blotting analysis (21).

Table 6   Interspecies Cross-reactivity of Weed Pollen Allergens

Species (common name)	Ragweed allergens	Remarks
Phleum pratense (Phl p 4, timothy grass)	Amb a 1	Basis for cross-reactivity between grass and weed allergens
Chamaecyparis obtusa (Cha a I, Japanese cypress)	Amb a 1	46–49% sequence identity
	Amb a 2	
Cryptomeria japonica (Cry j 1, Japanese cedar)	Amb a 1	46–49% sequence identity
	Amb a 2	
Zea mays (corn)	Amb a 1	Sequence homology
Partheniurn histerophorus (American feverfew)	Amb a	82–94% cross-inhibition

analyses of pollen proteins from different ragweeds that have demonstrated both intra- and interspecies cross-reactivity among ragweed allergens (21). Table 6 summarizes interspecies cross-reactivity of weed pollen allergens, especially considering Amb a 1 and Amb a 2 sequence homology. The results of these studies showed that the Amb a 1 and Amb a 2 allergens of short ragweed not only share significant homologies with each other, but also share homologies with the equivalent allergens from different ragweed species (21). Thus, these two allergens have not diverged significantly throughout the evolution of different ragweed species. Similarly, Amb a 5 and Amb t 5 share about 49% identity in their amino acid sequences (28).

In addition to the cross-reactivity among related ragweeds, the cross-reactivity of ragweed allergens and the allergens of other plants have been reported. Some of these studies are listed in Table 6. Analysis by RAST and immunoblotting inhibition revealed cross-reactivity between sunflower pollen and other pollen of the Compositae family (mugwort, marguerite, goldenrod, and short ragweed). Mugwort pollen exhibited the greatest degree of allergenic homology with sunflower pollen, whereas at the other end of the spectrum, short ragweed showed fewer cross-reactive epitopes (64). Another study showed that there is no cross-allergenicity between mugwort and ragweed pollen (65). However, it has been reported that mugwort and ragweed pollen contain a number of cross-reactive allergens, among them the major mugwort allergen Art v 1 and profilin (66).

Skin tests and tests for IgE antibodies of ragweed-sensitive subjects are usually positive to a number of different pollens, frequently from taxonomically diverse species, which are assumed to be allergenically non–cross-reactive (67–70). Cross-reactivity has also been reported between ragweed and a number of vegetables, including fennel, parsley, and carrot (71). Parthenium, a weed introduced from the United States to India, is the major aeroallergen in southern India. Parthenium allergens are cross-reactive with short ragweed pollen (72). Thus, the presence of pollen-reactive IgE antibodies may not necessarily identify the sensitizing pollen species. This information is clinically important in view of the increased migration of people among different continents.

LTPs have been identified as major allergens of the Rosaceae fruits (peach, apple, apricot, and cherry) in patients from the Mediterranean area, and many of these patients show cosensitization to mugwort pollen. In vitro and in vivo studies suggest that sensitization to the cross-reactive mugwort LTP (Art v 3) may extend the recognition pattern of these patients to more distantly related species (40,41). Although Par j 1 and Par j 2 are also related to the LTP family, an association between sensitization to *Parietaria* and Rosaceae fruits has not been demonstrated. It is worth mentioning that sensitization to *Parietaria* normally means sensitization to several species of this genus, since a strong cross-reactivity among the major allergens from different species has been demonstrated (73).

As far as English plantain is concerned, a 30-kDa allergen cross-reactive with the grass Group 5 allergens has been identified, yet this cross-reactivity shows little or no clinical relevance (44). In the same way, despite the structural similarity between Pla l 1 and Ole e 1, a rather limited allergenic cross-reactivity between these allergens has been found (46).

VII. RAGWEED IMMUNOTHERAPY

The effectiveness of ragweed immunotherapy for hay fever was established in the 1960s, at much the same time as the allergenic composition of the extract was being determined (74–76). There have been attempts, however, to investigate the efficacy and safety of variations in the approach to immunotherapy. In an effort to increase the safety of allergen immunotherapy, some clinical studies have been done using chemically modified (77) or peptidic fragments of ragweed vaccine (78), or encapsulated allergens (79). However, none of these modified products are utilized in clinical practice. The original immunotherapy protocols for ragweed-allergic subjects have remained unchanged, except that ragweed allergens used today are standardized with respect to the content of Amb a 1, the major ragweed allergen (75,79). Similarly, methods to determine the concentration of the major allergens from *Parietaria*, mugwort, and English plantain pollens have been devised, and some companies market allergenic products of these species that are standardized on this basis (73,80–82).

VIII. SALIENT POINTS

1. A large number of weed species, not all of which are clinically important, contribute to the seasonal increases in weed pollen allergens in the air. The most important allergenic pollens are derived from ragweed and its relatives, mugwort, and pellitory.
2. The identification of local and regional weed plants and weed pollens is important for clinical practice.
3. The cross-reactivity of weed allergens should be considered in the management of weed-allergic subjects.
4. The most important allergens of short ragweed are the major allergens, Amb a 1 and Amb a 2. These two major allergens and three minor short ragweed allergens, as well as allergens from other weeds, such as mugwort, pellitory, plantain, and lamb's quarters, have been characterized in terms of their molecular structure and cross-reactivity.
5. Many weed pollen allergens are cross-reactive. Amb a 1, the major allergen of ragweed, cross-reacts with some other allergens of ragweed pollen, but also cross-reacts with allergens from other taxonomically diverse genera and species. On the basis of cross-reactivity, weed allergens can be categorized into

three classes: (1) ragweeds and related plants, including *Parthenium*; (2) mugwort and sunflower; and (3) *Parietaria*.

6. The immunotherapy of weed-allergic subjects is conducted with ragweed allergen vaccines standardized with respect to Amb a 1 content. Allergenic products of pellitory, English plantain, and mugwort standardized in some areas of the world on the basis of major allergens content are also available.

REFERENCES

1. Holm, Doll J, Holm E, Pancho J, Herberger J. World Weeds: Natural Histories and Distributions. New York: John Wiley & Sons, 1949.
2. Wodenhouse RP. Pollengrains: Their Structure, Identification and Significance in Science and Medicine. New York: Hafner, 1965.
3. Agriculture Research Service of the Department of Agriculture. Common Weeds of the United States. New York: Dover, 1971.
4. Gutman AA, Bush RK. Allergens and other factors important in atopic disease. In: Allergic Diseases: Diagnosis and Management, 4th ed. (Patterson R, Crammer LC, Greenberger PA, Zeiss CR, eds.). Philadelphia: J. B Lippincott, 1993: 93–158.
5. Agarwal MK, Swanson MC, Reed CE, Yuninger JW. Airborne ragweed allergens: Association with various particle sizes and short ragweed plant parts. J Allergy Clin Immunol 1984; 74:687–693.
6. Spieksma FTM, von Wahl PG. Allergenic significance of *Artemisia* (mugwort) pollen. In: Allergenic Pollen and Pollinosis in Europe (D'Amato G, Spieksma FTM, Bonini S, eds.). Oxford: Blackwell Scientific, 1991: 121–124.
7. Bernton HS. Plantain hay fever and asthma. J Am Med Assoc 1925; 84:944–946.
8. D'Amato G, Ruffilli A, Sacerdoti G, Bonini S. *Parietaria* pollinosis: A review. Allergy 1992; 47:443–449.
9. Frenz DA, Palmer MA, Hokanson JM, Scamehorn RT. Seasonal characteristics of ragweed pollen dispersal in the United States. Ann Allergy Asthma Immunol 1995; 75(5):417–422.
10. Spieksma FTM, Charpin H, Nolard N, Stix E. City spore concentrations in the European Economic Community (EEC): IV. Summer weed pollen (*Rumex, Plantago, Chenopodiaceae, Artemisia*) 1976 and 1977. Clin Allergy 1980; 10:319–329.
11. Subiza J, Jerez M, Jiménez JA, Narganes MJ, Cabrera M, Varela S, Subiza E. Allergenic pollen and pollinosis in Madrid. J Allergy Clin Immunol 1995; 96:15–23.
12. Krilis S, Baldo BA, Basten A. Analysis of allergen-specific IgE responses in 341 allergic patients: Associations between allergens and between allergen groups and clinical diagnoses. Aust N Z J Med 1985; 15:421–426.
13. Holgate ST, Jackson L, Watson HK, Ganderton MA. Sensitivity to *Parietaria* pollen in the Southampton area as determined by skin-prick and RAST tests. Clin Allergy 1988; 18:549–556.
14. Kaufman HS. *Parietaria*: An unrecognized cause of respiratory allergy in the United States. Ann Allergy 1990; 64:293–296.
15. D'Amato G, Lobefalo G. Allergenic pollens in the southern Mediterranean area. J Allergy Clin Immunol 1989; 83:116–122.
16. King T, Norman PS, Connell TJ. Isolation and characterization of allergens from ragweed pollen: II. Biochemistry 1964; 3:458–468.
17. King T, Norman PS, Lichtenstein LM. Isolation and characterization of allergens from ragweed pollen: IV. Biochemistry 1967; 6:1992–2000.
18. Rogers BL, Bond JR, Morgenstern JP, Counsell CM, Griffith IJ. Immunochemical characterization of the major ragweed allergens Amb a I and Amb a II. In: Pollen Biotechnology, Gene

Expression and Allergen Characterization (Mohapatra SS, Knox B, eds.). New York: Chapman & Hall, 1996: 211–234.

19. Rafnar T, Griffith IJ, Kuo MC, Bond JF, Rogers BL, Klapper DG. Cloning of Amb a I (Antigen E), the major allergen family of short ragweed pollen. J Biol Chem 1991; 266:1229–1236.

20. Smith JJ, Olson JR, Klapper DG. Monoclonal antibodies to denatured ragweed pollen allergen Amb a I: Characterization, specificity for the denatured allergen, and utilization for the isolation of immunogenic peptides of Amb a I. Mol Immunol 1988; 125:355–365.

21. Rogers BL, Bond JF, Morgenstern JP, Counsell CM. Griffith IJ. Immunological characterization of the major ragweed allergens Amb a I and Amb a 2. In: Pollen Biotechnology: Gene Expression and Allergen Characterization. (Mohapatra SS, Knox B, eds.). New York: Chapman & Hall, 1996: 211–234.

22. Rogers BL, Morgenstern JP, Griffith IJ, Yu XB, Counsell CM, Brauer AW, King TP, Garman RD, Kuo MC. Complete sequence of the allergen Amb a II: Recombinant expression and reactivity with T cells from ragweed allergic patients. J Immunol 1991; 147:2547–2552.

23. Klapper DG, Goodfriend L, Capra JD. Amino acid sequence of ragweed allergen, Ra3. Biochemistry 1980; 19:5729–5734.

24. Adolphson CR, Goodfriend L, Gleich GJ. J Allergy Clin Immunol 1978; 62:197.

25. Atassi MZ, Atassi H. Antibody and T-lymphocyte recognition regions on ragweed allergen Amb a III (Ra3). In: Epitopes of Atopic Allergens (Sehon A, Kraft D, Kunkel G, eds.). Brussels: UCB Institute of Allergy, 1990: 33–40.

26. Roebber M, Klapper DG, Goodfriend L, Bias WB, Hsu SH, Marsh DG. Immunochemical and genetic studies of Amb t V (Ra5G), an Ra5 homologue from giant ragweed pollen. J Immunol 1985; 134:3062–3069.

27. Goodfriend L, Choudhury AM, Klapper DG, Coulter KM, Dorval G, DelCarpio J, Osterland CK. Ra5G, a homologue of Ra5 in giant ragweed pollen: Isolation, HLA-DR-associated activity and amino acid sequence. Mol Immunol 1985; 22:899–906.

28. Ghosh B, Perry MP, Rafnar T, Marsh DG. Cloning and expression of immunologically active recombinant Amb a V allergen of short ragweed (*Ambrosia artemisiifolia*) pollen. J Immunol 1993; 150:5391–5399.

29. Metzler WJ, Valentine K, Roebber M, Friedrichs M, Marsh DG, Mueller L. Solution structures of ragweed allergen Amb t V. Biochemistry 1992; 31:5117–5127.

30. Metzler WJ, Valentine K, Roebber M, Marsh DG, Mueller L. Proton resonance assignments and three-dimensional structure of the ragweed allergen Amb a V by nuclear magnetic resonance spectroscopy. Biochemistry 1992; 31; 8697–8705.

31. Rafner T, Metzler WJ, Marsh DG. The Amb V allergens from ragweed. In: Pollen Biotechnology: Gene Expression and Allergen Characterization (Mohapatra SS, Knox B, eds.). New York: Chapman & Hall, 1996: 235–244.

32. Lubahn B, Klapper DG. Cloning and characterization of ragweed allergen Amb a VI (abstr). J Allergy Clin Immunol 1993; 91:338.

33. Pilyavskaya A, Wieczorek M, Jones SW, Gross K. Isolation and characterization of a new basic antigen from short ragweed pollen (*Ambrosia artemisiifolia*). Mol Immunol 1995; 32(7):523–529.

34. Rogers BL, Pollock J, Klapper DG, Griffith IJ. Sequence of the proteinase-inhibitor cystatin homologue from the pollen of *Ambrosia artemisiifolia* (short ragweed). Gene 1993; 133(2):219–221.

35. Ipsen H, Formgren H, Lowenstein H, Ingemann L. Immunochemical and biological characterization of a mugwort (*Artemisia vulgaris*) pollen extract. Allergy 1985; 40:289–294.

36. de la Hoz F, Polo F, Moscoso del Prado J, Sellés JG, Lombardero M, Carreira J. Purification of *Art v* I, a relevant allergen of *Artemisia vulgaris* pollen. Mol Immunol 1990; 27:651–657.

37. Himly M, Jahn-Schmid B, Dedic A, Kelemen P, Wopfner N, Altmann F, van Ree R, Briza P, Richter K, Ebner C, Ferreira F. Art v 1, the major allergen of mugwort pollen, is a modular

glycoprotein with a defensin-like and a hydroxyproline-rich domain. FASEB J 2003; 17:106–108.

38. Jahn-Schmid B, Kelemen P, Himly M, Bohle B, Fischer G, Ferreira F, Ebner C. The T cell response to Art v 1, the major mugwort pollen allergen, is dominated by one epitope. J Immunol 2002; 169:6005–6011

39. Nilsen BM, Sletten K, Paulsen BS, O'Neill M, van Halbeek H. Structural analysis of the glycoprotein allergen Art v II from the pollen of mugwort (*Artemisia vulgaris L.*). J Biol Chem 1991; 266:2660–2668.

40. Díaz-Perales A, Lombardero M, Sánchez-Monge R, García-Sellés FJ, Pernas M, Fernández-Rivas M, Barber D, Salcedo G. Lipid-transfer proteins as potential plant panallergens: Cross-reactivity among proteins of *Artemisia* pollen, Castanea nut and Rosaceae fruits, with different IgE-binding capacities. Clin Exp Allergy 2000; 30:1403–1410.

41. García-Sellés FJ, Díaz-Perales A, Sánchez-Monge R, Alcántara M, Lombardero M, Barber D, Salcedo G, Fernández-Rivas M. Patterns of reactivity to lipid transfer proteins of plant foods and *Artemisia* pollen: An in vivo study. Int Arch Allergy Immunol 2002; 128:115–122.

42. Wopfner N, Willeroidee M, Hebenstreit D, van Ree R, Aalbers M, Briza P, Thalhamer J, Ebner C, Richter K, Ferreira F. Molecular and immunological characterization of profilin from mugwort pollen. Biol Chem 2002; 383(11):1779–1789.

43. Baldo BA, Chensee QJ, Howden ME, Sharp PJ. Allergens from plantain (*Plantago lanceolata*): Studies with pollen and plant extracts. Int Arch Allergy Appl Immunol 1982; 68:295–304.

44. Asero R, Mistrello G, Roncarolo D, Casarini M. Detection of allergens in plantain (*Plantago lanceolata*) pollen. Allergy 2000; 55:1059–1062.

45. Calabozo B, Barber D, Polo F. Purification and characterization of the main allergen of *Plantago lanceolata* pollen, Pla l 1. Clin Exp Allergy 2001; 31:322–330.

46. Calabozo B, Díaz-Perales A, Salcedo G, Barber D, Polo F. Cloning and expression of biologically active *Plantago lanceolata* pollen allergen Pla l 1 in the yeast *Pichia pastoris*. Biochem J 2003; 372:889–896.

47. Corbí AL, Carreira J. Identification and characterization of *Parietaria judaica* allergens. Int Arch Allergy Appl Immunol 1984; 74:318–323.

48. Ford SA, Baldo BA, Geraci D, Bass D. Identification of *Parietaria judaica* pollen allergens. Int Arch Allergy Appl Immunol 1986; 79:120–126.

49. Polo F, Ayuso R, Carreira J. HPLC purification of the main allergen of *Parietaria judaica* pollen. Mol Immunol 1990; 27:151–157.

50. Oreste U, Coscia MR, Scotto d'Abusco A, Santonastaso V, Ruffilli A. Purification and characterization of Par o I, major allergen of *Parietaria officinalis* pollen. Int Arch Allergy Appl Immunol 1991; 96:19–27.

51. Kahlert H, Weber B, Teppke M, Wahl R, Cromwell O, Fiebig H. Characterization of major allergens of *Parietaria officinalis*. Int Arch Allergy Immunol 1996; 109:141–149.

52. Ayuso R, Carreira J, Lombardero M, Duffort O, Peris A, Basomba A, Polo F. Isolation by mAb based affinity chromatography of two Par j I isoallergens: Comparison of their physicochemical, immunochemical and allergenic properties. Mol Immunol 1993; 30:1347–1354.

53. Costa MA, Colombo P, Izzo V, Kennedy H, Venturella S, Cocchiara R, Mistrello G, Falagiani P, Geraci D. cDNA cloning, expression and primary structure of Par j I, a major allergen of *Parietaria judaica* pollen. FEBS Lett 1994; 341:182–186.

54. Duro G, Colombo P, Costa MA, Izzo V, Porcasi R, Di Fiore R, Locorotondo G, Cocchiara R, Geraci D. Isolation and characterization of two cDNA clones coding for isoforms of the *Parietaria judaica* major allergen Par j 1.0101. Int Arch Allergy Immunol 1997; 112:348–355.

55. Duro G, Colombo P, Costa MA, Izzo V, Porcasi R, Di Fiore R, Locorotondo G, Mirisola MG, Cocchiara R, Geraci D. cDNA cloning, sequence analysis and allergological characterization of Par j 2.0101, a new major allergen of the *Parietaria judaica* pollen. FEBS Lett 1996; 399:295–298.

56. Colombo P, Kennedy D, Ramsdale T, Costa MA, Duro G, Izzo V, Salvadori S, Guerrini R, Cocchiara R, Mirisola MG, Wood S, Geraci D. Identification of an immunodominant IgE epitope of the *Parietaria judaica* major allergen. J Immunol 1998; 160:2780–2785.

57. Asturias JA, Arilla MC, Gómez-Bayón N, Martínez A, Martínez J, Palacios R. Recombinant DNA technology in allergology: Cloning and expression of plant profilins. Allergol Immunopathol (Madr) 1997; 25:127–134.

58. Hoz de la F, Melero JA, González R, Carreira J. Isolation and characterization of allergens from *Helianthus annuus* (Sunflower pollen). Allergy 1994; 49:1848–1854.

59. Jiménez A, Moreno C, Martínez J, Martínez A, Bartolomé B, Guerra F, Palacios R. Sensitization to sunflower pollen: Only an occupational allergy? Int Arch Allergy Immunol 2002; 105:297–307.

60. Barderas R, Villalba M, Lombardero M, Rodriguez R. Identification and characterization of Che a 1 allergen from *Chenopodium album* pollen. Int Arch Allergy Immunol 2002; 127:47–54.

61. Carnés J, Fernández-Caldas E, Casanovas M, Lahoz C, Colás C. Immunochemical characterization of *Salsola kali* pollen extracts (abstr). Allergy 2001; 56(suppl 68):274.

62. Gupta N, Martin BM, Metcalfe DD, Rao PV. Identification of a novel hydroxyproline-rich glycoprotein as the major allergen in *Parthenium* pollen. J Allergy Clin Immunol 1996; 98(5 pt 1):903–912.

63. Weber RW, Nelson HS. Pollen allergens and their interrelationships. Clin Rev Allergy IQSS 1985; 3:291–318

64. Fernández C, Martín-Esteban M, Fiandor A, Pascual C, Lopez Serrano C, Martínez Alzamora F, Díaz Pena JM, Ojeda Casas JA. Analysis of cross-reactivity between sunflower pollen and other pollens of the Compositae family. J Allergy Clin Immunol 1993; 92(5):660–667.

65. Park HS, Kim MJ, Moon HB. Antigenic relationship between mugwort and ragweed pollens by crossed immunoelectrophoresis. J Kor Med Sci 1994; 9(3):213–217.

66. Hirschwehr R, Heppner C, Spitzauer S, Sperr WR, Valent P, Berger U, Horak F, Jager S, Kraft D, Valenta R. Identification of common allergenic structures in mugwort and ragweed pollen. J Allergy Clin Immunol 1998; 101:196–206.

67. Fischer S, Grote M, Fahlbusch B, Muller WD, Kraft D, Valenta R. Characterization of Phl p 4, a major timothy grass (*Phleum pratense*) pollen allergen. J Allergy Clin Immunol 1996; 98(1):189–198.

68. Astwood JD, Mohapatra SS, Hill RD. Pollen allergen homologues in barley and other crop species. Clin Exp Allergy 1995; 25:66–72.

69. Mohapatra SS. Determinant spreading, implications for vaccine design of atopic disorders. Immunol Today 1994; 15:596–597.

70. Turcich MP, Hamilton OA, Mascarenhas JP. Isolation and characterization of pollen-specific maize genes with sequence homology to ragweed allergens and pectate lyases. Plant Mol Biol 1993; 23(5):1061–1065.

71. Bonnin JP, Grezard P, Cohn L, Perrot H. A very significant case of allergy to celery cross-reacting with ragweed (French). Allergie Immunol 1995; 27(3):91–93.

72. Sriramarao P, Rao PV. Allergenic cross-reactivity between *Parthenium* and ragweed pollen allergens. Int Arch Allergy Immunol 1993; 100(1):79–85.

73. Ayuso R, Carreira J, Polo F. Quantitation of the major allergen of several *Parietaria* pollens by an anti–Par 1 monoclonal antibody–based ELISA: Analysis of crossreactivity among purified Par j 1, Par o 1 and Par m 1 allergens. Clin Exp Allergy 1995; 25:993–999.

74. Creticos PS. Efficacy parameters. In: Immunotherapy: A Practical Guide to Current Procedures (Creticos PS, Lockey RF, eds.). Milwaukee: American Academy of Allergy and Immunology, 1994: 1–19.

75. Helm RM, Gauerke MB, Baer H, Lowenstein H, Ford A, Levy DA, Norman PS, Yunginger JW. Production and testing of an international reference standard of short ragweed pollen extract. J Allergy Clin Immunol 1984; 73:790–800

76. Norman PS, Winkenwerder WL, Lichtenstein LM. Immunotherapy of hay fever with ragweed antigen U: Comparison with whole pollen extract placebos. J Allergy 1968; 42:93–108.

77. Grammer LC, Zeiss CR, Suszko IM, Shaughnessy MA, Patterson. K. A double blind, placebo-controlled trial polymerized whole ragweed for immunotherapy of ragweed allergy. J Allergy Clin Immunol 1982; 69:494–499.

78. Litwin A, Pesce AJ, Fisher T, Michael M, Michael JO. Regulation of the human immune response to ragweed pollen by immunotherapy: A controlled trial comparing the effect of immunosuppressive peptic fragments of short ragweed with standard treatment. Clin Exp Allergy 1991; 21:457–465

79. Litwin A, Flanagan M, Entis G, Gottschlich G, Esch R, Gartside P, Michael JG. Immunologic effects of encapsulated short ragweed extract: A potent new agent for immunotherapy. Ann Allergy Asthma Immunol 1996, 77:132–138.

80. García Villalmanzo I, Hernández MD, Campos A, Giner AM, Polo F, Cortés C, Basomba A. Immunotherapy with a mass unit *Parietaria judaica* extract: A tolerance study with evidence of immunological changes to the major allergen Par j 1. J Investig Allergol Clin Immunol 1999; 9:321–329.

81. Jimeno L, Duffort O, Barber D, Polo F. ELISA con anticuerpos monoclonales para la cuantificación de un alergeno mayoritario de *Artemisia vulgaris* (abstr). Alergol Inmunol Clin 2002; 17(extr 2):243–244.

82. Calabozo B, Duffort O, Carpizo JA, Barber D, Polo F. Monoclonal antibodies against the major allergen of *Plantago lanceolata* pollen, Pla l 1: Affinity chromatography purification of the allergen and development of an ELISA method for Pla l 1 measurement. Allergy 2001; 56:429–435.

13

Fungal Allergens

HARI M. VIJAY

Health Canada, Ottawa, Ontario, Canada

VISWANATH P. KURUP

Medical College of Wisconsin, Milwaukee, Wisconsin, U.S.A.

I. INTRODUCTION

Fungi are eukaryotic, non-chlorophyllus, mostly spore-bearing organisms, that exist as saprophytes or as parasites of animals and plants (1). Fungi constitute unicellular to multicellular organisms, and their presence in the environment is dependent on the climate, vegetation, and other ecological factors. The presence and prevalence of fungi indoors depends on the moisture content, ventilation, and the presence or absence of carpets, pets, and houseplants (2). Fungi grow in most substrates, including glass and plastic surfaces, and at low temperatures, such as in refrigerators and cold rooms. Colonies of *Aspergillus fumigatus, Alternaria alternata, Cladosporium herbarum, Penicillium,* and *Fusarium* are the universally present molds in our environment (Fig. 1). The development of allergies to fungi follows the same biological principles as allergies to other environmental agents.

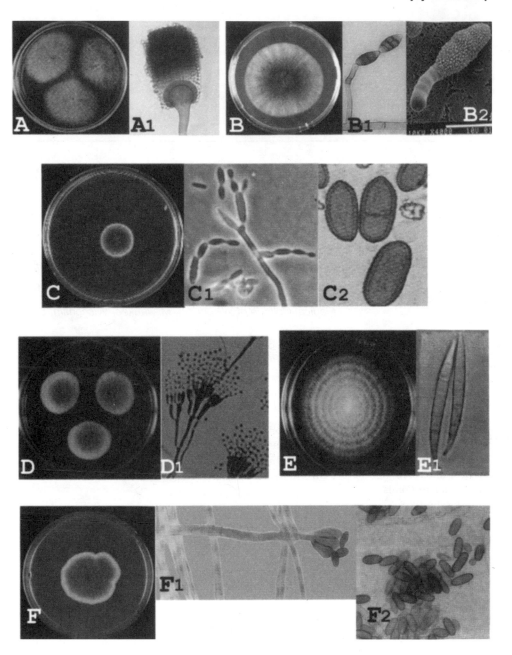

Figure 1   Colonies of (*A*) *Aspergillus fumigatus*, (*B*) *Alternaria alternata*, (*C*) *Cladosporium herbarum*, (*D*) *Penicillium chrysogenum*, (*E*) *Fusarium solani*, and (*F*) *Stachybotrys chartarum*; (*A1*) conidiospores of *A. fumigatus*; (*B1*) *A. alternata*, showing vertical and horizontal septa; (*B2*) scanning electron micrograph of *A. alternata*; (*C1, C2*) conidiophores and conidia of *C. herbarum*; (*D1*) broom-shaped sporophores of *Penicillium* sp.; (*E1*) spores (macor conidia) of *Fusarium* sp.; and (*F1, F2*) conidiophores and conidia of *S. chartarum*.

Fungi are associated with a number of allergic diseases in humans. The prevalence of respiratory allergy to fungi is estimated as 20–30% in atopic individuals and up to 6% in the general population (2–4). The major allergic manifestations induced by fungi are asthma, rhinitis, allergic bronchopulmonary mycoses, and hypersensitivity pneumonitis (5–10). These diseases can result from exposure to either spores, vegetative cells, or metabolites of the fungi. The spores of the fungi and vegetative hyphae are shown in Fig. 1. Because the spores are small (usually less than 5 μm), a majority of them can penetrate the airways of the lung and mediate allergic reactions. The conidia and fungal spores associated with the immediate type of hypersensitivity are usually larger than 5 μm, while those associated with the delayed type of hypersensitivity are considerably smaller and can penetrate the smaller airways (5). The site of deposition of spores also depends on whether spores enter the respiratory tract as propagules or as aggregates. The clusters of small conidia of *Aspergillus* and *Penicillium* are usually deposited in the upper respiratory tract, while the smaller individual spores reach the lower airways. On bronchial provocation tests, spores and fungal extracts cause both early and late-phase reactions in patients. More than 80 genera of the major fungal groups have been associated with symptoms of respiratory tract allergy (5,11). Ascomycetes and Deuteromycetes include the largest number of fungal species; however, only a few fungi such as *Aspergillus, Penicillium, Alternaria*, and *Cladosporium* have been investigated systematically for their role in causing allergy (2,12–14). Exposure to the toxigenic fungi such as *Aspergillus flavus* and *Stachybotrys chartarum* present in agricultural materials has been reported to be particularly dangerous (15). A strong association has been noted between reported dampness, mold content in homes, and respiratory symptoms among children (16).

The allergens of fungi are a highly heterogeneous complex and are partly or completely shared by a number of fungi. Understanding the antigens associated with allergy are very important both in diagnosis and in understanding the pathogenesis. Well-characterized relevant antigens are essential for reliable immunodiagnosis, and antigens and allergens with known structure and properties are also essential for understanding their role in the immunopathogenesis and for developing specific immunotherapy. Furthermore, the specificity of the skin test and serological results can be ascertained only by understanding the cross-reactivity of the allergens. Thus, standardized allergens are essential for reliable and dependable immunological assays. Although there are a number of well-characterized fungal allergens, acceptable standard allergens for immunoassays are not currently approved or designated.

II. CLASSIFICATION OF FUNGI

Molds belong to the fungal kingdom and include yeasts, mildews, and mushrooms (17). Mold is defined in the Oxford English Dictionary as a furry growth of microscopic fungi and has been used incorrectly as a synonym for fungi. Classification schemes for fungi have been undergoing continuous revisions to develop a more acceptable and easier-to-follow system (18–20). Since the fungi constitute a very large and diverse group of organisms, their taxonomy is complicated (21). The hyphae, which is the basic structural unit in most fungi (Fig. 1) is typically branched with tubular filaments possessing a definite cell wall composed of chitin and other complex carbohydrates. These hyphae may be divided by cross-walls called septa into individual cells. Some fungi exist exclusively as single-celled yeast forms, while others demonstrate extensive hyphae. Mushrooms belong to the group Basidiomycetes, where aggregation of mycelium results in the development of large macroscopic structures of diverse color and shape. The pleomorphism of fungi further complicates their classification, affects their antigenicity, and poses problems in identification (22,23).

Because of the lack of chlorophyll, fungi are usually heterotrophic in nature. The various modes of fungal reproductions include fragmentation, fission, budding, and spore production. Most fungi produce both sexual and asexual spores. The taxonomy of fungi is based to a large degree on spore characteristics including spore size, shape, color, surface ornamentation, and ontogeny (24). Fungi are named in accordance with guidelines of the International Code of Botanical Nomenclature (ICBN). Fungi are eukaryotic, unicellular or multicellular organisms with absorptive nutrition and have been classified traditionally as members of the plant kingdom. They have been reclassified under a new kingdom, named Myceteae.

Myceteae are divided into the standard taxonomic categories of division, class, order, family, genus, and species, and each of these categories may contain further subdivisions, subclasses, and suborders. The kingdom Myceteae has been divided into three major divisions, namely Gymnomycota, Mastigomycota, and Amastigomycota (25,26). The organisms belonging to Gymnomycota are referred as the "true plasmodium slime molds." The fungi belonging to Mastigomycota produce flagellated cells at some part in their life cycle, whereas Amastigomycota produce extensive well-developed mycelia, consisting of either septate or aseptate hyphae (27). Some single-celled organisms are also included in Amastigomycota. In a recent classification, the group of fungi producing airborne spores are divided into three divisions, Dikaryomycota, Zygomycota, and Oomycota. Three classes, Ascomycetes, Basidiomycetes, and Deuteromycetes, are included in Dikaryomycota. The fungi associated with allergic reactions in humans are listed in Table 1. The fungi belonging to the class Deuteromycetes are of considerable interest and importance in human diseases, including allergies (28).

The organisms belonging to Deuteromycetes are also designated as "fungi imperfecti," which, as the name indicates, is an artificial group consisting of those fungi known to reproduce only by asexual means. The conidial stages of many deuteromycetous fungi are similar to those of Ascomycetes and, in some cases, to those of Basidiomycetes. The members of the group fungi imperfecti are also believed to represent Ascomycetes and Basidiomycetes, whose sexual stages have not been identified or have been excluded from the life cycle during their evolution. Fungi in buildings can be divided according to their damage-causing ingredients and the microenvironments. Fungi grown on surfaces cause discoloration and the "moldy" smell. Common types of fungi that decay buildings and building materials are *Penicillium, Aspergillus, Rhizopus* spp., *Botrytis, Alternaria, Cladosporium*, and others.

III. IDENTIFICATION OF FUNGI

The most important group of air-disseminated fungi that cause respiratory allergic diseases in humans are the conidial fungi, which compose the form-class Deuteromycetes. The spores produced by the imperfect fungi vary in shape, size, texture, color, number of cells, thickness of the cell wall, and methods by which they attach to each other and to their conidiophores. The identification of the common fungi is difficult, as their fungal colony characteristics and even microscopic characteristics vary according to the medium on which the fungus is grown, the temperature of incubation, and the strain variation and pleomorphic nature of the spores (29).

Table 1 Taxonomic Distribution of Allergenic Fungi

Phycomycetes	Deuteromycetes (fungi imperfecti)
Phytophthora	*Acremonium*
Plasmophora	*Alternaria*
Mucor	*Aspergillus*
Rhizopus	*Aureobasidium*
Ascomycetes	*Botryotrichum*
Chaetomium	*Botrytis*
Claviceps	*Cephalosporium*
Daldinia	*Chrysosporium*
Didymella	*Cladosporium*
Erysiphe	*Coniosprium*
Eurotium	*Curvularia*
Microsphaera	*Cylindrocarpon*
Zylaria	*Drechslera*
Yeasts	*Epicoccum*
Candida	*Fusarium*
Rhodotorula	*Gliocladium*
Saccharomyces	*Helminthosporium*
Basidiomycetes	*Monilia*
Agaricus	*Neurospora*
Calvatia	*Nigrospora*
Cantharellus	*Paecilomyces*
Cyathus	*Penicillium*
Ganoderma	*Phoma*
Geastrum	*Pyrenochaeta*
Lentinus	*Scopulariopsis*
Merulius	*Sporotrichum*
Phollogaster	*Stachybotrys*
Pleurotus	*Stemphylium*
Polyporus	*Torula*
Psilocybe	*Trichoderma*
Puccinia	*Trichophyton*
Tilletia	*Ulocladium*
Urocystis	*Wallemia*
Ustilago	
Xylobolus	

Within the Hyphomycetes, two principal types of classification have been proposed. The first is based on spore morphology using the characteristics of color and septation (Fig. 1). Thus, *Alternaria* has dark "dictyospores," with both horizontal and vertical septae (Fig. 1, B1 and B2). *Fusarium* has colorless "phragmospores" (horizontal septae) (Fig. 1, E1). *Aspergillus* and *Penicillium* have bright-colored "amerospores" (Fig. 1, A1 and D1), with no septation at all. Some fungi, however, have several different methods of spore production within each life cycle. The second approach emphasizes details of asexual spore production as in *Alternaria*, where the porospores are formed by extrusion of protoplasm through the tiny pores of special spore-bearing hyphae or sporophores, and the phialospores of *Penicillium* and *Fusarium* formed within a specialized hyphal cell called the phialide (Fig. 1, D1) (30).

The chemical composition of the cell wall may also help in classifying different fungal allergens and their role in causing allergic responses of patients. The cell wall of yeasts is composed mostly of a chitin-glucan combination, contrasting with the predominantly chitin in mycelial fungi. Some fungi can change from yeast to mycelial form, depending on environmental conditions (31). Another aspect of vegetative morphology commonly used for identification purposes is color. The allergenic fungi have been mainly classified into two large groups based on whether the mycelium and asexual spores are brown (Dematiaceae) or colorless (Moniliaceae).

In addition to the major interest in proteins and glycoproteins of fungi as allergens, in recent years the attention of researchers has been directed toward understanding the role of mycotoxins produced by molds in causing human diseases, including acute toxicosis. These mycotoxins have been shown to occur in mycelia, spores, and matrix in which molds grow. There is an adequate evidence that inhalation of fungi, particularly those that produce mycotoxins, results in immunological disregulation, with potential neurological effects (32) (Table 2). There is probably one important mechanism: interference with pulmonary macrophage function. Important mycotoxins produced by species of *Fusarium, Aspergillus*, and *Penicillium*—T2 toxin, deoxynivalenol (DON), fumonisin, and aflatoxin—are involved in toxicoses of humans and/or animals (33). Regardless of the type of damage caused by acute exposures to these toxins, chronic exposure shows that all are immunosuppressants of varying potency. Trichothecenes are the most potent known inhibitors of protein synthesis by one or two orders of magnitude (34,35). Aflatoxin is the most potent carcinogen known. Conidia of a number of molds have been demonstrated to contain concentrations of toxins from 1 to 650 µg/g.

IV. FUNGAL ALLERGENS

The spores of fungi are ubiquitous in nature. The number of fungal species present in the environment is estimated to be at least 1 million, which include different classes and families of fungi (24). Some genera of airborne fungal spores such as *Alternaria, Aspergillus, Penicillium*, and *Cladosporium* are found throughout the world. The airborne spores of these fungi are generally considered to be important causes of allergic diseases such as allergic rhinitis, allergic asthma, allergic bronchopulmonary mycoses, and hypersensitivity pneumonitis (5,36,37).

Diagnosis of allergic disease is mainly based on clinical symptoms of the patients, skin test reaction, detection of allergen-specific serum IgE antibodies, (RAST, ELISA, etc.), and in some cases provocative inhalation challenge testing (5). The effective in vivo and in vitro diagnosis of fungal allergies depends on the availability of well-characterized allergen preparations. Aerobiological identification and assessment of fungi in outdoor and indoor environments is necessary to determine their role in causing allergic diseases. Aerobiological surveys conducted in different parts of the world, and skin tests and in vitro tests for specific mold allergies identified predominant mold allergens. Based on such results, extracts from *Alternaria alternata, Aspergillus fumigatus, Cladosporium herbarum, Epicoccum purpurascens, Fusarium roseum*, and *Penicillium chrysogenum* have been made available commercially. The selection of species and strains of fungi with allergenicity is crucial for obtaining a representative antigen. Since the prevalence of fungi and their allergenicity varies, relevant allergenic fungi need to be identified for consistent results.

Because of the variability among strains and species in their morphology, biochemistry, and allergenicity, it is difficult to obtain antigens and allergens with consistent

Table 2 Some Toxigenic Fungi and Secondary Chemical Metabolites and Associated Health Effects

Fungus	Chemical metabolite	Health effects
Penicillium (>150 species)	Patulin	Hemorrhage of lung, brain disease
	Citrinin	Renal damage, vasodilatation, bronchial constriction, increased muscular tone
	Ochratoxin A	Nephrotoxic, hepatotoxic
	Citroviridin	Neurotoxic
	Emodin	Reduced cellular oxygen uptake
	Gliotoxin	Lung disease
	Verraculogen	Neurotoxic: trembling in animals
	Secalonic acid D	Lung, teratogenic in rodents
Aspergillus species	Patulin	Hemorrhage of lung, brain disease
A. flavus and *A. parasiticus*	Aflatoxin B1	Liver cancer, respiratory system cancer, cytochrome P-450 monooxygenase disorder
A. versicolor	Sterigmatocystin	Carcinogen
A. ochraceus	Ochratoxin A	Nephrotoxic, hepatotoxic
Stachybotrys chartarum	Trichothecenes[a] (more than 170 derivatives known)	Immune suppression and dysfunction, cytotoxic bleeding, dermal necrosis; high-dose ingestion lethal (human case reports); low-dose, chronic ingestion potentially lethal; teratogenic abortogenic (in animals)
	T2	Alimentary toxic aleukia reported in Russia and Siberia
	Nivalenol	Staggering wheat in Siberia
	Deoxynivalenol	Red mold disease in Japan
	Diacetoxyscirpenol	Neurotoxic/nervous system and behavior abnormality
	Satratoxin H	
	Spirolactone	Anticomplement function
Fusarium species	Zearalenone	Phytoestrogen may alter immune function, stimulates growth of uterus and vulva, atrophy of ovary
Claviceps species	Ergot alkaloids	Prolactin inhibitor, vascular constriction, uterus contraction promoter

[a] Trichothecenes are also produced by species of *Myrothecium, Trichoderma, Trichothecium,* and *Gibberella* (teleomorph of some *Fusarium* species).

reactivity from these fungi. In addition, considerable cross-reactions exist among various taxonomically and antigenically related strains, species, and even genera. With some fungi it is almost impossible to grow two consecutive cultures with similar antigenic profiles (38). Factors contributing to the variability of commercial and laboratory-made extracts are (1) variability of stock cultures used to prepare allergenic extracts and to their proper identification, (2) usage of mycelial-rich material as the source of allergens, (3) conditions under which molds are grown and extracts prepared, (4) the stability of the extracts, and (5) the quality control measures used. It is now possible to grow allergenic fungi in synthetically defined media rather than in complex media containing macromolecules.

These allergenic extracts show less variability and demonstrate specific reactivity with patients (39,40). However, complex media components are essential for the broth and production of certain relevant antigens by fungi. Two-to-3-week-old cultures are a rich source of culture filtrate antigens, while reliable mycelial antigens for immunoassay can be obtained from short-term fungal growth of aerated culture (41).

The extraction procedures for inhalant allergens should reflect the pattern in which the allergens are released under natural conditions. The extraction procedure for each species and strain should be optimized for consistent results by the use of suitable extraction buffer, length of extraction time, appropriate cell disruption method, and the use of protease inhibitors and preservatives (42,43). The allergenic activity of an extract or fraction can be evaluated by skin testing allergic subjects. Either prick tests or intradermal tests can be used. The intradermal method is, however, more quantitative and sensitive than the prick test (44,45). The most common in vitro tests for allergenic activity are RAST and ELISA. Both RAST and ELISA correlate well with allergen-specific IgE in the sera (46). In recent years, semi-automated specific IgE assays such as Immuno-CAP have been evaluated for a number of allergens including mold allergens (47).

Antibody response to allergens and their specificity can also be studied by competitive inhibition assays of various serological methods. Patients' sera are incubated with varying dilutions of the allergens to be tested before the sera are added to the solid-phase–bound reference allergens. Immunoassay, namely RAST or ELISA, can be performed and the percentage inhibition of binding of the pre-adsorbed sera to the reference allergen determined. A 50% inhibition in binding of the patient's IgE to the reference allergen is taken as a measure of potency of the test allergen. Direct challenge of allergic patients by inhalation of small doses of various fungal extracts has been used in patient evaluation studies; however, the use of mold allergens for inhalation studies is controversial because of the possibility of late-phase reactions and other adverse effects. Furthermore, exposure to novel antigens present in fungal extracts may result in new sensitizations.

The stability of allergenic extracts depends on the type and quality of the allergen, the storage temperature, and the presence of preservatives and other nonallergic materials in the mixture. For most extracts, lyophilization is the best method to maintain the allergenic potency, but some allergens may be permanently altered and inactivated by this process. The loss of potency of any extract may be due to degradation of a specific allergen rather than a general reduction in activity of all allergens. Moreover, reconstituted extract must contain a stabilizer such as human serum albumin, glycerol, phenol, or ε-aminocaproic acid to preserve the integrity of allergenic extracts (48).

V. DISTRIBUTION OF INDOOR AND OUTDOOR FUNGAL ALLERGENS

Fungi grow on any material if enough moisture is available. A large number of airborne spores are usually present in outdoor air throughout the year, frequently exceeding the pollen population by 100- to 1000-fold, depending on environmental factors such as water, nutrients, temperature, and wind (6,49). Most fungi commonly considered allergenic, such as *Alternaria, Cladosporium, Epicoccum*, and *Ganoderma*, have a seasonal spore-releasing pattern (2,50).

Indoor fungi are a mixture of those that have entered from outdoors and those that grow and multiply indoors (51,52). *Aspergillus* and *Penicillium* are less common outdoors and are usually considered the major indoor fungi. Recently, *Aternaria* species have been found in house dust samples in the absence of environmental mold spores (53). All studies have found good correlation between outdoor spore counts and clinical symptoms. There is not much information on the effect of the indoor spore concentration and allergic symptoms (50,54). Dampness, excess moisture, and mold growth in buildings are associated with an increased prevalence of respiratory symptoms such as asthma and bronchitis. The indoor air fungal flora may differ from that of outdoor air, both quantitatively and qualitatively. Most of the time, outdoor concentrations of fungal spores outnumber those of indoor environments. The ratio of indoor/outdoor concentration (I/O) of spores is usually less than 1, and it is of concern when this ratio reverses. The intramural sourcesof fungi result in a different composition of indoor airborne fungi compared with the outdoor air (55). The health effects caused by fungal propagules may be irritative, allergic, or infectious. These effects could be caused by viable and nonviable fungal spores and hyphal particles. The overall concentration of both viable and nonviable propagules may give a more accurate estimate of the actual exposure.

Once fungi have been detected growing in the building, other types of exposure-induced diseases may also be considered. Moist conditions in buildings seem to favor the growth of toxigenic fungi (Table 2). An example of this is *Stachybotrys chartarum*, a toxigenic fungus that grows on moist-surface materials containing cellulose. Mycotoxins produced by the fungi, which have high concentrations of the toxins in spores, cause severe symptoms (56). The concentration of both spores and their volatile metabolites may become significantly higher in indoor as opposed to outdoor environments. Since people spent most of their time indoors, they are in continuous contact with the airborne spores and toxins, to which exposure may become remarkable even if the toxin concentrations are low (57).

Most studies of the presence of mold spores in indoor air have been performed with discontinuous viable samplers. Surveys on outdoor mold spores are mostly done with continuous nonviable techniques (58). The spectrum of airborne mold spores indoors, such as in homes, offices, and other workplaces, differs from place to place due to the influx of spores from outdoor air through ventilation systems and air exchangers, which may influence the quality and quantity of indoor spores. Hence, it is difficult to arrive at any significant conclusion on the role of the indoor mold spore in the allergic response. Spieksma reported that the 10 most common types of outdoor atmospheric mold spores are present in all distant regions of Europe (59).

Distributions of indoor and outdoor mold spore counts reported from different parts of the world are given in Table 3 (58,60–62). The fungal spore count in outdoor air is usually about 230/m^3 while the indoor count may vary from 100 to 1000/m^3 (58,60). A spore count of 10–100/m^3 is a substantially high antigen load for exposed individuals. Recently, Garrett and colleagues (63), in their studies of airborne fungal spores in southeastern Australian homes, found that the most common fungal genera/groups were *Cladosporium, Penicillium*, and yeast, both indoors and outdoors in winter and late spring. Outdoor levels were higher than those indoors throughout the year, and significant seasonal variation in spore levels was seen both indoors and outdoors, with an overall maximum in summer. Contrary to this trend, the levels of *Aspergillus, Cephalosporium, Gliocladium*, and yeasts were higher in winter. *Penicillium* was detected more commonly indoors than outdoors. Outdoor spore levels do have a significant influence on the indoor levels of spores. The composite airborne spore load and the associated allergen levels remain incompletely characterized.

Table 3 Distribution of Indoor and Outdoor Allergenic Fungi

		Range spores/m^3			
	Indoor[a]	Indoor summer[b]	Indoor winter[b]	Outdoor summer[b]	Outdoor summer[c]
Penicillium	0–4737	0–7900	0–480	0–95	15,000
Cladosporium	12–4637	0–160	0–160	11–430	600,000
Botrytis	0–54	—	—	—	12,000
Yeasts	0–5	0–74	0–78	0–790	10,000
Aspergillus	0–306	0–76	0–19	0–11	15,000
Alternaria	0–282	—	—	—	7500
Rhizopus	0–24	—	—	—	—
Nonsporulating mycelium	0–14,194	0–1700	0–200	19–9300	—
Epicoccum	0–155	—	—	—	—
Fusarium	0–47	—	—	—	7500

[a] Ref. 60. Studies carried out in Southern California homes.
[b] Ref. 58. Studies carried out in Finnish homes.
[c] Ref. 61. Studies carried out in European homes.

VI. CROSS-REACTIVITY OF FUNGAL ALLERGENS

The term "cross-reactivity" refers to the antigenic determinants shared by different molecules from different fungi (64). Studies of cross-reactivity with techniques such as immunoprecipitation, immunoblotting, and RAST inhibition has contributed to our understanding of this phenomenon. Cross-reactivity should be distinguished from parallel, independent sensitization to multiple fungal allergens (64). The degree of cross-reactivity between different species and strains of fungi depends on the number of antigenic components that cross-react, the immunogenicity of epitopes, and the method used to detect the reactivity (65). The presence of cross-reactive epitopes among allergens is advantageous for the diagnosis because it reduces the number of antigens required in the panel of extracts used for testing (14). However, this may lack specificity and necessitate secondary testing to determine the specific sensitizing mold. Cross-reactive antigens are more advantageous for immunotherapy due to their broad-spectrum effect with fewer numbers of allergens.

There are shared allergenic and antigenic components from cytoplasmic and cell wall antigens of a number of fungi. The cell wall antigens usually contain carbohydrates, which may contribute to the cross-reactivity. Several related genera of fungi share similar proteins. For example, *Aspergillus* and *Penicillium* species share a number of proteases, and these proteins usually cross-react with antibodies. Even unrelated fungi also share some of these antigens, with low to high levels of cross-reactivity with antibodies.

It has been shown that allergens from unrelated sources can also show cross-reactivity. Mold-latex allergy is an example of this. A number of minor and major allergens from *Hevea brasiliensis* latex share partial homology with fungal allergens (66). These allergens show some degree of cross-reactivity and thereby complicate the specific diagnosis. However, further research is needed to establish the importance and degree of allergen cross-reactivity for specific diagnosis and for devising a desensitization therapy regimen. As fungal extracts are variable, several batches of antigens should be used for cross-reactivity studies to prevent inaccurate conclusions. By the use of monoclonal antibodies and recombinant allergens, cross-reactivity among fungal allergens can be understood more precisely. A better understanding of cross-reactivity between different fungi is clinically very important, as such information may be relevant for diagnosis and in devising control measures.

VII. ISOLATION AND CHARACTERIZATION OF FUNGAL ALLERGENS

Because information available on allergens is restricted to only a few species of fungi, in the present discussion we have selected only the predominant fungi associated with IgE-mediated allergy. A number of allergens from *Aspergillus, Alternaria, Penicillium, Cladosporium, Malasezzia, Trichophyton*, and species belonging to Basidiomycetes fungi and yeasts have been isolated and characterized.

A. *Aspergillus*

Aspergillus fumigatus is one of the predominant fungi implicated in the pathogenesis of allergic diseases in humans. Besides *A. fumigatus*, the principal etiological agent of allergic bronchopulmonary aspergillosis (ABPA), other species such as *A. nidulans, A. oryzae, A. terreus, A. flavus*, and *A. niger* have also been reported as causing allergic diseases in man (7,67,68). All these organisms are freely distributed in most environments, although in certain conditions they grow much faster and liberate numerous spores.

A. fumigatus antigens are diverse in their physicochemical and immunological characteristics (69). A number of protein and glycoprotein antigens react with specific antibodies in the sera from patients with allergic aspergillosis (70). Four antigens (Ag 3, Ag 5, Ag 7, and Ag 13) were purified by size exclusion chromatography (71–73). Ag 7, of 150–200 kDa, and Ag 13, of 70 kDa, bound to Con-A and reacted with sera from ABPA patients. Ag 5 and Ag 3, the thermolabile peptides having molecular masses of 35 and 18 kDa, respectively, were also useful for detecting antibodies in patients with ABPA. Two allergens (18 and 20 kDa) purified by conventional purification techniques were compared with other allergens of *A. fumigatus*. The crossed immunoelectrophoretic pattern of 18 kDa is similar to that of Ag 3 or Ag 10, described earlier, whereas the 20-kDa allergen is a Con-A nonbinding glycoprotein and appears to be different from the other known allergens of *A. fumigatus*. Another glycoprotein allergen, designated as gp 55, was sensitive to protease treatment but not to deglycosylation (74). The amino terminal sequence of protein gp 55 did not show sequence homology with other allergens. Two nonglycosylated 18-kDa (Asp f1) and 24-kDa allergens of *A. fumigatus* were purified using monoclonal antibody affinity chromatography and showed strong IgE binding with ABPA patient sera (75,76).

Several recombinant allergens from *A. fumigatus* have been identified and purified from cDNA and phage display libraries of *A. fumigatus* (Table 4). The majority of these proteins showed specific binding to IgE from asthmatic and ABPA patients. The molecular structures cover a wide range of functional proteins including toxins, enzymes, heat shock proteins, and several unique proteins lacking homology to any of the known proteins. Asp f 1, a ribotoxin that inhibits protein translation, was shown to be toxic to EBV-transformed PHA-stimulated peripheral blood mononuclear cells (PBMCs). This allergen showed positive skin test reactivity in 80% of ABPA patients and 50% of asthmatic patients. This allergen also demonstrated IgE antibody in 68–83% of patients with skin test positivity to *Aspergillus* allergens (77,78). However, because of the high toxicity and reactivity with skin test–positive asthmatics and some normals, the usefulness of this allergen in the diagnosis is questioned. This allergen demonstrated 13 linear

Table 4 Fungi Allergens Approved by the Allergen Nomenclatural Committee[a]

Fungus	Mol. size (kDa)	Biological activity	Sequence accession number
Alternaria alternata			
Alt a 1	28		U82633
Alt a 2	25		U62442
Alt a 3		Heat shock protein 70	U87807
Alt a 4	57	Prot. disulfidisomerase	X84217
Alt a 6	11	Acid. ribosomal protein P2	X-78222
Alt a 7	22	YCP4 protein	X-78225
Alt a 10	53	Aldehyde dehydrogenase	X-78227
Alt a 11	45	Enolase	U82437
Alt a 12	11	Acid. ribosomal protein P1	X84216
Cladosporium herbarum			
Cla h 1	13		
Cla h 2	23		
Cla h 3	53	Aldehyde dehydrogenase	X-78228
Cla h 4	11	Acid. ribosomal protein P2	X-78223
Cla h 5	22	YCP4 protein	X-78224
Cla h 6	46	Enolase	X-78226
Cla h 12	11	Acid. ribosomal protein P1	X85180
Aspergillus flavus			
Asp fl 13	34	Alkaline serine protease	
Aspergillus fumigatus			
Asp f 1	18	Ribonuclease	M-83781
Asp f 2	37		U-56938
Asp f 3	19	Peroxisomal protein	U20722
Asp f 4	30		AJ001732
Asp f 5	40	Metalloproteinase	Z-30424
Asp f 6	26.5	Mn superoxide dismutase	U53561
Asp f 7	12		AJ-223315
Asp f 8	11	Ribosomal protein P2	AJ224333
Asp f 9	34		AJ223327
Asp f 10	34	Aspartic proteinase	X85092
Asp f 11	24	Peptidyl prolyl isomerase	
Asp f 12	90	Heat shock protein P90	
Asp f 13	34	Alkaline serine proteinase	
Asp f 15	16		AJ002026
Asp f 16	43		g3643813
Asp f 17			AJ224865
Asp f 18	34	Vacuolar serine proteinase	
Asp f 22w	46	Enolase	AF284645
Aspergillus niger			
Asp n 14	105	Beta-xylosidase	AF108944
Asp n 18	34	Vacuolar serine protease	
Asp n ?	85		Z84377
Aspergillus oryzae			
Asp o 13	34	Alkaline serine protease	X17561
Asp o 21	53	TAKA amylase A	D00434

(*Continued*)

Table 4 Continued

Fungus	Mol. size (kDa)	Biological activity	Sequence accession number
Penicillium brevicompactum			
Pen b 13	33	Alkaline serine protease	
Penicillium chrysogenum			
Pen ch 13	34	Alkaline serine proteinase	
Pen ch 18	32	Vacuolar serine proteinase	
Pen ch 20	68	*N*-acetyl glucosaminidase	
Penicillium citrinum			
Pen c 3	18	Peroxisomal membrane protein	
Pen c 13	33	Alkaline serine proteinase	
Pen c 19	70	Heat shock protein P70	U64207
Pen c 22w	46	Enolase	AF254643
Penicillium oxalicum			
Pen o 18	34	Vacuolar serine protease	
Fusarium culmorum			
Fus c 1	11	Ribosomal protein P2	AY077706
Fus c 2	13	Thioredoxin-like protein	AY077707
Trichophyton rubrum			
Tri r 2			
Tri r 4		Serine protease	
Trichophyton tonsurans			
Tri t 1	30		
Tri t 4	83	Serine protease	
Candida albicans			
Cand a 1	40		
Cand a 3	29	Peroxisomal protein	AY136739
Candida boidinii			
Cand b 2	20		J04984
Psilocybe cubensis			
Psi c 1			
Psi c 2	16	Cyclophilin	
Coprinus comatus			
Cop c 1	11	Leucine zipper protein	AJ132235
Cop c 2			AJ242791
Cop c 3			AJ242792
Cop c 5			AJ242793
Cop c 7			AJ242794
Rhodotorula musilaginosa			
Rho m 1	47	Enolase	
Malassezia furfur			
Mala f 2	21	MF1, peroxisomal membrane protein	AB011804
Mala f 3	20	MF2, peroxisomal membrane protein	AB011805
Mala f 4	35	Mitochondrial malate dehydrogenase	AF084828

(Continued)

Table 4 Continued

Fungus	Mol. size (kDa)	Biological activity	Sequence accession number
Malassezia sympodialis			
Mala s 1			X96486
Mala s 5	18		AJ011955
Mala s 6	17		AJ011956
Mala s 7			AJ011957
Mala s 8	19		AJ011958
Mala s 9	37		AJ011959
Epicoccum purpurascens			
Epi p 1	30	Serine protease	P83340

[a] http://www.allergen.org (124) (IUIS Allergen List).

epitopes binding to IgE. Asp f 1 also showed TH1- and TH2-specific epitopes when studied in a murine model of allergic aspergillosis (79,80).

Another major allergen, a 37-kDa protein of *A. fumigatus* (Asp f 2), has been cloned, expressed, and characterized (81). Recombinant Asp f 2 exhibits specific IgE binding with sera of ABPA patients and discriminates ABPA with serological confirmation and no evidence of central bronchiectasis (ABPA-S) from ABPA with definitive central bronchiectasis (ABPA-CB).

The Af gene encoding a polypeptide fragment of a heat shock protein (HSP) 90 family has been expressed and its allergenicity confirmed (82). The heat shock protein Asp f 12 has homologous counterparts in *Candida albicans*, *Saccharomyces*, *Trypanasoma*, housefly, mouse, and humans because of the extremely conserved HSP gene. Asp f 16 has no known biological functions and showed strong binding to IgG from ABPA patients (83). This antigen showed sequence homology with Asp f 9 and a membrane protein from *Saccharomyces*. A few other minor allergens isolated from *A. fumigatus* and related *Aspergillus* species demonstrated binding to IgE antibody from ABPA and allergic asthma patients (Table 4). Several of these *A. fumigatus* allergens also exhibited high sequence homologies with the known functional proteins and enzymes of other fungi (84–87). Alkaline serine proteinases with allergenic properties such as Asp f 13, Asp fl 13, and Asp o 13 from *A. fumigatus, A. flavus*, and *A. oryzae*, respectively, have been reported (87,88). Similar serine proteinases Pen b 13, Pen c 13, and Pen ch 13 with sequence homology to *Aspergillus* proteinases have also been identified from various species of *Penicillium* (89,90). Recently, another group of homologous vacuolar serine proteinases—Asp f 18, Asp n 18, Pen ch 18, and Pen o 18—with conserved sequence have been reported from *Aspergillus* and *Penicillium* (85,91). *A. flavus* extracts demonstrated IgE antibody binding in 44% of asthmatic patients studied by immunoblotting (92). Recently a 34-kDa alkaline serine proteinase, Asp fl 13, with signficant IgE antibody binding was purified and its enzyme activity ascertained (92).

A phage display method has recently been used to express allergenic proteins from Af (93). The expressed proteins from a cDNA library from Af have been displayed on the surface of filamentous phage M13 and screened with sera from ABPA patients for IgE-binding antibodies to the phage surface protein. The Af proteins selected from the phage display library that bound IgE were in the range of 20–40 kDa. A 26.7-kDa manganese superoxide dismutase, cloned and expressed from Af, reacted with IgE antibodies in sera from patients with allergic aspergillosis and stimulated their peripheral blood lymphocytes (47,94).

B. *Alternaria alternata*

Alternaria alternata, a member of the imperfect fungi, is one of the most important among the allergenic fungi (95). The spores produced by imperfect fungi vary in shape, size, texture, color, number of cells, and thickness of the cell wall. This species is known to be an important cause of bronchospasm in a significant number of patients with bronchial asthma (96,97). Hypersensitivity pneumonitis, a condition that has been linked with precipitating antibodies of the IgG class, may also be caused by sensitization to *Alternaria* (98). Most fungi, including *A. alternata* amd *C. herbarum*, have a seasonal spore-releasing pattern. Recently *Alternaria*, a predominantly outdoor fungus, has been reported in house dust samples in spite of its absence in the environment (53). Although other *Alternaria* species are probably also relevant clinally, most research has been directed toward *A. alternata* (65).

The first allergen of *A. alternata* (ATCC 6663) was a mycelial allergen partially purified by gel chromatography. This glycoprotein fraction was named Alt-1, had an apparent molecular weight between 25 and 50 kDa, and contained at least five isoelectric variants between pI 4.0 and 4.5 (99). The two variants of Alt-1, namely Ag 1 and Ag8, have molecular masses of 60 and 35–40 kDa and pI of 4.0 and 4.3–4.65, respectively (100).

Hybridoma technology has been employed to produce murine monoclonal antibodies (MAbs) to *A. alternata*. Vijay et al. reported the purification of a 31-kDa protein of *A. alternata* using MAb affinity chromatography (101). In immunoblots, this protein reacted with human atopic IgE antibodies. Sanchez and Bush (102) reported purification of *Alternaria* allergens of 62 kDa by IgE immunoblot using MAbs. Similarly, Portnoy et al. purified an allergen of 70 kDa (gp 70) using MAbs (103). Of the 16 subjects positive to skin tests with *Alternaria* extract, 11 reacted with gp 70, although purified allergen was less potent than the crude extract in skin tests. Lepage et al. produced 11 MAbs that reacted with antigenic determinants at 200-, 65-, and 45 kDa regions that reacted with IgE antibody (104).

Subsequently, several groups isolated the major allergenic component of *Alternaria*. Two groups of investigators used anion exchange chromatography to purify Alt a 1 from mycelium (105,106). Paris and co-workers designated the allergen Alt a 1_{1563} (31 kDa, pI 4.0–4.5), determined to be heat-stable glycoproteins containing 20% carbohydrate (107). Deards and Montague designated this allergen Alt a BD 29k (pI 4.2, 29 kDa) and determined that it is composed of 15-kDa subunits (105). Matthiesen et al. and Curran et al. have reported purification of Alt a 1 of molecular weights 28 kDa and 29 kDa, respectively (107,108). These authors have established that a reduced form of Alt a 1 produced a doublet pattern on SDS-PAGE with molecular weights of 14.5 and 16 kDa. In immunoblot with human atopic serum, this doublet was confirmed as allergenic. These polypeptide chains are closely related, since their N-terminal sequences are virtually identical. In immunoblots, it was demonstrated that 29-kDa protein and its reduced form reacted with 92% of the human atopic sera tested (108).

Bush and Sanchez determined the amino acid sequence of 60-kDa *A. alternata* allergen and established the partial cDNA sequence for another *A. alternata* allergen (109). Another partially purified allergen that has been designated as a basic peptide (pI 9.5, 6 kDa) is able to induce a wheal-and-flare skin reaction in sensitized subjects (110). Eighteen of 20 (90%) skin test–positive subjects reacted to this basic peptide, which was designated Alt a II d.

Tremendous advances in the molecular characterization of *A. alternata* allergens have been made during the past few years. Allergens that have been cloned and expressed as IgE-binding proteins include a subunit of the major allergen Alt a 1 (111,112). Recombinant Alt a 1 secreted into the media of *Pichia pastoris* cultures appeared as a dimer, similar to the natural allergen from *A. alternata* culture medium or mycelium. Recombinant Alt a 1, like the natural allergen in *A. alternata*, is reactive with serum IgE antibodies from *A. alternata*–sensitive patients (111). Several groups have isolated and characterized minor allergens of *A. alternata* Alt a 2 (25 kDa), Alt a 3 (hsp 70), Alt a 4 (57 kDa), Alt a 6 (ribosomal P2 protein, 11 kDa) Alt a 7 (22 kDa), Alt a 10 (aldehyde dehydrogenase, 53 kDa), Alt a 11 (45 kDa), and Alt a 12 (11 kDa) (Table 4) (109,111–113). Alt a 7, a 22-kDa allergen, has been reported to have 70% sequence homology with the YCP4 protein of *Saccharomyces cerevisiae*, while Alt a 6, the 11-kDa protein, has been determined to have homology with ribosomal P2 protein. They also have homology with *Cladosporium herbarum* allergens.

Recently, Alt a 1, the major allergen of *A. alternata*, was studied for its IgE-binding linear epitopes using overlapping decapeptides spanning the whole Alt a 1 sequence. The reactivity of the synthesized peptides was studied using serum IgE from *Alternaria*-allergic patients (114). The two peptides (K41–P50 and Y54–K63) reacted strongly with all the patients studied.

C. *Cladosporium herbarum*

Cladosporium herbarum is widely distributed in our environment and is a major source of fungal inhalant allergen (115). *A. alternata* is a major allergen in houses as well as outdoor air in humid climates, such as the southern part of United States, while *Cladosporium* is the leading allergenic mold in cooler climates, such as Scandinavia (113). About 60 antigens from *C. herbarum* have been identified by crossed immunoelectrophoresis (CIE), and 36 of them have been shown to react with IgE antibodies from patients' sera (38). Three major *C. herbarum* allergens have been purified and characterized (Table 4). Cla h 1 is a small 13-kDa acidic allergen composed of five isoallergens (pI 3.4–4.4) (116), and Cla h 2, a slightly larger molecule with a size of 23 kDa less acid (pI 5.0), is a glycoprotein that contains 50% carbohydrates (116–118). The protein part retained the IgE-binding property even after carbohydrate moieties were removed, and the binding was stronger than shown by the native Cla h 2. Cla h 4, a ribosomal P2 protein, is a low-molecular-weight (11 kDa) acidic allergen (pI 3.94) with high alanine and serine content and shares 60% sequence homology with other ribosomal P2 proteins (119). Breitenbach et al. (120) recently reported purified recombinant *Cladosporium* enolase (Cla h 6, 48 kDa), which has strong binding to IgE antibodies by immunoblots in 20% of patients allergic to *Alternaria*. Enolase has been found to be a highly conserved major allergen in most fungi and may contribute to allergen cross-reactivity in mold allergy. About 20% of the serum IgE from patients allergic to *Alternaria* and *Cladosporium* showed binding to enolase. An allergenic HSP-70 has also been isolated from the organism (120).

D. *Penicillium* Species

Species belonging to the genus *Penicillium* are prevalent indoor fungi (5,6). Inhalation of *Penicillium* spores in quantities comparable with those encountered by natural exposure can induce both immediate and late asthma in sensitive persons (52). Among more than a hundred different *Penicillium* species, *P. citrinum*, together with *P. chrysogenum* (*P. notatum*), *P. oxalicum, P. brevicompactum*, and *P. spinulosum*, were the five most frequently recovered species of *Penicillium* in the United States, while *P. citrinum* was the most prevalent *Penicillium* species reported from Taiwan (121,122).

About 12 antigens from *P. citrinum* and 11 antigens from *P. chrysogenum* have been shown to react with IgE from patients' sera by immunoblotting (90). Recently, several *Penicillium* allergens have also been characterized at the molecular level (Table 4). Among the *Penicillium* allergens, the 32–34-kDa alkaline and/or vacuolar serine proteases were identified as the major allergens of *P. citrinum, P. brevicompactum, P. chrysogenum*, and *P. oxalicum* (123). They have been designated as Group 13 for alkaline serine protease and Group 18 for vacuolar serine protease allergens as recommended by the Allergen Nomenclature Subcommittee (88,124). Immunoblotting data showed that IgE antibodies against components of these prevalent *Penicillium* species could be detected in the sera of about 16–26% of asthmatic patients (88). Majority of the positive serum samples tested showed IgE binding to the 32–34-kDa serine proteinase(s) with a frequency >80% in different fungal species tested. The cDNA of the alkaline serine protease allergens from *P. citrinum* (Pen c 13) and *P. chrysogenum* (Pen ch 13), and the vacuolar serine proteases from *P. citrinum* (Pen c 18), *P. oxalicum* (Pen o 18), and *P. chrysogenum* (Pen ch 18) have recently been cloned (84–86). The mature Pen ch 13 allergens are formed by the removal of the preprosequence of the precursor molecule (84). Besides N-terminal cleavage, the mature Pen c 18 and Pen o 18 also undergo C-terminal processing (85). The IgE cross-reactivity between the allergens in *Penicillium* and *Aspergillus* species has been detected (84,85,87,90,91,123,125). In addition to reactivity with IgE antibody serine proteases, Pen ch 13 also demonstrated histamine-releasing activity from peripheral blood leukocytes of asthmatic patients (84).

Besides the serine protease allergens, a 68-kDa allergen *N*-acetyl glucosaminidase and an allergenic heat shock protein belonging to the HSP-70 family have also been identified from *P. chrysogenum* and *P. citrinum*, respectively (89). The Allergen Nomenclature Subcommittee has designated them Pen ch 20 and Pen c 19, respectively (124) (Table 4). An 18-kDa peroxisomal membrane protein (Pen c 3) similar to Asp f 3 and an enolase (Pen c 22) similar to Asp f 22 were also identified from *P. citrinum* (92,126). Cross-reacting IgE antibodies have been reported against these allergens (92,126).

E. Basidiomycetes

Basidomycetes are physically the largest and morphologically most complex fungi. Most of these are considered microfungi. Basidiomycetes fungi number over 20,000 species, including mushrooms, puffballs, bracket fungi, rusts, and smuts. Although microfungi unquestionably are important allergen sources, reports now indicate that basidiospores occur in the air in high concentration in many parts of the world, and positive skin tests, RAST, and bronchial reactivity to their extracts has been detected in hypersensitive subjects (127,128).

Calvatia species are seasonally occurring puffballs that produce a large number of spores. Immunoprints of crude and fractionated extracts of *Calvatia cyathiformis* have indicated that allergens (pI 9.3 and 6.6) reacted with 68% and 63%, respectively, of serum samples from 19 patients who showed positive skin tests to this mold antigen (129). These allergens are designated Cal cBd q3 and Cal cBd 6.6 (124).

For *Coprinus quadrifidus* spores and *Coprinus commatus* mycelium extracts, skin test and RAST have demonstrated that most reactive fractions of each extract were in the same size range (10.5–12 kDa) (130).

F. *Ganoderma*

Ganoderma are important wood-decaying fungi that produce large shelflike fruiting bodies called brackets or conks. Spores of *Ganoderma* occur widely and are easily demonstrable in air-sampling surveys (131,132). The allergenicity of *Ganoderma* has been well studied by more laboratories than is the case for other Basidiomycetes. Despite the fact that several extracts are reasonably well characterized, no allergens have yet been isolated. Western blots of *G. meredithae* spore and cap extracts with atopic serum revealed 10 allergens (14 to >66 kDa and pI <3.5 to 6.6). *G. applanatum* spore and fruiting body extracts tested by crossed-line immunoelectrophoresis (CLIE) also demonstrated common antigens (133). In another study of *G. applanatum* spores, 14 antigens were detected by CIE and immunoblots (134). This study also revealed that IgE binding bands are mostly between 18 and 82 kDa. However, no purified antigens have been obtained as yet.

G. *Candida albicans*

Ten of 120 *Candida* species cause significant human infections. *C. albicans* is the most frequently isolated pathogenic species (28). Although IgE reactivity of *C. albicans* allergens has been reported on several occasions, the view that *C. albicans* is a major inhalant allergen remains controversial. A 40-kDa *C. albicans* allergen has been cloned, and sequence identity revealed 70% homology with alcohol dehydrogenase (135,136).

H. Yeasts

Yeasts are true fungi belonging to the group Ascomycetes. Most yeasts are single-celled and reproduce by budding. Various species within Ascomycetes, Basidiomycetes, and fungi imperfecti have yeast forms (28,137). Yeasts are reported to cause chronic urticaria and respiratory allergic diseases (138).

I. *Malassezia furfur*

Malassezia furfur (as *Pityrosporum orbiculare*) extracts induce positive skin tests and leukocyte histamine release in subjects with atopic dermatitis (139). SDS-PAGE immunoblots of *Malassezia furfur* extracts showed dominant allergens at 9, 15, 25, and 72 kDa (140). The 9- and 15-kDa components are mostly carbohydrates. Mabs have been raised against the 67-kDa allergen of *M. furfur* (141). These Mabs do not cross-react with *Candida albicans* extracts and hence may be useful to detect whether patients with atopic dermatitis are sensitized initially to *M. furfur* or the yeasts.

J. *Trichophyton* Spp.

Trichophyton species induce classic delayed-type or cell-mediated hypersensitivity. The possible role of *Trichophyton* spp. in IgE-mediated urticaria, asthma, and rhinitis has been suggested; the relevance of these species in causing allergy remains controversial. IgE antibodies to *Trichophyton tansurans* have been found in skin test–positive subjects (142). A 30-kDa hydrophobic major allergen of *Trichophyton tansurans* (Tri t 1) has been purified by gel filtration and hydrophobic interaction chromatography, and the sequence for 30 N-terminal amino acids was determined (143). The Mabs that recognize distinct epitopes on Tri t 1 have been prepared. Studies with these Mabs should help understand the importance of *Trichophyton* spp. as an allergen.

K. Other Fungi

Aerobiological study performed in different countries demonstrated the presence of *Botrytis, Phoma, Helminthosporium, Fusarium* and *Epicoccum, Puccinia, Ustilago, Cephalosporium*, and *Saccharomyces*, and these fungi have been implicated in allergic disorders in humans (Table 1). However, careful evaluation has not been carried out due to the lack of appropriate, reliable antigens and diagnostic methods to ascertain the results.

VIII. CONCLUSIONS AND FUTURE DIRECTIONS

There has been significant progress in fungal allergen standardization, particularly since 1990, as a result of the availability of partially purified and well-characterized antigens. Monoclonal antibodies serve as a useful immunoprobe for studying epitopes responsible for allergic diseases. These antibodies also help to understand the cross-reactivity between the antigens of different fungi. Most important, Mabs are extremely useful for obtaining pure antigenic and allergenic proteins for diagnosis and immunotherapy. Several IgE-binding allergens of *A. alternata, C. herbarum, A. fumigatus*, and *Penicillium* spp. have been obtained using molecular cloning techniques. The complete amino acid and DNA sequences of these allergens have been reported. Large quantities of these purified allergens can be produced in appropriate expression systems. Two epitopes of Asp f 2, a major allergen of *A. fumigatus*, showed strong IgE binding and cross-reactivity with related species of *Aspergillus*, but not with allergens from unrelated taxa. Two major epitopes of Alt a 1, major allergen of *A. alternata*, show strong IgE binding and no identity with any of the known allergens. Hence, these epitopes can be safely and efficiently used as immunotherapeutic agents for managing fungal allergies. Similarly, mutants engineered from allergens may be of value in immunotherapy.

The information obtained from the screening of indoor mold allergens and the detection of atopic antibodies in patients using cloned allergens will help us in developing safety codes for buildings and enhancing the health of the occupants. The availability of well-characterized recombinant allergens may lead to the development of standardized allergens.

IX. SALIENT POINTS

1. Progress in the standardization of mold vaccines has been impeded by the wide variation in biological potency among mold allergen extracts.
2. Fungi may mutate, producing morphologically different forms. As fungal taxonomy is based largely on microscopic appearance of fungi, particularly their spores, striking differences exist among mycologists in terms of the identity of the fungi. Once the fungal isolate is correctly identified, the question arises whether spores, mycelia, or culture filtrate should be used for the preparation of the antigen. Most extracts are prepared from mycelia and contain

little or no spore material. The inherent variability among extracts is a major problem.

3. Fungal spores are structurally very different from pollens since inhaled particles consist of entire living cells, capable of growing and secreting allergens in vivo.

4. Apart from *Alternaria, Aspergillus, Penicillium, Cladosporium*, and a few other species of the fungi, purified and standardizable antigens are not available from fungal species. Hence, the use of fungal antigens for diagnosis or for use as vaccines may not be comparable due to their variability.

5. Many common fungi still await clinical evaluation and testing.

6. Cloning of allergen genes will facilitate desirable epitope identification and provide safer and more effective treatment for fungal allergy.

7. Some mold allergens, such as glycopeptides, share common antigenic determinants with related and sometimes even unrelated species.

8. Although the fungal spores in the outdoor air are seasonal, most of the mold-sensitive patients have perennial symptoms. This is the result of growth and sporulation of the outdoor fungi in the indoor environment.

9. Production of more well-characterized allergens at the molecular level for immunological evaluation of patients, combined with engineered allergens, synthetic peptides, conjugated allergens with CpG-motif, and DNA vaccines will lead to better understanding of the mechanisms of allergy to fungi as well as information for improved management of the diseases they provoke.

ACKNOWLEDGMENTS

This study was supported by the U.S. Veterans Affairs Medical Research. The editorial assistance of Drs. Makonnen Abebe and Serdal Sevinc, is gratefully acknowledged.

REFERENCES

1. Ainsworth GC. Ainsworth and Bisby's Dictionary of the Fungi, 6th ed. Kew, England: Commonwealth Mycological Institute, 1971.

2. Portnoy J, Chapman J, Burge H. Muieleberg M, Solomon W. Epicoccum allergy: Skin reaction patterns and spore/mycelium disparities recognized by IgG and IgE ELISA inhibition. Ann Allergy 1987; 59:39–43.

3. Wuethrich B. Epidemiology of allergic diseases: Are they really on the increase? Int Arch Allergy Appl Immunol 1989; 90:3–10.

4. Hagy GW, Settipane GA. Bronchial asthma, allergic rhinitis, and allergy skin tests among college students. J Allergy 1969; 44:323–332.

5. Kurup VP, Fink JN. Fungal allergy. In: Fungal Infection and Immunity Responses (Murphy JW, Friedman H, Bendinelli M, eds.). New York: Plenum Press, 1993: 393–404.

6. Burge HA. Airborne-allergenic fungi. Immunol Allergy Clin North Am 1989; 9:307 319.

7. Greenberger PA. Allergic bronchopulmonary aspergillosis and fungoses. Clin Chest Med 1988; 9:599–608.

8. Fink JN. Allergic bronchopulmonary aspergillosis. Hosp Pract 1988; 23:105–128.

9. Katzenstein A, Sale SR, Greenberger PA. Allergic *Aspergillus* sinusitis: A newly recognized form of sinusitis. J Allergy Clin Immunol 1983; 72:89–98.

10. Kurup VP. Hypersensitivity pneumonitis due to sensitization with thermophilic actinomycetes. Immunol Allergy Clin North Am 1989; 9:285 306.

11. Bierman WC, Van Arsdel PP Jr. Clinical evaluation of the patient with allergic and immunologic disease. In: Principles of Immunology and Allergy (Lockey RF, Bukantz SC, eds.). Philadelphia: WB Saunders, 1987: 1–26.

12. Kurup VP, Kumar A. Immunodiagnosis of aspergillosis. Clin Microbiol Rev 1991; 4:439–459.

13. Patterson R, Greenberger PA, Roberts ML. Allergic Bronchopulmonary Aspergillosis. Providence, RI: Oceanside, 1996.

14. Horner WE, Helbling A, Salvaggio JE, Lehrer SB. Fungal allergens. Clin Microbiol Rev 1995; 8:161–179.

15. Ganassini A, Cazzadori A. Invasive pulmonary aspergillosis complicating allergenic bonchopulmonary aspergillosis. Respir Med 1995; 89:143–145.

16. Johannine E, Morev PR, Jarvis BB. Clinical-epidemiological investigation of health effects caused by *Stachybotrys atra* building contamination. In: Indoor Air 93: Proceedings of the 6th International Conference on Indoor Air Quality and Climate, vol. I: Health Effects (Jaakola JJK, Ilmarinen R, Sepanen S, eds.). Helsinki: Institute of Occupational Health 1993; 225–230.

17. Margulis L, Schwartz K. Five Kingdoms: An Illustrated Guide to the Phyla of Life on Earth, (2nd ed.) New York: W.H. Freeman, 1988.

18. Hawksworth DL, Kirk PM, Sutton BC, Ainsworth GC. Ainsworth & Bisby's Dictionary of the Fungi. Cambridge: CAB International, 1995.

19. Miller OK, Fair DF. An Index of the Common Fungi of North America: Synonyms and Common Names. Vaduz, Liechtenstein: J. Cramer, 1990.

20. Alexopoulos C, Mims C, Blackwell M. Introductory Mycology. New York: John Wiley & Sons, 1996.

21. Ainsworth GC. Introduction and keys to higher taxa. In: The Fungi (Ainsworth GC, Sparrow FK, Sussman AS, eds.). New York: Academic Press, 1973.

22. Carmichael JW. Pleomorphism. In: Biology of Conidial Fungi (Cole GT, Kendrick B, eds.). New York: Academic Press, 1981.

23. Weresub LK, Pirozynski KA. Pleomorphism of fungi as treated in the history of mycology and nomenclature. In: The Whole Fungus (Kendrick B, ed.). Ottawa: National Museums of Canada, 1979.

24. Bold HC, Alexopoulos CJ, Delevoryas T. Morphology of Plants and Fungi. New York: Harper & Row, 1973.

25. Alexopoulos CJ, Mims CW. Introductory Mycology, 3rd ed. New York: John Wiley & Sons, 1979.

26. Talbot PHB. Principles of Fungal Taxonomy. New York: St. Martin's Press, 1971.

27. Loomis WF. *Dictyostelium discoideum*: A Developmental System. New York: Academic Press, 1975.

28. Kendrick B. The Fifth Kingdom. Waterloo, Ontario, Canada: Mycologue, 1985.

29. Kendrick B. The history of conidial fungi. In: Biology of Conidial Fungi (Cole GT, Kendrick B, eds.). New York: Academic Press, 1981.

30. Kendrick B, Nag Raj TR. Morphological terms in fungi imperfecti. In: The Whole Fungus (Kendrick B, ed.). Ottawa: National Museums of Canada, 1979.

31. Wicklow ET, Carroll GC. The Fungal Community: Its Organization and Role in the Ecosystem. New York: Marcel Dekker, 1981.

32. Etzel HA, Montana E, Sorenson W, Kullman GJ, Allan TM, Olson OR, Jams B, Miller JO, Dearborn DG. Acute pulmonary hemorrhage in infants associated with exposure to *Stachybotrys atra*. Arch Pediatr Adolesc Med 1998; 152:757–762.

33. Dveraetova I. Aflatoxin inhalation and alveolar cell carcinoma. Br Med J 1976; 111:691.

34. Ueno Y. Toxicological features of T-2 toxin and related trichothecenes. Fund Appl Toxicol 1984; 4:S124–S132.

35. Smoragiewicz W, Cosselle B, Boutard A, Krzystyniak K. Trichothecene mycotoxins in the dust of ventilation systems in office buildings. Int Arch Occup Environ Health 1993; 65:113–117.

36. Latge JP, Paris S. The fungal spore: Reservoir of allergens. In: The Fungal Spore and Disease Initiation in Plants and Animals (Cole GT, Moch HC, eds.). New York: Plenum Press, 1991: 379–401.

37. Yunginger JW, Jones RT, Gleich GJ. Studies on *Alternaria* allergens: II. Measurement of the relative potency of commercial *Alternaria* extracts by the direct RAST and by RAST inhibition. J Allergy Clin Immunol 1976; 58:405–413.

38. Aukrust L. Cross radioimmunoelectrophoretic studies of distinct allergens in two extracts of *Cladosporium herbarum*. Int Arch Allergy Appl Immunol 1979; 58:375–390.

39. Kim SJ, Chaparas SD. Characterization of antigens from *Aspergillus fumigatus*: I. Preparation of antigens from organism grown in completely synthetic medium. Am Rev Respir Dis 1978; 118:547–551.

40. Kurup VP, Fink JN, Scribner GH, Falk J. Antigenic variability of *Aspergillus fumigatus* strains. Microbios 1977; 19:191–204.

41. Van der Heide SH, Kauffman HF, de Vries K. Cultivation of fungi in synthetic and semi-synthetic liquid medium: I. Growth characteristics of the fungi and biochemical properties of the isolated antigenic material. Allergy 1985; 40:586–591.

42. Chapman MD. Monoclonal antibodies as structural probes for mite, cat and cockroach allergens. In: Advances in Biosciences, Allergy and Molecular Biology (Shami AE, Merrett TG, eds.). New York: Pergamon Press, 1989: 281–295.

43. Lehrer SB, Salvaggio JE. Allergens: Standardization and impact of biotechnology—a review. Allergy Proc 1990; 11:197–208.

44. Aas K, Backman A, Belin L, Weeke B. Standardization of allergen extracts with appropriate methods. Allergy 1978; 33:130–137.

45. Dreborg S, Agrell B, Foucard T, Kjellman NIM, Kolvikka A, Nilsson S. A double-blind, multicenter immunotherapy trial in children, using a purified and standardized *Cladosporium herbarum* preparation. Allergy 1986; 41:131–140.

46. Turner KJ, Stewart GA, Sharp AH, Czarny D. Standardization of allergen extracts by inhibition of RAST, skin test and chemical composition. Clin Allergy 1980; 10:441–450.

47. Kurup VP, Banerjee B, Hemmann S, Greenberger PA, Blaser K, Crameri R. Selected recombinant *Aspergillus fumugatus* allergens bind specifically to IgE in ABPA. Clin Exp Allergy 2000; 30:988–993.

48. Weber RW. Allergen immunotherapy and standardization and stability of allergen extracts. J Allergy Clin Immunol 1989; 84:1093–1095.

49. Lehrer SB, Aukrust L, Salvaggio JE. Respiratory allergy induced by fungi. Clin Chest Med 1983; 4:23–41.

50. Beaumont F, Kauffman HF, Sluiter HJ, De Vries K. Sequential sampling of fungal air spores inside and outside the homes of mold sensitive, asthmatic patients: A search for a relationship to obstructive reactions. Ann Allergy 1985; 55:740–746.

51. Burge HA. Fungus allergens. Clin Rev Allergy 1983; 3:319–329.

52. Licorish K, Novey HS, Kozak P, Fairshter RD, Wilson AF. Role of *Alternaria* and *Penicillium* spores in the pathogenesis of asthma. J Allergy Clin Immunol 1985; 76:819–825.

53. Becker AB, Muradia G, Vijay HM. Immunoreactive *Alternaria* allergens in house dust in the absence of environmental mold (abstr 151). J Allergy Clin Immunol 1996; 97(suppl 1): 220.

54. Malling HJ. Diagnosis and immunotherapy of mold allergy: IV. Relation between asthma symptoms, spore counts and diagnostic tests. Allergy 1986; 41:342–350.

55. Lehtonen M, Reponen T, Nevalainen A. Every day activities and variation of fungal spore concentrations in indoor air. Int Biodeterior Biodegradation 1993: 31:25–39.

56. Miller JD. Fungi as contaminants in indoor air. Atmos Environ 1992; 26A:2163–2172.

57. Yocom JE, McCarthy SM. Measuring indoor air-quality. Chichester: John Wiley & Sons, 1991.

58. Nevalainen A, Rautiala S, Hyvarinen A, Reponen T, Husman T, Kalliokoski P. Exposure to fungal spores in mouldy houses: Effect of remedial work. In: Recent Trends in Aerobiology, Allergy and Immunology (Agashe SN, ed.). New Delhi. Oxford GIBII, 1994: 99 107.

59. Spieksma F Th M. Aerobiology of common environmental allergens: Sizes of allergen carrying particles. Asian Pac J Allergy Immunol 1993; 11(suppl 1):93–94.

60. Kozak PP Jr, Gallup J, Cummins LH, Gillman SA. Factors of importance in determining the prevalence of indoor molds. Ann Allergy 1979; 43:88–94.

61. D'Amato G, Spieksma FThM. Aerobiologic and clinical aspects of mould allergy in Europe. Allergy 1995; 50:870–877.

62. Solomon WR. A volumetric study of winter fungus prevalence in the air of Midwestern homes. J Allergy Clin Immunol 1976; 57:46.

63. Garrett MH, Hooper BM, Cole FM, Hooper MA. Airborne fungal spores in 80 homes in Latrobe Valley, Australia: Levels, seasonality and indoor-outdoor relationship. 1997; 13:121–126.

64. Vijay HM, Hughes DH, Young NM. The allergens of *Alternaria* species. Current Persp Palynol Res 1990; 91:387–397.

65. Aukrust L, Borch SM. Cross-reactivity of moulds. Allergy 1985; 40(suppl 3):57–60.

66. Wagner S, Sowka S, Mayer C, Crameri R, Focke M, Kurup VP, Scheiner O, Breiteneder H. Identification of a *Hevea brasiliensis* latex manganese superoxide dismutase (Hev b 10) as a cross-reactive allergen. Int Arch Allergy Immunol 2001; 125:120–127.

67. Shimada, Matsumura K. A case of probable allergic bronchopulmonary aspergillosis due to *Aspergillus niger*. Nippon Kyobu-Shikkan Zasshi 1995; 33:336–341.

68. Laham MN, Allen RC, Greene JC. Allergic bronchopulmonary aspergillosis (ABPA) caused by *Aspergillus terreus*: Specific lymphocyte sensitization and antigen-directed serum opsonic activity. Ann Allergy 1981; 46:74–80.

69. Hearn VM, Wilson EV, Latge JP, Mackenzie DWR. Immunochemical studies of *Aspergillus fumigatus* mycelial antigens by polyacrylamide gel electrophoresis and Western blotting techniques. J Gen Microbiol 1990; 136:1525–1535.

70. Kurup VP, Ramasamy M, Greenberger PA, Fink JN. Isolation and characterization of a relevant *Aspergillus fumigatus* antigen with IgG and IgE binding activity. Int Arch Allergy Appl Immunol 1988; 86:176–182.

71. Longbottom JL, Austwick PKC. Antigens and allergens of Aspergillus fumigatus: 1. Characterization by quantitative immunoelectrophoretic techniques. J Allergy Clin Immunol 1986; 78:9–17.

72. Longbottom JL, Harvery C, Taylor ML, Austwick PKC, Fitzharris P, Walken CA. Characterization of immunologically important antigens and allergens of *Aspergillus fumigatus*. Int Arch Allergy Appl Immunol 1989; 88:185–186.

73. Taylor ML, Longbottom JL. Partial characterization of a rapidly released antigenic/allergenic component (Ag 5) of *Aspergillus fumigatus*. J Allergy Clin Immunol 1988: 81:548–557.

74. Teshima R, Ikebuchi H, Sawader J, Miyachi S, Kitani S, Iwama M, Irie M, Ichinol M., Terao T. Isolation and characterization of a major allergenic component (gp 55) of *Aspergillus fumigatus*. J Allergy Clin Immunol 1993; 92:698–706.

75. Kumar A, Kurup VP, Greenberger PA, Fink JN. Production and characterization of a monoclonal antibody to a major Concanavalin A–nonbinding antigen of *Aspergillus fumigatus*. J Lab Clin Med 1993; 121:431–436.

76. Arruda KL, Platts-Mills TAE, Fox JW, Chapman MD. *Aspergillus fumigatus* allergen 1, a major IgE-binding protein, is a member of the mitogillin family of cytotoxins. J Exp Med 1990; 172:1529–1532.

77. Arruda LK, Mann BJ, Chapman MD. Selective expression of a major allergen and cytotoxin, Asp f 1, in *Aspergillus fumigatus*: Implications for the immunopathogenesis of *Aspergillus* related diseases. J Immunol 1992; 149:3354–3359.

78. Moser M, Crameri R, Menz G, Schneider T, Dudler T, Virchow C, Gmachl M, Blaser K, Suter M. Cloning and expression of recombinant *Aspergillus fumigatus* allergen I/a (rAsp f I/a) with IgE binding and type I skin test activity. J Immunol 1992: 149:454–460.

79. Kurup VP, Vijay H, Guo J, Murali PS, Resnick A, Krishnan M, Fink JN. *Aspergillus fumigatus* peptides differentially express Th1 and Th2 cytokines. Peptides 1996; 17:183–190.

80. Kurup VP, Banerjee B, Murali PS, Greenberger PA, Krishnan M, Vijay H, Fink JN. Immunodominant peptide epitopes of allergen Asp f I from the fungus *Aspergillus fumigatus*. Peptides 1998; 19:1469–1477.

81. Banerjee B, Kurup VP, Phadnis S, Greenberger PA, Fink JN. Molecular cloning and expression of a recombinant *Aspergillus fumigatus* protein Asp f 2 with significant Immunoglobulin E reactivity in allergic bronchopulmonary aspergillosis. J Lab Clin Med 1996; 127:253–262.

82. Kumar A, Reddy LV, Sochanik A, Kurup VP. Isolation and characterization of a recombinant heat shock protein of *A. fumigatus*. J Allergy Clin Immunol 1993; 91:1024–1030.

83. Banerjee B, Kurup VP, Greenberger PA, Johnson BD, Fink JN. Cloning and expression of *Aspergillus fumigatus* allergen Asp f 16 mediating both humoral and cell-mediated immunity in allergic bronchopulmonary aspergillosis (ABPA). Clin Exp Allergy 2001; 31:761–770.

84. Chou H, Lai HY, Tarn MF, Chou MY, Wang SR, Han SH, Shen HD. cDNA cloning biological and immunological characterization of the alkaline serine protease major allergen from *Penicillium chrysognum*. Int Arch Allergy Immunol 2002; 127:15–26.

85. Shen HD, Wang CW, Lin WL, Lai HY, Tarn MF, Chou H, Wang SR, Han SH. CDNA cloning and immunological characterization of *Pen o* 18, the vacuolar serine protease major allergen of *Penicillium oxalicum*. J Lab Clin Med 2001; 137:115–124.

86. Su NY, Yu CJ, Shen HD, Pan FM, Chow LP. Pen c I, a novel enzymic allergen protein from *Penicillium citrinum*: Purification, characterization, cloning and expression. Eur J Biochem 1999; 261:115–123.

87. Shen HD, Lin WL, Tarn MF, Wang SR, Tsaj JJ, Chou H, Han SH. Alkaline serine proteinase: A major allergen of *Aspergillus oryzae* and its cross-reactivity with *Penicillium citrinum*. Int Arch Allergy Immunol 1998; 116:29–35.

88. Shen HD, Tarn MF, Chou H, Han SH. The importance of serine proteinases as aeroallergens associated with asthma. Int Arch Allergy Immunol 1999; 119:259–264.

89. Shen HD, Au LC, Lin WL, Liaw SF, Tsai JJ, Han SH. Molecular cloning and expression of a *Penicillium citrinum* allergen with sequence homology and antigenic cross-reactivity to a hsp 70 human heat shock protein. Clin Exp Allergy 1997; 27:682–690.

90. Shen HD, Lin WL, Tsai JJ, Liaw SF, Han SH. Allergenic components in three different species of *Penicillium*: Cross-reactivity among major allergens. Clin Exp Allergy 1996; 26:444–451.

91. Shen HD, Lin WL, Tarn MF, Chou H, Wang CW, Tsai JJ, Wang SR, Han SH. Identification of vacuolar serine proteinase as a major allergen of *Aspergillus fumigatus* by immunoblotting and N-terminal amino acid sequence analysis. Clin Exp Allergy 2001; 31:295–302.

92. Lai HY, Tarn MF, Tang RB, Chou H, Chang CY, Tsai JJ, Shen HD. cDNA cloning and immunological characterization of a newly identified enolase allergen from *Penicillium citrinum* and *Aspergillus fumigatus*. Int Arch Allergy Immunol 2002; 127:181–19.

93. Crameri R, Jaussi R, Menz G, Blaser K. Display of expression products of cDNA libraries on phage surfaces. Eur J Biochem 1994; 226:53–58.

94. Crameri R, Faith A, Hemmann S, Jaussi R, Ismail C, Menz G, Blaser K. Humoral and cell-mediated autoimmunity in allergy to *Aspergillus fumigatus*. J Exp Med 1996; 184:265–270.

95. Durham OC. Incidence of air-borne fungus spores: I. *Alternaria*. J Allergy 1937; 8:480–490.

96. Aas K. Bronchial provocation tests in asthma. Arch Dis Child 1970; 45:221–228.

97. Bronsky EA, Ellis EF. Inhalation bronchial challenge testing in asthmatic children. Pediat Clin North Am 1969; 16:85–94.

98. Schlueter DP, Fink JN, Hensley GT. Wood-pulp worker's disease: A hypersensitivity pneumonitis caused by *Alternaria*. Ann Intern Med 1972; 77:907–914.

99. Yunginger JW, Jonen RT, Nesheim ME, Gieller M. Studies on *Alternaria* allergens: III. Isolation of major allergenic fraction (*ALT-1*). J Allergy Clin Immunol 1980; 66:138–147.

100. Nyholm L, Lowenstein H, Yunginger JW. Immunochemical partial identity between two independently identified and isolated major allergens from *Alternaria alternata* (*ALT-1* and *Ag1*). J Allergy Clin Immunol 1983; 71:461–467.

101. Vijay HM, Muradia G, Young NM, Gidney MAJ, Curran IHA. Characterization of monoclonal antibodies of *Alternaria alternata* (abstr). J Allergy Clin Immunol 1993; 91(suppl 1):273.

102. Sanchez H, Bush RK. Purification of *Alternaria* (ALT) allergens by use of monoclonal antibody (abstr). J Allergy Clin Immunol 1988; 81:184.

103. Portnoy J, Olson I, Pacheco F, Barnes C. Affinity purification of a major *Alternaria* allergen using a monoclonal antibody. Ann Allergy 1990; 65:109–114.

104. Lepage D, Boutin Y, Vrancken ER. Allergenic determinants of *Alternaria* extracts defined by monoclonal antibodies (abstr). J Allergy Clin Immunol 1989; 83:216.

105. Deards MJ, Montague AE. Purification and characterization of a major allergen of *Alternaria alternata*. Mol Immunol 1991; 28:409–415.

106. Paris S, Debeaupuis JP, Prevost MC, Casotto M, Latge JP. The 31 kD major allergen, ALT a I$_{1563}$, *Alternaria alternata*. J Allergy Clin Immunol 1991; 88:902–908.

107. Matthiesen F, Olsen M, Lowenstein H. Purification and partial sequenization of the major allergen of *Alternaria alternata* Alt a1 (abstr 386). J Allergy Clin Immunol 1992; 89:241.

108. Curran IHA, Young NM, Burton M, Vijay HM. Purification and characterization of Alt a-29 from *Alternaria alternata*. Int Arch Allergy Immunol 1993; 102:267–275.

109. Bush RK, Sanchez H. cDNA sequence of an *Alternaria* allergen. In: Molecular Biology and Immunology of Allergens (Kraft D, Sehon A, eds.). Boca Raton, FL: CRC Press, 1993: 271–273.

110. Budd TW, Kuo CY, Yoo TJ, McKenna WR, Cazin J. Antigens of *Alternaria*: I. Isolation and partial characterization of a basic peptide allergen. J Allergy Clin Immunol 1983; 71:277–282.

111. DeVouge MW, Thaker AJ, Curran IHA, Zhang L, Muradia G, Rode H, Vijay HM. Isolation and expression of cDNA clone encoding an *Alternaria alternata* Alt a1 subunit. Int Arch Allergy Immunol 1996; 111:385–395.

112. DeVouge MW, Thaker AJ, Zhang L, Muradia G, Rode H, Vijay HM. Molecular cloning of IgE-binding fragments of *Alternaria alternata* allergens. Int Arch Allergy Immunol 1998; 116:261–268.

113. Achatz G, Oberkofler H, Lechenauer E, Simon B, Unger A, Kandler D, Ebner C, Prillinger H, Kraft D, Breitenbach M. Molecular cloning of major and minor allergens of *Alternaria alternata* and *Cladosporium herbarum*. Mol Immunol 1995; 32(suppl 3):213–227.

114. Kurup VP, Vijay HM, Kumar V, Castillo L, Elms N. IgE binding synthetic peptides of Alt a1, major allergen of *Alternaria alternata* peptides (in press).

115. Solomon WR, Matthews KP. Aerobiology and inhalant allergens. In: Allergy: Principles and Practice, 3rd ed. (Middleton E, Reed CE, Ellis EF, Adkinson NF, Yunginger JW, eds.). St. Louis: C.V. Mosby, 1989: 312–372.

116. Aukrust L, Borch SM. Partial purification and characterization of two *Cladosporium herbarum* allergens. Int Arch Allergy Appl Immunol 1979; 60:68–79.

117. Sward-Nordmo M, Wold JK, Paulsen BS, Aukrust L. Purification and partial characterization of the allergen Ag54 from *Cladosporium herbarum*. Int Arch Allergy Appl Immunol 1985; 78:249–255.

118. Sward-Nordmo M, Paulsen BS, Wold JK. Immunological studies of glycoprotein allergen Ag-54 (Cla h II) in *Cladosporium herbarum* with special attention to the carbohydrate and protein moieties. Int Arch Allergy Appl Immunol 1989; 90:155–161.

119. Zhang L, Muradia G, Curran IHA, Rode H, Vijay HM. A cDNA clone coding for a novel allergen, Cla h III, of *Cladosporium herbarum* identified as a ribosomal P2 protein. J Immunol 1995; 154:710–716.

120. Breitenbach M, Simon B, Probst G, Oberkofler H, Ferreira F, Briza P, Achatz G, Unger A, Ebner C, Kraft D, Hirschwehr R. Enolases are highly conserved fungal allergens. Int Arch Allergy Immunol 1997; 113:114–117.

121. Muilenberg M, Burge H, Sweet, T, Solomon W. *Penicillium* species in and out of doors in Topeka KS. J Allergy Clin Immunol 1990; 85:247.

122. Wei DL, Chen JH, Jong SC, Shen HD. Indoor airborne *Penicillium* species in Taiwan. Curr Microbiol 1993; 26:137–140.

123. Shen HD, Lin WL, Liaw SF, Tarn MF, Han SH. Characterization of the 33-kilodalton major allergen of *Penicillium citrinum* by using MoAbs and N-terminal amino acid sequencing. Clin Exp Allergy 1997; 27:79–86.

124. IUIS Allergen Nomenclature Subcommittee. Official List of Allergens, http://www.allergen.org

125. Chou H, Lin WL, Tarn MF, Wang SR, Han SH, Shen HD. Alkaline serine proteinase is a major allergen of *Aspergillus flaus*—a prevalent airborne *Aspergillus* species in the Taipei area. Int Arch Allergy Immunol 1999; 119:282–290.

126. Shen HD, Wang CW, Chou H, Lin WL, Tarn MF, Huang MH, Kuo ML, Wang SR, Han SH. cDNA cloning and immunological characterization of a new *Penicillium citrinum* allergen (Pen c 3). J Allergy Clin Immunol 2000; 105:827–833.

127. Vijay HM, Thaker AJ, Banerjee B, Kurup VP. Mold allergens. In: Allergens and Allergen Immunotherapy (Lockey RF, Bukantz C, eds). New York: Marcel Dekker, 1998: 133–154.

128. Kurup VP, Shen H-D, Banerjee B. Respiratory fungal allergy. Microbes Infect 2000; 2:1101–1110.

129. Horner WE, Ibanez MD, Lehrer SB. Immunoprint analysis of *Calvatia cyathiformis* allergens: I. Reactivity with individual sera. J Allergy Clin Immunol 1989; 83:784–792.

130. Davis WE, Horner WE, Salvaggio JE, Lehrer SB. Basidiospore allergens: Analysis of *Coprinus quadrifidus* spore, cap, and stalk extracts. Clin Allergy 1988; 18:261–267.

131. Tarlo SM, Bell B, Srinivasan J, Dolovich J, Hargreave FE. Human sensitization to *Ganoderma* antigen. J Allergy Clin Immunol 1979; 64:43–49.

132. Cutteon AEC, Hasnain SM, Segedin BP, Bai TR, McKay EJ. The basidiomycete *Ganoderma* and asthma: Collection, quantitation and immunogenicity of the spores. N Z Med J 1988; 101:361–363.

133. Horner WE, Helbling A, Lehrer SB. Basidiomycete allergens: Comparison of three *Ganoderma* species. Allergy 1993; 48:110–116.

134. Vijay HM, Comtois P, Sharma R, Lemieux R. Allergenic components of *Ganoderma applanatum*. Grana 1991; 30:167–170.

135. Ishiguro A, Homma M, Torii S, Tanaka K. Identification of *Candida albicans* antigens reactive with immunoglobulin E antibody of human sera. Infect Immun 1992; 60:1550–1557.

136. Shen HD, Choo KB, Lee HH, Hsieh JC, Lin WL, Lee WR, Han SH. The 40 kD allergen of *Candida albicans* is an alcohol dehydrogenase: Molecular cloning and immunological analysis using monoclonal antibodies. Clin Exp Allergy 1991; 21:675–681.

137. Baldo BA, Baker RS. Inhalant allergies to fungi: Reactions to baker's yeast and identification of baker's yeast enolase as an important allergen. Int Arch Allergy Appl Immunol 1998; 86:201–208.

138. Koivikko A, Kalimo K, Nieminen E, Savolainen J, Viljanen M, Viander M. Allergenic cross-reactivity of yeasts. Allergy 1988; 43:192–200.

139. Jensen-Jarolim E, Poulsen LK, With H, Kieffer M, Ottevanger V, Stahl Skov P. Atopic dermatitis of the face, scalp, and neck: Type I reaction to the yeast *Pityrosporum ovale*? J Allergy Clin Immunol 1992; 89:44–51.

140. Zargari A, Doekes G, van Ieperen-van Dijk AG, Landberg E, Harfast B, Scheynius A. Influence of culture period on the allergenic composition of *Pityrosporum orbiculare* extracts. Clin Exp Allergy 1995; 25:1235–1245.

141. Zargari A, Harfast AB, Johansson S, Johansson SGO, Scheynius A. Identification of allergen components of the opportunistic yeast *Pityrosporum orbiculare* by monoclonal antibodies. Allergy 1994; 49:50–56.

142. Woodfolk JA, Wheatley LM, Piyasena RN, Benjamin DC, Platts-Mills TAE. Trichophyton antigens associated with IgE antibodies and delayed type hypersensitivity: Sequence homology to two families of serine proteinases. J Biol Chem. 1998; 273:489–496.

143. Deuell B, Arruda LK, Hayden ML, Chapman MD, Platts-Mills TA. *Trichophyton tonsurans* allergen. I. Characterization of a protein that causes immediate but not delayed hypersensitivity. J Immunol 1991; 147:96–101.

14

Mite Allergens

ENRIQUE FERNÁNDEZ-CALDAS

C.B.F. LETI, S.A., Tres Cantos, Madrid, Spain

LEONARDO PUERTA and LUIS CARABALLO

University of Cartagena, Cartagena, Colombia

RICHARD F. LOCKEY

University of South Florida College of Medicine and James A. Haley Veterans' Hospital, Tampa, Florida, U.S.A.

I. INTRODUCTION

Domestic mites, the main source of allergens in house dust, produce potent allergens that are capable of inducing sensitization and respiratory and cutaneous diseases. The most common species belong to the families Pyrogyphidae, Acaridae, Glycyphagidae, Echymopodidae, Chortoglyphidae, Cheyletidae, and Tarsonemidae. These microarthropods have a worldwide distribution. The most important species are *Dermatophagoides pteronyssinus, D. farinae, D. siboney, D. microceras, Euroglyphus maynei, Acarus siro, Suidasia medanensis, Aleuroglyphus ovatus, Tyrophagus putrescentiae, Glycyphagus domesticus, Lepidoglyphus destructor, Blomia tropicalis, Chortoglyphus arcuatus, Cheyletus* spp., and *Tarsonemus* spp. (Fig. 1).

Storage mites belong to a wide range of families, genera, and species and are found in stored grain, barns, hay, and straw. Exposure to these mites and their allergens can also

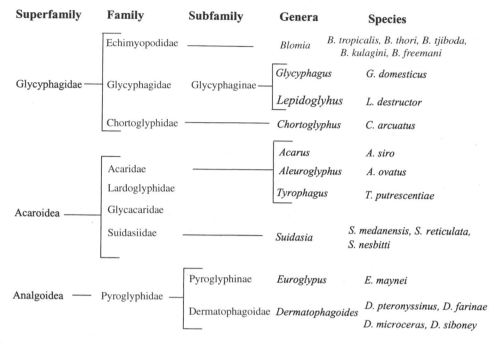

Figure 1 Taxonomic classification of the most important domestic mite species.

occur in homes. Several species of storage mites have been identified in house dust world-wide. The term "domestic mites" applies to all mite species that can be found in the indoor environment and to which type I allergic sensitization has been demonstrated.

In 1964, the role of a species of the genus *Dermatophagoides* in the etiology of bronchial asthma produced by the inhalation of house dust was proposed (1). Sensitization to domestic mites and asthma has since been recognized as a worldwide clinical problem. Cutaneous sensitivity to mite allergens has been demonstrated in 50% to 90% of asthmatic individuals (2,3). Several groups have identified nasal and bronchial reactivity in response to direct challenge with mite allergens in humans, supporting the idea that mite allergens play an important role in the pathogenesis of allergic respiratory diseases (4–9). High specific IgE titers to mite, cat, and cockroach allergens are also highly prevalent among asthmatic individuals treated in emergency rooms in the southeastern United States and the Caribbean (10–13).

Domestic mite extracts contain many allergens, which are grouped according to their homologies, or order of description. So far, approximately 19 groups of mite allergens have been characterized and/or sequenced.

II. TAXONOMY OF MITES

Mites belong to the phylum Arthropoda, class Arachnida, subclass Acari. They vary considerably in their anatomy and habitat; some feed on plants, while others have developed complex parasitic relationships with other animals. More than 30,000 species have been identified. They have an exoskeleton, jointed appendages, and a blood-filled body cavity (hemocoel). The life cycle of house dust mites and some storage mites consists of

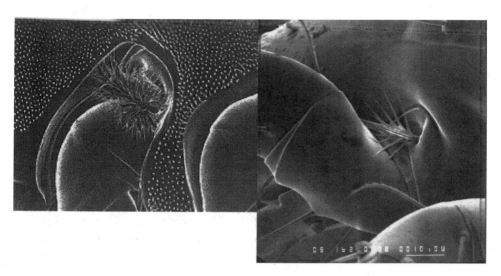

Figure 2 Supracoxal gland in the mite species *L. destructor* (*left*) and *T. putrescentiae* (*right*).

five stages (egg, larva, protonymph, tritonymph, and adult). Each stage consists of an active feeding period followed by a short, nonfeeding, inactive period before the next stage emerges from the exoskeleton. Mites are distinguished from insects because in the adult stage they have four pairs of legs, instead of three; only the larvae have three pairs of legs.

Mites have a well-developed digestive tract, including mouth parts (chelicerae and pedipalps), salivary glands, and gut consisting of esophagus, midgut with a large cecum, hindgut, and an anus (14). Their digestive system produces spherical fecal pellets (approximately 20 μm in diameter) wrapped in a peritrophic membrane. Their respiration is cutaneous, and the skin serves as a barrier to exchange gas and water vapor. The water loss of the body regulates colonization and population growth. House dust mites extract water vapor from the air by means of a hygroscopic salt solution in the supracoxal gland (Fig. 2). If the humidity falls below the critical level of 50%, the salt crystallizes, obstructs the entrance of the gland, and slows down the rate of dehydration. For the successful completion of their life cycle, mites require an optimal relative humidity ranging from 70% to 90%. The process of water uptake also depends on the temperature. A temperature of approximately 25°C is required for their successful reproduction. The development on bare floors is slower than in warmer locations, such as mattresses or couches. The development of *D. farinae* and *D. pteronyssinus* from egg to adult takes from 19 to 33 days between 22°C and 32°C and at 75% relative humidity (15,16). In tropical countries, *S. medanensis* and *B. tropicalis* need shorter periods of time to reach the adult stages (17).

Most domestic mites belong to the suborder Astigmata. Free-living (mite species that primarily live in the outdoor environment and are not parasitic) Astigmata commonly live in decaying organic matter and in nests of birds, insects, and mammals. Many of these mites infest stored food, and certain species are of economic importance because of the damage they inflict to stored grains. Several species in this group are capable of producing respiratory allergic disease as well as contact dermatitis. Some have heteromorphic deutonymphs (hypopus), which invade hair follicles or subcutaneous tissues of mammals or birds and cause cutaneous lesions. The name "house dust mites" has been used to include those members of the family Pyroglyphidae (pyroglyphid mites) that live permanently in house dust. Important nonpyroglyphid species, distributed globally, include several species that have been traditionally regarded as storage mites, such as Acaridae, Chortoglyphidae, and Glycyphagidae (18), which also inhabit homes and accumulate in house dust.

III. HOUSE DUST COLLECTION AND MITE IDENTIFICATION

Mite identification and counting requires expertise. Several publications are available to assist in preparing samples for identification and counting (19,20). House dust can be collected by brushing, sweeping, and vacuum cleaning. The most important sampling sites are bedding (mattress cover, sheets, pillows and pillow casings, and blankets), bedroom and living room carpets, floor, and sofas. Closets, basement carpets, clothes (21), human scalps (22), and air ducts can also be sampled using a modified vacuum cleaner. In the event that linoleum or tile floors must be sampled, brushing or sweeping of the entire surface is indicated, and the collected dust is placed in a plastic or glass container. Dust samples should not be stored at room temperature, since mature, live mites could start or continue reproduction and change the collected mite count. The amount of dust collected using any of the aforementioned methods should be large enough to allow sieving and counting (minimum of 100 to 200 mg of fine dust). Other methods developed for collecting dust mites include the heat escape and the passive transfer (mobility test) methods. In both techniques, a piece of adhesive tape is placed on a carpet and mites are forced to migrate upward by heat (37°C) or by their natural space requirements. After several hours, the adhesive tape is removed and the mites present are counted and expressed as mites per area sampled. These methods yield a higher number of live mites than brushing and vacuuming.

A. Morphological Analysis of House Dust Samples

Suspension, flotation, sedimentation, and heat extraction are the methods most commonly used to separate mites from house dust. These methods include those described by Arlian et al. (23), Hart and Fain (24), Korsgaard and Hallas (25), and Fernández-Caldas et al. (26). Using any of the previous methods, mites are collected with a fine needle under a dissecting microscope and mounted in two drops of Hoyer's medium on microscope slides for species identification and counting. Hoyer's medium consists of a mixture containing 50 ml of distilled water, 30 g of Arabic gum, 200 g of chloral hydrate, and 20 ml of glycerin. These ingredients are mixed in this sequence at room temperature. Ideally, all mites extracted from dust samples should be washed, cleared, and mounted on microscope slides for identification and counting under the microscope. Once the mites have been isolated, temporary or permanent preparations can be made. Temporary preparations can be established by mounting the mites directly in two drops of 50–100% lactic acid. The lowest concentration should be used for the weakly sclerotized species. The slide can be warmed over an electric bulb or on a hot plate at about 60°C. Once the mites are cleared, they should be kept in the cold. Mites can be mounted in lactophenol in place of lactic acid or in lactic acid colored with lignin pink. Permanent preparations are usually made in Hoyer's medium. Living mites make better preparations for study. Specimens are placed in two drops of Hoyer's medium on a microscope slide. After the cover slip has been placed over the drops, the slide may be heated gently to hasten clearing, expand the specimens, and set the mounting material. If the storage of unmounted specimens is desirable, mites can be preserved indefinitely in 70–80% ethanol or in Oudemans' fluid, which consists of 87 parts of ethanol, 5 parts of glycerin, and 8 parts of glacial acetic acid.

IV. DISTRIBUTION OF MITES AND THEIR ALLERGENS

Mite allergens can be detected in many areas of the home, including beds, carpets, upholstered furniture, and clothing. Leather-covered couches, wood furniture, and bare floors contain fewer mites than the aforementioned locations. Beds are the ideal habitat for mites, since they provide the ideal temperature, food, and moisture for their proliferation. Mites can be found deep inside mattresses and pillows, especially when they are old. They can act as a source of reinfestation when the surface of the mattress is vacuumed or cleaned. Mite allergens are present in mite bodies, secreta, and excreta, and fecal particles contain the greatest proportion of mite allergen (27). Mite levels between 100 (2 µg of Group 1 allergen/g) and 500 mites per gram of dust (10 µg of Group 1 allergen/g) can be considered risk factors for sensitization and asthma. Any mite species present in the human environment in large enough quantities (>100/g of dust) could be considered a potential allergen with sensitizing capabilities. This sensitizing capability may be due to the presence of potent proteolytic enzymes, which could be implicated in the sensitization process acting as an adjuvant of the immune response.

Various mite species can be found in house dust. Species belonging to the Pyroglyphidae family, *D. pteronyssinus, D. farinae,* and *E. maynei,* are the most frequently reported, followed by *Cheyletus* spp., *B. tropicalis, T. putrescentiae, G. domesticus, Tarsonemus* spp., *L. destructor, Suidasia* spp., and *C. arcuatus*. The prevalence of these species varies depending on the geographical location and may be found in large quantities in a specific environment.

Mite densities and allergen levels are usually greater in humid locations than in those at high altitudes. In Switzerland, above 1200 m, the mite fauna decreases in numbers and in species, most likely due to a decrease in temperature and absolute humidity. Similar results have been obtained in Colorado (28). However, in humid mountain regions of the Andes, such as Peru or Colombia, mite growth takes place even at such high altitudes. The geographical distribution of mites is variable, and although several species can coexist, usually one mite species tends to predominate (29).

The main domestic mite species in the United States are *D. pteronyssinus, D. farinae, E. maynei,* and *B. tropicalis* (30). Most ecological studies in temperate climates have demonstrated that *D. pteronyssinus* (originally known as the European house dust mite) and *D. farinae* (American house dust mite) are the predominant house dust mites worldwide. In tropical and subtropical areas of the world, *B. tropicalis* occurs with a very high frequency, and in some regions it is present at the same rate as *D. pteronyssinus* (31). Several species of allergologically important mites have been described in Europe (32) including *D. pteronyssinus, D. farinae, E. maynei, G. domesticus, T. putrescentiae,* and *L. destructor*. New technologies and sensitive immunoassays are now available to detect minimal concentrations of mite allergens in settled and airborne dust. ELISA, RIA, RAST-inhibition, and guanine detection are used for the determination of allergens from the main mite species. A two-site monoclonal antibody-based ELISA is the most popular method to quantify levels of mite allergens. The assay uses a monoclonal antibody coated to plastic microtiter wells, which binds to a specific epitope on an allergen. Bound allergens are detected using a second antibody directed against a different epitope on the molecule, either enzyme or ^{125}I labeled. The quantification is performed using reference preparations containing known amounts of a given allergen. The total allergenic content in a house dust sample can also be quantified by RAST inhibition. Based on these measurements, allergen levels that represent a risk factor for sensitization and asthma have been proposed (2). Exposure to 2 µg of Der p 1 and/or Der f 1 per gram of dust can be considered a risk factor for sensitization; exposure to 10 µg/g of dust can be considered a major risk factor for sensitization and asthma in genetically predisposed individuals. Allergen levels in excess of 10 µg/g of dust have been identified in many parts of the world. There seems to be no difference between mite allergen levels in homes of mite-allergic asthmatic and nonallergic control individual.

Airborne mite allergens can also be detected. It has been suggested that mite fecal pellets may occasionally enter the lung and cause inflammation and bronchoconstriction. Fergusson and Broide (33) demonstrated the presence of Der p 1 in bronchial alveolar lavage fluids of asthmatic children after an overnight exposure to Der p 1 levels of 13.4 and 27.3 µg of Der p 1 in carpets and mattresses, respectively. A mean value of 3.4 ng of Der p 1/ml was recovered from bronchial alveolar lavage fluids. In the same study, endobronchial provocations with 5–60 ng of Der p 1 induced pulmonary eosinophilia.

Mite allergens are consistently higher in the air during cleaning activities than in undisturbed conditions. Furthermore, Der p 1 seems to be airborne in larger quantities than Der p 2 (34,35). Studies using volumetric samples equipped with sizing devices have shown that mite allergens remain airborne for a short period of time. Allergenic activity has been detected in particles smaller than 1 µm and in particles larger than 10 µm. Mite allergens settle more rapidly than cat allergens, which remain airborne for longer periods of time and can be detected in air samples collected in homes under disturbed and undisturbed conditions.

V. MOLECULAR CHARACTERISTICS OF MITE ALLERGENS

There has been considerable progress in the study of the molecular characteristics of mite allergens. Mite allergens have been purified from aqueous extracts or produced as recombinant proteins, of which nucleotide and amino acid sequences have been obtained. Molecular cloning provides an efficient way of obtaining pure polypeptides, which in their native sources form complex mixtures and are often present in very small amounts. The cloning of allergen provides pure proteins to map B- and T-cell epitopes and permits the identification of these binding sites. Sequence similarity searches have identified the biological function of many mite allergens. When sequence homologies with known proteins have not been found, the biological function of these allergens remains unknown. Sequence polymorphisms have been identified for several allergens. These polymorphisms influence antibody binding and T-cell recognition.

The number of purified allergens has increased significantly over recent years. Most of the well-characterized allergens have an ascribed biological function based on the similarity with other proteins of known functions. Most have been placed in groups based on their chronological characterization and/or homology with previously purified *Dermatophagoides* allergens.

Originally, purified allergens were named according to the first three letters of the genus, the first letter of the species, and a number indicating the order of purification (Der p 1). Later on, as more allergens were purified and sequenced, homologies in their sequences were identified. It was then agreed that allergens with a similar biological function and a high degree of homology would be placed in the same group, e.g., Group 1,

Group 2, etc. Mite allergens that belong to a certain group all have the same biological function.

A. Allergens with Enzymatic Activity: Groups 1, 3, 4, 6, 8, 9, and 15

Group 1 allergens are glycoproteins with sequence homology and thiol protease functions similar to the enzymes papain, actinidin, bromelain, and cathepsins B and H (36). There is a 30% homology between the primary structure of Der p 1 and cathepsins B and H, papain, bromelain, and actinidin. Regions near the active catalytic site show 100% homology.

Der p 1 cleaves the low-affinity IgE receptor (CD23) from the surface of human B-cell lymphocytes (37). Soluble CD23 promotes IgE production, and therefore fragments of CD23 released by the Der p 1 allergen may enhance IgE synthesis. It has also been suggested that Der p 1 cleaves the α subunit of the IL-2 receptor (IL-2R or CD25) from the surface of human peripheral blood T-cells, and as a result, these cells show markedly diminished proliferation and IFN-γ secretion in response to potent stimulation by anti-CD3 antibody (38). The authors concluded that since IL-2R is pivotal for the propagation of Th1 cells, its cleavage by Der p 1 may consequently bias the immune response toward Th2 cells. The cleavage of CD23 and CD25 by Der p 1 enhances its allergenicity by creating an allergic microenvironment (39). Studies have also demonstrated that the proteolytic activity of Der p 1 enhances the IgE antibody response to bystander antigens. It has been shown that the cysteine protease activity of Der p 1 seems to selectively enhance the IgE response and that the proteolytic activity of Der p 1 conditions T-cells to produce more IL-4 and less IFN-γ (40,41). The enzymatic activity of Der p 1, and other mite allergens, may also contribute to their immunogenicity by increasing mucosal permeability. The peptidase activity creates conditions that favor delivery of any allergen to antigen-presenting cells by a process that involves cleavage of tight junctions that regulate paracellular permeability (42).

Blo t 1 of *B. tropicalis* has also been characterized. This allergen is 35% identical to Der p 1 and Der f 1 and shows 61% of specific IgE binding in the serum of *B. tropicalis*–allergic patients (43). Eur m 1 is an important allergen of *E. mainey* and has an amino acid sequence homology of approximately 85% with Der p 1 and Der f 1 (44). Der s 1, a major allergen of *D. siboney*, purified using cross-reacting monoclonal antibodies directed against Group 1 allergen from *Dermatophagoides* spp., has an 89% frequency of specific IgE binding (45).

Group 3 has a trypsin-like serine protease activity and 50% homology with other serine proteases, including chymotrypsin (46). The sequence of Der p 3 has 81% sequence identity with Der f 3, and both have a 41% sequence identity with bovine trypsin. A frequency of IgE binding between 51% and 90% for Der p 3 and between 42% and 70% for Der f 3 has been described (47). Blo t 3, which also has a trypsin-like protease activity, has also been characterized (48).

Der p 4, an enzyme similar to carbonic anhydrases, shows significant homology with mammalian α-amylase (49). It is recognized as an allergen by 25% to 46% of mite-allergic individuals. Der p 6 is a chymotrypsin-like serine protease that shows a 40% to 60% frequency of IgE binding. It has 37% homology with Der p 3 (50). Der p 8 is a 26-kDa allergen with strong homology with rat and mouse glutathione-S-transferase. Approximately 40% of mite-allergic subjects tested with recombinant (r) Der p 8 bound specific IgE to this allergen (51). Der p 9 is a 24-kDa protein, as indicated by mass spectroscopy, with collagenolytic serine protease activity and a frequency of IgE reactivity higher than 80% (52). Der f 15 is homologous to insect chitinases. It is a major allergen recognized by dogs and cats (53) and by the sera of approximately 70% of mite-allergic humans.

B.   Allergens with Ligand-Binding Activity: Groups 2, 13, 14, and 16

Der p 2 and Der f 2 are heat- and pH-stable proteins of 14 kDa (54,55). These allergens have 88% homology. In their native stage and expressed as a fusion protein, both have an 83% frequency of specific IgE recognition (56). The amino acid sequences of Der p 2 and Lep d 2 have 28% and 26.4% homology with the epididymis-specific human HEI gene product, respectively. These proteins seem to arise from secretions of the male mite reproductive tract (57). Der p 2 and Der f 2 show a significant degree of sequence polymorphism. The polymorphic residues are also found in regions containing T-cell epitopes (58). Crystallographic studies suggest that Der p 2 is a lipid-binding protein (59).

The existence of Eur m 2 in *E. maynei* and of Tyr p 2 in *T. putrescentiae* has also been demonstrated (60,61). Gly d 2, the Group 2 allergen of *G. domesticus*, has also been cloned (62). Blo t 13 is homologous to cytosolic fatty acid–binding proteins found in many species (63). Lipid-binding assays confirmed the fatty acid–binding properties of this allergen (64). Another homologous allergen has been identified in *Acarus siro* (65) and *L. destructor* (66). A frequency of IgE binding of 11%, 23%, and 13% has been reported for Blo t 13, Aca s 13, and Lep d 13, respectively. ELISA inhibition assays with monoclonal antibody specific for Blo t 13 suggest that the homologous allergen Der s 13 is also present in *D. siboney* (67). A report suggests the presence of Der f 13 in *D. farinae* (68), confirming the presence of Group 13 to the *Dermatophagoides* spp.

Group 14 is an apolipophorin-like lipid transport protein, isolated by molecular cloning from *Dermatophagoides* spp. (69,70). Group 16 includes calcium-binding proteins. An amino acid similarity search revealed that the predicted Der f 16 polypeptide sequence showed similarity to gelsolin, a Ca2+- and polyphosphoinositide 4,5-biphosphate (PIP2)-regulated actin filament severing and capping protein. Der f 16 showed an IgE-binding frequency of 47.1% using sera of allergic individuals (71). Skin test and IgE-binding studies showed that 62% (skin test) and 50% (specific IgE binding) of mite-sensitive asthmatic patients recognized Der f 16 as an allergen.

C.   Allergens with Activity on the Cytoskeleton: Groups 10 and 11

These groups are composed of tropomyosin and paramyosin, respectively. They are involved in muscle contraction in invertebrates and are present in low concentrations in mite extracts. The invertebrate tropomyosins are allergenic in man with high IgE cross-reactivity and therefore have been referred to as pan-allergens. Der f 10 is a 32-kDa allergen with significant homology with tropomyosins from different species (72). Der p 10 may be involved in the cross-reactivity process between mites, shrimp, and insects in shrimp-allergic patients (73). Blo t 10 was isolated using mouse anti–Der p 10 antibodies. The allergenicity of the cloned Blo t 10 was confirmed by skin prick test and enzyme-linked immunosorbent assay. The cloned Blo t 10 shared approximately 96% of amino acid identity with tropomyosin of other mite species. Skin tests and specific IgE determinations demonstrated a sensitization rate to r Blo t 10 of 20% to 29% in atopic subjects. Some allergic individuals recognized unique IgE-binding epitopes on Blo t 10. Although Blo t 10 and Der p 10 are highly conserved (95% amino acid identity) and significantly cross-reactive, unique IgE epitopes do exist (74).

Der f 11 has 34% to 60% sequence identity with other known paramyosins (75). Skin test and IgE-binding studies showed that 62% and 50% of mite-sensitive asthmatic patients reacted with recombinant Der f 11 (76), respectively. It has been shown that Blo t 11, a paramyosin identified in *B. tropicalis*, binds specific IgE with frequency of 52% in allergic patients (77).

D. Allergens of Unknown Biological Activity: Groups 5, 7, and 12

Der p 5 is a 15-kDa allergen with an estimated IgE-binding prevalence of 50% (78). Blo t 5 from *B. tropicalis* has also been characterized by molecular cloning (79,80). It has approximately 40% sequence homology with Der p 5. This allergen is recognized by 60% to 70% of *B. tropicalis*–sensitive patients, especially those residing in tropical areas. Der p 7 and Der f 7 have 86% sequence homology. Recombinant Der f 7 reacted with 46% of sera from asthmatic children (81). The allergenicity of r Der p 7 has been demonstrated by direct specific IgE binding and skin testing; about 50% of mite-allergic individuals analyzed were sensitized to this allergen (82). Group 12 has only been described by cDNA cloning from *B. tropicalis*. Blo t 12 has a mature sequence of 14 kDa, binds specific IgE with a 50% frequency, and does not show homology with other known proteins (83).

E. Other Cloned Mite Allergens: Groups 17, 18, and 19

Several allergens have been recently entered in the IUIS database but have not been widely studied (84). These allergens include Der f 17, Der f 18, and Blo t 19. Der f 17 is a calcium-binding protein that binds IgE in 35% of the sera from mite-allergic patients (85).

Der f 18 is a 60-kDa-molecular-weight chitinase that is a strong allergen for dogs and also reacts with 60% of mite-allergic humans. Blo t 19 has a molecular weight of 7 kDa, is homologous to an antimicrobial peptide, and only reacts with the serum of 10% of mite-allergic individuals.

VI. MITE ALLERGEN CROSS-REACTIVITY

Allergenic cross-reactivity occurs when different proteins have a certain degree of homology and contain identical or similar specific IgE-binding epitopes. Cross-reactivity is a common feature among mite allergens, especially in those from taxonomically related species. The allergenicity of the house dust mite *D. pteronyssinus, D. farinae*, and *E. maynei* is documented, but the extent to which their allergens are unique or cross-react with mite allergens or other genera has not been completely delineated. *E. maynei, D. pteronyssinus*, and *D. farinae* show significant allergenic cross-reactivity, in which several allergens are involved, including Der p 2 (86).

In vitro cross-reactivity studies between whole extracts of *B. tropicalis* and other mite species have demonstrated that these mites share common, as well as species-specific, allergens. Puerta et al. (87) demonstrated a greater degree of cross-reactivity between *B. tropicalis* and *L. destructor* than between *B. tropicalis* and *Dermatophagoides* spp. Arlian et al. (88) demonstrated that the majority of the allergens present in *B. tropicalis* are species-specific. Only three allergens are common with *D. farinae* body and faeces extracts, two and one with body and faeces extracts of *D. pteronyssinus*, respectively, using immunoelectrophoresis. Morgan et al. (89) demonstrated corresponding IgE-binding proteins of 105, 75, 57, 18, and 14 kDa in extracts of *E. maynei* and *B. tropicalis*. However, the majority of IgE-binding proteins did not show corresponding bands in both extracts.

The authors concluded that *E. maynei* and *B. tropicalis* are the source of both species-specific and cross-reactive allergens, and that most allergens in each extract were species-specific. Several allergens of *B. tropicalis* have been cloned and sequenced. Some of them have shown sequence homology with purified allergens of *D. pteronyssinus* such as Blo t 5, a homologue of Der p 5; Blo t 13, a fatty acid–binding protein; Blo t 11, homologous to paramyosin; Blo t 10, homologous to tropomyosin and Der p 10; Blo t 3, a trypsin-like protease (18); and Blo t 1, homologous to cysteine proteases. All these studies have confirmed a low to moderate degree of cross-reactivity. Several studies have focused on the in vitro cross-reactivity of purified Blo t 5 and Der p 5 (90,91) and Blo t 10 and Der p 10 (tropomyosin). Most Group 5 studies demonstrated low to moderate cross-reactivity at the molecular level. Less information is available about Group 10 allergens.

The allergenic cross-reactivity between *L. destructor* and *B. tropicalis* was initially demonstrated by specific IgE inhibition studies using whole allergen extracts. The participation of Group 2 in the cross-reactivity between these two species has also been suggested (92). Cross-reactivity among Group 2 allergens from nonpyroglyphid mites, such as *L. destructor*, *T. putrescentiae*, and *G. domesticus*, is greater than with Der p 2. Homologous allergens to Blo t 13 have also been identified in *L. destructor*. These allergens may also contribute to the high degree of cross-reactivity among nonpyroglyphid mites. Group 13 also seems to contribute to the cross-reactivity between *B. tropicalis* and *D. siboney*. Der p 10 and Blo t 10 share 95% of amino acid identity and have a significant degree of cross-reactivity. However, they have unique IgE-binding epitopes. The results suggest the potential deficiency of using only one of these highly conserved allergens as diagnostic or therapeutic reagents.

Dermatophagoides ssp.–allergic individuals may experience allergic symptoms after consumption of crustaceans and mollusks. Der f 10 and Der p 10 proteins with homology to tropomyosin from various animals is involved in the cross-reactivity among *Dermatophagoides* spp., mollusks, and crustaceans. The 36-kDa cross-reactive tropomyosin present in mites, various insects (chrinomids, mosquito, and cockroach), and shrimp (93) is responsible for cross-reactivity among different arthropods (94). In addition, a 25-kDa allergen present in several arthropod groups seems to be involved in this cross-reactivity.

Immunochemical studies have demonstrated that allergens from snails, crustaceans, cockroaches, and chironomids cross-react with house dust mite allergens. However, house dust mites are usually the primary source of sensitizing allergens.

The nematode *Anisakis simplex*, a common fish parasite, can act as a hidden food allergen inducing IgE-mediated reactions. Allergic cross-reactivity between this nematode and the domestic mites *A. siro*, *L. destructor*, *T. putrescentiae*, and *D. pteronyssinus* has been reported, in which tropomyosin seems to be involved. The clinical relevance of this cross-reactivity needs to be further investigated (95).

The feather mite *Dipleagidia columbae* is a major source of clinically relevant allergens for pigeon breeders. The results of RAST inhibition experiments suggest that this feather mite cross-reacts with *D. pteronyssinus* (96). Arlian et al. demonstrated that antigens of the parasitic mite *Sarcoptes scabiei* cross-react with antigens of *D. pteronyssinus* (97). Proteins with homology to different groups of mite allergens also have been identified by molecular cloning in the parasitic mites *S. scabiei* (98) and *Soroptes ovis* (99). The clinical relevance of these finding remains to be established.

However, it is well established that mites contain species as well as cross-reactive allergens. The degree and nature of the exposure and the genetic background of the individuals may dictate the degree of cross-reactivity that may be expected in a certain patient.

In the event of patients with skin test sensitivities to multiple mite species, conjunctival, nasal, or bronchial challenges may be indicated for a more precise diagnosis and more effective treatment.

VII. ENVIRONMENTAL CONTROL

Environmental control is the matter of current debate and has been the subject of a meta-analysis. Several studies have shown negative results (100,101), while others have shown significant improvement in symptoms and a reduction in respiratory symptoms (102). The main conclusion of environmental control studies is that they are difficult to conduct and that an absolute reduction in allergen exposure is needed in order to be clinically effective. The placebo effect also seems to be important in these kinds of studies.

A meta-analysis has attempted to determine whether mite-sensitive asthmatics benefit from measures designed to reduce their exposure to dust mite allergens in homes (103). It concluded that current chemical and physical methods aimed at reducing exposure to dust mite allergens seem to be ineffective and cannot be recommended for mite-sensitive asthmatics. Only 4 of 23 trials achieved a reduction in mites/allergen levels, were sufficiently long to show an effect on outcomes, and showed evidence of clinical benefit (104).

Allergen avoidance for children should begin as early as possible, even before birth, especially if one of the parents is allergic. Some studies suggest that avoidance of ingested and inhaled allergens and tobacco smoke delays the onset of allergy and allergy-associated diseases, including asthma (105,106). It has also been shown that admission of dust mite–sensitive asthmatics to a hospital with low mite allergen levels decreases bronchial hyperreactivity (107). A pronounced improvement in nonspecific airway responsiveness has also been shown after allergen avoidance, suggesting a reduction in airway inflammation following avoidance of aeroallergens (108–110). There is good evidence that sensitization to house dust mites is a major independent risk factor for asthma in all areas where climate is conducive to mite population growth (111–113). For other allergens, the relationship depends mainly on the climate and socioeconomic characteristics of the community. There is a significant dose-response relationship between exposure to mite allergens and subsequent sensitization (114–116). Another important consideration is that many mite allergens are potent enzymes. A study has suggested that exposure to house dust mite antigen can induce airway epithelial shedding even in subjects with low eosinophil airway infiltration, thus supporting the idea that epithelial damage in asthmatics sensitized to *Dermatophagoides* may be due to a proteolytic activity of the mite allergens (117).

Although indoor allergen control measures to reduce symptoms in individuals allergic to mites have produced controversial results, environmental allergen avoidance is today one of the four primary goals of asthma management recommended in several guidelines of asthma treatment (118). Exposure to high indoor aeroallergen levels, especially to house dust mite allergens, is an important environmental risk factor for allergic sensitization and the subsequent development and exacerbation of asthma. Several studies have demonstrated that effective aeroallergen avoidance, using a combination of methods, is of clinical use to prevent and treat allergic diseases (119–121).

Environmental control can be used in several stages of the sensitization and disease process. It can be used to prevent or delay sensitization or to control symptoms once an individual has been sensitized. Excessive exposure to allergens in the first months of life increases the risk of sensitization and the subsequent development of allergic asthma. The institution of allergen avoidance measures early in life has reduced the frequency of aller-

Table 1   Ideal Environmental Control Measures

Most important
1. Thoroughly vacuum mattresses and bases of the beds.
2. Encase mattresses, washable pillows, and box springs in plastic covers.
3. Wash sheets and mattress pads in hot water (>139°F) weekly, or use a liquid acaricide and cold water.
4. Blankets should be washed at least once a month.
5. Remove carpets, drapes, toys, books, and other objects, where possible, that may collect dust in the bedroom.
6. Vacuum carpets and stuffed furniture with a double-bagged potent vacuum cleaner once a week.
7. Fix humidity problems in the home.

Difficult-to-institute measures
1. Apply an acaricide and/or a denaturing agent (tannic acid).
2. Dehumidify the entire home or the bedroom to less than 50% relative humidity.
3. Keep air conditioning set at the lowest possible level.
4. Remove carpets throughout the house.

Of questionable importance
1. Use room air cleaners and central air filter systems.
2. Regularly clean air ducts.

gic symptoms in infancy. Admission of house dust mite–sensitive asthmatics to a hospital with low mite allergen levels decreases bronchial hyperreactivity. Therefore, effective aeroallergen avoidance, using a combination of methods, is of clinical use to prevent and treat allergic diseases. Additional information is needed about the dynamics of production of indoor allergens, decay rate, and environmental factors that promote or create the sources of indoor allergen exposure. Environmental control depends upon such knowledge. Each indoor environment is unique, and allergen levels may vary from room to room. Therefore, recommendations on indoor environmental control measures are incomplete and less effective without a thorough investigation of the indoor environment.

The fundamental objectives of environmental control are (1) to prevent or minimize occupant exposure that can be deleterious and (2) to provide for the comfort and well-being of the occupants. Table 1 contains the main methods used to reduce mite allergen exposure.

A. Cleaning

Mites attach themselves to the fibers in furniture and carpets, making it difficult to remove them by vacuuming. However, vacuuming does remove surface dust and fecal pellets that otherwise would become airborne.

B. Acaricides

Various chemicals have been used to control mite populations. Products containing benzyl benzoate, benzoic acid, pyrethroids, and pirimiphos methyl, among others, are effective acaricides. Denaturating agents, such as tannic acid, reduce allergen levels in carpets but do not kill mites.

C. Use of Covers

Plastic covers are used to control mites and their allergens in mattresses, pillows, and blankets. They are an effective barrier against mites and their allergens and reduce exposure to mite allergens in the bedroom.

D. Modifying Indoor Climatic Conditions

Humidity and temperature are the most important factors influencing the geographical distribution, seasonal fluctuation, reproduction, and survival of house dust mites. Mite populations are affected by seasonal changes. Peak domestic mite population densities in temperate climates occur during the summer and are lowest during the late winter. A seasonal rise in mite numbers occurs with increased humidity. In the tropics, mite allergen levels experience less variation. Mite-allergic patients should be advised to control the humidity in their homes. Inadequate ventilation, a consequence of home energy efficiency, and damp housing conditions are important risk factors in temperate regions for mite sensitization and exacerbation of allergic diseases.

E. Air Filtration

Group 1 and 2 mite allergens become airborne during domestic and cleaning activities. The efficacy of air filtration in alleviating mite-induced allergic respiratory symptoms remains to be established.

VIII. SALIENT POINTS

1. Domestic mites have a worldwide distribution.
2. Sensitization to their allergens is an etiological risk factor for allergic asthma and rhinitis.
3. Major domestic mite allergens have been sequenced and cloned. Some of them are enzymes involved in the digestion process, which may amplify the immune response.
4. Domestic mites have species-specific and unique allergenic epitopes. The degree of cross-reactivity is greater among pyroglyphid mites than between *Dermatophagoides* spp. and storage mites.
5. Allergens with similar biological functions exist in most mite species that have been analyzed.
6. Mite extracts containing other than *Dermatophagoides* spp. should be considered for diagnosis and treatment in regions where mites species, such as *B. tropicalis*, occur and induce sensitization.
7. Fecal particles easily become airborne during turbulence due to their small size. Mite allergens are consistently higher in the air during cleaning activities.
8. Mite allergen avoidance is the first line of treatment once sensitization has been demonstrated and should be instituted to reduce the risk of sensitization early in life and later on to reduce the risk of developing mite-induced allergic disease and exacerbation of symptoms.
9. Effective house dust mite allergen avoidance will not be achieved using a single control measure; many methods are required to affect the multiple factors that facilitate high mite allergen levels.

REFERENCES

1. Voorhorst R, Spieksma-Bozeman MIA, Spieksma FTHM. Is a mite (*Dermatophagoides* spp.) the producer of the house dust allergen? Allergie Asthma 1964; 10:329.
2. Platts-Mills TAE, De Weck A. Dust mite allergens and asthma—A world wide problem. Bull WHO 1989; 66:769–780.
3. Fernández-Caldas E, Baena-Cagnani CE, Lopez M, Patiño C, Neffen HE, Sanchez-Medina M, Caraballo LR, Huerta López J, Malka S, Naspitz CK, Lockey RF. Cutaneous sensitivity to 6 mite species in asthmatic patients from 5 Latin American countries. J Investig Allergol Clin Immunol 1993; 3:245–249.
4. Stanaland BE, Fernández-Caldas E, Jacinto CM, Trudeau WL, Lockey RF. Positive nasal challenges with *Blomia tropicalis*. J Allergy Clin Immunol 1996; 97:1045–1049.
5. García Robaina JC, Sánchez Machín I, Fernández-Caldas E, Vázquez Moncholi C, Bonnet Moreno C, de la Torre Morín F. Skin tests, conjunctival and bronchial challenges with extracts of *Blomia tropicalis* and *Dermatophagoides pteronyssinus* in patients with asthma and/or rhinoconjunctivitis. Int Arch Allergy Immunol 2003. In press.
6. Arshad SH, Hamilton RG, Adkinson NF Jr. Repeated aerosol exposure to small doses of allergen: A model for chronic allergic asthma. Am J Respir Crit Care Med 1998; 157:1900–1906.
7. Ronborg SM, Mosbech H, Poulsen LK. Exposure chamber for allergen challenge: A placebo-controlled, double-blind trial in house-dust-mite asthma. Allergy 1997; 52:821–828.
8. Horak F, Toth J, Hirschwehr R, Marks B, Stubner UP, Jager S, Berger U, Schleinzer K, Gunczler P. Effect of continuous allergen challenge on clinical symptoms and mediator release in dust-mite-allergic patients. Allergy 1998; 53:68–72.
9. Van Der Veen MJ, Jansen HM, Aalberse RC, van der Zee JS. Der p 1 and Der p 2 induce less severe late asthmatic responses than native *Dermatophagoides pteronyssinus* extract after a similar early asthmatic response. Clin Exp Allergy 2001; 31:705–714.
10. Nelson RP Jr, DiNicolo R, Fernández-Caldas E, Seleznick MJ, Lockey RF, Good RA. Allergen-specific IgE levels and mite allergen exposure in children with acute asthma first seen in an emergency department and in nonasthmatic control subjects. J Allergy Clin Immunol 1996; 98:258–263.
11. Caraballo L, Puerta L, Fernández-Caldas E, Lockey RF, Martínez B. Sensitization to mite allergens and acute asthma in a tropical environment. J Investig Allergol Clin Immunol 1998; 8:281–284.
12. Gelber LE, Seltzer LH, Bouzoukis JK, Pollart SM, Chapman MD, Platts-Mills, TA. Sensitization and exposure to indoor allergens as risk factors for asthma among patients presenting to hospital. Am Rev Resp Dis 1993; 147:573–578.
13. Duff AL, Pomeranz ES, Gelber LE, Price GW, Farris H, Hayden FG, Platts Mills TAE, Heymann PW. Risk factors for acute wheezing in infants and children: Viruses, passive smoke, and IgE antibodies to inhalant allergens. Pediatrics 1993; 92:535–540.
14. Spieksma FTM. Domestic mites from an acarologic perspective. Allergy 1997; 52:360–368.
15. Arlian LG, Rapp CM, Ahmed SG. Development of *Dermatophagoides pteronyssinus* (Acari; Pyrologyphidae). J Med Entomol 1990; 27:1035–1040.
16. Colloff MJ. Differences in development, time, mortality and water loss between egg from laboratory and wild populations of *Dermatophagoides pteronyssinus* (Trouessart 1987) (Acari; Pyrologyphidae). Exp Appl Acarol 1987; 3:191–200.
17. Mercado D, Puerta L, Caraballo L. Life-cycle of *Suidasia medanensis* (Pontifica) (Acari:Suidasiidae) under laboratory conditions in a tropical environment. Exp Appl Acarology 2001; 25:751–755..
18. O'Connor BM. Astigmata. In: Synopsis and Classification of Living Organisms, Vol 2. (Parker S, ed.). New York: McGraw Hill, 1982:146–169.
19. Huges AM. The mites of stored food. Her Majesty's Stationary Office, Minister of Agriculture and Fisheries, Technical Bulletin No. 9, London, 1961.

20. Colloff MJ, Spieksma FThM. Pictorial keys for the identification of domestic mites. Clin Exp Allergy 1992; 22:823–830.

21. Tovey ER, Mahmic A, McDonald LG. Clothing—An important source of mite allergen exposure. J Allergy Clin Immunol 1995; 96:999–1001.

22. Naspitz CK, Diniz C, Rizzo MC, Fernández-Caldas E, Solè D. Human scalps as a reservoir of domestic mites. Lancet 1997; 349:404.

23. Arlian LG, Bernstein IL, Gallagher JS. The prevalence of house dust mites, *Dermatophagoides* spp., and associated environmental conditions in homes in Ohio. J Allergy Clin Immunol 1982; 69:527–532.

24. Hart BJ, Fain A. A new technique for the isolation of mites exploiting the differences in density between ethanol and saturated NaCI: Qualitative and quantitative studies. Acarologia 1987; 28:251–254.

25. Korsgaard J, Hallas TE. Tarsonemid mites in Danish house dust. Allergy 1979; 34:225–232.

26. Fernández-Caldas E, Puerta L, Mercado D, Lockey RF, Caraballo L. Mite fauna, *Der p* I, *Der f* I and *Blomia tropicales* allergen in a tropical environment. Clin Exp Allergy 1993; 23:292–297.

27. Tovey ER, Chapman MD, Platts-Mills TAE. Mite feces are a major source of house dust allergens. Nature 1982; 289:592–593.

28. Nelson H, Fernández-Caldas E. The prevalence of house dust mites in the Rocky Mountain states. Ann Allergy 1995; 337–339.

29. Fernández-Caldas E, Andrade J, Trudeau WL, Souza Lima E, Souza Lima I, Lockey RF. Serial determinations of Der p 1 and Der f 1 show predominance of one *Dermatophagoides* ssp. J Invest Allergol Clin Immunol 1998; 8:27–29.

30. Arlian L, Bernstein D, Bernstein L, Friedman S, Grant A, Lieberman P, Lopez M, Metzger J, Platts-Mills T, Schatz M, Spector S, Wasserman S, Zeiger S. Prevalence of dust mites in the homes of people with asthma living in eight different geographic areas of the United States. J Allergy Clin Immunol 1992; 90:292–300.

31. Fernández-Caldas E, Fox R, Bucholtz G, Truedeau W, Ledford, Lockey R. House dust mite allergy in Florida: Mite survey in households of mite sensitive individuals in Tampa, Florida. J Allergy Clin Immunol 1990; 11:263–267.

32. Fernández-Caldas E. Mite species of allergologic importance in Europe. Allergy 1997; 52:383–387.

33. Fergusson P, Broide DH. Environmental and bronchoalveolar lavage *Dermatophagoides pteronyssinus* antigen levels in tropic asthmatics. Am J Respir Crit Care Med 1995; 151:71–74.

34. Swanson MC, Agarwal MK, Reed CE. An immunochemical approach to indoor aeroallergen quantitation with a new volumetric air sampler. Studies with mite, roach, cat, mouse, and guinea pig antigens. J Allergy Clin Immunol 1985; 76:724.

35. Sakaguchi M, Inouye H, Yasueda H, Irie T, Yoshizawua S, Shida T. Measurement of allergen associated with dust mite allergy II: Concentration of airborne mite allergen (Der I and Der II) in the house. Int Arch Allergy Appl Immunol 1989; 90:190.

36. Chua KY, Stewart GA, Thomas WR, Simpson RJ, Dilworth RJ, Plozza TM, Turner KJ. Sequence analysis of cDNA coding for a major house dust mite allergen, Der p I homology with cysteine proteases. J Exp Med 1988; 167:175–182.

37. Hewitt CR, Brown AP, Hart BJ, Pritchard DI. A major house dust mite allergen disrupts the immunoglobulin E network by selectively clearing CD23: Innate protection by antiproteases. J Exp Med 1995; 182:1537–1544.

38. Schulz O, Sewell HF, Shakib F. Proteolytic cleavage of CD25, the α subunit of the human T cell Interleukin 2 receptor, by Der p 1, a major mite allergen with cystein protease activity. J Exp Med 1998; 187:271–275.

39. Shakib F, Schulz O, Sewell H. A mite subversive: Cleavage of CD23 and CD25 by Der p 1 enhances allergenicity. Immunology Today 1998; 19:313–316.

40. Gough L, Sewell HF, Shakib F. The proteolytic activity of the major dust mite allergen Der p 1 enhances the IgE antibody response to a bystander antigen. Clin Exp Allergy 2001; 31:1594–1598.

41. Ghaemmaghami AM, Robins A, Gough L, Sewell HF, Shakib F. Human T cell subset commitment determined by the intrinsic property of antigen: The proteolytic activity of the major mite allergen Der p 1 conditions T cells to produce more IL-4 and less IFN-gamma. Eur J Immunol 2001; 31:1211–126.

42. Wan H, Winton HL, Soeller C, Taylor GW, Gruenert DC, Thompson PJ, Cannell MB, Stewart GA, Garrod DR, Robinson DC. The transmembrane protein occluding of epithelial tight junctions is a functional target for serine peptidases from faecal pellets of *Dermatophagoides pteronyssinus*. Clin Exper Allergy 2001; 31:279–294.

43. Mora C, Flores I, Montealegre F, Díaz A. Cloning and expression of Blo t 1, a novel allergen from the dust mite *Blomia tropicalis*, homologous to cysteine proteases. Clin Exp Allergy 2003; 33:28–34.

44. Kent NA, Hill MR, Keen NJ, Holland PWH, Hart BJ. Molecular characterization of group I allergen Eur m I from house dust mite Euroglyphus meynei. Int Arch Allergy Immunol 1992; 99:150–152.

45. Ferrándiz R, Casas R, Dreborg S, Einarsson R, Bonachea I, Chapman M. Characterization of allergenic components from house dust mite *Dermatophagoides siboney*. Purification of Der s I and Der s 2 allergens. Clin Exp Allergy 1995; 25:922–928.

46. Stewart GA, Ward LD, Simpson RJ, Thompson PJ. The group III allergen from the house dust mite *Dermatophagoides pteronyssinus* is a trypsin-like enzyme. J Immunol 1992; 75:29–35.

47. Stewart GA, Thompson PJ. The biochemistry of common aeroallergens. Clin Exp Allergy 1996; 26:1020–1044.

48. Flores I, Mora C, Rivera E, Donnelly R, Montealegre F. Cloning and molecular characterization of a cDNA from *Blomia tropicalis* homologous to dust mite group 3 allergens (trypsin-like proteases). Int Arch Allergy Immunol 2003;130:12–16.

49. Lake FR, Ward LD, Simpson RJ, Thompson PJ, Stewart GA. House dust mite derived amylase: Allergenicity and physicochemical characterization. J Allergy Clin Immunol 1991; 87:1035–1042.

50. Bennett BJ, Thomas WR. Cloning and sequencing of the group 6 allergen of *Dermatophagoides pteronyssinus*. Clin Exp Allergy 1996; 26:1150–1154.

51. O'Neill GM, Donavan GR, Baldo BA. Cloning and characterization of a major allergen of the house dust mite, *Dermatophagoides pteronyssinus*, homologous with glutathione-S-transferase. Biochim Biophys Acta 1994; 1219:521–528.

52. King C, Simpson RJ, Moritz RL, Reed GL, Thompson PJ, Stewart GA. The isolation and characterization of a novel collagenolitic serine protease allergen (Der p 9) from the dust mite *Dermatophagoides pteronyssinus*. J Allergy Clin Immunol 1996; 98:739–747.

53. McCall C, Hunter S, Stedman K, Weber E, Hillier A, Bozic C, Rivoire B, Olivry T. Characterization and cloning of a major high molecular weight house dust mite allergen (Der f 15) for dogs. Vet Immunol Immunopathol 2001; 10;78(3–4):231–247.

54. Ovsyannikova IG, Vailes LD, Li Y, Heymann PW, Chapman MD. Monoclonal antibodies to group II *Dermatophagoides* spp. allergens: Murine immune response, epitope analysis, and development of a two-site ELISA. J Allergy Clin Immunol 1994; 94:537–546.

55. Lombardero M, Heymann PW, Platts-Mills TA, Fox JW, Chapman MD. Conformational stability of B cell epitopes on group I and group II *Dermatophagoides* spp. allergens: Effect of thermal and chemical denaturation on the binding of murine IgG and human IgE antibodies. J Immunol 1990; 144:1353–1360.

56. Chua KY, Doyle CR, Simpson RJ, Turner KJ, Stewart GA, Thomas WR. Isolation of cDNA coding for the major mite allergen Der p 2 by IgE plaque immunoassay. Int Arch Allergy Appl Immunol 1990; 91:118–123.

57. Thomas WR, Chua KY. The major mite allergen Der p 2—A secretion of the male mite reproductive tract? Clin Allergy 1995; 25:666–669.

58. Chua KY, Huang CH, Shen HD, Thomas WR. Analysis of sequence polymorphism of a major mite allergen, Der p 2. Clin Exp Allergy 1996; 26:829–837.

59. Derewenda U, Li J, Derewenda Z, Dauter Z, Mueller GA, Rule GS, Benjamin DC. The crystal structure of a major dust mite allergen, Der p 2, and its biological implications. J Mol Biol 2002; 318:189–197.

60. Morgan MS, Arlian LG, Barnes KC, Fernández-Caldas E. Characterization of the allergens of the house dust mite *Euroglyphus maynei*. J Allergy Clin Immunol 1997; 100:222–228.

61. Eriksson TL, Johansson E, Whitley P, Schmidt M, Elsayed S, van Hage-Hamsten M. Cloning and characterisation of a group II allergen from the dust mite *Tyrophagus putrescentiae*. Eur J Biochem 1998; 251:443–447.

62. Gafvelin G, Johansson E, Lundin A, Smith AM, Chapman MD, Benjamin DC, Derewenda U, van Hage-Hamsten M. Cross-reactivity studies of a new group 2 allergen from the dust mite *Glycyphagus domesticus*, Gly d 2, and group 2 allergens from *Dermatophagoides pteronyssinus*, *Lepidoglyphus destructor*, and *Tyrophagus putrescentiae* with recombinant allergens. J Allergy Clin Immunol 2001; 107:511–518.

63. Caraballo L, Puerta L, Jimenez, S, Martinez B, Mercado D, Avjioglu A, Marsh D. Cloning and IgE binding of a recombinant allergen from the mite *Blomia tropicalis*, homologous with fatty acid-binding proteins. Int Arch Allergy Immunol 1997; 112:341–347.

64. Puerta L, Kennedy M, Jiménez S, Caraballo L. Structural and ligand binding analysis of recombinant Blo t 13 allergen from *Blomia tropicalis* mite, a fatty acid binding protein. Int Arch Allergy Immunol 1999; 119:181–184.

65. Eriksson T, Whitley P, Johanson E, van Hage-Hamsten M, Gafvelin G. Identification and characterization of two allergens from the dust mite *Acarus siro*, homologous with fatty acid-binding proteins. Int Arch Allergy Immunol 1999; 119:275–281.

66. Eriksson TL, Rasool O, Huecas S, Whitley P, Crameri R, Appenzeller U, Gafvelin G, van Hage-Hamsten M. Cloning of three new allergens from the dust mite *Lepidoglyphus destructor* using phage surface display technology. Eur J Biochem 2001; 268:287–294.

67. Labrada M, Uyema K, Sewer M, Labrada A, Gonzalez M, Caraballo L, Puerta L. Monoclonal antibodies against Blo t 13, a recombinant allergen from *Blomia tropicalis*. Int Arch Allergy Immunol 2002; 129:212–218.

68. Lim SH, Chew FT, Ong ST, Tsai LC, Le BW. Identification of new *Dermatophagoides* allergens and isoforms from an expressed sequence tag database showing homology to other known allergens. ACI International 2000; suppl 2:175.

69. Epton MJ, Dilworth RJ, Smith W, Thomas WR. Sensitisation to the lipid-binding apolipophorin allergen Der p 14 and the peptide Mag-1. Int Arch Allergy Immunol 2001; 124:57–60.

70. Epton MJ, Dilworth RJ, Smith W, Hart BJ, Thomas WR. High-molecular-weight allergens of the house dust mite: An apolipophorin-like cDNA has sequence identity with the major M-177 allergen and the IgE-binding peptide fragments Mag1 and Mag3. Int Arch Allergy Immunol 1999; 120:185–191.

71. Kawamoto S, Suzuki T, Aki T, Katsutani T, Tsuboi S, Shigeta S, Ono K. Der f 16: A novel gelsolin-related molecule identified as an allergen from the house dust mite, *Dermatophagoides farinae*. FEBS letter 2002; 516:234–238.

72. Aki T, Kodama T, Fujikawa A, Miura K, Shigeta S, Wada T, Jyo T, Murooka, Y, Oka S, Ono K. Immunochemical characterization of recombinant and native tropomyosin as a new allergen from the house dust mite, *Dermatophagoides farinae*. J Allergy Clin Immunol 1995; 96:74–83.

73. Witteman A, Akkerdaas J, Leeuwen J, van der Zee J, Aalberse RC. Identification of a cross-reactive allergen (presumably tropomyosin) in shrimp, mite and insects. Int Arch Allergy Immunol 1994; 105:56–61.

74.   Yi FC, Cheong N, Shek PC, Wang DY, Chua KY, Lee BW. Identification of shared and unique immunoglobulin E epitopes of the highly conserved tropomyosins in *Blomia tropicalis* and *Dermatophagoides pteronyssinus*. Clin Exp Allergy 2002; 32:1203–1210.

75.   Tsai LC, Chao P, Hung MW, Sun YC, Kuo IC, Chua KY, Liaw SH. Protein sequence analysis and mapping of IgE and IgG epitopes of an allergenic 98-kDa Dermatophagoides farinae paramyosin, Der f 11. Allergy 2000: 55:141–147.

76.   Tsai LC, Sun YC, Chao PL, Ng HP, Hung MW, Hsieh KH, Liaw SH, Chua KY. Sequence analysis and expression of a cDNA clone encoding a 98-KDa allergen in *Dermatophagoides farinae*. Clin Exp Allergy 1999; 29:1606–1613.

77.   Ramos J, Nge C, Wah LB, Chua KY. cDNA cloning and expression of Blo t 11, the *Blomia tropicalis* allergen homologous to paramyosin. Int Arch Allergy Immunol 2001; 126:286–293.

78.   Lin KL, Hsieh KH, Thomas WR, Chiang BL, Chua KY. Characterization of Der p 5 allergen, cDNA analysis and IgE-medicated reactivity of the recombinant protein. J Allergy Clin Immunol 1995; 94:989–996.

79.   Arruda K, Vailes LD, Platts-Mills AE, Fernández-Caldas E, Montealegre F, Lin K, Chua KY, Rizzo MC, Naspitz CK, Chapman MD. Sensitization to *Blomia tropicalis* in patients with asthma and identification of allergen Blo t 5. Am J Respir Crit Care Med 1997; 155:343–350.

80.   Caraballo L, Mercado D, Jiménez S, Moreno L, Puerta L, Chua KY. Analysis of the cross-reactivity between BtM and Der p 5, two group 5 recombinant allergens from *Blomia tropicalis* and *Dermatophagoides pteronyssinus*. Int Arch Allergy Immunol 1998; 117:38–45.

81.   Shen HD, Chua KY, Lin WL, Hsieh KH, Thomas WR. Molecular cloning and immunological characterization of the house dust mite allergen Der f 7. Clin Exp Allergy 1995; 25:1000–1006.

82.   Shen HD, Chua KY, Lin KL, Hsieh KH, Thomas WR. Molecular cloning of a house dust mite allergen with common antibody binding specificities with multiple components in mite extracts. Clin Exp Allergy 1993; 23:934–940.

83.   Puerta L, Caraballo L, Fernández-Caldas E, Avjioglu A, Marsh DG, Lockey RF, Dao ML. Nucleotide sequence analysis of a complementary DNA coding for a *Blomia tropicalis* allergen. J Allergy Clin Immunol 1996; 98:932–937.

84.   Thomas WR, Smith WA, Hales BJ, Mills KL, O'Brien RM. Characterization and immunobiology of house dust mite allergens. Int Arch Allergy Immunol 2002; 129:1–18.

85.   Tategaki A, Kawamoto S, Aki. T, Jyo T, Suzukí O, Shigeta S, Ono K. Newly described house dust mite allergens. ACI Int 2000; suppl 1:64–66.

86.   Smith AM, Benjamin D, Hozic N, Derewenda U, Smith W, Thomas W, Gafvelin G, van Hage-Hamnsten M, Chapman M. The molecular basis of antigenic cross-reactivity between the group 2 mite allergens. J Allergy Clin Immunol 2001; 107:977–984.

87.   Puerta L, Fernández-Caldas E. Caraballo LR, Lockey RF. Sensitization of *Blomia tropicalis* and *Lepidogyphus destructor* in *Dermatophagoides* spp. allergic individuals. J Allergy Clin Immunol 1991; 88:943–950.

88.   Arlian LG, Vyszenski-Moher DL, Fernández-Caldas E. Allergenicity of the mite, *Blomia tropicalis*. J Allergy Clin Immunol 1993; 91:1042–1050.

89.   Morgan MS, Arlian LG, Fernández-Caldas E. Cross-allergenicity of the house dust mites *Euroglyphus maynei* and *Blomia tropicalis*. Ann Allergy Asthma Immunol 1996; 77:386–392.

90.   Simpson A, Green R, Custovic A, Woodcock A, Arruda LK, Chapman MD. Skin test reactivity to natural and recombinant *Blomia* and *Dermatophagoides* spp. allergens among mite allergic patients in the UK. Allergy 2003; 58:53–56.

91.   Kuo IC, Cheong N, Trakultivakorn M, Lee BW, Chua KY. An extensive study of human IgE cross-reactivity of Blo t 5 and Der p 5. J Allergy Clin Immunol 2003; 111:603–609.

92.   Johansson E, Schmidt M, Johansson SGO, Machado L, Olsson S, van Hage-Hamsten M. Allergenic cross-reactivity between *Lepidoglyphus destructor* and *Blomia tropicalis*. Clin Exp Allergy 1997; 27:691–699.

93. Witteman AM, Akkerdaas JH, van Leeuwen J, van der Zee JS, Aalberse RC. Identification of a cross-reactive allergen (presumably tropomyosin) in shrimp, mite and insects. Int Arch Allergy Immunol 1994; 105:56–61.

94. van Ree R, Antonicelli L, Akkerdaas JH, Pajno GB, Barberio G, Corbetta L, Ferro G, Zambito M, Garritani MS, Aalberse RC, Bonifazi F. Asthma after consumption of snails in house-dust-mite-allergic patients: A case of IgE cross-reactivity. Allergy 1996; 51:387–393.

95. Johansson E, Aponno M, Lundberg M, van Hage-Hamsten M. Allergenic cross-reactivity between the nematode *Anisakis simplex* and the dust mites *Acarus siro, Lepidoglyphus destructor, Tyrophagus putrescentiae*, and *Dermatophagoides pteronyssinus*. Allergy 2001; 56:660–666.

96. Colloff MJ, Merrett TG, Merrett J, McSharry C, Boyd G. Feather mites are potentially an important source of allergens for pigeon and budgerigar keepers. Clin Exp Allergy 1997; 27:60–67.

97. Arlian LG, Vyszenski-Moher DL, Ahmed SG, Estes SA. Cross-antigenicity between the scabies mite, *Sarcoptes scabiei*, and the house dust mite, *Dermatophagoides pteronyssinus*. J Invest Dermatol 1991; 96:349–354.

98. Fisher K, Holt DC, Harumal P, Currie BJ, Walton SF, Kemp DJ. Generation and characterization of cDNA clones from *Sarcoptes scabiei* var. *homonis* for an expressed sequence tag library: Identification of homologues of house dust mite allergens. Am J Trop Med Hyg 2003; 68:61–64.

99. Temeyer KB, Soileau LC, Pruett JH. Cloning and sequence analysis of a cDNA encoding Pso II, a group II mite allergen of the sheep scab mite (Acari:Psoroptidae). J Med Entomol 2002; 39:384–391.

100. Woodcock A, Forster L, Matthews E, Martin J, Letley L, Vickers M, Britton J, Strachan D, Howarth P, Altmann D, Frost C, Custovic A. Medical Research Council General Practice Research Framework. Control of exposure to mite allergen and allergen-impermeable bed covers for adults with asthma. N Engl J Med 2003, Jul 17; 349(3):225–236.

101. Terreehorst I, Hak E, Oosting AJ, Tempels-Pavlica Z, de Monchy JG, Bruijnzeel-Koomen CA, Aalberse RC, Gerth van Wijk R. Evaluation of impermeable covers for bedding in patients with allergic rhinitis. N Engl J Med 2003, Jul 17; 349(3):237–246.

102. Platts-Mills TA. Allergen avoidance in the treatment of asthma and rhinitis. N Engl J Med 2003, Jul 17; 349(3):207–208.

103. Gotzsche PC, Hammarquist C, Burr M. House dust mite control measures in the management of asthma: Meta-analysis. BMJ 1998; 317:1105–1110.

104. Custovic A, Murray CS, Gore RB, Woodcock A. Controlling indoor allergens. Ann Allergy Asthma Immunol. 2002; 88:432–441.

105. Arshad SH, Matthews S, Gant C, Hide DW. Effect of allergen avoidance on development of allergic disorders in infancy. Lancet 1992; 339:1493–1497.

106. Hide DW, Matthews S, Matthews L, Stevens M, Ridout S, Twiselton R, Grant C, Arshad SH. Effect of allergen avoidance in infancy on allergic manifestation at age two years. J Allergy Clin Immunol 1994; 93:842–846.

107. Platts Mills TAE, Tovey ER, Mitchell EB, Moszoro H, Nock P, Wilkins SR. Reduction of bronchial hyperreactivity during prolonged allergen avoidance. Lancet 1982; 2:675–678.

108. van Velzen E, van den Bos JW, Benckhuijsen JA, van Essel T, de Bruijn R, Aalbers R. Effect of allergen avoidance at high altitude on direct and indirect bronchial hyperresponsiveness and markers of inflammation in children with allergic asthma. Thorax 1996; 51(6):582–584.

109. Benckhuijsen J, van den Bos JW, van Velzen E, de Bruijn R, Aalbers R. Differences in the effect of allergen avoidance on bronchial hyperresponsiveness as measured by methacholine, adenosine 5′-monophosphate, and exercise in asthmatic children. Pediatr Pulmonol 1996; 22:147–153.

110. Grootendorst DC, Dahlen SE, Van Den Bos JW, Duiverman EJ, Veselic-Charvat M, Vrijlandt EJ, O'Sullivan S, Kumlin M, Sterk PJ, Roldaan AC. Benefits of high altitude

allergen avoidance in atopic adolescents with moderate to severe asthma, over and above treatment with high dose inhaled steroids. Clin Exp Allergy 2001; 31:400–408.

111. Custovic A, Smith A, Woodcock A. Indoor allergens are the major cause of asthma. Eur Respir Rev 1998; 8:155–158.

112. Squillace SP, Sporik RB, Rakes G, Couture N, Lawrence A, Merriam S, Zhang J, Platts Mills TAE. Sensitisation to dust mites as a dominant risk factor for asthma among adolescents living in Central Virginia: Multiple regression analysis of a population-based study. Am J Respir Crit Care Med 1997; 156:1760–1764.

113. Peat JK, Tovey E, Mellis CM, Woolcock A. House-dust mite allergens: An important cause of childhood asthma. Aust N Z J Med 1994; 24:473.

114. Kuehr J, Frischer T, Meinert R, Barth R, Forster J, Schraub S, Urbanek R, Karmaus W. Mite allergen exposure is a risk for the incidence of specific sensitisation. J Allergy Clin Immunol 1994; 94:44–52.

115. Lau S, Falkenhorst G, Weber A, Werthmann I, Lind P, Buettner-Goetz P, Wahn U. High mite-allergen exposure increases the risk of sensitization in atopic children and young adults. J Allergy Clin Immunol 1989; 84:718–725.

116. Wahn U, Lau S, Bergmann R, Kulig M, Forster J, Bergmann K, Bauer CP, Guggenmoos H, Holzmann I. Indoor allergen exposure is a risk factor for sensitisation during the first three years of life. J Allergy Clin Immunol 1997; 99:763–769.

117. Piacentini GL, Vicentini L, Mazzi P, Chilosi M, Martinati L, Boner AL. Mite-antigen avoidance can reduce bronchial epithelial shedding in allergic asthmatic children. Clin Exp Allergy 1998; 28:561–567.

118. Platts-Mills TA, Vaughan JW, Carter MC, Woodfolk JA. The role of intervention in established allergy: Avoidance of indoor allergens in the treatment of chronic allergic disease. J Allergy Clin Immunol 2000; 106(5):787–804.

119. Eggleston PA, Bush RK. Environmental allergen avoidance: An overview. J Allergy Clin Immunol 2001; 107:S403–S405.

120. Arlian LG, Platts-Mills TAE. The biology of dust mites and the remediation of mite allergens in allergic disease. J Allergy Clin Immunol 2001; 107:S406–S413.

121. Tovey E, Marks G. Methods and effectiveness of environmental control. J Allergy Clin Immunol 1999; 103:179–191.

Cockroach and Other Inhalant Insect Allergens

RICKI M. HELM

University of Arkansas for Medical Sciences, Little Rock, Arkansas, U.S.A.

ANNA POMÉS

INDOOR Biotechnologies, Inc., Charlottesville, Virginia, U.S.A.

I. INTRODUCTION

Inhalant sensitivity to airborne allergens of animal and plant origin is a significant problem. The varieties and distribution of insects and the accumulation of debris associated with heavy infestations vary significantly from place to place, from year to year, and by geographic location. The allergens may be extremely potent and can be found indoors, outdoors, in the home, and at the workplace. Sensitization due to occupational exposures, encountered by professionals such as research entomologists, provide examples of allergy to inhaled insect allergens. Involuntary exposure to wind-borne insect emanations in house dust also induces sensitization to insect aeroallergens in a significant population of individuals. Inhalant insect allergy is widespread and has been reported in the United States, Japan, Australia, Taiwan, Pakistan, United Kingdom, Germany, France, Sudan, and Egypt.

In the animal kingdom, the phylum Arthropoda constitutes 75% of the known animal species that can contribute significant organic material for airborne dispersal. Three major taxonomic groups, Insecta, Crustacea, and Arachnida, are of major concern as allergen producers. This chapter focuses on the class Insecta: insects that have bodies divided into a head, thorax, and abdomen; with one or two pairs of wings or wingless; and with three pair of legs. Cockroaches, mayflies, caddis flies, moths, butterflies, flies, fleas, midges, ants, bees, and vespids are representative members of this class. "Caddis fly" and "mayfly" are generic terms used by laity and professionals; each has several species. Caddis flies are more commonly called sedges by insectologists. The diversity of foraging strategies of these insects, the aeroallergens they produce, and the association with allergic disease can be phenomenal.

In urban or inner city areas, the sera of 40% to 60% of patients with asthma have IgE to cockroach allergens. In certain locales, inhalant insect dust is clearly visible in association with the emergence of caddis flies in May, June, and July. In Japan, documented sensitization to moths and butterflies is as common as sensitization to house dust mite. Chironomidae larvae and midges cause allergic reactions in approximately 20% of workers environmentally exposed to insect larvae and subjects living in affected areas. Exposure to large numbers of the "green nimitti" midge in Sudanese communities is associated with an increased incidence of both asthma and allergic rhinitis. Honeybees produce "bee dust," which causes inhalant allergy in beekeepers, and subjects extracting bee venom can develop inhalant allergy to phospholipase C. Wherever allergenic exposure (onset, intensity, and frequency) and adjuvant forces (ozone, NO_2, tobacco smoke, viruses, etc.) are present in the environment, allergic symptoms can develop, particularly in those with a genetic atopic predisposition.

Inhalation of occupational and environmental allergens derived from other classes of arthropods also causes IgE antibody responses in exposed and susceptible individuals. The subphylum Crustacea includes crabs, shrimp, lobster, and crayfish, members regarded to be among aquatic insects, where allergen exposure primarily occurs orally. This group includes several other species that have not been identified as sources of allergens, e.g., zooplankton, sow bugs, and slaters. They contain allergens that cross-react with insect-derived allergens. The class Arachnida represents animal species that are wingless and possess four pairs of legs. This class includes spiders and mites (including the house dust mite) (Chapter 14).

Insect allergy (i.e., IgE-mediated sensitivity) may be induced by a wide variety of insect-derived allergens in the environment either on a seasonal (vast aquatic insect emergences, such as caddis flies, mayflies, and midges) or a perennial basis (terrestrial pests, such as cockroaches). Cockroaches, which evolved over 350 million years ago, represent some of the oldest and most primitive of insects. Over 4000 species of cockroach are described worldwide, the majority of which are not directly associated with humans in their home and work environments. Cockroaches can be categorized as domestic, peridomestic, or feral. Feral species are those that survive independent of humans and represent 95% of all species worldwide. Seventy-four species occur in the United States, some of which have been introduced from other parts of the world. Domestic species include the

German and brown-banded cockroaches, which live almost exclusively indoors and depend on human refuse (harborage food and water) for survival. Their ideal environment is warm and humid, making indoor households their primary dwelling places; however, some species live outdoors. Peridomestic species include those that survive in or around domestic environments. This group is represented by American, Australian, brown and smoky brown, Oriental, and woods cockroaches. These were introduced into North America over the past two centuries and have been very successful in establishing habitats throughout the world, including industrialized/highly developed countries where insect infestation is better controlled.

The desire to control the indoor climate with air-conditioning units to mitigate extremes of temperature, moisture, and airflow sets the stage for several cockroach species to infest and inhabit homes. The presence of some domestic species in dwellings, such as the German or brown-banded cockroach, is often a sign of poor sanitation or substandard housekeeping. Survival of these species is enhanced by crowded living, as in apartment complexes, where associated clutter and accumulation of organic debris is often present. An overpopulation of peridomestic American or Oriental cockroaches in their native habitats, such as municipal sewage systems and septic tank areas, facilitates their entrance into nearby homes through crawl spaces, construction joints, and attic vents, causing infestation of even the best-kept homes and workplaces. The species that infest household structures typically have a high reproduction potential, which results in accumulation of relatively high dust levels of cockroach airborne allergenic proteins derived from shed exoskeletons (cast skins) and feces.

II. TAXONOMY OF COCKROACHES

Cockroaches belong to the phylum Arthropoda, class Insecta, and there are five cockroach families in the order Blattaria: Blattidae, Blattellidae, Blaberidae, Cryptocercidae, and Polyphagidae. The first two families contain the most common peridomestic pests found throughout the world (Table 1). A more detailed taxonomy of cockroaches can be found in Atkinson et al. (1) and Koehler et al. (2).

Table 1 Taxonomy of Cockroaches

Phylum:	Arthropoda	
Class:	Insecta	
Order:	Blattaria	

Family	Genus/species	Common name
Blaberidae	*Leucophaea maderae*	Maderia
Blattidae	*Periplaneta americana*	American
	Periplaneta australasiae	Australian
	Periplaneta brunnea	Brown
	Periplaneta fuliginosa	Smoky brown
	Blatta orientalis	Oriental
Blattellidae	*Blatella germanica*	German
	Blatella asahinai	Asian
	Supella longipalpa	Brown-banded

III. COCKROACH IDENTIFICATION

Cockroaches are characterized by having an exoskeleton, a segmented body (head, thorax, and abdomen), three pairs of legs, and one or two pairs of wings or none. An Asian and a German female cockroach, both carrying egg cases, are shown in Fig. 1. The possession of an exoskeleton gives the insect its form and attachment points for muscles, and provides a hardened protective covering that requires molting for growth. The old exoskeleton is discarded as exuviae (cast skins), allowing the insect to enlarge before a new exoskeleton hardens. These cast skins and fecal material contribute to the release of large amounts of amorphous airborne particles. Cockroaches are omnivorous and will consume any organic material, including fresh and processed foods, stored products, and even bookbindings and paste found on stamps and in wallpaper. In times of food shortage, some species will become cannibalistic to maintain a colony.

Infestations of cockroaches in primary dwellings (Fig. 2) and workplaces represent one of the most intimate and chronic associations of pests with humans. All cockroach species are adept crawlers; however, their flight ability varies. The two most common species of cockroach are the American *Periplaneta* (*P. americana*) and German *Blattella* (*B. germanica*). Adult *Periplaneta* occasionally fly and may be attracted to lights. German cockroaches are incapable of flight and are primarily nocturnal species; they characteristically avoid light. Asian (*B. asahinai*) cockroaches, which are closely related to German cockroaches, are particularly strong fliers and will fly indoors and outdoors at twilight toward light-colored or brightly lit surfaces (Fig. 3). A brief description of the five major cockroach species associated with humans and their immediate environment is provided in Table 2.

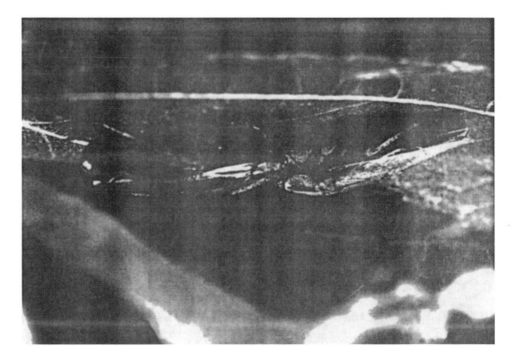

Figure 1 Asian (*left*) and German (*right*) female cockroaches carrying egg cages.

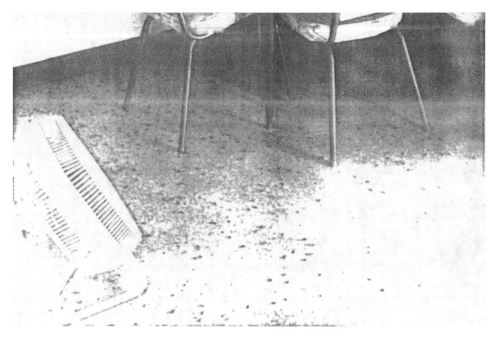

Figure 2 Kitchen floor cluttered with dead cockroaches following an insecticide treatment.

IV. DISTRIBUTION OF COCKROACHES AND PUBLIC HEALTH IMPORTANCE

Bernton and Brown made the first reports of cockroach sensitization in the 1960s (3). The incidence of patients suffering with asthma who are sensitized to cockroach allergens ranges from 40% to 70% depending on the geographical location. Kang and colleagues showed that 60% of patients with asthma in the Chicago area had positive skin tests, serum IgE antibodies, or positive bronchial challenge tests to *B. germanica* allergens (4). The National Cooperative Inner-City Asthma Study, consisting of eight major inner-city areas (Bronx, East Harlem, St. Louis, Washington D.C., Baltimore, Chicago, Cleveland, and Detroit), undertook a comprehensive analysis of factors that might be associated with the severity of asthma in inner-city children. Of 476 children with asthma (age 4–7 years) from these eight inner-city areas, 36.8% were allergic to cockroach allergen (5). Children who were both allergic to cockroach allergen and exposed to high levels of this allergen had 0.37 hospitalizations and 2.56 unscheduled medical visits for asthma per year as compared with 0.11 and 1.43, respectively, for other children. Southeast Asia (Taiwan, Thailand, Singapore), Central America (Costa Rica), the Caribbean (Puerto Rico and the Dominican Republic), India, South Africa, and Europe are among other parts of the world reporting an important association between cockroach infestations and asthma. Occupational asthma has been reported among research entomologists and laboratory personnel as well as personnel working in agricultural research centers that have cockroach-breeding programs. It appears that cockroaches and/or evidence of their infestations can be detected wherever critical evaluation of the pests is made. Reports have been made of cockroach infestations and allergic sensitization in Egypt, Japan, Brazil, and Mexico.

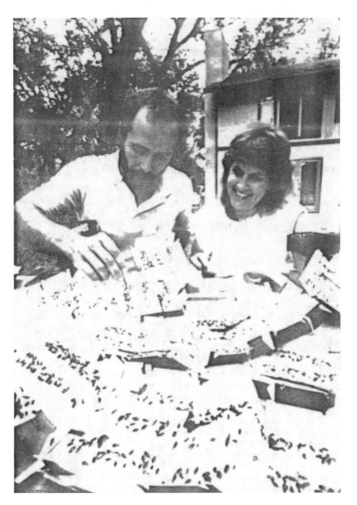

Figure 3 Dr. Richard Brenner (*left*), research entomologist, with homeowner in Florida showing Asian cockroaches, estimated at 103,000/acre, collected in this homeowner's backyard using sticky traps.

Cockroaches may adversely affect human health in several ways through biting, psychological stress, and contamination of food with excrement, associated pathogens, and allergy. At least 32 species of bacteria in 16 genera have been isolated from field-collected cockroaches; however, isolation of pathogens may simply be indicative of the natural flora and fauna in the domestic environment. Documentation of biting is limited. Early literature citations report that sometimes in the night when heavy infestations occurred, cockroaches fed on food residues around human faces and on human skin (lips, fingernails, eyebrows). Reports of biting were also reported on wooden sailing vessels. Bites of Oriental cockroaches and contact with cockroach excretions have resulted in blisterlike lesions and inflammation associated with mild dermatitis. Psychological stress is most often associated with the magnitude of the infestation and the size of the cockroach. Dense populations produce a characteristic odor that nauseates some individuals. Consuming foods that have become contaminated with excrement may cause vomiting and diarrhea.

Table 2 Cockroach Identification

Common name	Morphology	Features	Habitat
German *Blattella germanica*	16 mm long, brown, parallel dark bands along axis of body	Incapable of flight, nocturnal. Varying degrees of pesticide resistance. Most prominent pest. Strictly domestic.	Kitchens, pantries, bathrooms, bedrooms
Asian *Blattella asahinai*	16 mm long, light brown, requires taxonomist for differentiation from German	Capable of flight, attracted to light. Wild and peridomestic. Introduced in Tampa and Lakeland, Florida, 1986. Interbreed with German.	Rich ground cover, citrus groves of Florida, leaf litter, manicured lawns
American *Periplaneta americana*	34–53 mm long, reddish brown with variation light	Capable of flight. Mostly cosmopolitan. Peridomestic.	Landfills, crawl spaces, sewage systems, storm drains, septic tanks, attics, dark tree holes, caves, mines
Oriental *Blatta orientalis*	25–35 mm long, light brown	May or may not fly. Commonly known as waterbug.	Dark, damp conditions, water meter boxes, garbage chutes
Smoky brown *Periplaneta fuliginosa*	25–33 mm long, dark brown	Major southern U.S. pest. Peridomestic, majority are wild.	Tree holes, palm trees, loose mulch (pine bark, straw), firewood piles soffits, panel walls, block wall interstices, false ceilings
Brown-banded *Supella longipalpa*	13–14.5 mm long, dark band across abdomen	Capable of flight, attracted to light	Nonfood areas, bedrooms, closets, living rooms

Infestations by domiciliary cockroaches are largely dependent on housing conditions (6), and hypersensitivity is dependent on exposure (7). Americans now spend more than 95% of their time indoors in homes that are better insulated and temperature controlled while outdoor air exchange has been drastically reduced, if not eliminated, creating conditions that support pest growth and associated dust accumulation in the home. Marginal housekeeping and inadequate pesticides are also conducive to pest infestations. Cockroach allergy in American cities is typically higher in urban than in rural populations, especially in low-income housing, where there are greater cockroach infestations for prolonged periods of time (5–11). A study by Barnes and Brenner (12) suggests that in the tropics, individuals living in well-built concrete households show a higher incidence of positive skin tests to cockroach than atopics residing in wooden homes.

In the last 10 to 15 years, cockroach hypersensitivity has played an increasingly important role in allergic disease, especially asthma (13). Allergy to cockroach species can result from initial sensitization to the allergen though inhalation, ingestion, dermal abrasion, or injection. Potential sources of relevant cockroach allergens in the environment include whole bodies, cast skins, secretions, egg casings, or fecal material. Aerosolized particles containing allergens of cockroaches are rapidly being recognized as significant indoor allergens, second only to the house dust mite. Helm et al. (14) using the Air Sentinel (Rochester, MN), and polytetrafluoroethylene (PTFE) membranes to capture airborne particulates from living colonies of *P. americana* and *B. germanica*, demonstrated that aerosolized cockroach allergens were present in amorphous dust particles from living cockroach colonies. Mild to moderate symptoms induced by cockroach allergen inhalation include sneezing and rhinorrhea, skin reactions (mild dermatitis), and eye irritation, with difficulty in breathing and anaphylactic episodes occurring in more severely allergic individuals.

V. IDENTIFICATION OF COCKROACH ALLERGENS

Allergenic material with molecular weights (MWs) ranging from 6 to 120 kDa has been identified by several investigators from a variety of source materials using serum IgE from cockroach-sensitive individuals. Cockroach-sensitive individuals show a wide variation in their IgE binding patterns to extracts of crude whole-body German cockroaches (Fig. 4). Richman et al. (15) identified allergenic activity in whole-body and cast-skin extracts of the German cockroach and suggested that eggshells and feces were less important sources of allergen. Cockroach allergens, such as Bla g 1 and Bla g 2, are secreted into the feces. These allergens may be important for digestion of food by the cockroach, although their function remains unknown and no proteolytic activity has been described for either of them. A group of investigators in New Orleans established a high correlation ($r = 0.882$, $p < 0.001$) of RAST activity between German whole-body and fecal extracts (16). They were able to identify five allergens with approximate MWs of 67, 60, 50, 45, and 36 kDa that demonstrate IgE-binding reactivity in 50% to 80% of 37 subjects' sera tested. Twarog et al. (11), using column chromatography, identified three major allergens: CRI (MW 25 kDa); CRII (MW 63–65 kDa), which elicited skin test reactivity in 70% of individuals sensitive to American or German whole-body crude extracts; and CRIII (MW < 10 kDa), which elicited positive skin test reactivity in 30% of sensitive individuals. Helm et al. (17), using SDS-PAGE and Western IgE immunoblotting, identified a 36-kDa protein, GCR3, as a principal allergen of German cockroach whole-body extracts. This allergen was not present in extracts of armyworm, caddis fly, lake fly, or other insects. However, a 55-kDa

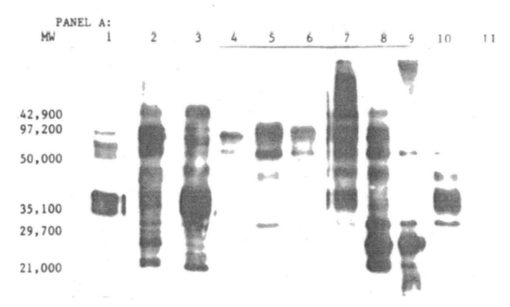

Figure 4 Representative autoradiograph of 10% SDS-PAGE/immunoblot analysis of German cockroach proteins incubated with serum IgE from cockroach-sensitive individual followed by radiolabeled anti-IgE. Lane 1 = pooled serum from eight cockroach-sensitive individuals; lanes 2–11 = individual serum samples from known cockroach-sensitive individuals. Note the wide variation in both the intensity and different patterns of IgE binding.

protein, identified in German cockroach extract and in the true armyworm, honeybee, and lake fly extracts, demonstrated that IgE from German cockroach–sensitive patients reacts with proteins from other insect species. The clinical relevance of cross-sensitization or allergenicity via cross-reacting cockroach allergens was not confirmed in these studies.

Crude extracts of whole-body American cockroach were shown to contain at least 29 antigenic components, of which 18 were identified as allergens by crossed immunoelectrophoresis (CIE) and crossed radioimmunoelectrophoresis (CRIE) (18,19). Two of these allergens, with molecular weights of 78 and 72 kDa, were identified as major allergens, since they were bound to IgE in 100% of the sera (12/12) of individuals tested and could cause T-cell proliferation of peripheral blood cells from cockroach-allergic patients (20). Monoclonal antibodies to both allergens have been generated (21). Using an immunofluorescent test on whole-body cockroach cryostat sections, Zwick et al. (22) found that proteins derived from the epithelial cells of the intestinal tract were present in the feces as well as in whole-body sections and could represent important cockroach allergens. Several groups have used conventional physicochemical techniques to identify and characterize cockroach allergens; however, the allergenic and antigenic relationships are less well studied. Cloning and in vitro expression of new cockroach allergens by using molecular biology techniques enables production of enough quantities of allergens to perform detailed antigenic studies.

Visual assessment of cockroach infestations correlates with skin test results. However, the best way to assess environmental concentration of cockroach allergens is by using enzyme-linked immunoassays. Two allergens from the German cockroach, Bla g 1 and Bla g 2, have been purified using monoclonal antibodies and protein purification techniques (9). Bla g 1 was shown to be a 25-kDa acidic, cross-reacting allergen previously identified by Twarog et al. (11), and Bla g 2 a 36-kDa species-specific allergen. Sandwich

ELISA using monoclonal antibodies against Bla g 1 and Bla g 2 (10A6 and 7C11, respectively) as capture antibodies, and specific polyclonal antibodies against the allergens have been produced to quantify both allergens (23). Specific immunoassays for both allergens monitor environmental cockroach exposure (9,23–25). A sandwich ELISA based on a monospecific rabbit antibody preparation reactive with determinants shared by Per a 1, a 25- to 35-kDa acidic allergen isolated from *P. americana*, and Bla g 1, had also been suggested for use in environmental assays (25). Studies in Atlanta and Tampa detected 10 to 10,000 units/ml of Bla g 1 in house dust collected from infested homes. Other monoclonal antibodies to important allergens in high- and low-molecular-weight fractions from American cockroach extracts have also been produced (21,26) and will permit isolation, purification, and standardization of these allergens. They will also allow development of assays to measure cockroach allergen load in dust samples that will be very useful to establish clinically relevant levels of cockroach exposure. These will certainly prove to be an important tool for further identification and characterization of cockroach-specific allergens with a potential application for diagnosis and treatment of cockroach-allergic patients. The relevance of better allergen characterization has been established by Patterson and Slater (27), who demonstrated that currently available cockroach extracts are very inconsistent in their allergenic potencies.

VI. OTHER SOURCES OF INSECT ALLERGENS

Arthropods that have been most studied as sources of allergens include crustaceans (mussels, snails, squids), insects (caddis flies, mayflies, moths and butterflies, chironomid midges, and cockroaches) and arachnids (mites). A number of other arthropods, including the houseflies (usually "housefly" implies plural species), ants, spiders, locusts and grasshoppers, bees, and silverfish (in this case it is a single genus and species; each of the other groups consists of several known species with allergen activity), have also been reported to cause sensitization either in the home or occupational setting.

The role of insects as providing inhalant allergens is further supported by data showing positive bronchial or nasal challenge with crude insect extracts. Airborne insect-derived particles include shed hairs, scales, excreta, and bits of disintegrated body parts, which contribute to amorphous dust. The composition of dust is influenced by geographical location, diligence and thoroughness of cleaning, use of insecticides, and both qualitative and quantitative sampling. The widespread incidence of swarming insects outdoors and the presence of mites in house dust samples and their related allergenicity have been firmly established. Less certainty exists for other insect allergens serving as allergen source material in dust samples.

Dogs and cats contribute dander, hair, and body secretions to allergenic loads in household dust. Not widely known is the contribution of the common flea. When dogs and cats are present in the house, the dog fleas, *Ctenocephalides* (*C.*) *canis*, and the cat fleas, *C. felis*, can reach pest proportions. Although most flea allergenicity has been attributed to bites from these insects, Trudeau et al. (28) were able to detect IgE antibodies in only 16 of 48 cat flea skin test–positive sera of individuals in the Tampa Bay area of Florida. Furthermore, using their in-house flea extract, flea allergens were quantified in eight house dust samples using RAST inhibition assays. Increasing evidence such as this indicates that insects are a significant source of both indoor and outdoor inhalant allergens.

The preparation and characterization of allergenic components in silverfish (*Lepisma saccharina*) suggest that additional care should be taken in selecting extraction media (29). Several allergenic components were shown to be insoluble at normal pH ranges used during extraction, with IgE-binding components identified in both supernatant and precipitated fractions.

In the ongoing debate of environmental, geographical, and genetic susceptibility to increases in the prevalence of asthma symptoms in fruit-cultivating farmers, environmental exposure to spider mites (*Tetranychus urticae*), an arachnid, was regarded to be a significant risk factor (30). Similarly, in forestry workers, investigations into exposure to the pine processionary caterpillar (*Thaumetopoea pityocampa*) and IgE-binding profiles led to the identification of a 15-kDa protein with no known biological function or sequence homology to other insect allergens (31).

VII.   COCKROACH ALLERGEN CROSS-REACTIVITY

A.   Inter-Cockroach Species Cross-Reactivity

Allergen cross-reactivity refers to concordance of skin or RAST reactivity between two or more crude extracts (i.e., the ability of one crude extract to inhibit a heterologous RAST, or the relative affinity of two nearly identical molecules for specific IgE-binding). Allergenic cross-reactivity is due to the sharing of IgE-binding epitopes by homologous proteins from different species. Skin test or in vitro test panels are unlikely to identify primary sources of sensitization without adequate histories and evidence of exposure. In the attempt to control allergic disease by reducing allergen exposure, it is necessary to minimize exposure to all sources of the sensitizing allergens and cross-reacting allergens. Cross-reactivity studies clarify exposure patterns that are reflected in skin or in vitro test results and define important shared or unique allergens for further study.

Although most of the cloned cockroach allergens from *B. germanica* (Bla g 2, Bla g 4, Bla g 5, and Bla g 6) and *P. americana* (Per a 3) are species specific, allergen cross-reactivity among American and German cockroach proteins has been established (32–35). Several clinical studies have confirmed cross-reactivity between the two cockroach species. Skin tests of atopic asthmatics may be positive to whole-body and fecal extracts of both American and German cockroaches (36). Twarog and colleagues (11) showed a good concordance of skin test reactivity to crude American and German cockroach extracts, which they explained as either simultaneous exposure or cross-reacting antigens. Stankus et al. (34) identified two major acidic cockroach allergens from *P. americana* and *B. germanica* that shared allergenic activity using physicochemical techniques and immunoprinting studies. Helm et al. (32) used RAST inhibition and SDS-PAGE immunoblot analysis to identify common IgE-binding components in crude extracts of *B. germanica*, *B. asahinai*, *P. americana*, and *Blatta orientalis*. An analysis of 45 antigens in *P. americana* and 29 antigens in *B. germanica* by crossed immunoelectrophoresis and immunoblots identified Per a 1 and Bla g 1 as cross-reactive homologous allergens from *P. americana* and *B. germanica*, respectively (33). Investigations conducted by Chaudhry et al. (37) revealed that the two sexes of *P. americana* contained specific as well as cross-reactive allergenic components. Bla g 1 was initially purified as a 25-kDa acidic allergen previously identified by Twarog et al. (11). Subsequent molecular cloning and protein expression revealed that Bla g 1 is a mixture of allergenic proteins of different sizes (6, 21, 32, 43 kDa up to 90 kDa) (38,39). A sequence homology of 70–72% amino acid identity between Bla g 1 and Per a 1 reveals the molecular basis of allergenic cross-reactivity between the two allergens (38,40–42).

Apart from the Group 1 cockroach allergens, it is likely that other not-yet-cloned allergens are also responsible for the cross-reactivity among different cockroach species. For example, the allergen tropomyosin was cloned from *P. americana* and named Per a 7 (43,44). Per a 7 cross-reacts with tropomyosin from other non-cockroach species (see later section). In April 2000 Jeong K.Y. and Yong T.-S. submitted to the Genbank (accession number AF260897) (Genbank is a nucleotide sequence database that can be accessed at http://www.ncbi.nlm.nih.gov/PubMed) a tropomyosin sequence from *B. germanica* that shares approximately 98% amino acid sequence identity with Per a 7. Although the allergenic nature of this protein is unknown, it is likely that tropomyosin is another inter–cockroach-species cross-reactive allergen. Continued recognition and identification of cockroach allergens responsible for initiating cockroach allergy will help to understand and guide the proper management of cockroach-induced atopic disease. For example, when known IgE-binding epitopes from shrimp tropomyosin were used to query a structural database of allergenic proteins, similar sequences in shellfish and insect allergens were identified that were consistent with clinical observations (45).

B. Extra Species Cross-Reactivity

Initial reports on the relationship between arthropod allergens, cockroaches in particular, and storage dust mites (*Dermatophagoides* (*D.*) *pteronyssinus* and *D. farinae*) were contradictory. Kang et al. (46), using hyperimmune rabbit serum, showed that crude cockroach extracts did not contain antigenic fractions, that cross-reacted with extracts of house dust or house dust mite. Cross-reactions among other insect species have been suggested, including the cat flea, housefly, spider, and stinging insects. However, in most of these reports, detailed studies using RAST inhibition or allergen purification and sequence homology studies were not performed to verify cross-reacting proteins.

In 30% of house dust mite–allergic patients in the Netherlands, Witteman et al. (47) showed that IgE antibodies in patients' sera reacted with silverfish, cockroach, and/or chironomid extracts. RAST inhibition studies identified a cross-reactive allergen among members of the groups Crustacea, Arachnida (*D. pteronyssinus*), and Insecta (*B. germanica*) (48). Tropomyosin, a protein involved in muscle contraction, was also identified as a cross-reactive allergen among members of the phyla Arthropoda and Mollusca (49–51). The Arthropoda producing allergenic tropomyosin include species from Crustacea (shrimp, crab, lobster, crawfish), Arachnida (dust mites), and Insecta (cockroaches, chironomids). The Mollusca include Bivalvia (oysters, mussels, scallops, clams, pen shells), Gastropoda (snails, abalones, whelks), and Cephalopoda (squids, octopus, and cuttlefish). For example, tropomyosin may be the cross-reactive allergen in IgE-binding components between boiled Atlantic shrimp and German cockroach in the studies performed by Crespo et al. (52), or between cockroaches and crustacea in the studies by O'Neil et al. (53) using immunoelectrophoretic techniques and RAST inhibition. These invertebrate tropomyosins share an ~80% amino acid sequence homology, whereas they are only ~45% homologous to human and edible meat (chicken, beef, pork, lamb, etc.) tropomyosins. This may explain why humans do not develop allergies to edible meat tropomyosin (54). Interesting observations have been reported emphasizing the clinical relevance of tropomyosin cross-reactivity: Exposure and sensitization to a particular food tropomyosin (dietary source) may lead to reactivity to aeroallergen exposure, and vice versa—increased exposure to aeroallergens (such as mite tropomyosin during immunotherapy) may result in reactivity to cross-reacting seafood tropomyosin (55).

In investigations of crustacean foods and stinging insects, Koshte et al. (56) found IgE antibodies to cross-reacting carbohydrate determinants (CCDs) and other cross-reacting antibodies to homologous proteins in extracts of mussels, oysters, shrimps, crabs, and honeybee and yellow jacket venoms. An IgE-reactive determinant has been proposed to be the alpha-1,3-fucosylation site of the innermost *N*-acetyl glucosamine residue of *N*-glycoproteins, which are common in insects and plants. This structural element may explain some of the major causes of broad allergenic cross-reactivity among various allergens from insects and plants. IgE antibodies against nonmammalian *N*-glycans, alpha-1,3-fucose and beta-1,2-xylose, can result in extensive cross-reactivity to plant and invertebrates (57). Whether these substitutions play a prominent clinical role as dominant IgE epitopes or in the synthesis of allergen-specific IgE in vivo has not yet been determined.

Precautions must be taken to avoid assuming that positive RAST to an allergen is evidence of exposure to that allergen. Indoor, outdoor, and workplace exposure to large numbers of insect species in different geographic regions make it extremely difficult to determine whether multiple sensitivities are explained by multiple exposures or by insect allergen cross-reactivity. From the clinical and immunological findings, allergy to a single arthropod is uncommon and cross-reactivity can extend to foods and other arthropods. The term "pan-allergy," sensitization to one or a few insect proteins with allergenic similarities that may extend to other, noninsect members of the phylum Arthropoda, may well define this phenomenon (58).

VIII. MOLECULAR CHARACTERISTICS OF COCKROACH ALLERGENS

Molecular cloning techniques have been used to sequence several cockroach allergens and to investigate their biochemical activities and biological roles. American and German cockroach cDNA expression libraries have been screened with human IgE antibodies or murine monoclonal antibodies to identify clones expressing the allergen. This approach allows for the rapid determination of allergen primary structure and production of recombinant allergen proteins for detailed characterization of linear B- and T-cell epitopes.

Helm et al. (40) showed that approximately 0.2% of the clones from a cDNA expression library constructed from German cockroaches bound IgE from a single patient with cockroach sensitivity. One of the largest clones, representing a 4-kb insert, expressed a recombinant protein with an apparent MW of 90 kDa (Bla g 90 kDa) and bound to sera from 17 of 22 individuals with cockroach hypersensitivity. DNA sequence analysis showed that the gene encoding Bla g 90 kDa consisted of seven 5876-bp tandem repeats with a shorter unique region at each end. Molecular cloning, using monoclonal antibodies against purified German cockroach allergen Bla g 1, produced several Bla g 1 isoforms, including Bla g 90 kDa (38). Each of the tandem nucleotide repeats encodes for two consecutive amino acid repeats of approximately 100 residues. Sequence homology among repeats shows that Bla g 1 originated by gene duplication and subsequent mutagenesis of a mitochondrial energy transfer domain (38). The same tandem-repeated structure was also found in the cross-reactive homologous allergen from *P. americana*, Per a 1 (41,42).

Previous studies of 106 sera from cockroach-allergic patients showed Bla g 1 and Bla g 2 to have an IgE antibody prevalence of 30% and 58%, respectively (59). Molecular cloning techniques revealed that Bla g 2 was an aspartic proteinase specific to *B. germanica*. Aspartic proteinases are a widely distributed group of digestive enzymes with a bilobal structure. Their catalytic activity is dependent on a couple of amino acid triads (DTG) at the bottom of the cleft (Fig. 5). Bla g 2, however, has important amino acid substitutions in the catalytic site, especially at the level of the triads (DST and DTS) that make this molecule enzymatically inactive (60). Study results have led to the proposal that allergens with proteolytic activity may achieve access to antigen-presenting cells in the absence of inflammation by damaging the epithelium and facilitating their own access and penetration into the mucosa (54). For example, proteolytic activity of mite allergens (Der p 1, Der p 3, Der p 6) may contribute to allergenicity. However, Bla g 2 is an excellent example of a proteolytically inactive and potent allergen, inducing sensitization at exposure levels that are one or two orders of magnitude lower than for other allergens such as Der p 1. This indicates that proteolytic activity is not necessary for allergenicity (60–62).

Bla g 4 is another *B. germanica*–specific allergen that belongs to the family of proteins called lipocalins (63). Most of the known mammalian allergens are lipocalins: Bos d 2 (cow), Equ c 1 (horse), Mus m 1 (mouse), Rat n 1 (rat), and Can f 1 and Can f 2 (dog) (54). The milk allergen β-lactoglobulin (Bos d 5) is also a lipocalin. The structure of these allergens is very stable and consists of a C-terminal α-helix and a β-barrel enclosing an internal hydrophobic cavity that binds small ligands such as retinoids, glucocorticosteroids, and pheromones (Fig. 6) (64). The homology of Bla g 4 (calycin) with rodent urinary proteins raises the possibility of pheromones and/or pheromone transport proteins as representing potential families of inhalant arthropod allergens, especially the aggregation

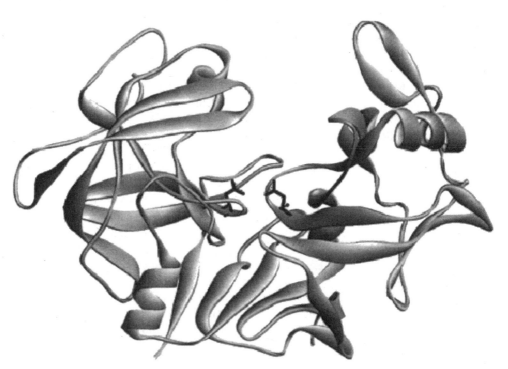

Figure 5   Ribbon representation of the Bla g 2 molecular model, based on the crystallographic structures of porcine pepsin and bovine chymosin. Aspartates in positions 32 and 215, corresponding to the catalytic amino acids triads of aspartic proteinases, are shown in black.

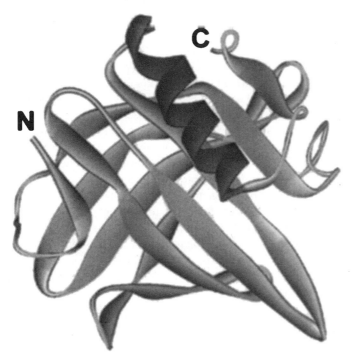

Figure 6   Ribbon representation of the molecular model of the dog lipocalin Can f 2 obtained using Swiss-Model (84-46). The C-terminal α-helix is shown in dark grey, and the β-barrel in light grey.

and sex pheromones. Soluble pheromone-binding proteins have been identified in several moth species, with an apparent molecular weight of 15 kDa and pI of 4.7 (65), which places them well within the realm of candidate allergens. The pathophysiological and allergic relevance of these proteins needs further investigation to determine their role in allergic sensitization.

Five additional cockroach clones were subsequently obtained from the *B. germanica* cDNA library by IgE antibody screening. Two recombinant proteins have been sequenced and shown to have sequence homology to *Drosophila* glutathione S-transferase (Bla g 5) and a muscle protein, troponin (Bla g 6) (66,67). The biological activity of glutathione S-transferase is to catalyze the reaction between xenobiotics and glutathione in the detoxification of xenobiotics to mercapturic acids. Troponins represent a minor protein component of the thin filaments of striated muscle. Troponins and tropomyosins include a diverse group of proteins with distinct isoforms found in muscle, brain, and some nonmuscle tissue. Structurally, tropomyosins are elongated two-stranded proteins wound around each other with dimeric alpha-helical coiled structures along their length (68,69). Although tropomyosins are highly homologous, structural forms do exist, which correspond to function domains of the proteins: actin-binding sites, troponin-binding regions, and head-to-tail polymerization sequences. Molecular biology techniques have allowed the cloning and sequencing of tropomyosins from different species. For example, Pen a 1, the major shrimp allergen, has been identified as a muscle tropomyosin and shown to have significant homology (87%) with tropomyosin of the fruit fly (*Drosophila melanogaster*) (70). As mentioned in Section VII, the considerable homology of tropomyosins from different species may explain a great deal of the allergenic cross-reactivity among arthropods and mollusks.

Several cDNA clones of the major *P. americana* allergen Per a 3 have a high degree of sequence identity (20.1–36.4%) to insect hemolymph proteins (71). Isoallergenic variants Per a 3.0202 (C13) and Per a 3.0203 (C28) of the allergen Per a 3.0201 (C20) showed significant differences in skin reactivity (26.3 and 94.7%, respectively), suggesting a high degree of polymorphism among the allergens and the potential usefulness of the isovariants in elucidating specific allergenic determinants (72). Other circulatory fluids or proteins, including hemolymph and hemoglobins, may contribute to the repertoire of insect allergens. The similarity of a lipopolysaccharide-binding protein from hemolymph of the American cockroach with other insect hemolymph proteins and with animal lectins also suggests that this class of proteins may be allergenic (73). Hemoglobins of the Diptera (insect) family of Chironomidae have been identified as causative agents in asthmatic patients living in regions where large swarms of nonbiting midges occur. Chi t 1, the hemoglobin from the European midge species (*Chironomus thummi*), represents the major allergenic component causing rhinitis, conjunctivitis, and bronchial asthma in exposed populations. There is considerable immunological cross-reactivity between hemoglobins of the same and closely related Chironomidae species; these results suggest that hemoglobins and hemocyanins of insects may also represent an important source of arthropod allergens (74). A list of the cockroach allergens and properties identified thus far is shown in Table 3.

Hypersensitivity reactions and clinical symptoms occur shortly after contact of soluble allergen with its corresponding IgE antibody bound to mast cells or basophils. The characterization of IgE antibody-binding epitopes on cockroach allergens may permit a better understanding of the immunopathogenic mechanisms involved in insect

Table 3 Properties of Cockroach Allergens

Source	Allergen	MW(kDa)	Identification[a]	Accession number
B. germanica	Bla g 1.0101	6–90	Unknown	AF072219
	Bla g 1.0102 (= Bla g 90 kDa)	90	Unknown	L47595
	Bla g 1.02	6–90	Unknown	AF072220
	Bla g 2	36	Inactive aspartic proteinase	U28863
	Bla g 4	21	Lipocalin	U40767
	Bla g 5	25	Glutathione transferase	U92412
	Bla g 6	~25	Troponin	Not available
P. americana	Per a 1.0101	26–51	Unknown	AF072222
	Per a 1.0102	26–51	Unknown	U78970
	Per a 1.0103	26–51	Unknown	U69957
	Per a 1.0104	26–51	Unknown	U69261
	Per a 1.02	26–51	Unknown	U69260
	Per a 3.01	79	Insect hemolymph	L40818
	Per a 3.0201	76	Insect hemolymph	L40820
	Per a 3.0202	56	Insect hemolymph	L40819
	Per a 3.0203	47	Insect hemolymph	L40821
	Per a 7	33	Tropomyosin	Y14854, AF106961

[a] Based on nucleotide-derived amino acid sequence homology.

hypersensitivity. The analysis of specific amino acids necessary for IgE binding will provide information on conserved or nonconserved regions important to binding and may lead to more sensitive and specific diagnostic tools and the design of novel therapeutic agents that can be used to modify the allergic response.

Overall, the use of recombinant cockroach allergens that retain IgE binding may provide the basis for improving diagnosis and therapy of individuals suffering with cockroach hypersensitivity. Sequence homology searches of databases will be used to investigate the biological function of cockroach allergens such as those identified by Chapman and his group. As more sequences become available, it will be possible to compare biological function and allergenicity, as well as allergen expression in different species, and to localize the source of allergens. Although a great deal is still unknown about the identification and biological role of insect allergens, the continued study of recombinant allergens identified from cDNA libraries will certainly benefit the understanding of the immune response and its prevention and control.

IX. MECHANISMS RELATED TO COCKROACH ALLERGEN SENSITIZATION

A mechanism for increased sensitization to cockroach allergens has been proposed by Antony et al. (75). American cockroach extracts (lacking serine and aspartic proteinase activity) induced the release of a vascular permeability factor (VEGF) to bronchial airway epithelial cells, causing endothelial barrier abnormalities and increased microvascular permeability. It is suggested that this barrier breakdown facilitates allergen entry into the bronchial airways, causing both sensitization and the allergic response. In contrast, Bhat et al. (76) demonstrated that German cockroach extracts contain a serine protease activity that has a direct inflammatory effect on airway epithelial cells. Serine protease activity in German cockroach extract had previously been reported (60). Using cultured human epithelial cells, German cockroach extracts synergistically increased TNF-α–induced transcription from the IL-8 promoter (76). Moreover, the IL-8 expression was dependent on a serine protease activity, sensitive to protease inhibitors but not induced with the endotoxin levels of the cockroach extracts. Rullo et al. (77) investigated the levels of endotoxin and mite and cockroach allergen levels in schools and suggested that the endotoxin, which has a strong pro-inflammatory property, may be capable of inducing airway inflammation and worsening asthma. Thus, environmental control of both allergen and endotoxin levels in environments where both are present may modify sensitization and allergic response. More work should be performed to determine the underlying mechanisms for cockroach sensitization.

X. DIAGNOSIS AND IMMUNOTHERAPY

A. Diagnosis

The health impact of allergens from indoor sources such as house dust and animal dander is greater than that from outdoor allergens associated with perennial allergic inflammation. This is due in large part to prolonged allergen exposure in confined climate-controlled homes. Cockroaches have received increased attention in the last several years as an important source of indoor allergens second only to the dust mite. Questionnaires have repeatedly found that few patients with allergy/asthma are aware of a direct relationship between specific allergen exposure and acute asthma attacks. In a routine diagnosis of asthma, multiple factors that may induce attacks in patients with inflamed lungs include ozone, passive smoke, cold air, and rhinovirus infections. Atopic individuals who live in cockroach-infested housing become sensitized by inhalation of potent cockroach allergens in amorphous dust and produce a vigorous IgE antibody response with high allergen-specific and total IgE levels.

Skin testing, using crude whole-body extracts, has been the gold standard to diagnose cockroach allergy. RAST, basophil histamine release, and total IgE have all been shown to be poor predictors of subsequent bronchial provocation results. RAST has been shown to have an approximately 50% false-negative rate. At present, cockroach extracts used for skin testing are not standardized, and those commercially marketed are prepared from whole-body extracts of the three most common species: American, German, and Oriental. The use of recombinant allergens, which can be produced as pure solutions using in vitro expression systems, should allow diagnosis of sensitization to specific allergens in the future. Serologic studies suggest that a cocktail of *B. germanica* allergens—Bla g 1, Bla g 2, Bla g 4, and Bla g 5—would diagnose 95% of U.S. patients with cockroach allergy (78).

Measurement of cockroach allergen exposure may allow prediction of sensitization. As with other indoor aeroallergens, airborne particles carrying allergens cannot be readily identified or counted. There is no equivalent of a pollen count. Counting numbers of cockroaches and mites may be a reasonable guide to the quantity of allergen; however, the best measurements are obtained using immunochemical assays of major allergens in extracts of dust collected from natural sources. Emergency room studies showed that individuals with a positive RAST to cockroach of >40 units/ml (U/ml) had Bla g 2 levels of >2 U/g in house dust samples. Current evidence suggests that >2 U/g Bla g 2 or Bla g 1 be established as the "threshold" allergen level for cockroach sensitization (8,79,80). The risk levels for asthmatic symptoms are 8 U/g Bla g 1 (5). Assays using monoclonal antibodies specific for Bla g 1 and Bla g 2 have shown differences of up to 200-fold in allergen levels in six commercial extracts, ranging from 4.7 to 1085 U/ml for Bla g 1 and only two with detectable Bla g 2 (248 and 324 U/ml) (9). These immunochemical measurements represent only a relative concentration of allergen in dust particles (2–20 μm in size), and measuring the concentration of a specific allergen in dust samples is not a direct measurement of allergen entering the lungs. An animal model developed by Kang et al. (81) shows that simple aerosolized cockroach contamination in chambers makes guinea pigs cockroach sensitive and asthmatic. In the guinea pig model, cockroach allergen did not appear to enhance other allergen sensitizations.

B. Immunotherapy

Allergen immunotherapy is an effective therapeutic modality for patients with insect sting hypersensitivity. Knowledge of the underlying mechanisms of effective immunotherapy is hampered by a lack of detailed understanding of the basic principles of immunological nonresponsiveness. Activation of CD4+ T-cells requires cross-linking of specific T-cell antigen receptors by peptide fragments attaching to the combining sites on MHC-II class molecules exposed on the surface of antigen-presenting cells. The ability to disrupt these interactions offers the opportunity to modulate the allergic immune response. Two approaches are currently under investigation: (1) presentation of specific antigen in the absence of costimulatory signals that inhibit function of T-cells and (2) administration of nonstimulating peptides that can compete with and prevent binding of dominant T-cell epitopes to MHC-II class molecules.

Because allergen immunotherapy can regulate the specific IgE response and the cellular response to allergens, treatment of cockroach-sensitive individuals with immunotherapy can now be studied. As with any other allergy therapy, cockroach allergy therapy should consist of three possible treatment methods: (1) environmental control (avoidance), (2) pharmacotherapy, and (3) immunotherapy with the appropriate allergens. The predominant hypothesis is that specific allergen immunotherapy will alter the balance of cytokines released from T lymphocytes in the respiratory tract with a shift toward interferon-gamma–producing cells (TH1) and a reduction in the TH2 pattern of cytokines (IL-4 and IL-5) associated with immediate-type allergic inflammation. Whether or not this can be accomplished by a single purified allergen or a combination of allergens is still a matter of intense investigation. In the meantime, drug therapy combined with allergen avoidance remains the recommended approach to asthma management overall.

In a single study, allergen immunotherapy using cockroach vaccines in sensitive individuals was shown to decrease symptom scores and medication requirements, to increase specific IgG levels, and to decrease basophil histamine release in response to cockroach antigen (82). The use of recombinant cockroach allergens that retain IgE-recognizable epitopes has been envisioned to provide the basis for improving therapy for persons suffering cockroach hypersensitivity. Benefits include better control of batch-to-batch variability and the assurance of representation of minor allergens in standard amounts. Additionally, immunotherapy with specific hypoallergenic recombinant allergens or peptides lacking IgE-binding epitopes rather than crude allergen vaccine mixtures could prove to be a more effective regimen to avoid anaphylactic reactions. Specific immunotherapy with recombinant cockroach allergens, unlike with cat and mite allergens, has yet to be performed.

XI. ENVIRONMENTAL CONTROL

Advances in integrated pest management include preventing or minimizing populations within structures. Manipulations of microclimates in discrete areas of new homes can and does reduce infestation. Methods include incorporation of nontoxic repellents in the structures to deny access to specific areas such as beneath sinks in kitchens and bathrooms. As in any management scheme, recognition of the risks, environmental control, and reduction in allergen level are the main objectives for asthma-related illness management. The development of new means of quantitating allergens will enable evaluation of the effect of reduction in allergen exposure. Monitoring allergen levels in individuals' homes should improve their understanding of the role of allergens in asthma and improve compliance with future avoidance measures.

For most inhalant allergens, the actual amount of allergen inhaled in natural exposures is low, but the inhaled particles, <10 μm, are very concentrated in terms of specific allergen content. Thus, for environmental control, it is mandatory not only to remove cockroaches but to remove dust-containing particles carrying the allergen. Control measures that can be taken should include removal of food and water sources from the natural habitat areas. Increased airflow, maintenance of dryness, and removal of any potential food sources will facilitate environmental control in kitchen cabinets, under sinks, and on kitchen floors where high concentrations of cockroach allergen are found.

Although these recommendations are sound for some dwellings, heavily infested homes and buildings that contain multiple apartments will be more difficult. Reinfestation from neighboring apartments, failure to get management to provide proper eradication and prevention measures, and poor construction and sanitation are obstacles that may be difficult to control. A significant problem is in determining the allergen levels; assays currently being used must be standardized to define the relationship between different cockroach species and other cross-reacting allergen sources.

Cockroaches have been controlled using a variety of chemicals, including organophosphates, carbamates, and botanicals such as pyrethrins and pyrethroids, which disrupt the insect's nervous system, causing locomotion and respiratory failure. Other materials, including wettable powders, emulsified concentrates, aerosols, and baits, have been added to the pesticide management of these pests. Ingestion of boric acid leads to damage of the epithelial cells in the gut, precluding nutrient absorption and causing subsequent starvation. Newer formulations containing active ingredients that interfere with metabolic activity and growth regulation are being used as baits for foraging cockroaches. Although currently available pesticides (abamectin, hydramethylon) can reduce populations by 93% to 100%, cockroach allergen in feces, cast skins, and body parts remain as accumulated dust. Sarpong et al. (83), using several rooms in a college dormitory as a model for home extermination studies, showed that Bla g 2 allergen levels of dust of 5.2 U/g could be reduced to 0.95 U/g following an extermination regimen and regular vacuuming. However, sustained removal of cockroach allergens is difficult to achieve, and the levels remain above those reported to be clinically significant (reviewed in 78). Pesticide treatment should be rotated to reduce the risk of resistant strains, and careful cleaning and maintenance are essential to remove and/or reduce the allergen load.

The current recommendations for cockroach control include both physical and chemical measures. Table 4 identifies several cockroach control techniques. An integrated pest management strategy consisting of sanitation, landscape management, and a perimeter insecticide treatment applied according to label directions is the best control measure possible. Although extensive measures are available to control cockroach populations, neither the effectiveness of control procedures for reducing allergen levels nor the extent of cockroach allergen stability and allergen persistence in the environment following cockroach eradication measures is known.

XII. SALIENT POINTS

1. Sensitization to indoor inhalant allergens is strongly associated with the development of asthma. In urban and inner-city areas, 40–60% of patients with asthma have IgE antibody to cockroach allergens.
2. Infestations of domiciliary cockroaches are largely dependent on housing conditions, and hypersensitivity is dependent on exposure. The average American spends approximately 95% of the time indoors in controlled environments, which leads to continued low-dose allergen exposure.
3. Amorphous cockroach particles containing allergens are recognized as a significant source of indoor allergens second only to the dust mite.
4. Cross-reactivity of arthropod allergens can be identified among members of the taxonomic groups Crustacea, Arachnida, and Insecta, which has been described as "pan-allergy."

Table 4 Cockroach Control Measures

I. Physical measures
  A. Reduce access to food
    1. Store food in sealed containers
    2. Eliminate sources of organic debris
  B. Reduce access to water
    1. Repair leaking faucets
    2. Wrap pipes to prevent condensation
    3. Eliminate damp areas beneath sinks
    4. Repair damp, damaged wood
  C. Improve ventilation by eliminating clutter beneath sinks
  D. Eliminate hiding places and access points
    1. Caulk and seal cracks and crevices in foundations
    2. Caulk around water pipe entry into house and beneath sinks
    3. Eliminate clutter within household (e.g., remove all newspaper and magazine storage areas)
II. Chemical measures
    1. Pyrethrum or pyrethroids
    2. Boric acid powders and baits
    3. Orange Guard (d-limonene)
    4. Maxforce Roach Bait Station (Fipronil)
    5. RoachFree TMSystem (food source and boric acid)
    6. Hydramethylnon (Combat)
    7. Abamectin (Roach Ender)
    8. Others: Sulfuramid, xanthine, oxypyrinol)

The composition of environmental dust can include every component of the biosystem and, given the widespread distribution of insects, their involvement in allergic reactions will more than likely continue to be of major social, economic, and medical importance.

5. The cloning of several cockroach and other insect allergens has been accomplished using molecular biology techniques. These studies offer the basis for investigating the relationship between allergen function/structure and allergenicity.

6. Recombinant cockroach allergens that retain IgE binding may provide new tools for improving the diagnosis and/or therapy for individuals suffering cockroach hypersensitivity.

7. Environmental control of cockroach infestations is essential to control cockroach allergen–induced allergic diseases.

8. Future directions for research should include cockroach reduction strategies, development of specific assays to detect clinically relevant allergens, and measures to reduce exposure to environmental allergens that include patient education for pest management and the safe use of insecticides and nontoxic traps.

ACKNOWLEDGMENTS

Research described in this chapter was supported in part by the National Institute of Health Grants AI 32557 and AI 34607, and by Philip Morris U.S.A., Inc.

REFERENCES

1. Atkinson TH, Koehler PG, Paterson RS. Catalog and atlas of the cockroaches (*Dictyoptera*) of North America and Mexico. Misc Pub Entomol Soc Am 1991; 78:1–86.

2. Koehler PG, Patterson RS, Brenner RJ. Cockroaches. In: Handbook of Pest Control, 7th ed. The Behavior, Life, History and Control of Household Pests (K. Storey, ed.) Cleveland: Franzak & Foster, 1995: 100–175.

3. Bernton H, Brown H. Insect allergy: Preliminary studies of the cockroach. J Allergy 1964; 35:506–513.

4. Kang B, Sulit N. A comparative study of prevalence of skin hypersensitivity to cockroach and house dust antigens. Ann Allergy 1978; 41:333–336.

5. Rosenstreich DL, Eggleston P, Kattan M, Baker D, Slavin RG, Gergen P, Mitchell H, McNiff-Mortimer K, Lynn H, Ownby D, Malveaux F. The role of cockroach allergy and exposure to cockroach allergen in causing morbidity among inner-city children with asthma. N Engl J Med 1997; 336(19):1356–1363.

6. Koehler PG, Patterson RS, Brenner RJ. German cockroach (Orthoptera: Blattellidae) infestations in low-income apartments. J Econ Entomol 1987; 80:446–450.

7. Kang B, Jones J, Johnson J, Kang U. Analysis of indoor environment and atopic allergy in urban populations. Ann Allergy 1989; 62:30–34.

8. Gelber LE, Seltzer LH, Bouzoukis JK, Pollart SM, Chapman MD, Platts-Mills TAE. Sensitization and exposure to indoor allergens as risk factors for asthma among patients presenting to hospital. Am Rev Respir Dis 1993; 147:573–578.

9. Pollart SM, Mullins DE, Vailes LD, Hayden ML, Platts-Mills TAE, Sutherland WM, Chapman MD. Identification, quantification, and purification of cockroach allergens using monoclonal antibodies. J Allergy Clin Immunol 1991; 87:511–521.

10. Bernton HS, Brown J. Cockroach allergy: The relation of infestation to sensitization. South Med J 1967; 60:852–855.

11. Twarog FJ, Picone FJ, Strunk RS, So J, Colten HR. Immediate hypersensitivity to cockroach: Isolation and purification of the major antigens. J Allergy Clin Immunol 1977; 59:154–160.

12. Barnes KC, Brenner RJ. Quality of housing and allergy to cockroaches in the Dominican Republic. Int Arch Allergy Immunol 1996; 109:68–72.

13. Arruda LK, Vailes LD, Ferriani VP, Santos AB, Pomés A, Chapman MD. Cockroach allergens and asthma. J Allergy Clin Immunol. 2001; 107(3):419–428.

14. Helm RM, Burks AW, Williams LW, Milne DE, Brenner RI. Identification of cockroach aeroallergens from living cultures of German or American cockroaches. Int Arch Allergy Immunol 1993; 101:359–363.

15. Richman P, Kan HA, Turkeltaub PC, Malveaux Fl, Baer H. The important sources of German cockroach allergens as determined by RAST analysis. J Allergy Clin Immunol 1984; 73:590–595.

16. Musmand JJ, Horner WE, Lopez M, Lehrer SB. Identification of important allergens in German cockroach extracts by sodium dodecyl sulfate-polyacrylamide gel electrophoresis and Western blot analysis. J Allergy Clin Immunol 1995; 95:877–885.

17. Helm RM, Bandele EO, Swanson MC, Campbell AR, Wynn SR. Identification of a German cockroach-specific allergen by human IgE and rabbit IgG. Int Arch Allergy Appl Immunol 1988; 87:230–238.

18. Lan JL, Lee DT, Wu CH, Chang CP, Yeh CL. Cockroach hypersensitivity: Preliminary study of allergic cockroach asthma in Taiwan. J Allergy Clin Immunol 1988; 82:736–740.

19. Wu CH, Lan JL. Cockroach hypersensitivity: Isolation and partial characterization of major allergens. J Allergy Clin Immunol 1988; 82:727–735.

20. Jeng KCG, Liu MT, Wu CH, Wong DW, Lan JL. American cockroach CR-PI allergen induces lymphocyte proliferation and cytokine production in atopic patients. Clin Exp Allergy 1996; 26:349–356.

21. Wu CH, Chiang BT, Fann MC, Lan JL. Production and characterization of monoclonal antibodies against major allergen of American cockroach. Clin Exp Allergy 1990; 20:675–681.

22. Zwick H, Popp W, Sertl K, Rauscher H, Wanke T. Allergenic structures in cockroach hypersensitivity. J Allergy Clin Immunol 1991; 87:626–630.

23. Pollart SM, Smith TF, Morris EC, Gelber LE, Platts-Mills TA, Chapman MD. Environmental exposure to cockroach allergens: Analysis with monoclonal antibody–based enzyme immunoassays. J Allergy Clin Immunol 1991; 87(2):505–510.

24. Chapman MD. Monoclonal antibodies as structural probes for mite, cat, and cockroach. Adv Biosci 1989; 74:281–295.

25. Schou C, Fernández-Caldas E, Lockey RF, Lowenstein H. Environmental assay for cockroach allergens. J Allergy Clin Immunol 1991; 87:828–834.

26. Wu CH, Hsieh MJ, Huang JH, Luo SF. Identification of low molecular weight allergens of American cockroach and production of monoclonal antibodies. Ann Allergy Asthma Immunol 1996; 76:195–203.

27. Patterson ML, Slater JE. Characterization and comparison of commercially available German and American cockroach allergen extracts. Clin Exp Allergy 2002; 32:721–727.

28. Trudeau WL, Fernández-Caldas E, Fox RW, Brenner R, Bucholtz GA, Lockey RF. Allergenicity of the cat flea (*Ctenocephalides felis*). Clin Exp Allergy 1993; 23:347–349.

29. Barletta B, Puggioni EMR, Afferni C, Butteroni C, Iacovacci P, Tinghino R, Ariano R, Panzani RC, DiFelice G, Pini C. Preparation and characterization of silverfish (*Lepisma saccharina*) extract and identification of allergenic components. Int Arch Allergy Immunol 2002; 128:179–186.

30. Kim YK, Chang YS, Lee SC, Bae JM, Jee YK, Chun BR, Cho SH, Min KU, Kim YY. Role of environmental exposure to spider mites in the sensitization and the clinical manifestation of asthma and rhinitis in children and adolescents living in rural and urban areas. Clin Exp Allergy 2002; 32:1305–1309.

31. Moneo I, Vega JM, Caballero ML, Vega J, Alday E. Isolation and characterization of Tha p 1, a major allergen from the pine processionary caterpillar *Thaumetopoea pityocampa*. Allergy 2003; 58:34–37.

32. Helm RM, Squillace DL, Jones RT, Brenner RI. Shared allergenic activity in Asian (*Blattella asahinai*), German (*Blattella germanica*), American (*Periplaneta americana*), and Oriental (*Blatta orientalis*) cockroach species. Int Arch Allergy Appl Immunol 1990; 92:154–161.

33. Shou C, Lind P, Fernández-Caldas E, Lowenstein H. Identification and purification of an important cross-reactive allergen from American (*Periplaneta americana*) and German (*Blattella germanica*) cockroach. J Allergy Clin Immunol 1990; 86:935–946.

34. Stankus RP, Homer WE, Lehrer SB. Identification and characterization of important cockroach allergens. J Allergy Clin Immunol 1990; 86:781–787.

35. Wu C-H, Luo S-F, Wong DW. Analysis of cross-reactive allergens from American and German cockroaches by human IgE. Allergy 1997; 52:411–416.

36. Menon P, Menon V, Hilman B, Stankus R, Lehrer SB. Skin test reactivity to whole body and fecal extracts of American (*Periplaneta americana*) and German (*Blattella germanica*) cockroaches in atopic asthmatics. Ann Allergy 1991; 67:573–577.

37. Chaudhry S, Jhamb S, Chauhan UP, Gaur SN, Agarwal HC, Agarwal MK. Shared and specific allergenic and antigenic components in the two sexes of American cockroach—*Periplaneta americana*. Clin Exp Allergy 1990; 20:59–65.

38. Pomés A, Melén E, Vailes LD, Retief JD, Arruda LK, Chapman MD. Novel allergen structures with tandem amino acid repeats derived from German and American cockroach. J Biol Chem 1998; 273:30801–30807.

39. Pomés A, Vailes LD, Helm R, Chapman MD. IgE reactivity of tandem repeats derived from cockroach allergen, Bla g 1. Eur J Biochem 2002; 269:1–7.

40. Helm R, Cockrell G, Stanley SI, Brenner RI, Burks AW, Bannon GA. Isolation and characterization of a clone encoding a major allergen (Bla g 90K) involved in IgE mediated cockroach hypersensitivity. J Allergy Clin Immunol 1996; 98:172–180.

41. Melén E, Pomés A, Vailes LD, Arruda LK, Chapman MD. Molecular cloning of Per a 1 and definition of the cross-reactive Group 1 cockroach allergens. J Allergy Clin Immunol 1999; 103:859–864.

42. Wu CH, Wang NM, Lee MF, Kao CY, Luo SF. Cloning of the American cockroach Cr-PII allergens: Evidence for the existence of cross-reactive allergens between species. J Allergy Clin Immunol 1998; 101(6 pt 1):832–840.

43. Asturias JA, Gómez-Bayón N, Arilla MC, Martínez A, Palacios R, Sánchez-Gascón F, Martínez J. Molecular characterization of American cockroach tropomyosin (*Periplaneta americana* allergen 7), a cross-reactive allergen. J Immunol 1999; 162(7):4342–4348.

44. Santos ABR, Chapman MD, Aalberse RC, Vailes LD, Ferriani VPL, Oliver C, Rizzo MC, Naspitz CK, Arruda LK. Cockroach allergens and asthma in Brazil: Identification of tropomyosin as a major allergen with potential cross-reactivity with mite and shrimp allergens. J Allergy Clin Immunol 1999; 104:329–337.

45. Ivancuic O, Schein CH, Braun W. Data mining of sequences and 3D structures of allergenic proteins. Bioinformatics 2002; 18:1358–1364.

46. Kang BC, Chang JL, Johnson I. Characterization and partial purification of the cockroach antigen in relation to housedust and housedust (*D.f.*) antigens. Ann Allergy 1989; 63:207–212.

47. Witteman AM, van den Oudenrijn S, van Leeuwen J, Akkerdaas J, van der Zee JS, Aalberse RC. 19B antibodies reactive with silverfish, cockroach and chironomid are frequently found in mite-positive allergic patients. Int Arch Allergy Immunol 1995; 108:165–169.

48. Witteman AM, Akkerdaas JH, Leeuwen J, van der Zee JS, Aalberse RC. Identification of a cross-reactive allergen (presumably tropomyosin) in shrimp, mite and insects. Int Arch Allergy Immunol 1994; 105:56–61.

49. Leung PSC, Chow WK, Duffey S, Kwan HS, Gershwin ME, Chu KH. IgE reactivity against a cross-reactive allergen in crustacea and mollusca: Evidence for tropomyosin as the common allergen. J Allergy Clin Immunol 1996; 98:954–961.

50. Ayuso R, Reese G, Leong-Kee S, Plante M, Lehrer SB. Molecular basis of arthropod cross-reactivity: IgE-binding cross-reactive epitopes of shrimp, house dust mite and cockroach tropomyosins. Int Arch Allergy Immunol 2002; 129(1):38–48.

51. Reese G, Ayuso R, Lehrer SB. Tropomyosin: An invertebrate pan-allergen. Int Arch Allergy Immunol 1999; 119(4):247–258.

52. Crespo IF, Pascual C, Helm R, Sanchez-Pastor S, Ojeda I, Romualdo L, Martin-Esteban M, Ojeda JA. Cross-reactivity of IgE-binding components between boiled Atlantic shrimp and German cockroach. Allergy 1995; 50:918–924.

53. O'Neil CE, Stankus RP, Lehrer SB. Antigenic and allergenic cross-reactivity between cockroach and seafood extracts. Ann Allergy 1985; 55:374.

54. Pomés A, Smith AM, Grégoire C, Vailes LD, Arruda LK, Chapman MD. Functional properties of cloned allergens from dust mite, cockroach and cat—Are they relevant to allergenicity? Allergy Clin Immunol Int, 2001; 13:162–169.

55. Van Ree R, Antonicelli L, Akkerdaas JH, Garritani MS, Aalberse RC, Bonifazi F. Possible induction of food allergy during mite immunotherapy. Allergy 1996; 51(2):108–113.

56. Koshte VL, Kagen SL, Aalberse RC. Cross-reactivity of 19B antibodies to caddis fly with Arthropoda and Mollusca. J Allergy Clin Immunol 1989; 84:174–183.

57. Van Ree R. Carbohydrate epitopes and their relevance for the diagnosis and treatment of allergic diseases. Int Arch Allergy Appl Immunol 2002; 129:189–197.

58. Baldo BA, Panzani RC. Detection of IgE antibodies to a wide range of insect species in subjects with suspected inhalant allergies to insects. Int Arch Allergy Appl Immunol 1988; 85:278–287.

59. Arruda KL, Vailes LD, Mann BI, Shannon J, Fox JW, Vedvick TS, Hayden ML, Chapman MD. Molecular cloning of a major cockroach (*Blattella germanica*) allergen, Bla g 2: Sequence homology to aspartic proteases. J Biol Chem 1995; 270:19563–19568.

60. Pomés A, Chapman MD, Vailes LD, Blundell TL, Dhanaraj V. Cockroach allergen Bla g 2: Structure, function and implications for allergic sensitization. Am J Respir Crit Care Med 2002; 165:391–397.

61. Chapman MD, Smith AM, Vailes LD, Arruda LK, Dhanaraj V, Pomés A. Recombinant allergens for diagnosis and therapy of allergic disease. J Allergy Clin Immunol 2000; 106:409–418.

62. Pomés A. Intrinsic properties of allergens and environmental exposure as determinants of allergenicity. Allergy 2002; 57:673–679.

63. Arruda LK, Vailes LD, Hayden ML, Benjamin DC, Chapman MD. Cloning of cockroach allergen, Bla g 4, identifies ligand-binding proteins (calycins) as a cause of IgE antibody responses. J Biol Chem 1995; 270:31196–31201.

64. Flower DR. The lipocalin protein family: Structure and function. Biochem J 1996; 318:1–14.

65. Krieger I, Raming K, Breer H. Cloning of genomic and complementary DNA encoding insect pheromone binding proteins: Evidence for microdiversity. Biochem Biophys 1991; 1088:277–284.

66. Arruda LK, Vailes LD, Platts-Mills TA, Hayden ML, Chapman MD. Induction of IgE antibody responses by glutathione S-transferase from the German cockroach (*Blattella germanica*). J Biol Chem 1997; 272(33):20907–20912.

67. Arruda LK, Vailes LD, Benjamin DC, Chapman MD. Molecular cloning of German cockroach (*Blattella germanica*) allergens. Int Arch Allergy Immunol 1995; 107:295–297.

68. Smillie LB. Structure and functions of tropomyosins from muscle and non-muscle sources. Trends Biochem Sci 1979; 4:151–155.

69. Sodek J, Hodges RS, Smillie LB, Jurasek L. Amino-acid sequence of rabbit skeletal tropomyosin and its coiled-coil structure. Proc Natl Acad Sci USA 1972; 69(12):3800–3804.

70. Daul CB, Slattery M, Reese G, Lehrer SB. Identification of the major brown shrimp (*Penaeus aztecus*) allergen as the muscle protein tropomyosin. Int Arch Allergy Immunol 1994; 105:49–55.

71. Wu CH, Lee MF, Liao SC, Luo SF. Sequencing analysis of cDNA clones encoding the American cockroach Cr-PI allergens: Homology with insect hemolymph proteins. J Biol Chem 1996; 271:17937–17943.

72. Wu CH, Lee MF, Wang NM, Luo SF. Sequencing and immunochemical characterization of the American cockroach Per a 3 (Cr-PI) isoallergenic variants. Mol Immunol 1997; 34:1–8.

73. Iomori T, Natori S. Molecular cloning of cDNA for lipopolysaccharide-binding protein from the hemolymph of American cockroach, *Periplaneta americana*. J Biol Chem 1991; 266:13318–13323.

74. Baur X. Chironomid midge allergy. Arerugi 1992; 41:81–85.

75. Antony AB, Tepper RS, Mohammed KA. Cockroach extract antigen increases bronchial airway epithelial permeability. J Allergy Clin Immunol 2002; 110(4):589–595.

76. Bhat RK, Page K, Tan A, Hershenson MB. German cockroach extract increases bronchial epithelial cell interleukin-8 expression. Clin Exp Allergy 2003; 33(1):35–42.

77. Rullo VE, Rizzo MC, Arruda LK, Sole D, Naspitz CK. Daycare centers and schools as sources of exposure to mites, cockroach, and endotoxin in the city of Sao Paulo, Brazil. J Allergy Clin Immunol 2002; 110(4):582–588.

78. Arruda LK, Ferriani VP, Vailes LD, Pomes A, Chapman MD. Cockroach allergens: Environmental distribution and relationship to disease. Curr Allergy Asthma Rep 2001; 1(5):466–473.

79. Sporik R, Squillace SP, Ingram JM, Rakes G, Honsinger RW, Platts-Mills TA. Mite, cat, and cockroach exposure, allergen sensitization, and asthma in children: A case-control study of three schools. Thorax. 1999; 54(8):675–680.

80. Eggleston PA, Rosenstreich D, Lynn H, Gergen P, Baker D, Kattan M, Mortimer KM, Mitchell H, Ownby D, Slavin R, Malveaux F. Relationship of indoor allergen exposure to skin test sensitivity in inner-city children with asthma. J Allergy Clin Immunol 1998; 102(4 pt 1):563–570.

81. Kang BC, Kambara T, Yun DK, Hoppe IF, Lui Y-L. Development of cockroach allergic guinea pig by simple room air contamination. Int Arch Allergy Immuno 11995; 107:569–575.

82. Kang BC, Johnson J, Morgan C. The role of immunotherapy in cockroach asthma. J Asthma 1988; 25:205–218.

83. Sarpong SB, Wood RA, Eggleston PA. Short-term effects of extermination and cleaning on cockroach allergen Bla g 2 in settled dust. Ann Allergy Asthma Immunol 1996; 76:257–260.

16

Mammalian Allergens

TUOMAS VIRTANEN and RAUNO MÄNTYJÄRVI

University of Kuopio, Kuopio, Finland

I. INTRODUCTION

People come into contact with animals in many different occupations and activities. In the indoor environment, household animals are significant sources of allergens. Cat and dog allergens have been especially recognized as being associated with allergic disorders, including asthma. Exposure to these allergens is perennial and is not limited to immediate contact with the animals. As people in industrialized countries spend some 90% of their time indoors, it is not surprising that sensitization is common.

Progress in allergy research has revealed intriguing aspects of allergy to animals. One of these is that almost all important mammalian respiratory allergens belong to the lipocalin family of proteins, with the exception of Fel d 1 of cat (1). This observation raises the question whether lipocalin allergens have intrinsic properties that would explain the phenomenon (2). It seems clear, however, that the allergenicity of lipocalin allergens cannot be explained by simple physicochemical characteristics. Another important observation, which will probably influence the recommendations on allergen avoidance in the future, is that early-life exposure to pets may actually protect against allergy to them (3,4). It was proposed that this effect may be based on a modified T helper type 2 (TH2) response (3).

II. TAXONOMY OF MAMMALS

The taxonomical classification created by Carl von Linné (1707–1778) sorts mammalian animals in the class of Mammalia into the subphylum Vertebrata of the phylum Chordata. The class of Mammalia comprises 17 orders, each divided consecutively into one or more suborders, superfamilies, and families. Figure 1 shows, in a condensed form, the taxonomical location of the eight mammals emitting allergens identified at the sequence level. The list reflects more the significance of the animals as sources of allergens for man than the quality or amount of allergens they emit. In addition to the animals in Fig. 1, sensitization to other members of Artiodactyla (e.g., reindeer, *Rangifer tarandus* in the family of Cervidae, and pig, *Sus scrofa domestica* in the family of Suidae) has been described. Apparently, several members of the Felidae family, in addition to the house cat, are also possible sources of allergens because hair extracts from these animals ("big cats," e.g., puma, lion, and jaguar) contain allergens similar to and cross-reacting with the house cat allergen Fel d 1. Although mouse, rat, and guinea pig are the only rodents included in the current list of allergens (http://www.allergen.org/List.htm, March 17, 2003), hamsters

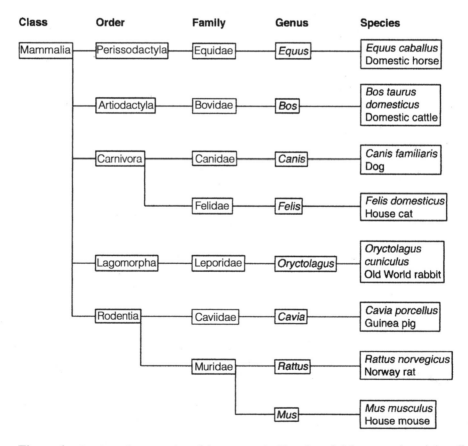

Figure 1   Condensed presentation of the taxonomical location of eight mammals emitting allergens.

(Muridae family) are also known to be significant causes of allergy both in home and in occupational environments.

III. HUMAN CONTACT WITH OTHER MAMMALS

People come into direct contact with mammalian animals in many ways (Fig. 2). Household pets, especially cats and dogs, are found in many (30–50%) homes in industrialized countries. Consequently, high levels of Can f 1 or Fel d 1 occur in the homes of dog or cat owners,

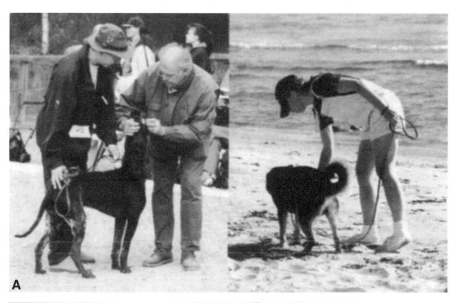

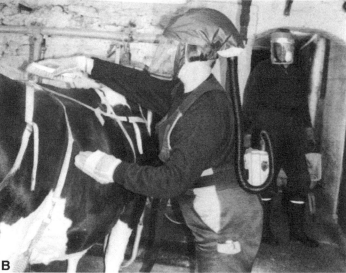

Figure 2   People come into contact with mammalian animals in several ways, in free time (A) and in the working environment (B). A ventilated, motorized helmet allows a person sensitized to cows to continue working with animals.

although variations of several orders of magnitude between houses has been observed. The effects of the exposure depend on a complex array of environmental and genetic factors. One intriguing question concerns the effect of household pets on primary sensitization. Contact with pets in early childhood may have a protective effect, as was indicated by a study quantifying the level of exposure to Fel d 1 in correlation with sensitization (3). The highest level of sensitization was found in children exposed to "intermediate" levels of Fel d 1 (1.7–23.0 μg/g of dust). The finding suggests that the dose-response relationship between exposure to cat and sensitization may be bell-shaped or flattened. A protective effect has also been described for exposure to dog (4). For persons already sensitized, the levels of Fel d 1 and Can f 1 considered significant for causing symptoms are 8–10 μg/g of dust (5). Ten- to 100-fold higher levels are found in homes with dogs or cats. Another interesting observation is the apparent beneficial effect of a farming environment against sensitization (6). Factors other than allergens, e.g., endotoxin, may be responsible for this effect.

Exposure to pet allergens is not limited to direct contact. Dog and cat allergens have a tendency to stick to clothing, and they are consistently found in homes without pets, in public buildings including schools and day care centers, and in public transport vehicles. The concentrations are low but may be high enough to cause sensitization and symptoms in sensitized persons (7).

Mice, hamsters, guinea pigs, and gerbils are also popular household pets, and handling the pets and cleaning their cages exposes children to allergens. The presence of rodent allergens in the home depends not only on the presence of pets but also on the living conditions: Mus m 1 is detectable in mouse-infested apartments. Horse allergy is not a very common health problem in children, but horseback riding as a hobby may cause sensitization and clinical illness.

Several occupations bring people into contact with animals. Sensitization associated with the handling of laboratory animals is a worldwide occupational problem. The exposure occurs through the respiratory tract and conjunctiva and by skin contact. One review of seven studies found that 15.6% of workers in laboratory animal facilities had work-related symptoms and 22.5% were skin-prick-test positive for animal allergens (8). The common laboratory animals (mouse, rat, guinea pig, hamster, rabbit, and dog) are all equally effective as sensitizers (9). The level of exposure varies according to the task concerned. The highest concentrations of airborne allergens are encountered during the emptying and cleaning of the cages. In addition to the personnel, scientists doing animal experiments are exposed to animal allergens at varying frequencies and durations.

An example of work-related allergy caused by domestic animals is the occupational asthma in Finnish dairy farmers. One interesting feature of this is the prolonged exposure time (median 22 years) before cattle asthma becomes clinically evident (10). In contrast, symptoms of laboratory animal allergy appear within 2–3 years of exposure in 70–80% of cases (9).

IV. MOLECULAR CHARACTERISTICS OF MAMMALIAN ALLERGENS

A. Protein Families of Mammalian Allergens

1. Lipocalins

Lipocalins are a large protein group comprising proteins from vertebrate and invertebrate animals, plants, and bacteria (http://www.expasy.org/cgi-bin/nicesite.pl?PS00213). They include mammalian respiratory allergens, milk allergen Bos d 5 (β-lactoglobulin), cockroach

Table 1 Internet Resources Referred to in the Text

Description	Address
GenBank, a genetic sequence database	http://www.ncbi.nlm.nih.gov/Genbank/index.html
Lipocalin family, documentation in the PROSITE protein database	http://www.expasy.org/cgi-bin/nicedoc.pl?PDOC00187
Lipocalins, general information and the list of lipocalins in the PROSITE protein database	http://www.expasy.org/cgi-bin/nicesite.pl?PS00213
List of allergens by Allergen Nomenclature Subcommittee of International Union of Immunological Societies	http://www.allergen.org/List.htm
Protein Data Bank, PDB, a databank for three-dimensional biological macromolecular structure data	http://www.rcsb.org/pdb/
Serum albumin family, documentation in the PROSITE protein database	http://us.expasy.org/cgi-bin/nicedoc.pl?PDOC00186
SWISS-PROT protein database	http://us.expasy.org/sprot/

allergen Bla g 4, and a "kissing bug" (*Triatoma protracta*) allergen. Together with fatty acid–binding proteins, avidins, a group of metalloproteinase inhibitors, and an insect salivary protein called triabin, lipocalins form the calycin superfamily (11). A protein should fulfill the requirements for sequence homology, biological function, and structural similarity to be included in the family (http://www.expasy.org/cgi-bin/nicedoc.pl?PDOC00187) (Table 1).

Although the overall amino acid identity between lipocalins is usually below 20%, they contain one to three characteristic conserved sequence motifs (structurally conserved regions, SCR) (11). The first motif, containing the triplet glysine-x-tryptophane, is present in all lipocalins (Fig. 3). While kernel lipocalins contain all three motifs, outlier lipocalins contain only one or two. In some cases, the sequential identity between animal species can be well above 20%. For example, human tear lipocalin (von Ebner's gland protein) exhibits a 57% identity with dog Can f 1, and human putative major urinary protein (MUP)–like lipocalin a 40–50% identity with rodent MUPs [the SIB BLAST network service (SBNS) at the Swiss Institute of Bioinformatics, Jan. 16, 2003 (12)]. Lipocalins exist as both monomers and dimers, and they can be either glycosylated or nonglycosylated (Table 2).

Despite the low sequential identity, lipocalins share a common three-dimensional structure (Fig. 4) (11). The central β-barrel of lipocalins is composed of eight antiparallel β-strands, and it encloses an internal ligand-binding site (Figs. 3 and 4). At the N-terminus, there is a 3_{10} helix, whereas at the C-terminus, there is an α-helix. The three-dimensional structures of several lipocalin allergens have been resolved (Table 2).

Lipocalins are typically small, extracellular proteins with the capacity (a) to bind small, principally hydrophobic molecules, (b) to attach to specific cell-surface receptors, and (c) to form covalent and noncovalent complexes with soluble macromolecules (11). Most of the mammalian lipocalins are produced in the liver or secretory glands. Although they were originally characterized as transport proteins for diverse molecules, such as odorants, steroids, and pheromones, they have been shown to be involved in a wide range of other biological functions.

Some lipocalins show immunomodulatory activity. One such protein, glycodelin (placental protein 14) has been observed to exert its anti-inflammatory activity by elevating

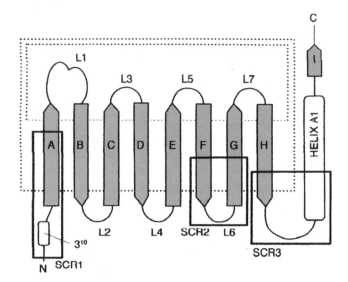

Figure 3 Schematic structure of the lipocalin fold. The nine β-strands of the antiparallel β-sheet are shown as arrows and labeled from A to I (shaded). The C-terminal α-helix A1 and N-terminal 3_{10}-like helix are also marked. Connecting loops are shown as solid lines and labeled L1–L7. A pair of dotted lines indicates the hydrogen-bonded connection of two strands. One end of the lipocalin β-barrel has four loops (L1, L3, L5, and L7); the opening of the internal ligand-binding site is here, and so it is called the Open end of the molecule. The other end has three β-hairpin loops (L2, L4, and L6); the N-terminal polypeptide chain crosses this end of the barrel to enter strand A via a conserved 3_{10} helix closing this end of the barrel (the Closed end of the molecule). Those parts that form the three main structurally conserved and sequence-conserved regions (SCRs) of the fold (SCR1, SCR2, and SCR3) are marked as heavy boxes. SCR3 corresponds closely to the sequence-conserved region rather than the structurally conserved region. (Reprinted from Ref. 11 with permission from Elsevier Science.)

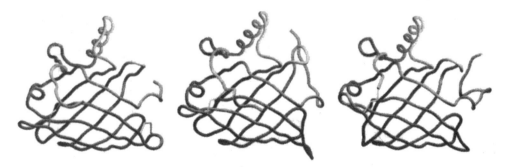

Figure 4 Similarity of the three-dimensional molecular structures of lipocalins shown by the ribbon models of lipocalin allergens, bovine Bos d 2, horse Equ c 1, and mouse Mus m 1. (Courtesy of Juha Rouvinen, Department of Chemistry, University of Joensuu, Joensuu, Finland.)

the T-cell activation threshold and, possibly, in this way favoring the TH2 deviation of immune response (13). Some lipocalins can also be enzymes, such as glutathione-independent prostaglandin D_2 synthase. Two other lipocalins, β-lactoglobulin (Bos d 5) and tear lipocalin, have been reported to have nonspecific endonuclease activity (14). The glutamic acid at position 128 in tear lipocalin, important for the activity, is present in

Table 2 Physicochemical Characteristics of Mammalian Lipocalin Allergens Causing Respiratory Sensitization[a]

Allergen	Animal	MM[b], kDa	Amino acids	Isoelectric point	Glycosylation	Oligomeric state	SWISS-PROT accession #[c]	Structure, PDB ID code[d]	Key reference
Bos d 2	Cow	20	156	4.2	No	M	Q28133	1BJ7	(42)
Can f 1	Dog	22–25	156	5.2	Putative		O18873		(34)
Can f 2	Dog	22–27	162	4.9	Putative		O18874		(34)
Cav p 1[e]	Guinea pig	20					P83507		(54)
Equ c 1	Horse	22	172	3.9	Yes	D	Q95182	1EW3	(38)
Equ c 2[e]	Horse	16		3.4–3.5	No		P81216 P81217		(40)
Mus m 1	Mouse	18–21	162	4.6–5.3	No	M	P02762	1MUP	(49)
Ory c 1[e,f]	Rabbit	17–18			Yes				(56)
Ory c 2[e,f]	Rabbit	21							(56)
Rat n 1	Rat	17–21	162	4.2–5.5	Yes	M	P02761	2A2U	(49)

[a] Practically all mammalian respiratory allergens belong to the lipocalin family of proteins.
[b] Molecular mass
[c] SWISS-PROT database, http://us.expasy.org/sprot/
[d] Protein Data Bank, http://www.rcsb.org/pdb/
[e] Only N-terminus known
[f] Tentatively named

several lipocalin allergens, such as Bos d 2, Mus m 1, Rat n 1, Equ c 1, and Can f 1. Interestingly, the amino acid is situated at or adjacent to the immunodominant T-cell epitope in Bos d 2 (15). Can f 1 has also been proposed to act as a cysteine proteinase inhibitor because of its sequential homology with tear lipocalin. Whether this is the case is not known, but the motifs crucial for the function are only partially conserved in Can f 1. Lipocalins also participate in the regulation of cell growth and proliferation.

As it is basically unknown why TH2 responses arise against inert inhaled antigens, the allergenicity of lipocalins also remains a mystery. One property associated with the allergenicity of a protein is that it is effectively dispersed in the environment. Lipocalin allergens appear to fulfill this requirement since they are found in animal dander and excretions. However, the crucial element in the sensitization to a protein is its recognition by the immune system. In this respect, allergens seem to differ from infectious agents, since the latter contain conserved pathogen-associated molecular patterns, the recognition of which favors the TH1 deviation of immune response.

We have observed an unexpected characteristic of the bovine lipocalin allergen Bos d 2. The peripheral blood mononuclear cells (PBMC) from highly allergic cow dust–asthmatic patients with positive skin prick test reactions to Bos d 2 proliferated very weakly upon stimulation with the allergen; the stimulation indices were mainly below two (15). In parallel with this finding, Bos d 2 was observed to be a weak immunogen for several inbred mouse strains (16). A weak stimulatory capacity is also a characteristic of another animal-derived (nonlipocalin) allergen, cat Fel d 1 (17,18).

It has been observed in studies with peptide analogues (altered peptide ligands) that the outcome of T-cell response is influenced by the extent of T-cell receptor (TCR) ligation: Weak stimulation favored TH2-type responses, whereas stronger stimulation favored TH1-type responses (19). As lipocalins can exhibit considerable amino acid identity between species, it is possible that high-avidity lipocalin allergen-reactive T-cells have been deleted during thymic maturation (1,2), as is the case with high-avidity self-reactive T-cells. The remaining T-cell population with low-avidity TCRs might recognize exogenous lipocalin allergens in a suboptimal way. Further studies are needed to assess whether T-cell recognition plays a role in the allergenicity of lipocalins (2).

2. Other

Albumins constitute another protein family containing mammalian respiratory allergens (http://us.expasy.org/cgi-bin/nicedoc.pl?PDOCØØ186). Albumin is produced in the liver, and it is a major constituent of plasma. It is involved in transporting various molecules and in maintaining the colloidal osmotic pressure of blood. The molecular mass of albumins is around 67 kDa (20). Albumins show about 80% amino acid identity between mammals (20). For cross-reactivity between albumins, see below.

B. Allergenic Proteins from Mammals

1. Cat

Fel d 1. Cat dander contains several IgE-binding components, the most important being Fel d 1 [accession numbers P30438, P30439, and P30440 at the SWISS-PROT protein database (http://us.expasy.org/sprot/)]. Fel d 1, formerly cat-1, is a potent allergen sensitizing over 90% of cat-allergic persons (21). It is also responsible for 80–90% of the IgE-binding capacity of cat allergen extracts (21). The removal of Fel d 1 from a dander extract decreases the histamine-releasing capacity of the preparation 200- to 300-fold

Fel d 1 is a glycoprotein with a molecular mass of 35–39 kDa (22). It is a tetramer composed of two noncovalently linked heterodimers with molecular masses of about 18 kDa. These dimers comprise a 4-kDa chain 1 (α-chain) and 14-kDa chain 2 (β-chain), which are linked together covalently by a disulfide bond. The primary structures of the Fel d 1 chains are known (23,24): Chain 1 contains 70 and chain 2 90–92 amino acids. Chain 1 exhibits about 25% amino acid identity with rabbit and human uteroglobin (Clara cell protein), but considerably higher identities (up to 50%) can be observed with other proteins, mostly rodent androgen-binding proteins (SBNS, Jan. 30, 2003). Chain 1 is classified as a member of the uteroglobin family. Chain 2 shows various degrees of amino acid identity with several proteins, up to 39% with a human protein in a segment of 40 amino acids (SBNS, Jan. 30, 2003), but it is not known to belong to any protein family. Fel d 1 can be produced in a recombinant form, the chains combined and refolded (21). The three-dimensional structure of Fel d 1 has recently been resolved.

Genes encoding Fel d 1 chains are expressed in the salivary glands and in the skin (24). Fel d 1 is found in hair roots and sebaceous glands, in dander and saliva, and in high concentrations in anal glands. The biological function of Fel d 1 is unknown, but it may be related to the protection of epithelia (23). Fel d 1 has been proposed to have enzymatic activity (25).

Most of the IgE-binding epitopes on Fel d 1 are conformational, and glycosylation present in chain 2 does not play a major role in IgE binding (22). Analyses with overlapping synthetic peptides suggested that IgE-binding epitopes are localized at residues 25–38 and 46–59 in chain 1 and at residues 15–28 in chain 2 (26). Among the sera tested, the highest percentage of positive reactions (46%) was against peptide 25–38.

The proliferative response of cat-allergic subjects' PBMC induced by Fel d 1 is in general not strong (17,18). In contrast, Fel d 1–specific T-cell clones and lines have been reported to proliferate vigorously upon stimulation with Fel d 1 (27,28). In two studies, T-cell response against Fel d 1 exhibited no correlation with human leukocyte antigen (HLA) phenotypes (17,27), while a third study found a possible excess of HLA-DR1 (odds ratio=2, p=0.002) among subjects with Fel d 1–specific IgE (29). In another study, no association was found between specific IgE and the alleles of the loci examined (including HLA-DRB1) (30). Human T-cell epitopes were detected in several regions of Fel d 1, but T-cell reactivity was more pronounced against chain 1 than against chain 2 of the molecule (17,28). In chain 1, most of the reactivity concentrated in the N-terminal half of the molecule, in amino acids 18–42, while in chain 2 the most reactive region was the C-terminus, amino acids 74–92. Two peptides, Fel-1 (IPC-1) and Fel-2 (IPC-2), amino acids 7–33 and 29–55 of chain 1, respectively, were shown to stimulate T-cells but to bind IgE only at low levels, which suggested that they could be suitable for peptide-based allergen immunotherapy (17). Ninety-eight percent of Fel d 1–specific T-cell lines were responsive to one or both of these peptides (17). The pattern of T-cell epitope recognition did not distinguish subjects allergic to Fel d 1 from the nonallergic, although the recognition was not identical between the groups (28).

Fel d 2. Fel d 2, cat serum albumin (P49064 at SWISS-PROT), is a minor allergen with IgE reactivity in about 20% of cat-allergic individuals (21). Its role in cat allergy is unclear, in that dominant IgE response against it was found in only 2% of cat-allergic individuals (21). Moreover, the significance of cat albumin as a primary sensitizer is difficult to assess (21), since albumins exhibit cross-reactivity across animal species (31). In accordance with IgE determinations, polyclonal T-cell lines raised with cat dander extract proliferated only weakly upon stimulation with cat albumin, whereas the response was strong against Fel d 1 (27).

Fel d 3.   Fel d 3, cystatin (Q8WNR9 at SWISS-PROT), was cloned from cat skin (32). The prevalence of IgE reactivity among cat-allergic subjects was about 10% when it was measured using *E. coli*–produced recombinant protein in a solid-phase ELISA (32).

Fel d 3 is an 11-kDa protein containing 98 amino acids. There is one potential N-linked glycosylation site in the sequence. Fel d 3 exhibits nearly 80% amino acid identity with bovine and human cystatin A. As endogenous protease inhibitors, cystatins control the function of cysteine proteases. Fel d 3 contains the signature motif conserved in cysteine protease inhibitors. Dog allergens Can f 1 and Can f 2, which are lipocalins, exhibit some degree of conservation with the sequence motif.

2. Dog

Can f 1.   The major allergen of dog, Can f 1, formerly called Ag 8, Ag 13, or Ag X, sensitizes over 70% of dog-allergic subjects (33,34). It accounted for about 50% of the IgE-binding capacity of dog hair and dander extract (33) and for 60–70% of the IgE-binding capacity of dog saliva preparation (35). Can f 1 belongs to the lipocalin family of proteins (34). Its physicochemical characteristics are shown in Table 2.

Can f 1 is mainly found in dog saliva, but it is also present in dog dander (35). It is absent or in a very low concentration in serum, urine, and feces. The allergen could be detected in the hair extracts of nine dog breeds, with variable amounts between individual dogs within a breed (35). Can f 1 has been cloned from the parotid gland and has been produced in a recombinant form (34). It is homologous to von Ebner's gland proteins (see above, Lipocalins). Can f 1 mRNA is expressed in tongue epithelial tissue but not in skin or liver.

Except for its IgE-binding capacity, the immunological characteristics of Can f 1 are poorly known. In two studies, no association between the Can f 1–specific IgE response and the HLA class II genotype was observed (29,30).

Can f 2.   Can f 2, formerly called dog allergen 2 or Dog 2, is a minor allergen sensitizing 25% of dog-allergic subjects (34). Dog-allergic subjects' average IgE response against Can f 2 was estimated to be 23% of that against dog dander extract (35). Can f 2 also belongs to the lipocalin family of proteins (34).

Can f 2 is found in dog dander and in saliva, whereas urine or feces contain very little of the allergen (35). The amount of Can f 2 in the hair extracts of nine dog breeds varied widely. It has been cloned from the parotid gland and produced as a recombinant protein (34). Can f 2 exhibits the highest level of amino acid identity, 36%, with trichosurin, a milk-derived lipocalin from the brush-tailed possum (SBNS, Jan. 30, 2003). Identities at the level of 30% are observed with rodent urinary proteins (34). Can f 2 mRNA is predominantly expressed in the parotid gland and to a lesser extent in tongue tissue (34). It is not found in skin or liver. The immunological properties of Can f 2 have not been studied in detail.

Can f 3.   Thirty-five percent of dog-allergic patients have IgE against Can f 3, the dog serum albumin (36), although both lower and higher figures have also been reported. In individual patients, a major part of dog-specific IgE is directed to Can f 3 (36). Dog albumin (P49822 at SWISS-PROT) has been cloned from dog liver and produced as a recombinant protein (20).

Other Dog Allergens.   Dog can be a source of up to 20 allergens. An analysis of hair and dander extract by electrophoresis and immunoblotting yielded a total of 11 allergens in the molecular mass range of 14–68 kDa. One of these was an immunoglobulin.

3. Horse

Equ c 1. IgE against Equ c 1, probably the formerly named Ag 6, was found in 76% of horse-allergic subjects' sera (37). According to one study, Ag 6 accounts for 55% of skin-prick-test reactivity to horse hair and dandruff extract. The physicochemical characteristics of Equ c 1, a lipocalin allergen (38), are shown in Table 2.

In addition to horse dander (37), Equ c 1 is found in a high concentration in saliva, while urine contains little of the allergen. Equ c 1 mRNA expression is about 100-fold higher in sublingual salivary glands than in submaxillary salivary glands or liver (38). The allergen has been cloned from sublingual salivary glands and produced in a recombinant form (38). Equ c 1 exhibits about 50% amino acid identity with rodent major urinary proteins (38) and a 37% identity with a human putative MUP-like lipocalin (SBNS, Jan. 16, 2003). There are several isoforms of the allergen. Equ c 1, unlike some other allergens, such as Equ c 2, was observed to have a surfactant-like property (39).

An analysis of the IgE-binding epitopes of Equ c 1 suggested that the dominant epitopes are localized in a restricted region of the molecule. Carbohydrates did not have a major impact on IgE binding (39).

Equ c 2. The N-terminal sequences of two horse dander allergens with slightly different isoelectric points (pI) were identical, and the allergens were named Equ c 2.0101 and Equ c 2.0102 (40). A 29-amino-acid fragment exhibited a 44% identity with bovine Bos d 2 and also contained the highly conserved GXW motif of lipocalins. Analyses of the amino acid compositions of the allergens also suggest that they are lipocalins. Up to 50% of horse-allergic patients have IgE against Equ c 2 (40).

Equ c 3. As with albumins from other mammals, the significance of horse serum albumin (P35747 at SWISS-PROT) as an allergen is not clear. The prevalence of IgE reactivity against it has been reported to be between 20% (41) and 50%.

Other Horse Allergens. Horse dander contains more than ten IgE-binding proteins (40). Equ c 4 and Equ c 5 have been partially characterized (39). Like Equ c 1, these allergens have surfactant-like properties. Equ c 4 (P82615 at SWISS-PROT) is a 19-kDa glycoprotein with a pI of 3.8 (39). Its partial sequence shows a 100% identity with horse latherin, a surfactant protein (Q8SPI9 at SWISS-PROT). About 30% of horse-allergic individuals have IgE against Equ c 4. Equ c 5 (P82616 at SWISS-PROT), a 17-kDa protein with a pI of 5.3, is not glycosylated (39). Its fragments show considerable homology with Equ c 4 and latherin (SBNS, Feb. 7, 2003). In one study, 77% of horse-allergic patients had IgE against this allergen (39).

The nomenclature of the horse allergens described here has been ambiguous to some extent but has now been clarified (39).

4. Cow

Bos d 2. Bos d 2, a lipocalin allergen (42), also known as Ag 3 or BDA20, is the major respiratory allergen in cow dander (Table 2). About 90% of dairy farmers with asthma of bovine origin react to Bos d 2, analyzed by IgE immunoblotting (43) or by bronchial allergen challenge (10). Both Ag 3 (Bos d 2) and Ag 1 account for about 70% of the IgE-binding capacity of cow hair and dander extract. Together they bind about 80% of the IgE.

Bos d 2 is found in cow skin (44), although the same or an immunologically related allergen is present in urine (43). In skin, Bos d 2 is localized in the secretory cells of the apocrine sweat glands and the basement membranes of the epithelium and hair follicles. It is probably a pheromone carrier (44). There are several isoforms of Bos d 2. It has been cloned from cow skin (42) and produced as a recombinant protein (45). Bos d 2 exhibits amino acid identity with odorant-binding proteins and other lipocalins from other species at the level of 30–40% (SBNS, Dec. 19, 2002).

To reduce its IgE-binding capacity, Bos d 2 has been produced in fragments and in mutated forms. IgE binding was found to be highly dependent on an intact three-dimensional structure. The epitopes responsible for IgE binding appear to be localized in the C-terminal part of Bos d 2.

The PBMC response of highly Bos d 2–allergic patients upon stimulation with the allergen was exceptional in that it was very weak (15). Bos d 2 is also a weak immunogen for several mouse strains (16). The human T-cell response is directed to few epitopes on Bos d 2 (15). The total number of epitopes detected was seven and the maximal number an individual's T-cells could recognize was five. One of the epitopes, epitope G, situated at the C-terminal α-helix, was recognized by the T-cells of all the Bos d 2–allergic patients studied. The T-cell response against this epitope was Th2/0-deviated. For BALB/c mice, the same area of Bos d 2 contains the immunodominant epitope (16). It has been proposed (see above) that the poor recognition of Bos d 2 may contribute to its allergenicity (1,2).

Bos d 3.   Bos d 3 (Q28050 at SWISS-PROT), known also as BDA11, is a minor bovine respiratory allergen (46). According to the immunoblotting analysis with recombinant Bos d 3, about 40% of patients with cow dust–induced asthma had IgE against the allergen (46).

Bos d 3 is an 11-kDa protein with a predicted pI of 5.19 (46). This 101-amino-acid-long allergen belongs to the S-100 family of proteins and exhibits a 63% amino acid identity with human psoriasin (P31151 at SWISS-PROT), a calcium-binding keratinocyte protein highly upregulated in psoriatic skin. The calcium-binding motif in psoriasin containing the so-called EF hand is located in the segment which is almost identical to that of Bos d 3. It is possible that Bos d 3 is a bovine homologue of psoriasin. The expression of psoriasin is not limited to psoriasis, and it has been reported to have chemokine-like properties selective for CD4+ T-cells and neutrophils.

Other Bovine Respiratory Allergens.   Using crossed radioimmunoelectrophoresis, serum proteins, including albumin (Bos d 6; P02769 at SWISS-PROT) and IgG (Bos d 7), have been found to be allergens in cow hair and dander. By immunoblotting, up to 10 IgE-binding components were detected in the bovine dander extract and four in the urine preparation in the molecular mass range of 16 kDa to over 100 kDa (43). Two of the allergens with molecular masses of 20 kDa (Bos d 2) and 22 kDa were classified as major allergens (43). An 11-kDa protein showing an almost complete homology with the bovine oligomycin sensitivity-conferral protein of the mitochondrial adenosine triphosphate synthase complex (P13621 at SWISS-PROT) was identified as a minor allergen in cow dander (47).

5. Mouse

Mouse allergens induce allergic symptoms in about 26% of laboratory animal workers (9). In a U.S. study, 18% of inner-city children with asthma had a positive skin prick test result with mouse allergen.

Mus m 1.   Mus m 1, a major allergen, known also as Ag 1, prealbumin, or mouse allergen 1 (MA1) (48), is the mouse major urinary protein MUP6 in the SWISS-PROT data bank (Table 2). It accounts for the major part of the IgE-binding capacity of the crude male urine (48). Mus m 1 belongs to the lipocalin family of proteins (49).

Mus m 1 is found in mouse urine, serum, pelt, and especially in liver (48), where it is mainly produced (49). The production of MUPs is under hormonal control and influenced by androgens (49). Forms of MUPs are also expressed constitutively in the exocrine glands of mice and rats (49). Mus m 1 is found in about fourfold higher concentrations in male than in female urine (48). Mouse MUPs are encoded by about 35 genes, and 15 forms of MUPs can be detected in male urine. Mouse MUP has been produced as a recombinant protein. The amino acid identity between mouse and rat MUPs is about 65% (49). For the amino acid identity between other lipocalins and the biological function, see above, Lipocalins.

Other Mouse Allergens. The other major allergen of mouse, Ag 3, tentatively named Mus m 2, is a glycoprotein (50). It is found in mouse dander and fur. It is localized in the hair follicles, coating the hairs, and on the skin (50). Mouse albumin has also been identified as an allergen.

6. Rat

Rat n 1. About 60% of laboratory animal workers symptomatic to rat are sensitized to rat urinary proteins. Sixty-six percent of laboratory workers with asthma and rhinitis on exposure to rats had IgE against Rat n 1 (51). Rat n 1, also known as rat MUP, prealbumin, or α_{2u}-globulin (α_2-euglobulin), is closely related to the major urinary proteins of mouse (see above, Mus m 1) and belongs to the lipocalin group (49). Adult female rats excrete in urine about one-sixth of the amount of MUPs of male rats. For the amino acid identities between lipocalins and the biological function, see above, Mus m 1 and Lipocalins.

Rat urinary prealbumin and α_{2u}-globulin were considered distinct allergens in the 1980s. Later analyses of these strongly cross-reactive proteins (51) have shown that prealbumin is an isoform of α_{2u}-globulin. Therefore, a more appropriate name for prealbumin is Rat n 1.01, and for α_{2u}-globulin Rat n 1.02 (1). α_{2u}-globulin has been cloned and produced as a recombinant protein. One study suggests that the IgE-binding epitopes of Rat n 1.02 tend to be clustered towards the N- and C-terminal parts of the allergen.

Other Rat Allergens. Male rat urine contains a total of eight allergens in the molecular mass range of 17–75 kDa (52). About 20 allergens have been observed in rat fur and in saliva (53). Rat serum proteins, including albumin, transferrin, and IgG, have been described as allergens.

7. Guinea Pig

Guinea pigs sensitize personnel in laboratory animal facilities, the prevalence of symptoms being about 30% (9). Keeping guinea pigs as pets has been associated with a more than threefold increased risk of atopic eczema, an effect not seen with other pets such as cats, dogs, or hamsters.

Guinea pig allergens have been characterized only partially. Guinea pig dust contains 10 (54) or more IgE-binding components. The allergens are present in guinea pig dander, fur, urine, and saliva (55). Analysis of guinea pig hair extract and urine by immunoblotting showed that the molecular masses of the allergens fall in the range of 8 kDa to 67 kDa (54). The 8-kDa, 17-kDa, and 20-kDa components, present in both sources, proved to be major allergens. The prevalence of guinea pig allergic subjects' IgE reactivity against the 20-kDa allergen in hair extract was 70% compared with 87% in urine. The allergen, named Cav p 1, was purified from the hair extract. Its N-terminal sequence analysis showed that it is a lipocalin with a 57% amino acid identity with the major mouse allergen Mus m 1 (54).

The 17-kDa allergen, named Cav p 2, was included in the list of allergens (http://www.allergen.org/List.htm, March 17, 2003). About 55% of guinea pig–allergic subjects had IgE against this allergen (54). Guinea pig serum albumin was previously considered a major allergen, but in a recent study only 8% of guinea pig–allergic patients exhibited IgE reactivity to the probable serum albumin (54).

8. Rabbit

Rabbits induce allergic symptoms in about 30% of laboratory animal workers (9). Allergy against rabbit develops rapidly, and the prevalence of allergy to rabbit was the highest in comparison with allergy to other animal species among workers sensitized in less than one year of exposure. Rabbits are also kept as pets. In a clinical survey of consecutively recruited asthma patients, 35% of the patients exhibited skin-prick-test reactivity against rabbit. In another study, contact with rabbits was associated with an increased risk of atopic eczema.

Rabbit allergens have been characterized preliminarily. Rabbit urine, fur, and saliva extracts contain a total of 26 allergens with molecular masses from 8 kDa to 80 kDa (56). Saliva, which contained 12 allergens, was the most potent of the extracts according to RAST inhibition experiments (56).

Ag R1, tentatively also referred to as Ory c 1, is a 17–18-kDa glycoprotein found in saliva and to a slightly lesser extent in fur. It is present in dander in small amounts but not in urine. The sequence of the 20 N-terminal amino acids suggests that the allergen is a lipocalin with a 72% homology with rabbit odorant-binding protein-II. The N-terminus of another allergen of 21-kDa molecular mass exhibited an even higher homology with the odorant-binding protein. This protein could be Ag2, found in several source materials and tentatively also referred to as Ory c 2. Rabbit serum albumin has been considered to be of minor importance, although in individual cases sensitization can be strong (56,57).

9. Human Autoallergens

IgE antibodies against human proteins have been found in patients with allergic conditions. These autoantigens are proteins conserved in evolution, and many of them are homologues of recognized exogenous allergens.

In one study, using extracts from a human epithelial cell line, IgE autoantibodies against a variety of human proteins were found in 43% of patients with atopic dermatitis (58). Recombinant forms of several of the autoantigens induced histamine release from basophils and showed a positive skin prick test. IgE antibodies against one of them (Hom s 1) were found to correlate with the severity of atopic dermatitis. However, their role in the pathogenesis of allergic conditions remains unclear.

Hom s 1. Hom s 1 (Y14314 at GenBank; http://www.ncbi.nlm.nih.gov/Genbank/index.html) is one of the five autoallergens listed in the allergen nomenclature. Five out of 65 sera from atopic dermatitis patients had IgE antibodies against Hom s 1 (59). Deduced from the cDNA sequence, it has a molecular mass of 73 kDa. However, a rabbit antiserum against Hom s 1 detected proteins of varied sizes in extracts of human tissues (59). Immunohistochemistry revealed that Hom s 1 is a cytoplasmic protein, although SART-1, a protein with an almost complete sequence identity with Hom s 1, is located in nuclei of normal and malignant cells (60). A secondary structure analysis of the sequence of Hom s 1 suggested a high content of α-helices.

Hom s 2–5. Like Hom s 1, these four autoallergens were found by screening a cDNA library from a human epithelial cell line with IgE antibodies from patients with atopic dermatitis (58). The presence of IgE antibodies was restricted to a few dermatitis patients. All four were identified as intracellular proteins. cDNA of Hom s 2 (Q13765 at SWISS-PROT) encodes a protein of 10 kDa and has sequence identity with a portion of the α-chain of the nascent polypeptide complex. Hom s 3 cDNA (Q13845 at SWISS-PROT) corresponding to a protein of 20 kDa displayed sequence identity with the onco-protein BCL7B. Several expressed sequence tags were found in Hom s 4 (O75785 at SWISS-PROT) encoding a protein of 36 kDa. A calcium-binding domain in Hom s 4 may be related to its (unknown) function. The cDNA clone of Hom s 5 (P02538 at SWISS-PROT) corresponding to a polypeptide of 43 kDa is identical to a portion of cytokeratin type II.

Human Homologues of Exogenous Allergens.   Several fungal allergens are phylogenetically highly conserved, and the corresponding human proteins have been found to react with IgE antibodies from patients with severe fungal allergies. Asp f 6 is a manganese superoxide dismutase (MnSOD) allergen of *A. fumigatus*. Recombinant human MnSOD was found to react with IgE and to stimulate T-cells from patients with chronic *A. fumigatus* allergy (61). Acidic ribosomal phosphoprotein type 2 (P2 protein) is another conserved protein identified as an allergen in several molds including *A. fumigatus* (Asp f 8). Human P2 protein shares a 62% amino acid identity with Asp f 8, and it was recognized by IgE antibodies and T-cells from patients heavily sensitized to *A. fumigatus* (62). Profilins are another group of conserved proteins identified as allergens of several plants, e.g., Bet v 2 of birch. IgE from sera of patients sensitized to plant profilins showed cross-reactivity with human profilin (63).

V. ALLERGENIC CROSS-REACTIVITY AMONG MAMMALS

Patients allergic to nonhuman mammals may have IgE antibodies reacting against a number of albumins from different species (31). Inhibition experiments have shown that albumin-specific IgE is often cross-reactive, although patients exhibit individual variation in this respect (31,41). As pointed out for Fel d 2, the primary sensitizer can be difficult to identify (21). A study with three tryptic peptides from horse serum albumin identified regions involved in IgE cross-reactivity with dog albumin (64). Inhibition of a monoclonal antihuman albumin antibody with cat or dog albumin indicated that cat, dog, and human albumins have similar epitopes (20). In another study with monoclonal antibodies specific to cat or dog albumin, it was observed that the antibodies recognized the albumin of both species (65). The study also suggested that the monoclonal antibodies and human IgE recognized identical or closely related epitopes on cat and dog albumin.

IgE cross-reactivities between mammalian non-serum-derived allergens have also been characterized. In a study in which animal-allergic patients' sera were incubated with cat or dog hair/dander extracts before immunoblotting, IgE binding was substantially reduced against the other extract in more than half of the cases (66). Inhibition was also seen against the components representing the major cat and dog allergens. When the level of reciprocal inhibition was estimated with an immunochemical method using sera with no albumin reactivity, dog extract inhibited almost 90% of IgE binding to cat allergens whereas cat extract inhibited about 60% of IgE binding to dog allergens. In another study, cat and dog hair/dander extracts inhibited IgE binding in RAST to the other extract practically to the same extent, with individual variation ranging from 30–75% (41). These extracts were also observed to inhibit IgE binding to horse hair/dander extract more than

70% (41). However, the inhibition of IgE binding by horse hair/dander extract to cat extract was about 30% and to dog extract mostly insignificant. Some studies suggest that the taxonomical relationship between animals is probably a factor contributing to the cross-reactivity of IgE antibodies against them.

The cross-reactivity of the lipocalin allergen Cav p 1 was studied by IgE ELISA inhibition (54). Cat, mouse, and rat allergen preparations in a hundredfold excess were able to induce weak inhibition, which was maximal, below 10%, with rat hair extract. In another study, a monoclonal antibody raised against Bos d 5 (β-lactoglobulin), a bovine food allergen of the lipocalin family, was observed to react against human serum retinol-binding protein, another lipocalin (67). The core of the antibody-binding epitope, DTDY, is localized in the second structurally conserved region of lipocalins. The sequence is also found in glycodelin.

VI. ENVIRONMENTAL CONTROL

Exposure to indoor allergens can be reduced by control measures (Figs. 2B and 5). It is reasonable to assume that the primary prevention by avoiding contact with pets during childhood will restrain sensitization and the clinical manifestations of allergy. This paradigm has been questioned, however, in recent years in view of several studies reporting diverse, often conflicting, results of the effect of pet ownership (68). Especially intriguing have been the reports on the protective effect of a high-level exposure to cat and dog

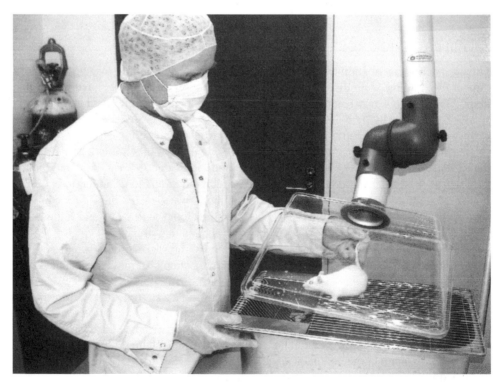

Figure 5 Control measures aimed at decreasing exposure to animal dust in a laboratory animal facility.

allergens (3,4). As a consequence, recommendations about pets and children in the same household, as far as primary sensitization is concerned, should be reconsidered.

The guidelines are more straightforward for persons who are already sensitized against mammalian allergens. Avoidance, or reduction of the exposure load when total avoidance is not possible, is the primary strategy to prevent or to alleviate allergic symptoms.

Allergen concentrations in homes with pets are several hundredfold higher than in homes without pets. As could be expected, removing the cat or dog from the household gradually reduces the allergen levels over time (69). In practice, families often try to keep their pets, and various measures have been proposed for reducing the exposure in those circumstances (69). These include keeping the pet out of the main living area, using air and vacuum cleaners with HEPA filters, and frequent washings of the pet. Although a reduction in the allergen levels can be achieved, the effect on clinical parameters is not well documented. However, a reduction of Fel d 1 concentrations with high-efficiency vacuum cleaners has been found to lead to a clinical improvement in cat-allergic asthmatics (70).

As the first line of prevention against laboratory animal allergy, persons with an atopic background, especially if they are already allergic to animals, should be discouraged from taking up occupations in animal care (71). Within laboratory animal facilities, the aims of preventive measures are to reduce the airborne allergen levels and make use of personal protection against exposure. Ideally, a comprehensive plan should be applied, starting from the designing of the facilities and the ventilation system. The use of individually ventilated cage systems has been shown to decrease ambient rodent allergen levels 250-fold or more under optimal conditions (72). To reduce the exposure of persons emptying and cleaning soiled cages, automated cage-handling machines have been developed. Handling animals during experimental procedures in Class II ventilated cabinets resulted in a >10-fold protection factor (72). Since the appearance of symptoms as well as sensitization in newly employed personnel are related to airborne allergen concentration (71), measures to reduce the allergen load are recommendable even if it is not possible to reach a zero level.

The most effective personal protection against airborne allergens is achieved by the use of ventilated, motorized helmets in which inhaled air is pumped through type P2 or P3 filters. Although somewhat inconvenient to use, the helmet allows even asthmatic persons to continue working with animals (Fig. 2B).

VII. SALIENT POINTS

1. Mammalian respiratory allergens are mainly dispersed in dander, saliva, and urine.
2. Exposure to mammalian allergens is not limited to immediate contacts with animals; these allergens are widely present in indoor environments.
3. Almost all important mammalian aeroallergens belong to the lipocalin family of proteins. Factors accounting for the allergenicity of lipocalins remain to be identified.
4. Environmental control measures can help symptomatic individuals, although avoidance of exposure is preferable.
5. High exposure to pets in early childhood may be protective against sensitization.
6. IgE cross-reactivity between animal serum albumins has been established; the issue is less clear with other animal allergens.

REFERENCES

1. Virtanen T, Zeiler T, Mäntyjärvi R. Important animal allergens are lipocalin proteins: Why are they allergenic? Int Arch Allergy Immunol 1999; 120:247–258.
2. Virtanen T, Zeiler T, Rautiainen J, Mäntyjärvi R. Allergy to lipocalins: A consequence of misguided T-cell recognition of self and nonself? Immunol Today 1999; 20:398–400.
3. Platts-Mills T, Vaughan J, Squillace S, Woodfolk J, Sporik R. Sensitisation, asthma, and a modified Th2 response in children exposed to cat allergen: A population-based cross-sectional study. Lancet 2001; 357:752–756.
4. Ownby DR, Johnson CC, Peterson EL. Exposure to dogs and cats in the first year of life and risk of allergic sensitization at 6 to 7 years of age. JAMA 2002; 288:963–972.
5. Ingram JM, Sporik R, Rose G, Honsinger R, Chapman MD, Plattsmills TAE. Quantitative assessment of exposure to dog (Can f 1) and cat (Fel d 1) allergens: Relation to sensitization and asthma among children living in Los Alamos, New Mexico. J Allergy Clin Immunol 1995; 96:449–456.
6. Lewis SA. Animals and allergy. Clin Exp Allergy 2000; 30:153–157.
7. Munir AKM, Einarsson R, Schou C, Dreborg SKG. Allergens in school dust.1. The amount of the major cat (Fel d I) and dog (Can f I) allergens in dust from Swedish schools is high enough to probably cause perennial symptoms in most children with asthma who are sensitized to cat and dog. J Allergy Clin Immunol 1993; 91:1067–1074.
8. Bush RK, Wood RA, Eggleston PA. Laboratory animal allergy. J Allergy Clin Immunol 1998; 102:99–112.
9. Aoyama K, Ueda A, Manda F, Matsushita T, Ueda T, Yamauchi C. Allergy to laboratory animals: An epidemiological study. Br J Ind Med 1992; 49:41–47.
10. Zeiler T, Taivainen A, Mäntyjärvi R, Tukiainen H, Rautiainen J, Rytkönen-Nissinen M, Virtanen T. Threshold levels of purified natural Bos d 2 for inducing bronchial airway response in asthmatic patients. Clin Exp Allergy 2002; 32:1454–1460.
11. Flower DR, North AC, Sansom CE. The lipocalin protein family: Structural and sequence overview. Biochim Biophys Acta 2000; 1482:9–24.
12. Altschul SF, Madden TL, Schaffer AA, Zhang J, Zhang Z, Miller W, Lipman DJ. Gapped BLAST and PSI-BLAST: A new generation of protein database search programs. Nucleic Acids Res 1997; 25:3389–3402.
13. Rachmilewitz J, Riely GJ, Huang JH, Chen A, Tykocinski ML. A rheostatic mechanism for T-cell inhibition based on elevation of activation thresholds. Blood 2001; 98:3727–3732.
14. Yusifov TN, Abduragimov AR, Gasymov OK, Glasgow BJ. Endonuclease activity in lipocalins. Biochem J 2000; 347:815–819.
15. Zeiler T, Mäntyjärvi R, Rautiainen J, Rytkönen-Nissinen M, Vilja P, Taivainen A, Kauppinen J, Virtanen T. T cell epitopes of a lipocalin allergen colocalize with the conserved regions of the molecule. J Immunol 1999; 162:1415–1422.
16. Saarelainen S, Zeiler T, Rautiainen J, Närvänen A, Rytkönen-Nissinen M, Mäntyjärvi R, Vilja P, Virtanen T. Lipocalin allergen Bos d 2 is a weak immunogen. Int Immunol 2002; 14:401–409.
17. Counsell CM, Bond JF, Ohman JL, Greenstein JL, Garman RD. Definition of the human T-cell epitopes of Fel d 1, the major allergen of the domestic cat. J Allergy Clin Immunol 1996; 98:884–894.
18. Marcotte GV, Braun CM, Norman PS, Nicodemus CF, Kagey-Sobotka A, Lichtenstein LM, Essayan DW. Effects of peptide therapy on ex vivo T-cell responses. J Allergy Clin Immunol 1998; 101:506–513.
19. Brogdon JL, Leitenberg D, Bottomly K. The potency of TCR signaling differentially regulates NFATc/p activity and early IL-4 transcription in naive CD4+ T cells. J Immunol 2002; 168:3825–3832.
20. Pandjaitan B, Swoboda I, Brandejsky-Pichler F, Rumpold H, Valenta R, Spitzauer S. *Escherichia coli* expression and purification of recombinant dog albumin, a cross-reactive animal allergen. J Allergy Clin Immunol 2000; 105:279–285.

21. van Ree R, van Leeuwen WA, Bulder I, Bond J, Aalberse RC. Purified natural and recombinant Fel d 1 and cat albumin in in vitro diagnostics for cat allergy. J Allerg Clin Immunol 1999; 104:1223–1230.

22. Duffort OA, Carreira J, Nitti G, Polo F, Lombardero M. Studies on the biochemical structure of the major cat allergen Felis domesticus I. Mol Immunol 1991; 28:301–309.

23. Morgenstern JP, Griffith IJ, Brauer AW, Rogers BL, Bond JF, Chapman MD, Kuo MC. Amino acid sequence of Fel d I, the major allergen of the domestic cat: Protein sequence analysis and cDNA cloning. Proc Natl Acad Sci U S A 1991; 88:9690–9694.

24. Griffith IJ, Craig S, Pollock J, Yu XB, Morgenstern JP, Rogers BL. Expression and genomic structure of the genes encoding FdI, the major allergen from the domestic cat. Gene 1992; 113:263–268.

25. Ring PC, Wan H, Schou C, Kristensen AK, Roepstorff P, Robinson C. The 18-kDa form of cat allergen Felis domesticus 1 (Fel d 1) is associated with gelatin- and fibronectin-degrading activity. Clin Exp Allergy 2000; 30:1085–1096.

26. van Milligen FJ, van't Hof W, van den Berg M, Aalberse RC. IgE epitopes on the cat (Felis domesticus) major allergen Fel d I—A study with overlapping synthetic peptides. J Allergy Clin Immunol 1994; 93:34–43.

27. van Neerven RJ, van de Pol MM, van Milligen FJ, Jansen HM, Aalberse RC, Kapsenberg ML. Characterization of cat dander-specific T lymphocytes from atopic patients. J Immunol 1994; 152:4203–4210.

28. Mark PG, Segal DB, Dallaire ML, Garman RD. Human T and B cell immune responses to Fel d 1 in cat-allergic and non-cat-allergic subjects. Clin Exp Allergy 1996; 26:1316–1328.

29. Young RP, Dekker JW, Wordsworth BP, Schou C, Pile KD, Matthiesen F, Rosenberg WMC, Bell JI, Hopkin JM, Cookson WOCM. HLA-DR and HLA-DP genotypes and immunoglobulin E responses to common major allergens. Clin Exp Allergy 1994; 24:431–439.

30. Howell WM, Standring P, Warner JA, Warner JO. HLA class II genotype, HLA-DR B cell surface expression and allergen specific IgE production in atopic and non-atopic members of asthmatic family pedigrees. Clin Exp Allergy 1999; 29:35–38.

31. Spitzauer S, Pandjaitan B, Söregi G, Mühl S, Ebner C, Kraft D, Valenta R, Rumpold H. IgE cross-reactivities against albumins in patients allergic to animals. J Allergy Clin Immunol 1995; 96:951–959.

32. Ichikawa K, Vailes LD, Pomes A, Chapman MD. Molecular cloning, expression and modelling of cat allergen, cystatin (Fel d 3), a cysteine protease inhibitor. Clin Exp Allergy 2001; 31:1279–1286.

33. Schou C, Svendsen UG, Løwenstein H. Purification and characterization of the major dog allergen, Can f I. Clin Exp Allergy 1991; 21:321–328.

34. Konieczny A, Morgenstern JP, Bizinkauskas CB, Lilley CH, Brauer AW, Bond JF, Aalberse RC, Wallner BP, Kasaian MT. The major dog allergens, Can f 1 and Can f 2, are salivary lipocalin proteins: Cloning and immunological characterization of the recombinant forms. Immunology 1997; 92:577–586.

35. de Groot H, Goei KG, van Swieten P, Aalberse RC. Affinity purification of a major and a minor allergen from dog extract: Serologic activity of affinity-purified Can f I and of Can f I-depleted extract. J Allergy Clin Immunol 1991; 87:1056–1065.

36. Spitzauer S, Schweiger C, Sperr WR, Pandjaitan B, Valent P, Mühl S, Ebner C, Scheiner O, Kraft D, Rumpold H, Valenta R. Molecular characterization of dog albumin as a cross-reactive allergen. J Allergy Clin Immunol 1994; 93:614–627.

37. Dandeu JP, Rabillon J, Divanovic A, Carmi-Leroy A, David B. Hydrophobic interaction chromatography for isolation and purification of Equ.c1, the horse major allergen. J Chromatogr B Biomed Appl 1993; 621:23–31.

38. Gregoire C, Rosinski-Chupin I, Rabillon J, Alzari PM, David B, Dandeu J-P. cDNA cloning and sequencing reveal the major horse allergen Equ c 1 to be a glycoprotein member of the lipocalin superfamily. J Biol Chem 1996; 271:32951–32959.

39. Goubran Botros H, Poncet P, Rabillon J, Fontaine T, Laval JM, David B. Biochemical characterization and surfactant properties of horse allergens. Eur J Biochem 2001; 268:3126–3136.

40. Bulone V, Krogstad-Johnsen T, Smestad-Paulsen B. Separation of horse dander allergen proteins by two-dimensional electrophoresis—Molecular characterisation and identification of Equ c 2.0101 and Equ c 2.0102 as lipocalin proteins. Eur J Biochem 1998; 253:202–211.

41. Cabanas R, Lopez-Serrano MC, Carreira J, Ventas P, Polo F, Caballero MT, Contreras J, Barranco P, Moreno-Ancillo A. Importance of albumin in cross-reactivity among cat, dog and horse allergens. J Investig Allergol Clin Immunol 2000; 10:71–77.

42. Mäntyjärvi R, Parkkinen S, Rytkönen M, Pentikäinen J, Pelkonen J, Rautiainen J, Zeiler T, Virtanen T. Complementary DNA cloning of the predominant allergen of bovine dander: A new member in the lipocalin family. J Allergy Clin Immunol 1996; 97:1297–1303.

43. Ylönen J, Mäntyjärvi R, Taivainen A, Virtanen T. IgG and IgE antibody responses to cow dander and urine in farmers with cow-induced asthma. Clin Exp Allergy 1992; 22:83–90.

44. Rautiainen J, Rytkönen M, Syrjänen K, Pentikäinen J, Zeiler T, Virtanen T, Mäntyjärvi R. Tissue localization of bovine dander allergen Bos d 2. J Allergy Clin Immunol 1998; 101:349–353.

45. Rouvinen J, Rautiainen J, Virtanen T, Zeiler T, Kauppinen J, Taivainen A, Mäntyjärvi R. Probing the molecular basis of allergy—Three-dimensional structure of the bovine lipocalin allergen Bos d 2. J Biol Chem 1999; 274:2337–2343.

46. Rautiainen J, Rytkönen M, Parkkinen S, Pentikäinen J, Linnala-Kankkunen A, Virtanen T, Pelkonen J, Mäntyjärvi R. cDNA cloning and protein analysis of a bovine dermal allergen with homology to psoriasin. J Invest Dermatol 1995; 105:660–663.

47. Parkkinen S, Rytkönen M, Pentikäinen J, Virtanen T, Mäntyjärvi R. Homology of a bovine allergen and the oligomycin sensitivity-conferring protein of the mitochondrial adenosine triphosphate synthase complex. J Allergy Clin Immunol 1995; 95:1255–1260.

48. Lorusso JR, Moffat S, Ohman JLJ. Immunologic and biochemical properties of the major mouse urinary allergen (Mus m I). J Allergy Clin Immunol 1986; 78:928–937.

49. Cavaggioni A, Mucignat-Caretta C. Major urinary proteins, α_{2U}-globulins and aphrodisin. Biochim Biophys Acta 2000; 1482:218–228.

50. Price JA, Longbottom JL. Allergy to mice. II. Further characterization of two major mouse allergens (AG 1 and AG 3) and immunohistochemical investigations of their sources. Clin Exp Allergy 1990; 20:71–77.

51. Platts-Mills TA, Longbottom J, Edwards J, Cockroft A, Wilkins S. Occupational asthma and rhinitis related to laboratory rats: Serum IgG and IgE antibodies to the rat urinary allergen. J Allergy Clin Immunol 1987; 79:505–515.

52. Gordon S, Tee RD, Taylor AJ. Analysis of rat urine proteins and allergens by sodium dodecyl sulfate-polyacrylamide gel electrophoresis and immunoblotting. J Allergy Clin Immunol 1993; 92:298–305.

53. Gordon S, Tee RD, Stuart MC, Newman Taylor AJ. Analysis of allergens in rat fur and saliva. Allergy 2001; 56:563–567.

54. Fahlbusch B, Rudeschko O, Szilagyi U, Schlott B, Henzgen M, Schlenvoigt G, Schubert H. Purification and partial characterization of the major allergen, Cav p 1, from guinea pig *Cavia porcellus*. Allergy 2002; 57:417–422.

55. Walls AF, Newman Taylor AJ, Longbottom JL. Allergy to guinea pigs: I. Allergenic activities of extracts derived from the pelt, saliva, urine and other sources. Clin Allergy 1985; 15:241–251.

56. Baker J, Berry A, Boscato LM, Gordon S, Walsh BJ, Stuart MC. Identification of some rabbit allergens as lipocalins. Clin Exp Allergy 2001; 31:303–312.

57. Warner JA, Longbottom JL. Allergy to rabbits. III. Further identification and characterisation of rabbit allergens. Allergy 1991; 46:481–491.

58. Natter S, Seiberler S, Hufnagl P, Binder BR, Hirschl AM, Ring J, Abeck D, Schmidt T, Valent P, Valenta R. Isolation of cDNA clones coding for IgE autoantigens with serum IgE from atopic dermatitis patients. FASEB J 1998; 12:1559–1569.

59. Valenta R, Natter S, Seiberler S, Wichlas S, Maurer D, Hess M, Pavelka M, Grote M, Ferreira F, Szepfalusi Z, Valent P, Stingl G. Molecular characterization of an autoallergen, Hom s 1, identified by serum IgE from atopic dermatitis patients. J Invest Dermatol 1998; 111:1178–1183.

60. Shichijo S, Nakao M, Imai Y, Takasu H, Kawamoto M, Niiya F, Yang D, Toh Y, Yamana H, Itoh K. A gene encoding antigenic peptides of human squamous cell carcinoma recognized by cytotoxic T lymphocytes. J Exp Med 1998; 187:277–288.

61. Flückiger S, Scapozza L, Mayer C, Blaser K, Folkers G, Crameri R. Immunological and structural analysis of IgE-mediated cross-reactivity between manganese superoxide dismutases. Int Arch Allergy Immunol 2002; 128:292–303.

62. Mayer C, Appenzeller U, Seelbach H, Achatz G, Oberkofler H, Breitenbach M, Blaser K, Crameri R. Humoral and cell-mediated autoimmune reactions to human acidic ribosomal P2 protein in individuals sensitized to *Aspergillus fumigatus* P2 protein. J Exp Med 1999; 189:1507–1512.

63. Valenta R, Duchene M, Pettenburger K, Sillaber C, Valent P, Bettelheim P, Breitenbach M, Rumpold H, Kraft D, Scheiner O. Identification of profilin as a novel pollen allergen; IgE autoreactivity in sensitized individuals. Science 1991; 253:557–560.

64. Goubran Botros H, Gregoire C, Rabillon J, David B, Dandeu JP. Cross-antigenicity of horse serum albumin with dog and cat albumins: Study of three short peptides with significant inhibitory activity towards specific human IgE and IgG antibodies. Immunology 1996; 88:340–347.

65. Boutin Y, Hebert J, Vrancken ER, Mourad W. Mapping of cat albumin using monoclonal antibodies: Identification of determinants common to cat and dog. Clin Exp Immunol 1989; 77:440–444.

66. Spitzauer S, Pandjaitan B, Mühl S, Ebner C, Kraft D, Valenta R, Rumpold H. Major cat and dog allergens share IgE epitopes. J Allergy Clin Immunol 1997; 99:100–106.

67. Reddy BM, Karande AA, Adiga PR. A common epitope of β-lactoglobulin and serum retinol-binding proteins: Elucidation of its core sequence using synthetic peptides. Mol Immunol 1992; 29:511–516.

68. Custovic A, Murray CS. The effect of allergen exposure in early childhood on the development of atopy. Curr Allergy Asthma Rep 2002; 2:417–423.

69. Custovic A, Simpson A, Chapman MD, Woodcock A. Allergen avoidance in the treatment of asthma and atopic disorders. Thorax 1998; 53:63–72.

70. Popplewell EJ, Innes VA, Lloyd-Hughes S, Jenkins EL, Khdir K, Bryant TN, Warner JO, Warner JA. The effect of high-efficiency and standard vacuum-cleaners on mite, cat and dog allergen levels and clinical progress. Pediatr Allergy Immunol 2000; 11:142–148.

71. Cullinan P, Cook A, Gordon S, Nieuwenhuijsen MJ, Tee RD, Venables KM, McDonald JC, Taylor AJ. Allergen exposure, atopy and smoking as determinants of allergy to rats in a cohort of laboratory employees. Eur Respir J 1999; 13:1139–1143.

72. Gordon S, Fisher SW, Raymond RH. Elimination of mouse allergens in the working environment: Assessment of individually ventilated cage systems and ventilated cabinets in the containment of mouse allergens. J Allergy Clin Immunol 2001; 108:288–294.

17

Food Allergens

WESLEY BURKS

Duke University Medical Center, Durham, North Carolina, U.S.A.

I. INTRODUCTION

A number of advances in the scientific knowledge concerning adverse food reactions have been made in the last several years. Current understanding is significantly different about the nature of the food allergen itself, the molecular characterization of the epitopes on these allergens, the pathophysiology of the clinical reaction, and the limitations of the diagnostic methods. Part of the difficulty in understanding adverse food reactions had resulted from the nomenclature used in this literature, but more-concise definitions are helping standardize the literature (1) (Table 1). An adverse food reaction is a generic term referring to any untoward reaction after the ingestion of a food. Adverse food reactions may be secondary to food allergy (hypersensitivity) or food intolerance. A food allergic reaction is the result of an immunologic mechanism induced by the ingestion of a food, while food intolerance is the result of nonimmunologic mechanisms (2).

The true prevalence of adverse food reactions is unknown. In American households, about one-third of the families believed some family member to be affected (3). The best

319

Table 1 Definitions of Adverse Food Reactions

Adverse food reaction—generic term referring to any untoward reaction after the ingestion of a food
Food allergy (hypersensitivity)—the result of an abnormal immunologic response after the ingestion of a food
Food intolerance—the result of nonimmunologic mechanisms after the ingestion of a food

---

studies to date indicate that approximately 6–8% of young children and 1% of adults have some type of food allergy (4).

II. TAXONOMY OF FOOD ALLERGENS

Foods are typically derived from animal and vegetable sources. Both animals and vegetables are classified botanically. Examples of animal groups include birds (e.g., chicken, duck), crustaceans (e.g., crab, lobster), and red meats (e.g., beef, veal). Examples of plant groups include the apple family (e.g., apple, pear), grass family (e.g., corn, wheat), legume family (e.g., lentil, peanut), and walnut family (e.g., black walnut, pecan).

Allergy to one member of some food groups may result in a variable degree of clinical reactivity to other members of the same group because of cross-reacting allergens. Much more is understood now about the differences between clinical sensitivity and clinical reactivity within a group of similar foods.

III. MOLECULAR CHARACTERISTICS OF FOOD ALLERGENS

Foods are composed of proteins, carbohydrates, and lipids. The major food allergens have been identified as water-soluble glycoproteins having molecular weights ranging from 10,000 to 60,000 daltons. Over the last several years it has been increasingly recognized that many food allergens occur naturally as dimers or trimers, making their molecular weight often 150,00 to 200,000 daltons (5). There are no known unique biochemical or immunochemical characteristics of food allergens. Comparisons of primary amino acid sequences of allergenic proteins have not revealed typical patterns. Food allergens tend to be resistant to usual food processing and preparation conditions. These proteins are comparatively resistant to heat and acid treatment, proteolysis, and digestion. The treatment of food allergens with acid concentrations simulating stomach acid conditions typically has little effect on the specific IgE binding of the allergen. There are, however, important exceptions, such as the major allergens in fresh fruits and some vegetables.

The food allergens, in general, are soluble in water and/or saline solutions, thus belonging to the classes known as albumins (water soluble) or globulins (saline soluble). Although the level of exposure to a specific protein necessary to sensitize an individual is unknown, individuals with preexisting IgE-mediated food allergies can respond adversely to extremely low levels of the offending food. Microgram to milligram quantities of peanut have elicited an adverse reaction in food challenges in selected individuals. The immunochemical or physicochemical properties that account for such unique allergenicity of food allergens are poorly understood.

IV. MAJOR AND MINOR FOOD ALLERGENS

The most common foods to cause documented IgE-mediated reactions in childhood are cow's milk, eggs, peanuts, soybeans, wheat, fish, and tree nuts (Table 2). Approximately

Table 2 Major Food Allergens in Children and Adults

Children	Adults
Milk	Peanuts
Egg	Tree nuts
Peanuts	Fish
Soybeans	Shellfish
Wheat	
Fish	
Tree nuts	

80% of these reactions are secondary to milk, eggs, and peanuts alone. In adulthood, the most common food allergens are peanuts, tree nuts, fish, and shellfish. Worldwide, there are some differences regarding which foods cause problems in both children and adults, primarily because of the diet of the population (6).

A. Cow's Milk

The prevalence of cow's milk allergy in infants and children, worldwide, is estimated at between 2.0% and 2.5% (7). Allergic symptoms related to cow's milk often begin in early childhood, but children typically lose their sensitivity in the first 3–5 years of life (8,9). Cow's milk is composed of a number of different proteins, traditionally divided into caseins, which compose 80% of the total protein, and whey proteins, which compose 20% of the total protein (10). Most patients allergic to cow's milk have specific IgE antibodies to more than one of the milk proteins. Caseins were originally defined as phosphoproteins that precipitate from raw skim milk upon acidification to pH 4.6 at 20°C; whey proteins are those proteins remaining in the milk after precipitation of caseins. The nomenclature of specific milk proteins utilizes a Greek letter with or without a subscript preceding the class name to identify the family of proteins. The genetic variant of the milk protein is indicated by an uppercase Arabic letter with or without a numerical superscript following the class name. Posttranslational modifications are added in sequence (Table 3).

A number of milk proteins have been identified as allergens in humans. By either skin prick testing or oral challenge, many patients have reactivity to multiple cow's milk proteins. Caseins and beta-lactoglobulin appear to be the major allergens in cow's milk. The caseins are a family of proteins (alpha, beta, and kappa) that are chemically related. The major alpha- and beta-caseins have a molecular weight of approximately 23 kDa. There are several genetic variants of each of these caseins. Beta-lactoglobulin (17 kDa), the most abundant whey protein, also has several genetic variants. Alpha-lactalbumin (14 kDa) and bovine serum albumin (67 kDa), both whey proteins, appear to be minor cow's milk allergens. Bovine serum albumin (BSA) has also been identified as a distinct milk allergen. This protein is heterogeneous in nature and has a molecular weight of 67 kDa composing approximately 1% of the total milk protein. Studies have identified the IgE-binding epitopes on the milk caseins (11) and on lactalbumin and lactoglobulin (12). Additionally, other studies have identified specific IgE-binding epitopes that may differentiate between patients with persistent and transient cow's milk allergy (13,14).

Table 3 Purified Antigens in Foods

Protein fraction	MW (daltons)
Cow's milk	
Caseins	19,000–24,000
α-casein	27,000
α_s-casein	23,000
β-casein	24,000
κ-casein	19,000
γ-casein	21,000
Whey	
β-lactoglobulin	36,000
α-lactoglobulin	14,400
Bovine serum albumin	69,000
Chicken egg white	
Ovalbumin	45,000
Ovomucoid	28,000
Ovotransferrin	77,700
Lysozyme	14,300
Peanut	
Ara h 1	63,500
Ara h 2	17,500
Ara h 3	60,000
Soybean	
Gly m 1	34,000
Soybean trypsin inhibitor	20,500
Fish	
Allergen M (Gad c 1)	12,328
Shrimp	
Antigen I	42,000
Antigen II	38,000
Pen a 1	36,000

B. Eggs

Egg allergy is one of the most commonly implicated causes of food allergic reactions both in the United States and Europe. Eggs from chickens (*Gallus domesticus*) are widely used for human consumption. Although there is extensive cross-reactivity among the various birds, hen eggs tend to be slightly more allergenic than duck eggs. Eggs are composed of egg white and egg yolk. The egg white (albumin) appears to be more allergenic than the yolk. The major protein in the egg white is ovalbumin, with other proteins including ovotransferrin, ovomucoid, ovomucin, and lysozyme. Egg yolk can be separated into two fractions using ultracentrifugation. This results in a granular fraction that contains primarily protein and a supernatant fraction that contains primarily lipid. The granular fraction contains lipovitellin, phosvitin, and low-density lipoprotein.

Several studies have documented the major allergens in eggs (15,16). Ovomucoid (Gal d 1), a glycoprotein with a molecular weight of 28 kDa and an acidic isoelectric point, has been implicated as the major allergen in egg (17). In that study, ovomucoid was found to be a more potent allergen than purified ovalbumin by skin prick testing and RAST in a group of 18 children with egg allergy. While previous studies had shown that ovalbumin was the major egg allergen, these studies demonstrated ovomucoid contamination in the ovalbumin. Ovalbumin (Gal d 2) is a monomeric phosphoglycoprotein with a molecular weight of 43 to 45 kDa and an acidic isoelectric point. Purified ovalbumin has three primary variants, A_1, A_2, and A_3. Because of ovomucoid contamination of ovalbumin, it is difficult to determine the exact role of this allergen (17). Ovotransferrin (Gal d 3) (conalbumin) has a molecular weight of 77 kDa and an acidic isoelectric point. It has antimicrobial activity and iron-binding properties. Lysozyme (Gal d 4) is a lower-molecular-weight allergen (14.3 kDa) that in some studies has appeared to be a major allergen but in other studies has been thought to be a minor allergen. Other minor allergens in eggs include apovitellin, ovomucin, and phosvitin. Additional studies have shown that the carbohydrate portion of the glycoproteins in eggs, particularly in ovomucoid, do not have a primary role in specific IgE binding. B- and T-cell epitopes have been mapped in a limited way for ovalbumin and ovomucoid. Similar to the milk allergens, the major IgE- and IgG-binding epitopes of ovomucoid have now been mapped (18).

C. Peanuts

The peanut is an annual plant in the family Leguminosae. In the United States, several varieties including the Virginia, Spanish, and runner are grown. Most of the peanut crop in the United States is used for production of peanut butter. Runner types are used most frequently for oil production and peanut butter. Children are increasingly being exposed to peanut products at an early age. Allergic reactions to peanuts are often very acute and severe, accounting for many of the cases of food-induced anaphylaxis documented each year.

Peanut proteins are customarily classified as albumins (water soluble) and globulins (saline soluble). The globulin proteins are made up of two major fractions, arachin and conarachin (also known as legumine and vicilin, respectively). Arachin in its native state exists as a molecule of at least 600 kDa and readily dissociates into a 340–360 kDa dimer and a monomer of approximately 170–180 kDa. Conarachin can be divided by ultracentrifugation into two fractions, one 2S and one 8.4S.

There have been a number of peanut allergens previously identified. Peanut-1 and concanavalin A-reactive glycoprotein (CARG) were some of the first peanut allergens partially characterized. Ara h 1 is a 63.5-kDa glycoprotein identified as a major peanut allergen using immunoblotting and ELISA (19). This allergen has an acidic isoelectric point and is relatively resistant to enzyme degradation. Molecular studies have identified multiple IgE binding sites in the amino acid sequence of Ara h 1. This peanut allergen has at least 23 specific IgE-binding epitopes along its amino acid sequence. Ara h 1 has been identified as a member of the vicilin family of seed storage proteins. Ara h 2 is a 17-kDa allergen with an acidic isoelectric point. This allergen has at least 10 specific IgE-binding epitopes along its amino acid sequence. Ara h 2 appears to be a member of the conglycinin family of seed storage proteins.

Other studies have identified the peanut allergen Ara h 3 as a glycinin seed storage protein with a molecular weight of 60,000 daltons. Approximately 45% of patients with peanut allergy have specific IgE to this allergen (20,21).

D. Soybeans

Soybeans, although not implicated as often as milk, eggs, and peanuts, are one of five major allergens in the United States causing allergic reactions in children. Soybean globulins are the major proteins of the soybean. The soybean globulins can be separated into ultracentrifugation components identified as 2S, 7S, 11S, and 15S fractions. Alpha-conglycinin is a primary protein of the 2S fraction, while beta-conglycinin is the primary fraction of the 7S component. The glycinin fraction is the primary component of the 11S ultracentrifugation fraction.

Soybeans, like peanuts, are legumes that have multiple allergens that have been identified (22,23). While examining specific IgE to the ultracentrifugation components, authors have primarily identified either the 2S or 7S fraction as containing the primary allergens. Gly m 1, a 30-kDa allergen, is a component of the 7S fraction. In one study, the majority of patients had soybean-specific IgE to Gly m 1 (24). Gly m 1 has an acidic isoelectric point. It has sequence homology to a soybean seed 34-kDa oil-body-associated protein (called soybean vacuolar protein P34). There appear to be at least 16 distinct soybean-specific IgE-binding epitopes along the amino acid sequence of this allergen. The Kunitz soybean trypsin inhibitor has been shown in several studies to bind soybean-specific IgE in soybean-allergic patients, although only in a minority of patients (making it likely a minor allergen).

E. Wheat

Although not the most common source of food allergy, wheat and other cereal grains are often implicated as food allergens, particularly in children (25). The proteins of wheat include the water-soluble albumins, the saline-soluble globulins, the aqueous ethanol-soluble prolamins, and the glutelins. It is not uncommon for children to have multiple positive prick skin tests to various cereal grains while having clinical reactivity to only one of the foods. There is extensive nonspecific IgE binding to the lectin fractions in cereal grains. Patients with wheat allergy apparently have specific IgE binding to wheat fractions of 47 kDa and 20 kDa (proteins not recognized by the serum from patients with grass allergy). Additional studies have shown the wheat alpha amylase inhibitor (15 kDa) to be a major wheat allergen. This protein did not bind IgE from any wheat-tolerant control patients, including those with grass allergy (26,27).

F. Fish

The consumption or inhalation of fish allergen is a common cause of IgE-mediated food reactions. The incidence of fish allergy is believed to be much higher in countries where fish consumption is greatest. For example, codfish allergy is extremely common in the Scandinavian countries (28). One of the most comprehensive descriptions of a food allergen has been the work by Aas and Elsayed on the codfish allergen, Gad c 1 (originally designated allergen M) (29). Gad c 1 belongs to a group of muscle proteins known as parvalbumins. The parvalbumins control the flow of calcium in and out of cells and are only found in the muscles of amphibians and fish. This allergen has an acidic isoelectric point and a molecular weight of 12 kDa. The tertiary structure of Gad c 1 has three domains. There are at least five IgE-binding sites on the allergen, and the carbohydrate moiety does not appear to be important in its allergenicity.

G. Tree Nuts

Tree nuts are occasional causes of food allergic reactions in both children and adults. Like allergic reactions to fish and peanuts, reactions to tree nuts may persist throughout the lifetime of an individual. Two major allergens have been identified in almonds. The allergens are a 70-kDa heat-labile protein and a 45–50-kDa heat-stable protein. Brazil nuts are another cause of food allergic reactions. Although several different proteins have been identified as allergens, the major allergen, Ber e 1, is a high-methionine protein (30). The 12-kDa protein has two subunits, a 9-kDa and a 3-kDa protein. Work with the walnut allergens has identified a major allergen as a 65-kDa glycoprotein (Jug r 2), similar to other plant vicilins, as well as another walnut allergen (Jug r 1), a 2S albumin seed storage protein (31).

H. Shrimp

Shrimp is the most studied of the crustacea allergens (32,33). The original two fractions characterized in shrimp were antigen I (45 kDa) and antigen II (38 kDa). SA-II was next characterized as a major allergen in shrimp. Further studies revealed that SA-II was similar to antigen I that had been previously described. Pen a 1 was identified as a major allergen from boiled brown shrimp (isolated in the boiled water) and was thus thought to be similar to SA-II. This allergen has a molecular weight of 36 kDa and constitutes 20% of the soluble protein in crude cooked shrimp. The protein has bound shrimp-specific IgE in over 85% of patients with shrimp allergy studied to date. Another shrimp allergen, Met e 1, has been isolated from another kind of shrimp and has a molecular weight of 34 kDa. Studies of these Pen a 1 and Met a 1 allergens have shown them to be highly homologous with tropomyosin from various species. The IgE-binding epitopes of the shrimp allergen Pen a 1 have now been identified (34,35).

V. FOOD ALLERGEN CROSS-REACTIVITY

A. Cow's Milk

Immunoblotting and crossed radioimmunoelectrophoresis studies have shown extensive milk-specific IgE cross-reactivity between milk proteins in cows, goats, and sheep (Table 4). Earlier studies showed that at least 50% of cow's milk–allergic individuals were also allergic to goat's milk. Clinical practice indicates that patients allergic to one type of milk protein will not tolerate milk proteins of other species.

Table 4 Food Allergen Cross-reactivity

	Specific IgE to multiple members of the family	Clinical reactivity
Milk	common	common
Legumes	common	uncommon
Wheat	common	uncommon
Fish	common	uncommon
Crustacea and mollusks	common	??
Tree nuts	common	uncommon
Egg and chicken	occasional	rare
Milk and beef	occasional	uncommon

B. Legumes

Extensive in vitro allergenic cross-reactivity in the legume family has been documented. A clinical study of 57 patients with legume sensitivity and in vitro cross-allergenicity with peanuts, soybeans, peas, and lima beans revealed that extensive IgE cross-reactivity did not indicate clinical reactivity (36). They found that 59% of skin-test-positive patients reacted to oral challenge and only 5% of the patients reacted in oral challenge to more than one legume. While patients with peanut-specific IgE may have clinical reactions to other legumes, these reactions are quite uncommon and should be evaluated on an individual basis.

C. Wheat

Serum from patients with cereal grain allergies exhibits extensive cross-reactivity in vitro among the different cereal grains. One hundred forty-five children with food sensitivity were found to have at least one positive prick skin test to one of the cereal grains (i.e., wheat, oat, rye, barley, corn, and rice) (26). Thirty-one children (21%) experienced clinical symptoms during food challenges: wheat, 26; rye, 4; barley, 4; oat, 5; rice, 1; and corn, 5. Of the children reacting to cereal grains, only 20% reacted to more than one. Approximately 70% of these patients also showed positive prick skin tests to grass pollens (i.e., timothy, orchard, and Bermuda). Overall, about 20% of patients with positive prick skin tests to cereal grains will react when ingesting the grain, and about 4% will react to more than one grain (26).

D. Fish

Several studies have assessed the reactivity of fish-allergic subjects to different species of fish. Of 11 children with a history of fish allergy with multiple positive skin tests to various fish, seven reacted to only one fish on oral blinded challenge, one reacted to two fish, two reacted to three fish, and one patient did not react to any fish (37). Similar in vitro cross-reactivity has been shown in other studies using immunoblotting techniques (27). Fish-allergic adults in general have more in vivo cross-reactivity than do children. Not only do adults have fish-specific IgE to multiple species of fish, they also are more likely to have adverse reactions to more than one species on oral challenges. Cooked salmon and tuna are allergenic fish, whereas canned salmon and tuna are generally nonallergenic.

E. Crustacea and Mollusks

Patients who have positive prick skin tests and/or RAST to the crustacea tend to react positively to multiple members of this family (38). In particular, individuals with shrimp allergy exhibit positive skin tests and RAST to other crustaceans. Studies have shown that extracts from shrimp, blue crab, and crawfish all inhibit Pen a 1 RAST to a similar extent. There is insufficient oral challenge data to know the extent of clinical reactivity among the different crustacea.

Although mollusks are much less commonly allergenic than crustacea, there are studies to show some in vitro cross-reactivity among the oyster (mollusks) and the crustacea. Shrimp, blue crab, spiny lobster, and crawfish were all highly cross-reactive with oyster. Again, the extent of clinical cross-reactivity has not been studied sufficiently. Clinical advice to patients must be individualized.

F. Tree Nuts

A variety of nuts have caused anaphylactic reactions in children and adults. In one study, 14 children underwent 19 blinded challenges to nuts; one patient reacted to five nuts, one to two nuts, and the remaining 12 children to one nut each (39). Overall, there were seven reactions to walnuts, six to cashews, three to pecans, two to pistachios, and one to filbert. Adults allergic to nuts generally do not need to avoid peanuts (a legume), and vice versa, although children with peanut allergy appear to be more likely to develop allergy to tree nuts than the general population.

G. Egg and Chicken

Egg-allergic patients older than 3 years of age may react (i.e., <5%) following the ingestion of chicken, and similarly chicken-allergic patients may react to eggs (40,41). An association also has been reported between allergic reactions to egg and respiratory symptoms in bird-keepers exposed to their birds (42).

H. Milk and Beef

Of 335 children with atopic dermatitis evaluated by blinded challenges for possible food hypersensitivity, 11 reacted to beef, eight of whom were also sensitive to milk on previous double-blind, placebo-controlled food challenge (DBPCFC). Three of the patients could tolerate well-cooked beef and only experienced symptoms when they ingested partially cooked beef (43). IgE immunoblots in these patients revealed the presence of both heat-labile and heat-stable protein fractions.

I. Tree Nuts and Pollen Allergy

Patients allergic to tree pollen may also have an allergic reaction upon the ingestion of nuts from the same tree. In one study, the observed patients with birch pollen–specific IgE also reacted to hazelnut (44). Through a series of elegant studies, it has been determined that a profilin with a molecular weight of 14 kDa is responsible for the cross-reactivity between a variety of fruits and vegetables (45,46). Profilins are highly conserved, ubiquitous proteins that are found in almost all eukaryotic organisms. Profilins have been isolated from a variety of pollens including timothy grass, rye grass, and mugwort. Pollen profilins also appear to share cross-reactivity with a number of foods. As an example, cross-reactivity has been demonstrated between mugwort pollen, and celery and carrot. Birch profilin has been associated with the fruits of rosaceae including apple, pear, cherry, and peach. For most of these studies, it is felt that exposure to tree pollens can lead to the development of IgE antibodies that recognize epitopes on a variety of food proteins that contain similar amino acid sequences. The primary sensitization appears to be to the pollen and not to the food.

J. Food—Nonpollen

A number of surveys have reported an association between latex allergy and allergic reaction to bananas, avocado, kiwi, chestnut, and papaya. In a series of 25 patients diagnosed with latex allergy (by history and prick skin tests), approximately one-half of these patients were diagnosed with food allergies (based on positive prick skin tests and history of at least two reactions within the previous 5 years) (47). Overall, 42 reactions were diagnosed in 13 patients (systemic anaphylaxis in 23): avocado, 9; chestnut, 9; banana, 7; kiwi, 5; and papaya, 3.

VI. DIAGNOSIS AND DIETARY CONTROL

As with all medical disorders, the diagnostic approach to the patient with a suspected adverse food reaction begins with the medical history and physical examination (40). Based upon the information derived from these initial steps, various laboratory studies may be helpful.

The true value of the medical history is largely dependent on the patient's recollection of symptoms and the examiner's ability to differentiate disorders provoked by food hypersensitivity and other etiologies. The history may be directly useful in diagnosing food allergy in acute events (e.g., systemic anaphylaxis following the ingestion of fish). In many series, though, less than 50% of reported food allergic reactions could be substantiated by DBPCFC (41). Several pieces of information are important to establish that a food allergic reaction occurred (Table 5): (1) the food suspected to have provoked the reaction, (2) the quantity of the food ingested, (3) the length of time between ingestion and development of symptoms, (4) a description of the symptoms provoked, (5) if similar symptoms developed on other occasions when the food was eaten, (6) if other factors (e.g., exercise) are necessary, and (7) the length of time since the last reaction. Any food may cause an allergic reaction, although only a few foods account for 90% of the reactions. In children, these foods are egg, milk, peanuts, soy, and wheat (fish in Scandinavian countries). In chronic disorders such as atopic dermatitis, the history is often an unreliable indicator of the offending allergen (48,49).

A diet diary has been frequently utilized as an adjunct to the medical history. Patients are asked to keep a chronological record of all foods ingested over a specified period of time and to record any symptoms they experience during this time. The diary can then be reviewed at a patient visit to determine if there is any relationship between the foods ingested and the symptoms experienced. It is uncommon to detect by this method an unrecognized association between a food and a patient's symptoms.

An elimination diet is frequently used in both diagnosis and management of adverse food reactions. If a certain food or foods are suspected of provoking the reaction, they are completely eliminated from the diet. The success of an elimination diet depends on several factors, including the correct identification of the allergen(s) involved, the ability of the patient to maintain a diet completely free of all forms of the possible offending allergen, and the assumption that other factors will not provoke similar symptoms during the study period. The likelihood of all of these conditions being met is often slim. For example, in a young infant reacting to cow's milk formula, resolution of symptoms following substitution

Table 5 Important Information from Medical History

---

(1) The food suspected to have provoked the reaction
(2) The quantity of the food ingested
(3) The length of time between ingestion and development of symptoms
(4) A description of the symptoms provoked
(5) If similar symptoms developed on other occasions when the food was eaten
(6) If other factors (e.g., exercise) are necessary
(7) The length of time since the last reaction

---

of cow's milk formula with a soy formula or casein hydrolysate formula (e.g., Alimentum, Nutramigen) is highly suggestive of cow's milk allergy but also could be due to lactose intolerance. Avoidance of suspected food allergens prior to blinded challenge is recommended so that the reactions occurring during the challenge may be heightened and more obvious. Elimination diets, though, are rarely diagnostic of food allergy, particularly in chronic disorders such as atopic dermatitis or asthma.

Allergy prick-puncture skin tests are highly reproducible and often utilized to screen patients with suspected IgE-mediated food allergies (41). The criteria established by May and Bock have proven useful to many investigators and clinicians. The glycerinated food extracts (1:10 or 1:20 w/v) and appropriate positive (histamine) and negative (saline) controls are applied by either the prick or puncture technique. A food allergen eliciting a wheal at least 3 mm greater than the negative control is considered positive; anything else is considered negative. A positive skin test to a food indicates only the possibility that the patient has symptomatic reactivity to that specific food (overall the positive predictive accuracy is less than 50%). A negative skin test confirms the absence of an IgE-mediated reaction (overall negative predictive accuracy is greater than 95%). Both of these statements are justified if appropriate and good-quality food extracts are utilized (50).

The prick skin test should be considered an excellent means of excluding IgE-mediated food allergies but only "suggestive" of the presence of clinical food allergies (51). There are some minor exceptions to the general statement: (1) IgE-mediated sensitivity to several fruits and vegetables (apples, oranges, bananas, pears, melons, potatoes, carrots, celery, etc.) is frequently not detected with commercial reagents, presumably secondary to the lability of the responsible allergen in the test food; (2) children less than 1 year of age may have IgE-mediated food allergy without a positive skin test, and children less than 2 years of age may have smaller wheals, possibly due to the lack of skin reactivity; and conversely (3) a positive skin test to a food ingested in isolation which provokes a serious systemic anaphylactic reaction may be considered diagnostic.

An intradermal skin test is a more sensitive tool than the prick skin test but is much less specific when compared with a blinded food challenge. In one study, no patient who had a negative prick skin test and a positive intradermal skin test to a specific food had a positive DBPCFC to that food. In addition, intradermal skin testing has a greater risk of inducing a systemic reaction than does prick skin testing.

Radioallergosorbent tests (RASTs) and similar in vitro assays (including enzyme-linked immunosorbent assays) are utilized for the identification of food-specific IgE antibodies. These tests are often used to screen for IgE-mediated food allergies. While slightly less sensitive than skin tests, one study comparing RASTs with DBPCFCs found prick skin tests and RASTs to have similar sensitivity and specificity when a RAST score of 3 or greater was considered positive. In this study, if a 2 were considered positive, there was a slight improvement in sensitivity, while the specificity decreased significantly. In general, in vitro measurement of serum food-specific IgE performed in high-quality laboratories provides information similar to prick skin tests (52).

Work with the CAP-fluorescent enzyme immunoassay (FEIA) system has now allowed patients to have a clinical diagnosis of food allergy without having a food challenge (53). Patients who have a positive skin test to the food can then have a CAP-FEIA done to that food allergen. For patients with specific IgE levels higher than the positive predictive values, the diagnosis of food allergy would be generally accepted (Table 6).

Basophil histamine release assays (BHR) have generally been reserved for research and academic settings. Newer, semiautomated methods utilizing small amounts of whole

Table 6   Food-Specific IgE Concentrations Predictive of Clinical Reactivity

Allergen	Decision point (KU$_A$/L)	Sensitivity	Specificity	PPV	NPV
Egg	7	61	95	98	38
Infants ≤2 yrs[b]	2		95		
Milk	15	57	94	95	53
Infants ≤2 yrs[c]	5		95		
Peanut	14	57	100	100	36
Fish	20	25	100	100	89
Soybean	30	44	94	73	82
Wheat	26	61	92	74	87
Tree Nuts[a]	~15	–	–	~95	–

PPV—Positive Predictive Value
NPV—Negative Predictive Value
[a]Tentative values
[b]Boyano MT, et al. Clin Exp Allergy 2001; 31(9):1464–1469.
[c]Garcia-Ara C, et al. J Allergy Clin Immunol 2001; 107(1):185–190.
Sampson HA. J Allergy Clin Immunol 2001; 107(5):891–896.
Definition of decision point: Above that value, you have the following sensitivity, specificity, etc.

blood have been developed and are being promoted for screening multiple food allergens. The use of whole blood in the assays should circumvent the problem of high spontaneous basophil histamine release seen in food-allergic individuals continuing to ingest the responsible allergen. One such method was employed in a study that compared BHR to prick skin tests, RASTs, food antigen–induced intestinal mast cell histamine release, and food challenges in suspected food-allergic children. As found in earlier studies, the food allergen–induced BHR correlated most closely with RAST results. The BHR did not appear to be any more predictive of clinical sensitivity than the prick skin test or RAST.

The intestinal mast cell histamine release (IMCHR) assay is primarily a research procedure performed with dispensed intestinal mast cells obtained from biopsy specimens. Food antigen is added in the assay to the mast cells and the percentage histamine release determined. Compared with prick skin tests, RASTs, and BHR, IMCHR correlated most closely to the outcome of oral food challenge when symptoms were confined to the gastrointestinal tract. This study implies that local IgE production may account for some gastrointestinal hypersensitivities not generally considered to be IgE-mediated.

Intragastral provocation under endoscopy (IPEC) was initially utilized for the diagnosis of food allergy over 50 years ago. In one study, small quantities of the suspected food extract (1:10 solution of food in normal saline) were applied to the gastric mucosa, and the site was observed and then scored. IPEC in patients with food allergy previously documented by DBPCFC provoked reactions on the gastric mucosa in all patients. The tissue histamine and stainable mast cells in biopsies of the site were decreased compared with pre-challenge samples. Other tests employed included prick skin tests and RASTs, which were positive in only one-half of these patients. One important item, the specificity of the test, has not been evaluated in skin-test-positive, nonreactive patients. Many patients experience systemic symptoms during the procedure, making it no safer than oral challenges.

DBPCFC has been labeled the "gold standard" for the diagnosis of food allergies (40). This test has been utilized successfully by many investigators in both children and adults for the last several years to examine a wide variety of food-related complaints. The foods to be tested in the oral challenge are based upon history and/or prick skin test (or RAST) results. Foods thought to be unlikely to provoke a food allergic reaction may be screened by open or single-blind challenges. It is necessary, though, except in very young infants, to confirm multiple positive reactions by DBPCFC. Prior to undertaking a DBPCFC, several conditions should be established: (1) Suspect foods should be eliminated for 7–14 days prior to challenge; (2) antihistamines should be discontinued long enough to establish a normal histamine skin test; (3) other medications should be minimized to levels sufficient to prevent breakthrough of acute symptoms; and (4) in some patients with asthma, short bursts of corticosteroids may be necessary to obtain adequate pulmonary reserve for testing ($FEV_1 > 70\%$ predicted).

The food challenge should be administered with the patient in a fasting state, starting the challenge with a dose of food unlikely to provoke symptoms (generally 125 mg to 500 mg of lyophilized food) (Table 7). This dose is then increased every 15 to 60 minutes, depending on the type of reaction that was suspected to occur. A similar scheme is followed with the placebo portion of the study. Clinical reactivity is generally ruled out when the patient who is blinded to the ingested food has tolerated 10 grams of lyophilized food in capsules or liquid. If the blinded portion of the challenge is negative, however, it must be confirmed by an open feeding under observation to rule out the rare false-negative challenge.

A DBPCFC is the best means of controlling for the variability of chronic disorders (e.g., chronic urticaria, atopic dermatitis), any potential temporal effects, and acute exacerbations secondary to reducing or discontinuing medications. In particular, psychogenic factors and observer bias are eliminated. There are the rare false-negative challenges in a DBPCFC, which may occur when a patient receives insufficient challenge material to provoke the reaction or when the lyophilization of the food antigen has altered the relevant allergenic epitopes (e.g., fish). Overall, the DBPCFC has proven to be the most accurate means of diagnosing food allergy at the present time.

DBPCFCs should be conducted in a clinic or hospital setting, especially if an IgE-mediated reaction is suspected. Trained personnel and equipment for treating systemic anaphylaxis should be present. If life-threatening anaphylaxis is suspected and the causative agent cannot be identified conclusively by history, a challenge should be conducted in the intensive care unit of a center frequently dealing with food allergic reactions (54). The evaluation of suspected "delayed" reactions can be conducted safely on an outpatient basis, provided the symptoms have not been severe and there is no concern about the patient breaking the blinding by opening capsules. There are some possible

Table 7 Sample Schedule for Double-Blind, Placebo-Controlled Food Challenge

Time (minutes)	Food	Time (hour of day)	Placebo
0:00	125–500 mg	3:00 P.M.	500 mg
0:15	1 g	3:15 P.M.	1 g
0:30	2 g	3:30 P.M.	2 g
0:45	3 g	3:45 P.M.	3 g
60	3.5 g	4:00 P.M.	3.5 g

Table 8   Practical Approach to Diagnosing Food Allergy

(1) Medical history
(2) Appropriate laboratory evaluation—selective prick-puncture skin tests and/or CAP-FEIA
(3) Exclusion diet based on above information
(4) Food challenge(s)
(5) Appropriate diet based on information generated above
(6) Adequate follow-up history and future challenges

adverse food reactions where the symptoms are largely subjective. Three crossover trials with reactions developing only during the allergen challenge are necessary to conclude that there exists a cause-and-effect relationship.

A.   Practical Approach to Diagnosing Food Allergy

The diagnosis of food allergy remains a clinical exercise that utilizes a careful history, selective prick skin tests followed by a CAP-FEIA (if an IgE-mediated disorder is suspected), an appropriate exclusion diet, and food challenges (55). (Table 8). Other diagnostic tests that do not appear to be of significant value include food-specific IgG or IgG4 antibody levels, food antigen-antibody complexes, evidence of lymphocyte activation (^{3}H-thymidine uptake, IL-2 production, and leukocyte inhibitory factor), and sublingual or intracutaneous provocation. Blinded challenges may not be necessary in suspected gastrointestinal disorders where pre- and post-challenge laboratory values and biopsies are often useful.

An exclusion diet eliminating all foods suspected by history and/or prick skin testing (or RASTs) for IgE-mediated disorders should be conducted for at least 1–2 weeks prior to challenge. Some gastrointestinal disorders, e.g., allergic eosinophilic gastroenteropathy, may need to have the exclusion diet extended for up to 12 weeks following appropriate biopsies. If no improvement is noted following the diet, it is unlikely that food allergy is involved. In the case of some chronic diseases, such as atopic dermatitis or chronic asthma, other precipitating factors may make it difficult to discriminate between the effects of the food allergen and other provocative factors.

Open or single-blind challenges (where the food being challenged is known only to the individuals administering the challenge) in a clinic setting may be helpful to screen suspected food allergens. Positive challenges should be confirmed by a DBPCFC unless a single "major" allergen (egg, milk, soy, wheat) provoked classic allergic symptoms. A patient with multiple food allergies is rare and, if suspected, should be confirmed by DBPCFC. Many dry foods can be obtained through grocery stores, health food stores, and camping outlets. The presumptive diagnosis of food allergy based on a patient's history and prick skin tests or RAST results is not acceptable. There are exceptions to this, such as patients with severe anaphylaxis following the isolated ingestion of a specific food, particularly peanuts, tree nuts, fish, and shellfish. It is important that the physician make an unequivocal diagnosis of food allergy so that the patient and family are aware of which foods they should specifically avoid.

After the diagnosis of food hypersensitivity is established, the only proven therapy is strict elimination of the offending allergen. It is important to remember that prescribing an elimination diet is like prescribing a medication; both can have positive effects and unwarranted side effects. Elimination diets may led to malnutrition and/or eating disorders, especially if they include a large number of foods and/or are utilized for extended periods. Patients and parents should be taught and given educational material to help them detect potential sources of hidden food allergens by appropriately reading food labels. Education of the patient and family is vital to the success of the elimination diet. Families should be given instructional material to help them remember what foods contain the allergen they are to avoid. As shown in Fig. 1, it is often difficult to determine what foods will contain an allergen without careful reading of the label. Studies in both children and adults indicate that symptomatic reactivity to food allergens is often lost over time, except possibly for peanuts, nuts, and seafood (56).

Symptomatic reactivity to food allergens is generally very specific. Patients rarely react to more than one member of a botanical family or animal species. Importantly, initiation of an elimination diet totally excluding only foods identified to provoke food allergic reactions will result in symptomatic improvement. This treatment generally will lead to resolution of the food allergy within a few years and is unlikely to induce malnutrition or other eating disorders.

VII. SALIENT POINTS

1. Adverse food reactions may be secondary to food allergy (hypersensitivity) or food intolerance. A food allergic reaction results from an immunologic response after the ingestion of a food, while food intolerance is the result of nonimmunologic mechanisms.

2. Foods are composed of proteins, carbohydrates, and lipids. In general, the major food allergens that have been identified are water-soluble glycoproteins that have molecular weights ranging from 10,000 to 60,000 daltons (naturally

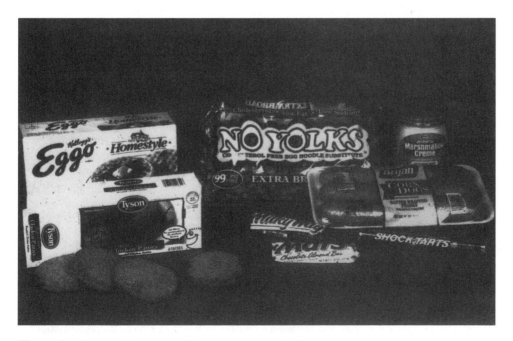

Figure 1 Groups of foods containing an unsuspected allergen, egg.

occurring 150,000 to 200,000 daltons). They are often stable to treatment with heat, acid, and proteases. However, other physicochemical properties that account for their unique allergenicity are poorly understood.

3. The major foods causing allergic reactions in different age groups are as follows:

Children	Adults
milk	peanuts
egg	tree nuts
peanuts	fish
soybeans	shellfish
wheat	
fish	
tree nuts	

4. Studies of the possible clinical cross-reactivity among various members of the legume family have shown that it is uncommon for patients to react in oral challenge to more than one legume. This is not to say that patients with peanut-specific IgE will not have clinical reactions to other legumes, but these reactions will be quite uncommon and should be evaluated on an individual basis.

5. Through a series of studies, it has been determined that a profilin (14 kDa) is responsible for the cross-reactivity between a variety of fruits and vegetables.

6. Several pieces of information are important to establish that a food allergic reaction occurred: (1) the food suspected to have provoked the reaction, (2) the quantity of the food ingested, (3) the length of time between ingestion and development of symptoms, (4) a description of the symptoms provoked, (5) if similar symptoms developed on other occasions when the food was eaten, (6) if other factors (e.g., exercise) are necessary, and (7) the length of time since the last reaction.

7. A positive skin test to a food indicates the possibility that the patient has symptomatic reactivity to that specific food (overall positive predictive accuracy is less than 50%). A negative skin test confirms the absence of an IgE-mediated reaction (overall negative predictive accuracy is greater than 95%).

8. A CAP-FEIA for specific food allergies is useful for patients with a positive prick skin test to diagnose patients with food allergy.

9. The presumptive diagnosis of food allergy based on a patient's history and prick skin tests or RAST results is not acceptable. There are exceptions to this, such as patients with severe anaphylaxis following the isolated ingestion of a specific food, as noted above. It is important that the physician make an unequivocal diagnosis of food allergy.

REFERENCES

1. Anderson JA, Sogn DD. Adverse food reactions that involve or are suspected of involving immune mechanisms: An anatomical categorization. American Academy of Allergy and Immunology Committee on Adverse Reactions to Foods. Washington, D.C.: National Institute of Allergy and Infectious Diseases, 1984: 43–102.

2. May CD. Objective clinical and laboratory studies of immediate hypersensitivity reactions to foods in asthmatic children. J Allergy Clin Immunol 1976, 58(4):500–515.

3. Sloan AE, Powers ME. A perspective on popular perceptions of adverse reactions to foods. J Allergy Clin Immunol 1986; 78(1 Pt 2):127–133.

4. Bock SA. Prospective appraisal of complaints of adverse reactions to foods in children during the first 3 years of life. Pediatrics 1987; 79(5):683–688.

5. Lemanske RF Jr, Taylor SL. Standardized extracts, foods. Clin Rev Allergy 1987; 5(1):23–36.

6. Strobel S, Mowat AM. Immune responses to dietary antigens: Oral tolerance. Immunol Today 1998; 19(4):173–181.

7. Host A, Halken S. A prospective study of cow milk allergy in Danish infants during the first 3 years of life: Clinical course in relation to clinical and immunological type of hypersensitivity reaction. Allergy 1990; 45(8):587–596.

8. May CD, Remigio L, Feldman J, Bock SA, Carr RI. A study of serum antibodies to isolated milk proteins and ovalbumin in infants and children. Clin Allergy 1977; 7(6):583–595.

9. May CD, Alberto R. In-vitro responses of leucocytes to food proteins in allergic and normal children: Lymphocyte stimulation and histamine release. Clin Allergy 1972; 2(4):335–344.

10. Gjesing B, Osterballe O, Schwartz B, Wahn U, Lowenstein H. Allergen-specific IgE antibodies against antigenic components in cow milk and milk substitutes. Allergy 1986; 41(1):51–56.

11. Busse PJ, Jarvinen KM, Vila L, Beyer K, Sampson HA. Identification of sequential IgE-binding epitopes on bovine alpha(s2)-casein in cow's milk allergic patients. Int Arch Allergy Immunol 2002; 129(1):93–96.

12. Jarvinen KM, Chatchatee P, Bardina L, Beyer K, Sampson HA. IgE and IgG binding epitopes on alpha-lactalbumin and beta-lactoglobulin in cow's milk allergy. Int Arch Allergy Immunol 2001; 126(2):111–118.

13. Jarvinen KM, Beyer K, Vila L, Chatchatee P, Busse PJ, Sampson HA. B-cell epitopes as a screening instrument for persistent cow's milk allergy. J Allergy Clin Immunol 2002; 110(2):293–297.

14. Chatchatee P, Jarvinen KM, Bardina L, Beyer K, Sampson HA. Identification of IgE- and IgG-binding epitopes on alpha(s1)-casein: Differences in patients with persistent and transient cow's milk allergy. J Allergy Clin Immunol 2001; 107(2):379–383.

15. Anet J, Back JF, Baker RS, Barnett D, Burley RW, Howden ME. Allergens in the white and yolk of hen's egg: A study of IgE binding by egg proteins. Int Arch Allergy Appl Immunol 1985; 77(3):364–371.

16. Hoffman DR. Immunochemical identification of the allergens in egg white. J Allergy Clin Immunol 1983; 71(5):481–486.

17. Bernhisel-Broadbent J, Dintzis HM, Dintzis RZ, Sampson HA. Allergenicity and antigenicity of chicken egg ovomucoid (Gal d III) compared with ovalbumin (Gal d I) in children with egg allergy and in mice. J Allergy Clin Immunol 1994; 93(6):1047–1059.

18. Mine Y, Wei ZJ. Identification and fine mapping of IgG and IgE epitopes in ovomucoid. Biochem Biophys Res Commun 2002; 292(4):1070–1074.

19. Burks AW, Cockrell G, Stanley JS, Helm RM, Bannon GA. Recombinant peanut allergen Ara h I expression and IgE binding in patients with peanut hypersensitivity. J Clin Invest 1995; 96(4):1715–1721.

20. Rabjohn P, West CM, Connaughton C, Sampson HA, Helm RM, Burks AW et al. Modification of peanut allergen Ara h 3: Effects on IgE binding and T cell stimulation. Int Arch Allergy Immunol 2002; 128(1):15–23.

21. Rabjohn P, Helm EM, Stanley JS, West CM, Sampson HA, Burks AW et al. Molecular cloning and epitope analysis of the peanut allergen Ara h 3. J Clin Invest 1999; 103(4):535–542.

22. Burks AW Jr, Brooks JR, Sampson HA. Allergenicity of major component proteins of soybean determined by enzyme-linked immunosorbent assay (ELISA) and immunoblotting in children with atopic dermatitis and positive soy challenges. J Allergy Clin Immunol 1988; 81(6):1135–1142.

23. Ogawa A, Samoto M, Takahashi K. Soybean allergens and hypoallergenic soybean products. J Nutr Sci Vitaminol (Tokyo) 2000; 46(6):271–279.

24. Ogawa T, Tsuji H, Bando N, Kitamura K, Zhu YL, Hirano H et al. Identification of the soybean allergenic protein, Gly m Bd 30K, with the soybean seed 34-kDa oil-body-associated protein. Biosci Biotechnol Biochem 1993; 57(6):1030–1033.

25. Sutton R, Hill DJ, Baldo BA, Wrigley CW. Immunoglobulin E antibodies to ingested cereal flour components: Studies with sera from subjects with asthma and eczema. Clin Allergy 1982; 12(1):63–74.

26. Jones SM, Magnolfi CF, Cooke SK, Sampson HA. Immunologic cross-reactivity among cereal grains and grasses in children with food hypersensitivity. J Allergy Clin Immunol 1995; 96(3):341–351.

27. James JM, Helm RM, Burks AW, Lehrer SB. Comparison of pediatric and adult IgE antibody binding to fish proteins. Ann Allergy Asthma Immunol 1997; 79(2):131–137.

28. Aas K. Studies of hypersensitivity to fish: A clinical study. Int Arch Allergy Appl Immunol 1966; 29(4):346–363.

29. Elsayed S, Apold J. Immunochemical analysis of cod fish allergen M: Locations of the immunoglobulin binding sites as demonstrated by the native and synthetic peptides. Allergy 1983; 38:449–459.

30. Nordlee JA, Taylor SL, Townsend JA, Thomas LA, Bush RK. Identification of a Brazil-nut allergen in transgenic soybeans. N Engl J Med 1996; 334(11):688–692.

31. Robotham JM, Teuber SS, Sathe SK, Roux KH. Linear IgE epitope mapping of the English walnut (Juglans regia) major food allergen, Jug r 1. J Allergy Clin Immunol 2002; 109(1):143–149.

32. Lehrer SB, Ibanez MD, McCants ML, Daul CB, Morgan JE. Characterization of water-soluble shrimp allergens released during boiling. J Allergy Clin Immunol 1990; 85(6):1005–1013.

33. Daul CB, Morgan JE, Waring NP, McCants ML, Hughes J, Lehrer SB. Immunologic evaluation of shrimp-allergic individuals. J Allergy Clin Immunol 1987; 80(5):716–722.

34. Teuber SS, Jarvis KC, Dandekar AM, Peterson WR, Ansari AA. Identification and cloning of a complementary DNA encoding a vicilin-like proprotein, jug r 2, from english walnut kernel (Juglans regia), a major food allergen. J Allergy Clin Immunol 1999; 104(6):1311–1320.

35. Reese G, Ayuso R, Leong-Kee SM, Plante MJ, Lehrer SB. Characterization and identification of allergen epitopes: Recombinant peptide libraries and synthetic, overlapping peptides. J Chromatogr B Biomed Sci Appl 2001; 756(1–2):157–163.

36. Bernhisel-Broadbent J, Sampson HA. Cross-allergenicity in the legume botanical family in children with food hypersensitivity. J Allergy Clin Immunol 1989; 83(2 Pt 1):435–440.

37. Bernhisel-Broadbent J, Scanlon SM, Sampson HA. Fish hypersensitivity. I. In vitro and oral challenge results in fish-allergic patients. J Allergy Clin Immunol 1992; 89(3):730–737.

38. Lehrer SB, Helbling A, Daul CB. Seafood allergy: Prevalence and treatment. J Food Safety 1992; 13:61.

39. Bock SA, Atkins FM. The natural history of peanut allergy. J Allergy Clin Immunol 1989; 83(5):900–904.

40. Sampson HA. Food allergy. J Allergy Clin Immunol 1989; 84(6 Pt 2):1062–1067.

41. Sampson HA, McCaskill CC. Food hypersensitivity and atopic dermatitis: Evaluation of 113 patients. J Pediatr 1985; 107(5):669–675.

42. Mandallaz M, DeWeck AL, Dahinden C. Bird-egg syndrome: Cross-reactivity between bird antigens and egg-yolk livetins in IgE-mediated hypersensitivity. Int Arch Allergy Immunol 1988; 87:143–150.

43. Werfel SJ, Cooke SK, Sampson HA. Clinical reactivity to beef in children allergic to cow's milk. J Allergy Clin Immunol 1997; 99(3):293–300.

44. Dreborg S, Foucard T. Allergy to apple, carrot and potato in children with birch pollen allergy. Allergy 1983; 38(3):167–172.

45. Valenta R, Duchene M, Ebner C, Valent P, Sillaber C, Deviller P et al. Profilins constitute a novel family of functional plant pan-allergens. J Exp Med 1992; 175(2):377–385.

46. van Ree R, Voitenko V, Van Leeuwen WA, Aalberse RC. Profilin is a cross-reactive allergen in pollen and vegetable foods. Int Arch Allergy Immunol 1992; 98(2):97–101.

47. Blanco C, Carrillo T, Castillo R, Quiralte J, Cuevas M. Latex allergy: Clinical features and cross-reactivity with fruits. Ann Allergy 1994; 73(4):309–314.

48. Sampson HA, Scanlon SM. Natural history of food hypersensitivity in children with atopic dermatitis. J Pediatr 1989; 115(1):23–27.

49. Sampson HA. Role of immediate food hypersensitivity in the pathogenesis of atopic dermatitis. J Allergy Clin Immunol 1983; 71(5):473–480.

50. Sampson HA. Comparative study of commercial food antigen extracts for the diagnosis of food hypersensitivity. J Allergy Clin Immunol 1988; 82(5 Pt 1):718–726.

51. Bock SA, Buckley J, Holst A, May CD. Proper use of skin tests with food extracts in diagnosis of hypersensitivity to food in children. Clin Allergy 1977; 7(4):375–383.

52. Sampson HA, Albergo R. Comparison of results of skin tests, RAST, and double-blind, placebo-controlled food challenges in children with atopic dermatitis. J Allergy Clin Immunol 1984; 74(1):26–33.

53. Sampson HA. Utility of food-specific IgE concentrations in predicting symptomatic food allergy. J Allergy Clin Immunol 2001; 107(5):891–896.

54. Yizinger JW, Sweeney KG, Sturner WQ, Giannandrea LA, Teigland JD, Bray M et al. Fatal food-induced anaphylaxis. JAMA 1988; 260(10):1450–1452.

55. Burks AW, Mallory SB, Williams LW, Shirrell MA. Atopic dermatitis: Clinical relevance of food hypersensitivity reactions. J Pediatr 1988; 113(3):447–451.

56. Bock SA. The natural history of food sensitivity. J Allergy Clin Immunol 1982; 69(2):173–177.

18

Hymenoptera Allergens

TE PIAO KING

Rockefeller University, New York, New York, U.S.A.

MILES GURALNICK

Vespa Laboratories, Inc., Spring Mills, Pennsylvania, U.S.A.

I. INTRODUCTION

Many insects can cause allergy in man (Table 1) (1). People can be exposed to insect body parts or their secretions by inhalation, to their venoms by stinging, and to their salivary gland secretions by biting. Examples of these routes of sensitization are, respectively, allergies to cockroaches of the order Orthoptera, to ants, bees, and vespids of the order Hymenoptera, and to flies and mosquitos of the order Diptera.

The importance of venoms as the allergen source in Hymenoptera allergy has been known for some time (2,3). All known insect venom allergens are proteins of 10–50 kDa containing 100–400 amino acid residues. The one exception is that the bee venom allergen melittin is a 26-residue peptide. But melittin is a minor allergen, active in less than one-third of bee-allergic patients (4). Nearly all these allergens have been

Table 1 Insects Reported to Cause Allergy in Man[a]

Order Coleoptera—beetles
Order Diptera—flies and mosquitos
Order Ephemeroptera—mayflies
Order Hemiptera—aphids, bed bugs, and kissing bugs
Order Hymenoptera—ants, bees, and vespids
Order Lepidoptera—moths and caterpillars
Order Orthoptera—cockroaches
Order Siphonaptera—fleas
Order Trichoptera—caddis flies

[a] *Source:* Ref. 1.

sequenced and/or cloned. Several of these allergens have been expressed in bacteria, insect, or yeast cells.

This chapter will review the immunochemical properties of known hymenopteran venom proteins and peptides and their relevance to our understanding and treatment of insect allergy.

II. TAXONOMY, GEOGRAPHIC DISTRIBUTION, AND IDENTIFICATION OF HYMENOPTERAN INSECTS

Essentially all insects responsible for causing insect sting allergic reactions belong to the order Hymenoptera. This is a large and diverse order comprising over 70 families (5) with over 100,000 species (6). Although many Hymenoptera are capable of stinging, only species belonging to three families sting people with a high degree of frequency. The usual perpetrators are social insects and belong to either the Apidae (bees), Formicidae (ants), or Vespidae (wasps). The medically important genera and their geographic distributions are outlined in Table 2. Four of these insects are shown in a photograph in Fig. 1.

Accurate identification of social stinging Hymenoptera to species level is a difficult task even for most entomologists. Although not definitive, there are several behavioral characteristics that can help provide clues as to a specimen's identity. For example, honeybees have a unique sting anatomy that causes worker bees to leave their sting apparatuses in the victim's skin. Although sting autotomy is almost exclusively attributed to honeybees, other stinging Hymenoptera will occasionally lose their sting. Conversely, honeybees will occasionally sting without autotomizing (7). Annoying wasps foraging around picnic foods, garbage, or fallen fruit are usually yellowjackets and belong to the genus *Vespula*. Large colonies of wasps living in subterranean nests are also usually of the genus *Vespula* (1). Since there are notable exceptions to the above, the only reliable means of obtaining a positive identification is to collect a specimen and have its identity determined by an entomologist with expertise in the social Hymenoptera.

III. BIOCHEMICAL STUDIES OF HYMENOPTERA VENOM PROTEIN ALLERGENS

Table 3 lists the venom protein allergens of bees, fire ants, and vespids that have been sequenced and/or cloned.

Table 2 Geographic Distribution and Medical Importance of Some Insects of Hymenoptera Order

Family/ subfamily	Genus and species	Common name	Geographic distribution within U.S.	Medical importance
Apidae/Apinae	*Apis mellifera*	honeybee	entire U.S.	major
	Bombus pennsylvanicus	bumblebee	entire U.S.	moderate
Formicidae/ Myrimicinae	*Solenopsis invicta*	fire ant	SE	major
	Solenopsis richteri	fire ant	Mississippi, Alabama	moderate
Vespidae/ Vespinae	*Vespa crabo*	European hornet	NE,SE	minor
	Dolichovespula maculata	white-face hornet (bald-face hornet)	entire U.S.	major
	Dolichovespula arenaria	yellow hornet (aerial yellow jacket)	NE,NW,SW	major
	Vespula flavopilosa	yellow jacket	NE,SE	major
	Vespula germanica	yellow jacket	NE	major
	Vespula maculifrons	yellow jacket	NE,E	major
	Vespula pennsylvanica	yellow jacket	NW,SW	major
	Vespula vulgaris	yellow jacket	NE,NW,SW	major
	Vespula squamosa	yellow jacket	NE,SE	major
	Vespula vidua	yellow jacket	NE	moderate
Polistinae	*Polistes annularis*	paper wasp	entire U.S.	major
	Polistes exclamans	paper wasp	entire U.S.	major
	Polistes fuscatas	paper wasp	entire U.S.	major

Only insects with known venom allergens are listed.
Data for geographic distribution and medical importance are taken from Ref. 1.

Vespid venoms each contain three to four known protein allergens. Three of them have been isolated from all vespids studied; they are antigen 5 of unknown biological function, hyaluronidase, and phospholipase A_1. The fourth one is a protease, and it has been characterized only from paper wasps.

Fire ant venom contains four known protein allergens: Sol i 1 to 4. Sol i 1 and 3 are homologous with vespid phospholipase and antigen 5, respectively (10).

Bumblebee venom has two protein allergens of known sequences: phospholipase A_2 and a protease. Honeybee venom has five allergens of known sequences. Four are proteins—acid phosphatase, hyaluronidase, phospholipase A_2, and protease—and the fifth one is a cytolytic peptide, melittin. The two bee venom phospholipases A_2 have sequence identity with each other but are not related to vespid phospholipase A_1 (12,19). Honeybee venom hyaluronidase has about 55% sequence identity with vespid hyaluronidases (14,19,30).

Several venom allergens have partial sequence identity with other proteins from diverse sources, and this is summarized in Table 4. As an example, the sequence identities of three vespid antigen 5s, fire ant antigen 5 (Sol i 3), human and mouse testis proteins, human glioma protein, and proteins from tomato, nematode, and lizard, in their C-terminal

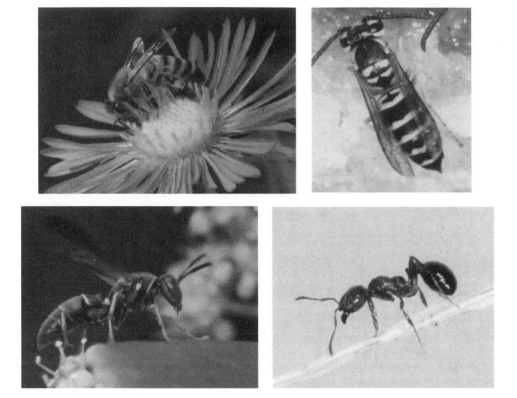

Figure 1 Common stinging insects. The photos, starting from top left and going clockwise, show respectively honeybee (*Apis mellifer*), yellow jacket (*Vespula maculifrons*), paper wasp (*Polistes fuscatus*), and fire ant (*Solenopsis invicta*). The approximate lengths of these insects in the order given are 16, 10, 19, and 3 mm. The photos are of different magnifications.

50-residue region, are given in Fig. 2. We may note in particular the partial sequence identity of venom allergens with proteins of male reproductive functions, antigen 5s with a mammalian testis protein (15), hyaluronidases with those from mammalian sperm and other tissues, phosphatase with a prostate enzyme (10), and protease with mammalian acrosin (12).

X-ray crystallography was used to determine the structures of bee venom hyaluronidase (39) and phospholipase A_2 (40) and that of antigen 5 from yellow jacket, *V. vulgaris* (41). Vespid phospholipase A_1 has sequence homology with porcine pancreatic lipase (38). As the structure of porcine lipase is known, the structure of vespid phospholipase can be obtained by modeling. Using the modeling approach, the structures of nearly all the proteins in Table 3 can be obtained.

The structures of a number of allergen proteins from different sources have been determined. No unusual structural features of these protein allergens are known (42).

IV. RECOMBINANT HYMENOPTERA VENOM PROTEIN ALLERGENS

Several of the allergens in Table 3 have been expressed in bacteria, insect, or yeast cells to yield recombinant proteins. The recombinant proteins that are expressed in the cytoplasm

Table 3 Some Insect Venom Allergens with Known Sequences and Structures

Allergen name[a]	Common name	Mol. size[b]	Structure[c]	Recombinant protein[d] Unfolded	Folded	References
		Honeybee, *Apis melifera*				
Api m 1[e]	Phospholipase A$_2$	16 kDa	++	+	+	8
Api m 2	Hyaluronidase	39 kDa	++	+	+	9
Api m 3	Acid phosphatase	43 kDa	–	–	–	10
	Protease					11
		Bumblebee, *Bombus pennsylvanicus*				
Bom p 1[e]	Phospholipase A$_2$	16 kDa	+	–	–	12
Bom p 4	Protease	28 kDa	–	–	–	12
		White-face hornet, *Dolichovespula maculata*				
Dol m 1	Phospholipase A$_1$	34 kDa	+	+	–	13
Dol m 2	Hyaluronidase	38 kDa	+	+	–	14
Dol m 5[f]	Antigen 5	23 kDa	+	+	+	15, 16
		European hornet, *Vespa crabo*				
Vesp c 1	Phospholipase A$_1$	34 kDa	+	–	–	10
Vesp c 5	Antigen 5	23 kDa	+	–	–	17
		Paper wasp, *Polistes annularis*				
Pol a 1	Phospholipase A$_1$	34 kDa	+	–	–	18
Pol a 2	Hyaluronidase	38 kDa	+	–	–	18
Pol a 5	Antigen 5	23 kDa	+	+	+	15
	Protease[g]					
		Yellow jacket, *Vespula vulgaris*				
Ves v 1[h]	Phospholipase A$_1$	34 kDa	+	+	–	19
Ves v 2	Hyaluronidase	38 kDa	+	+	–	19
Ves v 5	Antigen 5	23 kDa	++	+	+	20
		Fire ant, *Solenopsis invicta*				
Sol i 1	Phospholipase	37 kDa	+	–	–	10
Sol i 2		30 kDa	–	–	+	10, 21
Sol i 3	Antigen 5	23 kDa	+	–	+	22
Sol i 4		20 kDa	–	–	–	22

[a] Allergen names are designated according to an accepted nomenclature system (23).

[b] Several allergens are glycoproteins, and the molecular size given refers only to the protein portion.

[c] ++ and + signs refer respectively to structures determined directly or by modeling of structures of homologous proteins.

[d] + and – signs refer to the availability of recombinant proteins.

[e] Sequences of phospholipases A$_2$ from *A. crena, A. dorsata* (24), and *B. terrestris* (25) are known.

[f] Known sequences of other vespid antigen 5s are *D. arenaria, P. exclamans*, and *P. fuscatas* (15); *P. dominulus* (26); *V. flavopilosa, V. germanica, V. maculifrons, V. pensylvanica, V. squamosa*, and *V. vidua* (17); and *V. mandarinia* (27).

[g] Cloning of proteases from *P. dominulus* and *P. exclamans* were reported (28).

[h] Sequence of phospholipase A$_1$ from *V. maculifrons* is known (29).

of bacteria are usually unfolded, as they lack the disulfide bonds of the natural proteins and do not have the native conformation of the natural proteins. The cytoplasm of bacteria is a reducing environment, and any disulfide bonds that do form are reduced through the action of disulfide-reducing enzymes. Several recombinant proteins with disulfide bonds have been obtained in mutants of *E. coli* with decreased disulfide-reducing enzymes in their cytoplasm (43). In some cases, the unfolded recombinant proteins can be folded and

Table 4 Sequence Identity of Insect Allergens and Other Proteins

Insect allergens	Other proteins	Residues compared	% identity	References
Antigen 5s	Mammalian testis protein	130	35	31
	Human glioma PR protein	124	23	32
	Hookworm protein[a]	130	28	33
	Plant leaf PR protein[b]	130	28	35
	Mexican lizard toxin	130	28	35
Hyaluronidase	Mammalian sperm protein	331	50	30
Phosphatase	Mammalian phosphatase	343	16	10
Phospholipase A$_1$	Mammalian lipases	123	40	36
Phospholipase A$_2$	Mammalian phospholipases	129	20	
Protease	Mammalian acrosin	243	38	10
	Horseshoe crab enzyme	243	41	10

[a] Homologous worm proteins are present in other nematodes (cf 34).
[b] Homologous plant PR proteins are present in tobacco, tomato, barley, and maize (cf 35).

```
Dol m 5      VGHYTQMVWG KTKEIGCGSI KYIE.DNWYT H....YLVCN YGPGGNDFNQ
Pol a 5      IGHYTQMVWG KTKEIGCGSL KYME.NNMQN H....YLICN YGPAGNYLGQ
Ves v 5      TGHYTQMVWA NTKEVGCGSI KYIQ.EKWHK H....YLVCN YGPSGNFMNE
Sol i 3      VEHYTQIVWA KTSKIGCARI MFKEPDNWTK H....YLVCN YGPAGNVLGA
human tpx    VGHYTQLVWY STYQVGCGIA YCPNQDSLKY .....YYVCQ YCPAGNNMNR
mouse tpx    VGHYTQLVWY SSFKIGCGIA YCPNQDNLKY .....FYVCH YCPMGNNVMK
hum glioma   CGHYTQVVWA DSYKVGCAVQ FCPKVSGFDA LSNGAHFICN YGPGGNYPTW
tomato pr    CGHYTQVVWR NSVRVGCARV QC....NNGG Y....VVSCN YDPPGNYRGE
hookworm     IGHYTQMAWD TTYKLGCAVV FC....NDFT .....FGVCQ YGPGGNYMGH
lizard       IGHYTQVVWY RSYELGCAIA YCPDQPTYKY .....YQVCQ YCPGGNIRSR
```

Figure 2 Sequence identity of vespid antigen 5s and other proteins in their C-terminal region. The sequences shown from top to bottom are for antigen 5s from hornet, paper wasp, yellow jacket, and fire ant venoms, human and mouse testis-specific proteins, human glioma protein, tomato leaf pathogenesis-related protein, hookworm protein, and lizard venom protein, respectively. References for these proteins are given in Table 4. Bold characters indicate residues identical to those of vespid antigen 5s, and dots indicate blanks added for maximal alignment of sequences. The underlined peptide region was found to contain a dominant T-cell epitope of vespid antigen 5 (see text).

oxidized in vitro into their native conformation, e.g., bee venom hyaluronidase Api m 2, and phospholipase A$_2$ Api m 1 (8,30).

Recombinant proteins from insect or yeast cells have the native conformation of the natural proteins as they are folded during secretion into medium, e.g., Api m 2 (9), Sol i 2 (21), and vespid antigen 5s (16,20).

Recombinant allergens have many different applications. One application is for use as diagnostic reagents. For example, recombinant yellow jacket antigen 5 was used to show the frequency of patient response to three yellow jacket venom allergens. Ninety percent of the 26 patients tested were positive to antigen 5, and 70–80% were positive to hyaluronidase and phospholipase (44).

Another application is to prepare allergen hybrids with reduced allergenicity while retaining its immunogenicity. The hybrids contain a small segment of the guest allergen of interest and a large segment of a host protein. The host protein is homologous to the guest allergen, and they are poorly cross reactive as antigens. The host protein functions as a scaffold to hold the segment of the guest allergen in its native conformation, as homologous proteins of >30% sequence identity can have closely similar structures. In this way, the hybrids retain the discontinuous epitopes of the guest allergen but at a reduced density.

The above approach was demonstrated with hybrids of yellow jacket and wasp antigen 5s (45). These two antigens 5s have 59% sequence identity and are poorly cross-reactive in patients or in animals. Hybrids with 1/4 of yellow jacket antigen 5 and 3/4 of wasp antigen 5 showed 10^2–10^3-fold reduction in allergenicity when tested by histamine release assay in yellow jacket–sensitive patients. These hybrids retained the immunogenicity of antigen 5s for antibody responses specific for the native protein and for T-cell responses in mice. Therefore, the hybrids may be useful vaccines, as they may be used at higher doses than the natural allergen.

V. B-CELL EPITOPES OF HYMENOPTERA VENOM PROTEIN ALLERGENS

B-cell epitopes of proteins are of two types, continuous and discontinuous, and their sizes range from 6–17 amino acid residues. The continuous type consists of only contiguous amino acid residues in the molecule, while the discontinuous type consists of contiguous as well as noncontiguous residues which are brought together in the folded molecule. The majority of protein-specific antibodies, 90% or more, are of the discontinuous type. This is the case for venom allergen-specific IgEs in patients by comparative tests with natural or disulfide bond–reduced allergens, e.g., bee venom phospholipase A_2 (8) and fire ant Sol i 2 (21). Studies have shown that the same B-cell epitopes can induce both IgE and IgG responses.

Data in agreement with the above generalization were obtained with vespid allergen-specific mouse antisera, which contain mainly specific IgGs. Comparison of the data in Table 5 shows that vespid allergen-specific antisera bind natural allergens and bind poorly, if at all, reduced and unfolded allergens, which lack the discontinuous epitopes of the folded molecules. This is particularly the case for vespid hyaluronidases and phospholipases (14,19) and to a lesser extent for vespid antigen 5s (15,46).

Data in Table 5 also show that disulfide bond–reduced allergen-specific sera are more sensitive in the detection of antigenic cross-reactivities of homologous allergens than natural allergen-specific sera. This difference may result from the relative abundance of antibodies specific for continuous and discontinuous epitopes and/or the accessibility of epitopes in the disulfide bond–reduced allergen. The extent of cross-reactivity of the homologous allergens from hornets, yellow jackets, and paper wasps parallels their sequence identity in the order of hyaluronidases > antigen 5s > phospholipases. The data taken together suggest that there is greater cross-reactivity of these proteins from hornets and yellow jackets than those from paper wasps and yellow jackets.

The continuous B-cell epitopes can be mapped readily with a series of overlapping peptides of 7–20 residues in length. Multiple epitopes were found for the 204-residue hornet antigen 5, and only one was found for the 26-residue bee venom melittin (47). No unusual pattern of amino acid sequence was observed for these B-cell epitopes. Other studies have shown that the same B-cell epitopes can induce both IgE and IgG responses.

Bee venom phospholipase A_2 is a glycoprotein. Its oligosaccharide side chain has been demonstrated to function as a B-cell epitope for IgE and IgG responses in patients as

Table 5 Cross-reactivity of Vespid Allergens Detected with Natural or Reduced Allergen-Specific Mouse Sera

Solid-phase antigen 5	Natural or reduced antigen 5–specific sera								
	Hornet			Yellow jacket			Wasp		
Hornet	++	++	++	+	+	nd	+	–	nd
Yellow jacket	+	+	+	++	++	nd	±	–	nd
Wasp	+	+	+	+	+	nd	++	+	nd
Solid-phase hyaluronidase	Natural or reduced hyaluronidase-specific sera								
	Hornet			Yellow jacket			Wasp		
Hornet	++	±	++	++	+	++	±	–	nd
Yellow jacket	++	–	++	++	++	++	±	–	nd
Wasp	++	–	–	+	+	+	++	–	nd
Solid-phase phospholipase	Natural or reduced phospholipase-specific sera								
	Hornet			Yellow jacket			Wasp		
Hornet	++	±	++	–	–	+	–	–	+
Yellow jacket	±	–	+	++	±	++	±	–	+
Wasp	±	nd	–	±	nd	±	++	–	++

1. For each sera, there are three columns of results. The first column is from ELISA of natural allergen-specific sera on solid-phase natural allergen, and the second and third columns are from immunoblots of reduced allergen probed with natural allergen-specific or reduced allergen-specific sera, respectively.
2. The ++, +, ±, and – signs refer to relative titers of sera on ELISA, or intensities of bands on immunoblots when compared with that of the immunogen.
3. "nd" denotes not done.

well as in animals (48). Oligosaccharide side chains of closely similar sequences to that of bee venom protein are present in plant proteins, and this may be one explanation for the cross-reactivity of glycosylated allergens from diverse sources.

VI. T-CELL EPITOPES OF HYMENOPTERA VENOM PROTEIN ALLERGENS

T-cell epitopes are of interest because of the central role of T-cells in regulating the antibody class switch event of B-cells. This approach was tested recently in patients with T-cell peptides of bee venom phospholipase A_2 (49).

T-cell epitopes are peptides of about 15 residues in length formed following intracellular processing of antigens by antigen-presenting cells, and they do not depend on the secondary or tertiary structure of the antigen. This is the case with venom allergens as shown by the identical T-cell–stimulating activities of natural or recombinant allergens or reduced allergens, e.g., vespid antigen 5s, hyaluronidases, and phospholipases A_1 (19,46).

Bee venom phospholipase A_2 and hornet antigen 5 are found to have multiple T-cell epitopes distributed throughout the entire molecule by tests with a series of overlapping peptides in patients (50,51) or in mice (52,53). Because of MHC class II restriction, patients of different polymorphic background, or mice of different haplotypes, differ in their pattern of peptide recognition. Nonetheless, both insect allergens were found to have several dominant T-cell epitopes recognized by nearly all patients or mice tested.

One T-cell epitope–containing peptide of bee venom phospholipase was found to require the presence of its carbohydrate side chain for its activity (54).

No unusual features were observed for the dominant T-cell epitope peptides of insect venom allergens. Others have reported similar findings for T-cell epitopes of allergens from grass and tree pollens, cat dander, mites, and chicken ovalbumin (55). Both normal and atopic people were found to recognize the same T-cell epitope peptides of bee venom phospholipase (51) and the major birch pollen allergen (56); this was also shown for their IgG antibody responses.

One of the dominant T-cell epitope peptides of hornet antigen 5 was found to cross-react with a homologous peptide of a mouse testis protein. The cross-reactivity is not reciprocal as the corresponding peptide from mouse testis protein did not cross-react with hornet antigen 5–specific cells (57). When male or female mice were immunized with hornet antigen 5, indistinguishable antibody titers were obtained. The cross-reacting T-cell epitope peptide sequence of hornet antigen 5 is underlined in Fig. 2. It can be seen that there is a high degree of sequence identity in this region for vespid and fire ant antigen 5s, human and mouse testis-specific proteins, and hookworm, plant, and lizard proteins.

VII. ANTIGENIC CROSS-REACTIVITY OF HYMENOPTERA VENOMS

Insect-allergic patients often have sensitivity to multiple insects by skin test or RAST with venoms (3). This multiple sensitivity can be due to exposure to different insects and/or antigenic cross-reactivity of different venoms. This issue of multiple exposure or antigenic cross-reactivity is of importance in the choice of single or multiple venoms for immunotherapy of patients. RAST inhibition carried out with multiple venoms is one possible approach to resolve this issue of multiple sensitivity (58).

Bees, fire ants, and vespids each have unique as well as homologous venom allergens. One of the four known bee allergens is homologous to vespid hyaluronidases with about 50% sequence identity. Two of the four known fire ant allergens are homologous to vespid antigen 5s and phospholipases. Fire ant antigen 5 has about 35% sequence identity with vespid antigen 5s. Antigen 5s, or phospholipases, of hornets, yellow jackets, and wasps have 44–68% sequence identity, and their hyaluronidases have 73–92% sequence identity.

Protein allergens of different species within a species group of each genus generally have a higher degree of sequence identity than those of a different species group. For example, antigen 5s from five species of yellow jackets of the V. vulgaris group in Table 2 have about 95% sequence identity within the group and about 73% identity with antigen 5s of V. squamosa and V. rufa groups (17). Phospholipases A_1 from two species of yellow jackets, V. maculifrons and V. vulgaris, have 95% sequence identity and about 67% and 55% identity with white-face hornet and paper wasp proteins, respectively (13,19,29).

Data on the B- and T-cell epitopes of venom allergens, described in the preceding sections, indicate that cross-reactivity is detectable for homologous hyaluronidases of >90% sequence identity, and variable extents of cross-reactivity are detectable for homologous antigen 5s and phospholipases with about 70% sequence identity. The variable extents of cross-reactivity of antigen 5s and phospholipases probably reflect the degree of identity at the epitope sites.

The above considerations would indicate that sensitivity to multiple insects can be due to cross-reactivity of a single allergen, hyaluronidase in the case of bees and vespids or multiple allergens in other cases. For cross-reactivity of fire ants and vespids, or of different vespids, hyaluronidase again has the major role, with antigen 5 and phospholipase having secondary and negligent roles, respectively.

These considerations would also suggest that patients with sensitivity to multiple insects due to cross-reactivity of venoms be treated with the primary sensitizing venom. Treatment with a cross-reacting venom will provide immunity for only the venom being used and will not necessarily provide complete immunity for the sensitizing venom. Cross-reactivity of insect venoms and plant proteins due to their common oligosaccharide side chains is another example (59,60). Treatment of insect-allergic patients with cross-reactive plant proteins clearly will not result in immunity for insect proteins.

Several authors have reported that a sizable group of normal people who showed no clinical sensitivity to insects tested positive with insect venoms (61,62). These false-positive results may possibly represent cross-reactivity of insect venoms with other proteins to which people have been exposed. As noted earlier in Table 4, insect allergens have variable extents of sequence identity with proteins from diverse sources.

Investigators have observed that more men than women, in a ratio of about 2 to 1, had insect allergy as judged by their systemic and large local reactions or by their death statistics (63). It has been assumed that these results were primarily due to greater exposure because of work habits of men and women. Whether or not the partial sequence identity of venom allergens with proteins of male reproductive functions (Table 4) plays a role in these observations is not known.

VIII. BIOCHEMICAL STUDIES OF HYMENOPTERA VENOM PEPTIDES

In addition to proteins, hymenoptera venoms contain peptides, biogenic amines, such as histamine and dopamine, and other low-molecular-weight components (64). Table 6 lists the biological activities and the names of these venom peptides (65). These biological activities include mast cell degranulation, chemotaxis, kinin, and others. The most abundant peptides in bee and vespid venoms are melitin and mastoparan, respectively, and they have mast cell–degranulating activity. Bee venom contains another peptide, known as MCD, with a greater mast cell–degranulating activity than melitin.

Melitin and mastoparan are basic peptides with 26 and 14–15 residues, respectively. Both peptides were reported to be immunogenic in mice for antibody responses (66–68). Melitin was reported to be an allergen but not mastoparan (4).

Mastoparan was discovered for its activity to induce release of histamine and other mediators from mast cells (69). It binds to cell membranes (70,71) and it can act as a strong secretagogue for different cell types. For example, mastoparan is reported to stimulate the release of the inflammatory mediators TNF-α, IL-1β, nitrous oxide, and prostaglandin E_2 into peritoneal exudates of mice (72). These mediator releases are related to its diverse range of biochemical activities. They include stimulation of phospholipases A_2 (73), C (74), and D (75,76) and G-protein activation (77).

Mastoparan was found to have a weak adjuvant activity to enhance IgG1 and IgE responses to yellow jacket antigen 5 in mice (78). This adjuvant action may be related to its activity to induce the release of TH2 cell–associated mediators from basophils/mast cells, macrophages, and possibly other antigen-presenting cells. Melitin was not found to have adjuvant activity for Ves v 5–specific antibody response, although melitin has biological properties similar to mastoparan. Others found melitin to be an adjuvant for ovalbumin-specific IgE response in mice (66). The two different findings on melitin may

Table 6 Bioactive Peptides in Hymenoptera Venoms

Species	Kinin	Chemotaxis	Mast cell degranulation[a]	Others[a]
Apis mellifera	No	No	MCD	Melitin Apamin
Bombus spp.				Bombolitin
Polistes spp.	Yes	Yes	Mastoparan	
Vespa spp.	Yes	Yes	Mastoparan	Crabolin
Vespula spp.	Yes	Yes	Mastoparan	

[a] Peptide names are listed.

reflect that the experimental conditions used as IgE responses in mice are antigen-, dose-, and mice strain–dependent.

Yellow jacket venom was found to be lethal in mice when injected intraperitoneally but not subcutaneously (78). The toxic action was shown to require the synergistic action of the venom peptide mastoparan and the venom protein phospholipase A_1.

IX. STING REACTIONS

There are three types of reactions that individuals may experience from a Hymenoptera sting. The normal response is a *local cutaneous reaction* characterized by redness, swelling, and pain confined to the sting site. This is a toxic response. A *large local reaction* is thought to be IgE mediated and involves an extensive area of warmth, redness, and swelling contiguous with the site of the sting. Large local reactions typically develop in 1–3 days, may involve an entire extremity, and may persist for up to 5 days. An *allergic systemic reaction* usually occurs within half an hour of envenomization and includes symptoms remote from the site of the sting. Systemic allergic reactions may involve the skin, the respiratory system, the vascular system, or any combination thereof.

Minimal treatment is necessary for local cutaneous reactions. The sting site should be kept clean to avoid secondary infections, and ice packs may help to reduce local pain and swelling. Large local reactions may cause considerable discomfort and are frequently treated with analgesics, antihistamines, and glucocorticosteroids. Systemic allergic reactions can be quite serious and occasionally fatal.

X. SALIENT POINTS

1. The medically important stinging insects are fire ants, bees, and vespids (wasps). The vespids include hornets, paper wasps, and yellow jackets.
2. Insect venom allergens are proteins of 10–50 kDa. Nearly all known venom allergens have been cloned and expressed as recombinant proteins in different systems. However, some recombinant proteins are not properly folded.
3. Insect venom allergens have different biochemical functions. Their only known common feature is their partial sequence identity with proteins from other sources in our environment.
4. Each insect venom has unique allergen(s), as well as homologous allergen(s) with partial sequence identity.

5. Multiple sensitivity of patients to different insects, or to more closely related vespids, can be due to multiple exposures and/or antigenic cross-reactivity of venom allergen(s).
6. Detailed immunochemical knowledge of insect venom allergens is useful for monitoring the quality of insect venoms used for diagnosis and treatment and may lead to the development of new immunotherapeutic reagents.

REFERENCES

1. Guralnick MW, Benton AW. Entomological aspects of insect sting allergy. In: Levine M, Lockey R (eds). Monograph on Insect Allergy American Academy of Allergy and Immunology, Milwaukee, WI, 1995: 7–20.
2. Loveless MH, Fackeler WR. Wasp venom allergy and immunity. Ann Allergy 1995; 14:347–366.
3. Lichtenstein LM, Valentine MD, Sobotka AK. Insect Allergy: The state of the art. J Allergy Clin Immunol 1979; 64:5–12.
4. King TP, Sobotka AK, Kochoumian L, Lichtenstein LM. Allergens of honeybee venom. Arch Biochem Biophys 1976; 172:661–671.
5. Krombein KV, Hurd PV, Smith DR, Burks BD. Catalog of Hymenoptera in America North of Mexico. Washington, DC: Smithsonian Institute Press, 1979: v–vii.
6. Borror DJ, White RE. Sawflies, Ichneumons, Chalcids, Ants, Wasps, and Bees: Order Hymenoptera. Boston, MA: Houghton Mifflin Company, 1970: 312 p.
7. Mulfinger LM, Yorkinger JW, Styer WE, Guralnick MW, Lintner TJ. Sting mophology and frequency of sting autotomy among medically important vespids and the honey bee. J Med Entomol 1992; 29:325–328.
8. Dudler T, Chen W, Wang S, Schneider T, Annand RR, Dempcy RO, Crameri R, Gmachl M, Suter M, Gelb MH. High-level expression in Escherichia coli and rapid purification of enzymatically active honey bee venom phospholipase A2. Biochim Biophys Acta 1992; 1165:201–210.
9. Soldatova LN, Crameri R, Gmachl M, Kemeny DM, Schmidt M, Weber M, Mueller UR. Superior biologic activity of the recombinant bee venom allergen hyaluronidase expressed in baculovirus-infected insect cells as compared with Escherichia coli. J Allergy Clin Immunol 1998; 101:691–698.
10. Hoffman DR. Hymenoptera Venom Proteins. New York and London: Plenum Publishing Co., 1996; 169–186.
11. Winningham KM, Schmidt M, Hoffman DR. Honey bee venom allergy: Cloning of the Apis Mellifera venom protease J Allergy Clin Immunol 2001; 107:S221.
12. Hoffman DR, Jacobson RS. Allergens in Hymenoptera venom XXVII: Bumble bee venom allergy and allergens. J Allergy Clin Immunol 1996; 97:812–821.
13. Soldatova L, Kochoumian L, King TP. Sequence similarity of a hornet D. maculata venom allergen phospholipase A1 with mammalian lipases. FEBS Letters 1993; 320:145–149.
14. Lu G, Kochoumian L, King TP. Sequence identity and antigenic cross reactivity of white face hornet venom allergen, also a hyaluronidase, with other proteins. J Biol Chem 1995; 270:4457–4465.
15. Lu G. Villalba M, Coscia MR, Hoffman DR, King TP. Sequence analysis and antigen cross reactivity of a venom allergen antigen 5 from hornets, wasps and yellow jackets. J Immunol 1993; 150:2823–2830.
16. Tomalski MD, King TP, Miller LK. Expression of hornet genes encoding venom allergen antigen 5 in insects. Arch Insect Biochem Physiol 1993; 22:303–313.
17. Hoffman DR. Allergens in hymenoptera venom XXV: The amino acid sequences of antigen 5 molecules and the structural basis of antigenic cross-reactivity. J Allergy Clin Immunol 1993; 92:707–716.

18. King TP, Lu G. Genbank Accession No. AF174527 and AF174528, 1996.

19. King TP, Lu G, Gonzalez M, Qian NF, Soldatova L. Yellow jacket venom allergens, hyaluronidase and phospholipase: Sequence similarity and antigenic cross reactivity with their hornet and wasp homologs and possible implications for clinical allergy. J Allergy Clin Immunol 1996; 98:588–600.

20. Monsalve RI, Gang L, King TP. Recombinant venom allergen, antigen 5 of yellow jacket (Vespula vulgaris) and paper wasp (Polistes annularis) by expression in bacteria or yeast. Protein Expr Purif 1999; 16:410–416.

21. Schmidt M, McConnel TJ, Hofmann DR. Production of a recombinant imported fire ant venom allergen, Sol i 2, in native and immunoreactive form. J Allergy Clin Immunol 1996; 98:82–88.

22. Hoffman DR. Allergens in Hymenoptera venom XXIV: The amino acid sequences of imported fire ant venom allergens Sol i II, Sol i III and Sol i IV. J Allergy Clin Immunol 1995; 91:71–78.

23. King TP, Hoffman DR, Lowenstein H, Marsh DG, Platts-Mills TAE, Thomas WR. Allergen nomenclature. J Allergy Clin Immunol 1995; 96:5–14.

24. Hoffman DR, Schmidt JO. Phopholipases from Asian honeybees. J Allergy Clin Immunol 2000; 105:S56.

25. Hoffmann DR, El-Choufani E, Smith MM, de Groth H. Occupatinal allergy to bumblebees: Allergens of Bombus terrestris. J Allergy Clin Immunol 2001; 108:855–860.

26. Hoffman DR. Antigen 5 and phospholipase from Polistes dominulus differ significantly in amino acid sequence from those of North American Polistes venoms. J Allergy Clin Immunol 1997; 99:S377.

27. Hoffman DR, Schmidt JO. Amino acid sequences of allergens from Vespa mandarinia an Asian hornet. J Allergy Clin Immunol 1999; 103:S164.

28. Fitch CD, Hoffman DR, Schmidt M. Cloning of a paper wasp venom serine protease allergen. J Allergy Clin Immunol 2001; 107:S221.

29. Hoffman DR. Allergens in hymenoptera venom XXVI: The complete amino acid sequences of two vespid venom phospholipases. Int Arch Allergy Immunol 1994; 104:184–190.

30. Gmachl M, Kreil G. Bee venom hyaluronidase is homologous to a membrane protein of mammalian sperm. Proc Natl Acad Sci USA 1993; 90:3569–3573.

31. Kasahara M, Gutnecht J, Brew K, Spur N, Goodfellow PN. Cloning and mapping of a testis-specific gene with sequence similarity to a sperm-coating glycoprotein gene. Genomics 1989; 5:527–534.

32. Murphy EV, Zhang Y, Zhu W, Biggs J. The human glioma pathogenesis-related protein is structurally related to plant pathogenesis-related proteins and its gene is expressed specifically in brain tumors. Gene 1995; 159:131–135.

33. Hawdon JM, Jones BF, Hoffmann DR, Hotez PJ. Cloning and characterization of ancylostoma-secreted protein. J Biol Chem 1996; 271:6672–6678.

34. Ravi V, Ramachandran S, Thompson RW, Anderse JF, Neva FA. Characterization of a recombinant immunodiagnostic antigen (NIE) from Strongyloides Stercoralis L3 larvae. Mol Biochem Parasitol 2002; 125:73–81.

35. Morrissette J, Kratzschmar J, Haendler B, El-Hayek R, Mochca-Morales J, Martin BM, Patel JR, Moss RL, Schleuning W, Coronado R, Possani LD. Primary structure and properties of helothermine, a peptide toxin that blocks ryanodine receptors. Biophys J 1995; 68:2280–2288.

36. Lokeshwar VB, Schroeder GL, Carey RL, Soloway MS, Iida N. Regulation of hyaluronidase activity by alternative mRNA splicing. J Immunol 2002; 277:33654–33663.

37. Kreil G. Hyaluronidases—A group of neglected enzymes. Prot Sci 1995; 4:1666–1669.

38. Carriere F, Thirstrup K, Boel E, Berger R, Thim L. Structure-function relatioships in naturally occurring mutants of pancreatic lipase. Protein Eng 1994; 7:563–569.

39. Markovic-Housley Z, Miglierini G, Soldatova L, Rizkallah PJ, Muller U, Schirmer T. Crystal structure of hyaluronidase, a major allergen of bee venom. Structure Fold Des 2000; 8:1025–1035.

40. Scott DL, Otwinowski Z, Gelb MH, Sigler P. Crystal structure of bee venom phospholipase A2 in a complex with a transition-state analogue. Science 1990; 250:1563–1566.

41. Henriksen A, King TP, Mirza O, Monsalve RI, Meno K, Ipsen H, Larsen JN, Gajhede M, Spangfort MD. Major venom allergen of yellow jackets, Ves v 5: Structural characterization of a pathogenesis-related protein superfamily. Protein: Structure, Function and Genetics 2001; 45:438–448.

42. Aalberse RC. Structural biology of allergens. J Allergy Clin Immunol 2000; 106:228–238.

43. Bessette P, Aslund F, Beckwith J, Georgiou G. Efficient folding of proteins with multiple disulfide bonds in the Escherichia coli cytoplasm. Proc Natl Acad Sci 1999; 96:13703–13708.

44. Binder M, Fierlbeck G, King TP, Valent P, Buehring H. Individual hymnenoptera venom compounds induce upregulation of the basophil activation marker ectonuleotide pyrophos-phatase/phosphodiesterase 3 (CD203c) in sensitized patients. Int Arch Allergy Immunol 2002; 129:160–168.

45. King TP, Jim SY, Monsalve RI, Kagey-Sobotka A, Lichtenstein LM, Spangfort MD. Recombinant allergens with reduced allergenicity but retaining immunogenicity of the natural allergens: Hybrids of yellow jacket and paper wasp venom allergen antigen 5s. J Immunol 2001; 166:6057–6065.

46. King TP, Kochoumian L, Lu G. Murine T and B cell responses to natural and recombinant hornet venom allergen, Dol m 5.02 and its recombinant fragments. J Immunol 1995; 154:577–584.

47. King TP, Lu G, Agosto H. Antibody responses to bee melittin (Api m 4) and hornet antigen 5 (Dol m 5) in mice treated with the dominant T-cell epitope peptides. J Allergy Clin Immunol 1998; 101:397–403.

48. Tretter V, Altmann F, Kubelka V, Marz L, Becker WM. Fucose alpha 1,3-linked to the core region of glycoprotein N-glycans creates an important epitope for IgE from honeybee venom allergic individuals. Int Arch Allergy Immunol 1993; 102:259–266.

49. Muller U, Akdis CA, Fricker M, Akdis M, Blesken T, Bettens F, Blaser K. Successful immunotherapy with T-cell epitope peptides of bee venom phospholipase A2 induces specific T-cell tolerance in bee sting allergic patients. J Allergy Clin Immunol 1998; 101:747–754.

50. Dhillon M, Roberts C, Nunn T, Kuo M. Mapping human T cell epitopes on phospholipase A2: The major bee-venom allergen. J Allergy Clin Immunol 1992; 90:42–51.

51. Carballido JM, Carballido-Perrig N, Kagi MK, Meloen MH, Wuthrich B, Heusser CH, Blaser K. T cell epitope specificity in human allergic and non-allergic subjects to bee venom phospholipase A2. J Immunol 1993; 150:3582–3591.

52. Specht C, Kolsch E. The murine (H-2k) T-cell epitopes of bee venom phospholipase A2 lie outside the active site of the enzyme. Int Arch Allergy Immunol 1997; 112:226–230.

53. King TP, Lu G. Hornet venom allergen antigen 5, Dol m 5: Its T-cell epitopes in mice and its antigenic cross-reactivity with a mammalian testis protein. J Allergy Clin Immunol 1997; 99:630–639.

54. Dudler T, Altmann F, Carballido JM, Blaser K. Carbohydrate-dependent, HLA class II-restricted, human T cell response to the bee venom allergen phospholipase A2 in allergic patients. Eur J Immunol 1995; 25:538–542.

55. van Neerven RJJ, Ebner C, Yssel H, Kapsenberg Martien L, Lamb Jonathan R. T-cell responses to allergens: Epitope-specificity and clinical relevance. Immunol Today 1996; 17:526–532.

56. Ebner C, Schenk S, Najafian N, Siemann U, Steiner R, Fischer GW, Hoffmann K, Szepfalusi Z, Scheiner O, Kraft D. Nonallergic individuals recognize the same T cell epitopes of Bet v 1, the major birch pollen allergen, as atopic patients. J Immunol 1995; 154:1932–1940.

57. King TP, Lu G. Hornet venom allergen, Dol m 5; Its T cell epitopes in mice and its antigenic cross reactivity with a mammalian testis protein. J Allergy Clin Immunol 1997; 99:630–639.

58. Hamilton RG, Wisenauer JA, Golden DB, Valentine MD, Adkinson NJ. Selection of Hymenoptera venoms for immunotherapy on the basis of patient's IgE antibody cross-reactivity. J Allergy Clin Immunol 1993; 92:651–709.

59. Hemmer W, Focke M, Kolarich D, Wilson IB, Altman F, Wohrl S, Gotz M, Jarisch R. Antibody binding to venom carbohydrates is a frequent cause for double positivity to honeybee and yellow jacket venom in patients with stinging-insect allergy. J Allergy Clin Immunol 2001; 108:1045–1052.

60. van Ree R. Carbohydrate epitopes and their relevance for the diagnosis and treatment of allergic diseases. Int Arch Allergy Immunol 2002; 129:189–197.

61. Muller UR. Insect sting allergy. Gustav Fisher Stuttgart 1990; 54:54.

62. Zora JA, Swanson MC, Yuninger JW. A study of the prevalence and clinical significance of venom-specific IgE. J Allergy Clin Immunol 1988; 81:77–82.

63. Settipane GA, Chafee FH, Klein DE, Boyd GK, Sturam JH, Freye HB. Anaphylactic reactions to hymenoptera stings in asthmatic patients. Clin Allergy 1980; 10:659–665.

64. Habermann E. Bee and wasp venoms. Science 1972; 177:314–322.

65. Nakajima T. Biochemistry of vespid venom. In: Handbook of Natural Toxins (Tu AT, ed.). Marcel Dekker 1984; 109–133.

66. Kind LS, Ramaika C, Allaway E. Antigenic, adjuvant and permeability enhancing properties of melittin in mice. Allergy 1981; 36:155–160.

67. King TP, Kochoumian L, Joslyn A. Melittin-specific monoclonal and polyclonal IgE and IgG1 antibodies from mice. J Immunol 1984; 133:2668–2673.

68. Ho CL, Lin YL, Chen WC, Yu HM, Wang KT, Hwang LL, Chen CT. Immunogenicity of mastoparan B, a cationic tetradecapeptide isolated from the hornet (Vespa basalis) venom, and its structural requirements. Toxicon 1995; 33:1443–1451.

69. Hirai Y, Yasuhara T, Yoshida H, Nakajima T, Fujino M, Kitada C. A new mast cell degranulating peptide 'Mastoparan' in the venom of vespula lewisii. Chem Pharm Bull (Tokyo) 1979; 27:1942–1944.

70. Higashijima T, Wakamatus K, Takemitsu M, Fujino M, Nakajima T, Miyazawa T. Conformational change of mastoparan from wasp venom on binding with phospholipid membrane. FEBS Letters 1983; 152:227–230.

71. Whiles JA, Brasseur R, Glover KJ, Melacini G, Komives EA, Vold RR. Orientation and effects of mastoparan X on phospholipid bicelles. Biophys J 2001; 80:280–293.

72. Wu TM, Chou TC, Ding YA, Li ML. Stimulation of TNF-alpha, IL1-beta and nitrite release from mouse cultured spleen cells and lavaged peritoneal cells by mastoparan M. Immunol Cell Biol 1999; 77:476–482.

73. Agriolas A, Pisano JJ. Facilitation of phospholipase A2 activity by mastoparans, a new class of mast cell degranulating peptides from wasp venom. J Biol Chem 1983; 258:13697–13702.

74. Okano Y, Takai H, Tohmatsu T, Nakashima S, Kuoda Y, Saito K, Nozawa Y. A wasp venom mastoparan-induced polyphosphoinositide breakdown in rat peritoneal mast cells. FEBS Letters 1985; 188:363–366.

75. Mizuno K, Nakahata N, Ohizumi Y. Mastoparan-induced phosphatidylcholine hydrolysis by phospholipase D activation in human astrocytoma cells. British J Pharmacol 1985; 116:2090–2096.

76. Mizuno K, Nakahata N, Ohizumi Y. Characterization of mastoparan-induced histamine release RBL-2H3 cells. Toxicon 1998; 36:447–456.

77. Higashijima T, Burnier J, Ross EM. Regulation of Gi and Go by mastoparan, related amphiphilic peptides and hydrophobic amines. J Biol Chem 1990; 265:14176–14186.

78. King TP, Sui YJ, Wittkowski KM. Inflammatory role of two venom components of yellow jackets (Vespula Vulgaris): A mast cell degranulating peptide mastoparan and phospholipase A1. Int Arch Allergy Immunol 2003; 131:25–32.

19

Biting-Insect Allergens

DONALD R. HOFFMAN

*Brody School of Medicine at East Carolina University, Greenville,
North Carolina, U.S.A.*

I. INTRODUCTION

Allergic reactions to insect bites are much less common than reactions to insect stings. Several studies suggest that severe bite reactions occur about 50 times less commonly than severe sting reactions. Many of the clinical aspects of biting-insect allergy have been thoroughly discussed in a recent review (1). In this chapter, the main foci will be on which insects are important, the known allergens and salivary components, and the appropriate use of immunotherapy. There are more than 14,000 species from 400 genera of blood-feeding arthropods. The most important hematophagous insects belong to the orders Diptera (flies), Hemiptera (bugs), and Siphonaptera (fleas). Ticks of the order Acarina of the class Arachnida will also be considered, although they are not insects. Many other bugs of the order Hemiptera and some beetles, especially aquatic species, of the order Coleoptera occasionally bite man, but allergic reactions have not been reported. In addition, many larval forms may bite, but again allergic reactions to these bites are extremely rare. Allergic reactions to bites have been ascribed to other arachnids, but definitive evidence is lacking to demonstrate IgE antibodies against centipede and millipede bites. There probably are rare cases of IgE-mediated allergy to spider bites, but there are no published systematic studies.

II. TAXONOMY OF BITING INSECTS

A. Diptera, Flies

Many flies are hematophagous. In almost all cases, only the females bite, requiring a blood meal to develop eggs. The more common biting flies are outlined in Table 1. A blackfly, deerfly, and horsefly are illustrated in Figs. 1–3.

B. Hemiptera, Bugs

There are two important families of biting bugs in North America. The members of the first are variously called kissing bugs, assassin bugs, conenose bugs, vinchucas, or reduviid bugs and are members of the family Reduviidae. There are 39 genera, of which the most important are *Triatoma* (Fig. 4) and *Reduvius*. The Latin American genera *Rhodnius* and *Panstrongylus* are important members of this family. The second family of blood-sucking bugs is Cimicidae, or bedbugs. There are seven genera, and the species *Cimex lectularius* is the most infamous human bedbug.

C. Siphonaptera, Fleas

The fleas are almost all parasitic insects with 74% of species associated with rodent hosts and about 6% with avian hosts. The species associated with man are members of the superfamily Pulicoidea, family Pulicidae. The most common are the dog and cat fleas *Ctenocephalides canis* and *felis felis*. *Pulex irritans*, a parasite of carnivores, is sometimes called the human flea. Fleas of the genus *Tunga* are found in Central and South America.

D. Other Arachnids

Many species of hard and soft ticks and chiggers bite man. Allergic reactions to these bites are extremely rare, although they have been reported (2,3) from many regions.

Table 1 Biting Flies (Diptera)

Common name	Family	Genera
Mosquito	Culicidae	*Aedes, Culex, Anopheles*, others
Blackfly	Simuliidae	*Simulium, Prosimulium, Cnephia*
Biting midge	Ceratopogonidae	*Culicoides*, others
Horsefly	Tabanidae	*Tabanus, Hypomitra*
Deerfly, Yellow fly	Tabanidae	*Chrysops*
Sand fly	Psychodidae (Phlebotominae)	*Lutzomyia, Phlebotomus*
Bot and warble flies	Oestridae	*Dermatobia*, others
Stable fly	Muscidae	*Stomoxys, Haematobia*
Tsetse fly	Glossinidae (Muscidae)	*Glossina*

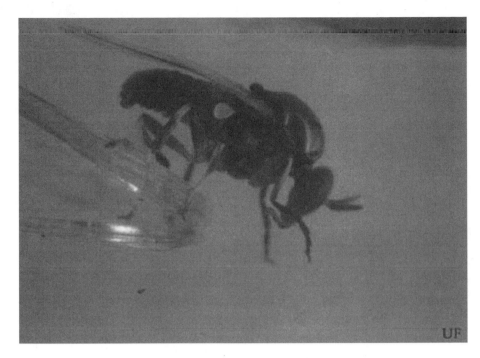

Figure 1 Photograph of a blackfly, *Simulium*; note the humped appearance. (Courtesy of Jerry F. Butler, University of Florida.)

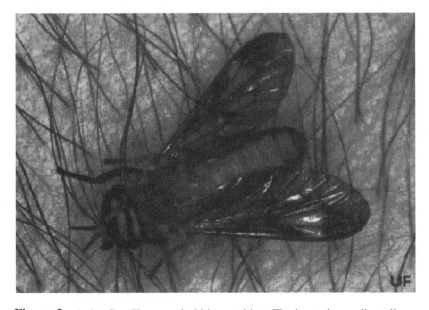

Figure 2 A deerfly, *Chrysops*, in biting position. The insect is usually yellow or green and the bite is painful. (Courtesy of Jerry F. Butler, University of Florida.)

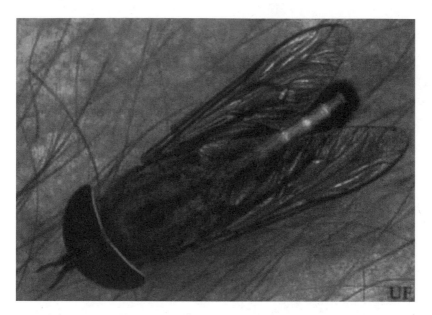

Figure 3 A horsefly, *Tabanus*, biting. Horseflies are typically larger than deerflies and have very noisy flight, and the bites are quite painful. (Courtesy of Jerry F. Butler, University of Florida.)

III. IDENTIFYING BITING INSECTS

The identification of biting insects can be extremely difficult, even with representative specimens. Deerflies, horseflies (see Fig. 1), and stable flies all cause immediate pain when they bite. Mosquitos can usually be recognized, but identification of species may require an expert. Identification of flea species is the realm of specialists. Kissing bugs typically bite painlessly, most commonly while the victim is sleeping. Useful identification guides with many illustrations are available for hobbyists, including the Peterson's Field Guide Series and the Audubon Society Series. The much more technical and comprehensive reference to insects of North America by Arnett (4) is recommended for those with a serious interest. Keys to various groups are available in the entomology literature and vary widely in quality and usability. Most states have official entomologists, usually with the Department of Agriculture, who are oftentimes willing to assist in insect identification for medical purposes. There are also entomologists at many land grant universities who are willing to assist with insect identification.

IV. GEOGRAPHIC DISTRIBUTION OF SOME BITING INSECTS

Mosquitos are cosmopolitan, with species found in almost all land areas of the world. Fleas are found in most areas of the world, excepting very dry climates. Blackflies are found in the northern United States and in most of Canada; in tropical areas they require the presence of rapidly running water to breed. Horseflies and deerflies are found in most areas of the United States. Tsetse flies are found only in tropical Africa and a few laboratories in the United States.

Ticks are found around wooded areas and are commonly carried by dogs, birds, and deer. Various species are found in different areas of the United States. Sand flies and biting midges are also found in many areas, especially around beaches and livestock.

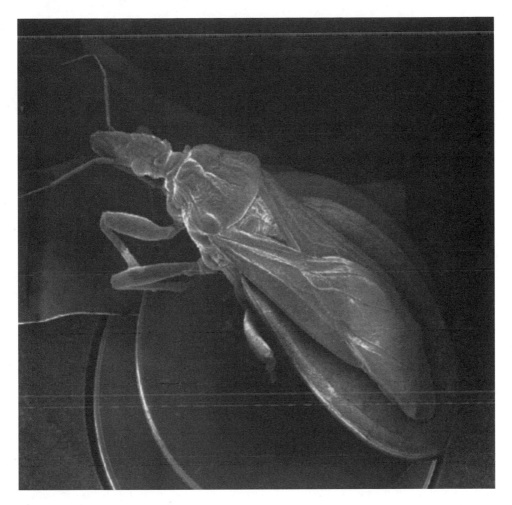

Figure 4 Scanning electron micrograph of a kissing bug, *Triatoma protracta*. Bites are painless, typically occurring while sleeping. The insect's definitive host is the wood rat. (Courtesy of C. Demetry and R. Biderman, Worcester Polytechnic Institute.)

Although bugs of the reduviid group are found in many areas, almost all cases of allergic reactions to bites are found in the southwestern United States, Hawaii, Mexico, and Central America. These insects are dependent upon the distribution of their hosts, for example, the wood rat in California for *Triatoma protracta*. Other species feed on dogs, cats, mice, opossums, and armadillos.

V. SALIVARY COMPONENTS AND ALLERGENS OF BITING INSECTS

According to Ribeiro (5), blood feeding evolved independently multiple times among hematophagous arthropods. A variety of anticlotting factors, platelet aggregation antagonists, and vasodilators developed to counter the host's hemostatic and immunomodulatory factors (6). In addition, arthropod salivas contain digestive enzymes (7) and hyaluronidase. One unsuspected property of some insect salivas is enhancement of infectivity of parasites carried

Table 2 Some Characterized Protein Components in Mosquito Salivas

Component	Molecular weight	Species[a]	Reference
Tachykinin		At, Ag	14
Catechol oxidase/peroxidase		Ag	14
Apyrase	61,800	Aa	15
Maltase-I	63,700	Aa	16
Amylase I	81,500	Aa	17
Esterase	65,000	Aa	18
Factor Xa inhibitor	35,500	Aa, 8 others	19
Protein D7	37,000	Aa, others	20

[a] Species: Aa—*Aedes aegypti*
Ag—*Anopheles gambiae* (genome sequence completed)
At—*Aedes triseriatus*

by the arthropod (8). Sand fly saliva decreases the minimum effective dose of *Leishmania major* in mice by several orders of magnitude. In 2002 the first complete genome sequence of a biting insect, the malaria mosquito, *Anopheles gambiae*, became available (9). The proteins expressed by the salivary glands have been named the sialome (10) and are being mapped for mosquitos (11,12) and ticks (13).

A. Mosquitos

There are at least eight characterized protein components of mosquito saliva, which are described in Table 2. All appear to be related to either digestive functions, such as maltase, amylase, and esterase, or inhibition of hemostasis, such as tachykinin, factor Xa inhibitor, purine nucleosidase, and apyrase or adenosine triphosphate diphosphohydrolase, which inhibits ADP-dependent platelet aggregation. Protein D7 contains two insect pheromone/odorant-binding protein domains and is expressed in a number of different sizes. D7 proteins appear to be major allergens in most species.

There are numerous published studies of IgE binding components of various mosquito extracts. Some are performed with "saliva," some with salivary gland extract, some with thorax extract and some with whole-body extract. Numerous species and at least four genera have been investigated. Table 3 is a compendium of the major and shared

Table 3 Molecular Weights of IGE Binding Components in Mosquito Extracts from Various Species

Aedes aegypti	*Aedes vexans*	*Aedes communis*	*Culex tarsalis*	*Culiseta inornata*
Major allergens				
65 kDa	65	36	43	65
48	43	30	17	40
34 = D7	38	22	15	34
31				
15				

Minor allergens shared by at least three species: 160, 110, 65, 62, 50, 46, 40, 32.5, 24, 17, 15.
(Allergens have not been purified; data mainly from immunoblot experiments. Some, e.g., D7, have been cloned or expressed.)
Source: Combined from Refs. 21–26.

allergens in immunoblot experiments for five species and thirteen species, respectively. It appears that D7 protein is an important allergen in *Aedes*, *Culex*, and related mosquitos and that apyrase may also be an allergen. None of the other IgE binding bands has been definitively characterized at the present time.

B. Blackflies

Studies on the saliva of blackflies are very limited. Cupp et al. (27,28) isolated and cloned a major protein of molecular weight 15,351 daltons with strong vasodilator activity manifested by rapid and persistent induction of erythema. The enzyme apyrase is also found in blackfly salivary gland secretions. Wirtz (29) demonstrated high contents of histamine, putrescine, spermine, N-monoacetyl-spermine, and spermidine, as well as the presence of proteins with esterase activity. Almost all reactions to blackfly bites are not IgE mediated, and the dermatologic reactions have been classified into six forms by Farkas (30). These are edematous, erythematous-edematous, "erysipeloid," inflammatory-indurative, hemorrhagic plaques, hemorrhagic nodules, and hemorrhagic vesicles.

C. Horseflies and Deerflies

Deerfly saliva contains chrysoptin, an inhibitor of ADP-induced platelet aggregation that inhibits fibrinogen binding to the glycoprotein IIb/IIIa receptor on platelets (31,32). The recombinant protein with a molecular mass of 65 kDa, the same as that of the natural protein, has been expressed in insect cells. This may be a protein similar to the 69-kDa IgE-binding protein found in immunoblots using sera from European patients who experienced anaphylaxis from Chrysops bites (33).

D. Sand Flies

Sand fly saliva contains a factor that enhances the infectivity of *Leishmania* by inhibiting the ability of interferon-gamma to activate macrophages and reduces nitric oxide production (34). A delayed-type hypersensitivity reaction to saliva components may also play a role in infectivity and adverse reactions (35). Sand fly saliva is also known to contain the potent vasodilator maxadilan, apyrase, 5′-nucleotidase, hyaluronidase, a carbohydrate-recognition domain anticlotting protein, and several proteins of unknown function.

E. Kissing Bugs and Bedbugs

The major salivary anticoagulant proteins of *Rhodnius prolixus* are named prolixins and consist of four related nitrophorin molecules (36), which are heme proteins that carry nitric oxide. The major component has a molecular weight of 19,689 daltons and inhibits factor VIII–mediated activation of factor X. Two proteins have been characterized from the saliva of *Triatoma pallipidipennis*, triabin of 15,620 daltons molecular weight, an inhibitor of thrombin-based hydrolysis of fibrinogen (37), and pallidipin (38) of 19,000 daltons molecular weight, an inhibitor of collagen-induced platelet aggregation. Functional studies of coagulation inhibition suggest that different species of Triatominae have functionally different mechanisms of coagulation inhibition and different SDS-PAGE profiles of salivary proteins (39). These proteins, along with proteins having histamine binding, platelet inhibition, anticoagulation, and nitric oxide transport, are all members of the lipocalin family (40). The three-dimensional structures of the nitrophorins NP1, 2, and 4 have been determined by X-ray crystallography. Many important vertebrate-derived allergens are also members of the lipocalin family. An activatable serine protease of 40,000 daltons molecular weight, named triapsin, with an arginine specificity has been isolated from saliva of *Triatoma infestans* (41).

Studies to characterize the allergenic proteins of *Triatoma protracta* indicate that the major allergens are of 18,000–20,000 daltons molecular weight, and almost all the allergenic activity was found between pI 6.7 and 7.3 and at pI 8.2 (42). This allergen, a member of the lipocalin family named procalin, has been identified, cloned, and expressed in yeast cells (43). The recombinant procalin reacts in ELISA assays with IgE antibodies from allergic patients and cross-reacts with native allergen. Antiserum against procalin was used in immunohistochemistry to localize procalin to the cytoplasm of cuboidal epithelium and the luminal contents of the salivary glands.

The saliva of the bedbug *Cimex lectularius* contains a nitrophorin (44) and also an inhibitor of activation of factor X to factor Xa in the tenase complex that does not directly inhibit factor VIII (45). The apparent molecular weight of this factor was 17,000 daltons. Bedbug saliva also contains apyrase.

F. Fleas

Very little work has been done applying contemporary methods to studies of flea saliva. The only characterized proteins in flea saliva are apyrase, which prevents ADP-induced platelet aggregation (46), platelet activating factor acetylhydrolase, and naphthyl esterases.

Diagnostic studies of allergy to flea bites in humans are complicated by the relatively more common occurrence of inhalant allergy to cat fleas. The major salivary allergen of cat fleas active in dogs is a protein of 18,000 daltons molecular weight and pI 9.3, termed Cte f 1 (47).

G. Ticks

There has been a great deal of interest in ticks with the recognition of Lyme disease and ehrlichiosis. Allergic reactions to tick bites are usually the result of bites by soft ticks, Ixodiae. Pigeon ticks, *Argas reflexus*, as well as deer ticks and paralysis ticks have all been reported to cause systemic allergic reactions. Tick salivas have been found to contain apyrase and antiplatelet activities (48) as well as numerous proteins from 18 to 160 kDa. Several proteins from 15 to 50 kDa were induced by feeding (49).

Five salivary allergens have been isolated from the Australian paralysis tick, *Ixodes holocyclus*, of molecular weights 28, 45, 50, 55, and 355 kDa (50). The allergens at 28 and 355 kDa appear to react with IgE from most patients, and SGA1 at 28 kDa is useful for skin prick testing and radioimmunoassay (51).

VI. CROSS-REACTIVITY AMONG BITING INSECTS

There is very limited experimental data on IgE cross-reactivity among biting insects. There are some common antigens exhibiting a limited degree of cross-reactivity among mosquito genera and species (21–23). However, typically clinical reactions including nonallergic responses are species-dependent for most individuals. There appears to be some cross-reactivity based upon RAST testing between horseflies and deerflies and sometimes also blackflies (1). It is not known if this is clinically relevant.

Allergic reactions to kissing bugs and bedbugs exhibit a strong species dependence, and it is rare to find patients either skin test positive or RAST positive to more than a single species (52).

There is no data on cross-reactivity with fleas in human subjects, but studies on dogs suggest species specificity. Reactions to sand flies, biting midges, ticks, tsetse flies, and other biting arthropods are probably species specific, but experimental data are lacking.

VII. BITING-INSECT CONTROL

The control of biting insects is a very difficult problem, as attempts at mosquito vector control in the tropical world have demonstrated. Use of most pesticides, especially large-area spraying, is best left to public health authorities. Spraying of yards is not recommended and is almost always of extremely limited value and may involve significant risk of pesticide exposure to children and pets.

Control of biting insects in the home should emphasize avoidance. Screens should be used on all doors and windows. Various forms of flypaper traps with and without attractants are effective and environmentally friendly. One highly recommended type is clear and is placed on glass doors and windows, and another uses 7-watt lightbulbs. Control of fleas from pets, particularly in warm and humid areas, can be extremely difficult. Veterinarians can recommend several programs, including the use of growth regulators that are fed to dogs and cats to prevent development of adult fleas and substances that are spotted onto the animal and absorbed through the skin or injected. The extensive use of anti-acetylcholinesterase pesticides is ineffective and leads to development of resistant fleas. Animals should be regularly washed and carpets and furniture regularly vacuumed to help control fleas.

Bedbug infestations should be eliminated by treatment with appropriate pesticides, preferably by a licensed professional. Reduviid bugs are primarily outdoor insects and are best controlled by eliminating their definitive hosts around houses. *Triatoma protracta* comes from wood rat nests, but other species have varied hosts. Professional assistance is recommended.

Horseflies, deerflies, and blackflies are primarily found around water. They can be extremely difficult to avoid in these areas. The almost ubiquitous mosquito is extremely difficult to avoid. The use of repellants containing DEET (*N,N'*-diethyl-*m*-toluamide) can help; these should be used with caution on small children. Many other repellants are less effective. Covering up as much exposed skin as possible and avoiding being outdoors at high-risk times such as early morning and evening can help. Avoidance of areas of high mosquito density should be practiced. Sources of standing water should be minimized or eliminated. Mosquito netting and the use of citronella candles can also reduce mosquito density. An ultraviolet bug light can also help, particularly after dark. Both electrocuting and trap models are available. Use of yellow or orange lightbulbs outdoors minimizes the attraction of insects to porches and garages.

VIII. IMMUNOTHERAPY

A. Evidence for Efficacy

There is very limited controlled-study evidence for the efficacy of immunotherapy in preventing life-threatening systemic reactions to insect bites. There are a significant number of anecdotal reports, most of which describe variants of large local reactions. The only challenge-verified trial with an insect salivary gland–derived vaccine was reported with *Triatoma protracta* in 1984 (53). Immunotherapy provided protection in all five patients with no significant side effects. Immunologic changes were also observed in parallel with protection as assessed by bite challenge.

A report of treatment with deerfly whole-body vaccine, although not controlled, suggests efficacy for patients with systemic reactions (54). Immunotherapy with whole-body extracts has been tried in cases of life-threatening allergy to mosquito bites (55). Results have been mixed, with some patients developing a higher tolerance to bites and some developing major complications.

It should be noted that in the United States and most other countries, there are no licensed extracts of insect saliva or salivary glands and that most whole-body extracts from biting insects are not approved for use in allergen vaccine therapy. These products should only be used under an investigational new drug application (IND), preferably as part of a controlled study. A recent study (56) demonstrated that it is possible to prepare substantially more potent vaccines from biting insects than are available in current commercial products.

Most cases of severe allergy to mosquito bites are best managed by prophylactic use of the antihistamine cetirizine (57). In controlled trials, cetirizine has been shown to reduce pruritis and significantly decrease large local reaction development, and it appears to also prevent systemic reactions (57,58). The antihistamine loratadine, used prophylactically, reduces whealing and pruritis from mosquito bites in children; it also reduces the size of bite lesions at 24 hours (59).

B. Known Risks

Immunotherapy with mosquito whole-body vaccine has been shown to cause local pain, swelling, and redness in a patient who tolerated injections at lower concentrations. Another patient in the same report developed arthralgias, myalgias, fatigue, weakness, and swelling of distal extremities, despite treatment with terfenadine, cimetidine, and prednisone (55). Life-threatening anaphylactic reactions have been observed in studies of experimental vaccines derived from mosquito cell tissue culture (60).

The use of other biting-insect vaccines has not been reported to cause unusual reactions, and the experiences reported in the literature correspond to those seen with other allergens routinely used in allergen vaccine therapy.

C. Potential Risks

The existence of species and genus specificity for many biting-insect reactions requires the use of more sophisticated diagnostic reagents than are currently commercially available. There is a significant risk of using an ineffective preparation and a potential risk of sensitization. Many hematophagous insects are vectors for serious diseases—parasitic, viral, rickettsial, and bacterial. Extracts prepared from salivary glands must be carefully monitored to be agent-free. It cannot be overemphasized that use of biting-insect extracts in allergen vaccine therapy is an experimental procedure, and that all proper safety procedures and regulations should be followed.

IX. SALIENT POINTS

1. There are a large variety of hematophagous insects and arachnids.
2. Many different arthropods can cause bite allergy.

3. Much, if not most, insect bite allergy is species and/or genus specific.
4. Insect saliva varies widely, but most species contain potent anticoagulants and digestive enzymes.
5. The best diagnostic reagents are insect saliva or salivary gland extract, but none are commercially available or licensed in the United States.
6. Immunotherapy has been shown to be effective prophylaxis for severe systemic reactions for *Triatoma protracta*, deerflies, and mosquitos.
7. Immunotherapy with mosquito whole-body vaccine has substantial risks.
8. Immunotherapy with biting-insect extracts—whole-body, salivary gland, and saliva—is still an experimental procedure.
9. Control of many biting insects is difficult, but risk of exposure to bites can be greatly reduced.
10. Reactions to mosquito bites are best managed by prophylaxis with cetirizine or loratadine.

REFERENCES

1. Hoffman DR. Allergic reactions to biting insects. In: Monograph on Insect Allergy, 3rd ed. (Levine MI, Cockey RF, eds.) Milwaukee, WI: American Academy of Allergy, Asthma and Immunology, 1995:99–108.
2. Van Wye JE, Hsu Y-P, Lane RS, Terr AI, Moss RB. IgE antibodies in tick bite induced anaphylaxis. J Allergy Clin Immunol 1991; 88:968–970.
3. Gauci M, Loh RKS, Stone BF, Thong YH. Allergic reactions to the Australian paralysis tick, *Ixodes holocyclus*. Diagnostic evaluation by skin test and radioimmunoassay. Clin Exp Allergy 1989; 74:279–283.
4. Arnett RH. American Insects. New York, NY: Van Nostrand Reinhold, 1985.
5. Ribeiro JM. Blood-feeding arthropods: Live syringes or invertebrate pharamcologists? Infect Agents Dis 1995; 3:143–152.
6. Tabachnik WJ. Pharmacological factors in the saliva of blood-feeding insects. Ann N Y Acad Sci 2000; 916:444–452.
7. Kerlin RL, Hughes S. Enzymes in saliva from four parasitic arthropods. Med Vet Entomol 1992; 6:121–126.
8. Theodos CM, Ribeiro JM, Titus RG. Analysis of enhancing effect of sand fly saliva on *Leishmania* infection in mice. Infect Immun 1991; 59:1592–1598.
9. Holt RA, Subramanian GM, Halpern A, et al. The genome sequence of the malaria mosquito *Anopheles gambiae*. Science 2002, Oct 4; 298:129–149.
10. Valenzuela JG, Pham VM, Garfield MK, Francischetti IM, Ribeiro JM. Toward a description of the sialome of the adult female mosquito *Aedes aegypti*. Insect Biochem Mol Biol 2002; 32:1101–1122.
11. Ribeiro JM, Francischetti IM. Role of arthropod saliva in blood feeding: Sialome and post-sialome perspectives. Annu Rev Entomol 2003; 48:73–88.
12. Valenzuela JG, Francischetti IM, Pham VM, Garfield MK, Mather TN, Ribeiro JM. Exploring the sialome of the tick *Ixodes scapularis*. J Exp Biol 2002; 205:2843–2864.
13. Francischetti IM, Valenzuela JG, Pham VM, Garfield MK, Ribeiro JM. Toward a catalog for the transcripts and proteins (sialome) from the salivary gland of the malaria vector *Anopheles gambiae*. J Exp Biol 2002; 205:2429–2451.
14. Ribeiro JM, Nussenzveig RH, Tortorella G. Salivary vasodilators of *Aedes triseriatus* and *Anopheles gambiae* (Diptera: Culicidae). J Med Entomol 1994; 31:747–753.
15. Champagne DE, Smartt CT, Ribeiro JM, James AA. The salivary gland-specific apyrase of the mosquito *Aedes aegypti* is a member of the 5′-nucleotidase family. Proc Nat Acad Sci U S A 1995; 92:694–698.

16. James AA, Blackmer K, Racioppi JV. A salivary gland-specific, maltase-like gene of the vector mosquito, *Aedes aegypti*. Gene 1989; 75:73–83.

17. Grossman GL, James AA. The salivary glands of the vector mosquito, *Aedes Aegypti*, express a novel member of the amylase gene family. Insect Mol Biol 1993; 1:223–232.

18. Argentine JA, James AA. Characterization of a salivary gland-specific esterase in the vector mosquito, *Aedes aegypti*. Insect Biochem Mol Biol 1995; 25:621–630.

19. Stark KR, James AA. A factor Xa-directed anticoagulant from the salivary glands of the yellow fever mosquito *Aedes aegypti*. Exp Parasitol 1995; 81:321–331.

20. James AA, Blackmer K, Marinotti O, Ghosn CR, Racioppi JV. Isolation and characterization of the gene expressing the major salivary gland protein of the female mosquito, *Aedes aegypti*. Mol Biochem Parasitol 1991; 44:245–253.

21. Peng Z, Li HB, Simon FER. Immunoblot analysis of IgE and IgG binding antigens in extracts of mosquitos *Aedes vexans, Culex tarsalis* and *Culiseta inornata*. Int Arch Allergy Immunol 1996; 110:46–51.

22. Li H, Simons FER, Peng Z. Immunoblot analysis of salivary allergens in 10 mosquito species with worldwide distribution and the human IgE responses to these allergens. J Allergy Clin Immunol 1998; 101:498–505.

23. Peng Z, Simons FE. Cross-reactivity of skin and serum specific IgE responses and allergen analysis for three mosquito species with worldwide distribution. J Allergy Clin Immunol 1997; 100:192–198.

24. Xu W, Lam H, Peng Z, Simons FER. Mosquito allergy: Expression, purification and characterization of Aed a 2, an *Aedes aegypti* salivary allergen. J Allergy Clin Immunol 1997; 99:S152 (abstract).

25. Brummer-Korvenkontio H, Kalkkinen N, Palusuo T, Reunala T. Molecular characterization of the major 22kD *Aedes communis* mosquito saliva allergen. J Allergy Clin Immunol 1997; 99:S353 (abstract).

26. Brummer-Korvenkonito H, Palusuo T, Francois G, Reunala T. Characterization of *Aedes communis, Aedes aegypti* and *Anopheles stephensi* mosquito saliva antigens by immunoblotting. Int Arch Allergy Immunol 1997; 112:169–174.

27. Cupp MS, Ribeiro JM, Cupp EW. Vasodilative activity in black fly salivary glands. Amer J Trop Med Hyg 1994; 50:241–246.

28. Cupp MS, Ribeiro JMC, Champagne DE, Cupp EW. Analyses of cDNA and recombinant protein for a potent vasoactive protein in saliva of a blood-feeding fly, *Simulium vittatum*. J Exp Biol 1998; 201:1553–1561.

29. Wirtz HP. Bioamines and proteins in the saliva and salivary glands of palaearctic blackflies (Diptera:Simuliidae). Trop Med Parasitol 1990; 41:59–64.

30. Farkas J. Simuliosis: Analysis of dermatological manifestations following blackfly (Simuliidae) bites as observed in the years 1981–1983 in Bratislava (Czechoslovakia). Derm Beruf Umwelt 1984; 32:171–173.

31. Grevelink SA, Youssef DE, Loscalzo J, Lerner EA. Salivary gland extracts from the deerfly contain a potent inhibitor of platelet aggregation. Proc Natl Acad Sci U S A 1993; 90:9155–9158.

32. Reddy VB, Kounga K, Mariano F, Lerner EA. Chrysoptin is a potent glycoprotein IIb/IIIa fibrinogen receptor antagonist present in salivary gland extracts of the deerfly. J Biol Chem 2000; 275:15861–15867.

33. Hemmer W, Focke M, Vieluf D, Berg-Drewniok B, Gotz M, Jarisch R. Anaphylaxis induced by horsefly bites: Identification of a 69kd IgE-binding salivary gland protein from *Chrysops* spp. (Diptera, Tabanidae) by western blot analysis. J Allergy Clin Immunol 1998; 101:134–136.

34. Hall LR, Titus RG. Sand fly vector saliva selectively modulates macrophage functions that inhibit killing of *Leishmania major* and nitric oxide production. J Immunol 1995; 155:3501–3506.

35. Belkaid Y, Valenzuela JG, Kamhawi S, Rowton E, Sacks DL, Ribeiro JM. Delayed-type hypersensitivity to *Phlebotomus papatasi* sand fly bite: An adaptive response induced by the fly? Proc Natl Acad Sci U S A 2000; 97:6704–6709.

36. Champagne DE, Nussenzveig RH, Ribeiro JM. Purification, partial characterization, and cloning of nitric oxide-carrying heme proteins (nitrophorins) from salivary glands of the blood sucking insect *Rhodnius prolixus*. J Biol Chem 1995; 270:8691–8695.

37. Noeske-Jungblut C, Haendler B, Donner P, Alagon A, Possani L, Schleuning WD. Triabin, a highly potent exosite inhibitor of thrombin. J Biol Chem 1995; 270:28629–28634.

38. Haendler B, Becker A, Noeske-Jungblut C, Kratzschmar J, Donner P, Schleuning WD. Expression, purification and characterisation of recombinant pallidipin, a novel platelet aggregation inhibitor from the hematophageous triatome bug *Triatoma pallidipennis*. Blood Coagul Fibrinolysis 1996; 7:183–186.

39. Pereira MH, Souza ME, Vargas AP, Martins MS, Penido CM, Diotaiuti L. Anticoagulant activity of *Triatoma infestans* and *Panstrongylus megistus* saliva (Hemiptera/Triatominae). Acta Trop 1996; 61:255–261.

40. Montfort WR, Weichsel A, Anderson JF. Nitrophorins and related antihemostatic lipocalins from *Rhodnius prolixus* and other blood-sucking arthropods. Biochim Biophys Acta 2000; 1482:110–118.

41. Amino R, Tanaka AS, Schenkman S. Triapsin, an unusual activatable serine protease from the saliva of the hematophagous vector of Chagas' disease *Triatoma infestans* (Hemiptera: Reduviidae). Insect Biochem Mol Biol 2001; 31:465–472.

42. Chapman MD, Marshall NA, Saxon A. Identification and partial purification of species-specific allergens from *Triatoma protracta* (Heteroptera:Reduviidae). J Allergy Clin Immunol 1986; 78:436–442.

43. Paddock CD, McKerrow JH, Hansell E, Foreman KW, Hsieh I, Marshall N. Identification, cloning and recombinant expression of procalin, a major triatomine allergen. J Immunol 2001; 167:2694–2699.

44. Valenzuela JG, Walker FA, Ribeiro JM. A salivary nitrophorin (nitric-oxide-carrying hemoprotein) in the bedbug *Cimex lectularius*. J Exp Biol 1995; 198:1519–1526.

45. Valenzuela JG, Guimaraes JA, Ribeiro JM. A novel inhibitor of factor X activation from the salivary glands of the bed bug *Cimex lectularius*. Exp Parasitol 1996; 83:184–190.

46. Ribeiro JM, Vaughn JA, Azad AF. Characterization of the salivary apyrase activity of three rodent flea species. Comp Biochem Physiol B 1990; 95:215–219.

47. McDermott MJ, Weber E, Hunter S, Stedman KE, Best E, Frank GR, Wang R, Escudero J, Kuner J, McCall C. Identification, cloning, and characterization of a major cat flea salivary allergen (Cte f 1). Mol Immunol 2000; 37:361–375.

48. Ribeiro JM, Endris TM, Endris R. Saliva of the soft tick, *Ornithodoros moubata*, contains antiplatelet and apyrase activities. Comp Biochem Physiol A 1991; 100:109–112.

49. Sanders ML, Scott AL, Glass GE, Schwartz BS. Salivary gland changes and host antibody responses associated with feeding of male lone star ticks (Acari:Ixodidae). J Med Entomol 1996; 33:628–634.

50. Gauci M, Stone BF, Thong YH. Isolation and immunological characterization of allergens from salivary glands of the Australian paralysis tick *Ixodes holocyclus*. Int Arch Allergy Appl Immunol 1988; 87:208–212.

51. Gauci M, Loh RKS, Stone BF, Thong YH. Evaluation of partially purified salivary gland allergens from the Australian paralysis tick, *Ixodes holocyclus* in diagnosis of allergy by RIA and skin prick test. Ann Allergy 1990; 64:297–299.

52. Marshall NA, Chapman MD, Saxon A. Species specific allergens from the salivary glands of Triatominae (Heteroptera:Reduviidae). J Allergy Clin Immunol 1986; 78:430–435.

53. Rohr AS, Marshall NA, Saxon A. Successful immunotherapy for *Triatoma protracta*-induced anaphylaxis. J Allergy Clin Immunol 1984; 73:369–375.

54. Wilbur RD, Evans R. An immunologic evaluation of deerfly hypersensitivity. J Allergy Clin Immunol 1975; 55:72.

55. McCormack DR, Salata KF, Hershey JN, Carpenter GB, Engler RJ. Mosquito bite anaphylaxis: Immunotherapy with whole body extracts. Ann Allergy Asthma Immunol 1995; 74:39–44.

56. Peng ZK, Simon FER. Comparison of proteins, IgE and IgG binding antigens, and skin reactivity in commercial and laboratory-made mosquito extracts. Ann Allergy Asthma Immunol 1996; 77:371–376.

57. Reunala T, Brummer-Korvenkontio H, Karppinen A, Coulie P, Palosuo T. Treatment of mosquito bites with cetirizine. Clin Exp Allergy 1993; 23:72–75.

58. Karppinen A, Rantala I, Vaalasti A, Palosuo T, Reunala T. Effect of cetirizine on the inflammatory cells in mosquito bites. Clin Exp Allergy 1996; 26:703–709.

59. Karppinen A, Kautianen H, Reunala T, Petman L, Reunala T, Brummer-Korvenkontio H. Loratadine in the treatment of mosquito-bite-sensitive children. Allergy 2000; 55:668–671.

60. Scott RM, Shelton AL, Eckels KH, Bancroft WH, Summers RJ, Russell PK. Human hypersensitivity to a sham vaccine prepared from mosquito cell culture fluids. J Allergy Clin Immunol 1984; 74:808–811.

20

Latex Allergens

JAY E. SLATER

U.S. Food and Drug Administration, Bethesda, Maryland, U.S.A.

I. INTRODUCTION

Over the past years, latex allergy has evolved from a curiosity to an important health care and patient management concern. Allergic reactions to *Hevea* latex proteins occur, for the most part, in members of well-defined risk groups. These include health care workers, rubber industry workers, and children with spina bifida (meningomyelocele) and urogenital abnormalities. The only common feature among these groups appears to be a high degree of exposure to natural rubber. Health care and rubber industry workers are exposed during the course of their occupations, and spina bifida patients through repeated surgery and, in some cases, fecal disimpaction and the repeated introduction of a latex catheter into the bladder.

The views expressed in this article are the personal opinions of the author and are not the official opinion of the U.S. Food and Drug Administration or the Department of Health and Human Services.

The prevalence of type I latex allergy in the general population is unknown, although the risk appears to be higher among atopic than among nonatopic individuals. One of the largest screening surveys was performed by Reinheimer and Ownby, who screened 200 consecutive sera sent to their laboratory for total IgE determination. In this group, 24 sera (12%) were positive using the AlaSTAT assay. Chart review suggested an identifiable risk group for only 2 of the 24 patients; 22 were probably atopic (1). In their analysis of the NHANES III data (1988 through 1991), Garabrant et al. found that the prevalence of latex-specific IgE (by AlaSTAT EIA) was between 8% and 37%, depending upon occupation; atopics [odds ratio (OR) of 2.53] and blacks (OR 1.41 for non-Hispanics, 2.25 for Hispanics) were at greater risk for latex-specific IgE (2). Buckland et al. found that 3/59 patients in the United Kingdom with chronic rhinitis were skin-test positive for latex (ALK-Abello reagent), and 2/3 of these patients reported symptoms associated with latex exposure (3). In another study, 9/100 atopic Danish children had either a positive skin test to latex (Stallergenes reagent) or a positive blood latex-specific IgE (Pharmacia CAP), but only one child, who had spina bifida, had experienced allergic reactions to latex products (4). In a sequential survey of patients in an urban American emergency room, 84/1027 patients had elevated latex-specific IgE (AlaSTAT EIA), and patients who were nonwhite or atopic were at even greater risk (ORs 4.7 and 7.4, respectively) (5). While the seroprevalence of latex-specific IgE appears to be high in the general population, true clinical reactivity appears to be relatively low. This discrepancy may be due to cross-reactivity and the relative nonspecificity of some of the assays currently in use (see below).

Early studies consistently indicated that health care workers had a 5% to 10% risk of clinical latex allergy (6–9). Other surveys of health care workers in Korea (10) and Japan (11) have confirmed these observations, using skin tests, questionnaires, and use tests. However, reviews of workers' compensation claims—which are based on clinical manifestations and not on specific testing—have failed to indicate that systemic reactions to latex gloves are an important cause of job-associated disability (12–15). Local reactions that are limited to the hands are an important source of claims, but not for lost work time, suggesting that the disability in these cases was usually minor. As the authors of these studies [and others (16,17)] have pointed out, these methods are likely to underestimate the true incidence of latex allergy among health care workers. On the other hand, serological data are likely to overestimate the problem. Thus, it is notable that the NHANES III data—which are based upon serological evidence of latex sensitization—suggests only a modest enhancement of risk among health care workers [OR 1.49 for those whose longest-held occupation had been in health care; OR 1.17 for current health care workers who use gloves; OR 2.53 for current health care workers who do not use gloves (2)]. Certain limitations of these analyses were acknowledged by the authors, among them that the lack of a dose response may have been due to the likelihood that clinically sensitive individuals will depart from jobs in which they experience heavy latex glove exposure. Others have suggested that the relatively poor specificity of the AlaSTAT EIA test for latex-specific IgE, as well as the inclusion of all adverse responses, such as nonallergic dermatitis and contact dermatitis, reduced the apparent differences attributable to health care worker status (18). Budnick noted another feature of the data that may have resulted in reducing the apparent risk associated with health care worker status: The period covered by NHANES III (1988–1991) preceded the 1992 mandate by the Occupational Safety and Health Administration that health care workers use gloves as a barrier against bloodborne infection (19).

For all their differences, the preceding studies share an important feature; they are all prevalence studies. One prospective assessment of the *incidence* of latex allergy is particularly illuminating (20). A cohort of 769 apprentices in three different fields were followed prospectively for the development of allergy (by questionnaire) and sensitization (by skin testing) over a period of up to 44 months after their entry into the apprenticeship programs. The trainees were in animal care, dental hygiene, and pastry-making programs. Aside from latex, allergens of interest included grains and animal proteins. Sensitization occurred to specific allergens among each of the three types of apprentices. Of particular interest is that 6.4% of the dental hygiene trainees developed new latex sensitivity over the period studied, and the annual incidence was 2.5%. These data are consistent with previous reports suggesting a prevalence of latex allergy of 5–10% in health care–related fields. The incidence of latex sensitization among pastry-makers was 1.6%, and among animal care apprentices, 0.4% (21). However, the annualized incidence of sensitization to program-specific allergens was greater among the animal care trainees (animal allergens, 8.9%) and the pastry-makers (grain allergens, 4.2%). Put in context, this analysis suggests two important novel conclusions. First, health care workers appear to be sensitized against latex allergens, but at rates only modestly greater than other workers with considerably less latex exposure. Second, the rate of latex sensitization among health care trainees may be less than the sensitization rate of other workers to protein allergens to which they are chronically exposed (20).

The prevalence of IgE-mediated latex allergy in children with spina bifida is much higher. Serologic surveys suggest sensitization rates of as high as 37% (22), and clinical latex allergy occurs in less than half of that number (22–24). In addition, children with other conditions requiring frequent surgery may be at risk. These conditions include bladder exstrophy, cerebral palsy, and spinal cord injury. Two related questions that have arisen are whether spina bifida is an independent risk factor for latex allergy and whether the risk of latex allergy rises with increasing numbers of operative procedures. Hochleitner et al. compared the prevalence of latex sensitization (latex-specific IgE and/or positive skin test to latex) in patients with ventriculo-peritoneal shunts with and without spina bifida. Multiple logistic regression analyses indicated that spina bifida, atopy, and the number of surgical interventions were independent risk factors (OR 6.76, 3.37, and 1.14/operation, respectively) (25). Two additional studies indicate that surgery—but not necessarily the number of procedures—is associated with an increase in latex sensitization (26,27). In one of these (27), the only patients with *clinical* latex allergy were those that had undergone greater than 10 prior procedures (5.6%; $p < 0.001$).

II. *HEVEA* LATEX PRODUCTION

Natural rubber (*cis*-1,4-polyisoprene) is a processed plant product that has found widespread use since the second half of the nineteenth century. Today, over 99% of natural rubber is derived from the *latex*, or milky sap, of the commercial rubber tree *Hevea brasiliensis*. Over 200 other species of plants produce rubber, but only *H. brasiliensis* and the guayule bush *Parthenium argentatum* produce rubber in commercially significant quantities.

Natural rubber was originally discovered by native peoples of Central and South America and the Caribbean basin. Its exploitation by Europeans as a commercial resource followed two developments: the discovery of vulcanization and the cultivation of *H. brasiliensis* in large plantations, which are today present in Africa and south Asia.

Vulcanization is a process by which latex is heated in the presence of sulfur, during which the elasticity and thermostability of rubber are vastly improved (28).

Latex is a delicate, complex intracellular product of a highly anastomosed system of cells that synthesize *cis*-1,4-polyisoprene. These cells are called laticiferous cells. The essential functional unit in latex is the rubber particle, a spherical droplet of polyisoprene, which ranges in diameter from 5 nm to 3 μm. These particles are internally homogeneous but are coated with a layer of protein, lipid, and phospholipid, that provides structural integrity. Among these surface proteins is prenyltransferase, which is found both free in the cytosol and in association with the rubber particles. Ultracentrifuged, fresh latex separates into three phases: (1) a white "cream" which contains virtually all the polyisoprene and a thin band of organelles called the Frey-Wyssling particles; (2) a translucent fluid called "C-serum," which corresponds to latex cytosol without polyisoprene; and (3) a bottom fraction containing organelles collectively called "lutoids" (29).

Rubber biosynthesis appears to occur in the following sequence (30). Three acetyl CoA molecules are converted into hydroxymethylglutaryl CoA, which is in turn reduced to mevalonic acid, and phosphorylated and decarboxylated to the five-carbon isopentenyl diphosphate. This so-called "isoprene" subunit forms the backbone of a bewildering array of biomolecules, from monoterpenes (two isoprene units) to diterpenes (four isoprene units) to sterols (six isoprene units). Prenyltransferase in several species can generate polymers as large as 10^5 Da; *Hevea* rubber ranges up to 10^6 Da. Rubber elongation factor (REF, Hev b 1) is tightly bound to rubber particles and allows prenyltransferase, which normally condenses fewer than three isoprene units, to elongate polyisoprene chains to lengths that run in the thousands in latex-producing species.

Mature, cultivated *H. brasiliensis* trees are tapped for latex, usually on alternate days. A spiral groove is cut in the bark of the tree, and a spout and cup are placed at the bottom of the groove to collect the latex. Ammonia, or some other preservative, is placed in the collection cup to prevent autocoagulation or bacterial contamination. Ammonia disrupts the rubber particles and produces a two-phase product that is about 30–40% solids. This is typically concentrated to 60% solids, producing *ammoniated latex concentrate*, which contains 1.6% ammonia by weight. This concentration is usually accomplished by centrifugation but may also occur by "creaming," in which controlled coagulation occurs by the addition of calcium alginate, a salt derived from seaweed. Low-ammonia latex concentrate, containing 0.15–0.25% ammonia, is also available. At low ammonia concentration, however, a secondary preservative is necessary to avoid coagulation and contamination. These may include sodium pentachlorophenate, tetramethylthiuram disulfide, sodium dimethyldithiocarbamate, and zinc oxide.

Latex concentrates are used for the production of dipped products, adhesives, foam, and carpet backing. Dipped products include gloves, balloons, and condoms. In dipping, porcelain molds are first coated with a coagulating salt (such as calcium alginate) and then dipped into the already vulcanized latex concentrate. After drying, the gloves are washed ("leeched"), coated with lubricating powder, and pulled off the mold. Natural rubber from latex concentrates is also found in toys, erasers, driveway sealants, sports equipment, clothing, elastic bands, and numerous medical and dental devices.

Trans-polyisoprene is a harder natural polymer with commercial and dental applications. The two sources of the *trans* polymer are gutta-percha, obtained from *Sapotaceae* trees, and balata, harvested from bushes and trees in South America. Synthetic rubbers are available in increasing quantity. Synthetic polyisoprene ("neoprene") is virtually identical to natural rubber in its physical properties but contains none of the protein allergens associated with the *Hevea* product. Other alternatives are commercially available as well and vary in their commercial applications.

III. *HEVEA* LATEX ALLERGENS

Table 1 lists currently identified, as of May 2003, latex allergens and isoallergens, their estimated molecular masses, and appropriate database references. There are two reasons that the identification of the specific inciting allergens is important: to guide specific avoidance strategies, and to establish sensitive and specific diagnostic techniques. Thus, the two most important features of any putative allergen are the degree of exposure and the prevalence of IgE-specific responses in the target population. Since tests for allergen-specific IgE can result from sensitization with cross-reactive allergens (see below), even exposure and seroprevalence data are not enough to prove causation with certainty; this can be accomplished only by demonstrating that avoidance of the allergen and/or specific immunotherapy with the allergen are curative. Such data are seldom available. Exposure, seroprevalence, and skin testing data, where known, are summarized in Tables 2A and 2B.

Table 1 Known Allergens from *Hevea brasiliensis*

Formal name	Common name	Mass	Database reference (if available)
Hev b 1	Elongation factor	58	A34309
Hev b 2	1,3-glucanase	34/36	U22147
Hev b 3		24	O82803
Hev b 4	Component of microhelix complex	100–115	Reference (121)
Hev b 5		16	U42640
Hev b 6.01	Hevein precursor	20	M36986, p02877
Hev b 6.02	Hevein	5	M36986, p02877
Hev b 6.03	C-terminal fragment	14	M36986, p02877
Hev b 7.01	Homologue: patatin from B-serum	42	U80598
Hev b 7.02	Homologue: patatin from C-serum	44	AJ223038
Hev b 8	Profilin	14	
Hev b 8.0101			Y15042
Hev b 8.0102			AJ132397
Hev b 8.0201			AF119365
Hev b 8.0202			AF119366
Hev b 8.0203			AF119367
Hev b 8.0204			AJ243325
Hev b 9	Enolase	51	AJ132580
Hev b 10	Mn superoxide dismutase	26	
Hev b 10.0101			L11707
Hev b 10.0102			AJ249148
Hev b 10.0103			AJ289158
Hev b 11	Class 1 chitinase		
Hev b 11.0101			AJ238579
Hev b 11.0102			AJ431363
Hev b 12	Lipid transfer protein	9.3	AY057860
Hev b 13	Esterase	42	P83269

Adapted from www.allergen.org/List.htm.

Table 2A Exposure, Seroprevalence, and Skin Test Data for Individual *Hevea* Latex Allergens (Hev b 1 through Hev b 5)

Allergen	Exposure	Ref	Seroprevalence	Ref	Skin test prevalence	Ref
Hev b 1	Mattresses	31	10% (Mixed A/C) 67% (S/cong)	32	23% (H)	33
	Breathing zone samplers; gloves	34	82% (S)	35		
	Gloves	36	13–32% (H) 54–100% (S)	37		
			52% (H) 81% (S)	36		
	Gloves	38	27% (C) 67% (S)	39		
Hev b 2					63% (H)	33
					7% (A)	40
			48–65% (H) 38–54% (S)	37		
Hev b 3			79% (S)	35	24% (H)	33
			83% (S)	41	7% (A)	40
			19–32% (H) 77–100% (S)	37		
			83% (S)	41		
Hev b 4			23–65% (H) 30–77% (S)	37	39% (H)	33
Hev b 5	Gloves	42			65% (H)	33
					62% (A)	40

A: adults; C: children; S: spina bifida; cong: congenital abnormalities; H: health care workers.

A. Cross-reactivity

Several reports have highlighted clinical and immunochemical cross-reactivity between latex and banana, chestnut, avocado, and other fruits [reviewed in (50)], and structural homologies between *Hevea* proteins and food proteins have been noted in several studies. Hev b 6 shares multiple domains with wheat germ agglutinin (51). The potato storage protein patatin (Sol t 1) contains a region with strong homology to Hev b 7 (52) and is cross-reactive to Hev b 7 by ELISA and immunoblotting (43). Hev b 5 is strongly homologous to the cDNA sequence in kiwi, pKIWI501 (53). Hev b 3 is homologous with a stress-related protein in red kidney bean (54). Lysozymes are present in *Hevea* latex and are ubiquitous; homologies among these may elicit some of the cross-reactions seen (55). Taken together, there is strong evidence that true cross-reactivity exists between *Hevea* latex allergens and several commonly eaten fruits and vegetables. However, it is important to remember that in vitro tests do not necessarily predict clinical sensitivity. Furthermore, it is not yet clear whether patients allergic to fruit constitute an independent risk group. Only one study has addressed the issue of latex sensitivity in a cohort of fruit- allergic patients. Among 57 individuals with clinical histories and testing consistent with IgE-mediated fruit allergy, 86% had positive skin test or serologic evidence of latex sensitization, while 11% had clinical evidence of latex sensitivity (56).

Table 2B Exposure, Seroprevalence and Skin Test Data for Individual *Hevea* Latex Allergens (Hev b 6 through Hev b 13)

Allergen	Exposure	Ref	Seroprevalence	Ref	Skin test prevalence	Ref
Hev b 6.01			64% (A+C)	32	63% (H)	33
			83% (S/cong)			
					66% (A)	40
			45–55% (H)	37		
			30–69% (S)			
			86% (C)	39		
			58% (S)			
Hev b 6.02			63% (C)	39		
			58% (S)			
Hev b 7.01			23–45% (H)	37	45% (H)	33
			15–77% (S)			
					41% (A)	40
Hev b 7.02			40% (S)	35		
			49% (A)	43		
			3% (C)			
Hev b 8.0101					3% (A)	40
			35% (S)	44	88% (S)	44
			50% (A)		100% (A)	
Hev b 8.0102			12% (S)	45		
			20% (H)			
			6% (S)	46		
			24% (H)			
Hev b 10.0102			27% (A)	47		
Hev b 10.0103			10% (S)	48		
			0% (H)			
Hev b 11.0102			25% (H)	49		
			80% (S)			
Hev b 13					63% (H)	33

A: adults; C: children; S: spina bifida; cong: congenital abnormalities; H: health care workers.

Hevea latex proteins may also have homologies with other common allergens. Hev b 9, an enolase, demonstrates IgE cross-reactivity with enolases from *Cladosporium herbarium* and *Alternaria alternata* (57). The latex profilin Hev b 8 is homologous and cross-reactive with profilins from other plant species, such as celery and birch (45,46). Likewise, the latex manganese superoxide dismutase Hev b 10 cross-reacts with homologous human and *Aspergillus* proteins (47,48).

Finally, homology and cross-reactivity between the latex proteins Hev b 1 and Hev b 3 (41,54,58) and between Hev b 6 and Hev b 11 (49) may obscure seroprevalence data and should be considered in the determination of immunologically relevant proteins.

A single case report describes a latex-allergic health care worker who experienced a local and systemic IgE-mediated reaction following the insertion of gutta-percha points into a maxillary molar (59). However, a RAST inhibition study indicated that raw gutta-balata, but not gutta-percha products, contained significant amounts of protein that is cross-reactive with *Hevea* latex (60).

B.   Routes of Exposure and Bioavailability

Latex antigen exposure can occur by cutaneous, percutaneous, mucosal, and parenteral routes, and the antigen can be transferred by direct contact and aerosol. Aerosol transmission of antigen has been documented (61–63). In another study, the amounts of latex antigen measured in air samples from different areas of the Mayo Clinic correlated well with the frequency of glove use and glove changes in those areas (64). Tomazic and colleagues have shown convincingly that the cornstarch powder with which some gloves are dusted is a potent carrier of latex proteins (65).

Although severe systemic reactions have occurred following cutaneous and respiratory exposure (66–69), it is clear that direct mucosal and parenteral exposure pose the greatest risk of anaphylaxis. Several reports highlight the hazards of patients with previously mild (and easily manageable) cutaneous or respiratory reactions who experience more severe reactions with mucosal or parenteral exposure (70–75).

Latex antigens appear to be readily bioavailable across the skin and mucosal surfaces; anaphylactic reactions have occurred following all types of exposure. However, it is not clear that all latex antigens are equally absorbed by all routes. Yeang et al. have suggested that Hev b 1 and Hev b 3, which are particle-bound proteins that appear to be less soluble than other latex antigens, elicit reactions predominantly in spina bifida patients, who are more likely to experience repeated mucosal contact with latex gloves than are health care workers who, in general, experience daily cutaneous exposure to gloves and respiratory contact to airborne allergens (76). This hypothesis needs to be tested by direct measurement of the specific allergen content of powder-bound protein, elutable protein, and nonelutable protein.

IV.   DIAGNOSIS

The diagnosis of latex allergy is based on the identification of patients with latex-specific IgE *and* symptoms consistent with IgE-mediated reactions to latex-containing devices. *The diagnosis of latex allergy should not be made on the basis of either of these criteria alone.* Patients who have laboratory findings indicating the presence of latex-reactive IgE antibody without clinical reactivity may have cross-reactive antibodies of no clinical significance. Likewise, patients with frankly anaphylactoid symptoms but no evidence of latex-specific IgE on serologic or skin testing may be reacting to other environmental allergens, and the diagnosis of latex allergy should be entertained only after a thorough evaluation of other possibilities. Risk group category alone is of no value in determining the diagnosis; however, it does affect the predictive value of the testing, especially of in vitro tests.

A.   Skin Tests

In literature reports, epicutaneous skin testing is safe, sensitive, specific, and economical. In all studies, epicutaneous testing appears to be quite sensitive, especially when two or more source materials are used (77–80). Among 907 health care workers, 18 were thought to be rubber allergic by questionnaire. All 18 were skin-prick-test positive with "prevulcanized" latex. Of the 889 history-negative patients, only six were skin-prick-test positive; one of these six was subsequently shown to be rubber allergic by challenge. Thus, in this series, percutaneous testing was 100% (18/18) sensitive and 99% (883/889) specific. The predictive value of a positive test was 80% (19/24), and the predictive value of a negative test was 100% (883/883) (81). In another series, the results were stratified further. Of 268 operating room nurses questioned, 102 reported urticaria, redness, or itching associated with latex glove use. Among the 197 who agreed to be skin-tested with a latex extract, only 21 nurses, all of whom were symptomatic, had positive tests. The highest percentage of positive tests (70%) was in atopic nurses with urticaria. Itching alone was least associated with a positive skin test (7). In Milwaukee, investigators examined 15 health care workers with latex allergy and 83 children with spina bifida. Eleven of the 15 health care workers were skin-test positive, as were 42 of the 83 spina bifida patients, some of whom had no clinical evidence of latex allergy. All patients who had experienced anaphylaxis were skin-test positive (82).

Epicutaneous testing with latex extracts has been associated with anaphylactic events (66,67,82–84). Although these reports form a distinctly small minority opinion among those investigators who have examined the use of skin tests, there is reason to be concerned. Anaphylactic events associated with skin testing have occurred without regard to risk group or prior history of anaphylaxis. Presumably, anaphylactic events may be attributed to antigen dose, antigen bioavailability, individual sensitivity, or all three factors. Since no standardized extracts were used in any of these studies, we do not know which of these factors were of greatest importance in these anaphylactic events. Comparisons of extracts made using different techniques indicate that the amount of protein extracts from a single glove can vary over twofold, depending on the extraction time (85); other factors, such as temperature, salt concentration, and detergent activity, can also affect extraction efficiency. The stability of the different latex antigens is also variable. Since the antigen content of gloves can vary several hundredfold, unstandardized extracts can contain vastly different amounts of latex protein. Furthermore, the measurable content of specific immunoreactive allergens is probably even more unpredictable. Thus, much of the danger of skin tests can probably be attributed to the use of uncharacterized extracts.

There is, at this time, no FDA-approved skin-test extract for rubber allergy. Western Allergy Services (Missisauga, Ontario), Stallergenes S.A. (Marseilles, France), Lofarma (Milan, Italy), and ALK Abello (Horsholm, Denmark) have latex extracts available for use outside the United States (74,75).

B. Serologic Tests

The predictive value of the in vitro measurement of latex-specific IgE is highly dependent on the population being studied. Spina bifida patients typically have such high specific IgE titers that most in vitro assays are adequately predictive. In the past, the in vitro diagnosis of latex allergy in health care workers and other adults with latex allergy has been considerably less predictive. The Pharmacia CAP and Hycor HyTECH systems are automated specific-IgE detection systems in which the antigen is bound to a solid phase prior to reaction with the test antibodies. In the DPC AlaSTAT assay, antigen and antibody interact in the liquid phase prior to solid-phase immobilization. Hamilton and colleagues have studied and reviewed these tests (86–88). The CAP and AlaSTAT assays appear to have diagnostic sensitivities of about 70–80% while the HyTECH assay has 90% sensitivity, when compared with a latex skin-test reagent. Conversely, the specificities of the CAP and AlaSTAT assays are greater (>90%) than the specificity of the HyTECH assay (about 70%). As is the case with skin tests, the composition of the allergen mixture is important. It is likely that the diagnostic performance of serologic tests is more a function of the molecular integrity and the biological relevance of the antigens in the allergen mixture than the technology employed to detect the bound IgE. Thus, Lundberg et al. have suggested that the sensitivity of the CAP assay could be increased by 1–2% by adding the Hev b 5 fusion protein to the crude latex mixture used in preparing the solid phase (89). The use of other recombinants, perhaps in combination with native extracts, may offer the best possibility of improved performance. Kurup et al. found that assays for IgE with a mixture of pure native Hev b 2 and recombinant Hev b 7 could detect 75% of latex-allergic health care workers and 91% of latex-allergic spina bifida patients, and that the addition of Hev b 3 increased the sensitivity to 100% for the spina bifida patients (37). A dipstick test for the detection of latex-specific IgE uses both ammoniated and nonammoniated latex as the allergen source, but the sensitivity was only 73.9% when compared with other serologic tests and skin tests with a panel of latex extracts (90).

C. Challenge Tests

Given the uncertainties that surround the diagnosis of latex allergy, it is understandable that challenge testing has been considered to be a "gold standard." Thus, the U.S. trial of a latex skin-test reagent included a glove provocation challenge to resolve discrepancies between the skin tests and clinical histories (88). Kurtz et al. developed a hooded exposure chamber technique in which subjects are exposed to a cloud of latex-adsorbed cornstarch for 3 minutes, followed by an assessment of peak expiratory flow and rhinoconjunctival symptoms (91). Quirce et al. designed a quantified environmental (glove) challenge in an enclosed space (92). Challenge techniques have the advantage of being useful in monitoring the natural history of latex allergy as well as responses to immunomodulatory intervention. As before, the utility of this technique will be limited by the relevance of the allergens used in the challenge. The task before the diagnostician—and the scientists that support the effort to develop accurate diagnostic techniques—remains to identify the correct allergens, generate them in an immunoreactive and stable formulation, and determine doses with which one can safely assess whether the patient is hypersensitive to the allergens.

V. TREATMENT STRATEGIES

A. Allergen Avoidance

Avoidance of latex products is the only measure that can avert a serious allergic reaction to latex. Given the ubiquity of latex in household and medical devices, complete latex avoidance is a daunting task. Holtzman introduced the rational concept of providing a "latex-safe" environment, rather than a "latex-free" one (93). In the FDA series, 79% of reported reactions to medical devices (excluding barium enema catheters, condoms, and diaphragms) were due to latex gloves or bladder catheters. Reported much less often were reactions to adhesive tape (5%), piston syringes (0.6%), intravascular administration sets (1.3%), and numerous other devices (94).

Latex avoidance practices vary from center to center. At a minimum, latex avoidance entails the stringent elimination of latex-containing gloves and bladder catheters from the immediate environment. Condom catheters and balloons also constitute a hazard in patient rooms and outpatient settings. Penrose drains, latex bandages, rubber dams, prophylaxis cups, and rubber anesthesia masks have also been directly associated with type I reactions. Adhesives have usually been associated only with local reactions, but prudence would suggest the use of alternative, nonlatex products.

Well-documented episodes of aerosol spread of latex antigen have raised levels of concern beyond the direct contact of the latex-allergic patient with an antigen-containing device. Care should be taken to avoid the presence of any latex implements near the patient, and all surgical or dental assistants, even those who do not anticipate direct contact with the patient, should wear nonlatex gloves. Powdered latex products are especially problematic due to the aerosolization of antigen. Some centers have set aside latex-free areas in surgical suites and dental clinics; others have found it sufficient to reserve the first morning time slot, when the latex aeroallergen level appears to be lowest, for procedures on latex-allergic patients. *The elimination of powdered latex gloves is probably the single most effective measure in the reduction of overall risk of sensitization and clinical reactions* (95).

Health care workers with latex allergy can usually stay at work by switching to nonlatex gloves and asking colleagues to use powder-free gloves; for some workers, more stringent measures may be required. Such workers should be warned that when they become patients, mucosal or parenteral exposure to latex may result in anaphylaxis, even if the reactions during occupational exposure had been relatively mild.

Otherwise-unexplained anaphylaxis in latex-allergic patients has suggested the possibility, first raised by Silverman (96), that antigens may be released from rubber medication stoppers and the injection ports of intravenous tubing. Kwittken et al. have reported such reactions in four children (97); other, similar reports have also appeared (98,99). In some centers, it has become the practice to eliminate multidose vials and remove latex injection ports from the operating theater when the patient is latex allergic. An attempt to extract measurable antigen from injection ports failed (100); however, latex vial stoppers appeared to release latex allergens (as determined by positive skin tests in highly allergic individuals) after 40 punctures (5 of 12 subjects positive) and even after incubation without puncture (2 of 12 subjects positive). No latex antigen could be measured in any of these solutions by RAST inhibition (101) . Thus, the presence and bioavailability of antigen in stoppers has been documented in a single study. The practice of removing stoppers should be balanced against the likelihood of microbial contamination and oxidative deterioration of the drug.

Latex condoms have been associated with local urticaria in both males and females (79) and a life-threatening anaphylactic reaction in a female (72). Polyurethane condoms for males (Avanti) and female (Reality) are currently available. In addition to decreasing the likelihood of allergic events (102), primary avoidance may decrease the incidence of latex allergen sensitization. The best evidence of this is in patients with spina bifida. In one study, the incidence of latex sensitization in patients with a comparable number of operative procedures was 8.1% in the exposed group and 2.1% in the avoidance group (103). In another study, the incidences were 8.1% and 0%, respectively (104). Avoidance programs have also reduced the incidence of latex allergy among health care workers in an Ontario teaching hospital (105) and in a national surveillance program in Germany (106).

B. Measurement of Latex Allergens in Devices and in the Environment

Optimal latex allergen avoidance is possible only when the latex allergen content of devices can be determined reliably. Several approaches have been advanced (reviewed in Ref. 107). For devices in which the protein content is likely to originate only from *Hevea* latex, a modified Lowry total-protein method is applicable (see, for example, protocol D5712–99 at the American Society for Testing and Materials Web site, www.astm.org). Direct assays with polyclonal animal hyperimmune sera (108), inhibition immunoassays with pooled human sera (109), and specific monoclonal antibodies (31,38,42) have all been used with success. The bioassay approach (101), while appealing, will not lend itself to ready usage. Commercial kits for the measurement of latex proteins in the environment are available (see, for example, www.inbio.com/FIT.html and www.indoorairtest.com/aboutedl.html).

C. Reducing the Allergen Content of Medical Devices

Latex medical devices need not contain protein antigens. The protein content of *Hevea* latex products can be reduced considerably by washing, heat treatment, chlorination, and enzyme digestion (110–114). Siler et al. have shown that natural rubber derived from alternative species (*Parthenium argentatum*) contains very little protein compared with *Hevea* rubber and has no cross-reactivity when measured with mouse and human polyclonal antisera (115).

D. Allergen Immunotherapy

Latex allergy is an IgE-mediated disorder, and specific immunotherapy should be curative. Case reports suggested that immunotherapy might be effective (116–118). Seventeen adult latex-allergic subjects with occupational exposure to latex were enrolled in a double-blind placebo-controlled trial. The subjects achieved their maximum tolerated dose of the Stallergenes latex extract (or placebo control) over a period of 2 days, followed by weekly, biweekly, and then monthly doses for a year. In comparison with the placebo group, the treatment group had significantly reduced symptom and medication scores and increased threshold doses for conjunctival provocation testing. Systemic reactions occurred in an appreciable percentage of injections, including rhinitis (15.2%), wheezing (2.7%), pharyngeal edema (1.2%), and urticaria (1.2%) (119). Sutherland et al., in their review of the options for the treatment of latex allergy with specific immunotherapy (120), highlight the importance of including the *Hevea* allergens Hev b 5, Hev b 6, and Hev b 7, because of prevalence of latex-allergic individuals who are sensitized—in many cases, monosensitized—to these allergens (Table 2) (40). Using an inhibition assay, Chen et al. concluded that 45% of latex-allergic spina bifida patients are monosensitized to Hev b 1 (36). At this time, because of the uncertainties about the optimal allergens and dosing, and because of the likelihood of systemic reactions in immunotherapy recipients, latex allergen immunotherapy must be considered an investigational procedure reserved for those individuals for whom all other approaches have failed.

VI. SALIENT POINTS

1. At this time, prevention is the only effective treatment for latex allergy.
2. Latex allergens are ubiquitous.
3. Gloves are the most important source of latex allergen in the health care environment. Deal with the gloves first. Catheters are also important.
4. All latex allergy tests, whether RAST, ELISA, skin tests, or challenges, are only as good as the allergens that are used. The allergens must be intact, and all significant specific allergens must be represented in the allergen mix used.
5. Testing is readily available now. The predictive value of testing *as a diagnostic tool* is excellent. However, the value of such tests *as a screening tool* is uncertain.
6. Premedication does not prevent antigen-induced anaphylaxis.

7. Consider food allergy.

8. There is probably no way to construct a latex-free environment in the health care setting, but it is certainly possible to construct a latex-safe environment. The degree of latex allergen avoidance required for latex-allergic health care workers to remain at work is variable.

9. All latex avoidance measures come with a price (money, resources, risk of contamination, diminished barrier protection). Latex avoidance should be consonant with the risk.

10. History alone is a poor predictor of latex allergy, but the predictive value of not obtaining a history is zero. *Asking your patients if they have symptoms consistent with latex allergy is simple and quick and should be part of routine screening for all medical and dental practitioners.*

REFERENCES

1. Reinheimer G, Ownby DR. Prevalence of latex-specific IgE antibodies in patients being evaluated for allergy. Ann Allergy Asthma Immunol 1995; 74:184–187.

2. Garabrant DH, Roth HD, Parsad R, Ying GS, Weiss J. Latex sensitization in health care workers and in the US general population. Am J Epidemiol 2001; 153(6):515–522.

3. Buckland JR, Norman LK, Mason PS, Carruth JA. The prevalence of latex allergy in patients with rhinitis. J Laryngol Otol 2002; 116(5):349–351.

4. Jensen VB, Jorgensen IM, Rasmussen KB, Prahl P. The prevalence of latex sensitisation and allergy in Danish atopic children. Evaluation of diagnostic methods. Dan Med Bull 2002; 49(3):260–262.

5. Grzybowski M, Ownby DR, Rivers EP, Ander D, Nowak RM. The prevalence of latex-specific IgE in patients presenting to an urban emergency department. Ann Emerg Med 2002; 40(4):411–419.

6. Turjanmaa K. Incidence of immediate allergy to latex gloves in hospital personnel. Contact Dermatitis 1987; 17:270–275.

7. Lagier F, Vervloet D, Lhermet I, Poyen D, Charpin D. Prevalence of latex allergy in operating room nurses. J Allergy Clin Immunol 1992; 90:319–322.

8. Bubak ME, Reed CE, Fransway AF, Yunginger JW, Jones RT, Carlson CA, Hunt LW. Allergic reactions to latex among health-care workers. Mayo Clin Proc 1992; 67:1075–1079.

9. Berky ZT, Luciano WJ, James WD. Latex glove allergy: A survey of the US Army Dental Corps. JAMA 1992; 268:2695–2697.

10. Hwang JI, Park HA. Prevalence of adverse reactions to latex gloves in Korean operating room nurses. Int J Nurs Stud 2002; 39(6):637–643.

11. Mitsuya K, Iseki H, Masaki T, Hamakawa M, Okamoto H, Horio T. Comprehensive analysis of 28 patients with latex allergy and prevalence of latex sensitization among hospital personnel. J Dermatol 2001; 28(8):405–412.

12. Horwitz IB, Arvey RD. Workers' compensation claims from latex glove use: A longitudinal analysis of Minnesota data from 1988 to 1997. J Occup Environ Med 2000; 42(9):932–938.

13. Horwitz IB, Kammeyer-Mueller JD, McCall BP. Assessing latex allergy among health care employees using workers' compensation data. Minn Med 2001; 84(3):47–50.

14. Horwitz IB, Kammeyer-Mueller J, McCall BP. Workers' compensation claims related to natural rubber latex gloves among Oregon healthcare employees from 1987–1998. BMC Public Health 2002; 2(1):21.

15. Horwitz IB, Kammeyer-Mueller JD. Natural rubber latex allergy workers' compensation claims: Washington State healthcare workers, 1991–1999. Appl Occup Environ Hyg 2002; 17(4):267–275.

16. Bonauto DK, Foley M, Baggs J, Kaufman J. Workers' compensation latex claims. J Occup Environ Med 2001; 43(7):589–590.

17. Petsonk EL, Liss GM. Workers' compensation claims from latex glove use. J Occup Environ Med 2001; 43(7):590–591.

18. Wartenberg D, Buckler G. Invited commentary: Assessing latex sensitization using data from NHANES III. Am J Epidemiol 2001; 153(6):523–526.

19. Budnick LD. Re: "Latex sensitization in health care workers and in the US general population". Am J Epidemiol 2001; 154(2):190–191.

20. Gautrin D, Ghezzo H, Infante-Rivard C, Malo JL. Incidence and determinants of IgE-mediated sensitization in apprentices: A prospective study. Am J Respir Crit Care Med 2000; 162(4 pt 1):1222–1228.

21. Garabrant DH, Franzblau A. Incidence of latex sensitization. Am J Respir Crit Care Med 2001; 163(6):1501–1502.

22. Tosi LL, Slater JE, Shaer C, Mostello LA. Latex allergy in spina bifida patients: Prevalence and surgical implications. J Pediatr Orthop 1993; 13:709–712.

23. Meeropol E, Kelleher R, Bell S, Leger R. Allergic reactions to rubber in patients with myelodysplasia [letter]. N Engl J Med 1990; 323:1072.

24. Meeropol E, Frost J, Pugh L, Roberts J, Ogden JA. Latex allergy in children with myelodysplasia: A survey of Shriners Hospitals. J Pediatr Orthop 1993; 13:1–4.

25. Hochleitner BW, Menardi G, Haussler B, Ulmer H, Kofler H, Reider N. Spina bifida as an independent risk factor for sensitization to latex. J Urol 2001; 166(6):2370–2373.

26. Hourihane JO, Allard JM, Wade AM, McEwan AI, Strobel S. Impact of repeated surgical procedures on the incidence and prevalence of latex allergy: A prospective study of 1263 children. J Pediatr 2002; 140(4):479–482.

27. Rueff F, Kienitz A, Schopf P, Hartl WH, Andress HJ, Zaak D, Menninger M, Pryzbilla B. Frequency of natural rubber latex allergy in adults is increased after multiple operative procedures. Allergy 2001; 56(9):889–894.

28. St Cyr DR. Rubber, natural. In: Encyclopedia of Chemical Technology (Kirk-Othmer, ed.). New York: John Wiley & Sons, 1982: 468–491.

29. d'Auzac J, Jacob J-L. The composition of latex from *Hevea brasiliensis* as a laticiferous cytoplasm. In: Physiology of Rubber Tree Latex (d'Auzac J, Jacob J-L, Chrestin H, eds.). Boca Raton, FL: CRC Press, 1989: 59–96.

30. Kekwick RGO. The formation of isoprenoids in *Hevea* latex. In: Physiology of Rubber Tree Latex (d'Auzac J, Jacob J-L, Chrestin H, eds.). Boca Raton, FL: CRC Press, 1989: 145–164.

31. Chardin H, Chen Z, Raulf-Heimsoth M, Mayer C, Senechal H, Desvaux FX, Senechol H, Peltre A. Identification of Hev b1 in natural latex mattresses. Int Arch Allergy Immunol 2000; 121:211–214.

32. Alenius H, Kalkkinen N, Yip E, Hasmin H, Turjanmaa K, Makinen-Kiljunen S, Reunnala T, Palosno T. Significance of rubber elongation factor as a latex allergen. Int Arch Allergy Immunol 1996; 109:362–368.

33. Bernstein DI, Biagini RE, Karnani R, Hamilton R, Murphy K, Bernstein C, Arifs A, Berendts B, Yeang HY. In vivo sensitization to purified *Hevea brasiliensis* proteins in health care workers sensitized to natural rubber latex. J Allergy Clin Immunol 2003; 111(3):610–616.

34. Poulos LM, O'Meara TJ, Hamilton RG, Tovey ER. Inhaled latex allergen (Hev b 1). J Allergy Clin Immunol 2002; 109:701–706.

35. Wagner B, Buck D, Hafner C, Sowka S, Niggemann B, Scheiner O, Breitender H. Hev b 7 is a *Hevea brasiliensis* protein associated with latex allergy in children with spina bifida. J Allergy Clin Immunol 2001; 108(4):621–627.

36. Chen Z, Cremer R, Posch A, Raulf-Heimsoth M, Rihs HP, Baur X. On the allergenicity of Hev b 1 among health care workers and patients with spina bifida allergic to natural rubber latex. J Allergy Clin Immunol 1997; 100(5):684–693.

37. Kurup VP, Yeang HY, Sussman GL, Bansal NK, Beezhold DH, Kelly KJ, Hoffman DR, Williams B, Fink JN. Detection of Immunoglobulin antibodies in the sera of patients using purified latex allergens. Clin Exp Allergy 2000; 30(3):359–369.

38. Raulf-Heimsoth M, Sander I, Chen Z, Borowitzki G, Diewald K, van Kanpen V, Baur X. Development of a monoclonal antibody-based sandwich ELISA for detection of the latex allergen Hev b 1. Int Arch Allergy Immunol 2000; 123(3):236–241.

39. Ylitalo L, Alenius H, Turjanmaa K, Palosuo T, Reunala T. IgE antibodies to prohevein, hevein, and rubber elongation factor in children with latex allergy. J Allergy Clin Immunol 1998; 102(4 pt 1):659–664.

40. Yip L, Hickey V, Wagner B, Liss G, Slater J, Breiteneder H, Sussman G, Beezhold D. Skin prick test reactivity to recombinant latex allergens. Int Arch Allergy Immunol 2000; 121(4):292–299.

41. Wagner B, Krebitz M, Buck D, Niggemann B, Yeang HY, Han KH, Scheiner O, Breitender H. Cloning, expression, and characterization of recombinant Hev b 3, a *Hevea brasiliensis* protein associated with latex allergy in patients with spina bifida. J Allergy Clin Immunol 1999; 104(5):1084–1092.

42. Sutherland MF, Drew A, Rolland JM, Slater JE, Suphioglu C, O'Hehir RE. Specific monoclonal antibodies and human immunoglobulin E show that Hev b 5 is an abundant allergen in high protein powdered latex gloves. Clin Exp Allergy 2002; 32(4):583–589.

43. Seppala U, Palosuo T, Seppala U, Kalkkinen N, Ylitalo L, Reunala T, Turjanmaak K, Reunala T. IgE reactivity to patatin-like latex allergen, Hev b 7, and to patatin of potato tuber, Sol t 1, in adults and children allergic to natural rubber latex. Allergy 2000; 55(3):266–273.

44. Nieto A, Mazon A, Boquete M, Carballada F, Asturias JA, Martinez J, Martinez A. Assessment of profilin as an allergen for latex-sensitized patients. Allergy 2002; 57(9):776–784.

45. Rihs HP, Chen Z, Rozynek P, Baur X, Lundberg M, Cremer R. PCR-based cloning, isolation, and IgE-binding properties of recombinant latex profilin (rHev b 8). Allergy 2000; 55:712–717.

46. Ganglberger E, Radauer C, Wagner S, Riordain G, Beezhold DH, Brehler R, Niggemann B, Scheiner O, Jensen H, Jarolim E, Breitender H. Hev b 8, the *Hevea brasiliensis* latex profilin, is a cross-reactive allergen of latex, plant foods and pollen. Int Arch Allergy Immunol 2001; 125:216–227.

47. Wagner S, Sowka S, Mayer C, Crameri R, Focke M, Kurup VP, Scheiner O, Becitender H. Identification of a *Hevea brasiliensis* latex manganese superoxide dismutase (Hev b 10) as a cross-reactive allergen. Int Arch Allergy Immunol 2001; 125:120–127.

48. Rihs HP, Chen Z, Rozynek P, Cremer R. Allergenicity of rHev b 10 (manganese-superoxide dismutase). Allergy 2001; 56:85–86.

49. Rihs HP, Dumont B, Rozynek P, Lundberg M, Cremer R, Bruning T, Raulf H, Heimsoth M. Molecular cloning, purification, and IgE-binding of a recombinant class I chitinase from *Hevea brasiliensis* leaves (rHev b 11.0102). Allergy 2003; 58(3):246–251.

50. Blanco C. Latex-fruit syndrome. Curr Allergy Asthma Rep 2003; 3(1):47–53.

51. Wright HT, Brooks DM, Wright CS. Evolution of the multidomain protein wheat germ agglutinin. J Mol Evol 1985; 21:133–138.

52. Beezhold DH, Sussman GL, Liss GM, Chang NS. Latex allergy can induce clinical reactions to specific foods. Clin Exp Allergy 1996; 26:416–422.

53. Slater JE, Vedvick T, Arthur-Smith A, Trybul DE, Kekwick RGO. Identification, cloning and sequence of a major allergen (Hev b 5) from natural rubber latex (*Hevea brasiliensis*). J Biol Chem 1996; 271:25394–25399.

54. Scheiner O, Wagner B, Wagner S, Krebitz M, Crameri R, Niggemann B, Yeang HY, Ebner C, Breitender H. Cloning and molecular characterization of Hev b 3, a spina-bifida-associated allergen from *Hevea brasiliensis* latex. Int Arch Allergy Immunol 1999; 118:311–312.

55. Yagami T, Sato M, Nakamura A, Shono M. One of the rubber latex allergens is a lysozyme. J Allergy Clin Immunol 1995; 96:677–686.

56. Garcia Ortiz JC, Moyano JC, Alvarez M, Bellido J. Latex allergy in fruit-allergic patients. Allergy 1998; 53(5):532–536.

57. Wagner S, Breiteneder H, Simon-Nobbe B, Susani M, Krebitz M, Niggemann B, Brehles R, Scheines O, Hoffman H, Sommergruben K. Hev b 9, an enolase and a new cross-reactive allergen from hevea latex and molds: Purification, characterization, cloning and expression. Eur J Biochem 2000; 267:7006–7014.

58. Banerjee B, Kanitpong K, Fink JN, Zussman M, Sussman GL, Kelly KJ, Kurup VP. Unique and shared IgE epitopes of Hev b 1 and Hev b 3 in latex allergy. Mol Immunol 2000; 37(12–13):789–798.

59. Boxer MB, Grammer LC, Orfan N. Gutta-percha allergy in a health care worker with latex allergy. J Allergy and Clin Immunol 1994; 93(5):943–944.

60. Costa GE, Johnson JD, Hamilton RG. Cross-reactivity studies of gutta-percha, gutta-balata, and natural rubber latex (*Hevea brasiliensis*). J Endod 2001; 27(9):584–587.

61. Baur X, Jager D. Airborne antigens from latex gloves [letter]. Lancet 1990; 335:912.

62. Lagier F, Badier M, Charpin D, Martigny J, Vervloet D. Latex as aeroallergen. Lancet 1990; 336:516–517.

63. Jaeger D, Kleinhans D, Czuppon AB, Baur X. Latex-specific proteins causing immediate-type cutaneous, nasal, bronchial, and systemic reactions. J Allergy Clin Immunol 1992; 89:759–768.

64. Swanson MC, Bubak ME, Hunt LW, Yunginger JW, Warner MA, Reed CE. Quantification of occupational latex aeroallergens in a medical center. J Allergy Clin Immunol 1994; 94:445–451.

65. Tomazic VJ, Shampaine EL, Lamanna A, Withrow TJ, Adkinson NF, Hamilton RG. Cornstarch powder on latex products is an allergen carrier. J Allergy Clin Immunol 1994; 93:751–758.

66. Spanner D, Dolovich J, Tarlo S, Sussman G, Buttoo K. Hypersensitivity to natural latex. J Allergy Clin Immunol 1989; 83:1135–1137.

67. Beuers U, Baur X, Schraudolph M, Richter WO. Anaphylactic shock after game of squash in atopic woman with latex allergy [letter]. Lancet 1990; 335:1095.

68. Chen MD, Greenspoon JS, Long TL. Latex anaphylaxis in an obstetrics and gynecology physician. Am J Obstet Gynecol 1992; 166:968–969.

69. Ber DJ, Davidson AE, Klein DE, Settipane GA. Latex hypersensitivity: Two case reports. Allergy Proc 1992; 13:71–73.

70. Leynadier F, Pecquet C, Dry J. Anaphylaxis to latex during surgery. Anaesthesia 1989; 44:547–550.

71. Turjanmaa K, Reunala T, Tuimala R, Karkkainen T. Allergy to latex gloves: Unusual complication during delivery. Br Med J 1988; 297:1029.

72. Taylor JS, Cassettari J, Wagner W, Helm T. Contact urticaria and anaphylaxis to latex. J Am Acad Dermatol 1989; 21:874–877.

73. Sussman GL, Tarlo S, Dolovich J. The spectrum of IgE-mediated responses to latex. JAMA 1991; 265:2844–2847.

74. Laurent J, Malet R, Smiejan JM, Madelenat P, Herman D. Latex hypersensitivity after natural delivery. J Allergy Clin Immunol 1992; 89:779–780.

75. Oei HD, Tjiook SB, Chang KC. Anaphylaxis due to latex allergy. Allergy Proc 1992; 13:121–122.

76. Yeang HY, Cheong KF, Sunderasan E, Hamzah S, Chew NP, Hamid S, Hamilton RG, Cardosa MJ. The 14.6 kD (REF, Hev b 1) and 24 kD (Hev b 3) rubber particle proteins are recognized by IgE from spina bifida patients with latex allergy. J Allergy Clin Immunol 1996; 98:628–639.

77. Wrangsjo K, Wahlberg JE, Axelsson IGK. IgE-mediated allergy to natural rubber in 30 patients with contact urticaria. Contact Dermatitis 1988; 19:264–271.

78. Turjanmaa K, Reunala T, Rasanen L. Comparison of diagnostic methods in latex surgical contact urticaria. Contact Dermatitis 1988; 19:241–247.

79. Turjanmaa K, Reunala T. Condoms as a source of latex allergen and cause of contact urticaria. Contact Dermatitis 1989; 20.360–364.

80. Pecquet C, Leynadier F, Dry J. Contact urticaria and anaphylaxis to natural latex. J Am Acad Dermatol 1990; 22:631–633.

81. Moneret-Vautrin DA, Laxenaire MC. Routine testing for latex allergy in patients with spina bifida is not recommended [reply]. Anesthesiology 1991; 74:391–392.

82. Kelly KJ, Kurup V, Zacharisen M, Resnick A, Fink JN. Skin and serologic testing in the diagnosis of latex allergy. J Allergy Clin Immunol 1993; 91:1140–1145.

83. Bonnekoh B, Merk HF. Safety of latex prick skin testing in allergic patients [letter]. JAMA 1992; 267:2603.

84. Nettis E, Dambra P, Traetta PL, Loria MP, Ferrannini A, Tursi A. Systemic reactions on SPT to latex. Allergy 2001; 56(4):355–356.

85. Fink JN, Kelly KJ, Elms N, Kurup VP. Comparative studies of latex extracts used in skin testing. Ann Allergy Asthma Immunol 1996; 76:149–152.

86. Hamilton RG, Biagini RE, Krieg EF. Diagnostic performance of Food and Drug Administration-cleared serologic assays for natural rubber latex-specific IgE antibody. The Multi-Center Latex Skin Testing Study Task Force. J Allergy Clin Immunol 1999; 103(5 pt 1):925–930.

87. Biagini RE, Krieg EF, Pinkerton LE, Hamilton RG. Receiver operating characteristics analyses of Food and Drug Administration-cleared serological assays for natural rubber latex-specific immunoglobulin E antibody. Clin Diagn Lab Immunol 2001; 8(6):1145–1149.

88. Hamilton RG, Peterson EL, Ownby DR. Clinical and laboratory-based methods in the diagnosis of natural rubber latex allergy. J Allergy Clin Immunol 2002; 110(suppl 2):S47–S56.

89. Lundberg M, Chen Z, Rihs HP, Wrangsjo K. Recombinant spiked allergen extract. Allergy 2001; 56:794–795.

90. Kutting B, Weber B, Brehler R. Evaluation of a dipstick test (Allergodip-Latex) for in vitro diagnosis of natural rubber latex allergy. Int Arch Allergy Immunol 2001; 126(3):226–230.

91. Kurtz KM, Hamilton RG, Schaefer JA, Adkinson NF Jr. A hooded exposure chamber method for semiquantitative latex aeroallergen challenge. J Allergy Clin Immunol 2001; 107(1):178–184.

92. Quirce S, Swanson MC, Fernandez-Nieto M, De Las HM, Cuesta J, Sastre J. Quantified environmental challenge with absorbable dusting powder aerosol from natural rubber latex gloves. J Allergy Clin Immunol 2003; 111(4):788–794.

93. Holzman RS. Latex allergy: An emerging operating room problem. Anesth Analg 1993; 76:635–641.

94. Dillard SF, MacCollum MA. Reports to FDA: Allergic reactions to latex containing medical devices. International Latex Conference: Sensitivity to latex in medical devices, 23. 1992.

95. Tarlo SM, Sussman G, Contala A, Swanson MC. Control of airborne latex by use of powder-free gloves. J Allergy Clin Immunol 1994; 93:985–989.

96. Silverman HI. Rubber anaphylaxis [letter]. N Engl J Med 1989; 321:837.

97. Kwittken PL, Becker J, Oyefara B, Danziger R, Pawlowski NA, Sweinberg S. Latex hypersensitivity reactions despite prophylaxis. Allergy Proc 1992; 13:123–127.

98. Schwartz HA, Zurowski D. Anaphylaxis to latex in intravenous fluids. J Allergy Clin Immunol 1993; 92(2):358.

99. Setlock MA, Cotter TP, Rosner D. Latex allergy: Failure of prophylaxis to prevent severe reaction. Anesth Analg 1993; 76:650–652.

100. Yunginger JW, Jones RT, Fransway AF, Kelso JM, Warner MA, Hunt LW, Reed CE. Latex allergen contents of medical and consumer rubber products. J Allergy Clin Immunol 1993; 91:241.

101. Primeau MN, Adkinson NF Jr, Hamilton RG. Natural rubber pharmaceutical vial closures release latex allergens that produce skin reactions. J Allergy Clin Immunol 2001; 107(6):958–962.

102. Bernstein DI, Karnani R, Biagini RE, Bernstein CK, Murphy K, Berendts B, Bernstein JA, Bernstein L. Clinical and occupational outcomes in health care workers with natural rubber latex allergy. Ann Allergy Asthma Immunol 2003; 90(2):209–213.

103. Nieto A, Mazon A, Pamies R, Lanuza A, Munoz A, Estornell F, Garcia-Ibarra F. Efficacy of latex avoidance for primary prevention of latex sensitization in children with spina bifida. J Pediatr 2002; 140(3):370–372.

104. Cremer R, Kleine-Diepenbruck U, Hering F, Holschneider AM. Reduction of latex sensitisation in spina bifida patients by a primary prophylaxis programme (five years experience). Eur J Pediatr Surg 2002; 12(suppl 1):S19–S21.

105. Tarlo SM, Easty A, Eubanks K, Parsons CR, Min F, Juvet S, Liss GM. Outcomes of a natural rubber latex control program in an Ontario teaching hospital. J Allergy Clin Immunol 2001; 108(4):628–633.

106. Allmers H, Schmengler J, Skudlik C. Primary prevention of natural rubber latex allergy in the German health care system through education and intervention. J Allergy Clin Immunol 2002; 110(2):318–323.

107. Tomazic-Jezic VJ, Lucas AD. Protein and allergen assays for natural rubber latex products. J Allergy Clin Immunol 2002; 110(suppl 2):S40–S46.

108. Beezhold DH, Kostyal DA, Tomazic-Jezic VJ. Measurement of latex proteins and assessment of latex protein exposure. Methods 2002; 27(1):46–51.

109. Baur X. Measurement of airborne latex allergens. Methods 2002; 27(1):59–62.

110. Leynadier F, Tran Xuan T, Dry J. Allergenicity suppression in natural latex surgical gloves. Allergy 1991; 46:619–625.

111. Dalrymple SJ, Audley BG. Allergenic proteins in dipped products: Factors influencing extractable protein levels. Rubber Developments 1992; 45:51–60.

112. Ab Aziz NA. Chlorination of gloves. Latex Protein Workshop of the International Rubber Technology Conference 1993.

113. Hashim MYA. Effect of leeching on extractable protein content. Latex Protein Workshop of the International Rubber Technology Conference 1993.

114. Perrella FW, Gaspari AA. Natural rubber latex protein reduction with an emphasis on enzyme treatment. Methods 2002; 27(1):77–86.

115. Siler D, Cornish K, Hamilton RG. Absence of cross-reactivity of IgE antibodies from subjects allergic to *Hevea brasiliensis* latex with a new source of natural rubber latex from guayule (*Parthenium argentatum*). J Allergy Clin Immunol 1996; 98:895–902.

116. Pereira C, Rico P, Lourenco M, Lombardero M, Pinto-Mendes J, Chieira C. Specific immunotherapy for occupational latex allergy. Allergy 1999; 54(3):291–293.

117. Nucera E, Schiavino D, Buonomo A, Roncallo C, Del Ninno M, Milani A, Pollastrani E, Patriarca G. Latex rush desensitization. Allergy 2001; 56(1):86–87.

118. Patriarca G, Nucera E, Buonomo A, Del Ninno M, Roncallo C, Pollastrini E, de Pasquale T, Milani A, Schiavind D. Latex allergy desensitization by exposure protocol: Five case reports. Anesth Analg 2002; 94(3):754–758.

119. Leynadier F, Herman D, Vervloet D, Andre C. Specific immunotherapy with a standardized latex extract versus placebo in allergic healthcare workers. J Allergy Clin Immunol 2000; 106(3):585–590.

120. Sutherland MF, Suphioglu C, Rolland JM, O'Hehir RE. Latex allergy: Towards immunotherapy for health care workers. Clin Exp Allergy 2002; 32(5):667–673.

121. Sunderasan E, Hamzah S, Hamid S, Ward MA, Yeang HY, Cardosa MJ. Latex B-serum b-1,3-glucanase (Hev b II) and a component of the microhelix (Hev b IV) are major latex allergens. J Nat Rubb Res 1995; 10:82–99.

21

Drug Allergens, Haptens, and Anaphylatoxins

VIVIAN P. HERNANDEZ-TRUJILLO and PHILLIP L. LIEBERMAN

University of Tennessee College of Medicine, Memphis, Tennessee, U.S.A.

BADRUL A. CHOWDHURY

U.S. Food and Drug Administration, Rockville, Maryland, U.S.A.

I. INTRODUCTION

An adverse reaction to a drug or biological agent is a significant problem in the practice of medicine. An adverse drug reaction is undesirable and usually unanticipated independent of its intended therapeutic or diagnostic purpose. Although the exact frequency of adverse reactions to drugs and biological agents is unknown, it is estimated that each year 1 to 2 million people in the United States experience a drug reaction. An adverse drug

---

Dr. Badrul Chowdhury writes this chapter in his private capacity and not in his capacity as an employee of the U.S. Food and Drug Administration. No official support or endorsement by the U.S. Food and Drug Administration is intended or should be inferred.

reaction is reported as the cause of admission in 2% to 5% of all hospitalizations in the United States (1). Also, it is estimated that about 30% of all hospitalized patients experience an adverse drug event (2). The most important form of drug reaction is the immunologically mediated allergic reaction, which is relatively common and occurs unpredictably in an otherwise normal individual. Fear of recurrent allergic reactions often leads to repeated avoidance of a drug of choice. Therefore, measures that prevent, minimize, or reverse allergic reactions to drugs can have a major impact on the effectiveness and cost of patient care (3).

This chapter reviews the central concept of drug reactions based on immunological mechanisms. However, in approaching the problem of drug allergy, the entire spectrum of adverse reactions must be kept in mind because the clinical presentations of many reactions may be similar, although the mechanisms differ. In this chapter the term "drug" is generically used, and incorporates small- as well as large-molecule drugs, either synthesized in the laboratory or produced in a living biological system. The latter are often referred to in the scientific literature as "biological agents."

A. Classification of Adverse Drug Reactions

Before proceeding with a detailed review of drug allergy, it is appropriate to place it in perspective with other adverse drug reactions. A simple classification of adverse drug reactions is given in Table 1. Adverse drug reactions may be divided into two major groups: predictable adverse reactions and unpredictable adverse reactions. Predictable adverse drug reactions are often dose dependent, are related to the known pharmacology of the drug, and occur in otherwise normal subjects. Unpredictable adverse drug reactions are usually dose independent, usually unrelated to the drug's pharmacology, and often related to a subject's immunological responsiveness or genetic susceptibility. Physicians should carefully analyze and determine the nature of the adverse drug reaction, because this will influence future use of the drug. For example, a drug-induced toxic effect may be corrected by dose reduction, while an allergic reaction may mean that the drug cannot be used in that subject or its use may require special considerations (4).

Predictable adverse drug reactions include toxic reactions, side effects, drug–drug interactions, and secondary effects. A *toxic reaction* or *drug overdose* is directly related to the dose administered, and toxicity may occur after an excessive dose or because of slow degradation or elimination of the drug. *Side effects* of drugs are therapeutically undesirable effects but are potentially unavoidable due to the pharmacological action of the particular drug. Most drugs have multiple effects, only a few of which are therapeutically desirable.

Table 1 Classification of Adverse Drug Reactions

Predictable reactions that can occur in all individuals (dose dependent)
    Overdose or toxic reactions
    Side effects
    Drug–drug interactions
    Secondary effects
Unpredictable reactions that occur only in certain susceptible individuals (dose independent)
    Intolerance
    Idiosyncratic reactions
    Immunological and allergic reactions

The nontherapeutic biological activities often produce the side effects. *Drug–drug inter-actions are predictable and involve the action of one drug on the metabolism, toxicity,* or effectiveness of another drug. The *secondary effects* are undesirable effects unrelated to the primary pharmacological action of the medication. A classic example is vaginal candidiasis resulting from administration of a broad-spectrum antibiotic.

Unpredictable adverse drug reactions include drug intolerance, idiosyncratic reactions, and immunologically mediated reactions. *Drug intolerance* is caused by an exaggerated reactivity or lowered threshold to the normal pharmacological action of a drug. Such reactions are qualitatively normal. An *idiosyncratic reaction* describes a qualitatively abnormal response to a drug that is not related to its pharmacological activity. These are uncommon and unpredictable and often confused with allergic reactions. Susceptible individuals may possess a genetic deficiency that is expressed only following exposure to a drug, and not under normal conditions; an example is primaquine- and other oxidant drug–induced hemolytic anemias occurring in patients whose erythrocytes lack the enzyme glucose-6-phosphate dehydrogenase. *Immunological and allergic* drug reactions depend on the ability of the drug or its metabolite to interact with the immune system to invoke a humoral or cellular immune response. The three major classes of immunologic drug reactions are the IgE-mediated drug allergic reaction, the non–IgE-mediated anaphylactoid reaction, and the drug-induced autoimmune reaction. The term "drug allergy" describes the type I hypersensitivity reaction induced by a drug or its metabolite that leads to activation of cells bearing the high-affinity IgE receptor, such as the mast cells and basophils, resulting in the release of histamine and other mediators. *Anaphylactoid drug reactions* clinically resemble anaphylaxis but result from non–IgE-mediated activation of mast cells and basophils. The clinical manifestations of anaphylactoid reactions may be similar to type I allergic reactions, as the mediators of the two may be identical.

B. Drugs as Allergens

Large-molecular-weight drugs, which are often complete proteins, such as insulin, heteroantisera, chymopapain, clotting factors, and cytokines, are complete antigens that can induce immune responses and elicit immunopathologic reactions. However, most drugs and their metabolites have molecular weights less than 1000 daltons and therefore are not able to elicit an immune response in their native state. These drugs act as haptens. For an immune response to occur, the drug or its metabolite must bind to a tissue or plasma carrier protein to produce a complete antigen. This process of drug coupling to a carrier molecule is called haptenation (5). The sensitization capacity of a drug is dependent on the formation of strong covalent bonds between the hapten drug and the protein carrier. Some drugs, such as penicillin, are directly chemically reactive in their native state as a result of the instability of their molecular structure. Most drugs, however, are not active in their native state. The reactive forms are usually a metabolic product of the native drug. Haptenation usually is accomplished through the formation of a covalent bond. In rare cases, the bond may be noncovalent but of sufficient affinity for the drug–protein complex to remain intact during antigen processing and presentation. Thus, drugs or drug metabolites that easily form covalent bonds will be more immunogenic than those that are relatively unreactive. Since a drug metabolite can be the hapten, thorough knowledge of the biotransformation products of a drug is critical in the evaluation of drug allergies. Unfortunately, for most drugs these products are not known. This limits the ability to predict the immunogenicity of a given drug and the ability to test for the presence of drug allergy (6,7). Some small-molecular-weight drugs, such as succinylcholine and other quaternary ammonium muscle relaxants, are exceptions and do not need haptenation. These drugs have sufficient distance between determinants (typically over 6 angstroms) to permit them to act as bivalent antigens without being conjugated to a carrier (1).

On initial exposure to an allergenic drug, a predisposed individual typically exhibits a period of 10 to 20 days before the onset of an hypersensitivity reaction. During this latency period, the drug or its metabolite complexes to a protein carrier, is processed by antigen-presenting cells, and initiates an immune response. In the case of IgE sensitization, IgE specific for the drug or its metabolite fixes to the surface of cells bearing high-affinity IgE receptors, such as mast cells and basophils. Once this sensitization has occurred, there is no latency period on reexposure. Maximum response to a small drug dose, including anaphylaxis, can occur within minutes.

C. Factors Influencing Drug Allergy

Immune responses to drugs occur in a small percentage of exposed patients. Several factors have been identified that influence the expression of immune responses and allergic reactions to drugs. These factors may be related to the drug, the host, and other, concurrent diseases or therapies.

Certain drugs are more likely to be associated with adverse reactions than others. According to hospital surveys, antimicrobial drugs, particularly the β-lactam antibiotics, are responsible for 42% to 53%, aspirin and other nonsteroidal anti-inflammatory drugs (NSAIDs) are responsible for 14% to 27%, and central nervous system depressants cause 10% to 12% of drug reactions (1). The drug dose, route, duration, and number of courses influence the incidence of drug allergy. Larger doses and frequent intermittent courses, rather than prolonged continuous treatment, are more likely to predispose an individual to an IgE-mediated reaction (7). However, for an IgG-mediated reaction, such as penicillin-induced hemolytic anemia, high and sustained blood levels are required. For IgE production, topical administration of drugs is usually associated with a higher incidence of sensitization than parenteral administration. Parenteral administration via the intramuscular route is more sensitizing than via the intravenous route. Once sensitization has occurred, an immune reaction may occur on administration of the drug by any route (4,8).

Certain host-related factors play a role in drug reactions. The incidence of cutaneous drug reactions is reported to be higher in women than in men (9). In most studies in adults, no correlation has been found between the risk of drug reactions and advancing age. The presence of other allergic diseases or an atopic family history does not increase the risk of allergic reaction to drugs (1). Genetic factors influence the expression of some drug reactions. The risk of hydralazine-induced lupus-like syndrome is increased in patients with the HLA-DR4 phenotype. Adverse reactions to insulin are higher in individuals with HLA-B7, HLA-DR3, and HLA-DR3 types. The rate of hepatic metabolism of drugs may influence the susceptibility to some drug reactions. Patients with the slow acetylator phenotype are at increased risk for developing drug-induced lupus in response to hydralazine and procainamide. Adverse reactions to sulfonamides are possibly also more severe in patients with the same phenotype (1,4).

Some medications and disease states can alter the expression of reactions to drugs. An increased risk and severity of anaphylaxis has been linked to concurrent use of β-adrenergic blocking drugs (10). The incidence of ampicillin-induced skin rash is increased in patients with Epstein-Barr virus (EBV) infections causing acute infectious mononucleosis. About 5% of the normal population develop a skin rash reaction to ampicillin. The incidence is increased to nearly 100% in infectious mononucleosis. The higher incidence may be due to an abnormal immunoregulatory effect of the virus (11). In human immunodeficiency virus (HIV) infection, a high frequency of reactions to drugs is seen. The incidence of skin rash in response to trimethoprim-sulfamethoxazole is reported to be about 10-fold higher in HIV-infected individuals than in the general population. Allergic reactions to other drugs also appear to be higher in HIV-infected patients (12). The mechanisms behind this increased susceptibility to drug reactions are not known. Clinically, the reactions generally resemble the ampicillin-induced skin rash seen during EBV infection, raising the possibility that the mechanism may be related to an altered immune response attributable to the virus. Altered hepatic drug metabolism in HIV-infected patients may also explain the increased incidence of drug reactions. Reduced hepatic glutathione levels, resulting from the requirement of the liver to metabolize the diverse medications often administered to HIV-infected patients, may contribute by favoring the formation of more reactive drug metabolites.

Epidemiological studies indicate that patients who are allergic to one drug are not only at increased risk to react to another drug of the same class, but also are more likely to develop allergic reactions to drugs of other classes. Patients allergic to penicillin are reported to have an approximately 10-fold greater chance of experiencing reactions to non–β-lactam antibiotics such as sulfonamides, tetracyclines, and aminoglycosides. The mechanism of this apparent multiple-drug allergy syndrome is not clear. It may be due to an innate propensity of some individuals to develop an immune response to haptens irrespective of drug class (13,14).

II. ANTIBIOTIC ALLERGENS AND CROSS-REACTIVITY

Allergy to β-lactam antibiotics is commonly reported, especially penicillin allergy. The most frequent manifestations of penicillin allergy are cutaneous, notably urticaria and maculopapular or morbilliform rash. However, anaphylaxis occurs rarely, with an incidence of 1 per 5000 to 10,000 treatment courses (15). Although penicillin-induced anaphylaxis is rare, it is still a common cause of anaphylaxis, accounting for approximately 75% of fatal anaphylaxis in the United States (16).

A. Penicillin and Other β-Lactam Antibiotics

Penicillin and other β-lactam antibiotics commonly cause all types of immunological drug reactions, including IgE-mediated hypersensitivity, IgG-mediated hemolysis, antigen-antibody complex–mediated serum sickness, T-cell–mediated contact dermatitis, and antibody-mediated cytolysis. The most common and life-threatening reactions are those resulting from the production of specific IgE.

The β-lactam antibiotics include the penicillins, cephalosporins, carbapenams, and monobactams (Fig. 1). The penicillins have a β-lactam ring conjugated to a five-sided thiazolidine ring. The cephalosporins have the same β-lactam ring conjugated to a six-sided sulfur-containing ring. The carbapenams have the β-lactam ring attached to a five-sided ring containing carbon or oxygen in place of the sulfur in penicillin. The monobactams do not have a second ring attached to the β-lactam ring.

B. Penicillin as an Allergen

Penicillins have been extensively studied from a drug allergy standpoint, and much is known about their immunochemistry. Allergic reaction to penicillin is a prototype example

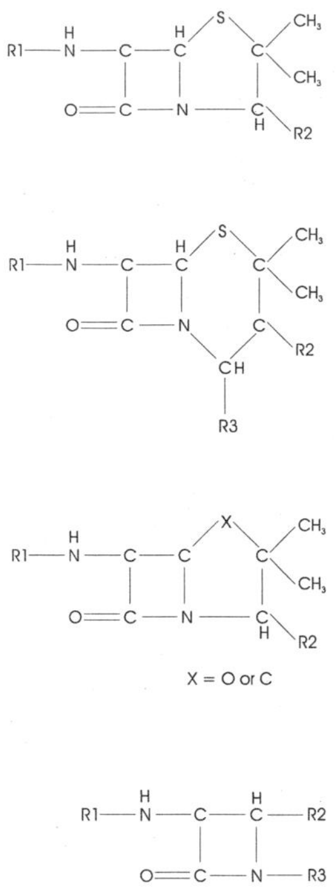

Figure 1 Structures of β-lactam antibiotics.

of direct haptenation. Penicillins contain a common β-lactam ring, a common thiazolidine ring, and a unique R side chain (Fig. 1). Unlike most other drugs, which must be metabolized before they react with proteins as a hapten, penicillins are intrinsically reactive because the β-lactam ring is unstable. The β-lactam ring of penicillin spontaneously opens under certain physiological conditions, allowing it to react as a hapten. Some of the haptens derived from penicillin are shown in Fig. 2. The most common penicillin-derived hapten is the penicilloyl moiety. The penicilloyl moiety is called the *major determinant* because approximately 95% (by weight) of the penicillin molecules that irreversibly combine with proteins are the penicilloyl moieties. In addition to penicilloyl, several other penicillin determinants, such as penicillenate and penicillamine, are also formed in the body, and these are also able to act as haptens and elicit IgE-mediated responses. These determinants are formed in smaller quantities and are therefore called the *minor determinants*. Some of the minor determinants are very unstable and formed transiently and their structures are not known (17).

The terms "major" and "minor" determinants refer to the abundance, not the clinical significance of any determinant, as all determinants, when present in sufficient quantity, can sensitize and initiate an allergic reaction. Antibodies to minor determinants usually mediate anaphylactic reactions, and antibodies to the major determinant generally mediate urticarial skin reactions. The major determinant, conjugated to a polylysine carrier to form penicilloyl-polylysine, is the only commercially skin-testing reagent for penicillin in the United States (17). Skin testing for diagnosing penicillin allergy is discussed further in Section VIII.

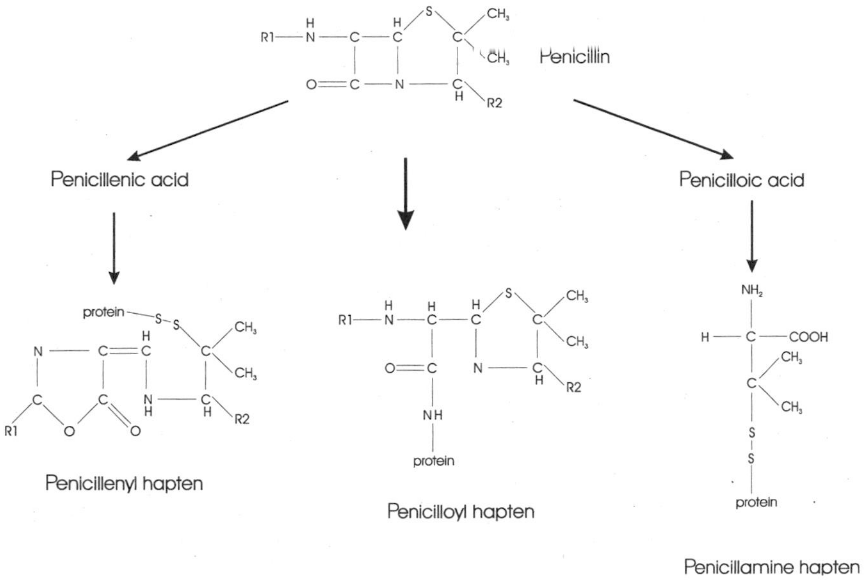

Figure 2 Haptens derived from penicillin.

In addition to the antigenic determinants formed from the β-lactam ring, the side chains that distinguish different penicillins also may elicit production of IgE antibodies that are clinically significant.

C. Immunologically Mediated Reactions to Penicillin

The most common and serious immunologically mediated reaction to penicillin is the *IgE-mediated type I hypersensitivity* reaction (Fig. 3). Estimates of incidence range from 1% to 10% of patients receiving penicillin. Of all the drugs, penicillin is the most frequent cause of anaphylaxis. Anaphylactic reactions can occur in all ages, although most are seen in adults between the ages of 20 and 50 years. High-dose intermittent use of penicillin is thought to be most sensitizing. Once an individual has been sensitized, a small dose of penicillin can produce a rapid and life-threatening response. The reaction may be localized to skin, presenting only as urticaria, or may be anaphylactic and potentially fatal

Penicillin-induced *hemolytic anemia* is rare. This is caused principally by IgG antibodies that develop usually after a prolonged course of high-dose parenteral penicillin. Penicillin and its metabolites are normally bound to red cell membranes. When IgG antibodies are produced against the penicillin, the red cells, the innocent bystanders, are destroyed by the complement pathway. In these patients, the antibody can be detected by a positive direct Coombs' test. However, a positive direct Coombs' test alone does not necessitate the discontinuation of penicillin, as almost 3% of patients receiving large parenteral doses of penicillin become Coombs' positive. Very rarely, patients may develop penicillin-induced *neutropenia* and *thrombocytopenia* via a mechanism analogous to that producing hemolytic anemia.

Penicillins can cause *acute interstitial nephritis*, and methicillin is the most commonly reported offender. The nephritis typically occurs in patients receiving a

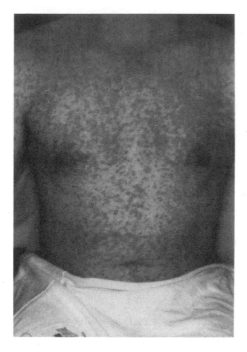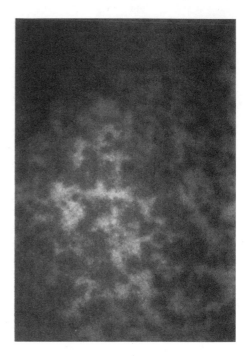

Figure 3 Morbilliform drug eruption from β-lactam antibiotic. Numerous erythematous macules and papules of varying size and symmetric distribution of the trunk are commonly seen, as in this patient shown in the left panel. In some areas the rash may become confluent, as is seen in a close-up picture of the same patient shown on the right panel. (Photograph courtesy of Dr. R. Rasberry, Division of Dermatology, University of Tennessee, Memphis.)

prolonged course of penicillin. Clinical manifestations include renal failure, fever, rash, arthralgia, hematuria, eosinophiluria, and peripheral eosinophilia. The mechanism of production of penicillin-induced interstitial nephritis is not known. Elevated IgE levels have been detected in some patients, suggesting that IgE-penicillin immune complexes contribute to the production of the nephritis.

D. Cross-Reactivity of Penicillin with Other β-Lactams

The structure of benzylpenicillin metabolites has been studied extensively, as described earlier. Similar information is not yet available for related antibiotics, such as the semisynthetic penicillins, cephalosporins, carbapenams, and monobactams. In vitro studies (RAST and ELISA inhibition assays) show that IgE antibody to benzylpenicillin cross-reacts with other β-lactam antibiotics. Therefore, if a patient reports allergy to one penicillin, allergy to all penicillins should be assumed. The only exception is the nonIgE mediated ampicillin-induced skin rash that occurs during EBV-induced infectious mononucleosis. Generally, cross-reactivity between penicillins is mostly due to shared β-lactam and thiazolidine rings. However, in vitro tests suggest that cross-reactivity between different penicillins may also be due to shared or similar side chain determinants (17).

Understanding of the immunochemistry of cephalosporins and of the cross-reactivity between cephalosporin and penicillin is limited. This is because understanding of cephalosporin antigenic determinants is lacking. Although penicillin and cephalosporins share a β-lactam ring, cephalosporins have a unique dihydrothiazide ring and unique side chains. The true incidence of clinical cross-reactivity between penicillins and cephalosporin has also been difficult to estimate. Early reports overestimated the degree of cross-reactivity, often claimed to be as high as 50%, because early cephalosporin antibiotic preparations contained trace amounts of penicillin. A review of the topic concluded that the risk of allergic reaction to cephalosporins in patients with a history of allergy to penicillin may be up to eight times as high as the risk in those with no history of allergy to penicillin. Patients with a history of allergy to penicillin and a positive skin test to penicillin should avoid cephalosporin because of possibility of cross-reactivity. However, patients with a history of allergy to penicillin, but negative skin tests to penicillin, do not appear to be at increased risk for allergy to cephalosporin (18).

Carbapenams like cephalosporins, also contain the β-lactam ring and cross-react with penicillin. However, monobactams do not contain the β-lactam ring and appear to lack cross-reactivity with penicillin (19). Sometimes patients with penicillin allergy produce IgE antibody to the side chain of the drug and not to the β-lactam ring, thus complicating the issue of cross-reactivity. Therefore, the similarity of the R1 and R2 side chains needs to be considered when determining cross-reactivity. Cross-reactions among cephalosporins may occur through R1 recognition of identical (cefaclor, cephalexin, cephaloglycin) or similar (cefaclor and cefadroxil) side chains, or through R2 recognition (cephalothin and cefotaxime) (20). Cross-reactions may also occur due to similarity of the side chains among different β-lactam antibiotics. For example, amoxicillin and cefadroxil contain the same side chain and thus cross-react (21). The monobactam aztreonam and the third-generation cephalosporin ceftazidime contain the same side chain. Piperacillin and cephapyrizone also contain an identical side chain. These drug pairs, therefore, may potentially cross-react. Independent anaphylaxis to cefazolin, with no cross-reactivity to other β-lactam antibiotics, has also been reported (22,23).

E. Sulfonamide Allergy

Reactions to sulfonamide antimicrobials are usually cutaneous in nature and commonly manifest as dermatitis or urticaria. Less common but more severe reactions include vasculitis, erythema multiforme, Stevens-Johnson syndrome, and toxic epidermal necrolysis (Figs. 4 and 5). Stevens-Johnson syndrome presents as a disseminated cutaneous eruption of discrete dark red macules, erosive stomatitis, and fever. In toxic epidermal necrolysis, there are extensive areas of epidermal necrolysis with loss of skin, giving a scalded appearance (24). The increased use of trimethoprim-sulfamethoxazole for a variety of infections, including its use for *Pneumocystis carinii* pneumonia (PCP) prophylaxis in AIDS, is partly responsible for a resurgence of drug reactions to sulfonamides. The incidence of reaction to trimethoprim/sulfamethoxazole is about 3% to 6% in hospitalized patients. In patients with AIDS, the incidence is about 10 times higher (19).

Sulfonamides are metabolized primarily by hepatic N-acetylation yielding nontoxic metabolites or, alternatively, by cytochrome P_{450}-catalyzed N-oxidation yielding reactive hydroxylamines. These hydroxylamines are then oxidized to reactive nitroso species, which are reduced by glutathione and excreted (25). When the capacity for glutathione conjugation is exceeded, the reactive metabolites may cause direct cytotoxic reactions or form immunogenic complexes by haptenation to protein carriers (26). One of the oxidative sulfonamide metabolites, $N4$-sulfonamidoyl, appears to be a major sulfonamide hapten. Multiple $N4$-sulfonamidoyl residues attached to a polytyrosine carrier have been reported to be useful as a skin test reagent. The clinical utility of this reagent is not yet

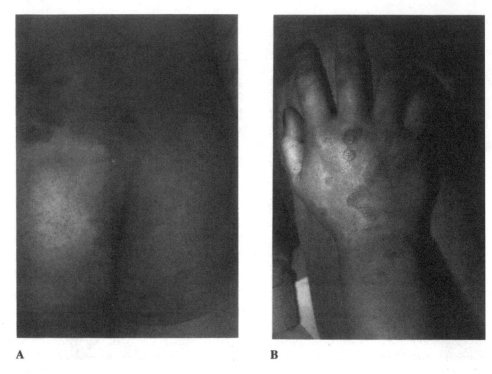

A   B

Figure 4   Erythema multiforme from sulfonamide antibiotic. Some lesions on the trunk and hand have targetlike appearance with a central erythematous dusky papule that may blister, a raised edematous middle ring, and an erythematous outer ring. Erythema multiforme may also occur with infections, especially herpes simplex and mycoplasma. Without mucosal involvement and systemic symptoms, this has a relatively benign course. (Photograph courtesy of Dr. R. Rasberry, Division of Dermatology, University of Tennessee, Memphis, TN.)

established. In HIV-infected patients, glutathione levels in the liver are reduced as a result of multiple infections and diverse prophylactic medication use. This retards the catabolism of the oxidative metabolites and may explain the increased incidence of sulfonamide allergy seen in HIV-infected patients.

The sulfonamide class of drugs includes the sulfonamide antibacterial agents and other non-antimicrobial drugs such as furosemide, thiazide diuretics, celecoxib, and sumatriptan. The frequency of cross-reactivity of members of this class is not known. However, sulfon-amides differ from other non-antimicrobials by their structure. The antimicrobial sulfano-mides have a substituted ring at N1 and an aromatic amine present at N4 (17). Because the N4-sulfamidoyl group allows haptenation to protein carriers, its absence in sulfonamide nonmicrobials may preclude formation of immune complexes. Patients sensitized to one sulfonamide may or may not react to another member of the class.

III.   ANESTHETIC ALLERGENS AND CROSS-REACTIVITY

A.   General Anesthetic Agents

Adverse reactions, including allergic reactions, can occur during induction and mainte-nance of general anesthesia. The estimated incidence of these reactions is between 1 in

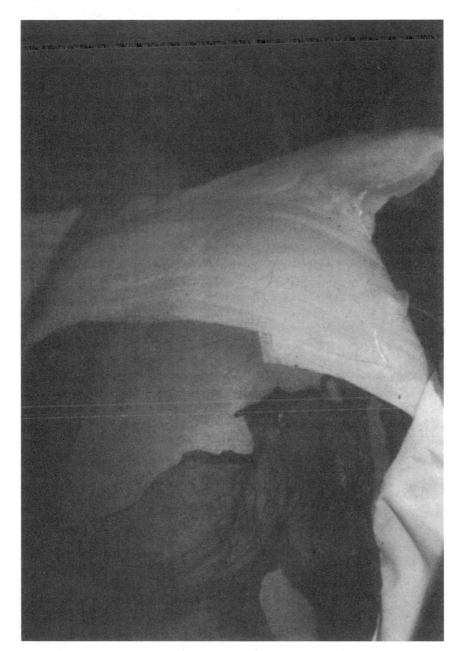

Figure 5 Toxic epidermal necrolysis from sulfonamide antibiotic. Extensive area of skin necrosis and sloughing is present. Initially the lesion presents with varying degrees of erythema; subsequently the dead skin is lost, resulting in skin ulcers giving the appearance of burn, as seen in this photo. Mortality is as high as 40%. (Photograph courtesy of Dr. R. Rasberry, Division of Dermatology, University of Tennessee, Memphis.)

5000 and 1 in 15,000, with fatalities reported to be about 5% (27). The majority of these reactions is due to the use of quaternary ammonium neuromuscular blocking agents, such as succinylcholine, tubocurarine, and pancuronium. Most frequently, reactions occur to vercuronium, atracurium, and suxamethonium (succinylcholine) (28). Anaphylaxis during surgical procedures is often difficult to diagnose. While the patient is under the effects of anesthesia, the clinician must rely on signs alone. The most common manifestations seen with anaphylactic reactions are bronchospasm and cardiovascular effects, whereas cutaneous signs are more frequent in anaphylactoid reactions (28). Since a single manifestation may occur, the clinician must be astute. Examination of the skin of a patient intraoperatively may be beneficial when cutaneous signs are present, but not visualized, while the patient is draped (28). Drugs of these groups contain small epitopes separated by a distance large enough to induce IgE production without haptenation. If anaphylaxis due to these neuromuscular blocking drugs is suspected, percutaneous skin testing with 1:10 to 1:100 wt/vol concentrations, or intradermal skin tests with 1:100 to 1:1,000 wt/vol concentrations, can be done. A positive skin test, with appropriate positive and negative controls, correlates with immediate hypersensitivity to these agents (27).

Latex allergy is an important cause of anaphylaxis during anesthesia (29). Reactions can manifest as urticaria, asthma, conjunctivitis, rhinitis, or anaphylaxis and can be fatal. A latex-free environment is essential when surgical or other procedures are performed on known latex-allergic individuals (see Chapter 20).

Opiates are known to cause direct (non–IgE-mediated) release of mast cell and basophil mediators. For this reason, skin prick testing may not predict opiate sensitivity, and wheals in opiate-sensitive patients may not significantly differ from the wheals in the control population. The wheals developed within 5 minutes of skin prick testing are likely due to direct release of histamine from mast cells. An assay for serum IgE specific for opiates is not commercially available, which makes it difficult to classify reactions as IgE mediated (30). Some reported reactions during general anesthesia may have been due to opiates (8,31).

B. Local Anesthetic Agents

Although allergic reactions to local anesthetic agents are commonly reported by patients and labeled as "allergic to caines," true allergic reactions to injected local anesthetics are exceedingly rare. Allergic mechanisms are often stipulated by patients, their dentists, or their physicians to explain reactions, which in reality are a pharmacological reaction to a large amount of absorbed drug or additive (such as epinephrine), vasovagal syncope, anxiety, or a hyperventilation reaction. The goal of management of these patients is to identify the very rare patient who is truly allergic by a safe testing and challenge protocol and to provide information relating to a local anesthetic that could be used safely in these patients.

1. Classification of Local Anesthetics and Cross-Reactivity

Despite the observation that the overwhelming majority of reactions to local anesthetics are not allergic in nature, the possibility of an immunological reaction must be considered in these patients who report an adverse reaction to the administration of a local anesthetic. Patients with such reported sensitivity are approached by drug selection based on chemical class and a testing and challenge protocol (32). Based on chemical structure, local anesthetics are classified into two groups, those that contain the para-aminophenyl derivatives and those that do not (Table 2). From an immunological standpoint, such classification has

Table 2 Classification of Local Anesthetics

Para-aminophenyl group present	Para-aminophenyl group absent
Procaine	Xylocaine
Proparcaine	Carbocaine
Tetracaine	Mepivacaine
Benzocaine	Proparacaine

some utility. Based on contact sensitivity cross-reactivity testing, para-aminophenyl derivatives cross-react with each other, whereas local anesthetics that do not contain the para-aminophenyl group do not cross-react with para-aminophenyl drugs or with each other. Therefore, during testing and challenge for a reaction due to a local anesthetic that does not contain the para-aminophenyl group, an agent from the non–para-aminophenyl–derived group, other than the drug associated with the reaction, should be used.

2. Approach to the Patient with Reported Local Anesthetic Sensitivity

The evaluation of a patient with a history of an adverse reaction to local anesthetics includes a complete history of the episode, skin testing, and subsequent drug challenge under careful observation. As with any allergy testing and challenge, only physicians experienced with the procedure and trained to treat possible allergic reactions should perform local anesthetic testing and challenge. A protocol for local anesthetic testing is given in Table 3.

The question of whether IgE-mediated reactions occur with local anesthetics is controversial. Prospective studies show that IgE-mediated reactions to local anesthetic perhaps do not occur (32,33) and the rare reactions are often due to preservatives in the local anesthetic preparation. In such cases, preservative-free local anesthetic should be used. Isolated case reports, on the other hand, have described allergic reactions to local

Table 3 Protocol for Local Anesthetic Provocative Dose Testing[a]

Route	Dilution	Dose
Prick test	Undiluted	1 drop
Intradermal test	1:100	0.02 ml
Subcutaneous challenge	1:100	0.1 ml
Subcutaneous challenge	1:10	0.1 ml
Subcutaneous challenge	Full strength	0.1 ml
Subcutaneous challenge	Full strength	0.5 ml
Subcutaneous challenge	Full strength	1.0 ml
Subcutaneous challenge	Full strength	2.0 ml

[a] Dosing and procedure may be used with any local anesthetic
The dilutions in the table are based on the usual therapeutic strength of the anesthetic (e.g., 1% xylocaine) that is commonly used. For testing, a local anesthetic free of both epinephrine and preservative should be used initially. The choice of anesthetic for testing is based on the anticipated use. The anesthetic that is anticipated to be used on the patient for a procedure should be used in testing. Xylocaine, because of its excellent safety profile and the fact that it is often the drug of choice for minor surgical and dental procedures, is quite often used for testing and challenge. Testing is performed by percutaneous, followed by intracutaneous, procedures. Subsequently, the drug is administered at 15-min intervals in incremental doses, until a dose that is anticipated to be used in the procedure (usually 2 ml) is given to the patient.

anesthetics. Two reports of allergic reactions to local anesthetics have been described, in both of which patients developed generalized urticaria. Each reacted to intradermal skin tests using three local anesthetics within the amide group, which is likely due to cross-reactivity among the agents (34,35). In another study, patients with a history of adverse reactions to local anesthetics, including cutaneous, cardiovascular, or respiratory manifestations, reacted positively to intradermal testing with local anesthetics compared with controls (36). From this study, it appears that skin testing may be useful in determining alternative local anesthetics to which patients may not react.

IV. ASPIRIN AND OTHER NONSTEROIDAL ANTI-INFLAMMATORY DRUGS

A. Types of Reactions

Aspirin and other nonsteroidal anti-inflammatory drugs (NSAIDs) produce a number of predictable adverse reactions based on pharmacological effects. These include gastritis, blood dyscrasia, nephrotoxicity, and hepatotoxicity. Toxic doses of the drugs cause tinnitus and metabolic acidosis.

Aspirin also can cause two types of unpredictable reactions. First, reactions may occur in patients with the aspirin triad or Samter syndrome (chronic hyperplastic pansinusitis with eosinophilic rhinitis, nasal polyps, and asthma), and second, reactions may manifest as urticaria, angioedema, and anaphylaxis. The mechanisms of each of these reactions are incompletely understood, but they are clearly different (37).

During the acute respiratory response to aspirin and all other NSAIDs in patients with the aspirin triad, there is both an overproduction of sulfidopeptide leukotrienes, such as LTE_4, as well as mast cell degranulation (38). Aspirin and other NSAIDs inhibit the cyclooxygenase pathway, thereby shunting arachidonic acid metabolism through the 5-lipoxygenase pathway, producing large amounts of vasoactive and bronchoconstrictive sulfidopeptide leukotrienes, such as LTC_4, LTD_4, and LTE_4. In the second type of reaction, patients are uniquely allergic to a specific NSAID and will not react to any other member of the class of drugs (i.e., drug specific rather than class specific). Their reaction may be urticaria and/or angioedema or an anaphylactoid reaction. This may be an IgE-mediated reaction (37).

B. Approach to the Patient with Reported Respiratory Tract Aspirin Sensitivity (Aspirin Triad)

Aspirin-sensitive individuals with respiratory reactions are sensitive to all nonselective COX-1 and COX-2 inhibitors (Table 4). The pharmacological effect shared by these drugs is inhibition of both the COX-1 and COX-2 cyclooxygenase pathways of arachidonic acid

Table 4 NSAIDs That Cross-React with Aspirin

Enolic acids	Piroxicam
Carboxylic acids	
Acetic acids	Indomethacin, sulindac, tolmentin
Propionic acids	Ibuprofen, naproxen, fenoprofen
Fenamates	Mefanamic acid, meclofenamate
Salicylates	Aspirin, choline magnesium trisalicylate

metabolism. The severity of the clinical reaction correlates with the drug's in vitro potency in inhibition assays of the COX 2 pathway; that is, NSAIDs that inhibit the enzyme at lower drug concentration are more potent inducers of the clinical response. The most potent NSAID in this regard is indomethacin. Most aspirin-sensitive patients can tolerate sodium salicylate and acetaminophen. However, in a small subpopulation of aspirin-sensitive asthmatics, large doses of these drugs (e.g., >1 g of acetaminophen or >2 g of salicylate) can produce respiratory tract reactions. Purported cross-reactivity between aspirin and tartrazine (FDC yellow dye No. 5) has not been substantiated in double-blind, placebo-controlled studies of aspirin-sensitive asthmatics or in patients with aspirin-induced urticaria (39,40). NSAID-sensitive patients with respiratory reactions can tolerate selective COX-2 inhibitors, a finding that has altered the approach to the patient with this disorder (39).

The diagnosis of aspirin sensitivity is made by history and does not usually require a challenge test to confirm the diagnosis. Stevenson et al. have developed a classification system to describe reactions to aspirin and NSAIDs (41). Patients with aspirin-sensitive respiratory disease are classified under NSAID-induced asthma and rhinitis. These patients typically present in the second or third decade of life with vasomotor rhinitis characterized by intermittent and profuse watery rhinorrhea (39). This is followed by persistent nasal congestion, anosmia, and mucopurulent nasal discharge. At this point, nasal polyps and acute, followed by chronic, sinusitis occurs. Nasal eosinophilia and peripheral blood eosinophilia are also present. Symptoms of asthma usually appear many months or years after the onset of upper airway symptoms, although inflammation may be present prior to the manifestations of symptoms and, in some patients, may occur simultaneously (39). For these patients, the respiratory disease is the main problem, which is exacerbated by nonselective NSAID ingestion (39). Asthma is usually severe and often requires systemic corticosteroids for optimal control. Occasional patients do not develop lower airway symptoms. Intolerance to aspirin and related drugs is usually noted after upper and lower airway symptoms are established. Until drug intolerance develops or is demonstrated by challenge, it is not possible to differentiate rhinosinusitis asthma that is related to aspirin from other causes.

An oral aspirin/NSAID challenge can be performed on patients in whom the diagnosis is unclear and in whom a specific diagnosis is necessary (39). In a controlled setting, with precautions for treating severe asthma, increasing doses of aspirin are given, usually starting at 3 or 30 mg and increasing at 3-hour intervals to 60, 100, 150, 325, and 650 mg. In sensitive individuals, reactions usually occur from 15 min to 3 h after aspirin ingestion, and include bronchospasm or naso-ocular reaction. Bronchospasm may last up to 24 h after the reaction begins (39). Medications that can be continued include theophylline, long-acting bronchodilators, oral and inhaled corticosteroids, and intranasal steroids. This is important in order to minimize potential bronchospasm.

In patients who must use aspirin, "desensitization" can be performed. Under close observation, patients should be monitored and, if necessary, admitted to an intensive care unit. Patients are desensitized to aspirin with increasing doses during oral challenges until 650 mg is tolerated without adverse signs or symptoms (see Chapter 32). After desensitization, patients are maintained at 650 mg aspirin twice daily. The desensitized state can be maintained at this dose of aspirin for long intervals. If the drug regimen is stopped, the patients revert to a sensitized state within 2 to 5 days. Long-term aspirin desensitization has been shown to improve control of rhinosinusitis and asthma, reduce steroid requirement for asthma control, and prevent polyp regrowth (42).

C. Approach to the Patient with Urticaria/Angioedema and/or Anaphylactoid Reaction to Aspirin

Stevenson et al. also described some patients with NSAID-induced urticaria/angioedema and/or anaphylactoid reaction, in whom the reaction is drug specific and probably does not go through the arachidonic acid metabolic pathway (41). The diagnosis is usually made after an acute reaction manifested by urticaria/angioedema and/or anaphylactoid reaction, shortly after NSAID ingestion. While asthmatic reactions are class specific, occur with any nonselective NSAID, and relate to the prostaglandin synthetase activity, urticaria/angioedema and/or anaphylactoid reactions are drug specific and are not related to the prostaglandin synthetase activity. For reactions consisting of urticaria/angioedema and/or anaphylactoid reactions, sensitivity to other NSAIDs is usually not an issue; drug-specific induced urticaria or angioedema follows ingestion of either aspirin or a specific NSAID. Cross-reactivity is not likely (38). Although we do not know the exact mechanism causing urticaria/angioedema, it is not believed to occur via the prostaglandin pathway.

Again, for patients in whom the diagnosis is unclear and in whom a specific diagnosis is necessary, oral aspirin/NSAID challenge can be done as described previously for patients with respiratory tract sensitivity (39). However, for cutaneous manifestation of aspirin sensitivity, the endpoint is the appearance of urticaria or angioedema (43). In contrast to NSAID-induced asthma, patients with NSAID-induced urticaria and angioedema cannot be desensitized. Attempts at desensitization uniformly result in severe flares of the skin that do not remit until aspirin is discontinued (43). Instead, starting alternative NSAIDs or COX-2 selective inhibitors are useful for patients with single drug-induced urticaria or angioedema (39).

There may be a genetic predisposition to this kind of NSAID reaction with cutaneous manifestations, as described in a study investigating HLA-DRB1 and HLA-DQb1 alleles (44). An association was seen between unrelated patients carrying the HLA-DR11 alleles and anaphylactoid reactions to NSAIDs.

D. Selective COX-2 Inhibitors

Selective COX-2 inhibitors have been used as an alternative treatment for aspirin- and NSAID-sensitive patients. COX-1 and COX-2 are enzymes that make up the prostaglandin H_2 synthase coenzyme (45). COX-1 catalyzes the synthesis of prostaglandin E_2, (PGE_2), which inhibits 5-lipoxygenase production. PGE_2 enhances mast cell stabilization and can, in this setting, be considered "anti-inflammatory" (45,46). COX-2 catalyzes the production of inflammatory prostanoids and is increased with inflammatory states. Three selective COX-2 inhibitors have been approved by the FDA (Table 5). There are ongoing investigations on other selective COX-2 inhibitors.

Rofecoxib has been tolerated by many patients with aspirin-sensitive asthma (45,47). In two double-blind, placebo-controlled studies, rofecoxib was tolerated by all

Table 5 FDA-Approved Selective COX-2 Inhibitors

Generic name	Brand name
Celecoxib	Celebrex
Rofecoxib	Vioxx
Valdecoxib	Bextra

patients, with no decrease in FEV_1 (45) and no rise in urinary leukotrienes or PGD_2 (47). In other studies, rofecoxib was useful in the treatment of cutaneous reactions to aspirin (46,48). Rofecoxib was tolerated by all patients with cutaneous reactions to NSAIDs, while almost half the patients reacted to nimesulide, which inhibits both COX-1 and COX-2 (48). Another study compared single-blinded oral challenge reactions in NSAID-sensitive patients with a history of cutaneous reactions (49). The reaction rate to rofecoxib was 3%, compared with a reaction rate of 17% to meloxicam, 21% to nimesulide, and 33% to celecoxib. One report described a group of patients with asthma and aspirin intolerance. All 27 patients tolerated treatment with celecoxib, with no bronchospasm observed (50). One case of anaphylaxis to celecoxib has been reported (51). While the patient described did not have sulfa allergy, celecoxib does contain a sulfa group and should be avoided by those known to have sulfa allergy. Selective COX-2 inhibitors offer a safe alternative to nonselective COX inhibitors in subjects with NSAID-induced asthma and may be safe for patients with NSAID-induced urticaria/angioedema.

V. OTHER DRUGS THAT CAUSE ALLERGIC REACTIONS

A. Insulin

Human insulin contains a total of 51 amino acids in two polypeptide chains, the alpha and beta chains, connected by a disulfide bond. The commercial insulin preparations used by diabetic patients are either the recombinant human insulin or purified animal insulin, such as bovine or porcine insulin. The primary amino acid sequence of human insulin differs from bovine insulin by three amino acids and from porcine by one amino acid. These amino acid differences may account for some of the immunogenicity of animal insulin. However, changes in tertiary structure occurring during insulin production also account for insulin immunogenicity. Reactions to recombinant human insulin appear to be due to alterations of tertiary structure (19). Commercially available animal insulin contain small amounts of noninsulin proteins such as C peptide, proinsulin, and intestinal and pancreatic polypeptides. Recombinant human insulin does not contain such contaminants, although it is possible that reactions may occur (52). Although about 6 million diabetics in the United States are on insulin, significant allergic reactions to insulin are uncommon (53). The reactions that occur are almost always related to the insulin molecule and not to the impurities or additives. In some patients protamine allergy may masquerade as insulin allergy, as described in a case report by Wessbecher et al. (54). This is described further in the next section. Allergic reactions are more common to animal insulin than to human insulin. Unlike other drugs, insulin is a complete antigen and does not require haptenation to be immunogenic. Virtually all patients receiving animal insulin develop antibodies to all classes of insulin. These antibodies are of low binding affinity and generally are of no clinical significance.

Allergic reactions to insulin can either be localized to the site of injection or become generalized (55). Local reactions are usually mild and consist of erythema, induration, burning, and pruritus at the injection site. These reactions usually occur within the first 2 to 4 weeks of starting insulin and disappear within 2 to 4 weeks of continued treatment with insulin. The IgE-mediated reaction typically occurs 15 to 30 min after insulin injection. Rarely, some patients also have a late-phase reaction 4 to 6 h later, presenting as induration, which persists for about 24 h (56). Most local reactions do not require any intervention. For persistent local reactions, dividing the dose of insulin, giving the doses at separate sites, and concomitant oral antihistamine administration is useful. Switching to another commercial insulin can also be helpful. Of patients with local reactions, only a small percentage ever progress to systemic responses.

Generalized urticaria and other systemic reactions to insulin are rare, with a reported incidence of 0.1% to 0.2% (53). Systemic reactions usually occur after interruption of insulin therapy (53,55). With resumption of insulin, a large dermal reaction develops, which may progress to a generalized reaction. In fact, most systemic reactions are preceded by progressively enlarging local reactions. Despite the decrease in frequency of reactions since the introduction of recombinant insulin, both local and systemic allergic reactions have been reported to the administration of recombinant DNA insulin (52). One report described a female with non–insulin-dependent diabetes mellitus and asthma who developed gestational diabetes during treatment with prednisone. The patient required treatment with insulin and developed a large local reaction after a dose of recombinant insulin, followed by diffuse urticaria during a prednisone taper. In an attempt to control the urticarial reactions, the insulin was discontinued. Following ingestion of glipizide, however, she continued to have generalized urticaria. It was hypothesized that the patient became sensitized to her endogenous insulin due to its similarities with recombinant insulin (52).

If the patient is seen within 24 to 48 hours of an insulin reaction, and the systemic reaction is mild, then insulin should not be discontinued. The next dose should be reduced to approximately one-third of the previous reactive dose and then slowly increased by 2 to 5 U per dose, until the desired dose is given. If 48 hours or more have elapsed since the systemic reaction, or if the reaction is severe, insulin skin testing followed by desensitization is necessary. All commercial insulin preparations—human, bovine, and porcine— should be used for intracutaneous skin testing. The least reactive insulin, typically the human insulin, should be used for desensitization. Negative skin test reactions to insulin at 1 U/ml or less rule out insulin-specific IgE as the cause of the reaction. A positive skin test does not confirm insulin allergy as the cause of the systemic reaction, as about 40% of diabetic patients on insulin develop insulin-specific IgE antibody without clinical symptoms of allergy. In patients with a suggestive history and a positive skin test, with no emergency, desensitization over several days can be done. A typical insulin desensitization schedule is described in Table 6, using regular insulin on the first four days and a sustained-acting insulin beginning on the fifth day. As with all cases of drug desensitization, close monitoring of the patient is necessary.

In diabetic ketoacidosis or hyperosmolar syndrome, more rapid desensitization is necessary, with dose escalation every 15 minutes, in addition to monitoring for anaphylaxis. The physician should also be prepared to treat hypoglycemia.

Analogs to human insulin, such as lispro or aspart, are another increasingly popular option for the treatment of insulin-dependent diabetics. Lispro carries a transposition between positions B28 and B29 (57). Several studies describe the use of lispro analogue in patients with a history of allergy to human insulin (57–59). The first case described its success in the treatment of a patient with generalized urticaria and angioedema following both human regular and lente insulin (57). Despite immediate positive responses to intradermal tests with three types of insulin, increasing doses of lispro insulin at 4-hour intervals, over a 3-day period, were tolerated. The ability of lispro to dissociate to monomers likely makes it less antigenic, since polymeric aggregates with numerous available epitopes are more apt to lead to histamine release (57,59). Other reports have described the use of continuous subcutaneous administration of insulin, via the pump, as a useful alter-

Table 6 Insulin Desensitization Schedule

Day	Time of dosage (given at 8-hour intervals)	Insulin (units)	Route
1	Morning	0.00001	Intradermal
	Afternoon	0.0001	Intradermal
	Evening	0.001	Intradermal
2	Morning	0.01	Intradermal
	Afternoon	0.1	Intradermal
	Evening	1.0	Intradermal
3	Morning	2.0	Subcutaneous
	Afternoon	4.0	Subcutaneous
	Evening	8.0	Subcutaneous
4	Morning	10.0	Subcutaneous
	Afternoon	12.0	Subcutaneous
	Evening	16.0	Subcutaneous
5	Morning	20.0	Subcutaneous
6	Morning	24.0	Subcutaneous

Example of an insulin desensitization schedule to be performed over 6 days. Regular insulin should be used on the first 4 days, and a sustained-acting insulin beginning on the fifth day.

native in the treatment of insulin allergy (59–61). Aspart insulin is another analogue that has been used in the treatment of insulin allergy. In this analog, the B28 locus carries aspartate. One study described a patient with allergy to several types of insulin, including lispro, who tolerated treatment with aspart analogue (62).

Insulin resistance, defined as insulin requirements over 100 to 200 U/day, often has an immunological basis. The immunological resistance is due either to high titers of circulating IgG antibodies to insulin or to autoantibodies to the insulin receptor (55,63). These patients often have other autoantibodies. The management of immunological insulin resistance is aimed at controlling the diabetes and waiting for spontaneous resolution. Corticosteroids can also be tried in these patients.

B. Biological Agents

Biological agents such as heterologous antiserum, IV immunoglobulin, and some vaccines are complete proteins. They can elicit an immune response without haptenation. Allergic reactions to some biological agents are relatively common.

Allergic reactions to *heterologous antisera* are common in patients allergic to animals, such as horses, as most of these are produced in these animals. These include antithymocyte globulin, antisera to rabies and snakes, and spider venoms. Before these materials are used, skin testing must be performed following the instructions on the package insert. Skin test–positive patients need to be desensitized.

Anaphylactic reactions to *IV immunoglobulin* are rare but can occur in patients with selective IgA deficiency or with common variable immunodeficiency, in which anti-IgA antibodies have developed prior to immunoglobulin infusions. In these patients, immunoglobulin free of IgA should be used. Nonallergic reactions to IV immunoglobulin are more common. These include chills, fever, headache, myalgia, and fatigue during or at the end of the infusion. Slowing the rate of the infusion or pretreatment with antihistamines or aspirin can prevent these reactions (64).

MMR vaccine is produced in chicken egg embryo fibroblasts. Trace amounts of ovalbumin such as egg proteins are present in these vaccines. On theoretical grounds, children allergic to eggs are considered to be at increased risk of anaphylaxis to these vaccines. The standard practice in the past was to skin-test these children with the vaccine and immunize them with incremental desensitizing doses. Controlled studies suggest that such skin testing and desensitization are not necessary. Children without history of egg or egg product anaphylaxis can be safely given the MMR vaccine without skin testing or other allergy evaluation. The MMR vaccine can also be safely administered in a single dose to children with allergy to eggs (65). Many allergic reactions to MMR vaccine previously attributed to egg hypersensitivity have been shown to be due to IgE antibody against porcine and bovine gelatin present in the vaccine (66).

Protamine, which is contained in some insulin preparations (e.g., NPH) and is used to reverse heparin anticoagulation, can cause IgE-mediated anaphylactic events. Protamine is extracted from fish (mainly salmon) testes. Patients at risk, therefore, include fish-sensitive individuals and men who have undergone vasectomy. Patients experiencing anaphylactic events during coronary bypass surgery often were previously sensitized via administration of protamine-containing insulin preparations, and occasionally, patients exhibiting reactions to protamine-insulin injections were sensitized during the previous administration of protamine (54). Protamine sensitivity can be confirmed by skin testing or in vitro assay (67).

Streptokinase is a protein derived from β-hemolytic streptococci. It is used as a thrombolytic agent to lyse coronary artery occlusions. The incidence of IgE-mediated allergic reactions to streptokinase is reported to be between 1% and 15%, with higher incidences on repeated use of the drug. The incidence of allergic reactions to streptokinase is on the decline because tissue plasminogen activator has become the thrombolytic of choice in myocardial infarction, particularly if repeated thrombolysis is needed.

VI. ANAPHYLACTOID DRUG REACTIONS

Anaphylactoid reactions are caused by the direct degranulation of mast cells and basophils without activation of these cells through the antigen-specific IgE–IgE receptor pathway. Although IgE production is not involved, the symptoms of anaphylactoid reactions and anaphylaxis are very similar. One characteristic of anaphylactoid reactions that theoretically distinguishes them from anaphylaxis is the first-dose phenomenon. As opposed to classic IgE-mediated anaphylaxis, the first exposure to a drug can cause an anaphylactoid reaction. Classic examples of drugs causing anaphylactoid reactions are radiocontrast media, opioids, vancomycin, and ciprofloxacin. The reason for the susceptibility of a portion of a treated population to an anaphylactoid reaction is not known.

Intravenous vancomycin infusion has been associated with pruritus and erythema over the upper body (the "red neck" or "red man" syndrome). Rarely, angioedema and cardiovascular shock have been described. The total dose of the drug, and the rate of infusion of vancomycin, influence the release of histamine and the development of signs and symptoms of the syndrome. Successful administration of the drug can be accomplished by a reduction of the rate of infusion. Vancomycin can also cause classic IgE-mediated anaphylactic reactions. When the reaction is anaphylactic, desensitization, rather than a reduction in infusion rate, is necessary (68). Ciprofloxacin can cause both IgE-mediated allergic and non–IgE-mediated anaphylactoid reactions, based on the observation that about half of acute reactions, including one reported case of death, have been first-dose reactions (69). On skin testing with ciprofloxacin at a dose of 100 µg/ml or higher, wheal and flare reactions can be elicited in normal human skin. This is similar to the wheal and flare produced by opiates and vancomycin. This suggests that ciprofloxacin, like the other drugs, can cause direct mast cell activation in a non-IgE mechanism.

VII. REACTIONS TO RADIOCONTRAST MEDIA

From the allergists' standpoint, the most important type of reaction to radiocontrast media (RCM) is the anaphylactoid event. Therefore, this section deals mainly with anaphylactoid reactions. However, a delayed-type reaction consisting of a macular-papular rash has been described after the administration of RCM. Unlike anaphylactoid reactions that have diminished in frequency with the introduction of relatively isosmolar RCM (70–76), the frequency of the delayed-type response has increased with the increased use of relatively isosmolar agents (77–80). Thus, delayed reaction is also discussed.

The relatively isosmolar agents consist of three molecular forms of radiocontrast: nonionic monomers, ionic dimers, and nonionic dimers (Fig. 6). These have replaced the hyperosmolar ionic monomers that were universally employed prior to the introduction of the first nonionic monomer, metrizamide (70). Metrizamide contained the same basic configuration as ionic monomers, except that the carboxyl was replaced by an amide linkage, thus eliminating ionization in solution. Shortly after the development of additional nonionic monomers came ioxaglate, the first iodinated dimer. In this dimer there are two benzene rings rather than one. Although this dimer is ionic, it resembles the nonionic monomers both in osmolality and in diminished side effects. Most recently introduced were the nonionic dimers such as iodixanol. In this instance, salts are added to bring the product to iso-osmolality.

Ionic monomers have an osmolality approximately five times that of plasma. The nonionic monomers, ionic dimers, and nonionic dimers have an osmolality close to that of plasma. With the reduction of osmolality came a marked reduction in the frequency of reactions. For example, in one report (71), the frequency of reactions was reduced from 0.7% to 0.2% with the exclusive use of more isosmolar agents. Nonetheless, such agents can cause life-threatening anaphylactoid events, and patients experiencing previous reactions who must receive RCM again are at increased risk (70).

1. Mechanism of Production of the Anaphylactoid Event

The anaphylactoid event is clearly related to mast cell degranulation, which appears to be due to direct histamine release in the vast majority of cases (70,81,82), although there have been isolated reports of IgE-mediated reactions (83). In addition, immediate skin test reactions have been reported in a small number of patients (84,85).

In addition, RCM reactions have been associated with activation of complement and the recruitment of other mediators via the contact system (70). Nonetheless, the most likely explanation for most anaphylactoid events is direct mast cell and, perhaps, basophil degranulation.

2. Approach to the Patient at Risk of an Anaphylactoid Reaction

The allergist/immunologist is involved, from a clinical standpoint, in anaphylactoid reactions to RCM when a patient who has experienced a previous reaction requires the readministration of radiocontrast. An in-depth review of the pretreatment protocol and those elements of the protocol that are controversial is contained in a reference article (70). The pretreatment protocol is summarized in Table 7.

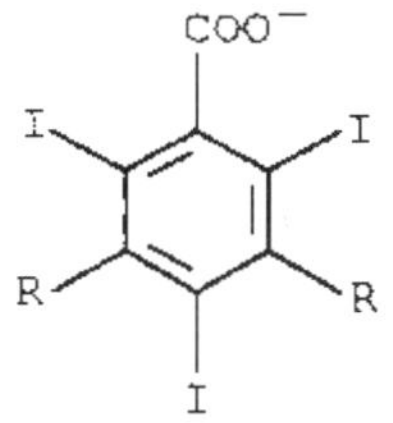

Ionic Monomer

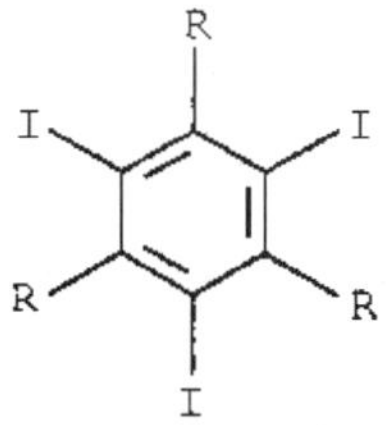

Nonionic Monomer

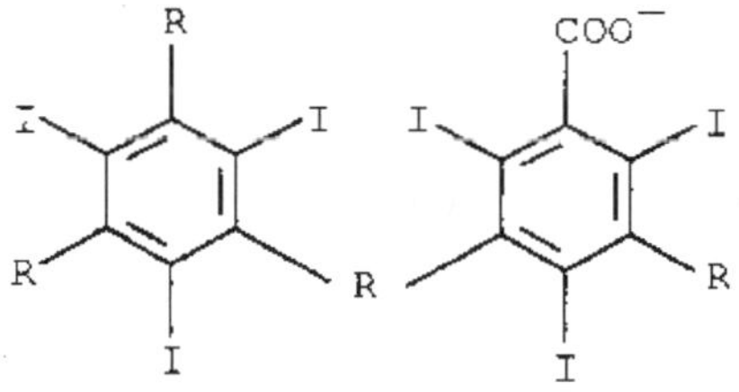

Ionic Dimer

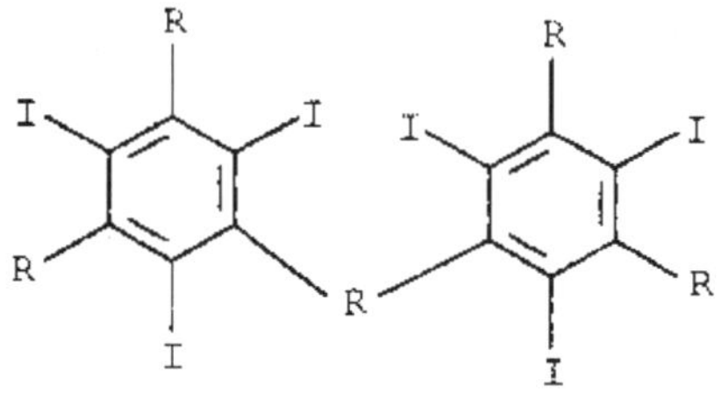

Nonionic Dimer

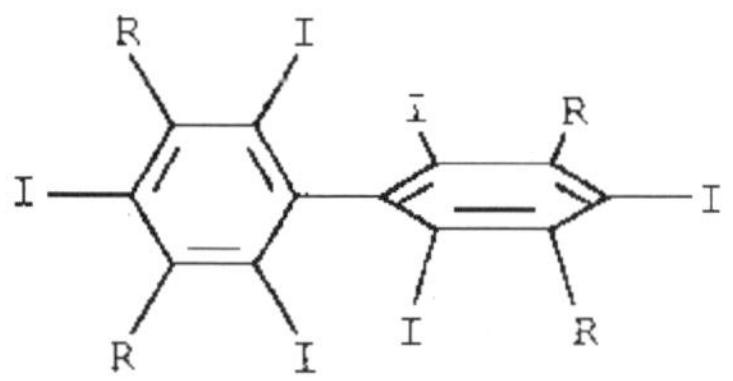

Compact Non-Ionic Dimer
(in Research)

Figure 6 Chemical structures of radiocontrast media

Table 7 Management of Patients Who Have Had a Previous Anaphylactoid Reaction to RCM and Require the Readministration of Radiocontrast

1. Confirm the necessity of the study.
2. Discuss the risk/benefit ratio with the patient and obtain consent.
3. Verify that the previous reaction was anaphylactoid and not due to noncardiogenic pulmonary edema.
4. Pretreat as follows:
   A. Diphenhydramine 50 mg intramuscularly 1 h before the procedure
   B. Prednisone 50 mg orally 15 h, 7 h, and 1 h before the procedure
   C. Ephedrine 25 mg orally 1 h before the procedure (when not contraindicated)
5. Use a lower osmolar agent.
6. If the patient is taking a β-adrenergic blocker, ACE inhibitor, or ACE blocker, discontinue the drug if possible. β-Adrenergic blocker medications should not be rapidly withdrawn.
7. A provocative dosage regimen can be used (at the discretion of the physician) if the previous reaction was life threatening.
8. The use of an H_2 antagonist is considered controversial and is employed at the discretion of the physician.

Several features of the pretreatment protocol deserve further explanation. The pretreatment regimen will not prevent noncardiogenic pulmonary edema (acute adult respiratory distress syndrome). It is therefore essential to determine the nature of the previous reaction. Although the adult respiratory distress syndrome or shock lung is rarely due to the administration of RCM, a number of cases have been reported (70). These reactions have occurred with both high and lower osmolar agents and are not prevented by standard pretreatment regimens. In such cases, readministration of RCM should be avoided if possible.

In previously life-threatening events, a provocative dosage regimen has been suggested (70) where gradually increasing amounts of RCM are administered along with the pretreatment protocol. This regimen has been studied only in a small number of patients and, of course, its disadvantage is the time it takes to perform. However, it can be used at the discretion of the physician seeing the patient in consultation. No data in this regard are available for lower osmolar agents, and it is not known whether such a procedure would enhance the safety of readministration of a lower osmolar preparation.

The use of an H_2 antagonist, such as ranitidine or cimetidine, along with prednisone, diphenhydramine, and ephedrine has been recommended by some investigators, but in the hands of others, an H_2 antagonist has actually increased the frequency of recurrent reactions (70). Therefore the use of an H_2 antagonist is considered optional and at the discretion of the physician. For a detailed review of the issues involved in this regard, the reader is referred to Ref. 70.

Anaphylactoid reactions can occur via any route of administration; nonvascular routes, such as are utilized for histosalpingograms, have caused anaphylactoid events. Therefore, regardless of the route of readministration, the patient must be pretreated.

Occasionally, a high-risk patient must undergo an emergency radiographic procedure when there is no time to use the standard pretreatment regimen, which requires 13 hours. An emergency pretreatment protocol has been devised for this purpose (86). This procedure consists of the administration of hydrocortisone 200 mg intravenously, immediately and every 4 hours until the procedure is performed. Diphenhydramine 50 mg intramuscularly is also given 1 hour before the procedure. Although there are no published data to validate the addition of ephedrine in this situation, it is likely that it would be helpful. A low osmolar agent should be used and, as noted earlier, the use of an H_2 antagonist remains an option, even though there are no data available regarding the effect of the addition of an H_2 antagonist. Theoretically, such as addition would be beneficial; however, based on a study showing the potential of repeat reactions (as noted previously), the decision to add an H_2 antagonist remains controversial.

There are other observations regarding anaphylactoid reactions to radiocontrast material that deserve mention. Gadopentetate dimeglumine is used as an imaging contrast medium for magnetic resonance imaging. It is associated with relatively few adverse reactions compared with radiopaque contrast media. However, reactions, including anaphylaxis, have been noted (70). The role of pretreatment in prevention of reactions to gadolinium-based contrast agents has not been evaluated. At this time, therefore, there are no clear-cut recommendations regarding their prevention. However, since the pretreatment anaphylactoid regimen presented in Table 7 has been used to prevent other types of anaphylactoid events, it seems reasonable to apply it to prevent repeat reactions to gadopentetate dimeglumine.

Anaphylactoid reactions to gastrointestinally administered contrast media may be unlike those due to intravenously administered RCM. The cause of the majority of these reactions remains unknown. However, they probably are heterogenous in nature and include reactions to latex, glucagon, carrageenan, and carboxymethylcellulose. Thus, agents administered through the gastrointestinal tract, including barium sulfate, as well as triiodinated benzene ring radiopaque agents, can also be problematic. For the barium sulfate–produced reactions, there are no data to support a pretreatment protocol; but as with gadopentetate, it seems reasonable to apply such a regimen if the patient requires a repeat study.

3. Delayed Reactions

The emergence of lower osmolar agents as the predominant radiocontrast medium has resulted in an increase in reports of delayed reactions to their administration (77–80). Although the clinical manifestations of these delayed reactions vary, the vast majority are cutaneous, and most are exanthematous (79). Many of these have been transient, but others have been severe and have required therapy.

The majority of delayed cutaneous reactions become apparent 3 to 48 hours after the administration of RCM, and subside within 1 to 7 days. Recurrences can occur after readministration of contrast medium.

As in acute reactions, a history of a previous reaction to RCM is a risk factor. The incidence of recurrent reactions has been reported to vary from 13% to 27% (79). Such reactions occur more frequently in females (87), and the simultaneous administration of IL-2 increases the frequency of such events (88).

The mechanism of late cutaneous reactions is unknown, but there is evidence incriminating many of the macular-papular reactions as T-cell mediated (79). The fact that previous reactors are at risk, that intradermal skin test lesions result in a delayed skin test reaction consistent with a T-cell–mediated reaction, and that patch tests have been positive in reactors, all support a T-cell–mediated immune response (89).

There has not yet been a large-scale study evaluating treatment or prevention of these delayed cutaneous responses. Severe cases have been treated with corticosteroids with varying success.

VIII. IN VIVO AND IN VITRO TESTS FOR DRUG ALLERGIES

A detailed history and in vivo and in vitro testing with the drug or its reactive metabolites are the key tools to confirm the diagnosis of drug allergy. The nature of the symptoms, a detailed knowledge of the drugs that the patient has taken, and the temporal relationship between the administration of the drug and the onset of symptoms are important elements of the history. The nature of the reaction often gives a clue to whether the symptoms were due to a drug reaction rather than to a disease process. Some drugs are more likely to produce an allergic reaction than others. For example, antibiotics are a common cause of drug allergy, whereas allergic reactions to digitalis glycoside are very rare. Knowledge of all drugs that the patient has taken in the past, and is taking currently, is important. Information on previous drug reactions, previous exposure to the same or a structurally related drug, and the effect of drug discontinuation give clues helpful in establishing a diagnosis. Medications should be considered with regard to their known propensity for causing allergic reactions. In general, agents that have been used for long periods of time before the onset of an acute reaction are less likely to be implicated than are agents recently introduced or reintroduced. Patients with a history of prior allergic drug reactions have an increased risk of subsequent adverse drug reactions, even to structurally unrelated medications. The temporal relationship between the institution of drug therapy and the onset of the reaction is important. Immunological reactions occur at different times following initiation of therapy. In individuals sensitized to a drug during a prior exposure, IgE antibody–mediated reactions typically occur within an hour of administration of the drug. Allergic contact dermatitis generally has a latency period of about 2 to 3 days, and serum sickness has a latency period of about a week. In individuals not sensitized to a drug by prior exposure, the reaction occurs after a longer latency period. For example, an IgE-mediated reaction generally occurs 7 to 10 days into the course of treatment with a new drug. In addition to the history, for some drug reactions, in vivo or in vitro tests can be done to confirm a suspected allergic drug reaction.

A. Skin Testing

Skin testing is used in allergy practice to diagnose IgE-mediated immediate hypersensitivity reactions to aeroallergens and Hymenoptera venom. The same principle can also be applied to diagnose drug allergy. However, the main limitation is the lack of availability of relevant drug and drug metabolites for testing. Among the small-molecular-weight drugs, skin test reagents are commercially available for only the major determinant of penicillin. The major determinant is conjugated to a weakly immunogenic polylysine carrier molecule to form penicilloyl-polylysine (PPL), which is useful as a skin test reagent for the detection of antibody to the major determinant. Since minor determinant products are labile and cannot be synthesized readily in multivalent form for commercial supply, skin testing for minor determinants can be reasonably accomplished using a mixture of benzylpenicillin, its alkaline hydrolysis product (benzylpenicilloate), and its acid hydrolysis product (benzylpenilloate) (19). Since minor determinants can cause severe anaphylactic reactions, patients at risk should be referred to special centers with access to and experience with the minor determinant mixture. Penicillin can be metabolized in vivo to multiple intermediates that may not be detected by a minor determinant mix. Therefore, a negative test cannot absolutely rule out the possibility of an IgE-mediated allergic reaction. In the clinical setting, penicillin skin testing is done with penicilloyl-polylysine, penicillin G, and, if available, the penicillin minor determinant mix. Initially a prick test followed by an intradermal test with increasing concentrations of each reagent are performed. A patient is considered to be allergic to penicillin if there is a reaction to any of the reagents at any dilution (15).

Skin testing to diagnose the presence of IgE antibody for other drugs such as cephalosporins, sulfonamides, muscle relaxants, chymopapain, insulin, latex, and protamine has also been reported (19). However, many of these are not standardized and interpretation is difficult.

B. Provocative Testing

Provocative testing gives the patient increasing doses of the drug, starting with a small dose, in an attempt to reach the full therapeutic dose. When an allergic reaction is observed, the drug is withdrawn. The protocols are designed following the desensitization schedules (as discussed in Section IX). This method is not without risk and should be considered only when no alternative medication is available, and the risks are fully understood.

C. In Vitro Testing for Allergen-Specific IgE

The radioallergosorbent test (RAST) and enzyme-linked immunoassay (ELISA) are the most common in vitro assays for detecting specific IgE against drugs. Both RAST and ELISA measure circulating allergen-specific IgE using a solid-phase immunoassay. In the assays, the allergen is attached to a solid-phase particle and incubated with the serum under study. After binding, the particle is washed and incubated again with a radiolabeled anti-IgE antibody (for RAST) or an enzyme-labeled antibody (for ELISA). The bound radioactivity- or enzyme-induced color changes are measured. These are proportional to the allergen-specific IgE antibody in the serum. Use of RAST and ELISA to diagnose drug allergy is limited by the lack of knowledge of the drug metabolites acting as haptens. The utility of RAST and ELISA is limited, as skin testing can provide the same and biologically more relevant information in a more rapid fashion.

D. Release of Mediators by Basophils

Basophils contain high-affinity IgE receptors to which specific IgE molecules are bound. Therefore, when basophils are incubated with a relevant antigen, the cells release histamine and other mediators that can be measured as an indicator of sensitivity. The test correlates with skin test, RAST, and ELISA results. However, the test has limited utility because it is labor intensive, requires fresh basophils, and is more expensive than skin testing.

E. Other In Vitro Tests

Drug-specific IgM and IgE antibodies are measured to diagnose drug-induced hemolytic anemia, neutropenia, and thrombocytopenia. Lymphocyte proliferation in response to a drug can be measured as radioactive thymidine uptake by lymphocytes cultured in the presence of a drug. This can be a predictor of a cell-mediated immune response to a drug. During or shortly after an allergic reaction to a drug, blood can be analyzed for the mediators of the allergic reaction, e.g., histamine, PGD_2, and tryptase. The presence of such mediators indicates mast cell and/or basophil degranulation.

IX. DESENSITIZATION

Patients who develop IgE antibody to a drug may develop an illness that can be effectively treated only with the drug to which they have become sensitive. Since anaphylaxis may occur with use of the drug in question, protocols have been developed to desensitize patients to the drug. Penicillin and other β-lactam antibiotics are the most common agents involved. In the past, when animal insulin was the only form of insulin available for treating diabetic patients, insulin desensitization was performed frequently. Today, sulfonamide allergy occurs more frequently, particularly in the HIV-infected patient. Therefore, in some settings sulfonamide desensitization is being performed more frequently than before.

The basic approach in all desensitization is to administer gradually increasing doses of the drug over a period of hours to days. The mechanism of the desensitization is not precisely known and may vary depending on the drug involved. For example, the mechanism of desensitization to prevent sulfonamide reactions, non–IgE-mediated events, differs from that to prevent reactions to penicillin, which are IgE-mediated events. In such IgE-mediated episodes, it is believed that mast cells and basophils are desensitized to the drug in an antigen-specific manner. That is, all IgE-antigen binding sites are gradually, but increasingly, bound until they are totally occupied by the incremental administration of antigen, at which time the drug can be given with impunity. The process is known as antibody neutralization. For maintenance of desensitization, continuous presence of the drug in the body is required. Also, desensitization is specific for the drug. For example, a patient desensitized to benzylpenicillin may still be reactive to other β-lactam antibiotics (4,90). Desensitization should always be conducted under close observation and, if necessary, in the intensive care setting.

Of all the antibiotics, experience with penicillin desensitization is most extensive (91). Penicillin desensitization has been performed clinically for over 50 years. Both oral and intravenous routes can be used for desensitization. The oral route of desensitization is preferred by some, as it is less likely to produce a systemic reaction and is therefore safer. Others prefer the parenteral route, since it allows more control over drug concentration and dosage, and is not dependent on absorption. Some prefer to begin with the oral route and then change over to the parenteral route, when the dose escalation has been completed. However, in this practice, the patient is at a theoretical risk of sudden exposure to a large dose of minor determinant, as some of them may not be adequately absorbed through the gastrointestinal tract during the oral dose escalation phase. Our choice is to desensitize via the route that will be ultimately used for the treatment of the infection. Various protocols for penicillin desensitization have been published (1,91). Desensitization is started with a very small dose, and a doubling dose is administered every 15 minutes until the therapeutic dose is achieved. An uncomplicated procedure usually takes 4 to 6 hours. The starting dose is empirical, based on skin testing results. Typically an intradermal skin test performed in duplicate by injecting 0.2 ml and employing a concentration of 1 mg/ml introduces about 400 μg of the drug. If these doses are tolerated with no systemic reaction, oral desensitization can be started with that dose. Parenteral desensitization is usually started at one-tenth or one-hundredth of the tolerated skin test dose.

The pandemic of HIV infection has led to the resurgence of sulfonamide use for treatment and prophylaxis of some HIV-related infection. Allergy to sulfonamides is reported at a higher frequency in the HIV-infected population than in the general population (as discussed in Section II). Successful empirical protocols have been developed to desensitize patients, including HIV-infected patients, to sulfonamide. Desensitization can be carried out over 10 days (92) or can be done in a few hours (93). A typical 10-day protocol is shown in Table 8. After successful desensitization, the patient should be maintained on the drug on a regular schedule. Patients with life-threatening skin reactions to sulfonamide or to any other drug, such as Stevens-Johnson syndrome, erythema multiforme, or toxic epidermal necrolysis, should not be desensitized, as reexposure to the same drug carries a substantial risk of mortality (24).

Desensitization to local anesthetics, aspirin, and insulin has been discussed in preceding sections.

X. AVOIDING DRUG ALLERGIES

As with any other illness, prevention is the most effective way to minimize the morbidity and mortality of drug reactions. In choosing a drug, avoid using drugs that are very likely to cause sensitization. Drugs such as heterologous antisera (eg. anti-thymocyte globulin) and streptokinase can induce sensitization in a large percentage of the population. Therefore, if the need arises for reuse of the same type of drug, it may be advisable to choose an alternative drug with similar efficiency or to skin-test the patient to rule out sensitivity. Intermittent use of large doses of a drug via the parenteral route is more sensitizing than continuous use. Penicillin is more likely to sensitize a predisposed individual if used intermittently. Insulin allergy is also more common after intermittent administration, as occurs during gestational diabetes in women with multiple pregnancies. After two or more pregnancies, some women become sensitized to insulin. During subsequent pregnancies, when insulin is needed again, allergic manifestations may appear. Therefore, if possible, intermittent use of large parenteral doses of drugs, particularly those that are reported to cause allergic reactions, should be avoided.

A detailed drug allergy history is valuable in preventing an allergic reaction to a drug. If a patient has had an adverse reaction to a drug, that particular drug as well as those that may cross-react with it should be avoided. If absolutely essential, appropriate in vivo

Table 8 Protocol for Oral Trimethoprim/Sulfamethoxazole (T/S) Desensitization

Day	Dose	Quantity
1	1 ml of 1:20 pediatric suspension of T/S[a]	0.4 mg/2 mg
2	2 ml of 1:20 pediatric suspension of T/S	0.8 mg/4 mg
3	4 ml of 1:20 pediatric suspension of T/S	1.6 mg/8 mg
4	8 ml of 1:20 pediatric suspension of T/S	3.2 mg/16 mg
5	1 ml of pediatric suspension of T/S	8 mg/40 mg
6	2 ml of pediatric suspension of T/S	16 mg/80 mg
7	4 ml of pediatric suspension of T/S	32 mg/160 mg
8	8 ml of pediatric suspension of T/S	64 mg/320 mg
9	1 tablet of T/S	80 mg/400 mg
10	1 tablet of double-strength T/S	160 mg/800 mg

This is followed by 1 tablet of double-strength T/S on Monday, Wednesday, and Friday for PCP prophylaxis, or two tablets a day for the treatment of isosporiasis.

[a] The concentration of the stock solution is 1 mg/ml.
This is an example of a protocol for trimethoprim/sulfamethoxazole desensitization. This can be performed over 10 days to obtain the therapeutic dose.

or in vitro testing and desensitization should be performed. In addition to the known cross-reactivity between the penicillins and cephalosporins, penicillins and carbapenams, and among the aminoglycosides, there is potential although unpredictable cross-reactivity among para-aminobenzoic acid derivatives (sulfonamide antibiotics, sulfonylurea hypoglycemics, thiazide diuretics, acetazolamide, and some angiotensin-converting enzyme inhibitors). Careful consideration of these factors will help reduce sensitization of a patient to a drug and subsequent allergic reaction.

XI. SALIENT POINTS

1. Although the IgE-mediated allergic reaction is the most common and important form of immunologically mediated drug reaction, in evaluating a patient with suspected drug allergy, the whole spectrum of adverse drug reactions must be considered.

2. Low-molecular-weight drugs, such as penicillin, are not complete antigens. These drugs bind to a carrier protein by a process called haptenation to produce allergic sensitization. Larger-molecular-weight drugs that are complete proteins, such as insulin, cause sensitization by themselves and do not need to be haptenated.

3. Penicillin is the most common cause of allergic reactions. IgE antibodies can be produced to determinants called the major and minor determinants. The nomenclature refers to abundance and not clinical significance. Antibodies to minor determinants usually mediate anaphylactic reactions, and antibodies to the major determinant generally mediate urticarial skin reactions. However, there are exceptions to this rule.

4. A high frequency of reactions to drugs occurs in human HIV infection. The incidence of skin rash to trimethoprim sulfamethoxazole is about 10-fold higher in HIV-infected individuals than in the general population.

5. COX-2–specific inhibitors are a clinically important alternative for patients with NSAID allergy.

6. Skin testing can be done to diagnose drug or other biological agent allergy. However, the main limitation is the lack of availability of relevant drugs and drug metabolites for testing.

7. Allergic patients can be desensitized to drugs by being given increasing concentrations of the drug. The procedure should be done under close observation, often in intensive care units.

8. Larger doses and frequent intermittent courses, rather than prolonged continuous treatment, are more likely to sensitize an individual for IgE-mediated reactions. However, for IgG reactions, such as penicillin-induced hemolytic anemia, high and sustained blood levels are required.

REFERENCES

1. Anderson JA. Allergic reactions to drugs and biological agents. J Am Med Assoc 1992; 268:2845–2857.
2. Classen DC, Pestotnik SL, Evans RS, Burke JP. Computerized surveillance of adverse drug events in hospitalized patients. J Am Med Assoc 1991; 266:2847–2851.
3. Patterson R, DeSware RD, Greenberger PA, Grammer LC, Brown JE, Choy AR. Drug allergy and protocols for management of drug allergies. Allergy Proc 1994; 15:239–264.

4. Ditto AM. Drug allergy: In Patterson's Allergic Disease (Grammer LC, Greenberger PA, eds.). Philadelphia: Lippincott Williams & Wilkins, 2002: 295–334.

5. Naisbitt DJ, Williams D, Pirmohamed M, Kitteringham NR, Park BK. Reactive metabolites and their role in drug reactions. Curr Opin Allergy Immunol 2001; 1:317–325.

6. Baldo BA, Harle DG. Drug allergenic determinants. Monogr Allergy 1990; 28:11–51.

7. DeWeck AL. Pharmacologic and immunochemical mechanisms of drug hypersensitivity. Immunol Allergy Clin North Am 1991; 11:461–474.

8. Van Arsdel PP Jr. Classification and risk factors for drug allergy. Immunol Allergy Clin North Am 1991; 11:475–492.

9. Bigby M, Jick S, Jick H, Arndt K. Drug-induced cutaneous reactions: A report from the Boston Collaborative Drug Surveillance Program on 15438 consecutive inpatients, 1975 to 1983. J Am Med Assoc 1986; 256:3358–3363.

10. Toogood JH. Risk of anaphylaxis in patients receiving beta blocker drugs. J Allergy Clin Immunol 1988; 81:1–5.

11. Hsu DH, deWaal Malefyt R, Fiorentine DF, Dang MN, Vieira P, deVries J, Spits H, Mosmann TR, Moore KW. Expression of interleukin-10 activity in Epstein-Barr virus protein BCRF1. Science 1990; 250:830–832.

12. Carr A, Cooper D, Penny R. Allergic manifestation of human immunodeficiency virus (HIV) infection. J Clin Immunol 1991; 11:55–64.

13. Kamada MM, Twarog F, Leung DYM. Multiple antibiotic sensitivity in a pediatric population. Allergy Proc 1991; 12:347–350.

14. Khoury L, Warrington R. The multiple drug allergy syndrome: A matched-control retrospective study in patients allergic to penicillin. J Allergy Clin Immunol 1996; 98:462–464.

15. Greenberger PA. Allergic reactions to individual drugs: Low molecular weight. In: Patterson's Allergic Disease Philadelphia: (Grammer LC, Greenberger PA, eds.). Lippincott Williams & Wilkins, 2002: 395–359.

16. Negut A. Ghatak A, Miller R. Anaphylaxis in the United States: An investigation into its epidemiology. Arch Intern Med 2001; 161:15–21

17. Gruchalla RS. Drug allergy. J Allergy Clin Immunol 2003; 111:S548–S559.

18. Kelkar PS, Li JT. Cephalosporin allergy. N Engl J Med 2001; 345:804–809.

19. Weiss ME. Drug allergy. Med Clin North Am 1992; 76:857–882.

20. Baldo BA. Penicillins and cephalosporins as allergens: Structural aspects or recognition and cross-reactions. Clin Exp Allergy 1999; 29:744–749.

21. Miranda A, Blanca M, Viga JM, Morena F, Carmona MJ, Garcia JJ, Segurado E, Justica JL, Juarez C. Cross-reactivity between a penicillin and a cephalosporin with the same side chain. J Allergy Clin Immunol 1996; 98:671–677.

22. Warrington RJ, McPhillips S. Independent anaphylaxis to cefazolin without allergy to other β-lactam antibiotics. J Allergy Clin Immunol 1996; 98:460–462.

23. Weber EA. Cefazolin specific side chain hypersensitivity. J Allergy Clin Immunol 1996; 98:849–850.

24. Roujeau JC, Stern RS. Severe adverse cutaneous reactions to drugs. N Engl J Med 1994; 331:1272–1284

25. Naisbitt D, Hough S, Gill H, Pirmohamed M, Kitteringham NR, Park BK. Cellular disposition of sulphamethoxazole and its metabolites: Implications for hypersensitivity. Br J Pharmacol 1999; 126:1393–1407.

26. Naisbitt D, Gordon S, Pirmohamed M, Burkhart C, Cribb AE, Pizhler WJ, Park BK. Antigenicity and immunogenicity of sulfamethoxaole: Demonstration of metabolism-dependent haptenation and T cell proliferation in vivo. Br J Pharmacol 2001; 133:295–305.

27. Moscicki RA, Sockin SM, Corsello BF, Ostro MG, Bloch KJ. Anaphylaxis during induction of general anesthesia: Subsequent evaluation and management. J Allergy Clin Immunol 1990; 86:325–332.

28. Lieberman P. Anaphylactic reactions during surgical and medical procedures. J Allergy Clin Immunol 2002; 110:S64–S69.

29. Slater JE. Latex allergy. J Allergy Clin Immunol 1994; 94:139–149.

30. Nasser SMS, Ewan PW. Opiate-sensitivity: Clinical characteristics and the role of skin prick testing. Clin Exp Allergy 2001; 31:1014–1020.

31. Van Arsdel PP Jr. Pseudoallergic drug reactions. Immunol Allergy Clin North Am 1991; 11:635–644.

32. Chandler MJ, Grammer LC, Patterson R. Provocative challenge with local anesthetics in patients with a prior history of reactions. J Allergy Clin Immunol 1987; 79:883–886.

33. Gall H, Kaufmann R, Kalveram CM. Adverse reactions to local anesthetics: Analysis of 197 cases. J Allergy Clin Immunol 1996; 97:933–937.

34. Cuesta-Herranz J, de las Heras M, Fernandez M, Lluch M, Figueredo E, Umpierrez A, Lahoz C. Allergic reaction caused by local anesthetic agents belonging to the amide group. J Allergy Clin Immunol 1997; 99:427–428.

35. Warrington RJ, McPhillips S. Allergic reaction to local anesthetic agents of the amide group. J Allergy Clin Immunol 1997; 100:855.

36. Hodgson TA, Shirlaw PJ, Challacombe SJ. Skin testing after anaphylactoid reactions to dental local anesthetics. Oral Surg Oral Med Oral Pathol 1993; 75:706–711.

37. Sainte-Laudy J, Vallon C. Nine cases of suspected IgE-mediated anaphylaxis induced by aspirin. ACI Int 2002; 14:220–222.

38. O'Sullivan S, Dahlen B, Dahlen S-E, Kumlin M. Increased urinary excretion of the prostaglandin D_2 metabolite $9\alpha,11\beta$-prostaglandin F_2 after aspirin challenge supports mast cell activation in aspirin-induced airway obstruction. J Allergy Clin Immunol 1996; 98:421–432.

39. Namazy JA, Simon RA. Sensitivity to nonsteroidal anti-inflammatory drugs. Ann Allergy 2002; 89:542–552.

40. Manning ME, Stevenson DD. Aspirin sensitivity. Postgrad Med 1991; 90:227–233.

41. Stevenson DD, Sanchez-Borges M, Szczeklik A. Classification of allergic and pseudoallergic reactions to drugs that inhibit cyclooxygenase enzymes. Ann Allergy 2001; 87:177–180.

42. Stevenson DD, Hankammer MA, Mathison DA, Christiansen SC, Simon RA. Aspirin desensitization treatment of aspirin-sensitive patients with rhinosinusitis-asthma: Long term outcomes. J Allergy Clin Immunol 1996; 98:751–758.

43. Stevenson DD, Simon RA. Sensitivity to aspirin and nonsteroidal anti-inflammatory drugs. In: Allergy: Principles and Practice, 4th ed. (Middleton E, Reed CE, Ellis EF, Adkinson NF, Yunginger JW, Busse WW, eds.). St. Louis: Mosby, 1993: 1747–1765.

44. Quiralte J, Sanchez-Garcia F, Torres MJ, Blanco C, Castillo R, Ortega N, de Castro FR, Perez-Aciego P, Carillo T. Association of HLA-DR11 with the anaphylactoid reaction caused by nonsteroidal anti-inflammatory drugs. J Allergy Clin Immunol 1999; 103:685–689.

45. Stevenson DD, Simon RA. Lack of cross-reactivity between rofecoxib and aspirin in aspirin-sensitive patients with asthma. J Allergy Clin Immunol 2001; 108:47–51.

46. Nettis E, DiPaola R, Ferrennini A, Tursi A. Tolerability of rofecoxib in patients with cutaneous adverse reactions to NSAID. Ann Allergy 2002; 88:331–334.

47. Szczeklik A, Nizankowska E, Bochenek G, Nagraba K, Mejza F, Swierszynska M. Safety of a specific Cox-2 inhibitor in aspirin-induced asthma. Clin Exp Allergy 2001; 31:219–225.

48. Quiralte J, Saenz de San Pedro B, Florido JJF. Safety of selective cyclooxygenase-2 inhibitor rofecoxib in patients with NSAID-induced cutaneous reactions. Ann Allergy 2002; 89:63–66.

49. Sanchez-Borges M, Capriles-Hulett A, Caballero-Fonseca F, Perez CR. Tolerability to new Cox-2 inhibitors in NSAID-sensitive patients with cutaneous reactions. Ann Allergy 2001; 87:201–204.

50. Dahlen B, Szczeklik A, Murray JJ. Celecoxib in patients with asthma and aspirin intolerance. N Engl J Med 2001; 344:142.

51. Levy MB, Fink JN. Anaphylaxis to celecoxib. Ann Allergy 2001; 87:72–73.

52. Alvarez-Thull L, Rosenwasser LJ, Brodie TD. Systemic allergy to endogenous insulin during therapy with recombinant DNA (rDNA) insulin. Ann Allergy 1996; 76:253–256.

53. Lieberman P. Difficult allergic drug reactions. Immunol Allergy Clin North Am 1991; 11:213–231.

54. Wessbacher R, Kiehn M, Stoffel E, Moll I. Management of insulin allergy. Allergy 2001; 56:919–920.

55. Blaiss MS, DeShazo RD. Drug allergy. Ped Clin North Am 1988; 35:1131–1147.

56. deShazo RD, Boehm TM, Kumar D, Galloway JA, Dvorak HF. Dermal hypersensitivity reaction to insulin: Correlations of three patterns to their histopathology. J Allergy Clin Immunol 1982; 69:229–237.

57. Kumar D. Lispro analog for treatment of generalized allergy to human insulin. Diabetes Care 1997; 20:1357–1359.

58. Lluch–Bernal M, Fernandez M, Herrera-Pombo JL, Sastre J. Insulin lispro, an alternative in insulin hypersensitivity. Allergy 1999; 54:186–187.

59. Eapen SS, Connor EL, Gern JE. Insulin desensitization with insulin lispro and an insulin pump in a 5-year-old child. Ann Allergy 2000; 85:395–397.

60. Nagai T, Nagai Y, Tomizawa T, Masatomo M. Immediate-type human insulin allergy successfully treated by continuous subcutaneous insulin infusion. Int Med (Tokyo) 1997; 36:575–578.

61. Naf S, Esmatjes, Recasens M, Valero A, Halperin I, Levy Z, Gomis R. Continuous subcutaneous insulin infusion to resolve an allergy to human insulin. Diabetes Care 2002; 25:634–635.

62. Yasuda H, Nagata M, Moriyama H, Fujihara K, Kotani R, Yamada K, Ueda H, Yokono K. Human insulin analog insulin aspart does not cause insulin allergy. Diabetes Care 2001; 24:2008–2009.

63. Moller DE, Flier JS. Insulin resistance: Mechanisms, syndromes, and implications. N Engl J Med 1991; 325:938–948.

64. Buckley R, Schiff R. The use of intravenous immune globulin in immunodeficiency disease. N Engl J Med 1992; 326:431–436.

65. James JM, Burks AW, Roberson PK, Sampson HA. Safe administration of the measles vaccine to children allergic to eggs. N Engl J Med 1995; 332:1261–1266.

66. Sakaguchi M, Nakayama T, Inouye S. Food allergy to gelatin in children with systemic immediate-type reactions, including anaphylaxis, to vaccine. J Allergy Clin Immunol 1996; 98:1058–1061.

67. Dykewicz MS, Kim HW, Orfan N, Yoo TJ, Lieberman P. Immunologic analysis of anaphylaxis to protamine component in neutral protamine hagedorn human insulin. J Allergy Clin Immunol 1994; 93:117–125.

68. Anne S, Middleton E, Reisman RE. Vancomycin anaphylaxis and successful desensitization. Ann Allergy 1994; 73:402–404.

69. Davis H, McGoodwin E, Reed TG. Anaphylactoid reactions reported after treatment with ciprofloxacin. Ann Intern Med 1989; 12:1041–1043.

70. Lieberman P, Seigle R. Reactions to radiocontrast material: Anaphylactoid events in radiology. Clin Rev Allergy Immunol 1999; 17:469–496.

71. Cochran ST, Bomyea K. Trends in adverse events from iodinated contrast media. Acad Radiol 2002; 9(suppl 1):S65–S68.

72. Palmer FJ. The RACR survey of intravenous contrast media reactions: Final report. Australas Radiol 1988; 32:426–428.

73. Katayama H, Yamaguchi K, Kozuka T, Takashima T, Seez P, Matsuura K. Adverse reactions to ionic and nonionic contrast media: A report from the Japanese Committee on the Safety of Contrast Media. Radiology 1990; 175:621–628.

74. Pedersen SH, Svaland MG, Reiss AL, Andrew E. Late allergy-like reactions following vascular administration of radiography contrast media. Acta Radiol 1998; 39:344–348.

75. Federle MP, Willis LL, Swanson DP. Ionic versus nonionic contrast media: A prospective study of the effect of rapid bolus injection on nausea and anaphylactoid reactions. J Comput Assist Tomogr 1998; 22:341–345.

76. Grant KL, Camamo JM. Adverse events and cost savings three years after implementation of guidelines for outpatient contrast-agent use. Am J Health Syst Pharm 1997; 54:1395 –1401.

77. Speck U, Bohle F, Krause W, Martin JL, Miklautz H, Schuhmann-Giampierl G. Delayed hypersensitivity to X-ray CM: Possible mechanisms and models. Acad Radiol 1998; 5(suppl 1):S162–S165.

78. Mikkonen R. Incidence and risk factors for delayed allergy-like reactions to X-ray contrast media in adult and pediatric populations. Pharmacoepidemiol Drug Saf 1998; 7:S11–S15.

79. Christiansen C, Pichler WJ, Skotland T. Delayed allergy-like reactions to X-ray contrast media: Mechanistic considerations. Eur Radiol 2000; 10:1965–1975.

80. Rydberg J, Charles J, Aspelin P. Frequency of late allergy-like adverse reactions following injection of intravascular non-ionic contrast media. Acta Radiol 1998; 39:219–222.

81. Laroche D, Almone-Gastin I, Dubois F, Huet H, Gerard P, Vergnaud MC, Monton-Faivre C, Gueant JL, Laxenaire MC, Bricard H. Mechanism of severe, immediate reactions to iodinated contrast material. Radiol 1998; 209:183–190.

82. Laroche D, Vergnaud MC, Lefrancois C, Hue S, Bricard H. Anaphylactoid reactions to iodinated contrast media. Acad Radiol 2002; 9(suppl 2):S431–S432.

83. Mita H, Tadokoro K, Akiyama K. Detection of IgE antibody to a radiocontrast medium. Allergy 1998; 53:1133–1140.

84. Dewachter P, Mouton-Faivre C, Felden F. Allergy and contrast media. Allergy 2001; 56:250–251.

85. Guillen TJ, Guido BR. Anamnesis and skin test to prevent fatal reactions to iodinated contrast media (Spanish). Rev Alerg Mex 2000; 47:22–25.

86. Greenberger PA, Halwig JM, Patterson R, Wallemark CB. Emergency administration of radiocontrast media in high-risk patients. J Allergy Clin Immunol 1986; 77:630–635.

87. Mikkonen R, Kontkanen T, Kivisaari L. Acute and late adverse reactions to low-osmolal contrast media. Acta Radiol 1995; 36:72–76.

88. Choyke PL, Miller DL, Lotze MT, Whiteis JM, Ebbitt B, Rosenberg SA. Delayed reactions to contrast media after interleukin-2 immunotherapy. Radiology 1992; 183:111–114.

89. Gall H, Pillekamp H, Peter R-U. Late-type allergy to the X-ray contrast medium Solutrast (iopamidol). Contact Dermatitis 1999; 40:248–250.

90. MacGlashan D, Lichenstein LM. Basic characteristics of human lung mast cell desensitization. J Immunol 1987; 139:501–505.

91. Lin R. A perspective on penicillin allergy. Arch Intern Med 1992; 152:930–937.

92. Absar N, Daneshvar H, Beall G. Desensitization to trimethoprim-sulfamethoxazole in HIV-infected patients. J Allergy Clin Immunol 1994; 93:1001–1005.

93. Nguyen MT, Weiss PJ, Wallace MR. Two day oral desensitization to trimethoprim-sulfamethoxazole in HIV-infected patients. AIDS 1995; 9:573–75.

22

Standardized Allergen Extracts in the United States

JAY E. SLATER

U.S. Food and Drug Administration, Bethesda, Maryland, U.S.A.

I. INTRODUCTION

Allergen extracts and other biological agents were first regulated in 1902 by the Hygienic Laboratory of the Public Health and Marine Hospital Service, renamed the National Institute (singular) of Health (NIH) in 1930. The NIH continued to regulate biologics from 1955 to 1972 through its Division of Biologics Standards. Regulatory authority over biologics was transferred in 1972 to the Bureau of Biologics at the Food and Drug Administration (FDA). In 1982, the FDA merged the Bureau of Biologics and the Bureau of Drugs into a single Center for Drugs and Biologics and 5 years later separated the entities that regulated drugs and biologics again, and the Center for Biologics Evaluation and Research (CBER) assumed responsibility for allergenics regulation (1,2).

The views expressed in this article are the personal opinions of the author and are not the official opinion of the U.S. Food and Drug Administration or the Department of Health and Human Services.

CBER's authority to regulate allergen extracts derives from two laws enacted by Congress, the Food, Drug, and Cosmetic Act of 1938 and the Public Health Service Act of 1944. The specific regulations which govern CBER's regulation of allergens appear in part 680 of Title 21 of the Code of Federal Regulations (21 CFR 680), although other parts of 21 CFR also apply to allergen regulation. Over the past 20 years, two features of CBER's regulatory program have had a significant impact on allergen manufacturers and enhanced the safety of allergen extracts marketed to the American public. The first is the enforcement of current good manufacturing practice (cGMP) standards (21 CFR 210, 211, and 600–680) on the manufacture of allergen products. cGMPs include requirements regarding organization and personnel, buildings and facilities, equipment, control of components and drug product containers and closures, production and process controls, holding and distribution, quality control, laboratory controls, and records and reports. cGMPs have been in effect since the 1960s. A second feature is allergen standardization. 21 CFR 680.3(e) specifies that when a potency test has been developed for a specific allergenic product, and when CBER has notified manufacturers that the test exists, manufacturers are required to use the test (or an equivalent alternative test) to determine the potency of each lot of the product prior to release. Since the 1980s, 19 allergen extracts have been standardized (see Table 1). This chapter focuses on these standardized products and the tests used to ascertain extract potency.

II. ALLERGEN EXTRACTS CURRENTLY ON THE MARKET (STANDARDIZED AND NONSTANDARDIZED)

Allergen extracts, which are manufactured and sold worldwide for the diagnosis and treatment of IgE-mediated allergic disease, are complex mixtures of natural biomaterials. Each extract contains proteins, carbohydrates, enzymes, and pigments, of which the allergens—presumably the active ingredients—may constitute only a small proportion (3). Traditionally, allergen extracts have been labeled either with a designation of extraction ratio (w/v) or with a protein unit designation which is determined using the Kjeldahl method (protein nitrogen units/ml). However, there is little correlation between these two designations and biological measures of allergen potency (4,5).

In the absence of a concerted effort to maintain product consistency, lot-to-lot variations in allergen content may be considerable. Product consistency may be affected by quality of the raw materials; for example, pollen and mite extracts (6) generally have greater lot-to-lot consistency than mold, house dust, and insect extracts (7). In addition, manufacturers can increase the consistency of their products by controlled collection, storage, and processing of the raw materials; by reproducible and optimized extraction and manufacturing techniques; and by establishing expiration dates based on real-time stability data. However, consistency can be assured only by measuring the potency of each lot of extracts and by marketing only those lots whose potency falls within an acceptable range.

FDA's allergen standardization regulation mandates that when an appropriate potency test exists, manufacturers must test each lot of an allergen extract for potency prior to sale. This regulation takes product consistency one step further by establishing a U.S. standard of potency for each standardized product. The purpose of allergen standardization is to ensure that the extracts are well characterized in terms of allergen content and that variation between lots is minimized even among different manufacturers (8). Since standardized extracts are compared to a single national potency standard, patients and their physicians can switch from one manufacturer's product to another with minimized risk of adverse reaction.

Table 1 Standardized Allergen Extracts Currently Licensed in the United States

Allergen vaccine	Current lot release tests	Labeled unitage
Dust mite (*Dermatophagoides farinae*)	Competition ELISA	AU/ml (equivalent to BAU/ml)
	Protein[a]	
Dust mite (*Dermatophagoides pteronyssinus*)		
Cat pelt (*Felis domesticus*)	Fel d 1 (RID)	BAU/ml
Cat hair (*Felis domesticus*)	IEF	5–9.9 Fel d 1 U/ml = 5000 BAU/ml
	Protein	10–19.9 Fel d 1 U/ml = 10,000 BAU/ml
BermTuda grass (*Cynodon dactylon*)	Competition ELISA	BAU/ml
Redtop grass (*Agrostis alba*)	IEF	
June (Kentucky blue) grass (*Poa pratensis*)	Protein[a]	
Perennial ryegrass (*Lolium perenne*)		
Orchard grass (*Dactylis glomerata*)		
Timothy grass (*Phleum pratense*)		
Meadow fescue grass (*Festuca elatior*)		
Sweet vernal grass (*Anthoxanthum odoratum*)		
Short ragweed (*Ambrosia artemisiifolia*)	Amb a 1 (RID)	Amb a 1 units
Yellow hornet (*Vespa* spp.)	Hyaluronidase & phospholipase activity	μg protein
Wasp (*Polistes* spp.)		
Honeybee (*Apis mellifera*)		
White-faced hornet (*Vespa* spp.)		
Yellow jacket (*Vespula* spp.)		
Mixed vespid (*Vespa* + *Vespula* spp.)		

[a] Test for informational purposes only. IEF: isoelectric focusing; RID: radial immunodiffusion.

There are 19 standardized allergen extracts currently available from manufacturers in the United States (Table 1). For each of these extracts, there is a U.S. standard of potency to which each lot of the vaccine is compared prior to release for sale to the public. The potency measures, and the assays used to determine them, are specified in the approved product license applications of each manufacturer for each product. Manufacturers may use the methods described in CBER's Methods of the Allergen Products Testing Laboratory (9) or may seek approval to use alternative test methods that provide equally reliable measures of product potency and meet regulatory requirements. The level of quality control for the 19 standardized allergen extracts is the exception rather than the rule. In vitro potency tests that correlate with in vivo clinical responses have not been developed for the hundreds of nonstandardized extracts available in U.S. product lines. Thus, for most allergen extracts manufactured in the United States, consistency cannot be assured by potency testing.

III. THE BASIS OF ALLERGEN STANDARDIZATION

Allergen standardization is dependent upon two important requirements: 1) the selection of a reference preparation of allergenic extract and 2) the selection of the procedures to compare manufactured products to the selected reference (10–12). In the United States, the use of a biological model of allergen standardization has permitted the assignment of bioequivalent allergen units (BAUs) for most standardized allergens (11). Once a specific unitage is assigned to a reference, all allergen extracts from the same source can be assigned units based on its relative potency (RP) with respect to the reference using an established quantitative in vitro potency method (13).

In theory, standardizing an allergen extract might involve purifying each allergen in the extract and establishing with precision the importance of each allergen. However, most allergen extracts are complex mixtures of numerous relevant allergens of as-yet-undetermined immunodominance. In addition, an individual allergen may be less "allergenic" in a particular lot due to instability or denaturation. The choice of the best potency test depends on the allergen extract to be standardized. In the absence of data supporting the safety of potency designations based on single allergen content, a measure of overall allergenicity may be a better predictor of safe dosing. For short ragweed and cat hair, data support the use of single allergen determinations (Amb a 1 and Fel d 1, respectively); for cat pelt, the presence of both Fel d 1 and albumin are ascertained; for Hymenoptera venoms, hyaluronidase and phospholipase A2 are verified for each lot; and for dust mites and grass pollen, overall allergenicity is determined.

For initial overall allergenicity assessment, CBER developed a method using erythema size following serial intradermal testing of highly allergic individuals. Intradermal testing was chosen over prick/puncture testing to achieve greater dosing accuracy; erythema size was chosen over wheal size to achieve greater accuracy in reaction measurements (14). This method, called "Intra Dermal dilution for 50 mm sum of Erythema determines the bioequivalent ALlergy units" ($ID_{50}EAL$), is used to compare the allergenicity of extracts regardless of source. Subsequent comparisons of extracts from the same source material are made by a variant analysis called the parallel line bioassay. Both of these methods are described in CBER's Methods of the Allergenic Products Testing Laboratory (9) and are discussed below.

In the $ID_{50}EAL$ method, allergenic extracts are evaluated in subjects maximally reactive to the respective reference concentrates. Each subject is tested with serial three-fold dilutions of the reference extract. After 15 minutes, the sum of the longest and midpoint orthogonal diameters of erythema (ΣE) is determined at each dilution, and the log dose producing a 50 mm ΣE response (D_{50}) is calculated (13). Extracts that produce similar D_{50} responses can be considered bioequivalent and are assigned similar units, the bioequivalent allergy unit (BAU). Because the modal D_{50} of a series of extracts was 14 (a 3^{-14} or 1:4.8 million dilution), extracts with a mean D_{50} of 14 were arbitrarily assigned the value of 100,000 BAU/ml (11). Thus, the formula for the determination of potency from the D_{50} is

$$\text{Potency} = 3^{-(14-\text{mean } D_{50})} \times 100,000 \text{ BAU/ml}$$

By a similar technique and analysis, bioequivalent doses of test extracts from the same source as the reference extract can be determined by the parallel-line bioassay (14). The inverse ratio of the doses of test extract required to produce identical D_{50} responses to a reference extract is the RP of that extract. This analysis requires that the log dose-response curves of the test extract and the reference extract be parallel; if the two dose-response lines are not parallel, then the ratio of skin test doses for identical responses—and the RP—will vary with the dose. In this situation, which strongly suggests compositional differences between the two extracts, the distance between the two lines is different at each dose and a meaningful RP cannot be determined (10,15) (Fig.1).

In the original 1994 protocol, the mean D_{50} for 15 highly allergic individuals was used to determine the D_{50} for the extract. In a recent reanalysis of the statistical considerations underlying such potency studies, Rabin et al. (16) applied the following formula for the number of study subjects, n, that would be required:

$$n = 2\,(\sigma/\delta)^2\,(z_{1-\alpha} + z_{1-\beta/2})^2$$

where σ is the standard deviation of the measurement, δ is the acceptable difference in D_{50}s of two equivalent products, and the z values are the critical values from the cumulative normal distribution table for a significance level α and a power of $1 - \beta$ (17). From this formula, n is a function of the *squares* of σ and δ. The value of n will depend on the particular allergen to be tested, but as may be seen in sample calculations represented in Table 2, n will usually be larger than 15.

Although skin testing is an essential component of the allergen standardization program, it is not intended for routine use in the testing of manufactured lots of extracts

PANEL A

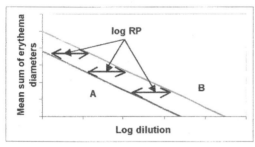

PANEL B

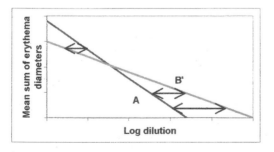

Figure 1 Hypothetical parallel-line bioassay curves. In panel A, the bioassay curves are parallel, and the difference of log dilutions resulting in the same diameters is constant at all diameters. The log relative potency (log RP) of test sample B compared with reference A is represented by the difference. In panel B, the curves are not parallel, and the differences vary with the strength of the reaction. Thus, the log RP of B′ compared with A cannot be calculated.

Table 2 Estimates of Sample Size n from the Formula $n = 2 \, (\sigma/\delta)^2 \, (z_{1-\alpha} + z_{1-\beta/2})^2$ to Demonstrate Equivalence at the $\alpha=0.05$ Level by the TOST Formalism for a Variety of β, Tolerance Intervals δ, and Standard Deviations σ ($z_{0.975} = 1.96$; $z_{0.95} = 1.645$; $z_{0.90} = 1.282$)

σ/δ	β	n
1.0	0.05	26
	0.10	22
	0.20	18
1.5	0.05	59
	0.10	49
	0.20	39
2.0	0.05	104
	0.10	87
	0.20	69

prior to release. In vitro potency assays that accurately predict the in vivo activity of extracts have been developed (15). Once an in vivo assay has been utilized to assign unitage to a reference extract, an appropriate surrogate in vitro assay can be used to assign units to test extracts from the same sources. These methods can be based on quantitation of the total protein content (Hymenoptera venoms), the specific allergen content within the allergen extracts (short ragweed and cat), or the inhibition of the binding of IgE from pooled allergic sera to reference allergen (grasses, mites) (18). For the Hymenoptera venom allergens, the potency determination is also based on the content of the known principal allergens within the extract, hyaluronidase and phospholipase, which is determined by enzyme activity (Table 1).

The potency units for short ragweed extracts were originally assigned based on their Amb a 1 content. Subsequent data suggested that 1 unit of Amb a 1 is equivalent to 1 µg of Amb a 1, and 350 Amb a 1 units/ml is equivalent to 100,000 BAU/ml. However, the original unitage has been retained. Grass pollen extracts are labeled in BAU/ml, based on $ID_{50}EAL$ testing. In some cases, the assignment of potency units to standardized allergenic extracts in the United States has changed as better bioequivalence data have become available (13). Cat extracts were originally standardized based on their Fel d 1 content, with arbitrary unitage (AU/ml) tied to the Fel d 1 determinations. Subsequent $ID_{50}EAL$ testing suggested that the 100,000 AU/ml cat extracts, which contained 10–19.9 Fel d 1 U/ml, should be relabeled as 10,000 BAU/ml (19). In addition, 20% of individuals allergic to cat were found to have antibody to non–Fel d 1 proteins (20), and the identification of a cat albumin band on IEF was added as a requirement for cat pelt extracts. Dust mite extracts were originally standardized (in AU/ml) based on RAST inhibition assays. Subsequent $ID_{50}EAL$ testing indicated that the arbitrary unitage was statistically bioequivalent to BAU/ml (21); in this case, the original unitage was retained (22).

The identity of an allergen extract may be verified by visualizing the separated allergen proteins based on their size and isoelectric points (3). The isoelectric focusing (IEF) assay is an important safety test in the lot release of grass pollen and cat extracts. The patterns produced by the crude allergen mixtures are reproducible enough to consistently indicate the presence of known allergens, to identify possible contaminants present in the extracts, and to check lot-to-lot variation in the extracts (23). In addition, IEF is used to verify the presence of cat albumin in cat pelt extracts.

IV. TESTS CURRENTLY APPLIED TO STANDARDIZED ALLERGENS

Several in vitro tests have been established for testing the potency and identity of standardized allergens (Table 1). Tests for potency include assays for the specific allergen content, for the RP, and for the enzyme activity of allergenic extracts. In addition, the identity of standardized extracts may be tested by the qualitative assessment of allergen content.

The specific allergen content of certain allergenic extracts can be measured by the radial immunodiffusion assay (RID). This assay is currently applied to two standardized allergenic extracts, short ragweed and cat, in which the immunodominant allergens (Amb a 1 and Fel d 1, respectively) have been identified and defined. In this assay, monospecific antiserum is added to an agar solution, which is allowed to solidify. Wells are then cut into the agar; test allergen is placed in the wells. As the specific allergen diffuses out into the agar, a precipitin ring forms, which delineates the equivalence zone for antigen-antibody binding. The radius of the precipitin ring can then be measured. Since the antibody concentration in the agar is constant, the antigen concentration decreases with increasing distance from the well and is proportional to the log of the concentration of the applied test allergen in comparison to the reference extract.

The potency of those standardized allergen extracts for which the immunodominant components have not been identified with certainty may be estimated using assays for IgE-antigen binding that compare the overall IgE binding properties of test and reference extracts, using pooled allergic sera. Initially, a RAST inhibition assay was used for this purpose; CBER adopted the competition ELISA as its standard assay because of its greater precision and convenience. After coating the wells of the polystyrene microtiter plate with the reference allergen and blocking the wells with bovine albumin, a mixture of the allergen extract to be tested and a reference serum pool is added to the wells. The greater the amount of immunoreactive allergen in the mix, the less free IgE antibody will be available from the serum pool to bind to the immobilized allergen on the plate. Once again, the concentration of the allergens in the allergen extract is determined by comparison to the reference allergen extract. However, since this assay does not explicitly measure a specific allergen, the allergen concentration is expressed as RP, with the reference extract assigned an arbitrary RP of 1.0. Early studies showed an excellent correlation between RP assigned by titration skin testing and RP determined by RAST inhibition (11); subsequent studies showed the competition ELISA to be equivalent as well (24).

Hymenoptera venoms contain multiple glycoprotein enzymes, the most important of which are hyaluronidase and phospholipases A1 and A2. Venom allergen extracts are standardized using enzymatic assays, which estimate hyaluronidase and phospholipase content based on their enzymatic activity. In these assays, an agar solution is prepared with the appropriate enzymatic substrate and test samples are then added to cut wells. As the enzyme present in the sample diffuses into the agar, it digests the substrate, forming clearing zones around the wells. The radius of the clear zones is then measured and calculated as the log of the concentration of the enzyme present in the sample.

In addition to determining the potency of these allergen extracts, manufacturers are expected to confirm the identity of certain standardized extracts (see Table 1) by IEF. This technique separates the proteins in the test extract based on their isoelectric points. The profile obtained in this technique is compared with the CBER standard to confirm the stated identity of the allergen extract (23).

In the past, manufacturers were required to perform ninhydrin protein assays on most standardized allergen extracts. CBER developed and adopted a modification of the more cumbersome ninhydrin technique for protein determination (25) in response to concerns about the inaccuracy of the more standard protein estimation techniques. However, release limits were not established for the total protein content of standardized allergen extracts. Rather, the results of the ninhydrin assay were required for information only. When the results were checked as part of CBER's lot release program, CBER required that the results of the CBER assay be within 40% of the manufacturer's result.

In effect, the protein assay requirement was a quality control test; in this phase of the allergen standardization program, CBER did not have data on the protein content of the standardized allergens, or the effect of the protein content on potency assays. The requirement that manufacturers perform the ninhydrin assay on their standardized allergen extracts was reexamined (26). As a result of these considerations, CBER no longer requires the use of the ninhydrin assay for standardized mite and grass allergen extracts. However, as part of ongoing quality control, manufacturers should continue to perform a validated protein assay on each lot of material, and CBER continues to require this information as part of its lot release program. The choice of protein assay is left to the manufacturer. Currently approved protein assay methods for other allergens (standardized cat, short ragweed, and Hymenoptera venoms) are unchanged.

V. HOW SHOULD RELEASE LIMITS BE CHOSEN?

Fundamental to the standardization process is establishing an acceptable range of comparability or equivalence. Limits that are too broad lead to unacceptable risk to patients (anaphylaxis when the physician changes from one bottle to another or changes to a different manufacturer), while limits that are too narrow lead to unacceptable risk for manufacturers (the rejection of a large percentage of safe and effective lots of product). In the competition ELISA, potency limits have been set according to the precision of the test; the candidate extracts are expected to be *statistically equivalent to the reference extract*, at a specified level of confidence with a specified test. Mite and grass pollen extracts are currently expected to be identical to reference at the 98% confidence level, using three replicates of a validated competition ELISA; the standard deviation σ in log (RP) for a single replicate is 0.1375 (24). The 98% confidence interval is given by $10^{\pm 2.326\sigma/\sqrt{3}}$. Consequently, a lot whose RP falls in the range 0.654–1.530 is within the 98% confidence interval and is approved for release. This criterion also implies that, on average, 2% of lots submitted to CBER will fall outside of the release limits even if they are identical to the reference extract. Lots that are not identical to the reference would fail at predictably higher rates, while a small fraction of lots whose RP is outside the limits (as could be established by more exhaustive testing) will pass release testing.

An alternative approach would be to base the potency limits on acceptable ranges established in clinical studies. Three criteria would appear to be important. The first, *therapeutic equivalence*, addresses the efficacy of allergen vaccines for immunotherapy. Thus, an RP range will have the property of therapeutic equivalence if, for the allergen vaccine in question, lots with RPs anywhere in that range have an equal likelihood of effecting clinical improvement in an immunotherapy trial. Likewise, *diagnostic equivalence* addresses the efficacy of allergen extracts for in vivo diagnostics. Finally, *safety equivalence* reflects the likelihood of the safe administration of the vaccine for either diagnostic or therapeutic indications. The acceptable limits should fall within the narrowest of the equivalence ranges established by these criteria.

The aggregate consistency of manufactured lots might also be taken into account when developing testing methods and limits. For example, if typical lot-to-lot consistency is very high and well within clinical limits, then testing protocols could be adjusted to eliminate outliers while rarely failing lots whose RP is close to 1. On the other extreme, if the distribution of lots is broad, equivalence to the reference would be imposed. This would narrow the distribution, but at a cost: At 95% equivalence, 5% of lots whose RP equals 1 would fail release.

In an analysis of studies using ragweed and dust mite allergens (6), it was found that the range of therapeutic equivalence was at least tenfold, and the ranges of diagnostic equivalence and safety equivalence were approximately fourfold. In the same study, the lot-to-lot consistency of 412 lots of grass pollen extracts and 91 lots of dust mite extracts was analyzed. The variability of the samples was comparable to the assay variability. Furthermore, it was determined that the mean ratio (in RP) of two randomly selected lots of allergen would be 1.12 (for mites) and 1.18 (for grass pollen). The calculated 95th percentile ratios were 1.48 and 1.8, respectively. Thus, the equivalence ranges appear to be considerably broader than the current lot release limits (twofold) and the expected variations in product potency using current manufacturing and quality control practices. Based on these estimates, CBER has proposed to broaden the internal release limits for standardized dust mite and grass pollen allergen extracts to 0.5–2.0 (27).

VI. FUTURE STANDARDIZATION EFFORTS

The effort to standardize allergens in the United States has resulted in the development of a core group of highly used allergen extracts that are better characterized and more consistent than their nonstandardized predecessors. Standardized allergens also facilitate accurate and informative scientific studies of the efficacy, safety, and mechanisms of allergen immunotherapy and will be essential for the study of novel immunotherapeutic products in the future. In spite of these clear advantages, most allergens marketed in the United States remain unstandardized. At a minimum, all allergen extracts should be subject to potency testing and compared with a reference extract, whether manufacturer-specific, industry-wide, national, or international. CBER continues to work with the allergen extract industry to establish and maintain U.S. standards of potency for an increasing number of allergen extracts and to improve the consistency of those products that are not standardized. In this section, the criteria that will be used to choose standardization targets are discussed, as well as the ways in which allergen standardization will be implemented in the future.

Standardization targets will be selected to maximize the public health benefit of greater allergen consistency. Criteria for allergen selection include the following:

1. Availability of stable, preferably lyophilized, material for use as long-term reference extracts.
2. Consistency of currently marketed product.
3. Widespread use as a diagnostic and/or therapeutic reagent in the United States.
4. Number of manufacturers producing the product.
5. Potential use in immunotherapy or diagnostics.
6. Public health impact of correct diagnosis and/or adequate treatment.

These impact criteria are meant to help establish priorities and are not intended to be exclusionary. Thus, for example, an extract produced by only one manufacturer might still be a standardization target if other impact criteria are met. Likewise, CBER might decide to move forward with a little-used product of great public health importance, the standardization of which might enhance its availability and quality in the United States.

As an example of these considerations, CBER investigators published a study in which American and German cockroach allergen extracts manufactured in the United States were determined to be of variable and low potency (7). Based on this study, as well as other evidence that exposure to cockroach allergens may be associated with asthma in the inner city (28), CBER has initiated studies to standardize these allergen extracts.

Once an allergen standardization target is selected, the marketed products that contain the allergen will be examined and compared with the best products available worldwide. Biological potency will be established using the $ID_{50}EAL$ method, and a surrogate test will be identified for lot release purposes. CBER intends to pursue these goals with the full knowledge and, ideally, active participation of the allergen extract industry and scientific investigators. When a test for a standard of potency exists, FDA notifies manufacturers [under 21 CFR 680.3(e)]. The regulation requires that manufacturers comply with the standard and test each lot of the specified extract prior to release for sale.

VII. SALIENT POINTS

1. Allergen standardization in the United States is based upon skin test responses in highly allergic individuals.
2. Most allergen extracts in the United States are not standardized.
3. Nonstandardized allergens are labeled in units (PNU/ml or w/v) that may be unrelated to potency.
4. All U.S. allergen extracts, whether standardized or nonstandardized, must be manufactured in accordance with current good manufacturing practices (cGMPs).
5. The number of individuals needed to establish the potency of a product by skin testing is related to the *square of the ratio* of the standard deviation (σ) of the skin test results and the acceptable difference (δ) in potency between two identically labeled products.
6. The unitage adopted for standardized allergens is based upon the best available scientific understanding of the specificity of responses in allergic individuals.
7. The potencies of individual lots of standardized allergen extracts are determined by specific surrogate in vitro tests that have been determined to correlate with the skin test results.
8. Release limits for lots of standardized allergens are established based upon manufacturing capabilities, potency assay performance, and clinical data.
9. The acceptable equivalence ranges for allergen extracts may be different when analyzed on the basis of diagnostic, therapeutic, or safety considerations.
10. New candidates for allergen standardization are chosen based upon specific impact criteria.

REFERENCES

1. Harden VA. A short history of the National Institutes of Health. http://www.history.nih.gov/exhibits/history/. 2000.
2. Milestones in U.S. food and drug law history. http://www.fda.gov/opacom/backgrounders/miles.html. 2000.
3. Yunginger JW. Allergenic extracts: Characterization, standardization and prospects for the future. Pediatr Clin North Am 1983; 30:795–805.
4. Baer H, Maloney CJ, Norman PS, Marsh DG. The potency and Group I antigen content of six commercially prepared grass pollen extracts. J Allergy Clin Immunol 1974; 54(3):157–164.
5. Baer H, Godfrey H, Maloney CJ, Norman PS, Lichtenstein LM. The potency and antigen E content of commercially prepared ragweed extracts. J Allergy 1970; 45(6):347–354.
6. Slater JE, Pastor RW. The determination of equivalent doses of standardized allergen vaccines. J Allergy Clin Immunol 2000; 105(3):468–474.
7. Patterson ML, Slater JE. Characterization and comparison of commercially available German and American cockroach allergen extracts. Clin Exp Allergy 2002 May 1932;721–727.
8. Yunginger JW. Allergens: Recent advances. Pediatr Clin North Am 1998; 35:981–993.
9. Methods of the allergenic products testing laboratory (Docket 94N-0012). Federal Register. 11–23–1994.
10. Turkeltaub PC. In-vivo standardization. In: Allergy, Principles and Practice (Middleton EJ, Reed CE, Ellis EF, eds.). St. Louis, MO: C.V. Mosby, 1988: 388–401.
11. Turkeltaub PC. Biological standardization of allergenic extracts. Allergol Immunopathol (Madr) 1989; 17(2):53–65.
12. Turkeltaub PC. Biological standardization. Arb Paul Ehrlich Inst Bundesamt Sera Impfstoffe Frankf A M 1997; (91):145–156.
13. Turkeltaub PC. Allergen vaccine unitage based on biological standardization: Clinical significance. In: Allergens and Allergen Immunotherapy (Lockey R, Bukantz SC, eds.). New York, NY: Marcel Dekker, 1999: 321–340.
14. Turkeltaub PC, Rastogi SC, Baer H, Anderson MC, Norman PS. A standardized quantitative skin-test assay of allergen potency and stability: Studies on the allergen dose-response curve and effect of wheal, erythema, and patient selection on assay results. J Allergy Clin Immunol 1982; 70(5):343–352.
15. Turkeltaub PC. In vivo methods of standardization. Clin Rev Allergy 1986; 4:371–387.
16. Rabin RL, Slater JE, Lachenbruch P, Pastor RW. Sample size considerations for establishing clinical bioequivalence of allergen formulations. Arb Paul Ehrlich Inst Bundesamt Sera Impfstoffe Frankf A M. In press.
17. Schuirmann DJ. A comparison of the two one-sided tests procedure and the power approach for assessing the equivalence of average bioavailability. J Pharmacokinet Biopharm 1987; 15(6):657–680.
18. Platts-Mills TAE, Rawle F, Chapman MD. Problems in allergen standardization. Clin Rev Allergy 1985; 3:271–290.
19. Matthews J, Turkeltaub PC. The assignment of biological allergy units (AU) to standardized cat extracts. J Allergy Clin Immunol 1992; 89:151.
20. Turkeltaub PC, Matthews J. Determination of compositional differences (CD) among standardized cat extracts by in vivo methods. J Allergy Clin Immunol 1992; 89:151.
21. Turkeltaub PC, Anderson MC, Baer H. Relative potency (RP), compositional differences (CD), and assignment of allergy units (AU) to mite extracts (Dp and Df) assayed by parallel line skin test (PLST). J Allergy Clin Immunol 1987; 79:235.
22. Turkeltaub PC. Use of skin testing for evaluation of potency, composition, and stability of allergenic products. Arb Paul Ehrlich Inst Bundesamt Sera Impfstoffe Frankf A M 1994; 87:79–87.
23. Yunginger JW, Adolphson CR. Standardization of allergens. In: Manual of Clinical Laboratory Immunology (Rose NR, de Macario EC, Fahey JL, Friedman H, Penn GM, eds.). Washington, DC: American Society for Microbiology, 1992: 678–684.

24. Lin Y, Miller CA. Standardization of allergenic extracts: An update on CBER's standardization program. Arb Paul Ehrlich Inst Bundesamt Sera Impfstoffe Frankf A M 1997; (91):127–130.

25. Richman PG, Cissel DS. A procedure for total protein determination with special application to allergenic extract standardization. J Biol Stand 1988; 16(4):225–238.

26. Slater JE, Gam AA, Solanki MD, Burk SH, Pastor RW. Statistical considerations in the establishment of release criteria for allergen vaccines. Arb Paul Ehrlich Inst Bundesamt Sera Impfstoffe Frankf A M 1993; 93:47–56.

27. Guidance for Reviewers: Potency Limits for Standardized Dust Mite and Grass Allergen Vaccines: A Revised Protocol. http://www.fda.gov/cber/gdlns/mitegrasvac.pdf. 11-10-2000.

28. Rosenstreich DL, Eggleston P, Kattan M, Baker D, Slavin RG, Gergen P, Mitchell H, McNiff-Mortimer K, Lynn H, Ownby D, Malveaux F. The role of cockroach allergy and exposure to cockroach allergen in causing morbidity among inner-city children with asthma. N Engl J Med 1997; 336(19):1356–1363.

23

Manufacturing and Standardizing Allergen Extracts in Europe

JØRGEN NEDERGAARD LARSEN, CHRISTIAN GAUGUIN HOUGHTON, and HENNING LØWENSTEIN

ALK-Abelló, Hørsholm, Denmark

MANUEL LOMBARDERO

ALK-Abelló, Madrid, Spain

I. INTRODUCTION

A. History of Standardization in Europe

Specific allergy treatment, i.e., specific immunotherapy or specific allergy vaccination, has been performed for almost a century, since it was first described by Noon in 1911 (1). The discovery in 1966 of the IgE molecule (2,3) and the central role of IgE in allergy facilitated a better understanding of the immunological mechanisms, led to an improvement of diagnostic tools, and consolidated the concept of specific allergy diagnosis and treatment. Scientific methods were introduced to standardize allergen extracts in the seventies and eighties (4) and, in combination with gradual improvement of the clinical procedures, established specific allergy treatment as a scientifically based, reproducible, and safe treatment for allergic diseases.

The first international initiative on allergen standardization was based on the Danish Allergen Standardization 1976 program and was published as the Nordic Guidelines in 1989 (5,6). These guidelines established the first regulatory demands for allergen extracts. The guidelines introduced the biological unit (BU), based on skin testing, for

433

potency measures. Each manufacturer was instructed to produce an In-House Reference Preparation (IHRP), adjust the potency in BU, and use the IHRP for batch-to-batch control using scientifically based laboratory testing. The significance of using the major allergen content for the biological activity was recognized in the early nineties and is now established in the WHO recommendations (7) and in the European Pharmacopoeia (8). This chapter describes important issues in the control of source materials and in the preparation of extracts as part of the standardization process the way it is performed in Europe. This differs from the procedures used in the United States, as does the selection of extracts for vaccination in common allergy practice.

B. Standardization of Allergen Extracts

Allergen extracts/vaccines are used for specific diagnosis and treatment of allergic diseases and indirectly for the detection of environmental allergens. Allergen extracts are aqueous solutions of allergenic source materials, such as pollen, animal hair and dander, dust mite bodies or cultures, insect venoms, or mold mycelia and spore particles. Since no structural feature defining an allergen has hitherto been described, the definition of an allergen is based upon the functional criterion of being able to elicit an IgE response in susceptible individuals. All allergens are proteins and are readily soluble in water. Airborne allergens are carried by particles in the μm range, a characteristic that is compatible with the concept that the particle carrying the allergen is inhaled and the allergen is deposited on the mucosal surface of the lower airways, thereby stimulating the immune system. The allergen is thus defined by the immune system of the individual patient.

By this definition, any immunogenic protein (antigen) has allergenic potential, even though most allergic patients have IgE specific for a relatively limited number of "major" allergens. Analysis of a larger number of patients leads to the identification of still more IgE-binding proteins (Fig. 1). Thus, the number of allergens in a given source material converge toward the total number of antigens, and any antigen has the potential to elicit an IgE response.

A major objective in the manufacture of allergen extracts, therefore, is to secure an adequate complexity reflecting the composition of water-soluble components of the allergenic source material. Another important matter of batch-to-batch control is standardization of potency, i.e., the overall IgE-binding capacity, which is a reflection of the anaphylactic potential of the preparation. The third important aspect of allergen extract manufacturing is controlling the major allergen content. The major allergens have distinct importance for the activity of allergen extracts/vaccines in diagnosis as well as treatment.

All aspects of the manufacturing procedure, from selection and collection of raw materials, extract preparation, and storage to validation of assays and reagents, have impact on extract quality and should be considered part of the standardization procedure.

II. PREPARATION OF ALLERGEN EXTRACTS

A. Source Materials

Inhalant allergens are present in airborne particles derived from a natural allergen source. The particles are inhaled and constitute the material to which humans are exposed. The

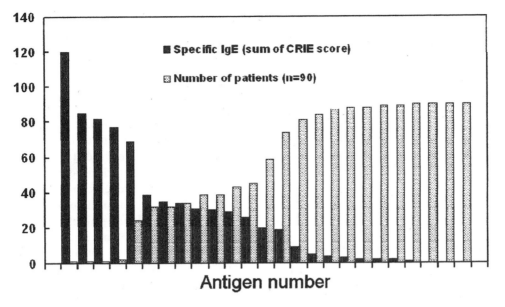

Figure 1 Complexity of patients' responses to allergen extracts. Serum samples from 90 grass-allergic patients were analyzed by crossed radioimmunoelectrophoresis (CRIE) using timothy grass, *Phleum pratense*, allergen extract. Labeled precipitates were assigned an arbitrary score for each patient depending on the staining intensity of the autoradiogram. In this way, a graduated score for the specific IgE reactivity of each individual patient with each individual allergen was obtained. The scores were summed for each allergen, and the antigens were arranged in ascending order and depicted on the ordinate axis. The score is depicted in the dark columns. The light column represents the cumulative number of patients having all their IgE specificities covered by the antigen in question and all other antigens to the left of the antigen in question.
Examples: A hypothetical extract containing the six most important allergens will cover all IgE specificities for 32 of the patients. Twenty-two allergens are needed to cover all IgE specificities of all 90 patients.

aim of selecting raw materials for allergen extract production is to gather materials containing the same active allergens in a manageable form. In most cases, the optimal source material is rather obvious, but in some cases, the allergen source is still debated, e.g., cat saliva/pelt/hair and dander or mouse urine/hair and dander.

The source materials should be selected with attention to the need for specificity and for inclusion of all relevant allergens in sufficient amounts (9). The collection of the source materials should be performed by qualified personnel, and reasonable measures must be employed by the producer of allergen extracts to ensure that collector qualifications and collection procedures are appropriate to verify the identity and quality of the source materials. This means that only specifically identified allergenic source materials that do not contain avoidable foreign substances should be used in the manufacture of allergen extracts. Means of identification and limits of foreign materials should meet established acceptance criteria for each source material. Where identity and purity cannot be determined by direct examination of the source materials, other appropriate methods should be applied to trace the materials from their origin. This includes complete identity labeling and certification from competent collectors. The processing and storage of source materials should be performed in a way to ensure that no unintended substances, including microbial organisms, are introduced into the materials. When possible, source materials should be fresh or stored in a manner that minimizes or prevents decomposition. Records should describe source materials in as much detail as possible, including the particulars of collection, pretreatment, and storage.

1. Pollen

The natural source of inhalant allergens from plants is the pollen. Pollen may be obtained either by collection in nature or from cultivated fields or greenhouses. The collection may be performed by several methods, such as vacuuming or drying flower heads followed by grinding. Furthermore, pollen may be cleaned either by passing it through sieves of different mesh sizes or by flotation. Finally, pollen is dried under controlled conditions and stored in sealed containers at –20°C. The maximum level of accepted contamination with pollen from other species is 1%. It should also be devoid of flower and plant debris, with a limit of 5% by weight. Pollen may show large variation in quantitative composition depending on season and location of growth, and in order to achieve a relatively constant composition, harvests from different years and sites of collection should be pooled for the production of allergen extracts.

2. Acarids

For the production of allergen extracts of house dust mites, the mites are grown in pure cultures. Source materials are either pure mite bodies (PMB) or whole mite cultures (WMC). The advantage of the WMC extract is that it contains all the material to which a mite-allergic patient is exposed under natural conditions, whereas the advantage of the PMB extract is a higher homogeneity and lot-to-lot consistency and avoidance of contamination debris from the culture medium. The WMC extract includes material from mite bodies, eggs, larvae, and faecal particles as well as mite decomposition material and contaminants from the culture medium that should not be allergenic. The PMB extract contains only material extracted from mite bodies, including eggs and faecal particles. The relative concentration of Group 1 and 2 allergens is dependent on the source materials, but clinical trials comparing vaccines based on WMC and PMB have shown both types to have similar clinical efficacy in specific allergy vaccination (10).

3. Mammals

Allergens of mammalian origin may emanate from various sources, i.e., hair, dander, serum, saliva, or urine. The allergens to which humans are exposed depend on the normal behavior of the animal. Therefore, the optimal source of allergens from mammals cannot be generalized and, in many cases, is still debated. Whether derived from dander or deposited from body fluids, however, most allergens are present in the pelt. Source materials should be collected only from animals that are declared healthy by a veterinarian at the time of collection. When sacrificed animals are used, the conditions for storing should minimize postmortem decomposition until the source materials can be collected. The optimal source materials are often dander, which should be free from visible traces of blood, serum, or other extractable materials. Hair proteins are insoluble, and thus it is not practical to use hair alone in the manufacture of mammalian allergen extracts. Likewise, the choice of whole pelt would increase the proportion of serum proteins, which are generally of low allergenic activity.

Due to the quantitative differences in the yield of the various allergens from different dog breeds, a mixture of material from a minimum of five different breeds is recommended. Furthermore, the same combination of dog breeds should be used from batch to batch.

4. Insects

The optimal source for insect allergens is dependent on the natural route of exposure, i.e., inhalation, bite, or sting. Where whole insects or insect debris are inhaled, the whole insect body is selected as the allergen source. In the case of stinging insects, venom is the ideal allergen source. With biting insects, saliva would be ideal since it contains the relevant allergens.

5. Fungi

Raw materials are obtained by growing the fungi under controlled conditions. The harvested raw materials should consist of mycelia and spores. Due to difficulties in maintaining a constant composition of fungal cultures, an extract should be derived from at least five independent cultures of the same species. Production of the source material should be conducted under aseptic conditions to reduce the risk of contamination by microorganisms or other fungi. The inoculum should be obtained from established fungal culture banks, i.e., American Type Culture Collection (ATCC), Manassas, Virginia (http://www.atcc.org), or Centraalbureau voor Schimmelcultures (CBS), Utrecth, The Netherlands (http://www.cbs.knaw.nl/CBSHOME.HTML). The cultivation medium should be synthetic or at least devoid of antigenic constituents, i.e., proteins. Controls performed in fungal allergen extract production must include tests for suspected toxins.

6. Foods

Foods constitute a diversified area, and the market for standardized allergen extracts is scarce. Foods are often derived from various subspecies grown under a broad variety of conditions reflecting geographical regions worldwide. In addition, foods are often cooked prior to ingestion, and cooking unpredictably affects the allergenicity of the foods. Consequently, the source of allergen exposure, qualitative as well as quantitative, is highly variable (11).

Ideally, source materials for food allergen extracts should reflect local subspecies, conditions, and habits for the cultivation, harvesting, storing, and cooking of the foods. However, ingested foods are increasingly derived from distant parts of the world. The best solution to these problems may be to combine materials from as many sources as possible to reflect variation in as many parameters as possible.

A further problem in food allergen extract production is the presence in many foods of natural or microbial toxins, pesticides, antibiotics, preservatives, and other additives that may be concentrated in the manufacturing process. The use of organic source material should therefore be preferred.

B. Aqueous Allergen Extracts

1. Preparation of Allergen Extracts

The production process of allergen extracts imposes a number of constraints upon both selection of source materials and the physicochemical conditions used during the extraction procedure. The process must neither denature the proteins/allergens nor significantly alter the composition, including the quantitative ratio between soluble components. The extraction should be performed under conditions resembling the physiological conditions in the human airways, e.g., pH and ionic strength, and suppressing possible proteolytic degradation and microbial growth (12). The optimal extraction time is always a compromise between yield and degradation/denaturation of the allergens, but extraction and processing should be performed at low temperatures and time should be minimized.

Low-molecular-weight materials (below 5000 Da) often include irritants, such as histamine, and should be removed from the final extract. This can be accomplished by dialysis, ultrafiltration, or size exclusion chromatography. Any substance excluded from the final extract should be verified nonallergenic. The production procedure should include assessment of known toxins, viral particles, microorganisms, and free histamine, verifying their concentration below defined thresholds.

The final extract should be stored under conditions that impede deterioration of the allergenic activity either by lyophilizing or by storing it at low temperatures ($-20°C$ to $-80°C$), possibly in the presence of stabilizing agents such as 50% glycerol or a nonallergenic protein (certified human serum albumin).

The most widely used extraction media are aqueous buffer systems of pH 6 to 9 and ionic strength 0.05 to 0.2. In general, nonaqueous solvents should be avoided due to the risk of protein denaturation. Table 1 lists the most important allergen extracts in Europe and the United States.

C. Modified Allergen Extracts/Vaccines

1. Introduction

The efficacy of traditional immunotherapy, i.e., specific allergen vaccination, is related to the dose of vaccine administered, but the inherent allergenic properties of the vaccine imply a risk of inducing anaphylaxis. The risk for such a reaction is minimized by administering repeated injections of increasing size over extended time periods. Physical or chemical modification of the extract can further reduce this risk. Physical modification involves adsorption of the allergens to inorganic gels, such as aluminum hydroxide or alum, for the purpose of attaining a depot effect characterized by a slow release of the allergens. Chemical modification includes cross-linking of the allergens by treatment with agents, such as formaldehyde ("allergoids"), for the purpose of reducing allergenic reactivity without compromising immunizing capacity. Other types of modification include use of partly degraded allergens or chemical coupling to polymers such as polyethylene glycol. Modified allergen vaccines are used for allergy vaccination but are not used for diagnosis since they were intentionally modified to reduce interaction with IgE.

2. Physical Modification of Allergens

Physical modification of allergens involves adsorption of the allergen extract with insoluble complexes of inorganic salts, such as aluminum hydroxide or calcium phosphate. Aluminum hydroxide, $Al(OH)_3$, is especially useful for vaccination purposes and is used for that purpose in both human and veterinary medicine (13). Its advantages are based on two characteristics of the complexes: the depot effect and the adjuvant effect. The allergens bind firmly to the inorganic complexes, giving rise to slow release of the proteins, thereby lowering the concentration of allergen in the tissue and reducing the risk of systemic side effects. Furthermore, the depot effect reduces the number of injections needed in the course of specific allergy vaccination. Although the significance of the adjuvant effect is unclear, higher levels of IgG antibodies have been observed when alum-adsorbed vaccines were used in specific allergy vaccination compared with aqueous vaccine (14). Compared with aqueous vaccines, patients receiving depot preparations seem to experience fewer systemic side effects (15), particularly severe early reactions. The number of late reactions, which seem to be milder and can be managed by the patient, is reduced to a lesser extent, especially in asthmatic patients (16).

Table 1 Most Important Allergen Extracts

Europe		North America	
Temperate grasses	*Lolium perenne* *Phleum pratense* *Poa pratensis* *Festuca pratensis* *Dactylis glomerata* *Secale sereale*	House dust mites	*Dermatophagoides pteronyssinus* *Dermatophagoides farinae*
House dust mites	*Dermatophagoides pteronyssinus* *Dermatophagoides farinae*	Temperate and subtropical grasses	*Lolium perenne* *Phleum pratense* *Poa pratensis* *Festuca pratensis* *Dactylis glomerata* *Cynodon dactylon*
Trees	*Alnus glutinosa* *Betula verrucosa* *Corylus avellana*	Ragweed	*Ambrosia* spp.
Parietaria	*Parietaria* spp.	Cat	*Felis domesticus*
Olive	*Olea europea*	Dog	*Canis familiaris*
Yellow jacket	*Vespula* spp.	Lambs quarter	*Chenopodium* spp.
Mugwort	*Artemisia vulgaris*	Mugwort	*Artemisia* spp.
Molds	*Alternaria* spp. *Cladosporium* spp. *Aspergillus* spp. *Penicillium* spp.	Pigweed	*Amranthus* spp.
Cat	*Felis domesticus*	Plantain	*Plantago* spp.
Honeybee	*Apis mellifera*	Molds	*Alternaria* spp. *Cladosporium* spp. *Aspergillus* spp. *Penicillium* spp.
Dog	*Canis familiaris*	Hymenoptera venoms	*Apis mellifera* *Vespula* spp.

The two most important allergen sources in the world are the house dust mites and the grass pollens. Patients often cross-react between the two important mite species, i.e., *D. pteronyssinus* and *D. farinae*, and between several species of the grasses. Commercial extracts are often based on mixtures of species within these groups. Important worldwide are also the indoor allergens from cat, dog, and molds, as well as the extracts derived from Hymenoptera venoms. In local regions other species may dominate. Examples are ragweed in large parts of the United States, birch in northern Europe, and *Parietaria* and olive in southern Europe.

Preparation of Aluminum Hydroxide–Adsorbed Extract. Aluminum hydroxide is available as a stable viscous homogeneous gel with a high capacity for noncovalent coupling of proteins. The adsorption is performed simply by mixing the aqueous extract and the gel. After a few minutes at room temperature, the adsorption is complete. Buffer conditions need to be controlled, as the binding capacity varies with buffer composition, ionic strength, pH, and additives (17).

Standardization of the allergen extract must be completed prior to adsorption, as the insoluble complex is difficult to analyze. Therefore, it is difficult to verify the amount of protein adsorbed. In practice, a known amount of standardized allergen extract is adsorbed, and the amount of unbound protein is determined following precipitation of the complex by centrifugation. Manufacturers must specify criteria to withdraw batches above certain thresholds, as different allergens are bound to the complex with different efficiency. Thus, if a large fraction of the allergen extract is unbound, the relative composition of the vaccine may not reflect the composition of the standardized extract.

The binding capacity of Alhydrogel (Brenntag, Denmark) was investigated using a 1000-donor human serum pool (18). Binding capacities of 14 individual serum proteins varied between 0.5 and 100 µg per mg of Alhydrogel for IgM and IgG, respectively. There was no correlation between the binding capacity and net charge, molecular weight, or carbohydrate content of the proteins. The adsorption capacity may reflect the surface density of pairs of neutralizing amino acids (carboxyl-guanidinium and carboxyl-ε amino groups). This parameter is very rarely known and cannot be predicted, even from the primary sequence of the allergen. Therefore, in each case, the binding capacity has to be empirically determined.

3.   Chemically Modified Allergens

The idea behind chemical modification of allergen extracts is based on the observation that successful allergy vaccination is accompanied by an increase in allergen-specific IgG. Thus, if the allergen could be modified in such a way as to reduce allergenic reactivity, e.g., IgE binding, while preserving immunogenicity, higher doses could be administered without the risk of systemic reactions, leading to higher levels of allergen-specific IgG and improved outcome of specific allergy vaccination (19).

Formaldehyde had been used for extract development in detoxification of bacterial toxins, when Marsh and coworkers successfully applied formaldehyde treatment of allergens for allergy vaccination (19). The allergens are incubated with formaldehyde yielding the "allergoids," high-molecular-weight covalently coupled allergen complexes. Compounds with similar immunological properties can be produced using glutaraldehyde instead of formaldehyde; this section will describe the formaldehyde-derived allergoids. The rationale behind the reduced allergenicity of allergoids is threefold: (1) The large polymeric structures would contain concealed antigenic determinants (epitopes) unable to react with IgE, (2) polymeric antigens would have a lower "epitope concentration" and thus reduced ability to cross-link IgE on mast cells, and (3) high-molecular-weight polymers would diffuse more slowly through tissue.

Preparation of Chemically Modified Allergens.   Several allergens are heat-labile and thus not readily applicable to the standard procedure of incubation with formaldehyde at elevated temperatures. Instead, a two-step procedure has been applied (20). The first step is incubation with 2 M formaldehyde at 10°C in aqueous buffer at pH 7.5, yielding a stabilized intermediate. After 16 days, the reaction is diluted fourfold and incubated another 16 days at 32°C. The first step at low temperature results in limited inter- and intramolecular cross-linking, thus stabilizing the native conformation of the allergens with minimal thermal denaturation even of heat-labile allergens. The conformation of the intermediate is stable and can be cross-linked further at elevated temperature. Residual formaldehyde is removed by dialysis, and the allergoid is distributed either stabilized by addition of 50% glycerol, lyophilized, or coupled to aluminum hydroxide.

4.   Other Modifications

Approaches have been taken to reduce the allergenicity of allergen extracts by disruption of the tertiary structure of allergen molecules using denatured or degraded antigens or peptides, but with reduced efficacy in allergy vaccination compared with native allergens.

Such molecules do have reduced IgE binding activity but also substantially reduced immunizing capacity leading to insufficient stimulation of a protective immune response, the beneficial effect of which is indicated by the rise in specific IgG accompanying successful allergy vaccination.

Another approach has been based on allergens chemically coupled to biodegradable polymers, such as (methoxy)-polyethylene glycol, (m)-PEG, or D-glutamic acid, D-lysine (DGL) copolymer, or other nonimmunogenic polymers. From mouse experiments, such compounds were expected to suppress IgE biosynthesis in humans (21). However, clinical studies in humans were discouraging, and the effect is possibly due to high dosing, mediated by a mechanism similar to the peptide-mediated "anergy" induction of T-cells described in vitro in mouse models (22). A common aspect of these approaches is the use of extremely high doses, rendering their clinical use in humans problematic.

The employment of structural and molecular biology has revealed molecular details to the atomic level of several important major allergens. Biotechnology may facilitate the development of safer allergen molecules in the form of mutated recombinant allergens, which can be standardized as chemical entities, obviating the problems of current allergen standardization (23).

5. Standardization of Modified Allergen Extracts

Most of the techniques used to characterize and standardize aqueous allergen extracts are not applicable to modified ones. It is therefore recommended that standardization be completed using the intermediate allergen preparation (IMP) prior to modification and that the reproducibility of the modification process be documented by methods specific to the procedure in question. Standardization of aqueous allergen extracts is discussed elsewhere in this chapter. A brief discussion of the methods suitable for the documentation of the modification processes in aluminum hydroxide–adsorbed and formaldehyde-treated allergen extracts follows.

Protein content in itself is not a suitable standardization parameter but may be a useful measure in terms of normalization of other activities—for example, RAST inhibition capacity per Lowry unit of protein. Determination of the reduction in primary amino groups is a good indication of the degree of modification in aldehyde-treated allergen extracts, since aldehydes react preferentially with primary amino groups. This measure can also be used for stability monitoring of the allergoid, as a reversal of the coupling will lead to an increase in the number of primary amino groups.

It is essential to verify that all protein is bound for adsorbed allergen vaccines. The acceptable level of allergen in the supernatant following centrifugation should be considerably below the initial dose used in the up-dosing schedule of allergy vaccination.

Electrophoretic techniques, such as acrylamide gel electrophoresis and isoelectric focusing possibly combined with immunoblotting, are widely used for allergen characterization. For analysis of allergens liberated from adsorbed complexes, acrylamide gel electrophoresis is preferred. However, for allergoids, acrylamide gel electrophoresis is not useful because of the high molecular weight. As formaldehyde preferentially reacts with primary amino groups, the pI of the allergoid is more acidic relative to the allergens. The shift in pI can be monitored by isoelectric focusing. Size exclusion chromatography, preferably conducted by high-performance liquid chromatography (HPLC), is suited to control for the increase in molecular weight of allergoids relative to the allergens.

Crossed (radio-)immunoelectrophoresis cannot be used to analyze modified allergen extracts. RAST inhibition or related techniques, however, are readily applicable to both alum-adsorbed allergen extracts and allergoids for the purpose of assessing the reduction in allergenicity. These methods are also suited for stability studies.

In vivo testing in patients to standardize modified allergen vaccines is theoretically attractive; however, it is not practical. First, it would not be ethically acceptable to base production of all batches of extracts on routine in vivo assays. There are also large differences in the immune responses of individual patients necessitating large patient panels for such assays. Second, in vivo tests are expensive in terms of labor, time, and money.

6. Comparison of Modified Extracts

Allergen extracts contain a variety of enzymatic activities, including proteolytic activities, resulting in reduced stability of aqueous extracts when stored in solution. However, the chemical cross-linking in modified extracts destroys practically all enzymatic activity, thereby increasing the stability of allergoid preparations; however, the modification process is slow and may permit proteolytic breakdown. In addition, both physical (aluminum hydroxide) and chemical (formaldehyde) modification result in reduced allergenicity.

Several clinical studies demonstrate that modified allergen extracts are safer than aqueous allergen vaccines and equally effective in treatment of allergic diseases. Acquired immune responses are driven by contact with epitopes, which are structural elements of the allergens (antigens). T-cell epitopes are linear fragments of its polypeptide chain, whereas B-cell epitopes (antibody-binding epitopes) are sections of the surface structure present only in the native conformation of the allergen (Figs. 2 and 3). Both T-and B-cell epitopes are essential for effective initiation and stimulation of immune responses; however, the repertoire of epitopes functional in any individual is highly heterogeneous (24,25).

Whereas the modification introduced by aluminum hydroxide adsorption is biologically reversible, the chemical modification of individual amino acids will irreversibly inactivate B-cell epitopes (and possibly also T-cell epitopes). This chemical effect decreases

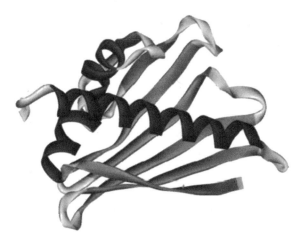

Figure 2   Molecular structure of the major allergen from birch, Bet v 1. The main feature of the structure is a 25-amino-acid-long α-helix surrounded by a seven-stranded antiparallel β-sheet. A most unusual feature of the structure is a large internal cavity with three openings to the surface. This is the first experimentally determined structure of a clinically important inhalant major allergen (26).

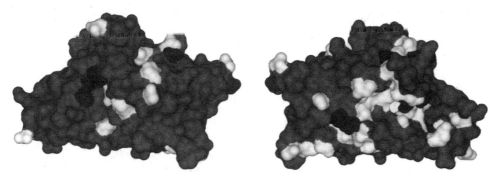

Figure 3 The molecular basis of cross-reactivity. Front and back view of the molecular structure of Bet v 1. Grey patches represent areas on the surface that are completely conserved among the homologous major allergens of alder, birch, and hazel. Conservative substitutions occur in dark gray areas. The conserved areas represent potential highly cross-reactive IgE epitopes on the protein surface.

the number of epitopes and hence allergenicity as well as immunogenicity, explaining why higher doses of allergoid are needed to achieve clinical efficacy. The chemical modifications are not randomly distributed, as ε amino groups on lysine residues are preferentially modified. Some epitopes are consequently more sensitive to modification than others, which may enhance the patient-to-patient variation when allergoids are analyzed by in vivo assays or used for allergy vaccination.

Contrary to expectation, the chemical modification by formaldehyde did not increase safety. This was documented in a report from the German Federal Agency for Sera and Vaccines which analyzed all reported adverse reactions to allergen vaccines over a 10-year period, 1991 to 2000, including 555 life-threatening, nonfatal events (27).

III. STANDARDIZATION OF ALLERGEN EXTRACTS

Allergen extracts are complex mixtures of antigenic components. They are produced by extraction of naturally occurring source materials that are known to vary considerably in composition depending on time and place. Without intervention, this variation would be reflected in the final products.

The purpose of standardization is to minimize the variation in composition, qualitative as well as quantitative, of the final products for the purpose of obtaining a higher level of safety, efficacy, accuracy, and simplicity for allergy diagnosis and allergen vaccination. Standardization of allergen extracts can never be absolute; standardization should be progressively improved as new methodologies and technologies are developed and the understanding of the properties of the allergens and of the immune responses of allergic patients increases. The benefits for the clinician from improved standardization of allergen vaccines include easier differentiation between allergic and nonallergic subjects, a more precise definition of the specificity and degree of allergy, and a more reliable and reproducible outcome of specific allergy vaccination.

Standardization of allergen extracts is complicated due to their complexity, the allergen molecules, and their epitopes. Allergens are complex mixtures of isoallergens and variants, differing in amino acid sequence (Fig. 4). Some allergens are composed of two or more subunits, the association and dissociation of which will affect IgE binding.

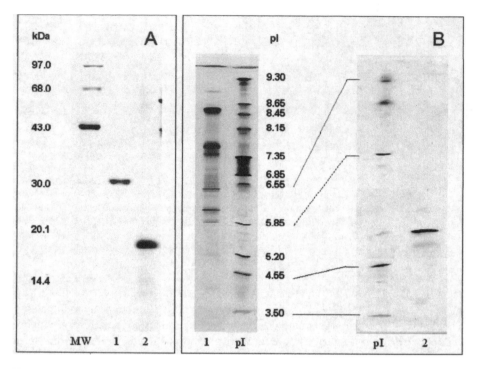

Figure 4 Isoallergenic variation. Allergens are mixtures of isoallergenic variants differing in amino acid sequence, whereas recombinant allergens are homogeneous. Panel A shows a silver-stained SDS gel; lane MW, molecular weight markers; lane 1, purified natural Phl p 1; lane 2, purified recombinant Bet v 1. Panel B shows silver-stained isoelectric-focusing gels of pI markers and the same preparations of purified allergens (lanes 1 and 2).

In addition, partial denaturation or degradation, which may be imposed by physical or chemical conditions in the production process, is difficult to assess and has a significant effect on the IgE binding activities of the allergens. The B-cell epitopes that bind to IgE are largely conformational by disposition, meaning that they will be missing from the extract if the allergens are irreversibly denatured.

Another complicating aspect is the complexity of the immune responses of individual patients. Patients respond individually to allergen sources with respect to both specificity and potency. Allergens are proteins, and all proteins are potential allergens. A major allergen is defined as an allergen that is frequently recognized by patients' serum IgE when a large panel of patient sera is analyzed. A minor allergen binds IgE less frequently (below 50%) (28). Furthermore, patients respond individually to B- and T-cell epitopes and hence to isoallergens and variants.

A major objective of allergen extract standardization is to ensure an adequate complexity in their composition. Knowledge of all essential allergens is a precondition for the safety of ensuring their presence in the final products (Fig. 5).

The other important aspect of standardization is the control of the total allergenic potency. The total IgE binding activity is intimately related to the content of major allergen (29), and for an optimal standardization procedure, control of the content of major allergen is essential.

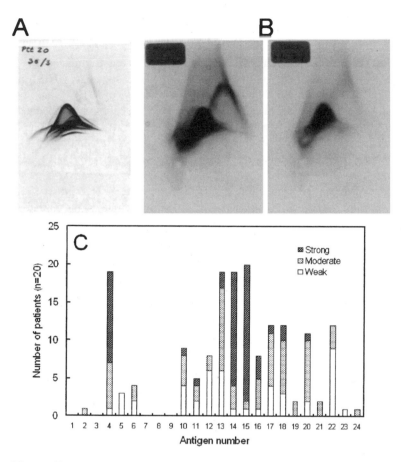

Figure 5 Complexity of allergen extracts. Crossed (radio-)immunoelectrophoresis used for the determination of important allergens. Panel A shows a crossed immunoelectrophoresis plate of a *Dermatophagoides pteronyssinus* allergen extract. Each bell-shaped precipitate represents the reaction of an antigen in the extract with the corresponding antibody present in a rabbit antiserum, raised by repeated immunization with the extract. Panel B shows an autoradiogram of similar plates after incubation with patient's serum and a radio-labeled anti-IgE antibody. Stained precipitates represent allergens. Precipitates from panel A are arbitrarily numbered, and the number of sera in a patient panel showing IgE reactivity with each precipitate is recorded and displayed in an allergogram, Panel C. Der p 1 corresponds to antigen number 15, Der p 2 to antigen 14.

A variety of techniques are available to assess allergen extract complexity and potency. Most techniques use antibodies as reagents, adding another level of complexity to the standardization procedure. Both human IgE and antibodies raised by immunization of animals are subject to natural variation and, in addition, may change over time.

These problems are handled by the establishment of reference and control extracts. International collaboration is necessary to ensure that manufacturers, government authorities, clinicians, and research laboratories worldwide can refer to the same preparations when comparing the results of quality control studies and potency estimates for different allergen extracts. Ideally, standards for reagents should also be established to promote and assist international collaboration.

A.   Standards, References, and Controls

1.   The Establishment and Use of International Standards

Guidelines for the establishment of international standards (IS) were formulated by a subcommittee under the International Union of Immunological Societies (IUIS) in 1980–1981. It was assumed that the collaboration and joint authority of WHO would be essential for international acceptance. In the following years, the subcommittee selected, characterized, and produced international standards from several allergenic sources. These included *Ambrosia artemisiifolia* (short ragweed) (30), *Phleum pratense* (timothy grass) (31), *Dermatophagoides pteronyssinus* (house dust mite) (32), *Betula verrucosa* (birch) (33), and *Canis familiaris* (dog) (34). Additional standards were planned for *Alternaria alternata* (a mold) (35), *Cynodon dactylon* (Bermuda grass) (36), *Lolium perenne* (rye grass) (37), *Felis domesticus* (cat), and *Dermatophagoides farinae* (house dust mite). This initiative failed because of a lack of consensus and acceptance, primarily due to the differences in practical standardization between Europe and the United States (see page 32).

Each of these standard reference extracts has been thoroughly investigated in collaborative studies involving laboratories and clinics worldwide. The results of the characterization and comparison of several coded extracts, which were made available by allergen manufacturers on a voluntary basis, as well as the selection of the international standards, have been published and are available to all interested parties. Each international standard has been produced in 3000 to 4000 lyophilized, glass-sealed ampules, which can be obtained from the National Institute of Biological Science and Control, NIBSC, Herts, U.K.

The content of each ampule is defined by the arbitrary assignment of 100,000 IU. This means that each ampule contains 100,000 IU of any included individual allergen and 100,000 IU of potency measured by any relevant method. Potency estimates will depend on methods and reagents, which must be stated, whereas IUs are independent of methods and reagents.

It is important to realize that the international standards are only recommended for use as calibrators (standards for measurement of relative potency). They are not recommended for use as prototypes, materials to which an extract is to be matched in all respects. None of the international standards have been tested in clinical trials of specific allergy vaccination, and no potency measures of their therapeutic effect have been established.

2.   Purified Allergens as International Standards

The WHO-IUIS Allergen Standardization Committee has started the initiative, called the "Development of Certified Reference Materials for Allergenic Products and Validation of Methods for Their Quantification" (CREATE Project), to develop certified reference materials (CRMs) based on purified natural and recombinant allergens. The project is funded by the European Union and involves the collaboration between academic researchers and pharmaceutical companies throughout Europe (38). Eight major allergens have been initially selected from the four most important allergen sources: birch, grass and olive pollen, and house dust mites. Recombinant allergens will be compared physicochemically and immunologically with their natural counterparts, and candidate CRMs will be selected to serve as primary standards for immunoassays. In addition, mAb-based ELISAs for measurement of the allergens will be evaluated and validated. Providing international allergen references and reference assays enables a common unitage system in absolute mass units of major allergen.

The existence and availability of allergen CRMs will enable the assignment of a major allergen content in common units to the internal reference preparations (see below), which are in use in different laboratories of manufacturers, allergen research groups, or control authorities. A common unit facilitates the collaboration of these groups and improves safety in practical allergy vaccination for the benefit of all involved parties, especially allergic individuals undergoing treatment.

3. The Establishment and Use of In-House Reference Preparations (IHRP)

Having established a production process, including control of raw material, batch-to-batch standardization is performed relative to an In-House Reference Preparation (IHRP). The IHRP must be thoroughly characterized by in vitro laboratory methods to demonstrate an adequate complexity as well as an appropriate content of relevant major allergen(s). The potency of the IHRP must be determined by in vivo methods, such as skin testing, and the content of major allergen(s) must be determined in absolute amounts. Furthermore, the IHRP should prove efficacious in clinical trials of specific allergy vaccination.

The IHRP serves as a blueprint of the allergy extract to be matched in all aspects by each and every following batch. Specific activities of the in-house reference preparations should be compared with international standards. In this way, measures from different manufacturers can be compared and consistency in internal standardization achieved (6).

B. Strategy for Standardization

It is impossible to assess the clinical efficacy of each and every batch in the production of routine batches of allergen extracts. In practice, the batches are compared with the IHRP using a combination of different in vitro techniques to achieve a uniform composition, content of major allergen, and potency of extracts. The standardization can be performed using the following three-step procedure:

1. Determination of allergen composition to ensure that all important allergens are present
2. Quantification of specific allergens to ensure that essential allergens are present in constant ratios
3. Quantification of the total allergenic activity to ensure that the overall potency of the extract is constant (in vivo and/or in vitro)

C. Methods for the Assessment of Allergen Extract Quality

The quality of an allergen extract is a measure of the complexity of the composition, including the concentration of each constituent. Having established careful control of raw materials and a robust production process, a relatively constant ratio between individual components can be achieved independently by quantifying only one or two components, i.e., the major allergens.

The complexity of the composition of allergen extracts can be assessed by several techniques. These techniques are standard biochemical and immunochemical separation techniques. Polyacrylamide gel electrophoresis with sodium dodecylsulfate (SDS-PAGE) (39) is a widely used high-resolution technique available in rapid and partly automated systems. The proteins are separated, but only after denaturation, according to size. Densitometric scanning has been reported, but this technique is not quantitative due to differences in staining intensities. It should only be used for a qualitative assessment of the allergen extract. In combination with electroblotting (40), the proteins can be immobilized on protein-binding membranes, such as nitrocellulose, and stained using a variety of dyes or labeled antibodies (immunoblotting), thereby considerably increasing the sensitivity. Some allergens, however, are irreversibly denatured by SDS treatment and may escape detection by IgE immunoblotting (41).

Isoelectric focusing (IEF) (42) is a qualitative electrophoretic technique that separates proteins according to charge [isoelectric points (pI)]. Individual allergens are difficult to identify, as many proteins form several bands due to charge differences between isoallergens and variants.

Crossed immunoelectrophoresis (CIE) (43) is a technique by which individual antigens are distinguished in agarose gels in the form of bell-shaped antigen–antibody precipitates. The technique is dependent on the availability of broadly reactive polyspecific rabbit antibodies, but the method yields information on the relative concentrations of several important antigens in a single experiment. In crossed radioimmunoelectrophoresis (CRIE) (44), the plates are incubated with patient serum for the identification of allergens.

D. Quantification of Specific Allergens

Having determined an adequate complexity in composition, an allergen extract may still theoretically be deficient in the content of major allergen (Fig. 6). It is important to independently assess the content of major allergen(s), especially for allergen vaccines used for allergy vaccination. The maintenance dose in effective allergy vaccination contains a defined amount of major allergen (5–20 µg, regardless of vaccine), and the major allergen content is therefore a usable measure relating vaccine potency and therapeutic effect (Table 2).

The importance of controlling individual allergens, where possible, in extracts is gaining more importance among government regulators and clinicians. Allergen extract manufacturers today have access to the published purification procedures of most major allergens. The purified major allergens can be used to produce antibodies for independent quantification, even in complex mixtures, such as allergen extracts. Polyspecific or mono-

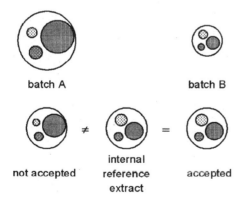

Figure 6 Standardization of allergen extracts. Complexity of allergen extracts represented by a model with three major allergens. The area of shaded circles represents the relative potency of individual components. The area of outer circles represents the total allergenic potency of the extracts. The total allergenic potency of batch A and B may be adjusted by dilution or concentration, but the composition of the extracts still may vary, accentuating the significance of the measurement of individual components.

Table 2   Maintenance Doses in Effective Specific Allergy Vaccination

Allergen source	Major allergen	Major allergen in maintenance dose	Approximate equivalent FDA potency	References
Cat				53–56
Felis domesticus	Fel d 1	14.6 µg	2500 BAU	45–48
House dust mite				10, 49
Der. pteronyssinus	Der p 1	9.8 µg	740 AU	
Der. farinae	Der f 1	13.8 µg	2628 AU	
Ragweed				50
Ambrosia artemisiifolia	Amb a 1	10.0 µg	3000 AU	
Grasses				51–53
Lolium perenne	Lol p 5	12.5 µg	3948 BAU	
Phleum pratense	Phl p 5	20.2 µg	5220 BAU	
Dactylis glomerata	Dac g 5	12.0 µg	2956 BAU	
Festuca pratense	Fes p 5	18.6 µg	12,568 BAU	

Discrepancy between diagnostic and therapeutic potency illustrated by the recommended maintenance doses of various clinical studies. For the average patient, the recommended maintenance dose contains 5–20 µg of major allergen.

specific polyclonal rabbit antibodies or murine monoclonal antibodies are most often used for this purpose.

Several immunoelectrophoretic techniques might be applied for the quantitative determination of individual allergens. These techniques are referred to as quantitative immunoelectrophoresis (QIE) (43), and they are convenient and reliable techniques to measure allergen concentrations relative to an in-house standard.

The area of a diffusion ring formed by the precipitated antigen in the monospecific antibody-containing gel can be correlated to the amount of antigen applied in single radial immunodiffusion (SRID), also known as the Mancini technique. The area of the precipitate, alternatively, the height of the precipitate, formed by electrophoresis of the antigen into the agarose gel containing the monospecific antibody, is proportional to the antigen concentration in rocket immunoelectrophoresis (RIE) or quantitative CIE. Both SRID and RIE are dependent on monospecific antibodies, whereas CIE is dependent on polyspecific antibodies.

The ELISA technique (54), in which the allergen is directly bound to a microtiter plate or captured using a monoclonal or polyclonal, monospecific antiserum coated to the plate and subsequently detected using a monoclonal or polyclonal, monospecific antiserum, is a technique offering the possibility of multisample testing and partial automation. When optimized properly, the technique is very accurate. Monoclonal antibody-based ELISA is the most widely used technique for allergen measurement in mass units (55), and a number of validated ELISAs for major allergens from the main allergenic sources are available. The standard format is a two-site sandwich assay. An allergen-specific mAb is coated to the microtiter plate, and upon incubating the allergen vaccine, the allergen molecules are captured and subsequently detected using a second mAb or a polyclonal antiserum. An in-house reference, calibrated against a purified allergen preparation, is used as standard. The advantages of mAb-based ELISAs are their suitability for automation, well-defined specificity and an inexhaustible reagent supply, precise quantification in mass units of allergen, detection limits in the range of 0.1–5 ng/ml, and good reproducibility (intra-assay coefficient of variation in the 10–15% range).

A potential problem of mAb-based ELISAs is the specificity of the mAb(s) used. Allergens are heterogeneous mixtures of isoallergens and variants, and in some cases it has been shown that specific mAb reacts to individual subsets of isoallergens (56) introducing a bias in the allergen measurement. A solution to this problem is to use a cocktail of mAbs on the solid phase of the ELISA and a polyclonal antibody as the second reagent.

E. Allergen Extract Potency

The potency of an allergen extract is the total allergen activity, i.e., the sum of the contribution to allergenic activity from any individual IgE molecule specific for any epitope on any molecule in the allergen extract. It follows that potency measures will always depend on the serum pool or patient panel selected as well as the methodology used. The potency of an allergen extract may be expressed mathematically as the sum of the activities of all individual allergens:

$$a = \sum_{i=1}^{n} f_i c_i$$

where a is the total allergen activity, and c_i and f_i are the concentration and activity coefficient, respectively, of molecule number i.

Methods used for the assessment of allergen extract potency may be divided in two: in vitro or in vivo techniques. The dominating in vitro technique for the estimation of relative allergenic potency is RAST inhibition (57) or related methods. A standardized reference extract is coupled to a solid phase, paper discs, sepharose gels, or magnetic particles. A serum pool is added, and bound IgE is detected using labeled anti-IgE. In RAST inhibition, the binding of IgE to the solid phase is inhibited by the simultaneous addition of a dilution series of the allergen extract subject to testing. The activity is determined relative to the reference extract itself; parallel inhibition curves indicate similar composition, whereas nonparallel curves indicate that the extracts differ both qualitatively and quantitatively.

The results are dependent upon the patient panel selected. The serum pool is a critical reagent and should contain sera from 20 or more different patients with clinically established allergy to the allergen source in question. A large serum pool should be made in order to ensure continuity, and care should be taken when the control serum pool is changed. Techniques based on ELISA using microtiter plastic trays as a solid phase may be applied using the same principles.

Tests of histamine release from washed human leukocytes utilize the quantification of histamine liberated from allergic patients' leukocytes upon stimulation with allergen (58). The tests are dependent on freshly drawn blood samples from a panel of allergic individuals, thus diminishing the practical applicability in routine allergen extract potency determination.

Direct skin testing of human allergic subjects is the main in vivo method to assess allergen extract potency (59). However, it is impractical to use in vivo testing as a routine assay for production batch release. However, production batches can be compared with internal reference extracts by suitable in vitro methods, the in vivo activity of which has been already established. Therefore, the patient selection criteria for the original in vivo assay are important since all in vivo methods will ultimately be dependent on the selected patient panel.

Skin testing in humans is the principle underlying the establishment of biological units of allergen extract potency. Several units are used. In Europe, the potency unit is based on the dose of allergen that results in a wheal comparable in size to the wheal produced by a given concentration of histamine. This unit was originally called histamine equivalent potency (HEP). The Nordic Guidelines introduced the biological unit (BU), which is used today. One thousand BU is the equivalent of 1 HEP.

F. Determination of Clinical Efficacy

The potency of allergen extracts used for specific allergy vaccination should ideally be expressed in units describing clinical efficacy rather than just skin-test potency. Approaches to relate extract potency and clinical efficacy have been performed in the United States and Europe and commented on by the WHO. For several standardized vaccines, various trials have established an optimal maintenance dose. This dose corresponds to 5–20 µg of major allergen (Table 2), which is a useful measure for quantification.

However, determinations of clinical efficacy are extremely laborious. They can be performed only by using highly standardized vaccines, which have been described in detail with respect to composition and in vitro and in vivo potency.

G. Standardization and Allergy Vaccination in Europe and in the United States

Standardization of allergy extracts in Europe, regulated by the European Pharmacopoeia, is different from the United States, where it is regulated by the Food and Drug Administration (FDA). Whereas allergy extract consistency in Europe is maintained primarily through the use of in-house standards and international references, this goal is achieved by the FDA by mandating detailed standardization procedures and reagents for use by all manufacturers. An advantage of the European system is that it provides options for the doctor to choose from different products and for manufacturers to continuously improve quality and incorporate new methodology in analysis and control of the extracts. The advantage of the American system is that it results in a higher degree of consistency of extracts among manufacturers. Another difference between Europe and the United States is in the formulation of the extracts used for allergy vaccination. Physicians in the United States primarily use aqueous vaccines, whereas in Europe, alum-adsorbed vaccines, either chemically modified or native, are most often used (Table 3).

IV. CONCLUSION

There are different methods to determine the in vivo allergenic activity of in-house reference preparations, meaning that different biological units are used. Furthermore, biological units in current use are based primarily on skin reactivity measurements, which may not be relevant to therapeutic efficacy. Since there is a remarkable coherence between the content of major allergen in the optimal maintenance dose comparing various allergen sources, the content of major allergen for many allergens could be used as a marker relating vaccine potency to therapeutic efficacy. The CREATE initiative will facilitate the major allergen measure, providing certified standards and assays for convenient major allergen determination. However, major allergen content in and of itself does not completely determine potency of current allergen vaccines, since other allergens, which may vary between extracts, also contribute to their biological potency. It is therefore still necessary to assess biological potency to avoid the misunderstanding that extracts/vaccines, even though they have equal major allergen content, are interchangeable.

Table 3 Major Differences Between United States and Europe in Allergen Vaccine
Standardization and Performing of Specific Allergy Vaccination

United States	Europe
Standardization of allergen vaccines	
FDA selects representative extract as FDA reference (FDAR).	Manufacturer selects representative extract as in-house reference preparation (IHRP) according to the European Pharmacopoeia.
Biological activity (in vivo and in vitro potency/total allergen activity) relative to FDAR.	Biological activity (in vivo and in vitro potency/total allergen activity) relative to IHPR.
Concentration of major allergen molecules (FDA optional) relative to FDA major allergen reference.	Concentration of major allergen molecules (cf. WHO recommendations) relative to IHPR.
Methods and reagents selected and distributed by the FDA.	Methods and reagents selected and developed by manufacturer.
Performing specific allergy vaccination	
Predominantly aqueous vaccines.	Predominantly aluminum hydroxide–adsorbed vaccines.
Nonmodified vaccine.	Nonmodified or chemically modified vaccines.
Vaccines are mixed for multi-allergic patients.	Vaccines are predominantly injected separately.

V. SALIENT POINTS

1. All allergens are proteins and all water-soluble proteins are potential allergens.
2. Allergen extracts are complex biological mixtures, and standardization is essential to ensure safety and efficacy of diagnosis and treatment.
3. The process of extraction is highly dependent on physicochemical conditions. Extreme conditions are likely to destroy allergen epitopes and affect activity.
4. Statistically, patients' IgE binds to some antigens more frequently than to others, thereby defining major allergens.
5. The effective maintenance dose in specific allergy vaccination for the average patient is proportional to the content of major allergen in an allergen vaccine.
6. Major allergen content alone is not a sufficient measure of extract potency.
7. Chemically modified allergen extracts are deficient in specific epitopes.
8. The existence and use of internal as well as external standards are essential for standardization and control of allergen extracts.
9. The quality of an allergen extract is dependent on the qualitative as well as quantitative composition.
10. The potency of an allergen extract is determined by the combination of the concentration of one or more major allergens and the composition, qualitative as well as quantitative, of the allergen extract.

REFERENCES

1. Noon, L. Prophylactic inoculation against hay fever. Lancet 1911; 1:1572–1573.
2. Ishizaka K, Ishizaka T, Hornbrook MM. Physicochemical properties of reaginic antibody. V. Correlation of reaginic activity with gamma-E-globulin antibody. J Immunol 1966; 97:840–853.

3. Johansson SG, Bennich H. Immunological studies of an atypical (myeloma) immunoglobulin. Immunology 1967; 13:381–394.

4. Løwenstein H. Report on behalf of the International Union of Immunological Societies (I.U.I.S.) Allergen Standardization Subcommittee. Arb Paul Ehrlich Inst 1983; 78:41–48.

5. Nordic Council on Medicines. Registration of allergen preparations: Nordic guidelines. NLN Publ 1989; no 23:1–34.

6. Løwentstein H: Physico-chemical and immunochemical methods for the control of potency and quality of allergenic extracts. Arb Paul Ehrlich Inst 1980; 75:122–132.

7. Bousquet J, Lockey RF, Malling HJ (eds.). WHO Position Paper—Allergen immunotherapy: Therapeutic vaccines for allergic diseases. Geneva: January 27–29, 1997. Allergy 1998; 53(suppl 44):1–42.

8. Council of Europe. European Pharmacopoeia. European Treaty Series 50. Strasbourg, 2001.

9. Løwenstein H. Selection of reference preparation. IUIS reference preparation criteria. Arb Paul Ehrlich Inst 1987; 80:75–78.

10. Wahn U, Schweter C, Lind P, Løwenstein H. Prospective study on immunologic changes induced by two different *Dermatophagoides pteronyssinus* extracts prepared from whole mite culture and mite bodies. J Allergy Clin Immunol 1988; 82:360–370.

11. Lemanske RF, Taylor SL. Standardized extracts, foods. Clin Rev Allergy 1987; 5:23–36.

12. Løwenstein H, Marsh DG. Antigens of *Ambrosia elatior* (short ragweed) pollen. I. Crossed immunoelectrophoretic analyses. J Immunol 1981; 126:943–948.

13. Butler NR, Voyce MA, Burland WL, Hilton ML. Advantages of aluminium hydroxide adsorbed combined diphtheria, tetanus and pertussis vaccines for the immunization of infants. Br Med J 1969; 1:663–666.

14. Norman PS, Lichtenstein LM. Comparisons of alum-precipitated and unprecipitated aqueous ragweed pollen extracts in the treatment of hay fever. J Allergy Clin Immunol 1978; 61:384–389.

15. Mellerup MT, Hahn GW, Poulsen LK, Malling H. Safety of allergen-specific immunotherapy. Relation between dosage regimen, allergen extract, disease and systemic side-effects during induction treatment. Clin Exp Allergy 2000; 30:1423–1429.

16. Tabar AI, Garcia BE, Rodriguez A, Olaguibel JM, Muro MD, Quirce S. A prospective safety-monitoring study of immunotherapy with biologically standardized extracts. Allergy 1993; 48:450–453.

17. al-Shakhshir RH, Regnier FE, White JL, Hem SL. Contribution of electrostatic and hydrophobic interactions to the adsorption of proteins by aluminium-containing adjuvants. Vaccine 1995; 13:41–44.

18. Weeke B, Weeke E, Løwenstein H. The adsorption of serum proteins to aluminium hydroxide gel examined by means of quantitative immunoelectrophoresis. In: Quantitative immunoelectrophoresis, new developments and applications (Axelsen NH, ed.) Scand J Immunol 1975; suppl 2:149–154.

19. Marsh DG, Lichtenstein LM, Campbell DH. Studies on 'allergoids' prepared from naturally occurring allergens. I. Assay of allergenicity and antigenicity of formalinized rye group I component. Immunol 1970; 18:705–722.

20. Marsh DG, Norman PS, Roebber M, Lichtenstein LM. Studies on allergoids from naturally occurring allergens. III. Preparation of ragweed pollen allergoids by aldehyde modification in two steps. J Allergy Clin Immunol 1981; 68:449–459.

21. Lee WY, Sehon AH. Abrogation of reaginic antibodies with modified allergens. Nature 1977; 267:618–619.

22. Yssel H, Fasler S, Lamb JR, de Vries JE. Induction of non-responsiveness in human allergen-specific type 2 T helper cells. Curr Opin Immunol 1994; 6:847–852.

23. Løwenstein H, Larsen JN. Recombinant allergens/allergen standardization. Curr Allergy Asthma Rep 2001; 1:474–479.

24. Larsen JN. Isoallergens—Significance in allergen exposure and response. ACI News 1995; 7:141–146.

25. van Neerven RJJ, Ebner C, Yssel H, Kapsenberg ML, Lamb JR. T-cell responses to allergens: Epitope-specificity and clinical relevance. Immunol Today 1996; 17:526–532.
26. Gajhede M, Osmark P, Poulsen FM, Ipsen H, Larsen JN, van Neerven RJJ, Schou C, Løwenstein H, Spangfort MD. X-ray and NMR structure of Bet v 1, the origin of birch pollen allergy. Nat Struct Biol 1996; 3:1040–1045.
27. Lüderitz-Püchel U, Keller-Stanislawski B, Haustein D. Neubewertung des Risikos von Test- und Therapieallergenen. Bundesgesundheitsblatt 2001; 44:709–718.
28. King TP, Hoffman D, Løwenstein H, Marsh DG, Platts-Mills TAE, Thomas W. Allergen Nomenclature. J Allergy Clin Immunol 1995; 96:5–14.
29. Dreborg S, Einarsson R. The major allergen content of allergenic preparations reflects their biological activity. Allergy 1992; 47:418–423.
30. Helm RM, Gauerke MB, Baer H, Løwenstein H, Ford A, Levy DA, Norman PS, Yunginger JW. Production and testing of an international reference standard of short ragweed pollen extract. J Allergy Clin Immunol 1984; 73:790–800.
31. Gjesing B, Jäger L, Marsh DG, Løwenstein H. The international collaborative study establishing the first international standard for timothy (*Phleum pratense*) grass pollen allergenic extract. J Allergy Clin Immunol 1985; 75:258–267.
32. Ford A, Seagroatt V, Platts-Mills TAE, Løwenstein H. A collaborative study on the first international standard of *Dermatophagoides pteronyssinus* (house dust mite) extract. J Allergy Clin Immunol 1985; 75:676–686.
33. Arntzen FC, Wilhelmsen TW, Løwenstein H, Gjesing B, Maasch HJ, Stromberg R, Einarsson R, Backman A, Makinen-Kiljunen S, Ford A. The international collaborative study on the first international standard of birch (*Betula verrucosa*) pollen extract. J Allergy Clin Immunol 1989; 83:66–82.
34. Larsen JN, Ford A, Gjesing B, Levy D, Petrunov B, Silvestri L, Løwenstein H. The collaborative study of the international standard of dog, *Canis domesticus*, hair/dander extract. J Allergy Clin Immunol 1988; 82:318–330.
35. Helm RM, Squillace DL, Yunginger JW, members of the international collaborative trial. Production of a proposed international reference standard *Alternaria* extract II. Results of a collaborative trial. J Allergy Clin Immunol 1988; 81:651–663.
36. Baer H, Anderson MC, Helm RM, Yunginger JW, Løwenstein H, Gjesing B, White W, Douglass G, Phillips PR, Schumacher M, Hewitt B, Guerin BG, Charpin J, Carreira J, Lombardero M, Ekramoddoullah AKM, Kisil F, Einarsson R. The preparation and testing of the proposed international reference (IRP) Bermuda grass (*Cynodon dactylon*)-pollen extract. J Allergy Clin Immunol 1986; 78:624–631.
37. Stewart GA, Turner KJ, Baldo BA, Cripps AW, Ford A, Seagroatt V, Løwenstein H, Ekramoddoullah AKM. Standardization of rye-grass pollen (*Lolium perenne*) extract. An immunochemical and physicochemical assessment of six candidate international reference preparations. Int Arch Allergy Appl Immunol 1988; 86:9–18.
38. van Ree R. A new start for allergen references and standardization based on purified/recombinant allergens and monoclonal and monospecific polyclonal antibodies. Ninth International Paul Ehrlich Seminar, Langen, Germany, Sept 9–11, 1999.
39. Laemmli UK. Cleavage of structural proteins during the assembly of the head of bacteriophage T4. Nature 1970; 227:680–685.
40. Kyhse-Andersen J. Electroblotting of multiple gels: A simple apparatus without buffer tank for rapid transfer of proteins from polyacrylamide to nitrocellulose. J Biochem Biophys Methods 1984; 10:203–209.
41. Ipsen H, Larsen JN. Detection of antigen-specific IgE antibodies in sera from allergic patients by SDS-PAGE immunoblotting and crossed radioimmunoelectrophoresis. In: Handbook of Immunoblotting of Proteins, vol II (Bjerrum O, Heegaard NHH, eds.). Boca Raton, FL: Chemical Rubber Company, 1988;159–166.

42. Brighton WD. Profiles of allergen extract components by isoelectric focussing and radioim-munoassay. Dev Biol Stand 1975, 29.302–369.
43. Løwenstein H. Quantitative immunoelectrophoretic methods as a tool for the analysis and isolation of allergens. Prog Allergy 1978; 25:1.
44. Weeke B, Søndergaard I, Lind P, Aukrust L, Løwenstein H. Crossed radio-immunoelec-trophoresis (CRIE) for the identification of allergens and determination of the antigenic specificities of patients' IgE. In Handbook of immunoprecipitation-in-gel techniques (Axelsen NH, ed.). Scand J Immunol 1983; 17(suppl 10):265–272.
45. Sundin B, Lilja G, Graff-Lonnevig V, Hedlin G, Heilborn H, Norrlind K, Pegelow K-O, Løwenstein H. Immunotherapy with partially purified and standardized animal dander extracts. I. Clinical results from a double-blind study on patients with animal dander asthma. J Allergy Clin Immunol 1986; 77:478–487.
46. van Metre TE, Marsh DG, Adkinson NF, Kagey-Sobotka A, Khattignavong A, Norman PS, Rosenberg GL. Immunotherapy for cat asthma. J Allergy Clin Immunol 1988; 82:1055–1068.
47. Hedlin G, Graff-Lonnevig V, Heilborn H, Lilja G, Norrlind K, Pegelow K, Sundin B, Løwenstein H. Immunotherapy with cat- and dog-dander extracts V. Effects of 3 years of treatment. J Allergy Clin Immunol 1991; 87:955–964.
48. Hedlin G, Heilborn H, Lilja G, Norrlind K, Pegelow K-O, Schou C, Løwenstein H. Long-term follow-up of patients treated with a three-year course of cat or dog immunotherapy. J Allergy Clin Immunol 1995; 96:879–885.
49. Haugaard L, Dahl R, Jacobsen L. A controlled dose-response study of immunotherapy with standardized, partially purified extract of house dust mite: Clinical efficacy and side effects. J Allergy Clin Immunol 1993; 91:709–722.
50. Creticos PS, Reed CE, Norman PS, Khoury J, Adkinson NF, Buncher CR, Busse WW, Bush RK, Gadde J, Li JT, Richerson HB, Rosenthal RR, Solomon WR, Steinberg P, Yunginger JW. Ragweed immunotherapy in adult asthma. N Engl J Med 1996; 334:501–506.
51. Østerballe O. Immunotherapy in hay fever with two major allergens 19, 25 and partially purified extract of timothy grass pollen. Allergy 1980; 35:473–489.
52. Varney VA, Gaga M, Frew AJ, Aber VR, Kay AB, Durham SR. Usefulness of immunotherapy in patients with severe summer hay fever uncontrolled by antiallergic drugs. Br Med J 1991; 302:265–269.
53. Durham SR, Walker SM, Varga EM, Jacobson MR, O'Brien F, Noble W, Till SJ, Hamid QA, Nouri-Aria KT. Long-term clinical efficacy of grass-pollen immunotherapy. N Engl J Med 1999; 341:468–475.
54. Engvall E, Perlmann P. Enzyme-linked immunosorbent assay, ELISA. III. Quantitation of specific antibodies by enzyme-labelled anti-immunoglobulin in antigen-coated tubes. J Immunol 1972; 109:129–135.
55. Carreira J, Lombardero M, Ventas P. New developments in in vitro methods. Quantification of clinically relevant allergens in mass units. Seventh International Paul Ehrlich Seminar, Langen, Germany, Sept 9–11, 1993.
56. Park JW, Kim KS, Jin HS, Kim CW, Kang DB, Choi SY, Yong TS, Oh SH, Hong CS. Der p 2 isoallergens have different allergenicity, and quantification with 2-site ELISA using monoclonal antibodies is influenced by the isoallergens. Clin Exp Allergy 2002; 32:1042–1047.
57. Ceska M, Eriksson R, Varga JM. Radioimmunosorbent assay of allergens. J Allergy Clin Immunol 1972; 49:1–9.
58. Siraganian RP. Automated histamine analysis for in vitro allergy testing. II. Correlation of skin test results with in vitro whole blood histamine release in 82 patients. J Allergy Clin Immunol 1977; 59:214–222.
59. Platts-Mills TAE, Chapman MD. Allergen standardization. J Allergy Clin Immunol 1991; 87:621–625.

24

Preparing and Mixing Allergen Vaccines

HAROLD S. NELSON

National Jewish Medical and Research Center and the University of Colorado Health Sciences Center, Denver, Colorado, U.S.A.

I.   COMMERCIALLY AVAILABLE ALLERGEN VACCINES

Allergen immunotherapy is appropriately performed with vaccines of inhalant allergens or the venom from stinging insects. These vaccines are prepared in the United States from standardized or unstandardized extracts in a variety of formulations: (1) lyophilized, adsorbed to aluminum or in solution; or (2) phosphate-buffered saline containing human serum albumin or glycerin with or without phenol. Potency is expressed in terms of bioequivalent allergen units (BAU), content of the major allergen, weight by volume (wt/vol), or protein nitrogen units (PNU) per ml.

A.   Standardized Extracts

The manufacturing and sale of allergen vaccines in the United States is regulated by the Center for Biologics Evaluation and Research (CBER) of the Food and Drug Administration (FDA) (1). CBER has established reference extracts and reference serum pools to be used by extract manufacturers to standardize certain allergen extracts. The

457

Table 1 Allergen Extracts: CBER Basis for Standardization

Cat hair: 10,000 BAU/ml contains 10.0–19.9 units Fel d 1/ml and "little" cat serum albumin by isoelectric focusing.

Cat pelt: 10,000 BAU/ml contains 10.0–19.9 units Fel d 1/ml and substantial amounts of cat serum albumin by isoelectric focusing.

Short ragweed: Designated weight by volume or PNU but with the Amb a 1 content in units/ml on the vial.

House dust mite: 5000, 10,000, and 30,000 BAU/ml (*D. pteronyssinus* and *D. farinae*) determined by quantitative skin testing.

Grasses: 10,000 and 100,000 BAU/ml determined by quantitative skin testing.

Hymenoptera: Expressed as the venom protein content (100 μg/ml) for each individual insect species (honeybee, yellow jacket, wasp, yellow- and white-faced hornet)

potency of the CBER standard extract has been established by titrated intradermal skin testing (2). In this method serial three-fold dilutions of the extract are tested on the backs of a group of patients highly sensitive to that inhalant. Based on the dilution that yields an area of erythema with a mean diameter of 25 mm (the D50), the extract is assigned a BAU. Extract companies then compare their extract to the CBER reference using radioallergosorbent test (RAST)- or enzyme-linked immunosorbent assay (ELISA) inhibition, and a potency is assigned.

Among the inhalant allergens there are currently standardized extracts (Table 1) for house dust mites (*Dermatophagoides pteronyssinus* and *Dermatophagoides farinae*), cat hair (which is low in cat serum albumin), and cat pelt (which contains substantial amounts of cat albumin), short ragweed (*Ambrosia elatior*), and eight grasses. In place of standardization by quantitative skin testing, the extracts of cat (3) and short ragweed (4) are standardized by their content of the major allergen expressed in arbitrary FDA units (Table 1).

While standardization of short ragweed, house dust mite, and cat resulted in, if anything, more consistently potent extracts than were previously available, the standardization in 1997 of the eight grasses resulted in a decrease—in some instances quite substantial—in the strength of the most potent extracts available. This resulted from a CBER decision to reduce these grass extracts to a maximum testing potency of 10,000 BAU/ml and for treatment to 100,000 BAU/ml, which is considerably less than the potency of many of the previously available grass pollen extracts (5).

A second group of standardized extracts are those of the stinging Hymenoptera (Table 1). These are standardized on the basis of venom protein content of 100 μg/ml for all the individual species, and 300 μg/ml for the mixed vespids.

B. Physical Form and Diluent of Available Allergen Extracts

Standardized extracts are available in a lyophilized state (cat and Hymenoptera venoms), in 50% glycerin-saline (grasses, short ragweed, cat, house dust mites), and in aqueous solution (short ragweed). Nonstandardized extracts are available in either a 50% glycerin or an aqueous solution. The 50% glycerin contains equal parts of glycerin and buffered saline. The aqueous extract consists of buffered saline and 0.4% phenol. Glycerin at 50% concentration inhibits microbial growth and maintains the potency of allergenic extracts. Phenol, which is added to aqueous extracts to inhibit bacterial and fungal growth, has an adverse effect on the potency of stored extracts. The choice between the two extracting and diluting fluids would be simple, were it not for the discomfort associated with injection of 50% glycerin (6).

A limited number of pollen extracts are available adsorbed to aluminum to delay their absorption from the injection site. When the initial extraction is performed with aqueous extracting fluids and the aluminum is subsequently added, the resulting vaccines have been shown to have clinical effectiveness comparable to that of aqueous vaccines (7) but with a decreased incidence of systemic reactions (8). However, aluminum-precipitated vaccines that have been initially extracted in pyridine have been shown to have markedly less potency than comparable aqueous vaccines (9,10).

C. Expressed Extract Potency

The traditional expressions of extract potency are weight by volume (wt/vol) and protein nitrogen units (PNU). Neither provides precise information regarding the allergenic potency of the extract. However, it is likely that within broad limits the initial potency of many extracts obtained from the same commercial supplier have reproducible batch-to-batch potency (11). Thus, it has been possible, as a general practice, to refill allergy treatment vaccines with new lots of the same stated potency from a given manufacturer without untoward reactions by reducing the first injection from the new vial by one-third to one-half of the previous dose.

Weight by volume is the simplest way to express the potency of allergen extracts. It is only necessary to weigh the material to be extracted and measure the volume of the extracting fluid. Thus, 10 g of pollen extracted in 100 ml of buffered saline yields a final concentration of 1:10 wt/vol. One advantage of this method is that the extract need not be further diluted to achieve the desired level of potency.

Protein nitrogen units were introduced in an attempt to more accurately express the allergen content of extracts (12). First, the protein nitrogen content is determined, and then the content is converted to units (with one unit equal to 0.00001 mg of protein nitrogen). The major allergens usually represent only a small percentage of the total protein content of allergen extracts. Therefore, PNU offers little advantage as an expression of allergenic potency over weight by volume. The distinct disadvantage of PNU is that extracts are commercially available in specific concentrations (e.g., 20,000–40,000 PNU/ml). This requires that the extract be diluted from the strength obtained during the extraction process, and therefore the most potent PNU extract available will be weaker than the most concentrated weight/volume measure for any given allergen.

The CBER bioequivalent allergen unit (BAU) is based on intradermal skin testing with serial threefold dilutions of the extract in at least 15 highly allergic individuals (2). The dilution of the extract that results in an erythema the largest orthogonal diameters of which add up to 50 mm is the endpoint. If the endpoint dilution is 9.0 to 10.9, the extract is considered to contain 1000 BAU/ml; if the endpoint dilution is 11.0 to 12.9, the concentration is 10,000 BAU/ml; and if the endpoint dilution is 13.0 to 14.9, it is 100,000 BAU/ml. Alternatively, the BAU potency can be determined by RAST or ELISA inhibition methods in comparison with the CBER reference product, whose BAU potency has been determined by quantitative intradermal skin testing. For a potency designation of 10,000 BAU/ml by the RAST inhibition method, the relative potency in relation to the reference product must be 0.47 to 2.12, and for the ELISA inhibition method 0.699 to 1.431. Thus, the required reproducibility of standardized products using the CBER method probably does not exceed the within-company reproducibility of many nonstandardized products. The

CBER-required reproducibility is greater when content of major allergen is used as a basis. For Amb a 1, the major allergen of ragweed, determinations by gel diffusion a range of ±25% is allowed, as opposed to ±100% for quantitative skin testing.

II. ADEQUATE DOSING FOR DEMONSTRATED EFFICACY

A. Studies with Vaccines Prepared from Unstandardized Extracts

Johnstone conducted a study of the efficacy of allergen immunotherapy employing a broad range of doses (13). New patients with perennial bronchial asthma referred to the pediatric allergy clinic of Strong Memorial Hospital for immunotherapy were randomly assigned to receive treatment with buffered saline, or all inhalable allergens to which the child reacted on skin testing but administered to maximum concentrations of $1:10^7$ wt/vol, 1:5000 wt/vol, or the highest tolerated dose up to a maximum of 1:250 wt/vol. Neither the child, the parent, or the evaluator knew to which group the patient was assigned. Two hundred children were randomized and 173 were available for evaluation during the winter of the fourth year of treatment. The results suggested that the degree of improvement steadily increased with increasing dosage of antigen (Table 2).

Franklin and Lowell demonstrated, in a study meeting all the requirements for adequate blinding, that immunotherapy with ragweed pollen vaccine was clinically effective (14). They then applied the same study design to examine the effect of two doses of ragweed pollen vaccine on seasonal rhinitis symptoms (15). Twenty-five ragweed-sensitive subjects were recruited who were still symptomatic during the ragweed pollen season despite receiving allergen immunotherapy that contained ragweed pollen vaccine. They were paired by severity of symptoms during the ragweed pollen season. One of each pair continued to receive ragweed vaccine at the customary level (median dose 0.3 ml of a 1:50 wt/vol concentration) while the other member of the pair received a dose reduced by 95% (median dose 0.3 ml of 1:1000 wt/vol). During the ensuing ragweed season, those receiving the reduced dose experienced significantly more symptoms of allergic rhinitis.

B. Studies with Vaccines Prepared from Standardized Extracts

One of the major advantages of using standardized vaccines is that information regarding treatment regimens that have proven successful in controlled studies can be applied by others to their clinical practices. There have been a number of double-blind, controlled studies employing the standardized extracts that are now available in the United States (Table 3). In some instances only one concentration was employed, but the clinical

Table 2 Immunotherapy Dose and Outcome of Asthma

Treatment group	Number evaluable	Wheezing with exertion	Wheezing with upper respiratory tract infections
Highest tolerated dose (maximum 1:250 wt/vol)	43	9%	9%
1:5000 wt/vol	39	31%	10%
1:10,000,000 wt/vol	49	45%	55%
Saline	42	64%	74%

Source: Ref. 13.

Table 3 Documented Optimal Effective Doses of Major Allergens

Allergen	Author	Optimal dose
Dermatophagoides	Ewan (16)	11.9 μg Der p I
	Haugaard (17)	7.0 μg Der p I
	Olsen (18)	7.0 μg Der p I
		10.0 μg Der f I
Cat dander	Van Metre (19)	13.8 μg Fel d
	Alvarez-Cuesta (20)	11.3 μg Fel d I
	Hedlin (21)	17.3 μg Fel d 1
	Varney (22)	15 μg Fel d I
	Ewbank (23)	15 μg Fel d 1
Grass	Varney (24)	18.6 μg Phl p V
	Dolz (25)	15 μg Dac q V, Lol p V, Phl p V
	Walker (26)	20 μg Phl p V
Short ragweed	Van Metre (27)	11 μg Amb a I
	Creticos (28)	12.4 μg Amb a I
	Creticos (29)	6 μg Amb a I
	Furin (30)	24 μg Amb a 1

benefit was prompt and clinically relevant. In other studies, more than one dose was employed, and a definite dose response was demonstrated. In all of these studies the dose of allergen employed was expressed in terms of the concentration of one of the major allergens, since this is the only method of standardization recognized internationally. To allow general application of this information to standardized extracts available in the United States, representative values for the major allergen content of specific lots of extracts standardized in bioequivalent allergen units are given in Table 4. It must be appreciated, however, that standardized extracts labeled in the same potency units by different manufacturers may contain different amounts of the major allergens.

1. House Dust Mites

The study by Ewan (16) demonstrated that a maintenance dose containing 11.9 μg Der p I was able to reduce symptoms and objective responses significantly after only 3 months, but with a high incidence of systemic reactions (approximately 15% of injections). The dose response study by Haugaard (17) demonstrated that there was marginal reduction in bronchial reactivity to mite allergen after 2 years of treatment with a maximum dose of 0.7 μg Der p I, but the reduction with a dose of 7 μg was significantly greater. Those receiving an even higher dose (21 μg) did not show any additional objective benefit, but incurred over twice as many systemic reactions per injection as the 7 μg/injection group (7.1% vs. 3.3%). Therefore, the investigators concluded that a maintenance dose of 7 μg Der p I per injection appeared to be near optimal, based on benefit/risk considerations. Olsen treated 23 adult patients with asthma for 1 year with a maintenance dose of 7.0 μg Der p I or 10.0 μg Der f I (18). Compared with patients who received placebo, those treated with mite vaccine had significantly reduced symptoms of asthma and a decreased need for β-adrenergic agonists and inhaled corticosteroids.

2. Cat Dander

Four studies have demonstrated significant improvement with employment of a narrow range of doses. Van Metre's (19) treatment with a maximum Fel d I dose of 13.8 μg reduced

Table 4 Representative Values for Major Allergen Content of U.S. Standardized Extracts[a]

Allergen extract (n = number of extracts tested)	Expressed concentration	Major allergen	Mean content of major allergen	Standard deviation	Maximum content of major allergen	Minimum content of major allergen
Orchard (n = 14)	100,000 BAU/ml	Dac g 5	918 µg/ml	±500	2414 µg	294 µg
Fescue (n = 12)	100,000 BAU/ml	Fes p 5	152 µg/ml	±138	204 µg	75 µg
Rye (n = 14)	100,000 BAU/ml	Lol p 5	337 µg/ml	±110	526 µg	157 µg
Kentucky (n = 15)	100,000 BAU/ml	Poa p 5	262 µg/ml	±57	338 µg	118 µg
Timothy (n = 12)	100,000 BAU/ml	Phl p 5	743 µg/ml	±294	1336 µg	354 µg
Short ragweed (n = 13)	1:10 wt/vol	Amb a 1	268 µg/ml	±109	458 µg	87 µg
Mixed ragweed (n = 10)	1:10 wt/vol	Amb a 1	174 µg/ml	±96	402 µg	56 µg
D. pteronyssinus (n = 28)	10,000 BAU/ml	Der p 1	172 µg/ml	±74	385 µg	68 µg
D. farinae (n = 18)	10,000 BAU/ml	Der f 1	44 µg/ml	±12	72 µg	30 µg
Cat hair (n = 12)	10,000 BAU/ml	Fel d 1	40 µg/ml	±7.2	52 µg	26 µg
Dog hair (n = 4)	1:10 wt/vol	Can f 1	5.4 µg/ml	±2.7	7.2 µg	2.7 µg

[a] Values provided by ALK-Abello. Sources are U.S. FDA reference extracts from ALK-Abello and other pharmaceutical firms that manufacture allergen extracts.
From Nelson HS. The use of standardized extracts in allergen immunotherapy. *J Allergy Clin Immunol* 2000; 106:41–45.

both bronchial and skin reactions to cat dander. Alvarez-Cuesta (20), treating with a maximum dose of 11.3 µg Fel d 1 for 1 year, noted decreased skin, conjunctival, and bronchial sensitivity, as well as a 90% reduction in symptom medication scores. Hedlin (21), treating with a maximum dose of 17.3 µg Fel d 1 for 3 years, not only reduced bronchial sensitivity to cat dander but also significantly reduced the response to bronchial challenge with histamine. Varney's (22) patients, treated with a maintenance dose of 15 µg Fel d I, had significantly reduced symptoms on exposure to a house contaminated with cat dander.

Ewbank (23) compared the response, shortly after achieving maintenance doses by a cluster build-up, of placebo to cat hair vaccines containing, at maintenance, either 0.6 µg Fed d 1, 3.0 µg Fel d 1, or 15 µg Fel d 1. The two higher doses of vaccine produced significant decreases in prick skin test sensitivity and increases in cat-specific IgG4, but only the vaccine containing a dose of 15 µg Fel d 1 produced a significant reduction in the percent of CD4+/ IL-4+ peripheral blood mononuclear cells. The conclusion was that a maintenance dose of cat vaccine containing 15 µg of Fel d 1 was optimal and superior to one containing 3 µg of Fel d 1.

3. Grass Pollen Vaccine
Varney conducted a preseasonal, double-blind trial of immunotherapy with timothy grass pollen vaccine in seasonal grass pollen allergic rhinitis (24). A maximum dose of 18.6 µg

Phl p 5 reduced symptoms and medication use over 50% compared with placebo, and also reduced conjunctival sensitivity and decreased the late cutaneous response to a timothy skin test. Dolz treated with 15 µg of the major allergens of a mixture of grasses for 3 years (25). He observed a progressive decrease in ocular, nasal, and pulmonary symptoms over the 3 years of the study. Walker treated subjects with both seasonal allergic rhinitis and asthma with a timothy vaccine containing, at maintenance, 20 µg of Phl p 5 (26). Immunotherapy not only diminished rhinitis but also markedly reduced chest symptoms and blocked the seasonal increase in methacholine sensitivity.

The lowest effective dose has not been determined for grass pollen vaccines, but a maintenance dose of 15 to 18.6 µg was effective.

4. Ragweed Pollen Vaccine

The most extensive experience with vaccines containing known amounts of the major allergens is with ragweed. Studies at Johns Hopkins University have included both single and cumulative maximum doses. However, the comparative-dose studies have been progressively increasing doses in the same individuals or the different doses have been administered for a different number of years. There have been no studies in which groups of subjects receive different maximum doses for the same duration of treatment. Nevertheless, it is clear that clinical and objective benefit is rapidly and regularly attained with maximum maintenance doses that contain 11 µg (27) to 24.8 µg (28) of the major ragweed allergen Amb a I. Similar benefit was observed in a group who had received a maintenance dose of 6 µg Amb a I for 3 to 5 years (29). However, the response to 0.6 µg (28) or to 2 µg (30) was inconsistent and less than that with the higher doses.

5. Hymenoptera Venom Vaccines

Immunotherapy for venom-sensitive patients with Hymenoptera venom was effective in blocking reactions to an intentional sting challenge (31). The original studies employed maximum doses of 100 µg of the venom proteins, an amount exceeding the 50 µg that is injected by the sting of the insect. Treatment with the 100-µg dose has been shown to be protective in the vast majority of sensitized subjects; therefore, there have been few studies of alternative dosing.

III. CONSIDERATIONS IN FORMULATING AN ALLERGEN VACCINE FOR TREATMENT

The considerations in formulating an allergen vaccine for immunotherapy are as follow:

1. Inclusion of an adequate dose of each extract in a vaccine to achieve an optimal response;
2. Utilization of allergenic relationships and cross-allergenicity to maintain balanced immunologic stimulation
3. Combination of the individual extracts in vaccines to ensure compatibility when they are combined in the treatment
4. Selection of the type of diluent to be employed

A. Adequate Doses of Each Allergen

The optimal maintenance doses of the major allergens that have proven effective in placebo-controlled studies are listed in Table 3, and the approximate contents of these major allergens in the U.S. standardized extracts are given in Table 4. From this information it is possible to estimate the amount of standardized extract in a vaccine to be given per injection to achieve the optimal dose. The amount will differ not only with different sources of the same extract but also with different extracts, as suggested by different BAU/ml values (e.g., grasses 100,000 BAU/ml, house dust mites 10,000 BAU/ml).

In order to formulate a 10-ml maintenance treatment vaccine containing sufficient concentrations of each standardized extract in an allergen vaccine so that the optimal amount would be delivered in a 0.5-ml maintenance injection, the mean effective dose for that vaccine in major allergen content is multiplied by 20 to give the total amount of major allergen required in the 10-ml vial. This amount is then divided by the mean major allergen content of the standardized vaccine. Clearly, there are a range of values for each extract depending on the major allergen content of that particular lot. An example of a vaccine mix containing optimal amounts of the standardized extracts is given in Table 5.

What of the majority of allergens for which there is no information on optimal doses and no standardized extracts? Here it is necessary to work with the best clinical information available. The study of Johnstone (13) indicated that for an inhalant allergen a mix containing 1:250 wt/vol of each allergen is better than one with 1:5000 wt/vol of each allergen, while the study of Franklin and Lowell (15) indicated that treatment with 1:50 wt/vol of ragweed was superior to treatment with 1:1000 wt/vol of ragweed. Limited data on major allergen content of nonstandardized pollen and mold extracts suggest a range of potencies similar to that of ragweed (see Table 6). This information would suggest that, at maintenance, a 1 to 10 dilution of the maximum concentration commercially available should be effective. Extracts that are less potent cannot be diluted to the same degree. Examples include cat dander and *D. farinae* extracts, for which substantially larger amounts of concentrate must be added to the maintenance vaccine to provide adequate potency compared with ragweed or timothy. The same consideration applies to such weak nonstandardized extracts as dog dander, fungi, and cockroach (Table 6). Twenty-four German and American cockroach extracts contained no measurable IgE binding in the aqueous extracts, while the relative potency of the 50% glycerin extracts of German

Table 5 Representative Prescription for an Optimal–Maintenance Dose Vaccine Using U.S. Standardized Extracts

Extract	Concentration	Optimal Dose of Allergen on Which Vaccine Contents Is Based	Amount (Assuming Mean Major Allergen Content in Table 4)
Timothy	100,000 BAU/ml	18.6 µg Phl p 5	0.5 ml
Short ragweed	1:10 wt/vol	12 µg Amb a 1	0.9 ml
House dust mite mix			
D. pteronyssinus	10,000 BAU/ml	3.5 µg Der p 1	0.4 ml[a]
D. farinae	10,000 BAU/ml	5 µg Der f 1	2.3 ml[a]
Cat dander	10,000 BAU/ml	15 µg Fel d 1	5.9 ml[b]
Diluent (to make 10 ml volume)			0

[a] Optimal dose of each reduced by 50% due to significant cross-reactivity.
[b] Optimal dosing would dictate 7.5 ml, but reduced to achieve 10 ml volume.
This prescription is based on the mean documented optimal effective doses (Table 3) and examples of the amounts of major allergens contained in U.S. standardized extracts (Table 4). Major allergen content will vary among manufacturers for extracts of the same labeled potency.

Table 6 Representative Values for Major Allergen Content of Nonstandardized Extracts

Allergen	Expressed concentration	Major allergen	Major allergen concentration	Reference
Birch	1:20 wt/vol 50% glycerin	Bet v 1	400 µg/ml	ALK-Abelló
English plantain	1:20 wt/vol 50% glycerin	Pla l 1	>40 µg/ml	ALK-Abelló
European olive	1:20 wt/vol 50% glycerin	Ole e 1	90 µg/ml	ALK-Abelló
European olive	1:10 wt/vol aqueous	Ole e 1	200 µg/ml	ALK-Abelló
Dog	1:10 wt/vol 50% glycerin	Can f 1	5–10 µg/ml	ALK-Abelló
Alternaria	1:20 wt/vol 50% glycerin	Alt a 1	1–5 µg/ml	ALK-Abelló
Alternaria alternaria	1:10 and 1:20 wt/vol, 50% glycerin ($n = 15$)	Alt a 1	<0.01 to 6.1 µg/ml	32
Aspergillus fumigatus	1:10 and 1:20 wt/vol, 50% glycerin ($n = 15$)	Asp f 1	<0.01 to 64.0 µg/ml	32

Source: Ref. 1.

Table 7 Representative Prescription for a Maintenance Vaccine Using Standardized and Nonstandardized Extracts

Extract	Concentration	Amount
Oak, white	1/10 wt/vol	1 ml
Elm, American	1/10 wt/vol	1 ml
Kochia	1/10 wt/vol	0.5 ml*
Russian thistle	1/10 wt/vol	0.5 ml*
Ragweed, short	1/10 wt/vol	0.5 ml*
Ragweed, giant	1/10 wt/vol	0.5 ml*
Timothy grass	100,000 BAU/ml	0.25 ml*
June grass	100,000 BAU/ml	0.25 ml*
Orchard grass	100,000 BAU/ml	0.25 ml*
Meadow fescue	100,000 BAU/ml	0.25 ml*
Diluent (to make 10 ml)	Saline with 0.03% HSA	5.0 ml

The final concentration for each nonstandardized allergen group is approximately 1:100 wt/vol. Those extracts marked with an asterisk (*) are included in reduced amounts to compensate for significant cross-allergenicity (34). The rationale for a target of 1:100 wt/vol or a 10-fold dilution from the strongest available stock extract is by analogy with clinical studies on standardized ragweed (27–30) extracts and published studies with nonstandardized pollen extracts (13,15).

cockroach was 10 to 782 BAU/ml and of American cockroach was 10 to 250 BAU/ml (33). It is unlikely that truly effective doses can be attained in vaccines with many of these weak extracts.

An example of a representative prescription for a maintenance vaccine containing nonstandardized vaccines is given in Table 7.

Table 8 Patterns of Botanical Cross-Allergenicity

• There is rarely significant cross-allergenicity between families.
• There is generally a degree of cross-allergenicity between tribes or genera of a family, but this is
  variable.
• There is generally a high degree of cross-allergenicity between species of the same genus.

B. Botanical Relationships and Cross-Allergenicity

In formulating the example of a maintenance vaccine (Table 7), only 50% of the projected
amounts of each of the two house dust mites were included. This reflects the high degree
of cross-allergenicity between these two species of *Dermatophagoides*. Cross-allergenicity among closely related plant pollen is also the rule (see Table 8). If these relationships
are not recognized, allergen vaccine mixtures may contain excessive amounts of some
groups of allergens, which is particularly likely to occur with the grasses, since most of the
prevalent species in the United States fall into two non–cross-reacting botanical subfamilies (34): the northern pasture grasses typified by timothy, and Bermuda and related
grasses. Other important cross-reacting groups are the individual members of the
Ambrosia tribe, the *Artemesia* genus, the Chenopod-Amaranth families of weeds, and
members of certain tree groups such as the genus *Populus*, containing aspen, poplar, and
cottonwood species (35). Also strongly cross-reactive are junipers and cedars of the family
Cupressaceae (36).

1. Patterns of Cross-Allergenicity

Trees.   Among the trees there are few cases of cross-allergenicity sufficiently strong to
restrict inclusion to only one representative in an allergen tree vaccine mix. These are
listed in Table 9.

Grasses.   Two non–cross-reacting subfamilies of grasses have been recognized. They are
represented by the northern pasture grasses and Bermuda, with its cross-reacting native
prairie grasses (34). There are also some regional grasses such as Bahia and Johnson that
are in distinct subfamilies. Although they share allergens with the northern pasture grasses
(Table 10), if locally important they should probably be added as additional components
of the grass vaccine.

   Immunotherapy with timothy and Bermuda grasses alone resulted in equivalent
suppression of prick skin test reactivity to 10 different grasses from all three of the
subfamilies listed in Table 10 (39). If more than one member of each of these subfamilies
of grasses is to be included in a vaccine, the amount of each grass should be reduced to
compensate for the marked cross-allergenicity.

Weeds.   There are three major groups of weeds (Table 11). Two are in the Compositae
family: Ambrosia, which includes the ragweeds and related species, and Artemesia, which
includes the sages, wormwoods, and mugworts. The Chenopod and Amaranth families
include many of the prominent weeds of the western United States. The major ragweeds
(short, giant, western, and false) are strongly cross-reactive, whereas southern and slender
ragweeds are allergenically distinct (40). There is no clinically important cross-allergenicity of the ragweeds with other members of the Ambrosia tribe, such as cocklebur and
burweed, nor is there significant cross reactivity between ragweeds and the other clinically
significant group in the Compositae family, the Artemesia (40). Within the Artemesia,

Table 9 Patterns of Significant Cross-allergenicity Among the Tree Pollens

Birch family (37)
  Birch
  Alder
  Hazelnut
  Hornbeam
Olive family (38)
  European olive
  Ash
  Privet
  Russian olive (unrelated)
Conifer family (36)
  Cedar
  Cypress
  Juniper
  Arbor vitae
Fagaceae family (35)
  Beech
  Oak
Genus *Carya* (35)
  Pecan
  Hickory
Genus *Populus* (35)
  Poplar
  Aspen
  Cottonwood

Table 10 Botanical and Allergenic Relationships Among the Grasses

Festucoideae: Northern pasture grasses: orchard, timothy, June, redtop, etc.
Eragrostoideae: Bermuda grass, grama, several western prairie grasses
Pancoideae: Bahia, Johnson

Source: Ref. 39.

however, there is strong cross-reactivity. The Chenopod-Amaranth families, which share some allergenicity, are best viewed as three groups: the Atriplex and the Amaranths, both of which are strongly cross-reactive, and the Chenopods, which share some allergens but are probably best included as a mix, rather than using only one representative, if several species are locally important. Locally important weeds such as sorrel, dock, and plantain should be treated as distinct allergens (35).

House Dust Mites. The house dust mites, *Dermatophagoides pteronyssinus* and *Dermatophagoides farina,* have been shown to be strongly cross-reactive (41). A mix of the two major species is probably best employed if both are locally important.

C. Components of Allergen Vaccines That May Have a Deleterious Effect on Other Extracts with Which They Are Mixed

Some extracts of pollen (42,43) contain enzymes that may cause autodigestion and contribute to loss of potency of a vaccine. Extracts of a number of fungi (molds) and insects contain proteases that are capable of disrupting allergenic proteins in other extracts

Table 11 Botanical and Allergenic Relationships Among the Weeds

---

Ambrosia
   Ragweeds
   Cocklebur
   Burweed
Artemesia
   Sages
   Wormwoods
   Mugworts
Chenopods
   Russian thistle
   Kochia (burning bush)
   Lamb's quarters
   Atriplex
Amaranths
   Pigweed
   Palmer's amaranth
   Western water hemp

From Ref. 35.

Table 12 Protease Content of Allergen Extracts

Extract	Protease content[a]	Potency of rye grass extract
Pollen		
Sagebrush	<1	1.18
Ragweed	<1	0.70
Oak	<1	0.89
Epithelia		
Cat	<1	0.95
Dog	<1	0.90
Insects/mites		
D. pteronyssinus	14	0.86
D. farinae	24	0.44
P. americana	168	0.17
Fungi		
Alternaria alternata	29	0.22
Penicillium notatum	242	0.19

[a] µg trypsin-equivalent units/ml.
The extract listed in the first column was mixed with perennial ryegrass extract and stored at 4°C for 1 month. Potency of the rye grass extract was compared with a reference preparation of 1.0. Potency of rye grass was determined by IgE ELISA inhibition.
From Ref. 44.

with which they may be mixed in a vaccine (44–47) (Table 12). Major allergens in American cockroach and house dust mites are gut derived and very likely are digestive enzymes. (44,48). Detectable trypsin-like proteolytic activity is absent from extracts derived from animal dander and pollen (44) (Table 12).

Grass pollen extracts are susceptible to these proteolytic enzymes (Fig. 1) (44,46,47,49). Birch pollen lost 70% of its allergenic potency over a period of 60 days

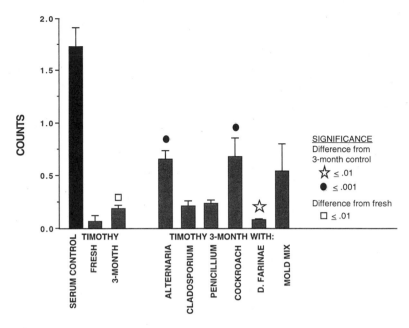

Figure 1 Stability of timothy grass alone and in mixtures. The potency of a 10-fold dilution of timothy grass stored under differing conditions was compared by ELISA inhibition with that of a freshly diluted aliquot. After 3 months the diluted timothy extract had a significant decrease in potency compared with the fresh. In addition, those aliquots of timothy stored in combination with *Alternaria*, cockroach, and a mixture of *Alternaria, Cladosporium, Penicillium*, and cockroach all showed significantly greater loss of potency than the timothy extract stored alone.

when mixed with *Fusarium* (47). In a systematic assessment (Table 13) a number of pollen and animal dander extracts lost potency when mixed with one or more protease-containing extracts while others were quite resistant (Fig. 2) (49). As illustrated in Table 13, the effect of mixing allergen extracts with potential protease-containing extracts is variable. *Alternaria* significantly reduced the potency of five of eight extracts, cockroach reduced the potency of three of eight and *Cladosporium* reduced the potency of only one extract. *Cladosporium* and cockroach reduced the potency of some extracts that were not affected by *Alternaria*. Furthermore, the effect of *Alternaria* extracts was inconsistent from lot to lot, suggesting that varying quantities of protease activity were present in different lots of *Alternaria* extract.

The extracts that have deleterious effects on the potency of other extracts include *Alternaria* (49), *Cladosporium* (49), cockroach (46,49), *Helminthosporium* (46), *Penicillium* (44), *Aspergillus* (44), and *Fusarium* (47). House dust mite extracts have had no effect on other extracts (46,49), despite their protease content (44). This possibly results from their having been tested in a diluent containing 25% glycerin. While no single inhibitor will protect against all proteases (45), glycerin has been shown to have protective effects against some (44).

The degree of loss of potency due to mixing extracts in a vaccine may be marked. Allergenic activity of perennial rye grass was reduced to 4% by mixing with *Helminthosporium* and to 11% by mixing with cockroach (46). Over 50% of timothy grass extract potency was lost within 3 days of being mixed with *Fusarium* (47). Some allergenic

Table 13 Effects of Mixing Extracts on Allergen Vaccines

Extract	Alt	Clad	PCN	CR	Mix	Mite	Overall p
Timothy	+	–	–	+	+	–	<0.0001
Bermuda	+	–	–	–	–	–	<0.0001
Short ragweed	–	–	–	–	–	–	0.64
Russian thistle							
1st	–	–	–	+	+	–	<0.0001
2nd	–	–	–	–	+	–	<0.01
White oak							
1st	+	–	–	–	–	–	<0.01
2nd	–	–	–	–	+	–	<0.02
Box elder							
1st	+	–	–	+	+	–	<0.0001
2nd	–	–	–	–	–	–	0.02
D. farinae							
1st	–	–	–	–	–	–	<0.01
2nd	–	ND	–	ND	ND	ND	0.49
Cat							
1st	–	+	–	–	–	–	<0.002
2nd	+	–	ND	ND	ND	ND	<0.001

Alt = *Alternaria*; Clad = *Cladosporium*; PCN = *Penicillium*; CR = cockroach; Mix = mixture of Alt, Clad, PCN, and CR; Mite = house dust mite; 1st = first of two studies with the same combinations; 2nd = second study; + = $p < 0.05$; – = $p > 0.05$; ND = not done.
The reference extracts listed on the ordinate were stored at a 10-fold dilution of the most concentrated forms available for 3 months either diluted in HSA-saline or combined with the extracts listed across the top of the table. After 3 months the residual allergenic activity of the reference allergen extract in the mixes was compared with that of the same extract stored alone. The p-value is the overall difference among the seven conditions of storage (alone and six different combinations with other allergenic extracts). A (+) indicates significant degradation of the reference allergen extract due to mixing.
Source: Ref. 49.

activity always remains, suggesting that not all allergens in these extracts are susceptible to proteolytic digestion. On mixing with *Fusarium*, Bet v 6 and Phl p 5 were almost entirely degraded, while Bet v 1 and Phl p 1 remained relatively stable (47). However, even though there may be a significant amount of overall allergenic activity remaining, the selective reduction in certain allergens will make the vaccine less suitable for treatment and may place patients at risk when they are treated with a freshly prepared vaccine that contains allergens no longer present in the mix that they had been receiving for immunotherapy.

In summary, many pollen and animal dander extracts are susceptible to accelerated loss of potency when mixed in a vaccine with protease-containing extracts. Pollen and dander extracts should not be included in a vaccine with cockroach or fungal extracts. House dust mite extracts in 25% glycerin appear neither to be susceptible to exogenous proteases nor to cause loss of potency due to their protease content. There are no good data on stability of mite extracts in vaccines of lower concentrations of glycerin. Degradation of fungal extracts by proteases in other fungal extracts contained in a vaccine has not been demonstrated, but has not been extensively investigated. Mixing cockroach, *Alternaria, Cladosporium*, and *Penicillium* extracts did not further reduce their potency in a vaccine (45). It is probable that the proteins susceptible to protease digestion had already been degraded by proteases in their own extract.

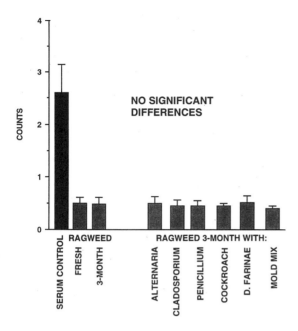

Figure 2 Stability of short ragweed alone and in mixtures. The potency of a 10-fold dilution of short ragweed stored under differing conditions was compared by ELISA inhibition to that of a freshly diluted aliquot. After 3 months the diluted short ragweed extract and those aliquots of ragweed stored in combination with *Alternaria, Penicillium, Cladosporium*, and cockroach alone and in combination were all equal in potency to the freshly diluted aliquot of short ragweed.

D. Diluents Employed in Mixing Allergen Vaccines

Because allergen extracts tend to lose potency with time, an effect that is enhanced by storage at higher temperatures and greater dilutions, a number of substances have been added to extracts both to preserve potency and to prevent growth of microorganisms. The most effective preservation of extract integrity and potency is achieved not by adding a preservative, however, but rather by lyophilization (50,51).

1. Glycerin

Glycerin is the most effective preservative for allergen extracts (52). It is very effective at a 50% concentration. At this concentration it inhibits some but not all proteolytic enzymes (44,46,51). This may contribute to, but does not completely explain, its effectiveness as a preservative. Decreasing effectiveness as a preservative has been demonstrated with 25% and 10% concentrations of glycerin (52,53); however, even 10% glycerin is as effective as 0.03% human serum albumin. It is possible that the presence of 25% glycerin accounted for the lack of proteolytic degradation of pollen extracts by the house dust mite extracts in several studies of mixing (46,49).

2. Human Serum Albumin

The preservative effect of human serum albumin is thought to relate to its protection against adsorption of allergenic protein to the vial surface (54) and to its protection against phenol denaturation (55). Human serum albumin has not been shown to have protective effects against proteolytic enzymes (44). Similar degrees of preservative effect were found with concentrations of 0.03%, 0.1%, and 1.0% HSA (52).

Concern has been expressed that patients may become sensitized by repeated injections of human serum albumin that may have been altered or aggregated in commercial processing (56). However, no cases of sensitization to human serum albumin in allergen vaccines have been reported, and one study that looked for evidence of positive skin tests or IgG antibodies directed toward human serum albumin was negative (57).

3. Phenol

Phenol is added to multidose vials of allergen extracts to prevent growth of microorganisms. Phenol denatures proteins, including those in allergen extracts (50), and the deleterious effect of phenol increases with increasing dilutions (52). Phenol degrades extracts in vaccines that are preserved in 50% glycerin (55,58). Human serum albumin is more protective than glycerin against the effect of phenol on extract potency (55,58).

4. Others

A number of other approaches to preserve extract potency have been suggested but have not found wide acceptance. Siliconization of vials has been suggested to decrease adsorption of proteins to their surface. Testing revealed this method to be without effect (52). Polysorbate 80 in concentrations of 0.002% to 0.2% had a slight effect in preserving potency, but it was less effective than HSA (52).

Epsilon-aminocaproic acid (EACA) has been suggested as a preservative (56), since pollens are known to contain enzymatic activity that may contribute to their loss of potency, and EACA is a potent enzyme inhibitor. However, EACA was found to be ineffective against a variety of fungal proteases (44). In studies on preservation of extract potency EACA was found to be less effective than glycerin (56). It was found to have less of a protective effect than human serum albumin on potency over the short term, perhaps because HSA works by blocking adsorption of allergenic proteins to the walls of the vial, whereas the protective effect of EACA is more on thermal denaturation that occurs over a longer period of time (56).

In the absence of preservatives, extracts stored in saline buffered with bicarbonate lost potency to a greater extent than those stored in phosphate-buffered saline or normal saline (51,52).

5. Mixing Extracts to Constitute a Vaccine

Single extracts that are stored combined with several other extracts retain their potency to a greater extent than the same extract, at the same dilution, stored alone (53). This preservative effect is probably related to total protein content. In this instance the proteins in the other extracts are functioning in a manner analogous to human serum albumin when combined in a vaccine.

IV. CONDITIONS OF STORAGE

Maintenance of potency of a therapeutic allergen vaccine is a function of the dilution, the diluent, the temperature of storage, and the presence of proteolytic enzymes that may degrade the allergenic proteins. The processes that lead to loss of vaccine potency and the measures that can be used to reduce the effect are given in Table 14.

A. Temperature

Allergen extracts and vaccines are susceptible to loss of potency if they are maintained at room rather than refrigerator temperature (53,58). Loss of activity with storage at room

Table 14 Mechanisms of Loss of Potency of Allergenic Extracts

Mechanism	Favored by	Avoided by
Adsorption	High dilution	Human serum albumin
	High surface to volume ratio	Glycerin
Thermal denaturation	High temperature	Storage at low temperature
Enzymatic autodigestion	Enzymes in extract	Glycerin
		Storage at low temperature

temperature is thought to be caused by the proteases (51), while loss of potency with brief exposure to even higher temperatures is thought to be related to heat lability of some of the allergenic proteins (59). Some extracts, such as cat (58), have been reported to be relatively resistant to this thermal effect. Other extracts, including white ash, elm, orchard grass, Bermuda grass (60), ragweed (59), and house dust mites (58), have been shown to lose some potency at high temperature. Since the loss of potency is a result of the presence in these extracts of either protease-susceptible or heat-labile proteins, the stored extract will have an altered pattern of specificity due to the preferential persistence of the resistant proteins, resulting in an altered pattern of skin test reactivity (59).

Less extreme temperature exposure of allergen extracts, such as exposure to room temp for 13 hours per week, resulted in significant loss of potency (53). The effect of repeated freezing and thawing on allergen extract potency has not been extensively studied, but it has been reported to reduce the potency of ragweed (42) and dilute *Lolium perenne* (56) extracts.

B. Dilution

Extracts are more susceptible to loss of potency when stored diluted than concentrated (49,52). The principal reason for the increased susceptibility of diluted extract is thought to be their lesser protein content and hence greater adsorption of allergens to the container wall (50,53,54). However, addition of human serum albumin does not completely protect, and all allergen extracts are not equally susceptible to this effect (49), suggesting that other factors may be involved.

Some studies of diluted extracts have reported unexpectedly preserved potency for prolonged periods. Thus, intradermal skin test concentrations of timothy, birch, cat, and house dust mite preserved with HSA showed preserved potency after 24 months storage at 6°C (58). The explanation for these apparently aberrant results is unclear, but perhaps relates to the pattern of sensitivity of the population studied.

Loss of potency is related to the total protein content of the extract. Not entirely filling a vial of extract has been reported to enhance loss of potency due to the greater surface area relative to the volume of extract from which protein is available for adsorption. This effect is diminished by including other extracts in a vaccine, thus increasing the total protein content (53). The same protective effect can be achieved by added extraneous protein, such as human serum albumin (53,54).

V. PATTERNS OF LOSS OF POTENCY

A. Assessment

A variety of methods have been employed to assess the residual potency of allergenic extracts (52). The two approaches most commonly employed, RAST or ELISA inhibition and skin testing, have been reported to yield similar results (53,61). In some studies residual activity has been greater by skin testing than by RAST inhibition (50,51). However, a careful comparison of titrated intradermal skin testing and ELISA inhibition yielded very similar results with multiple allergen extracts (46), suggesting that, the results with the two methods properly done, are comparable.

B. Individual Allergens

The stability of allergen extracts can vary due to differing heat susceptibility of their components, different total protein content affecting the percent adsorbed to the container wall, and content of proteolytic enzymes, which may cause auto-digestion (Figs. 3 and 4). They may be affected differently by the addition of phenol as well as by the presence of proteases in other extracts with which they are mixed in a vaccine. As would be expected, studies have shown differing loss of potency for different extracts stored under similar conditions. Therefore, it is best to follow general principles that will protect the potency of the most susceptible extracts. These include (1) avoiding mixing fungal and insect extracts with pollen and dander extracts in formulating a vaccine (an exception appears to be house dust mite extracts in 25% glycerin) (2) keeping the total protein content high by using concentrated extracts and adding human serum albumin to dilutions, and (3) keeping the extracts and vaccines at refrigerator temperature except when actually being used (for dilute vaccines left at room temperature, consider using a refrigerated tray when exposed to room temperatures).

With attention to these details, some diluted extracts will lose potency even after 3 months at concentrations used for maintenance immunotherapy (Figs. 1 and 3), whereas others will not lose any potency at the same dilution over the period of a year (Figs. 2 and 4).

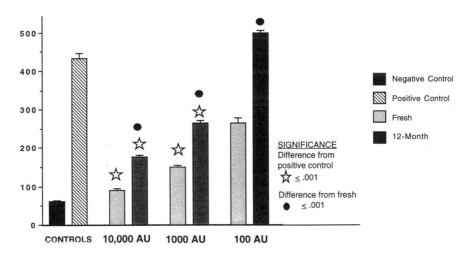

Figure 3 The potency of Bermuda grass extract stored at 4°C in concentrations of 100 AU/ml, 1000 AU/ml, and 10,000 AU/ml was compared after 12 months by ELISA inhibition with freshly diluted aliquots of the same Bermuda extract. There was, as indicated, significant loss of potency after 12 months in all dilutions. Negative control contained the Bermuda disc but no serum. Positive control contained Bermuda disc and mixed grass-allergic patients' serum, but no Bermuda extract, while the tested aliquoted contained Bermuda disc, Bermuda-allergic serum, and dilutions of Bermuda extract. AU = allergen units (former FDA terminology).

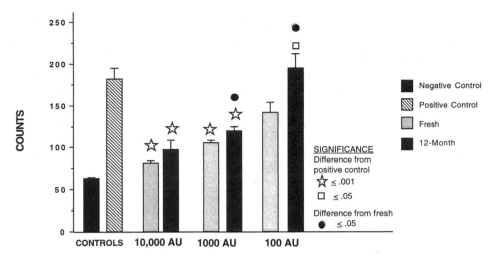

Figure 4 The potency of short ragweed extract stored at 4°C in concentrations of 100 AU/ml, 1000 AU/ml, and 10,000 AU/ml was compared after 12 months by ELISA inhibition to freshly diluted aliquots of the same short ragweed extract. There was no loss of potency after 12 months in the 10,000 AU/ml aliquot, but there was a significant loss of potency in the other two dilutions. Negative control contained the short ragweed disc but no serum. Positive control contained short ragweed disc and mixed ragweed-allergic patients' serum, but no short ragweed extract, while the tested aliquots contained short ragweed disc, ragweed-allergic serum, and dilutions of short ragweed extract. AU = allergen units (former FDA terminology).

Full-strength extracts and vaccines are probably stable at refrigerator temperature for their stated shelf life. Full-strength extracts in 50% glycerin, as used for prick skin testing, are certainly stable until their expiration date (52). Diluted extracts, used for intradermal skin testing, have been found to be stable for prolonged periods by some investigators (58) but not by others (52). Some allergen extracts are susceptible to rapid loss of potency at high temperatures (58–60), but the loss with exposure to room temperature is not rapid (53). It is unlikely that shipping allergen extracts and vaccines through the mail would result in exposure to temperatures that would be deleterious.

VI. SALIENT POINTS

1. Standardized extracts of cat pelt and hair, house dust mites, short ragweed, eight grasses, and the venoms of four Hymenoptera are commercially available in the United States.

2. Neither of the two expressions for potency used for nonstandardized extracts, weight by volume (wt/vol) or protein nitrogen units (PNU), adequately reflects the allergenic potency of a vaccine.

3. There are two immunotherapy studies that relate dose to outcome employing nonstandardized vaccines. In one study employing multiple allergens, the outcome with 1:250 wt/vol vaccines was better than with 1:5000 wt/vol. In the other study, results with 1:50 wt/vol ragweed vaccine were significantly better than with 1:1000 wt/vol.

4. Representative values for the major allergen content of U.S. standardized vaccines are listed in Table 4. However, the values in Table 4 are only representative and may vary significantly from one manufacturer to another.

5. Placebo-controlled studies demonstrating clinical effectiveness have been performed with house dust mites, cat dander, grass pollen, and ragweed vaccines. In each instance the effective dose of major allergen has been in the range of 7 to 20 µg (Table 3).

6. The information in Tables 3 and 4 allows formulation of an allergen vaccine mixture containing concentrations of the major allergens approximating those that have proven to be clinically effective (Table 5).

7. Vaccines should contain effective quantities of each aeroallergen. If two or more components of the allergen mixture cross-react, the amount of each should be decreased so that the sum of the cross-reacting aeroallergens is similar to the content of the other aeroallergens in the mixture.

8. Most fungal and whole-body insect extracts contain proteases that are capable of degrading allergenic proteins contained in other extracts when constituted together in a vaccine. Therefore, mixing fungal and cockroach extracts with pollen or dander extracts in a vaccine is to be avoided (Table 12).

9. Degradation of allergen extracts and vaccines is increased by dilution and by the time in which they are maintained at room temperature.

10. Glycerin is the most effective preservative but is poorly tolerated by injection. Human serum albumin is less effective but well tolerated. Glycerin or human serum albumin should be included in all dilute vaccines.

REFERENCES

1. de Weck AL. Allergen standardization at a crossroads? ACI Int 1997; 9:25–30.
2. Turkeltaub PC. In vivo standardization. In: Allergy: Principles and Practice, 3rd ed. (Middleton E Jr, Reed CE, Ellis EF, Adkinson NF Jr, Yunginger JW, eds.). St. Louis: C.V. Mosby, 1988: 388–401.
3. Allergy Update Vol. 1, No. 1. Le Noir, NC: Greer Laboratories, May 1992.
4. Technical Bulletin Vol. 1, No. 1. Spokane, WA: Hollister-Steir.
5. APMA. Letter to the President, American Academy of Allergy and Immunology. May 26, 1994.
6. Van Metre TE Jr, Rosenberg GL, Vaswani SK, Ziegler SR, Adkinson NF Jr. Pain and dermal reaction caused by injected glycerin in immunotherapy solutions. J Allergy Clin Immunol 1996; 97:1033–1039.
7. Norman PS, Winkenwerder WL, Lichtenstein LM. Trials of alum-precipitated pollen extracts in the treatment of hay fever. J Allergy Clin Immunol 1972; 50:31–44.
8. Nelson HS. Long-term immunotherapy with aqueous and aluminum-precipitated grass extracts. Ann Allergy 1980; 45:333–337.
9. Lichtenstein LM, Norman PS, Winkenwerder WL. Antibody response following immunotherapy in ragweed hay fever: Allpyral vs. whole ragweed extract. J Allergy 1968; 41:49–57.
10. Guerin B, Hewitt B. The effect of commonly used extracting media on the allergenic composition of cat fur extract. Ann Allergy 1981; 47:166–170.
11. Sherman WB. Hypersensitivity: Mechanisms and Management. Philadelphia: W.B. Saunders, 1968: 422.
12. Stull A, Cooke RA, Tennant J. The allergic content of pollen extracts: Its determination and its deterioration. J Allergy 1933; 4:455–467
13. Johnstone DE, Crump L. Value of hyposensitization therapy for perennial bronchial asthma in children. Pediatrics 1961; 27:39–44.

14. Lowell FC, Franklin W. A double-blind study of the effectiveness and specificity of injection therapy in ragweed hay fever. N Engl J Med 1965; 273:675–679

15. Franklin W, Lowell FC. Comparison of two dosages of ragweed extract in the treatment of pollenosis. J Am Med Assoc 1967; 201:915–917.

16. Ewan PW, Alexander MM, Snape C, Ind PW, Agrell B, Dreborg S. Effective hyposensitization in allergic rhinitis using a potent partially purified extract of house dust mite. Clin Allergy 1988; 18:501–508.

17. Haugaard L, Dahl R, Jacobsen L. A controlled dose-response study of immunotherapy with standardized, partially purified extract of house dust mite: Clinical efficacy and side effects. J Allergy Clin Immunol 1993; 91:709–722.

18. Olsen OT, Larsen KR, Jacobsen L, Svendsen UG. A 1-year, placebo-controlled double-blind house dust mite immunotherapy study in asthmatic adults. Allergy 1997; 52:853–859.

19. Van Metre TE Jr, Marsh DG, Adkinson NF Jr, Kagey-Sobotka A, Khattignavong A, Norman PS Jr, Rosenberg GL. Immunotherapy for cat asthma. J Allergy Clin Immunol 1988; 82:1055–1068.

20. Alvarez-Cuesta E, Cuesta-Herranz J, Puyana-Ruiz J, Cuesta-Herranz C, Blanco-Quiros A. Monoclonal antibody–standardized cat extract immunotherapy: Risk benefit effects from a double-blind placebo study. J Allergy Clin Immunol. 1994; 93:556–566.

21. Hedlin G, Graff-Lonnevig V, Heilbron H, Lilja G, Norrlind K, Pegelow K, Sundin B, Lowenstein H. Immunotherapy with cat- and dog-dander extracts: V. Effects of 3 years of treatment. J Allergy Clin Immunol 1991; 87:955–964.

22. Varney VA, Edward J, Tabbahk, Brewster H, Mavroleon G, Frey AJ. Clinical efficacy of specific immunotherapy to cat dander: A double-blind, placebo-controlled trial. Clin Exp Allergy 1997; 27:860–867.

23. Ewbank PA, Murray J, Sanders K, Curran-Everett D, Dreskin S, Nelson HS. A double-blind, placebo-controlled immunotherapy dose-response study with standardized cat extract. J Allergy Clin Immunol 2003; 111:155–161.

24. Varney VA, Gaga M, Frew AJ, Aber VR, Kay AB, Durham SR. Usefulness of immunotherapy in patients with severe summer hay fever uncontrolled by antiallergic drugs. Br Med J 1991; 302:530–531.

25. Dolz I, Martinez-Cocera C, Barlolome JM, Cimarra M. A double-blind, placebo-controlled study of immunotherapy with grass pollen extract Alutard SQ during a three-year period with initial rush immunotherapy. Allergy 1996; 51:489–500.

26. Walker SM, Pajno GB, Torres Lima M, Wilson DR, Durham SR. Grass pollen immunotherapy for seasonal rhinitis and asthma: A randomized, controlled trial. J Allergy Clin Immunol 2001; 107:87–93.

27. Van Metre TE Jr, Adkinson NF, Amodio FJ, Lichtenstein LM, Mardiney MR Jr, Norman PS, Rosenberg GL, Sobotka AK, Valentine MD. A comparative study of the effectiveness of the Rinkel method and the current standard method of immunotherapy for ragweed pollen hay fever. J Allergy Clin Immunol 1979; 66:500–513.

28. Creticos PS, Marsh DG, Proud D, Kagey-Sobotka A, Adkinson NF Jr, Friedhoff L, Naclerio RM, Lichtenstein LM, Norman PS. Responses to ragweed-pollen nasal challenge before and after immunotherapy. J Allergy Clin Immunol 1989; 84:197–205.

29. Creticos PS, Adkinson NF Jr, Kagey-Sobotka A, Proud D, Meier HL, Naclerio RM, Lichtenstein LM, Norman PS. Nasal challenge with ragweed pollen in hay fever patients: Effect of immunotherapy. J Clin Investig 1985; 76:2247–2253.

30. Furin MJ, Norman PS, Creticos PS, Proud D, Kagey-Sobotka A, Lichtenstein LM, Naclerio RM. Immunotherapy decreases antigen-induced eosinophil cell migration into the nasal cavity. J Allergy Clin Immunol 1991; 88:27–32.

31. Hunt KJ, Valentine MD, Sobotka AK, Benton AW, Amodio FJ, Lichtenstein LM. A controlled trial of immunotherapy in insect hypersensitivity. N Engl J Med 1978; 299:157–161.

32. Vailes L, Sridhara S, Cromwell O, Weber B, Breitenbach M, Chapman M. Quantitation of the major fungal allergens, Alt a 1 and Asp f1, in commercial allergenic products. J Allergy Clin Immunol 2001; 107:641–646.

33. Patterson ML, Slater JE. Characterization and comparison of commercially available German and American cockroach allergen extracts. Clin Exp Allergy 2002; 32:721–727.

34. Martin BG, Mansfield LE, Nelson HS. Cross-allergenicity among the grasses. Ann Allergy 1985; 54:99–104.

35. Weber RW, Nelson HS. Pollen allergens and their interrelationships. Clin Rev Allergy 1985; 3:291–318.

36. Yoo T-J, Spitz E, McGerity JL. Conifer pollen allergy: Studies of immunogenicity and cross antigenicity of conifer pollens in rabbit and man. Ann Allergy 1975; 34:87–93.

37. Valenta R, Breiteneder H, Pettenburger K, Breitenbach M, Rumpold H, Kraft D, Scheiner O. Homology of the major birch-pollen allergen, Bet v I, with the major pollen allergens of alder, hazel, and hornbeam at the nucleic acid level as determined by cross-hybridization. J Allergy Clin Immonol 1991; 87:677–682.

38. Kernerman SM, McCullough J, Green J, Ownby DR. Evidence of cross-reactivity between olive, ash, privet and Russian olive tree pollen allergens. Ann Allergy 1992; 69:493–496.

39. Leavengood DC, Renard RL, Martin B, Nelson HS. Cross allergenicity among grasses determined by tissue threshold changes. J Allergy Clin Immunol 1985; 76:789–794.

40. Leiferman KM, Gleich GJ, Jones RT. The cross-reactivity of IgE antibodies with pollen allergens: III. Analyses of various species of ragweed and other fall weed pollens. J Allergy Clin Immunol 1976; 58:140–148.

41. Heymann PW, Chapman MD, Aalberse RC, Fox JW, Platts-Mills TAE. Antigenic and structural analysis of group II allergens (Der f II and Der p II) from house dust mites (*Dermatophagoides* spp.). J Allergy Clin Immunol 1989; 83:1055–1067.

42. Center JG, Shuller N, Zeleznick LD. Stability of antigen E in commercially prepared ragweed pollen extracts. J Allergy Clin Immunol 1974; 54:305–310.

43. Bousquet J, Marty JP, Coulomb Y, Robinet-Levy M, Cour P, Michael FB. Enzyme determination and RAST inhibition assays for orchard grass (*Dactylis glomerata*): A comparison of commercial pollen extracts. Ann Allergy 1978; 41:164–169.

44. Esch RE. Role of Proteases on the Stability of Allergenic Extracts. Arbeiten aus dem Paul-Ehrlich-Institut. Stuttgart: Gustav Fischer Verlag, 1991: 171–179.

45. Wongtim S, Lehrer SB, Salvaggio JE, Horner WE. Protease activity in cockroach and basidiomycete allergen extracts. Allergy Proc 1993; 14:263–268.

46. Kordash TR, Amend MJ, Williamson SL, Jones JK, Plunkett GA. Effect of mixing allergenic extracts containing *Helminthosporium, D farinae*, and cockroach with perennial ryegrass. Ann Allergy 1993; 71:240–246.

47. Haff M, Krail M, Kastner M, Haustein D, Vieths S. *Fusarium culmorum* causes strong degradation of pollen allergens in extract mixtures. J Allergy Clin Immunol 2002; 109:96–101.

48. Stewart GA, Ward LD, Simpson RJ, Thompson PJ. The group III allergen from the house dust mite *Dermatophagoides pteronyssinus* is a trypsin-like enzyme. Immunol 1992; 75:29–35.

49. Nelson HS, Ikle D, Buchmeier A. Studies of allergen extract stability: The effects of dilution and mixing. J Allergy Clin Immunol 1996; 98:382–388.

50. Ayuso R, Rubio M, Herrera T, Gurbindo C, Carreira J. Stability of *Lolium perenne* extract. Ann Allergy 1984; 53:426–431.

51. Anderson MC, Baer H. Antigenic and allergenic changes during storage of a pollen extract. J Allergy Clin Immunol 1982; 69:3–10.

52. Nelson HS. The effect of preservatives and dilution on the deterioration of Russian thistle (*Salsola pestifer*), a pollen extract. J Allergy Clin Immunol 1979; 63:417–425.

53. Nelson HS. Effect of preservatives and conditions of storage on the potency of allergy extracts. J Allergy Clin Immunol 1981; 67:64–69.

54. Norman PS, Marsh DG. Human serum albumin and Tween 80 as stabilizers of allergen solutions. J Allergy Clin Immunol 1978; 62:314–319.

55. Naerdal A, Vilsvik JS. Stabilization of a diluted aqueous mite allergen preparation by addition of human serum albumin: An intracutaneous test study. Clin Allergy 1983; 13:149–153.

56. Van Hoeyveld EM, Stevens EAM. Stabilizing effect of epsilon-aminocaproic acid on allergenic extracts. J Allergy Clin Immunol 1985; 76:543–550.

57. Brown JS, Ledoux R, Nelson HS. An investigation of possible immunologic reactions to human serum albumin used as a stabilizer in allergy extracts. J Allergy Clin Immunol 1985; 76:808–812.

58. Niemeijer NR, Kauffman HF, van Hove W, Dubois AEJ, de Moncy GR. Effect of dilution, temperature, and preservatives on the long-term stability of standardized inhalant allergen extracts. Ann Allergy Asthma Immunol 1996; 76:535–540.

59. Baer H, Anderson MC, Hale R, Gleich GJ. The heat stability of short ragweed pollen extract and the importance of individual allergens in skin reactivity. J Allergy Clin Immunol 1980; 66:281–285.

60. Hale R, Grater WC, Haykik IB, McConnell LH, Santilli J Jr, Scherr MS, Zitt MJ. Report of the Committee on Standardization of Allergenic Extracts: A study of the heat stability of white oak, elm, orchard grass, and Bermuda grass. Ann Allergy 1985; 55:86–87.

61. Bousquet J, Djoukadar F, Hewitt B, Guerin B, Michel F-B. Comparison of the stability of a mite and a pollen extract stored in normal conditions of use. Clin Allergy 1985; 15:29–35.

25

Administration of Allergen Vaccines

PRIYANKA GUPTA and LESLIE C. GRAMMER

Northwestern University Medical School, Chicago, Illinois, U.S.A.

I. INTRODUCTION

Allergen immunotherapy has been practiced in the United States since its original description by Noon and Freeman in 1911 for the treatment of allergic symptoms due to inhalant allergens (1). In 1918, Dr. Robert Cooke suggested a mechanism of action for allergen injections as a "desensitization or hyposensitization." The more specific immunological basis for allergic disease was initially established by Prausnitz and Kustner, who demonstrated that the allergic sensitivity could be transferred by the serum of a sensitive person to the skin of a nonallergic person (2). Allergen immunotherapy is defined as the repeated administration of specific allergens to patients with IgE-mediated conditions for the purpose of providing protection against the allergic symptoms and inflammatory reactions associated with natural exposure to these allergens (3). The technique of allergen immunotherapy should be differentiated from the process of desensitization, which is the term applied to the rapid, progressive administration of an allergenic substance, usually a drug, to render effector cells less reactive.

In the United States, immunotherapy with inhalant allergens most commonly consists of once-or twice-weekly subcutaneous injections of aqueous allergen vaccines while the dose is being increased; once the highest dose (also called the maintenance dose) is achieved, the interval between injections is increased (4–6). In many other countries, the timing and route of administration are the same, but modified vaccines rather than aqueous vaccines are used. Numerous variations of inhalant immunotherapy are practiced relative to route of administration, timing, frequency, duration, and dosage.

II.   ADMINISTRATION OF INHALANT VACCINES

Immunotherapy for inhalant allergy is effective therapy for allergic asthma and allergic rhinoconjunctivitis. It has not proved to be effective for eczema, urticaria, or food allergies (7). Immunotherapy is effective treatment for allergic rhinitis due to a variety of pollen species, including grasses, ragweed, *Parietaria* species, and mountain cedar. Immunotherapy with house dust mite vaccines is effective treatment for both asthma and rhinitis (8). Fewer studies have reported that immunotherapy is effective for patients allergic to cats (9), *Alternaria* species (10), and *Cladosporium* species (11). Aeroallergens vary with geographic location; lists of pollen by geographic location and month are available in several standards texts (12–14). It is important to be familiar with the significant aeroallergens in a physician's geographic location in order to appropriately choose allergens for cutaneous testing and immunotherapy. Because the American population is relatively mobile, it is also important to be familiar with significant aeroallergens outside a physician's geographic region in order to appropriately test and treat with aeroallergens important in other areas of the country (15). For example, Bermuda grass is an important allergen in the southern United States but is not present in most northern climates. The clinical relevance of an aeroallergen depends on certain key properties: (1) its allergenicity, (2) its aerodynamic properties, (3) whether it is produced in large enough quantities to be sampled, (4) whether it is sufficiently buoyant to be carried long distances, and (5) whether the plant releasing the pollen is widely and abundantly prevalent in the region (16).

A.   Aqueous Vaccines

In the United States, aqueous vaccines are the most commonly administered inhalant vaccines. Aqueous extracts are prepared by extracting proteins from fresh source material at physiological pH and ionic strength, at low temperatures to delay proteolytic degradation and microorganism contamination. Some of the extracts are standardized by cutaneous endpoint titration and quantified by allergy units (AUs), such as dust mites, or biological allergen units (BAUs), such as grass pollen (15). However, many of them are labeled with protein nitrogen units (PNUs) or as weight/volume (w/v), neither of which is reliably associated with allergenic potency (17). One PNU is 10 ng protein nitrogen, and w/v refers to the weight (in grams) of the source material that is extracted in a given volume (in milliliters). In other parts of the world, other standard units are used to express allergenic potency. In Europe, especially in the Scandinavian countries, the biological unit (BU), which is based on comparative histamine skin testing, is used (18). Allergen standards developed by the International Union of Immunologic Societies (IUIS) are quantified in international units (IUs) (19).

The starting immunotherapy dose is usually 1000-fold to 10,000-fold less than the maintenance dose. For highly sensitive patients, the starting dose may be lower. The maintenance dose with standardized allergy vaccines is approximately 600 allergy units (AU) for dust mite or 4000 bioequivalent allergy units (BAU) for grass (Fig. 1). For nonstandardized vaccines, a suggested maintenance dose is 3000 to 5000 protein nitrogen units

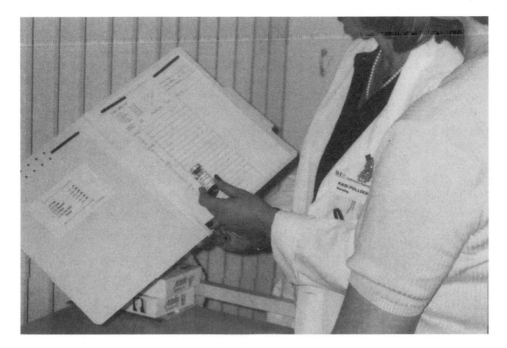

Figure 1 The patient, vial, dilution, and immunotherapy schedule are identified prior to administration of an injection.

(PNU) or 0.5 ml of a 1:100 weight/volume dilution of manufacturer's extract. If the major allergen concentration of the vaccine is known, a dose containing between 5 and 20 μg of the major allergen is a recommended maintenance dose (16). Whenever possible, standardized extracts should be used to prepare vaccine treatment sets. Some commonly used allergens are standardized. These include, as of 2003, cat hair, cat pelt, *Dermatophagoides pteronyssinus, Dermatophagoides farinae*, short ragweed, Bermuda grass, Kentucky bluegrass, perennial ryegrass, orchard grass, timothy grass, meadow fescue, red top, sweet vernal grass, and Hymenoptera venoms (yellow jacket, honeybee, wasp, yellow hornet, and white-faced hornet) (16).

    Allergen extracts should be maintained near labeled potency until used for diagnostic tests or immunotherapy. Because extracts/vaccines lose their potency when stored at room temperature and with freezing and thawing, specific steps must be taken to preserve their potency. Allergen extracts/vaccines should be kept at about 4°C. Dilutions of concentrated extracts/vaccines lose their potency more rapidly than the concentrates. Extracts that have lost potency—due to freezing and thawing, as an example—should be discarded (20).

B. Subcutaneous Immunotherapy

Administration of inhalant vaccines has usually been by subcutaneous injection. The first controlled study of the efficacy of immunotherapy, in 1949, administered house dust allergen by subcutaneous injection (21). Numerous subsequent studies have reported the efficacy of immunotherapy with tree (22,23), grass (24,25), and weed pollen (26,27); fungi (28,29); and house dust mite (30,31) aqueous vaccines administered by subcutaneous injection. Some studies support cat IT, whereas others indicate that there is only a transient beneficial effect. High-dose perennial immunotherapy is the time schedule of administration that results in the best efficacy (12–14). Of historical note, immunotherapy only during the pollen season, or coseasonal therapy, and immunotherapy only in the few months prior to the pollen season, or preseasonal therapy, are not recommended (13) in the United States but are used in other parts of the world.

When more than one inhalant allergen is required, the vaccines may be administered either individually or incorporated into a single vial. Since most patients would rather receive a single injection instead of multiple injections, this is generally preferable. There are data on house dust mite and fungal vaccines that suggest the enzymes in those vaccines might degrade proteins in them and in other vaccines with which they are mixed (32). There are, however, no data on efficacy of mixed vaccines as compared to individual vaccines to clarify the clinical relevance of the proteolytic potential of inhalant vaccines. There are occasional patients who are extremely sensitive to one inhalant allergen. In those cases, it may be warranted to administer that inhalant allergen in a separate injection. The dosage schedule for that allergen would be more conservative than the one employed for the other inhalant allergens administered.

1. Dosage Schedules

Three basic immunotherapeutic dosage schedules have been reported to be beneficial for the treatment of inhalant allergy: standard weekly immunotherapy, cluster immunotherapy, and rush immunotherapy (6). A generally accepted principle of immunotherapy is that the higher the cumulative dose, the greater the efficacy (26). The optimal dose is defined as the dose of allergen vaccine that induces a clinically relevant effect in the majority of patients without causing unacceptable side effects (33). Studies by investigators at Johns Hopkins reported that ragweed vaccines administered in annual cumulative doses of approximately 50 ug antigen E or Amb a 1 are likely to be effective (34). Effective cumulative doses for other vaccines are not as well defined; however, there have been studies of cat vaccines standardized by Fel d 1 content (35), mite vaccines standardized by Der p 1 content (36), and pollen standardized by BU (37) that support the hypothesis that higher cumulative doses of inhalant allergen are more likely to result in amelioration of symptoms of aeroallergen allergy.

Conventional Immunotherapy Regimens.   There are two phases of conventional immunotherapy administration: the initial buildup phase, when the dose and concentration of vaccine are slowly increased, and the maintenance phase, when the patient receives an optimal immunizing dose over a period of time (7). Perennial immunotherapy commonly follows a once- or twice-weekly dosage schedule (Table 1). If the extract/vaccine is labeled in AU or BAU, the initial concentration is generally 0.1–1 AU/ml or BAU/ml. The initial volume is usually 0.05 ml. In preparation for the buildup phase of immunotherapy, serial dilutions should be produced from each maintenance concentrate vaccine. Typically, these are 10-fold dilutions, although other dilutions are occasionally used. These dilutions should be labeled in terms of volume per volume to indicate that these are dilutions derived from the maintenance concentrate. For example, serial 10-fold dilutions from the maintenance concentrate would be labeled as 1:10 (vol/vol), 1:100 (vol/vol), and so on (16). Injections during the buildup phase are commonly administered once or twice weekly; when the maintenance dose is reached, the interval is generally increased to biweekly, triweekly, and finally monthly. The maintenance dose is usually administered at 2- to 4-week intervals provided that the injections are well tolerated and symptoms improve. If systemic reactions

Table 1 Illustrative Schedule for an Inhalant Allergen Vaccine

Dose	Dilution	ml	AU	wt/vol (approximate)
1	2 AU/ml	0.05	0.1	1:100,000
2		0.1	0.2	
3		0.2	0.4	
4		0.4	0.8	
5	20 AU/ml	0.05	1	1:10,000
6		0.1	2	
7		0.2	4	
8		0.4	8	
9	200 AU/ml	0.05	10	1:1000
10		0.10	20	
11		0.15	30	
12		0.20	40	
13		0.25	50	
14		0.30	60	
15		0.35	70	
16		0.40	80	
17		0.45	90	
18		0.50	100	
19	2000 AU/ml	0.05	100	1:100
20		0.10	200	
21		0.15	300	
22		0.20	400	
23		0.25	500	
24		0.30	600	
25		0.35	700	
26		0.40	800	
27		0.45	900	
28		0.50	1000	

or anaphylaxis occurs, the physician should review the patient's immunotherapy history and adjust the dose of immunotherapy accordingly. Subsequently, the dose is increased as tolerated at weekly or twice-weekly intervals. The maintenance vial is replaced with a newly prepared vial every 6 to 12 months, and the dose of the next injection is reduced by one-third to one-half with the first injection of the new vial. The dose is subsequently increased weekly or twice weekly to the routine maintenance dose (20).

Rush Immunotherapy Regimens.   Numerous schedules have been published for administration of allergen immunotherapy via a rush injection schedule. Initial doses are generally similar to those of more conventional schedules as listed in Table 1. A typical rush immunotherapy schedule entails multiple injections on the first day of treatment. On the second and third days, a lesser number of injections is administered, with the proportional increment of allergen also declining with each successive injection until a maintenance dose is reached in 3 to 7 days. During the first few days, injections are given at intervals of 30 minutes to 2 hours. Some rush protocols increase the dosages more rapidly than outlined in Table 1 with increases of 50–100% per injection. The obvious advantage of a rush schedule is that the patient can attain the maintenance dose and symptom relief more quickly (38). A disadvantage is the time commitment required during the first several days of therapy owing to the frequency and duration of visits. Another disadvantage is that rush immunotherapy is associated with a greater risk of systemic reaction than that entailed in conventional weekly immunotherapy; this increased reaction rate appears to be particularly significant in children (39). Premedication with prednisone, an H_1 histamine receptor antagonist, with or without an H_2 histamine receptor antagonist, before rush immunotherapy, has been reported to reduce the risk of systemic reaction in two studies (40,41). Efficacy and immunological changes have been reported to be similar to conventional immunotherapy with equivalent cumulative doses.

Cluster Immunotherapy. In cluster immunotherapy protocols, starting doses are similar to those of conventional immunotherapy (42). As with conventional protocols, weekly visits are necessary; however, at each visit more than one injection is administered with the interval between injections varying from 30 minutes to 2 hours. Once the maintenance dose has been achieved, the interval between visits is increased. The advantage of the cluster regimen is probably most obvious for the patient who must travel several hours in order to receive injections; receiving more than one injection per visit reduces overall travel time. Efficacy and immunological changes appear to be similar to conventional immunotherapy of equivalent cumulative dose. The disadvantage to cluster immunotherapy is that the reaction rate is generally higher than with conventional schedules (42).

2. Procedures for Subcutaneous Injection

Prior to administering inhalant immunotherapy, it is imperative that the patient, the immunotherapy vial(s) of the appropriate dilution, and the dosage schedule(s) be clearly identified. Error in dosage magnitude is a cause of serious systemic reactions to inhalant allergen injections (43). Careful documentation of the immunotherapy is extremely important. Information that should be noted in the medical record includes the concentration given; a record of the bottle's label and its contents; the volume of vaccine scheduled and given; which arm was used for the injection; peak expiratory flow before and, as indicated, 20 to 30 minutes before or after injection for high-risk patients; a history of reactions from previous shots; treatment of any reactions that occurred; and any adjustments from the standard schedule and the reasons for them (7). A copy of the AAAAI's suggested immunotherapy worksheet is shown in Fig. 1. If a patient's asthma is not controlled, the patient should be treated before an injection is administered due to the potential dangerous synergistic effects of asthma and anaphylaxis. Injections should be administered with a 0.5 to 1 milliliter syringe to ensure dosage measurement accuracy. The needle gauge should be more than 25, and the injection should be subcutaneous, not intradermal, intramuscular, or intravenous. The subcutaneous adipose tissue in the midportion posterior aspect of the arm (in the deltoid muscle) is the most common site for injections (Fig. 2). Prior to vaccine injection, the syringe plunger should be withdrawn to ensure that the needle is not intravenous. If blood appears in the syringe, it should be withdrawn and discarded, and a new needle and syringe should be used. After injections of inhalant allergen vaccines, the patient should be observed at least 20 to 30 minutes for reactions to injections and longer if they are at high risk for a reaction. (New practice parameters were published in the January 2003 issue of the Annals of Allergy, Asthma and Immunology.)

3. Reactions and Dosage Adjustment

Erythema and/or induration less than 2 cm, lasting less than 2 days, are common and of no consequence. Large local reactions, that is, induration greater than 2 cm lasting more than

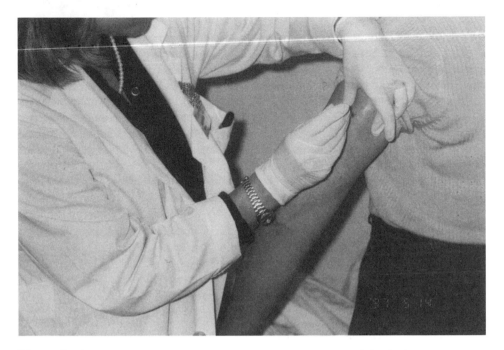

Figure 2   Proper technique for administration of an immunotherapy injection.

2 days, may require a repetition or decrease of the next dose. Reactions greater than 2 cm in diameter should be treated with topical application of ice to reduce local blood flow, oral antihistamine therapy, and possibly topical corticosteroid therapy. There are no data to indicate that large local reactions are harbingers of systemic anaphylactic reactions (20). Oral antihistamines and local application of ice are usually sufficient treatment for significant local reactions. Rarely, a local or biphasic local reaction may be so significant that a day or two of oral corticosteroids is indicated.

Anaphylaxis manifested by urticaria, angioedema, generalized pruritus and erythema, laryngeal edema, headache, nausea, vomiting, bronchospasm, hypotension, shock, and even death may occur following an injection of an allergen vaccine. Most systemic reactions occur during the buildup phase or in highly allergic individuals. Physicians who administer allergen immunotherapy vaccines must be prepared to treat these reactions. If a systemic reaction occurs, the subsequent dose should be reduced to one-half to one-tenth the dose that resulted in the systemic reaction, depending upon the severity of the reaction. After a systemic reaction, the rate of increase in dosage is usually reduced. After each systemic reaction, the risks and benefits of continuing immunotherapy should be reevaluated.

A common cause for dosage adjustment is a hiatus in therapy. Depending upon the patient's previous history of reactions and the length of the hiatus, compared with the usual frequency of injections, the dosage may be repeated or reduced. If a patient has a pattern of being unable to comply with the injection schedule, particularly if the maintenance dose has not been achieved, the risks and benefits of continuing immunotherapy should be reevaluated.

4. When to Stop Immunotherapy

Within a year of reaching the maintenance dose, patients should notice a reduction in symptoms and/or medications. If a patient has been on maintenance immunotherapy for a year and there has been no improvement, further immunotherapy is not likely to result in improvement and should be discontinued.

Approximately 90% of patients receiving optimal dose maintenance immunotherapy for a year will notice improvement. In a controlled study in which immunotherapy for grass pollen allergy was discontinued after 3 to 4 years of successful treatment, seasonal symptom scores and the use of rescue medication remained low for 3 to 4 years after the discontinuation of immunotherapy, and there was no significant difference between patients who continued and those who discontinued immunotherapy (44). There are no clear data to provide absolute indications for the optimal length of time to continue inhalant allergen immunotherapy. After 2 or 3 years of improvement, there should be consideration of discontinuing immunotherapy. In our experience, most patients whose inhalant allergen immunotherapy is discontinued at that time will continue to maintain their reduction of symptoms and/or medications. There is, however, a risk of relapse, and this should be discussed with the patient prior to stopping such therapy.

5. Subcutaneous Immunotherapy in Pregnancy

Allergen immunotherapy is effective in the pregnant patient, and maintenance doses may be continued during pregnancy. When a patient receiving immunotherapy reports that she is pregnant, the dose of immunotherapy usually is not increased; rather, the patient is maintained on the dose she is receiving at that time. Allergen immunotherapy is usually not initiated during pregnancy because of risks associated with a potential systemic reaction and its treatment. Systemic reactions are more likely to occur during the buildup phase of immunotherapy. Possible complications include spontaneous abortion, premature labor, and fetal hypoxia. The initiation of immunotherapy may be considered during pregnancy for the patient with life-threatening Hymenoptera sensitivity (16).

C. Modified Extracts/Vaccines

Despite the established efficacy of subcutaneous injection of conventional aqueous inhalant allergen vaccines, a variety of problems exist. First, they may induce systemic reactions that can be life-threatening. Second, the buildup phase of conventional immunotherapy generally requires 25–30 injections, each of which involves time and cost to the patient. Because of these problems, many investigators have attempted to modify inhalant allergen extracts to reduce the problems associated with aqueous vaccines (45). These modifications can be divided into three approaches: slowing absorption, inducing tolerance, and reducing allergenicity while retaining immunogenicity. Alum-precipitated extracts are an example of the slow absorption approach (46); they are the only modified extracts available in the United States. Ragweed, cat, and grass alum-precipitated vaccines have been studied and found to have the equivalent efficacy of aqueous vaccines. Systemic reactions are decreased; rarely, some patients experience a prolonged local reaction following administration of alum-precipitated vaccines (20). Aggregation of the proteins of an aqueous vaccine reduces the allergenicity while preserving the immunogenicity of the product. Two methods of modification have accomplished this goal: polyethylene glycol (PEG)–treated allergens and glutaraldehyde-treated allergens (polymerized allergen extracts). Regimens using the latter permit completion of an immunotherapy program with 10 to 15 injections with a less than 1% occurrence of systemic reactions (47). One trial of

Table 2 Example of Dosage Schedule for Polymerized Ragweed Injections

Week	ug Amb a 1 ml	Volume
1	25	0.10
2		0.25
3		0.50
4	250	0.10
5		0.25
6–15	250	0.50

immunotherapy with polymerized vaccines demonstrated clinical improvement lasting at least 4 years following a course of treatment. The FDA has not approved any modified extract other than alum-precipitated extracts. Most immunotherapy outside the United States employs modified extracts (4).

1. Dosage Schedules

A variety of dosage schedules have been published for modified vaccines. An example of an efficacious protocol for glutaraldehyde-polymerized vaccines is shown in Table 2. Most modified vaccines require fewer than half the injections necessary with standard aqueous immunotherapy.

2. Techniques

Most modified vaccines are marketed for usual subcutaneous injection at weekly intervals. However, modified dosage schedules such as rush or cluster schedules have been published (48).

3. Reactions and Dosage Adjustment

The package insert that accompanies modified vaccines generally advises physicians relative to the risk of reactions and dosage adjustment following reactions. For the most part, the reactions are similar to those with usual aqueous vaccines and the dosage adjustments are similar.

4. When to Stop

For glutaraldehyde-polymerized vaccines, 10 to 15 injections have been reported to result in efficacy for up to 6 years (49). Most other modified vaccines have not been studied as to persistence of efficacy after discontinuation of therapy. It should be noted that some forms of modification that reduce allergenicity can also denature the allergens; therefore, modified vaccines such as pyridine-extracted allergens should be used only if clinical efficacy has been demonstrated by appropriately controlled clinical trials. In general, package inserts accompanying modified allergen vaccines include recommendations relative to a course of therapy.

III. SALIENT POINTS

1. Allergen immunotherapy is defined as the repeated administration of specific allergens to patients with IgE-mediated conditions for the purpose of providing protection against the allergic symptoms and inflammatory reactions associated with natural exposure to these allergens.

2. The most commonly used form of inhalant allergen immunotherapy in the United States is subcutaneous injection of aqueous vaccines.

3. While various low-dose immunotherapy regimens have been published, optimal efficacy results from a high-dose immunotherapy schedule such as illustrated in Table 1.

4. Most systemic reactions occur during the buildup phase and in highly allergic patients.

5. Administering an incorrect dose can result in severe systemic reactions; the patient, vial, dilution, and immunotherapy schedule must be individually identified prior to administration of an injection of inhalant allergen. If there was a significant reaction to the previous immunotherapy dose or if the time interval is longer than designated, the dose may require adjustment.

6. If a patient has been on immunotherapy maintenance doses for more than a year without improvement, the immunotherapy should probably be discontinued. If improvement has occurred, the patient should be treated for 2 or 3 improved seasons before consideration of discontinuation.

7. Standardized extracts as of 2003 include cat hair, cat pelt, *Dermatophagoides pteronyssinus*, *Dermatophagoides farinae*, short ragweed, Bermuda grass, Kentucky bluegrass, perennial ryegrass, orchard grass, timothy grass, meadow fescue, red top, sweet vernal grass, and Hymenoptera venoms (yellow jacket, honeybee, wasp, yellow hornet, and white-faced hornet).

8. Allergen immunotherapy is effective in the pregnant patient, and maintenance doses may be continued during pregnancy. Allergen immunotherapy is usually not initiated during pregnancy because of risks associated with a potential systemic reaction and its treatment. Possible complications include spontaneous abortion, premature labor, and fetal hypoxia.

REFERENCES

1. Freeman J, Noon L. Further observation on the treatment of hayfever by hypodermic inoculations of pollen vaccine. Lancet 1911; 2:814–817.
2. Reisman R, Tronolone M. Immunotherapy: A practical review and guide. Immunol Allergy Clin North Am 2000; 20(3):469–478.
3. Bernstein IL, Nicklas RA, Greenberger PA, Pearlman D, Zeitz S, Blaiss M. Practice parameters for allergen immunotherapy. J Allergy Clin Immunol 1996; 98:1001–1011.
4. Grammer LC. Principles of immunologic management of allergic diseases due to extrinsic antigens. In: Patterson's Allergic Diseases: Diagnosis and Management (Grammer LC, Greenberger PA, eds.). Philadelphia, PA: J. B. Lippincott, 2002: 183–194.
5. Norman PS. Allergic rhinitis. In: Samter's Immunologic Diseases (Austen, Frank, eds.). Philadelphia, PA: Lippincott Williams and Wilkins, 2001; 817–824.
6. Nelson HS. Immunotherapy for inhalant allergens. In: Allergy: Principles and Practice (Middleton E, Reed CE, Ellis EF, Adkinson NF, Yuninger JW, Busse WW, eds.). St. Louis, MO: C. V. Mosby, 1998: 1050–1062.
7. Portnoy J. Immunotherapy for inhalant allergies—Guidelines for why, when and how to use this treatment. Postgrad Med 2001; 109:89–106.
8. Bousquet J, Michel FB. Specific immunotherapy in asthma: Is it effective? J Allergy Clin Immunol 1994; 94:1–11.
9. Alvarez-Cuesta E, Cuesta-Herranz J, Puyana-Ruiz J, Cuesta-Herranz C, Blanco-Quiros A. Monoclonal antibody-standardized cat extract immunotherapy: Risk-benefit effects from a double-blind placebo study. J Allergy Clin Immunol 1994; 93:556–566.

10. Horst M, Hejjaoui A, Horst V, Michel FB, Bousquet J. Double-blind, placebo-controlled rush immunotherapy with a standardized *Alternaria* extract. J Allergy Clin Immunol 1990, 85:460–472.

11. Malling HJ, Dreborg S, Weeke B. Diagnosis and immunotherapy of mold allergy. V. Clinical efficacy and side effects of immunotherapy with *Cladosporium herbarum*. Allergy 1986; 41:507–519.

12. Solomon WR, Platts-Mills TAE. Aerobiology of inhalant allergens. In: Allergy: Principles and Practice (Middleton E, Reed CE, Ellis EF, Adkinson NF, Yunginger JW, Busse WW, eds.). St. Louis, MO: C.V. Mosby, 1993: 469–528.

13. Chang WWY. Pollen survey of the United States. In: Allergic Diseases: Diagnosis and Management (Patterson R, Grammer LC, Greenberger PA, eds.). Philadelphia, PA: J.B. Lippincott, 1997: 131–166.

14. Sichere SH, Eggleston PA. Environmental allergens. In: Allergic Diseases: Diagnosis and Treatment (Lieberman P, Anderson JA, eds.). Totowa, NJ: Humana Press, 1997: 37–46.

15. Baer H. Potency units for allergenic extracts in the USA. Arb Paul Ehrlich Inst 1987; 80:167–168.

16. Li J, Lockey R, Bernstein L, Portnoy J, Nicklas RA. Allergen immunotherapy: A practice parameter. Ann Allergy Asthma Immunol 2003; 90:1–35.

17. Ipsen H, Klysner SS, Larsen JN, Lowenstein H, Matthiesen F, Schou C, Sparholt SH. Allergenic extracts. In: Allergy:Principles and Practice (Middleton E, Reed CE, Ellis EF, Adkinson NF, Yunginger JW, Busse WW, eds.). St. Louis, MO: C.V. Mosby, 1993: 529–553.

18. Dreborg S. Precision of biologic standardization of allergenic preparations. Allergy 1992; 47:291–294.

19. Helm RM, Gauerke MB, Baer H, Lowenstein H, Ford A, Levy DA, Norman PS, Yunginger JW. Production and testing of an international reference standard of short ragweed pollen extract. J Allergy Clin Immunol 1984; 73:790–800.

20. Tippet J. Comprehensive care in the allergy/asthma office. Immunol Allergy Clin North Am 1999; 19(1):129–148.

21. Bruun E. Controlled examination of the specificity of specific desensitization in asthma. Acta Allergol 1949; 2:122–128.

22. Pence HL, Mitchell DQ, Greely RL, Updegraff BR, Selfridge HA. Immunotherapy for mountain cedar pollinosis: A double-blind controlled study. J Allergy Clin Immunol 1976; 58:39–50.

23. Rak S, Hakanson L, Venge P. Immunotherapy abrogates the generation of eosinophil and neutrophil chemotactic activity during the pollen season. J Allergy Clin Immunol 1990; 86:706–713.

24. Ortolani C, Pestorello E, Moss RB, Hsu YP, Restuccia M, Joppolo G, Miadonna A, Cornelli V, Halpern G, Zanussi C.. Grass pollen immunotherapy: A single year double blind placebo controlled study in patients with grass pollen induced asthma and rhinitis. J Allergy Clin Immunol 1984; 73:283–290.

25. Reid MJ, Moss RB, Hsu YP, Kwasnicki JM, Commerford TM, Nelson BL. Seasonal asthma in northern California: allergic causes and efficacy of immunotherapy. J Allergy Clin Immunol 1986; 78:590–600.

26. Norman PS, Winkenwerder WL, Lichtenstein LM. Immunotherapy of ragweed hayfever with antigen E: Comparison with whole pollen extract and placebos. J Allergy 1968; 42:93–108.

27. Van Meter TE, Adkinson NF, Amodio FJ, Lichtenstein LM, Mardiney MR, Norman PS, Rosenberg GL, Kagey-Sobotka A, Valentine MD. A comparative study of the effectiveness of the Rinkel method and of the current standard method of immunotherapy for ragweed pollen hay fever. J Allergy Clin Immunol 1980; 66:500–513.

28. Horst M, Hejjaoui A, Horst V, Michel FB, Bousquet J. Double blind placebo controlled rush immunotherapy with a standardized *Alternaria* extract. J Allergy Clin Immunol 1990; 85:460–472.

29. Malling HJ, Dreborg S, Weeke B. Diagnosis and immunotherapy of mould allergy. V. Clinical efficacy and side effects of immunotherapy with *Cladisporium herbarum.* Allergy 1986; 41:507–519.

30. McHugh SM, Lavelle B, Kemeny DM, Patel S, Ewan PW. A placebo controlled trial of immunotherapy with two extracts of *Dermatophagoides pteronyssinus* in allergic rhinitis, comparing clinical outcome with antigen specific IgE, IgG, and IgG subclasses. J Allergy Clin Immunol 1990; 86:521–531.

31. Bousquet J, Hejjaoui A, Clauzel AM, Guerin B, Dhivert H, Skassa-Brociek W, Michel FB. Specific immunotherapy with a standardized *Dermatophagoides pteronyssinus* extract. II. Prediction of efficacy of immunotherapy. J Allergy Clin Immunol 1988; 78:971–977.

32. Nelson HS, Ikle D, Buchmeier A. Studies of allergen extract stability: The effects of dilution and mixing. J Allergy Clin Immunol 1996; 98:382–388.

33. Bousquet J, Lockey R, Malling H, WHO panel members. Allergen immunotherapy: Therapeutic vaccines for allergic diseases, a WHO position paper. J Allergy Clin Immunol 1998; 102:558–562.

34. Norman PS, Winkenwerder WL, Lichtenstein LM. Trials of alum-precipitated pollen extracts in the treatment of hayfever. J Allergy Clin Immunol 1972; 50:31–44.

35. Van Metre TE, Marsh DG, Adkinson NF, Kagey-Sobotka A, Khattignovong A, Norman PS, Rosenberg GL. Immunotherapy decreases skin sensitivity to cat extract.J Allergy Clin Immunol 1989; 83:888–899.

36. Bousquet J, Calvayrac P, Guerin B, Hejjaoui A, Dhivert H, Hewitt B, Michel FB. Immunotherapy with a standardized *Dermatophagoides pteronyssinus* extract. J Allergy Clin Immunol 1985; 76:734–744.

37. Bousquet J, Guerin B, Dotte A, Dhivert H, Djoukhadar F, Hewitt B, Michel FB. Comparison between rush immunotherapy with a standardized allergen and an alum adjuved pyridine extracted material in grass pollen allergy. Clin Allergy 1985; 15:179–193.

38. Bousquet J, Becker WM, Hejjaoui A, Chanal I, Lebel B, Dhivert H, Michel FB. Differences in clinical and immunologic reactivity of patients allergic to grass pollens and to multiple pollen species. II. Efficacy of a double blind, placebo controlled specific immunotherapy with standardized extracts. J Allergy Clin Immunol 1991; 88:43–53.

39. Hejjaoui JJ, Ferrando R, Dhivert H, Michel FB, Bousquet J. Systemic reactions occurring during immunotherapy with standardized pollen extracts. J Allergy Clin Immunol 1992; 89:925–933.

40. Portnoy J, Bagstad K, Kanarek H, et al. Premedication reduces the incidence of systemic reactions during inhalant rush immunotherapy with mixures of allergenic extracts. Ann Allergy 1994; 73:409–418.

41. Tankersley MS, Walker RL, Butler WK, et al. Safety and efficacy of an imported fire and rush immunotherapy protocol with and without prophylactic treatment. J Allergy Clin Immunol 2002; 109:556–562.

42. Van Metre TE, Adkinson NF, Amodio FJ, Lichtenstein LM, Mardiney MR, Norman PS, Rosenberg GL, Sobotka AK. A comparison of immunotherapy schedules for injection treatment of ragweed hayfever. J Allergy Clin Immunol 1982; 69:181–193.

43. Lockey RF, Benedict LM, Turkeltaub PC, Bukantz SC. Fatalities from immunotherapy (IT) and skin testing (ST). J Allergy Clin Immunol 1987; 79:660–677.

44. Durham SR, Walker SM, Varga EM, et al. Long-term clinical efficacy of grass-pollen immunotherapy. N Engl J Med 1999; 341:468–475.

45. Grammer LC, Shaughnessy MA, Patterson R. Modified forms of allergen immunotherapy. J Allergy Clin Immunol 1986; 76:297–301.

46. Varney VA, Gaga M, Frew AJ, Aber VR, Durham SR. Usefulness of immunotherapy in patients with severe hayfever uncontrolled by antiallergic drugs. Br Med J 1991; 302:265–269.

47. Marsh DG, Kiechtenstein LM, Campbell DN. Studies on allergoids, prepared from naturally occurring allergens. I. Assay of allergenicity and antigenicity of formalinized rye group 1 component. Immunology 1970; 18:705–710.

48. Bousquet J, Hejjaoui JA, Skassa-Brociek W, Guerin B, Maasch HJ, Dhivert H, Michel FB. Double blind placebo controlled immunotherapy with mixed grass pollen allergoids. I. Rush immunotherapy with allergoids and standardized orchard grass pollen extract. J Allergy Clin Immunol 1987; 80:591–598.

49. Grammer LC, Shaughnessy MA, Suszko IM, Shaughnessy JJ, Patterson R. Persistence of efficacy after a brief course of polymerized ragweed allergen: A controlled study. J Allergy Clin Immunol 1984; 73:484–489.

26

Immunotherapy for Allergic Rhinoconjunctivitis

HANS-JØRGEN MALLING

National University Hospital, Copenhagen, Denmark

I. INTRODUCTION

Allergic rhinitis, the most common allergic disease, affects about 20% of the adult population (1). The disease, which predominantly affects children and young adults, impairs both physical and cognitive functions and quality of life (2). Furthermore, allergic rhinitis constitutes a major risk factor for development of allergic asthma, with approximately 20% of patients with allergic rhinitis developing asthma later in life (2–4); patients with bronchial hyperreactivity are more likely to develop asthma (5,6). Management of allergic rhinoconjunctivitis is based on combining three essential interventions: allergen avoidance, pharmacological treatment, and allergen-specific immunotherapy with careful education of the patient on the nature of the disease. Education should include identification of triggers and relievers, step-ups and step-downs of drug treatment, and recognition of disease involvement of the lower airways (2). Nonspecific interventions are not restricted to the causative allergen, as is the case with pharmacological treatment and avoidance of nonspecific irritants. Specific interventions include avoidance of the causative allergen and allergen-specific immunotherapy. This chapter deals only with subcutaneous injection immunotherapy. Oral and inhaled routes of immunotherapy (local) are dealt with in Chapter 33.

II. TREATMENT STRATEGY

The treatment strategy for allergic rhinitis includes symptom reduction by drugs, attempts to interfere in the inflammatory cascade by anti-inflammatory drugs, and allergen-specific immunotherapy. The relative advantages of these interventions are unknown, but the combination of interventions at different levels should improve the clinical outcome. Allergen avoidance always is the first-line attempt and, even when not completely effective, may reduce the need for additional interventions (7). Drug treatment is often the next step to reduce disease severity, but for patients with a constant need for preventive (local steroids) pharmacotherapy, it is advantageous to institute immunotherapy early, while the severity of the disease is modest and when the possibility of preventing development of asthma is highest (8,9). Among the advantages of immunotherapy is its capacity to interfere with the pathophysiological mechanisms of allergic inflammation, with a potential for a prolonged effect or cure, compared with strictly pharmacological treatment, which only reduces symptoms during administration, with no long-term preventive capacity (8,9). Although drugs are highly effective and without important side effects, drugs represent a symptomatic treatment, while immunotherapy represents the only treatment that might alter the natural course of the disease (10). Using an appropriate allergen vaccine and correct indication, immunotherapy can significantly reduce the severity of the allergic disease, reduce the need for anti-allergic drugs, and consequently improve the quality of life for allergic patients (11).

A significant proportion of rhinitis patients have minimal persistent inflammation in the lower airways during allergen exposure (12), but symptoms from the lower airways seldom disturb the patients, and the inflammation is therefore rarely or insufficiently treated. Immunotherapy, as a solitary treatment, might ameliorate inflammatory reactions independently of the shock organ. Consequently, considering the allergen-IgE–mediated disease as a multi-organ disease, it is important to consider immunotherapy based on the allergen sensitization rather than on the disease or symptoms (9). Determining the advantages of combining allergen avoidance, immunotherapy, and drug treatment requires further investigations of single and combined treatment focusing on patient compliance, long-term preventive aspects, cost-effectiveness, and side effects.

The advantages of introducing disease-modifying interventions (allergen avoidance and immunotherapy) should be carefully evaluated in defining the treatment strategy for allergic diseases. It is obviously advantageous to apply a specific treatment to interfere with the activation of the immunological mechanisms involved in allergic diseases rather than to treat only symptoms. Furthermore, the exclusive use of drug treatment may affect the identification of specific allergen sensitization in the future. Basically, allergen identification is essential for prescribing specific treatment. The need to know the specific allergens to which a patient is sensitive is not essential for drug treatment, which is effective for both allergic and nonallergic symptoms. Not knowing the specific allergens might reduce the possibility of directly avoiding allergens responsible for inducing symptoms and exacerbations and interfere with the patient's recognition of factors inducing symptoms.

New insights into allergic inflammation are providing a platform for further investigations of the advantages and drawbacks of different intervention strategies and for the development of effective and safe treatment practices. Conventional immunotherapy using native allergen extracts to constitute vaccines may be replaced by a more refined and precisely targeted allergen-specific immunological intervention based on efficacy and side effect validation. While awaiting this development, allergists must continue to use the conventional allergen-specific intervention strategy.

III. CLINICAL EFFICACY

Allergic patients suffer from the clinical manifestations of the disease, i.e., rhinitis, conjunctivitis, and asthma. Consequently, the only parameter indicating the efficacy of a treatment is the reduction in symptoms and/or drug intake of a magnitude, from a clinical point of view, that significantly reduces the morbidity of allergic disorders (13). This can be estimated either by investigating the reduction in symptom/medication scores in relation to a pretreatment observation period (a season for seasonal allergies or a sufficiently long comparative period in the case of perennial allergies) or by comparing matched groups treated by active immunotherapy and by placebo. Changes in immunological parameters and challenge tests may be of interest in elucidating mechanisms but cannot replace clinical evaluation.

The magnitude of efficacy (minimal clinically relevant reduction in disease severity) may be debated. By including a high number of participants, statistically significant but clinically irrelevant differences might be observed. The magnitude of efficacy should be clinically relevant; i.e., the reduction in symptom scores and drug consumption should, from a clinical point, significantly reduce the morbidity of the disease. A review of 68 placebo-controlled, double-blind (PCDB) studies presenting symptom/medication scores (13) indicated that a reduction in disease severity >30% above the placebo effect was considered clinically relevant (and compatible with statistically significant differences). Depending on the risks of intervention, costs, and inconvenience, this figure is subject to change.

In evaluating the clinical efficacy of interventions it is critical that the study be designed to give conclusive answers. The primary and, when appropriate, secondary outcome measures should be clearly defined. The sample size should be large enough to provide a high probability (power) of detecting, as statistically significant, a clinically important difference of a given size if such a difference exists. Patients should be randomized to study groups to avoid bias in group characteristics, and the study should be a true placebo-controlled, double-blind trial.

The majority of studies evaluating clinical efficacy focus on short-term efficacy, i.e., efficacy obtained during active treatment, often after a rather short period of treatment for 6 months to 1 year. This degree of efficacy is important, but a major argument for instituting immunotherapy is to obtain long-term disease-modifying capacity (and to achieve preventive capacity).

A. Long-Term Efficacy

A fundamental objective in assessing the applicability of immunotherapy is to document its long-term efficacy and preventive capacity. Without long-term reduction in disease severity after termination of treatment and disease-modifying capability, immunotherapy may not be cost-effective, and consequently may not be a real alternative to pharmacological treatment (8). Some older studies indicate that the treatment may have a long-lasting effect. The PCDB study published by Durham et al. (14) is a continuation of a previous study documenting efficacy of the treatment (15). Patients with severe grass pollen rhinitis not controlled by standard anti-allergic drugs, including topical glucocorticosteroids, showed a reduction in symptoms and in the need for rescue drugs of >60% compared with placebo treatment after less than 1 year of grass pollen immunotherapy. After 3 more years of active treatment, patients were re-randomized to continue with active immunotherapy or to receive placebo. At termination of the study, no significant difference in symptom/medication scores between patients continuing and those discontinuing immunotherapy was found, and compared with a matched control group of patients not receiving immunotherapy, the reduction in disease severity was >75%. An open study compared 13 patients, 6 years after having been terminated following 3 years of grass pollen immunotherapy, with 10 patients of the former control group. Clinical symptoms and the use of rescue drugs in formerly immunotherapy-treated patients were significantly lower than in the control group (16).

B. Preventive Capacity

The capacity of immunotherapy to suppress the development of new sensitization was suggested by two large-scale studies in patients sensitized to one allergen only (17,18). The Purello-D'Ambrosio study (17) followed, in an open retrospective design, 7182 originally monosensitized (to a variety of allergens) patients treated with immunotherapy for 4 years and off immunotherapy for 3 years. The control group consisted of 1214 comparable patients followed for 7 years. The development of sensitization to new allergens at the 4 year follow-up was 68% in the control group versus 24% in the immunotherapy group. Corresponding figures at the 7-year follow-up were 78% and 27%, respectively. The difference between the control group and immunotherapy-treated group is statistically and clinically convincing. The Pajno study (18) followed 75 immunotherapy-treated children monosensitized to house dust mites and 63 comparable controls treated pharmacologically for 6 years. The results showed that 74% of the immunotherapy-treated patients versus 33% in the control group continued to be monosensitized (specific IgE to only one allergen).

Immunotherapy as a preventive measure against the progression of rhinitis to asthma has also been suggested in some historical studies. A multicenter study, the preventive allergy treatment study, investigated the capacity of immunotherapy for allergic rhinitis to prevent the disease progressing to asthma (19). Children with allergy to birch and grass pollens, without clinical evidence of lower airway hyperreactivity, were randomized to receive either immunotherapy or an optimal pharmacological treatment. After 3 years of treatment, the number of patients developing clinical asthma was statistically reduced in the immunotherapy group. The percentage of immunotherapy-treated patients with newly developed asthma was 24% versus 44% in the drug-treated group, indicating that the high risk of developing symptoms of the lower airways in allergic rhinitis patients may be diminished by immunotherapy. Furthermore, the study showed that careful evaluation for asthma uncovered 20% of unidentified mild seasonal asthma in the 205 children recruited for rhinitis. Bronchial hyperresponsiveness to methacholine decreased significantly in immunotherapy-treated patients, but only 2 out of 40 patients with asthma at inclusion were free of asthma after 3 years, indicating that immunotherapy has a greater capacity for preventing than for curing asthma.

IV. CONTROLLED STUDIES TO DEMONSTRATE EFFICACY

Published studies indicate that allergen-specific immunotherapy is an effective treatment for allergic rhinoconjunctivitis, under the conditions of careful selection of patients and the use of quality allergen extracts for treatment vaccines (13). In 1998 the author reviewed all double-blind, placebo-controlled immunotherapy studies (peer-reviewed full papers in English) published since 1980 providing symptom medication scores (13). The reason for not including older studies is that this arbitrary limit coincides with the general use of vaccines constituted from adequately standardized allergen extracts. Clinical efficacy was estimated by mean symptom medication scores or by measuring the area under the curve of symptom/medication scores during the registration period for the active group and the placebo group (Fig. 1). The magnitude of improvement induced by active treatment was calculated as the percentage reduction in disease severity (symptom medication scores) compared with placebo treatment. In 43 studies fulfilling the strict inclusion criteria, a mean clinical efficacy (i.e., an additional improvement in disease severity above the response to placebo injection) of 45% was observed in 1120 actively treated patients. An arbitrary lower limit for clinical efficacy of 30% improvement was chosen to balance clinically relevant efficacy with the inconvenience and risks of injection immunotherapy.

Using this approach, >75% of published studies documented the clinical value of immunotherapy. This magnitude of efficacy is equivalent to that for intranasal corticosteroids and better than that for antihistamines (2). Since the publication of the original review, five more double-blind, placebo-controlled studies evaluating the clinical efficacy of immunotherapy in rhinitis have been published (Table 1) (20–24). These studies

Symptom score

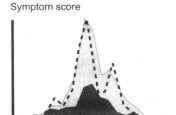

Medication score

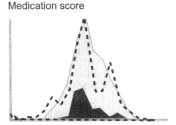

Figure 1 Magnitude of clinical efficacy estimated by measuring the area under the curve (AUC) of immunotherapy-treated patients (darkly shaded areas) as a percentage of placebo-treated patients (lightly shaded area). The median symptom score and medication score of the immunotherapy group was 39% and 28% of the placebo group, respectively, indicating a mean reduction in symptoms of 61% and of 72% in medication scores. The dotted line represents airborne grass pollen counts. Data adapted from Varney et al. (15).

Table 1 Placebo-Controlled, Double-Blind Immunotherapy Studies in Rhinitis Patients Published in 1998–2003

Author and year of publication	Age group	Allergen	Type of extract	Duration	Maximum dose	Number of patients		Significance	Clinical effect	Systemic side effects percentage of patients
						IT group	Placebo			
Belda (20), 1998	Ad	Tree pollen	Alum	7 W	1–3 μg Group 1	29	32	p < 0.03	39% improvement	4% Rh+U
Ariano (21), 1999	Ch+Ad	Parietaria	Allergoid Alum	12 M	10,000 AUeq	11	11	p = 0.02	47% improvement	15% As 23% Rh
Walker (22), 2001	Ad	Grass	Alum	24 M	20 μg Phl p 5	20	17	p < 0.01	48% improvement	20% mild
Leynadier (23), 2001	Ad	Grass	Calcium Ph	12 M	2.1 μg Phl p 5	15	12	p < 0.05	38% improvement	44% Rh+U 13% As
Bodtger (24), 2002	Ad	Birch	Alum	10 M	12 μg Bet v 1	17	17	p < 0.04	36% improvement	24% mild

Abbreviations: Ad = adults, Ch = children, W = weeks, M = months, As = asthma, Ax = anaphylaxis, Rh = rhinitis, U = urticaria.

Number of studies

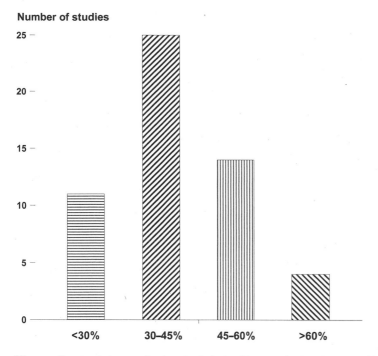

Figure 2 Graded magnitude of clinical efficacy of placebo-controlled, double-blind rhinitis immunotherapy studies published in 1980–2003, graded as efficacy <30% (no clinically relevant efficacy), efficacy 30–45% (low degree of efficacy), efficacy 45–60% (moderate degree of efficacy), and efficacy >60% (high degree of efficacy). The 48 clinical studies result in 54 groups comparable with placebo, as some studies include two actively treated groups.

confirm the conclusion of the initial review (13) but add birch and other tree pollens to the list of effective allergen vaccines. All studies are statistically significant compared with placebo, and the mean clinical effect is a reduction in disease severity of 42%, which is quite comparable to the 45% originally described. The additional number of actively treated patients is 92, bringing the total number of patients supporting the evidence of efficacy to about 1200. Adding these recently published studies to the original review (13), 80% of published studies document a clinically relevant clinical efficacy (Fig. 2). Looking at the allergens used in these studies, grass pollens make up almost 40%, and only about 10% of studies use non-pollen vaccines (house dust mites and *Alternaria*) (Fig. 3).

An interesting non–placebo-controlled, double-blind comparative study evaluated the clinical efficacy of birch pollen immunotherapy versus nasal glucocorticosteroid administered as budesonide, 400 µg daily (25). Symptom scores in the two groups were identical during the first 4 weeks of the 6-week season, and only during the final 2 weeks did nasal glucocorticosteroid–treated patients show fewer symptoms than the immunotherapy-treated group. No differences in medication scores were observed, indicating that a short course of preseasonal immunotherapy is almost as effective as high-dose intranasal glucocorticosteroid. An additional effect of immunotherapy, reinforcing that it represents a systemic treatment with effect on both the upper and the lower airways, was that seasonal peak expiratory flow values decreased significantly only in the nasal glucocorticosteroid–treated

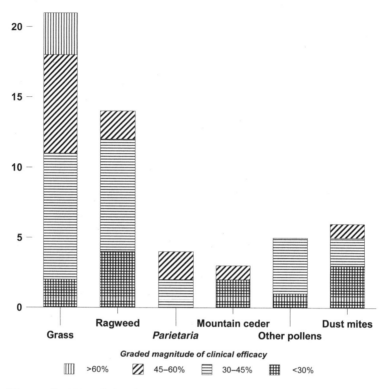

Number of studies

Figure 3 The relation between the allergen vaccines used in placebo-controlled, double-blind rhinitis immunotherapy studies published in 1980–2003 and the graded magnitude of clinical efficacy. One study with *Alternaria* (efficacy 75%) is not included.

patients and, furthermore, only immunotherapy prevented the seasonal bronchial hyperresponsiveness and eosinophil activation in asthmatic patients.

V. INDICATION AND CONTRAINDICATIONS

A. Indication

In defining the indication for immunotherapy for inhalant allergies, it is advantageous to recognize that the allergen-IgE reaction results in a multi-organ disease, with symptoms in many patients occurring in the eyes, nose, and lungs (9). Some patients have symptoms predominantly from one organ (which does not, however, indicate that they have no inflammation in other parts of the airways) (12). Consequently, all symptoms should be considered in selecting the most appropriate treatment of the allergic disease (9). Before instituting immunotherapy, the following must be considered: (1) the severity and duration of symptoms, (2) the requirement for and the effects of drugs, (3) the risk incurred by the treatment and by the disease, (4) psychological factors, and (5) the patient's attitude in relation to alleviating symptoms (drugs) versus trying to interfere with the pathophysiological background of the disease (specific treatment).

The indication for immunotherapy in allergic rhinoconjunctivitis relates to both the severity of the disease and the duration of the symptoms (8,9). Mild symptoms that respond adequately to oral or topical antihistamines are no indication for beginning immunotherapy. However, a need for repeated courses of topical glucocorticosteroids (applying to both a short or a long season) or symptoms lasting several months (even if these symptoms are rather mild and respond to pharmacological treatment) may favor initiating immunotherapy (8).

The number of drug doses needed to reduce symptoms and the frequency of daily administrations and the number of organs needing treatment have an important influence on the rationale for adding immunotherapy to the general treatment strategy (in an attempt to reduce the requirement for drugs optimally to a p.r.n. basis). It is a mistake to institute immunotherapy only in patients who do not respond to drug treatment or who develop side effects during drug treatment (8). Even though some guidelines recommend giving allergen immunotherapy only when all other forms of treatments fail, immunotherapy may be considered in patients with mild disease. Optimal results of immunotherapy are obtained in patients with mild disease, i.e., requiring a rather modest pharmacological treatment (26). Young patients (children) respond better to immunotherapy than adults (8), an effect that may be related to the age of the patient, but is more likely related to the duration of the disease. Attempts to interfere with the natural course of the disease should be introduced at a time when the patient has the capacity to respond positively, i.e., before the disease becomes a chronic, irreversible condition (27).

Risk/benefit assessments of both the disease and its possible treatments are important for evaluating the indication for immunotherapy (8,9). The disabling nature of rhinitis, which diminishes performance capacity in schoolwork, employment, and social contacts, is of great importance to the suffering patient (quality of life) (28). Of additional concern is that a number of rhinitis patients develop asthma in the course of the disease (29,30). Asthma is more severe in relation to acute attacks, hospital admissions, and days off work, and it may result in chronic pulmonary insufficiency. Therefore, inadequate treatment is associated with a considerably increased risk (27,31).

The hazards of immunotherapy are strictly related to the risk of inducing anaphylactic reactions. The rate of severe systemic reactions in patients with rhinitis treated with high-potency vaccines is approximately 5% of injections (32,33), primarily during the induction phase (8). Because in asthmatics the risk of systemic reactions is slightly higher, primarily due to bronchial obstruction, it is mandatory to monitor lung function before injections and to ensure an optimal anti-asthmatic pharmacological treatment in patients with symptoms of the lower airways (8,9). Systemic reactions represent a general limitation for the use of immunotherapy; therefore, the indication and possibly also the practical treatment must be the responsibility of a specialist who is aware of the risks of immunotherapy and capable of preventing systemic reactions and treating them when they occur (8,9).

Psychological factors include compliance with drug intake and the patient's assumption of a disease state due to constant use of medications. Studies of drug compliance in asthmatic patients show that only approximately half of the prescribed drugs are actually consumed (34,35). Drug compliance may be higher in rhinitis, due to the shorter duration of symptoms in seasonal allergic rhinitis, but patients tend to tolerate some symptoms (in a considerable number of patients, rather severe symptoms) without discontinuing the p.r.n.-based use of systemic or topical antihistamines and substituting the more effective topical glucocorticosteroids (36). It is important in treating allergic diseases to be aware of the patient's perception of disease severity and psychological motivation and the scientific understanding of the rationale for treating the allergic inflammation.

Based on their increased insight regarding the risks of taking medications, more patients are asking their physicians for a treatment modality with the potential to intervene in the natural cause of the disease (immunotherapy), in contrast to continuing medications that only reduce symptoms.

Several aspects of the treatment of allergic rhinitis require careful consideration: (1) About 10% of rhinitics experience symptoms of the lower airways—often not considered or treated as asthma; (2) those patients whose only presenting symptoms are from the upper airways have a significant risk of developing asthma; (3) patients with less intense symptoms need less symptomatic treatment, but on the other hand, intervention in the natural course of the disease is more successful. There are no definite rules for the institution of immunotherapy in rhinitis. The initiation of immunotherapy is based on careful balancing of its advantages and disadvantages, taking into consideration the patient's attitude to both the symptoms and possible treatments of the disease (8). Analyzed in this way, immunotherapy is not considered the ultimate treatment, but rather a supplement to drug treatment administration in the early phase of the disease (8,9). The considerations for initiating immunotherapy in allergic rhinitis (2,8,9) are listed in Table 2.

Table 2 Considerations for Initiating Immunotherapy in Allergic Rhinitis

---

1. IgE-mediated disease should be demonstrated by the presence of clinically significant positive skin test and/or serum-specific IgE.
2. Specific allergen sensitivity is responsible for clinical symptoms, and the specific sensitivity is responsible for the induction and the severity of symptoms.
   - Confirmed by appearance of symptoms after natural exposure to allergens identified by allergy testing, or
   - Confirmed, if required, by challenge with relevant allergen
3. Nonspecific triggers may play an additional but minimal role in the induction of symptoms.
4. Severity and duration of symptoms:
   - Involvement of lower airways
   - Symptoms induced by succeeding seasons or perennial exposure
5. Response of symptoms to non–disease-modifying intervention:
   - Response to allergen avoidance/reduction
   - Response to pharmacotherapy
6. The availability of standardized high-quality allergen extracts gives confidence in preparing efficacious vaccines for immunotherapy.
7. Clinical efficacy and safety of immunotherapy has been confirmed by randomized placebo-controlled, double-blind studies.
8. Psychological considerations:
   - Cost and effectiveness of intervention
   - Attitude toward pharmacotherapy
   - Impaired quality of life despite adequate pharmacotherapy
9. No relative contraindications.

Adapted from Refs. 8 and 9.

Generally, immunotherapy in allergic rhinoconjunctivitis is indicated for

> Patients with symptoms induced predominantly by allergen exposure
> Patients with a prolonged season or with symptoms induced by successive pollen seasons
> Patients with symptoms of the lower airways during peak allergen exposure
> Patients in whom antihistamines and topical medications insufficiently control symptoms
> Patients who do not want to be on pharmacotherapy
> Patients who do not want to be on constant or long-term pharmacotherapy
> Patients in whom pharmacotherapy induces undesirable side effects

B. Contraindications

In contrast to the multitude of aspects to consider in defining the indication for immunotherapy, relative contraindications are more straightforward (8,9). Relative contraindications include serious immunopathological and immunodeficiency diseases including malignancy, significant cardiovascular diseases (due to the risk of hypotension and the administering of epinephrine), treatment with beta-blockers (which reduces the effectiveness of epinephrine in the treatment of possible systemic reactions), severe asthma uncontrolled by pharmacotherapy and irreversible airway obstruction defined as FEV_1 consistently <70% of predicted value in spite of adequate drug treatment, severe psychological disorders, and lack of compliance. Other relative contraindications include pregnancy, due to the risk of anaphylactic reactions in the mother and consequently possible detrimental effects in the fetus. A well-tolerated and effective immunotherapy regimen may be continued if pregnancy occurs after initiation of immunotherapy. Age is a relative contraindication; in children <5 years of age, immunotherapy with inhalant allergens is rarely indicated due to the less dominant role of inhalation allergens in the total manifestation of the disease, due to the fact that some infants ultimately become asymptomatic, and due to an increased risk of inducing systemic side effects in very young children. When immunotherapy is performed in infants, it is necessary that the physician have extensive experience in the treatment of systemic reactions and be able to establish an intravenous line in that age group. In patients >50 years, the importance of possible allergen sensitization and the likelihood of successful immunotherapy should be carefully weighed against the risk of side effects (8,9).

Specific immunotherapy should be prescribed by specialists and administered by physicians trained in this special treatment and familiar with rescue treatment should anaphylaxis occur (9). The recommended equipment for settings where immunotherapy is administered includes epinephrine for injection; equipment for administering intravenous fluids and oxygen, including an oral airway; equipment for monitoring blood pressure; and glucocorticosteroids, antihistamine, and vasopressor for injection (8,9). When immunotherapy is administered far from intensive care units, additional rescue equipment may be appropriate. The prompt recognition of systemic reactions and the immediate administration of epinephrine, however, are the mainstays of therapy.

VI. DURATION OF IMMUNOTHERAPY

The international guidelines recommend perennial treatment because it achieves a higher cumulative allergen dose while reducing the side effects that are a problem predominantly during the induction phase (8,9). Injection of a high top allergen dose (in the range 5–20 μg major allergen) has been associated with efficacy and possibly also with long-term efficacy persisting after termination of immunotherapy (due to the immune-modulating capacity). Because there may be poorer patient compliance with perennial treatment, several short-term immunotherapy studies have been published (20,37). The problem with this design is that its preseasonal seven-injection regimen results in low-dose immunotherapy (due to a low cumulative allergen dose) and, consequently, the level of efficacy obtained relates only to the allergen season immediately following the preseasonal treatment. The observed immunological changes do not accomplish a fundamental change in the allergic phenotype and consequently do not imply a persistent suppression of the TH2 cytokine profile and do not induce long-term efficacy after termination of immunotherapy. This kind of treatment could be compared with symptomatic drug treatments, which also have a significant capability to suppress the clinical symptoms while being administered, but are without any long-term disease-modifying effect. In terms of at the cost-effectiveness profile, immunotherapy without documented long-term efficacy and preventive capacity is not attractive, especially considering the potential risk of anaphylactic side effects even with low-dose immunotherapy. A maintenance regimen consisting of the use of depot allergen vaccines, given six times per year with an interval of 8 weeks between injections, reduced the total number of injections of a perennial regimen, gave considerably higher doses of allergen, and minimized risks (38).

VII. DISCONTINUATION OF IMMUNOTHERAPY

Immunotherapy is usually intended as a treatment to be administered for a defined period of years. Efficacy is normally manifest after 1 year of treatment, and if no improvement is observed after 2 years of treatment, the probability of obtaining efficacy is low, and immunotherapy should be terminated (8). Short-term treatment has no protracted effect after the treatment is discontinued. Traditionally, immunotherapy (in responding patients) has been continued for 3 years. Given the relatively slow onset of action, and the recent knowledge of the likely mechanisms, there has been a tendency to extend the treatment period to 5 years, as is now used for venom allergy. This is not based on scientific data obtained by studies of inhalant allergies, but is rather an attempt to reduce the risk of relapses. However, when patients respond to treatment, discontinuing immunotherapy after less than 3 years results in a high frequency of relapses (39,40). In patients who improve with allergen administration and deteriorate following discontinuation, immunotherapy treatment could be prolonged. In nonresponders (i.e., patients showing marginal or no efficacy after 1 year of treatment) the indication for immunotherapy should be carefully reassessed, with a view to determining whether the development of concurrent sensitizations is responsible for the persisting symptoms (8). Patients not benefiting from immunotherapy should be discontinued after no more than 2 years of treatment. Likewise, in patients presenting with severe anaphylactic reactions, alternative treatments should be chosen, and this is also true for patients who are not compliant (41).

VIII. SALIENT POINTS

1. Immunotherapy for allergic rhinitis is well documented based on placebo-controlled, double-blind studies on an appropriate number of carefully selected

patients and the use of potent and standardized allergen vaccines in sufficiently high doses.

2. In daily clinical practice, immunotherapy should be performed only with allergen vaccines that in clinical trials have demonstrated clinical efficacy and safety.

3. The magnitude of clinical efficacy (reduction in symptom/medication scores) associated with immunotherapy is equivalent to or better than symptom reduction obtained with optimal pharmacological treatment.

4. The advantage of immunotherapy is the capacity to reduce symptoms and the need for drugs significantly, and to interfere with the natural course of the disease and consequently to prevent progression into more severe disease.

5. Allergen-specific immunotherapy is the only treatment that may alter the natural course of the disease, with a documented long-term efficacy after termination of treatment and preventive capacity.

6. Immunotherapy should be introduced at a time when the patient has the capacity to respond positively, i.e., before the disease deteriorates into a chronic, irreversible state. In this way, immunotherapy does not assume the position of an ultimate treatment principle, but represents a supplement to drug treatment used in the early phase of the disease.

7. Candidates for immunotherapy are rhinitis patients with symptoms almost exclusively induced by allergens, young patients, and especially those with signs of hyperresponsiveness of the lower airways.

8. Perennial subcutaneous immunotherapy is the treatment of choice in severe allergic rhinitis to reduce the development of asthma.

9. Immunotherapy should be continued for at least 3 and probably 5 years in order to obtain long-term persistent clinical efficacy.

REFERENCES

1. Sly RM. Changing prevalence of allergic rhinitis and asthma. Ann Allergy Asthma Immunol 1999; 82:233–248.

2. Bousquet J, Van Cauvenberge P, Khaltaev N. Allergic rhinitis and its impact on asthma. J Allergy Clin Immunol 2001; 108:S147–S334.

3. Linna O, Kokkonen J, Lukin M. A 10-year prognosis for childhood allergic rhinitis. Acta Paedriatr 1992; 81:100–102.

4. Settipane RJ, Hagy GW, Settipane GA. Long-term risk factors for developing asthma and allergic rhinitis: A 23-year follow-up study of college students. Allergy Proc 1994; 15:21–25.

5. Madonini E, Briatico-Vangosa G, Pappacoda A, Maccagni G, Cardani A, Saporiti F. Seasonal increase of bronchial reactivity in allergic rhinitis. J Allergy Clin Immunol 1987; 79:358–363.

6. Braman SS, Barrows AA, DeCotiis BA, Settipane GA, Corrao WM. Airway hyperresponsiveness in allergic rhinitis: A risk factor for asthma. Chest 1987; 91:671–674.

7. Gotzsche PC, Hammerquist C, Burr M. House dust mite control measures in the management of asthma: meta analysis. Br Med J 1998; 317:1105–1110.

8. Malling HJ, Weeke B. EAACI immunotherapy position papers. Allergy 1993; 48(suppl 14):9–35.

9. Bousquet J, Lockey RF, Malling H-J (eds.). Allergen immunotherapy: Therapeutic vaccines for allergic diseases (WHO position paper). Allergy 1998; 53(suppl 44):1–42.

10. Jacobsen L. Preventive allergy treatment as part of allergy disease management. J Investig Allergol Clin Immunol 1997; 7:367–368.

11. Bousquet J, Scheinmann P, Guinnepain MT, Perrin-Fayolle M, Sanvaget J, Tonnel AB, Pauli G, Caillaud D, Dubost R, Leynadier F, Vervloet D, Herman D, Galvaih S, Andre C. Sublingual-swallow immunotherapy (SLIT) in patients with asthma due to house-dust mites: A double-blind, placebo-controlled study. Allergy 1999; 54:249–260.

12. Ciprandi G, Buscaglia S, Pesce G, Pronzato C, Ricca V, Parmiani S, Bagnasco M, Canonica GW. Minimal persistent inflammation is present at mucosal level in patients with asymptomatic rhinitis and mite allergy. J Allergy Clin Immunol 1995; 96:971–979.

13. Malling H-J. Immunotherapy as an effective tool in allergy treatment. Allergy 1998; 53:461–472.

14. Durham SR, Walker SM, Varga EM, Jacobson MR, O'Brien F, Noble W, Till SJ, Hamid QA, Nouri-Aria KT. Long-term clinical efficacy of grass-pollen immunotherapy. N Engl J Med 1999; 341:468–475.

15. Varney VA, Gaga M, Frew AJ, Aber VR, Kay AB, Durham SR. Usefulness of immunotherapy in patients with severe summer hay fever uncontrolled by antiallergic drugs. Br Med J 1991; 302:265–269.

16. Eng PA, Reinhold M, Gnehm HPE. Long-term efficacy of preseasonal grass pollen immunotherapy in children. Allergy 2002; 57:306–312.

17. Purello-D'Ambrosio F, Gangemi S, Merendino RA, Isola S, Puccinelli P, Parmiani S, Ricciardi L. Prevention of new sensitizations in monosensitized subjects submitted to specific immunotherapy or not: A retrospective study. Clin Exp Allergy 2001; 31:1295–1302.

18. Pajno GB, Barberio G, de Luca Fr, Morabito L, Parmiani S. Prevention of new sensitizations in asthmatic children monosensitized to house dust mite by specific immunotherapy: A six-year follow-up study. Clin Exp Allergy 2001; 31:1392–1397.

19. Möller C, Dreborg S, Ferdousi HA, Halken J, Host A, Jacobsen L, Koivikko A, Koller DY, Niggemann B, Norberg LA, Urbanek R, Valovirta E, Wahn U. Pollen immunotherapy reduces the development of asthma in children with seasonal rhinoconjunctivitis (the PAT-study). J Allergy Clin Immunol 2002; 109:251–256.

20. Balda BR, Wolf H, Baumgarten C, Klime KL, Rasp G, Kunkel G, Muller S, Mann W, Hauswald B, Heppt W, Przybilla B, Amon U, Bischoff R, Becher G, Hummel S, Frosch PJ, Rustemeyer T, Jager L, Brehler R, Luger T, Schnitker J. Tree-pollen allergy is efficiently treated by short-term immunotherapy (STI) with seven preseasonal injections of molecular standardized allergens. Allergy 1998; 53:740–748.

21. Ariano R, Kroon AM, Augeri G, Canonica GW, Passalacqua G. Long-term treatment with allergoid immunotherapy with *Parietaria*: Clinical and immunologic effects in a randomized, controlled trial. Allergy 1999; 54:313–319.

22. Walker SM, Pajno GB, Torres Lima M, Wilson DR, Durham SR. Grass pollen immunotherapy for seasonal rhinitis and asthma: A randomized, controlled trial. J Allergy Clin Immunol 2001; 107:87–93.

23. Leynadier F, Banoun L, Dollois B, Terrier P, Epstein M, Guinnepain MT, Firon D, Traube C, Fadel R, Andre C. Immunotherapy with a calcium phosphate–adsorbed five–grass-pollen extract in seasonal rhinoconjunctivitis: A double-blind, placebo-controlled study. Clin Exp Allergy 2001; 31:988–996.

24. Bødtger U, Poulsen LK, Jacobi H, Malling H-J. The safety and efficacy of subcutaneous birch pollen immunotherapy: A one-year, randomised, double-blind, placebo-controlled study. Allergy 2002; 57:297–305.

25. Rak S, Heinrich C, Jacobsen L, Scheynius A, Venge P. A double-blinded, comparative study of the effects of short preseasonal specific immunotherapy and topical steroids in patients with allergic rhinoconjunctivitis and asthma. J Allergy Clin Immunol 2001; 108:921–928.

26. Bousquet J, Hejjaoui A, Clauzel AM, Guerin B, Dhivert H, Skassa-Brociek W, Michael FB. Specific immunotherapy with a standardized *Dermatophagoides pteronyssinus* extract: II. Prediction of efficacy of immunotherapy. J Allergy Clin Immunol 1988; 82:971–977.

27. Bousquet J, Chanez P, Lacoste JY, White R, Vic P, Godard P, Michael FB. Asthma: A disease remodeling the airways. Allergy 1992, 47.3–11.

28. Juniper EF, Guyatt GH, Griffith LE, Ferrie PJ. Interpretation of rhinocunjunctivitis quality of life questionnaire data. J Allergy Clin Immunol 1996; 98:843–845.

29. Strachan DP, Butland BK, Anderson HR. Incidence and prognosis of asthma and wheezing illness from early childhood to age 33 in a national British cohort. Br Med J 1996; 312:1195–1199.

30. Sly RM. Managed care: The key to quality of management of asthma. Ann Allergy 1996; 76:161–163.

31. Peat JK, Woolcook AJ, Cullen K. Rate of decline of lung function in subjects with asthma. Eur J Respir Dis 1987; 70:171–179.

32. Tabar AI, Garcia BE, Rodriguez A, Olaguibel JM, Muro MD, Quirce S. A prospective safety-monitoring study of immunotherapy with biologically standardized extracts. Allergy 1993; 48:450–453.

33. Rugosa FV, Passalacqua G, Gambardella R, Campanari S, Barbieri MM, Scordamaglia A, Canonica GW. Nonfatal systemic reactions to subcutaneous immunotherapy: A 10-year experience. Investig Allergol Clin Immunol 1997; 7:151–4.

34. Alessandro F, Vincenzo ZG, Marco S, Marcello G, Enrica R. Compliance with pharmacologic prophylaxis and therapy in bronchial asthma. Ann Allergy 1994; 73:135–140.

35. Yeung M, O'Connor SA, Parry DT, Cochrane GM. Compliance with prescribed drug therapy in asthma. Respir Med 1994; 88:31–35.

36. Bronsky EA, Dockhorn RJ, Meltzer EO, Shapiro G, Boltansky H, LaForce C, Ransom J, Weiler JM, Blumenthal M, Weakley S, Wisniewski M, Field E, Rogenes P. Fluticasone propionate aqueous nasal spray compared with terfenadine tablets in the treatment of seasonal allergic rhinitis. J Allergy Clin Immunol 1996; 97:915–921.

37. Klimek L, Wolf H, Mewes T, Dormann D, Reske-Kunz A, Schnitker J, Mann W. The effect of short-term immunotherapy with molecular standardized grass and rye allergens on eosinophil cationic protein and tryptase in nasal secretions. J Allergy Clin Immunol 1999; 103:47–53.

38. Malling H-J. Minimising the risks of allergen-specific injection immunotherapy. Drug Saf 2000; 23:323–332.

39. Des Roches A, Paradis L, Knani J, Hejjaoui A, Dhivert H, Chanez P, Bousquet J. Immunotherapy with a standardized *Dermatophagoides pteronyssinus* extract: V. Duration of efficacy of immunotherapy after its cessation. Allergy 1996; 51:430–433.

40. Hedlin G, Heilborn H, Lilja G, Norrlind K, Pegelow K-O, Schou C, Løwenstein H. Long-term follow-up of patients treated with a three-year course of cat or dog immunotherapy. J Allergy Clin Immunol 1995; 96:879–885.

41. Cohn JR, Pizzi A. Determinants of patient compliance with allergen immunotherapy. J Allergy Clin Immunol 1993; 91:734–737.

27

Allergen Immunotherapy: Therapeutic Vaccines for Asthma

JEAN BOUSQUET and FRANÇOIS-BERNARD MICHEL

Montpellier University, Montpellier, France

ANTONIO M. VIGNOLA

Palermo University, Palermo, Italy

I. INTRODUCTION

Specific immunotherapy (therapeutic vaccination) is the practice of administering gradually increasing quantities of an allergen vaccine to an allergic subject to ameliorate the symptoms associated with subsequent exposure to the causative allergen. Allergen immunotherapy was introduced to treat "pollinosis" or allergic rhinitis by Noon and Freeman in 1911 (1). There is evidence that injections of inhalant allergens to treat allergic rhinitis and asthma are clinically effective despite some risks. Other routes of vaccination have been proposed, and sublingual vaccination using high allergen doses appears to be effective and safe (2–4).

Allergen vaccination is not only effective in reducing symptoms and medication needs for the treatment of allergic rhinitis (5,6) and asthma (7,8), but it can also modify the natural course of the disease and has been shown to maintain efficacy for several years following cessation.

It may also be used for the secondary prevention of asthma and to prevent new sensitizations. Guidelines and indications for allergen vaccination with inhalant allergens have been published in collaboration with the World Health Organization (WHO) (5,9) following several other guidelines by the British Society for Allergy; the European Academy of Allergy; and the National Heart, Lung and Blood Institute of the NIH, U.S.A. (10–13).

II. OBJECTIVES OF ALLERGEN VACCINATION IN ASTHMA

Asthma is a multifactorial and complex disease in which allergic factors and nonallergic triggers interact and result in bronchial obstruction and inflammation (14). The inhalation of allergens leads to a complex activation of various cell types and the release of proinflammatory mediators; however, two different situations seem to exist. Although very few pollen grains can reach the lower airways, these allergens, carried on submicronic particles, frequently induce asthma via an IgE-mediated mechanism (15,16). Pollen-induced allergic reactions prolonged over several days almost always lead to nonspecific bronchial hyperreactivity (BHR), which is usually transient in patients allergic only to pollen, lasting from a few weeks to a few months after the end of the pollen season (8,17). House dust mites and other perennial allergens induce a long-sustained inflammation of the bronchi leading to a variable degree of BHR, and symptoms are due to allergens, inflammation, and BHR (14). It has been shown that patients with chronic asthma develop airway remodeling (18). Inflammation and airway remodeling may be involved in the "accelerated decline" of the pulmonary function characterized by a poorly reversible bronchial obstruction appearing after some decades of ongoing chronic asthma (19,20) as well as permanent bronchial wall alterations revealed by CT scans (21). However, the airway remodeling in asthma may differ according to the etiology of the disease.

The natural history of asthma in children is not completely known, but many children with episodic mild asthma outgrow it within several years whereas those with a more severe form of the disease continue to have asthma later in life (22,23). However, persistent inflammation occurs in some children who "outgrow" their asthma (24).

This suggests that (1) allergen vaccination may be more rapidly effective in patients allergic to pollen than in those sensitized to perennial allergens, (2) after a long course of the disease, patients with perennial asthma may have permanent airway abnormalities that cannot be reversed by vaccination, and (3) grass pollen allergy may be an ideal model to study the effects of vaccination in patients with normal bronchi. Vaccination in mite allergy may be used to examine the effects of treatment in patients with a variable degree of bronchial inflammation and remodeling (25).

The major objectives of immunological treatment are, in the short term, to reduce the allergic triggers precipitating symptoms and, in the long term, to decrease bronchial inflammation and BHR while it is not too severe and when bronchial damage is not prominent. Allergen vaccination appears to be the only treatment that might modify the course of the disease either by preventing the development of new sensitivities or by altering the natural history of asthma.

III. ASTHMA AND RHINITIS COEXIST IN THE SAME PATIENTS

The anatomy and physiology of nasal and bronchial mucosa are similar in many ways, and most patients with asthma also have rhinitis (26,27). Dysfunction of the upper and lower airways frequently coexist, suggesting a continuum of disease between rhinitis and asthma. Epidemiological (28), pathophysiological (29,30), quality-of-life (31), and clinical data suggest that a relationship exists between rhinitis and asthma. These data led to the concept that the upper and lower airways may be considered as a single entity influenced by a common and probably evolving inflammatory process, which may be sustained and amplified by intertwined mechanisms (32). The WHO initiative (ARIA: Allergic Rhinitis and Its Impact on Asthma) has been developed to assess the association between asthma and rhinitis, and it is important to consider asthma, rhinitis, and conjunctivitis as a single entity, especially when allergen vaccination is prescribed (5,33).

IV. MECHANISMS OF ALLERGEN VACCINATION IN ASTHMA

Allergen vaccination is specific for the antigen administered (34). Its mechanisms are complex (35,36) and may differ depending on the allergen, the target organ, and the route of immunization. Allergen vaccines are likely to act by modifying the T lymphocyte response to subsequent natural allergen exposure (35). Nonspecific bronchial hyperreactivity was found to be reduced during allergen vaccination (7,37,38). However, there are very few studies that have directly examined airway inflammation, and inconsistent results have been observed (39–42).

V. ALLERGEN VACCINATION ALTERS THE COURSE OF ALLERGIC DISEASES

Although medicines to treat asthma are highly effective and usually without important side effects, they represent only a symptomatic treatment. Allergen vaccination is the only treatment that may alter the natural course of the disease (9).

A. Long-Term Effects

Long-term efficacy of allergen vaccination after it has been discontinued has been demonstrated for subcutaneous vaccination (43–45). Durham et al. (45) conducted a randomized, double-blind, placebo-controlled trial of the discontinuation of vaccination for grass pollen allergy in patients in whom 3 to 4 years of treatment had previously been effective. Scores for seasonal symptoms and the use of rescue anti-allergic medication remained low after discontinuation, and there was no significant difference between patients who continued vaccination and those who discontinued it. However, in the study of Naclerio et al. (44), 1 year after discontinuation of ragweed vaccination, nasal challenges showed partial recrudescence of mediator responses even though reports during the season appeared to indicate continued suppression of symptoms. Long-term efficacy has still to be documented for local vaccination.

B. Prevention of New Sensitivities

Allergen vaccination may have preventive effects. Allergic sensitization usually begins early in life and symptoms often start within the first decade of life. Allergen vaccination is less effective in older patients than in children, and inflammation and remodeling of the airways in asthma reduce the effects of allergen vaccination. Several studies demonstrate that allergen vaccination prevents new sensitizations in patients sensitized to only one allergen (46–49). Therefore, if allergen vaccination is to be used as a preventive treatment, it should be started as soon as possible after allergy has been diagnosed (50).

C. Prevention of Asthma in Patients with Rhinitis

When allergen vaccination is introduced to patients who have only allergic rhinoconjunc-tivitis, it may prevent the development of asthma. The early study of Johnstone and Dutton (51) using several different allergens showed that after 3 years of treatment, children receiving pollen allergen vaccination developed less asthma than the control group. The Preventive Allergy Treatment study (PAT) (52) also showed that after 3 years of allergen vaccination, a significantly greater number of untreated children with rhinitis developed asthma compared with a group of matched children who received pollen vaccine. Another prospective study for 10 years, using sublingual vaccination with house dust mites, also showed prevention of asthma (53).

It is therefore proposed that allergen vaccination should be started early in the disease process in order to modify allergic inflammation and to prevent the onset of asthma (9,11,54).

VI. EFFICACY OF ALLERGEN VACCINATION IN ASTHMA

A. Evidence-Based Medicine

All recommendations should be established on an evidence-based model, of which one of the most commonly used is the guideline of Shekelle et al. (55). This is based on the qual-ity of clinical trials and meta-analyses (Table 1).

B. Randomized Controlled Trials of Injectable Vaccines in Asthma

1. Pollen Asthma

Several controlled studies have investigated the efficacy of allergen vaccination in pollen asthma. Some studies demonstrate that patients receiving vaccination have an improve-ment of the $PD_{20}FEV_1$ to allergen (56–58). Most double-blind, placebo-controlled clinical

Table 1   Classification Schemes of Statements of Evidence

Category of evidence
I.   a. Evidence for meta-analysis of randomized controlled trials
b. Evidence from at least one randomized controlled trial
II. a. Evidence from at lease one controlled study without randomization
b. Evidence from at least one other type of quasi-experimental study
III. Evidence from nonexperimental descriptive studies, such as comparative studies, correlation studies, and case-control studies
IV. Evidence from expert committee reports or opinions or clinical experience of respected authorities, or both
Strength of recommendation
A. Directly based on category I evidence
B. Directly based on category II evidence or extrapolated recommendation from category I evidence
C. Directly based on category III evidence or extrapolated recommendation from category I or II evidence
D. Directly based on category IV evidence or extrapolated recommendation from category I, II, or III evidence

Source: Ref. 55.

trials using aqueous or standardized vaccines or formaldehyde allergoids show that vaccination has a beneficial effect on bronchial symptoms, but only when optimal conditions are used (37,59–76). These conclusions were found in birch, grass, mountain cedar, *Parietaria*, and ragweed pollen allergy.

2. Mite-Induced Asthma

Bronchial challenges with mite extracts showed that the threshold dose eliciting an immediate bronchial obstruction was increased in many studies after treatment and that the late-phase reaction was inhibited in most (77–85) but not all studies (86). These studies suggest that vaccination is effective and may decrease inflammation since the late-phase reaction was decreased.

A review of the literature available indicates that vaccination with mites is more effective than with house dust. Although very few studies are conclusive (87), vaccination with house dust extracts should no longer be used owing to the great heterogeneity of house dust and the impossibility of appropriately standardizing house dust extracts (11,88,89).

Using aqueous or standardized *Dermatophagoides pteronyssinus* and/or *D. farinae* vaccines, many studies found a significant effect of allergen vaccination. However, some of the results are not impressive and, especially in adults, are sometimes negative. With other vaccines, results are even more variable (79,80,90–98). Haugaard and Dahl (99) examined the dose of allergen required to induce a significant clinical effect. Using a maximal dose of 7 μg of Der p I, patients presented a significant improvement in $PD_{20}FEV_1$, but the maximal effect was observed for a dose of 21 μg of Der p I. It appears that patients with severe asthma (FEV_1 under 70% of predicted values after optimal pharmacological treatment) present less improvement than those with milder asthma (100).

3. Other Allergens

A number of studies demonstrate significant improvement in bronchial sensitivity in patients with cat-allergic asthma following cat vaccination (101–111). Three studies have confirmed the clinical efficacy of cat vaccination leading to improvement in symptoms (106,111–113) and reduction of medication needs (113) in patients who kept their animal at home. Vaccination with dog is not fully validated (114,115).

Mold allergens often cause rhinitis and asthma. Multiple mold allergy is often present. The quality of mold extracts available in the past was often poor (116). However, vaccination with standardized *Cladosporium* and *Alternaria* vaccines was found to be highly effective in rhinitis and/or asthma in two studies (117,118) but less effective in one (119).

Only one double-blind, placebo-controlled study was reported in latex asthma (120). The treatment was effective, but the number of patients was too low to make clinical recommendations possible (see Chapter 20).

Efficacy of house dust immunotherapy is doubtful and the characterization of these extracts is poor. Double-blind, placebo-controlled studies of vaccination with bacterial vaccines for treatment of rhinitis and/or asthma did not show efficacy [for review see (121)]. There is no study of vaccination with *Candida albicans* and *Trichophyton*, and the characterization of the extracts is usually poor.

4. Multiple Allergens

A study reported a controlled trial of vaccination for treatment of mild to severe asthma in a nonselected population of allergic children (122). The children were closely supervised and given optimal medical therapy. The results showed no significant difference between the placebo and active-treatment groups. However, there are several methodological factors that may have led to the negative results. Among them, the study was carried out using mixtures of allergens including mold extracts, some important allergens such as cockroach were not used, and the population of asthmatic children was nonselected for optimal vaccination, whereas guidelines indicate that only highly selected asthmatic patients should receive allergen vaccination (13,89,123)

5. Meta-analysis

A meta-analysis using the Cochrane collaboration (7) found that allergen vaccination was effective. Fifty-four randomized controlled trials were analyzed. There were 25 trials of vaccination for house mite allergy, 13 pollen allergy trials, 8 animal dander allergy trials, 2 *Cladosporium* allergy trials, and 6 trials looking at multiple allergens. Concealment of allocation was assessed as clearly adequate in only 11 of these trials. Significant heterogeneity was present in a number of comparisons. Overall, there was a significant reduction in asthma symptoms and medication following allergen injections. There was also a significant improvement in asthma symptom scores (standardized mean difference –0.52, 95% confidence interval –0.70 to –0.35). People receiving allergen vaccines were less likely to report a worsening of asthma symptoms than those randomized to placebo (odds ratio 0.27, 95% confidence interval 0.21 to 0.35). People randomized to vaccination were less likely to require medication than those randomized to placebo (odds ratio 0.28, 95% confidence interval 0.19 to 0.42). Allergen vaccination reduced allergen-specific bronchial hyperreactivity, with some reduction in specific bronchial hyperreactivity as well. There was no consistent effect on lung function. The reviewer's conclusions were that "immunotherapy may reduce asthma symptoms and use of asthma medications, but the size of the benefit compared to other therapies is not known. The possibility of adverse effects (such as anaphylaxis) must be considered" (see Chapter 39).

C. Randomized Controlled Trials of Sublingual-Swallow Vaccines in Asthma

New routes of administration of immunotherapy are currently being explored: nasal, sublingual-swallow, and oral immunotherapy using high allergen doses (9).

High dose sublingual-swallow vaccination has been studied in a few controlled studies in mite allergy, and a significant reduction of symptoms and medication needs was found (124–129). In one study, FEV_1 was significantly improved by comparison to baseline values and the placebo group (126). Sublingual-swallow treatment with low doses is usually ineffective (130,131). Many studies had methodological flaws and were not considered scientifically sound, and thus were not included in many guidelines.

With pollen allergy, some studies reported a lower incidence of asthma cases in the vaccination group than in the placebo group (132), and there was one double-blind, placebo-controlled study of olive pollen allergy showing some effect (133). One controlled study examined the effect of sublingual-swallow vaccination in latex allergy and suggested efficacy (134). One double-blind, placebo-controlled study in sublingual-spit vaccination with a cat vaccine did not find an efficacy as determined by cat exposure in a cat room (135).

D. Recommendations for the Efficacy of Allergen Vaccination in Asthma

The level of evidence for the efficacy of subcutaneous vaccination in asthma, rhinitis, and conjunctivitis is A according to guidelines used by WHO (55) (Table 1). The level of

Table 2 Statement of Evidence for the Treatment of Rhinitis and Asthma by Immunotherapy

		Seasonal		Perennial	
		Children	Adults	Children	Adults
Subcutaneous	Rhinitis	A (Ib)	A (Ib)	A (Ib)	A (Ib)
	asthma	A (Ia)	A (Ia)	A (Ia)	A (Ia)
High-dose sublingual-swallow	Rhinitis	A (Ia)	A (Ia)	A (Ia)	A (Ia)
	Asthma	A (Ib)	A (Ib)	A (Ib)	A (Ib)

Evidence level according to Shekelle et al. (Table 1) (55).
Source: Ref. 5.

recommendation for sublingual-swallow vaccination in asthma is B since more studies are needed to reach a level A recommendation (Tables 1 and 2).

VII. SAFETY

A. Injectable Vaccines

The major risks of allergen vaccination are anaphylaxis and severe asthma (136–140). Therefore, allergen vaccination should be administered by or under the close supervision of a trained physician who can recognize early symptoms and signs of anaphylaxis and/or asthma, and administer emergency treatment (138). Recommendations to minimize risks of vaccination in asthmatics are included in Table 3.

Another possible risk of mite vaccination has been reported. Mites contain tropomyosin, which may be cross-reactive with snails; snail anaphylaxis, caused by ingestion, has been reported in patients receiving mite vaccination (141,142).

B. Sublingual Vaccines

With sublingual-swallow specific immunotherapy, some serious systemic side effects (asthma, urticaria, and gastrointestinal complaints) were observed in children in one study (124). However, in all other studies, only mild reactions were observed, even in children with asthma (125–127,132,133,143–152). Postmarketing surveillance of sublingual-swallow specific immunotherapy showed that this procedure appeared to be tolerated in children (153,154). Since local specific immunotherapy (sublingual swallow) is self-administered at

Table 3 Recommendations to Minimize Risk and Improve Efficacy of Allergen Vaccination

- Allergen vaccination needs to be prescribed by specialists and administered by physicians trained to manage systemic reactions if anaphylaxis occurs.
- Patients with multiple sensitivities may not benefit as much as patients with a single sensitivity from allergen vaccination. More data are necessary.
- Patients with nonallergic triggers will not benefit from allergen vaccination.
- Allergen vaccination is more effective in children and young adults than in older adults.
- It is essential for safety reasons that patients be asymptomatic at the time of the injections because lethal adverse reactions are more often found in asthma patients with severe airway obstruction.
- FEV_1 with pharmacological treatment should reach at least 70% of the predicted values, for both efficacy and safety reasons.

Source: International Consensus Report on Diagnosis and Management of asthma (89).

home, patients must be informed of the potential risks of a systemic reaction and how to treat such a reaction should it occur (9).

VIII. INDICATIONS FOR ALLERGEN VACCINATION IN ASTHMA AND RHINITIS

The treatment of allergic diseases is based on allergen avoidance, pharmacotherapy, allergen vaccination, and patient education. Physicians should know the local and regional aerobiology and be aware of potential allergens in the patient's indoor and outdoor environments. Only physicians with a training in allergology can select the clinically relevant allergen vaccines for therapy. Allergen vaccination, where appropriate, should be used in combination with other forms of therapy in the hope that the patient will become as symptom-free as medically possible.

Allergen vaccination by subcutaneous route is indicated for patients who have demonstrable evidence of specific IgE antibodies to clinically relevant allergens and whose allergic symptoms warrant the time and risk of allergen vaccination. Contraindications for inhalant allergen vaccination may be absolute or relative (11). Patient selection is important, and efficacy must always be balanced against the risk of side effects. The necessity of initiating allergen vaccination depends on the degree to which symptoms can be reduced by medication, the amount and type of medication required to control symptoms, and whether effective allergen avoidance is possible (Table 4).

Table 4 Considerations for Initiating Vaccination

---

1. Presence of a demonstrated IgE-mediated disease
   • Positive skin tests and/or serum-specific IgE
2. Documentation that specific sensitivity is involved in symptoms
   • Exposure to the allergen(s) determined by allergy testing related to appearance of symptoms
   • If required, allergen challenge with the relevant allergen(s)
3. Characterization of other triggers that may be involved in symptoms
4. Severity and duration of symptoms
   • Subjective symptoms
   • Objective parameters (e.g., work, loss, school absenteeism)
   • Pulmonary function (*essential* exclude patients with severe asthma)
   • Monitoring of the pulmonary function by peak flow
5. Response of symptoms to nonimmunological treatment
   • Response to allergen avoidance
   • Response to pharmacotherapy
6. Availability of standardized or high-quality extracts
7. Relative contraindications
   • Treatment with beta-blocker
   • Other immunological disease
   • Inability of patient to comply
8. Sociological factors
   • Cost
   • Occupation of candidate
   • Impaired quality of life despite adequate pharmacological treatment
9. Objective evidence of efficacy of vaccination for the selected patient (availability of controlled clinical studies)

Source: WHO position paper *Allergen Immunotherapy: Therapeutic Vaccines for Allergic Diseases.*

The use of allergen vaccination using the subcutaneous route requires specialist assessment, especially in children, because there are special problems and questions for this age group. Vaccination started early in the disease process may modify the long-term progress of the allergic inflammation and disease (11,54). It is rarely started before the age of 5 years.

In Europe sublingual-swallow vaccination has gained interest and in many countries represents an alternative to subcutaneous vaccination. The relative role of subcutaneous and sublingual vaccinations is still under scrutiny. However, only high doses of standardized extracts should be used. Specialist assessment is also needed due to the costs of treatment (155).

The indications for allergen vaccination in asthma and rhinitis have been separated in some guidelines (13,89,156), and this arbitrary separation has prompted unresolved questions (157,158), possibly because the IgE-mediated reaction has not been considered as a multiple organ disease. It is therefore important to consider allergen vaccination based on the allergen sensitization rather than on a particular disease manifestation.

IX. SALIENT POINTS

1. Vaccination for allergic rhinitis conjunctivitis is indicated (5,159) (1) when antihistamines and topical drugs insufficiently control symptoms, (2) in patients who do not wish to be on pharmacotherapy, (3) when pharmacotherapy produces undesirable side effects, (4) when the patient is concerned about long-term pharmacological therapy, and (5) if the season is prolonged or if polysensitized patients are exposed to several subsequent pollen seasons (i.e., tree, grass, and weed pollen sensitivity) (9). The risk/benefit ratio should be considered in every case.

2. One the major problems is the indication for allergen vaccination in asthma (8,160). Only patients with mild to moderate asthma should receive allergen vaccination (5). However, these patients do not usually require this form of treatment to control bronchial symptoms since drugs are effective at the doses required. Thus, if asthma only is considered, allergen immunotherapy is usually unnecessary. However, most asthmatics have rhinitis, and vaccines may be needed for persistent rhinitis. In these patients, immunotherapy will increase the control of asthma. Thus, allergen vaccination is important for patients with severe rhinitis and mild to moderate asthma (5).

3. Patients allergic to mites are candidates for mite allergen immunotherapy if they have significant symptoms of rhinitis or asthma when they are exposed to domestic mite allergens.

4. Avoidance is the treatment of choice for animal dander–induced allergic diseases. However, complete avoidance is often impossible due to exposure to animal allergens in environments where animals are not present (161). Allergen immunotherapy may be prescribed for patients who are unable to avoid animal contacts, for example, due to occupational exposure or refusal to evict an animal from the home.

5. For mold allergy, avoidance, where possible, of indoor mold allergens is the treatment of choice, although there are no data to support it. Some studies have demonstrated clinical improvement when well-characterized vaccines of *Cladosporium* or *Alternaria* have been used in the treatment of mold-induced

allergy. Patients with positive skin tests and symptoms when exposed to other relevant mold allergens may be considered for vaccination.

6. The duration of the treatment required to maintain improvement in clinical symptoms remains unknown. A duration of 3 years was found to be optimal for grass pollen vaccines (45). For those patients who respond to treatment, many clinicians advise 3 to 5 years of therapy. However, the decision on when to discontinue allergen vaccination should be individualized.

REFERENCES

1. Noon L. Prophylactic inoculation against hay fever. Lancet 1911; i:1572–1573.
2. Kagi MK, Wuthrich B. Different methods of local allergen-specific immunotherapy. Allergy 2002; 57(5):379–388.
3. Canonica GW, Passalacqua G. Noninjection routes for immunotherapy. J Allergy Clin Immunol 2003; 111(3):437–448, quiz 449.
4. Douglass J, O'Hehir R. Specific allergen immunotherapy: Time for alternatives? Clin Exp Allergy 2002; 32(1):1–3.
5. Bousquet J, Van Cauwenberge P, Khaltaev N. Allergic rhinitis and its impact on asthma. J Allergy Clin Immunol 2001; 108(suppl 5):S147–S334.
6. Malling HJ. Immunotherapy for rhinitis. Curr Allergy Asthma Rep 2003; 3(3):204–209.
7. Abramson M, Puy R, Weiner J. Immunotherapy in asthma: An updated systematic review. Allergy 1999; 54(10):1022–1041.
8. Bousquet J. Pro: Immunotherapy is clinically indicated in the management of allergic asthma. Am J Respir Crit Care Med 2001; 164(12):2139–2140, discussion 2141–2142.
9. Bousquet J, Lockey R, Malling H. Allergen immunotherapy: Therapeutic vaccines for allergic diseases. (WHO position paper). Allergy 1998; 53, suppl 54.
10. Frew AJ. Injection immunotherapy: British Society for Allergy and Clinical Immunology Working Party. Br Med J 1993; 307(6909):919–923.
11. Malling H, Weeke B. Immunotherapy: Position Paper of the European Academy of Allergy and Clinical Immunology. Allergy 1993; 48(suppl 14):9–35.
12. Malling H. Immunotherapy: Position Paper of the EAACI. Allergy 1988; 43, suppl 6.
13. Global Strategy for Asthma Management and Prevention: WHO/NHLBI Workshop Report. National Institutes of Health, National Heart, Lung and Blood Institute, Publication No. 95–3659. January 1995.
14. Platts-Mills TA. The role of allergens in the induction of asthma. Curr Allergy Asthma Rep 2002; 2(2):175–180.
15. Anto JM, Sunyer J. Thunderstorms: A risk factor for asthma attacks (editorial; comment) Thorax 1997; 52(8):669–670.
16. Knox RB. Grass pollen, thunderstorms and asthma. Clin Exp Allergy 1993; 23(5):354–359.
17. Sotomayor H, Badier M, Vervloet D, Orehek J. Seasonal increase of carbachol airway responsiveness in patients allergic to grass pollen: Reversal by corticosteroids. Am Rev Respir Dis 1984; 130(1):56–58.
18. Bousquet J, Jeffery P, Busse W, Johnson M, Vignola A. Asthma: From bronchospasm to airway remodelling. Am J Respir Crit Care Med 2000: (in press).
19. Lange P, Parner J, Vestbo J, Schnohr P, Jensen G. A 15-year follow-up study of ventilatory function in adults with asthma. N Engl J Med 1998; 339(17):1194–1200.
20. Ten Hacken NH, Postma DS, Timens W. Airway remodeling and long-term decline in lung function in asthma. Curr Opin Pulm Med 2003; 9(1):9–14.
21. Paganin F, Seneterre E, Chanez P, Daures JP, Bruel JM, Michel FB, et al. Computed tomography of the lungs in asthma: Influence of disease severity and etiology. Am J Respir Crit Care Med 1996; 153(1):110–114.

22. Gerritsen J, Koeter GH, Postma DS, Schouten JP, Knol K. Prognosis of asthma from childhood to adulthood. Am Rev Respir Dis 1989, 140(5):1325–1330.
23. van Den Toorn LM, Prins JB, Overbeek SE, Hoogsteden HC, de Jongste JC. Adolescents in clinical remission of atopic asthma have elevated exhaled nitric oxide levels and bronchial hyperresponsiveness. Am J Respir Crit Care Med 2000; 162(3 pt 1):953–957.
24. Warke TJ, Fitch PS, Brown V, Taylor R, Lyons JD, Ennis M, et al. Outgrown asthma does not mean no airways inflammation. Eur Respir J 2002; 19(2):284–287.
25. Bousquet J, Hejjaoui A, Michel FB. Specific immunotherapy in asthma. J Allergy Clin Immunol 1990; 86(3 pt 1):292–305.
26. Vignola AM, Chanez P, Godard P, Bousquet J. Relationships between rhinitis and asthma. Allergy 1998; 53(9):833–839.
27. Immunobiology of asthma and rhinitis: Pathogenic factors and therapeutic options. Am J Respir Crit Care Med 1999; 160(5):1778–1787.
28. Leynaert B, Bousquet J, Neukirch C, Liard R, Neukirch F. Perennial rhinitis: An independent risk factor for asthma in nonatopic subjects: Results from the European Community Respiratory Health Survey. J Allergy Clin Immunol 1999: 301–304.
29. Chanez P, Vignola AM, Vic P, Guddo F, Bonsignore G, Godard P, et al. Comparison between nasal and bronchial inflammation in asthmatic and control subjects. Am J Respir Crit Care Med 1999; 159(2):588–595.
30. Gaga M, Lambrou P, Papageorgiou N, Koulouris NG, Kosmas E, Fragakis S, et al. Eosinophils are a feature of upper and lower airway pathology in non-atopic asthma, irrespective of the presence of rhinitis (in process). Clin Exp Allergy 2000; 30(5):663–669.
31. Leynaert B, Neukirch F, Demoly P, Bousquet J. Epidemiologic evidence for asthma and rhinitis comorbidity. J Allergy Clin Immunol 2000; 106(5 pt 2):201–205.
32. Braunstahl GJ, Kleinjan A, Overbeek SE, Prins JB, Hoogsteden HC, Fokkens WJ. Segmental bronchial provocation induces nasal inflammation in allergic rhinitis patients. Am J Respir Crit Care Med 2000; 161(6):2051–2057.
33. Bousquet J, Demoly P, Michel FB. Specific immunotherapy in rhinitis and asthma. Ann Allergy Asthma Immunol 2001; 87(suppl 1):38–42.
34. Norman PS, Lichtenstein LM. Comparisons of alum-precipitated and unprecipitated aqueous ragweed pollen extracts in the treatment of hay fever. J Allergy Clin Immunol 1978; 61(6):384–389.
35. Durham SR, Till SJ. Immunologic changes associated with allergen immunotherapy. J Allergy Clin Immunol 1998; 102(2):157–164.
36. Akdis CA, Blaser K. Immunologic mechanisms of specific immunotherapy (in process). Allergy 1999; 56:31–32.
37. Rak S, Heinrich C, Jacobsen L, Scheynius A, Venge P. A double-blinded, comparative study of the effects of short preseason specific immunotherapy and topical steroids in patients with allergic rhinoconjunctivitis and asthma. J Allergy Clin Immunol 2001; 108(6):921–928.
38. Lombardi C, Gargioni S, Venturi S, Zoccali P, Canonica GW, Passalacqua G. Controlled study of preseasonal immunotherapy with grass pollen extract in tablets: Effect on bronchial hyperreactivity. J Investig Allergol Clin Immunol 2001; 11(1):41–45.
39. Foresi A, Pesci A, Pelucchi A, Gabrielli M, Mastropasqua B, Bertorelli G, et al. Bronchial inflammation in mite-sensitive asthmatic subjects after 5 years of specific immunotherapy. Ann Allergy 1992; 69(4):303–308.
40. Armentia-Medina A, Tapias JA, Martin JF, Ventas P, Fernandez A. Immunotherapy with the storage mite lepidoglyphus destructor. Allergol Immunopathol (Madr) 1995; 23(5):211–223.
41. Kohno Y, Minoguchi K, Oda N, Yokoe T, Yamashita N, Sakane T, et al. Effect of rush immunotherapy on airway inflammation and airway hyperresponsiveness after bronchoprovocation with allergen in asthma. J Allergy Clin Immunol 1998; 102(6 pt 1):927–934.
42. Silvestri M, Spallarossa D, Battistini E, Sabatini F, Pecora S, Parmiani S, et al. Changes in inflammatory and clinical parameters and in bronchial hyperreactivity of asthmatic children

sensitized to house dust mites following sublingual immunotherapy. J Investig Allergol Clin Immunol 2002; 12(1):52–59.

43. Des-Roches A, Paradis L, Knani J, Hejjaoui A, Dhivert H, Chanez P, et al. Immunotherapy with a standardized *Dermatophagoides pteronyssinus* extract: V. Duration of efficacy of immunotherapy after its cessation. Allergy 1996; 51:430–433.

44. Naclerio RM, Proud D, Moylan B, Balcer S, Freidhoff L, Kagey-Sobotka A, et al. A double-blind study of the discontinuation of ragweed immunotherapy. J Allergy Clin Immunol 1997; 100(3):293–300.

45. Durham SR, Walker SM, Varga EM, Jacobson MR, O'Brien F, Noble W, et al. Long-term clinical efficacy of grass-pollen immunotherapy (see comments). N Engl J Med 1999; 341(7):468–475.

46. Des-Roches A, Paradis L, Ménardo J-L, Bouges S, Daurès J-P, Bousquet J. Immunotherapy with a standardized *Dermatophagoides pteronyssinus* extract: VI. Specific immunotherapy prevents the onset of new sensitizations in children. J Allergy Clin Immunol 1997; 99:450–453.

47. Pajno GB, Barberio G, De Luca F, Morabito L, Parmiani S. Prevention of new sensitizations in asthmatic children monosensitized to house dust mite by specific immunotherapy: A six-year follow-up study. Clin Exp Allergy 2001; 31(9):1392–1397.

48. Purello-D'Ambrosio F, Gangemi S, Merendino RA, Isola S, Puccinelli P, Parmian S, et al. Prevention of new sensitizations in monosensitized subjects submitted to specific immunotherapy or not: A retrospective study. Clin Exp Allergy 2001; 31(8):1295–1302.

49. Eng PA, Reinhold M, Gnehm HP. Long-term efficacy of preseasonal grass pollen immunotherapy in children. Allergy 2002; 57(4):306–312.

50. Demoly P, Bousquet J, Michel FB. Immunotherapy in allergic rhinitis: A prevention for asthma? (in process). Curr Probl Dermatol 1999; 28:119–123.

51. Johnstone DE. Immunotherapy in children: Past, present, and future (part I). Ann Allergy 1981; 46(1):1–7.

52. Moller C, Dreborg S, Ferdousi HA, Halken S, Host A, Jacobsen L, et al. Pollen immunotherapy reduces the development of asthma in children with seasonal rhinoconjunctivitis (the PAT-study). J Allergy Clin Immunol 2002; 109(2):251–256.

53. Di Rienzo V, Marcucci F, Puccinelli P, Parmiani S, Frati F, Sensi L, et al. Long-lasting effect of sublingual immunotherapy in children with asthma due to house dust mite: A 10-year prospective study. Clin Exp Allergy 2003; 33(2):206–210.

54. Ownby DR, Adinoff AD. The appropriate use of skin testing and allergen immunotherapy in young children. J Allergy Clin Immunol 1994; 94(4):662–665.

55. Shekelle PG, Woolf SH, Eccles M, Grimshaw J. Clinical guidelines: Developing guidelines. Br Med J 1999; 318(7183):593–596.

56. McAllen M. Hyposensitization in grass pollen hay fever. Acta Allergol 1969; 24:421–431.

57. Ortolani C, Pastorello E, Moss RB, Hsu YP, Restuccia M, Joppolo G, et al. Grass pollen immunotherapy: A single year double-blind, placebo-controlled study in patients with grass pollen-induced asthma and rhinitis. J Allergy Clin Immunol 1984; 73(2):283–290.

58. Citron K, Frankland A, Sinclair J. Inhalation tests of bronchial hypersensitivity in pollen asthma. Thorax 1958; 13:229–232.

59. D'Amato G, Kordash TR, Liccardi G, Lobefalo G, Cazzola M, Freshwater LL. Immunotherapy with Alpare in patients with respiratory allergy to *Parietaria* pollen: A two year double-blind placebo-controlled study. Clin Exp Allergy 1995; 25(2):149–158.

60. Arvidsson MB, Lowhagen O, Rak S. Effect of 2-year placebo-controlled immunotherapy on airway symptoms and medication in patients with birch pollen allergy. J Allergy Clin Immunol 2002; 109(5):777–783.

61. Armentia-Medina A, Blanco-Quiros A, Martin-Santos JM, Alvarez-Cuesta E, Moneo-Goiri I, Carreira P, et al. Rush immunotherapy with a standardized Bermuda grass pollen extract. Ann Allergy 1989; 63(2):127–135.

62. Balda BR, Wolf H, Baumgarten C, Klimek L, Rasp G, Kunkel G, et al. Tree-pollen allergy is efficiently treated by short-term immunotherapy (STI) with seven preseasonal injections of molecular standardized allergens. Allergy 1998; 53(8):740–748.

63. Bodtger U, Poulsen LK, Jacobi HH, Malling HJ. The safety and efficacy of subcutaneous birch pollen immunotherapy: A one-year, randomised, double-blind, placebo-controlled study. Allergy 2002; 57(4):297–305.

64. Bousquet J, Becker WM, Hejjaoui A, Chanal I, Lebel B, Dhivert H, et al. Differences in clinical and immunologic reactivity of patients allergic to grass pollens and to multiple-pollen species: II. Efficacy of a double-blind, placebo-controlled, specific immunotherapy with standardized extracts. J Allergy Clin Immunol 1991; 88(1):43–53.

65. Bousquet J, Maasch HJ, Hejjaoui A, Skassa-Brociek W, Wahl R, Dhivert H, et al. Double-blind, placebo-controlled immunotherapy with mixed grass-pollen allergoids: III. Efficacy and safety of unfractionated and high-molecular-weight preparations in rhinoconjunctivitis and asthma. J Allergy Clin Immunol 1989; 84(4 pt 1):546–556.

66. Creticos PS, Reed CE, Norman PS, Khoury J, Adkinson N Jr, Buncher CR, et al. Ragweed immunotherapy in adult asthma. N Engl J Med 1996; 334(8):501–506.

67. Frankland A, Augustin R. Prophylaxis of summer hay fever and asthma: A controlled trial comparing crude grass pollen extract with the isolated main protein components. Lancet 1954; 1:1055–1058.

68. Hill DJ, Hosking CS, Shelton MJ, Turner MW. Failure of hyposensitisation in treatment of children with grass-pollen asthma. Br Med J Clin Res 1982; 284(6312):306–309.

69. Osterballe O. Immunotherapy in hay fever with two major allergens 19, 25 and partially purified extract of timothy grass pollen: A controlled double blind study. In vivo variables, season I. Allergy 1980; 35(6):473–489.

70. Machiels JJ, Buche M, Somville MA, Jacquemin MG, Saint-Remy JM. Complexes of grass pollen allergens and specific antibodies reduce allergic symptoms and inhibit the seasonal increase of IgE antibody. Clin Exp Allergy 1990; 20(6):653–660.

71. Machiels JJ, Somville MA, Jacquemin MG, Saint-Remy JM. Allergen-antibody complexes can efficiently prevent seasonal rhinitis and asthma in grass pollen hypersensitive patients: Allergen-antibody complex immunotherapy. Allergy 1991; 46(5):335–348.

72. Pastorello EA, Pravettoni V, Incorvaia C, Mambretti M, Franck E, Wahl R, et al. Clinical and immunological effects of immunotherapy with alum-absorbed grass allergoid in grass-pollen-induced hay fever. Allergy 1992; 47(4 pt 1):281–290.

73. Pence H, Mitchell D, Greenly R, Updegraft B, Selfridge H. Immunotherapy for mountain cedar pollinosis. A double-blind controlled study. J Allergy Clin Immunol 1976; 58:39–50.

74. Rak S, Hakansson L, Venge P. Eosinophil chemotactic activity in allergic patients during the birch pollen season: The effect of immunotherapy. Int Arch Allergy Appl Immunol 1987; 82(3–4):349–350.

75. Varney V. Hayfever in the United Kingdom. Clin Exp Allergy 1991; 21(6):757–762.

76. Walker SM, Pajno GB, Lima MT, Wilson DR, Durham SR. Grass pollen immunotherapy for seasonal rhinitis and asthma: A randomized, controlled trial. J Allergy Clin Immunol 2001; 107(1):87–93.

77. McAllen M, Assem E, Maunsell K. House-dust mite asthma: Results of challenge tests on five criteria with *Dermatophagoides pteronyssinus*. Br Med J 1970; 2:501–504.

78. Bousquet J, Calvayrac P, Guerin B, Hejjaoui A, Dhivert H, Hewitt B, et al. Immunotherapy with a standardized *Dermatophagoides pteronyssinus* extract: I. In vivo and in vitro parameters after a short course of treatment. J Allergy Clin Immunol 1985; 76(5):734–744.

79. Warner JO, Price JF, Soothill JF, Hey EN. Controlled trial of hyposensitisation to *Dermatophagoides pteronyssinus* in children with asthma. Lancet 1978; 2(8096):912–915.

80. Machiels JJ, Somville MA, Lebrun PM, Lebecque SJ, Jacquemin MG, Saint-Remy JM. Allergic bronchial asthma due to *Dermatophagoides pteronyssinus* hypersensitivity can be

efficiently treated by inoculation of allergen-antibody complexes. J Clin Investig 1990; 85(4):1024–1035.

81. Peroni DG, Piacentini GL, Martinati LC, Warner JO, Boner AL. Double-blind trial of house-dust mite immunotherapy in asthmatic children resident at high altitude. Allergy 1995; 50(11):925–930.

82. Van-Bever HP, Stevens WJ. Evolution of the late asthmatic reaction during immunotherapy and after stopping immunotherapy (see comments). J Allergy Clin Immunol 1990; 86(2):141–146.

83. Van-Bever HP, Stevens WJ. Effect of hyposensitization upon the immediate and late asthmatic reaction and upon histamine reactivity in patients allergic to house dust mite (*Dermatophagoides pteronyssinus*). Eur Respir J 1992; 5(3):318–322.

84. Garcia-Ortega P, Merelo A, Marrugat J, Richart C. Decrease of skin and bronchial sensitization following short-intensive scheduled immunotherapy in mite-allergic asthma. Chest 1993; 103(1):183–187.

85. Wahn U, Schweter C, Lind P, Lowenstein H. Prospective study on immunologic changes induced by two different *Dermatophagoides pteronyssinus* extracts prepared from whole mite culture and mite bodies. J Allergy Clin Immunol 1988; 82(3 pt 1):360–370.

86. Mosbech H. House dust mite allergy. Allergy 1985; 40(2):81–91.

87. Aas K. Hyposensitization in house dust allergy asthma. Acta Paediatr Scand 1971; 60:264–268.

88. The current status of allergen immunotherapy (hyposensitisation): Report of a WHO/IUIS working group. Allergy 1989; 44(6):369–379.

89. International Consensus Report on Diagnosis and Management of Asthma: International Asthma Management Project. Allergy 1992; 47(suppl 13):1–61.

90. Amaral-Marques R, Avila R. Results of a clinical trial with a *Dermatophagoides pteronyssinus* tyrosine adsorbed vaccine. Allergol Immunopathol Madr 1978; 6(3):231–235.

91. Basomba A, Tabar AI, de Rojas DH, Garcia BE, Alamar R, Olaguibel JM, et al. Allergen vaccination with a liposome-encapsulated extract of *Dermatophagoides pteronyssinus*: A randomized, double-blind, placebo-controlled trial in asthmatic patients. J Allergy Clin Immunol 2002; 109(6):943–948.

92. D'Souza M, Pepys J, Wells I, Tai E, Palmer F, Overell B, et al. Hyposensitization with *Dermatophagoides pteronyssinus* in house dust allergy: A controlled study of clinical and immunological effects. Clin Allergy 1973; 3:177–193.

93. Gaddie J, Skinner C, Palmer K. Hyposensitization with house dust mite vaccine in bronchial asthma. Br Med J 1976; 2:561–562.

94. Machiels JJ, Lebrun PM, Jacquemin MG, Saint-Remy JM. Significant reduction of nonspecific bronchial reactivity in patients with *Dermatophagoides pteronyssinus*–sensitive allergic asthma under therapy with allergen-antibody complexes. Am Rev Respir Dis 1993; 147(6 pt 1):1407–1412.

95. Newton D, Maberley D, Wilson R. House dust mite hyposensitization. Br J Dis Chest 1978; 72:21–28.

96. Pauli G, Bessot JC, Bigot H, Delaume G, Hordle DA, Hirth C, et al. Clinical and immunologic evaluation of tyrosine-adsorbed *Dermatophagoides pteronyssinus* extract: A double-blind placebo-controlled trial. J Allergy Clin Immunol 1984; 74(4 pt 1):524–535.

97. Pichler C, Marquardsen A, Sparholt S, Løwenstein H, Bircher A, Bischof M, et al. Specific immunotherapy with *Dermatophagoides pteronyssinus* and *D. farinae* results in decreased bronchial hyperreactivity. Allergy 1997; 52:274–283.

98. Pifferi M, Baldini G, Marrazzini G, Baldini M, Ragazzo V, Pietrobelli A, et al. Benefits of immunotherapy with a standardized *Dermatophagoides pteronyssinus* extract in asthmatic children: A three-year prospective study. Allergy 2002; 57(9):785–790.

99. Haugaard L, Dahl R, Jacobsen L. A controlled dose-response study of immunotherapy with standardized, partially purified extract of house dust mite: Clinical efficacy and side effects. J Allergy Clin Immunol 1993; 91(3):709–722.

100. Bousquet J, Hejjaoui A, Clauzel AM, Guerin B, Dhivert H, Skassa-Brociek W, et al. Specific immunotherapy with a standardized *Dermatophagoides pteronyssinus* extract: II. Prediction of efficacy of immunotherapy. J Allergy Clin Immunol 1988; 82(6):971–977.

101. Bertelsen A, Andersen JB, Christensen J, Ingemann L, Kristensen T, Ostergaard PA. Immunotherapy with dog and cat extracts in children. Allergy 1989; 44(5):330–335.

102. Bucur J, Dreborg S, Einarsson R, Ljungstedt-Pahlman I, Nilsson JE, Persson G. Immunotherapy with dog and cat allergen preparations in dog-sensitive and cat-sensitive asthmatics. Ann Allergy 1989; 62(4):355–361.

103. Hedlin G, Graff-Lonnevig V, Heilborn H, Lilja G, Norrlind K, Pegelow KO, et al. Immunotherapy with cat- and dog-dander extracts: II. In vivo and in vitro immunologic effects observed in a 1-year double-blind placebo study. J Allergy Clin Immunol 1986; 77(3):488–496.

104. Hedlin G, Graff-Lonnevig V, Heilborn H, Lilja G, Norrlind K, Pegelow K, et al. Immunotherapy with cat- and dog-dander extracts: V. Effects of 3 years of treatment. J Allergy Clin Immunol 1991; 87(5):955–964.

105. Lilja G, Sundin B, Graff-Lonnevig V, Hedlin G, Heilborn H, Norrlind K, et al. Immunotherapy with cat- and dog-dander extracts: V. Effects of 2 years of treatment. J Allergy Clin Immunol 1989; 83(1):37–44.

106. Ohman J, Jr., Findlay SR, Leitermann KM. Immunotherapy in cat-induced asthma: Double-blind trial with evaluation of in vivo and in vitro responses. J Allergy Clin Immunol 1984; 74(3 pt 1):230–239.

107. Rohatgi N, Dunn K, Chai H. Cat- or dog-induced immediate and late asthmatic responses before and after immunotherapy. J Allergy Clin Immunol 1988; 82(3 pt 1):389–397.

108. Sundin B, Lilja G, Graff-Lonnevig V, Hedlin G, Heilborn H, Norrlind K, et al. Immunotherapy with partially purified and standardized animal dander extracts: I. Clinical results from a double-blind study on patients with animal dander asthma. J Allergy Clin Immunol 1986; 77(3):478–487.

109. Taylor WW, Ohman J, Jr., Lowell FC. Immunotherapy in cat-induced asthma: Double-blind trial with evaluation of bronchial responses to cat allergen and histamine. J Allergy Clin Immunol 1978; 61(5):283–287.

110. Van-Metre TE J, Marsh DG, Adkinson N, Jr., Kagey-Sobotka A, Khattignavong A, Norman P, Jr., et al. Immunotherapy for cat asthma. J Allergy Clin Immunol 1988; 82(6):1055–1068.

111. Varney V, Edwards J, Tabbah K, Brewster H, Marvroleon G, Frew A. Clinical efficacy of specific immunotherapy to cat dander: A double-blind placebo-controlled trial. Clin Exp Allergy 1997; 27:860–867.

112. Haugaard L, Dahl R. Immunotherapy in patients allergic to cat and dog dander: I. Clinical results. Allergy 1992; 47(3):249–254.

113. Alvarez-Cuesta E, Cuesta-Herranz J, Puyana-Ruiz J, Cuesta-Herranz C, Blanco-Quiros A. Monoclonal antibody–standardized cat extract immunotherapy: Risk-benefit effects from a double-blind placebo study. J Allergy Clin Immunol 1994; 93(3):556–566.

114. Valovirta E, Koivikko A, Vanto T, Viander M, Ingeman L. Immunotherapy in allergy to dog: A double-blind clinical study. Ann Allergy 1984; 53(1):85–88.

115. Valovirta E, Viander M, Koivikko A, Vanto T, Ingeman L. Immunotherapy in allergy to dog. Immunologic and clinical findings of a double-blind study. Ann Allergy 1986; 57(3):173–179.

116. Salvaggio J, Aukrust L. Postgraduate course presentations: Mold-induced asthma. J Allergy Clin Immunol 1981; 68(5):327–346.

117. Horst M, Hejjaoui A, Horst V, Michel FB, Bousquet J. Double-blind, placebo-controlled rush immunotherapy with a standardized *Alternaria* extract. J Allergy Clin Immunol 1990; 85(2):460–472.

118. Malling HJ, Dreborg S, Weeke B. Diagnosis and immunotherapy of mould allergy: V. Clinical efficacy and side effects of immunotherapy with *Cladosporium herbarum*. Allergy 1986; 41(7):507–519.

119. Dreborg S, Agrell B, Foucard T, Kjellman NI, Koivikko A, Nilsson S. A double-blind, multi-center immunotherapy trial in children, using a purified and standardized *Cladosporium herbarum* preparation: I. Clinical results. Allergy 1986; 41(2):131–140.

120. Leynadier F, Herman D, Vervloet D, Andre C. Specific immunotherapy with a standardized latex extract versus placebo in allergic healthcare workers. J Allergy Clin Immunol 2000; 106(3):585–590.

121. Allergenic extracts made from bacteria. Federal Register, 42 FR 58266, 44 FR 1544 1979.

122. Adkinson N Jr, Eggleston PA, Eney D, Goldstein EO, Schuberth KC, Bacon JR, et al. A controlled trial of immunotherapy for asthma in allergic children. N Engl J Med 1997; 336(5):324–331.

123. Global strategy for asthma management and prevention. GINA. Update from NHLBI/WHO Workshop Report 1995, Revised 2002. NIH Publication No. 02-3659 2002.

124. Tari MG, Mancino M, Monti G. Efficacy of sublingual immunotherapy in patients with rhinitis and asthma due to house dust mite: A double-blind study. Allergol Immunopathol Madr 1990; 18(5):277–284.

125. Passalacqua G, Albano M, Fregonese L, Riccio A, Pronzato C, Mela G, et al. Randomised controlled trial of local allergoid immunotherapy on allergic inflammation in mite-induced rhinoconjunctivitis. Lancet 1998; 351:629–632.

126. Bousquet J, Scheinmann P, Guinnepain MT, Perrin-Fayolle M, Sauvaget J, Tonnel AB, et al. Sublingual-swallow immunotherapy (SLIT) in patients with asthma due to house-dust mites: A double-blind, placebo-controlled study (in process). Allergy 1999; 54(3):249–260.

127. Mungan D, Misirligil Z, Gurbuz L. Comparison of the efficacy of subcutaneous and sublingual immunotherapy in mite-sensitive patients with rhinitis and asthma: A placebo controlled study. Ann Allergy Asthma Immunol 1999; 82(5):485–490.

128. Pajno GB, Morabito L, Barberio G, Parmiani S. Clinical and immunologic effects of long-term sublingual immunotherapy in asthmatic children sensitized to mites: A double-blind, placebo-controlled study. Allergy 2000; 55(9):842–849.

129. Bahceciler NN, Isik U, Barlan IB, Basaran MM. Efficacy of sublingual immunotherapy in children with asthma and rhinitis: A double-blind, placebo-controlled study. Pediatr Pulmonol 2001; 32(1):49–55.

130. Hirsch T, Sahn M, Leupold W. Double-blind placebo-controlled study of sublingual immunotherapy with house dust mite extract (D.pt.) in children. Pediatr Allergy Immunol 1997; 8(1):21–27.

131. Lewith GT, Watkins AD, Hyland ME, Shaw S, Broomfield JA, Dolan G, et al. Use of ultra-molecular potencies of allergen to treat asthmatic people allergic to house dust mite: Double blind randomised controlled clinical trial. Br Med J 2002; 324(7336):520.

132. Clavel R, Bousquet J, Andre C. Clinical efficacy of sublingual-swallow immunotherapy: A double-blind, placebo-controlled trial of a standardized five-grass-pollen extract in rhinitis. Allergy 1998; 53(5):493–498.

133. Vourdas D, Syrigou E, Potamianou P, Carat F, Batard T, Andre C, et al. Double-blind, placebo-controlled evaluation of sublingual immunotherapy with standardized olive pollen extract in pediatric patients with allergic rhinoconjunctivitis and mild asthma due to olive pollen sensitization. Allergy 1998; 53(7):662–672.

134. Patriarca G, Nucera E, Pollastrini E, Roncallo C, Buonomo A, Bartolozzi F, et al. Sublingual desensitization: A new approach to latex allergy problem. Anesth Analg 2002; 95(4):956–960.

135. Nelson H, Oppenheimer J, Vatsia G, Buchmeier A. A double-blind, placebo-controlled evaluation of sublingual immunotherapy with standardized cat extract. J Allergy Clin Immunol 1993; 92:229–236.

136. Lockey RF, Benedict LM, Turkeltaub PC, Bukantz SC. Fatalities from immunotherapy (IT) and skin testing (ST). J Allergy Clin Immunol 1987; 79(4):660–677.

137. Stewart Gd, Lockey RF. Systemic reactions from allergen immunotherapy (editorial). J Allergy Clin Immunol 1992; 90(1 pt 1).567 570.
138. Personnel and equipment to treat systemic reactions caused by immunotherapy with allergenic extracts: American Academy of Allergy and Immunology. J Allergy Clin Immunol 1986; 77(2):271–273.
139. Bousquet J, Hejjaoui A, Dhivert H, Clauzel AM, Michel FB. Immunotherapy with a standardized *Dermatophagoides pteronyssinus* extract: III. Systemic reactions during the rush protocol in patients suffering from asthma. J Allergy Clin Immunol 1989; 83(4):797–802.
140. Bousquet J, Michel FB. Safety considerations in assessing the role of immunotherapy in allergic disorders. Drug Saf 1994; 10(1):5–17.
141. Peroni DG, Piacentini GL, Bodini A, Boner AL. Snail anaphylaxis during house dust mite immunotherapy. Pediatr Allergy Immunol 2000; 11(4):260–261.
142. Pajno GB, La Grutta S, Barberio G, Canonica GW, Passalacqua G. Harmful effect of immunotherapy in children with combined snail and mite allergy. J Allergy Clin Immunol 2002; 109(4):627–629.
143. Sabbah A, Hassoun S, Le-Sellin J, Andre C, Sicard H. A double-blind, placebo-controlled trial by the sublingual route of immunotherapy with a standardized grass pollen extract. Allergy 1994; 49(5):309–313.
144. Feliziani V, Lattuada G, Parmiani S, Dall'Aglio PP. Safety and efficacy of sublingual rush immunotherapy with grass allergen extracts: A double blind study. Allergol Immunopathol Madr 1995; 23(5):224–230.
145. Troise C, Voltolini S, Canessa A, Pecora S, Negrini AC. Sublingual immunotherapy in *Parietaria* pollen-induced rhinitis: A double-blind study. J Investig Allergol Clin Immunol 1995; 5(1):25–30.
146. Hordijk GJ, Antvelink JB, Luwema RA. Sublingual immunotherapy with a standardised grass pollen extract: A double-blind placebo-controlled study. Allergol Immunopathol 1998; 26(5):234–240.
147. Horak F, Stubner P, Berger UE, Marks B, Toth J, Jager S. Immunotherapy with sublingual birch pollen extract: A short-term double-blind placebo study. J Investig Allergol Clin Immunol 1998; 8(3):165–171.
148. La Rosa M, Ranno C, Andri C, Carat F, Tosca MA, Canonica GW. Double-blind placebo-controlled evaluation of sublingual-swallow immunotherapy with standardized *Parietaria judaica* extract in children with allergic rhinoconjunctivitis. J Allergy Clin Immunol 1999; 104(2 pt 1):425–432.
149. Passalacqua G, Albano M, Riccio A, Fregonese L, Puccinelli P, Parmiani S, et al. Clinical and immunologic effects of a rush sublingual immunotherapy to parietaria species: A double-blind, placebo-controlled trial (in process). J Allergy Clin Immunol 1999; 104(5):964–968.
150. Bousquet J. Local routes of immunotherapy. Arb Paul Ehrlich Inst Bundesamt Sera Impfstoffe Frankf A M 1999(93):121–127, discussion 128–129.
151. Andre C, Vatrinet C, Galvain S, Carat F, Sicard H. Safety of sublingual-swallow immunotherapy in children and adults. Int Arch Allergy Immunol 2000; 121(3):229–234.
152. Grosclaude M, Bouillot P, Alt R, Leynadier F, Scheinmann P, Rufin P, et al. Safety of various dosage regimens during induction of sublingual immunotherapy: A preliminary study. Int Arch Allergy Immunol 2002; 129(3):248–253.
153. Di Rienzo V, Pagani A, Parmiani S, Passalacqua G, Canonica GW. Post-marketing surveillance study on the safety of sublingual immunotherapy in pediatric patients. Allergy 1999; 54(10):1110–1113.
154. Lombardi C, Gargioni S, Melchiorre A, Tiri A, Falagiani P, Canonica GW, et al. Safety of sublingual immunotherapy with monomeric allergoid in adults: Multicenter post-marketing surveillance study. Allergy 2001; 56(10):989–992.
155. Nelson HS. Advances in upper airway diseases and allergen immunotherapy. J Allergy Clin Immunol 2003; 111(suppl 3):S793–S798.

156. International Consensus Report on Diagnosis and Management of Rhinitis: International Rhinitis Management Working Group. Allergy 1994; 49(suppl 19):1–34.

157. Norman P. Is there a role for immunotherapy in the treatment of asthma? Yes. Am J Respir Crit Care Med 1996; 154:1225–1228.

158. Barnes P. Is there a role for immunotherapy in the treatment of asthma? No. Am J Respir Crit Care Med 1996; 154:1227–1228.

159. Adkinson NF Jr. Immunotherapy for allergic rhinitis (editorial; comment). N Engl J Med 1999; 341(7):522–524.

160. Adkinson NF Jr. Con: Immunotherapy is not clinically indicated in the management of allergic asthma. Am J Respir Crit Care Med 2001; 164(12):2140–2141, discussion 2141–2142.

161. Custovic A, Green R, Taggart SC, Smith A, Pickering CA, Chapman MD, et al. Domestic allergens in public places: II: Dog (Can f 1) and cockroach (Bla g 2) allergens in dust and mite, cat, dog and cockroach allergens in the air in public buildings (see comments). Clin Exp Allergy 1996; 26(11):1246–1252.

28

Immunotherapy for the Prevention of Allergic Diseases

LARS JACOBSEN

ALK-Abelló, Hørsholm, Denmark

I. INTRODUCTION

Symptoms of allergic respiratory diseases are caused by exacerbation of an ongoing inflammatory process driven by basic immunological mechanisms related to antigen-mediated activation of mast cells, basophils, and eosinophils. Allergic patients can be described in relation to the complex interaction between the allergic condition and the allergic disease. It is important to understand the complexity of the allergic disease in order to offer the patient optimal treatment. The optimal treatment of allergy reduces the primary symptoms and the patient's need for medication, but may also influence the basic allergy syndrome by altering or modifying the immunological mechanism causing the disease. Giving appropriate drugs may decrease symptoms; however, the efficient diagnostic tools available today offer excellent possibilities for treating the patient in a specific way and changing the course of the disease. The optimal treatment of inhalant allergy should

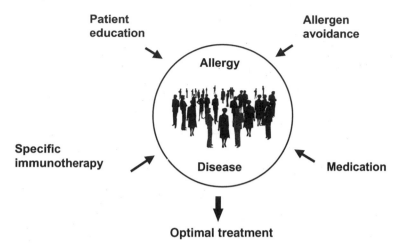

Figure 1   The concept of optimal treatment of the allergic patient. (From Ref. 25.)

include avoidance of airborne allergens, treatment of symptoms, and immunotherapy as the treatment of the immunological cause of the allergic disease together with education of the patient (Fig. 1).

Specific immunotherapy (SIT) is the only treatment that interferes with the basic pathophysiological mechanisms of the allergic disease (1). Controlled studies have generated important knowledge about the clinical efficacy of selecting an optimal dosage level of major allergens to influence the basic immunological mechanisms and inflammation causing the allergic disease (2). This recommended dosage level is between 5 and 20 μg of the major allergen per maintenance dose injected for those extracts so characterized. The fact that SIT acts by influencing basic immunological mechanisms has been documented in several studies. In birch pollen–allergic asthmatics, SIT suppressed the seasonal increase in eosinophilic cationic protein (3). During a 4-year period of SIT for grass-sensitive subjects, late-phase skin reaction was reduced in the active-treatment group compared with the placebo group following the clinical benefit (4), and there was a shift from a TH2- to a TH1-like response, which was maintained as a consequence of long-term treatment with SIT (5–8).

II. ALLERGY, HAY FEVER, AND ASTHMA

The link between hay fever and asthma has been described in several papers (9,10), and the comorbidity of upper and lower airway diseases was carefully described in collaboration with WHO (11). A European survey of 7000 allergy patients found that 80% of patients with typical asthma symptoms also reported nasal symptoms, and 40% of hay fever patients reported coexisting asthma (12). Allergic rhinitis is a major risk factor for later development of asthma (13,14). More than 20% of all children with hay fever develop asthma later in life (15,16), and rhinitis frequently precedes the onset of asthma (17,18). Many hay fever patients have increased bronchial hyperresponsiveness (BHR) during as well as outside the pollen season (19–21). Development of BHR and atopy may be significant factors influencing the increased prevalence of asthma seen over the last

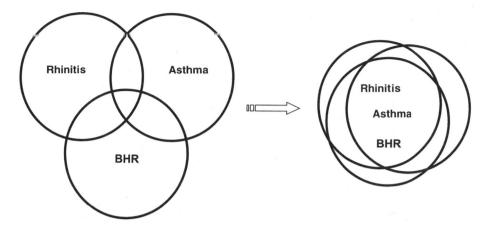

Figure 2 Illustration of the links between rhinitis, asthma, and bronchial hyperresponsiveness. (From Ref. 25.)

decades (19,22). Even when exposure to allergens is below the level of initiating symptoms, allergic patients have a constant minimal level of ongoing inflammation (23).

Hay fever, asthma, and bronchial hyperresponsiveness are closely related, and a systemic pathway, involving bloodstream and bone marrow, contributes to the interaction between upper and lower airways (24). This is important for the diagnosis of the allergic patient and for choosing between the various combinations of treatments available (25). The connection between hay fever, asthma, and BHR is illustrated in Fig. 2. How closely these different symptoms are intertwined remains to be described, but the more knowledge we get from epidemiological surveys, the more closely related the upper and lower airway diseases appear to be. Allergic sensitivities usually increase with age from childhood to adulthood, and monosensitized children are likely to become polysensitized with time (26).

III. CLINICAL BENEFITS OF SUBCUTANEOUS IMMUNOTHERAPY

Subcutaneous allergen-specific immunotherapy has been used for many years, but since characterized and standardized allergen extracts were introduced in the 1980s, careful clinical and immunological research has led to a much better understanding of its clinical benefit and the mechanisms by which it is accomplished. Subcutaneous immunotherapy is regarded as the "gold standard" for immunotherapy, although new knowledge about alternative administration routes of allergen vaccines has become available in recent years (see Chapter 35). The following discussion on the effects of immunotherapy is based on long-term high-dose subcutaneous administration of allergens, since the available documentation on the potential preventive capacity of the treatment is based on this concept. The documented efficacy of specific immunotherapy can be divided into four levels:

1. Early effect
   • Reduction in symptoms/need for medication
2. Persisting effect
   • Reduction in symptoms/need for medication

- Reduction in hyperresponsiveness/late-phase response
3. Long-term effect
   - Persistently reduced symptoms/need for medication
   - Persistently reduced hyperresponsiveness/late-phase response
4. Preventive effect
   - Prevention of new sensitivities and exacerbation of disease (rhinitis into asthma)

A. Early Effect

Eight to 12 weeks after initiation of the treatment, when patients have reached the maintenance dosage, they will experience a reduction in allergy symptoms and the need for rescue medication, as shown in several studies, including one for seasonal rhinoconjunctivitis (27) and one for cat asthma (28).

B. Persistent Effect

Persisting and potential increased benefits were achieved during a long-term treatment period of 3 to 5 years for grass (4) and cat and dog sensitivity (29). Continuing the treatment for more than 12 months introduces nonspecific efficacy parameters, seen as a decrease in the patient's nonspecific bronchial hyperresponsiveness (30). In this study the patients increased their tolerance to bronchial challenge with house dust mite allergen after 6 months, but it took up to 18 months to establish a persistent reduction in bronchial inflammation and hyperresponsiveness as measured by bronchial challenge with methacholine. Walker et al. observed, after 2 years of immunotherapy, that the treatment prevented the seasonal onset of bronchial hyperresponsiveness (31). A TH2/TH1 response back toward normal balance is associated with a positive clinical effect of immunotherapy. Grass pollen–allergic patients undergoing immunotherapy developed a significant change toward a TH1 response, measured by level of interferon-gamma in peripheral blood, after a 12-month treatment period. Despite documented clinical effect, the change toward a TH1 response was not yet present after 3 months (6).

C. Long-Term Effect

A persistent long-term clinical effect lasted for 6 years after termination of 2–3 years of SIT for grass pollen, tree pollen, as well as animal hair and dander and house dust mite (32–36). Cat-allergic patients with mild to moderate asthma not only reduced their reactivity to cat allergen following a 3-year course of immunotherapy, but specific as well as nonspecific hyperresponsiveness continued to be reduced during a 5-year follow-up period (36). A double-blind, placebo-controlled randomized long-term follow-up study of grass pollen immunotherapy patients demonstrated that the clinical improvement as well as decreased late-phase skin response to allergen challenge after a treatment period of 3 to 4 years persisted at least 3 years after termination of SIT (34).

D. Preventive Effect

The preventive effect of SIT, i.e., the potential to change the natural course of the allergic disease by preventing the exacerbation from hay fever to asthma and the onset of new sensitivities, is currently being investigated.

IV. PREVENTION OF ASTHMA

Johnstone and Dutton were the first to describe the potential of SIT to prevent the development of asthma in a long-term follow-up study in children. In their 14-year follow-up study, including 130 out of an initial group of 210 children treated with SIT or placebo, they found a highly significant reduction in the number of patients with asthma. At the time of follow-up, which corresponded to the time of the children's 16th birthdays, only 22% of the placebo-treated children were free of asthma, compared with 72% of the SIT-treated children (37). The children were initially treated for 4 years with individual mixtures of nonstandardized allergens. At inclusion in this study most of the children were from 2 to 10 years old, which means that the time from start of treatment to follow-up was individualized and represented a relatively large range of posttreatment follow-up periods. Another interesting observation in this study was that the clinical effect and potential prevention of asthmatic symptoms were dose related and most effective in children who were injected with relatively high doses of allergen.

Bauer demonstrated that fewer patients suffering only from hay fever develop nonspecific bronchial hyperresponsiveness if treated with SIT. In this study children with seasonal birch pollinosis were treated for 2 years with standardized birch pollen allergen vaccine and researchers found, after 1 year, a tendency toward reduction of seasonal bronchial hyperreactivity to histamine, which after 2 years of treatment was found to be highly significant (38).

To determine the effect of a 2-year placebo-controlled study of immunotherapy in patients with rhinoconjunctivitis caused by house dust mite allergy, Grembiale et al. selected children and adults with coexisting bronchial hyperresponsiveness. Immunotherapy reduced the provocative dose of methacholine fourfold in active patients compared with placebo. As a secondary outcome of the study, none of the SIT-treated patients developed symptoms of mild asthma during the 2-year study period, compared with 9% of the placebo-treated patients (39).

Jacobsen et al. studied 36 adult patients who received immunotherapy with standardized tree pollen allergen vaccines for 2 years. During the long-term follow-up, 6 years after termination of treatment, none of the patients initially suffering from only hay fever had developed asthma during the total study period of 8 years. These results were retrospective, but they indicate that immunotherapy not only influences the reduction in bronchial hyperresponsiveness, but also reduces the incidence of asthma (33).

PAT, the Preventive Allergy Treatment study (40), is the first prospective long-term follow-up study to test whether SIT can prevent the development of asthma in children suffering from seasonal allergic rhinoconjunctivitis caused by allergy to birch and/or grass pollen. The total immunotherapy treatment period was 3 years, after which the children were evaluated for development of asthma. The children were reevaluated after a total of 5 years, and will be evaluated again after another 5 years, resulting in a total study period of 10 years. Two hundred and eight children, 6–14 years old (mean 10.7 years), with grass and/or birch pollen allergy but without any other clinically important allergy from six pediatric allergy centers were included in this study. All had moderate to severe hay fever symptoms, but at inclusion, none reported asthma with need of daily treatment. After the initial season, two hundred and five children were stratified and randomized either to receive specific immunotherapy for 3 years or to become part of an open control group. Standardized depot allergen preparations were given every 6 weeks (±2 weeks). The content of major allergen per maintenance injection (Alutard SQ 100,000 SQ units/ml) corresponded to 20 μg Phl p V (grass) and 12 μg Bet v I (birch). Both groups received symptomatic treatment limited to loratadine, topical levocabastine, or sodium cromoglycate and, in cases unresponsive to these drugs, nasal budesonide. The development of asthma was monitored by clinical evaluation and a postseasonal visual analogue scale. Methacholine bronchial provocation tests were carried out during the relevant season(s) and during winter. Conjunctival provocation tests were done before SIT and then every year at the same time.

Although patients with perennial or seasonal asthma were excluded, it was found as a consequence of the careful study examination that 20% of the children had mild asthma symptoms during the base pollen season(s) and that more than one-third had a significant seasonal ongoing bronchial hyperresponsiveness measured by methacholine challenge. Those children with mild seasonal asthma would probably not have been diagnosed as asthmatics in daily routine practice. Among those without asthma before immunotherapy, the actively treated children had significantly less asthma after 3 years as evaluated by clinical symptoms (odds ratio 2.52; $p < 0.001$) (Fig. 3), visual analogue scale ($p < 0.001$–0.05), and seasonal as well as out-of-season methacholine bronchial provocation test ($p < 0.05$) (Fig. 4). Symptoms of hay fever and conjunctival provocation test results improved significantly in the specific immunotherapy group compared with the control group. At follow-up 2 years after termination of immunotherapy, the preventive capacity for development of asthma was confirmed by an odds ratio in favor of prevention of asthma at 2.68 (1.3–5.7) (41).

V. PREVENTION OF NEW ALLERGIES

The first study that showed the capacity of immunotherapy to reduce the risk of development of new allergies was published in 1961 (42). The researchers found that no children during a 4-year course of high-dose immunotherapy developed new IgE sensitivities, compared with 25% in the control group. In a low-dose treatment group included in this study, 23% of the children still developed new allergies.

Several studies have confirmed these findings. In 22 house dust mite–monosensitized children treated for 3 years with immunotherapy compared with 22 matched

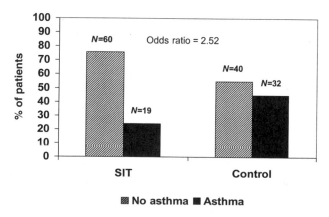

Figure 3 The percentage of children after 3 years of immunotherapy with and without asthma among those without asthma before treatment ($N = 151$). The absolute numbers of children are shown above the bars. (From Ref. 40.)

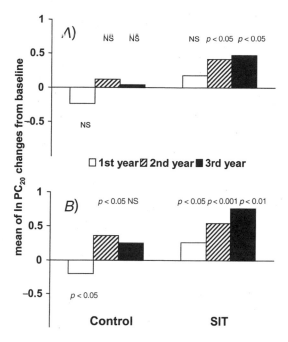

Figure 4　Development of bronchial hyperresponsiveness (methacholine challenge test) within each group (control/immunotherapy) measured as ln PC_{20} change from baseline (A) in the season of pollen exposure and (B) during winter. (From Ref. 40.)

nontreated open control children, a significant reduction in new allergies was found. In the immunotherapy-treated group approximately 45% (10 out of 22) of the patients did not develop any new sensitivities at all, whereas none of the control patients remained free of developing one or more new sensitivities by measure of skin prick test as well as allergen-specific IgE antibodies. The immunotherapy group was treated with a standardized house dust mite allergen vaccine (*Dermatophagoides pteronyssinus*) with a content of major allergen (Der p 1) corresponding to 2 μg per maintenance dose (43).

A controlled study including 138 monosensitized asthmatic children allergic to house dust mites confirms the potential of immunotherapy to prevent development of new allergic sensitivities. Seventy-five children were treated with a mixture of *Dermatophagoides pteronyssinus* and *Dermatophagoides farinae* (50/50) for a total of 3 years, and 63 children receiving only medical treatment acted as controls. The monthly maintenance dose given corresponded to approximately 6 μg (Der p 1/Der p 2) per injection. At follow-up examination 3 years after termination of immunotherapy, the researchers found that 75% of the control children had developed one or more new sensitivities by measure of skin prick test and specific IgE, compared with only 33% in the immunotherapy-treated group. The majority of new sensitivities that developed were against various pollens (44).

Also, for pollen-monosensitized allergic children it has been indicated that immunotherapy can reduce the risk of developing more allergies. Twenty-three children with seasonal hay fever caused by grass with or without coexisting allergy to trees were treated for 3 consecutive years with a preseasonal protocol using an allergoid modified grass pollen allergen vaccine. Thirteen patients were prospectively followed for 6 years after termination of immunotherapy and compared with an open control group. The result of this study was that all control patients developed one or more new sensitizations (skin prick test), compared with 61% in the immunotherapy group (45).

A large retrospective study including more that 8000 monosensitized patients suffering from rhinitis and/or asthma has confirmed the reduced risk of new sensitivities as a result of immunotherapy. For 4 years 7182 patients were treated with immunotherapy and 1214 were included as open controls treated only with symptomatic drugs. Almost half of the patients (44%) were monosensitized to either *Dermatophagoides pteronyssinus* or *Dermatophagoides farinae*; 53% were monosensitized to grasses or *Parietaria*; and 3% were monosensitized to mugwort, olive or trees. After the 4-year immunotherapy treatment, 68% of controls had developed one or more new sensitivities (skin prick test and specific IgE) compared with 24% in immunotherapy-treated patients. At follow-up 3 years after termination of the treatment period, 77% of controls had developed new sensitivities compared with 77% in the active group. Only 4% of the immunotherapy-treated patients developed a new sensitization in the follow-up period from termination of immunotherapy, compared with 27% of the controls (46).

VI. MECHANISMS OF PREVENTION

Although knowledge about the mechanisms of immunotherapy is available and intensive research continues, the preventive capacity is not yet fully understood. The fact that allergy is a systemic condition that may cause typical respiratory symptoms could explain why immunotherapy can prevent exacerbation of the disease. Immunotherapy does not limit its effect to a single shock organ. Through a reduction of the immune system's capacity to initiate the allergic cascade leading to a local inflammatory condition, immunotherapy may prevent development of hyperresponsiveness and inflammation in a not-yet-symptomatic organ. By modulating the immune response in allergic patients toward a "nonallergic" TH1 and regulatory T-cell response, symptoms that would have appeared in the unimmunized patient are prevented; i.e., the rhinitis patient does not develop asthma.

From what is known about the immunological mechanisms of immunotherapy, it is not clear how the risk of developing new sensitivities is reduced. The immunological response to immunotherapy is specifically related to the antigen with which the patient is treated. This means that the fact that patients appear with fewer positive IgE sensitivities may not be related to an allergen-specific mechanism but may be a consequence of reduced hyperresponsiveness. Allergen-induced hyperresponsiveness seems not to be related to only one organ type but is systemic and can occur in the nose, lungs, and skin. Durham has shown that immunotherapy results in fewer mast cells in the skin (47).

VII. CONCLUSION

Besides the very significant clinical effect and long-lasting benefit of specific immunotherapy, several controlled studies demonstrate that immunotherapy does reduce the risk of developing new allergic sensitivities and does reduce the risk of asthma in children suffering from hay fever.

The immunological mechanisms responsible for the preventive capacity remain to be investigated, but the investigation has to focus on the rationale for inability to initiate a new IgE response; the importance of reduced hyperresponsiveness in the nose, lungs, and skin; and the impact of immunotherapy on the T-cell response. Time of onset seems to be a very important factor in estimating the preventive potential of immunotherapy. The studies described in this paper show a preventive potential in children and adults. Most important is that in all studies referenced, the severity of the allergic symptoms were mild to moderate when such therapy was prescribed. Therefore, it is important to consider 3–5 years of high-dose immunotherapy early in the development of the allergic disease when the preventive potential is optimal and most of the disease is caused by the IgE-mediated reaction and inflammation (48).

VIII. SALIENT POINTS

1. Specific immunotherapy reduces allergic symptoms by initiation of an immunological change related to the basic pathophysiological mechanism of the allergic disease.
2. Symptoms of allergic hay fever and asthma often go together in the same patient and are caused by the same IgE-related immunological mechanism.
3. Allergic rhinitis is a risk factor for later development of asthma, and the number of allergic sensitivities in the individual patient usually increases with age.
4. The potential of immunotherapy to prevent the development of asthma in patients suffering from only rhinitis has been documented in prospective long-term follow-up studies.
5. In monosensitized patients, immunotherapy has shown to be effective in reducing the risk for development of new sensitivities as determined by skin testing.
6. Reduction in specific and nonspecific hyperresponsiveness as well as inflammatory potential related to a systemic immunological effector mechanism will not limit the treatment outcome to a single shock organ.

REFERENCES

1. Malling HJ, Weeke B. Immunotherapy: Position paper of the European Academy of Allergology and Clinical Immunology. Allergy 1993; 48:9–35.
2. Bousquet J, Lockey RF, Malling HJ (eds.). Allergen immunotherapy: Therapeutic vaccines for allergic diseases. WHO position paper. Allergy 1998; 53:1–42.
3. Rak S, Lowhagen O, Venge P. The effect of immunotherapy on bronchial hyperresponsiveness and eosinophil cationic protein in pollen-allergic patients. J Allergy Clin Immunol 1988; 82:470–480.
4. Walker SM, Varney VA, Gaga M, Jacobson MR, Durham SR. Grass pollen immunotherapy: Efficacy and safety during a 4-year follow-up study. Allergy 1995; 50:405–413.
5. Hamid QA, Schotman E, Jacobson MR, Walker SM, Durham SR. Increases in IL-12 messenger RNA+ cells accompany inhibition of allergen-induced late skin responses after successful grass pollen immunotherapy. J Allergy Clin Immunol 1997; 99:254–260.
6. Ebner C, Siemann U, Bohle B, Willheim M, Wiedermann U, Schenk S, Klotz F, Ebner H, Kraft D, Scheiner O. Immunological changes during specific immunotherapy of grass pollen allergy: Reduced lymphoproliferative responses to allergen and shift from TH2 to TH1 in T-cell clones specific for Phl p 1, a major grass pollen allergen (see comments). Clin Exp Allergy 1997; 27:1007–1015.
7. Wilson DR, Nouri-Aria KT, Walker SM, Pajno GB, O'Brien F, Jacobson MR, Mackay IS, Durham SR. Grass pollen immunotherapy: Symptomatic improvement correlates with

reductions in eosinophils and IL-5 mRNA expression in the nasal mucosa during the pollen season. J Allergy Clin Immunol 2001; 107:971–976.

8. Wachholz PA, Nouri-Aria KT, Wilson DR, Walker SM, Verhoef A, Till SJ, Durham SR. Grass pollen immunotherapy for hayfever is associated with increases in local nasal but not peripheral Th1:Th2 cytokine ratios. Immunology 2002; 105:56–62.

9. Togias A. Mechanisms of nose-lung interaction. Allergy 1999; 54(suppl 57):94–105.

10. Simons FE. Allergic rhinobronchitis: The asthma-allergic rhinitis link. J Allergy Clin Immunol 1999; 104:534–540.

11. Bousquet J, Van Cauwenberge P, Khaltaev N. Allergic rhinitis and its impact on asthma. In collaboration with the World Health Organization. Executive summary of the workshop report. 7–10 December 1999, Geneva, Switzerland. Allergy 2002; 57:841–855.

12. Jacobsen L, Chivato T, Andersen P, Valovirta E, Dahl R, de Monchy J. The co-morbidity of allergic hay fever and asthma in randomly selected patients with respiratory allergic diseases. Allergy 2002; 57:23.

13. Leynaert B, Neukirch F, Demoly P, Bousquet J. Epidemiologic evidence for asthma and rhinitis comorbidity. J Allergy Clin Immunol 2000; 106:S201–S205.

14. Guerra S, Sherrill DL, Martinez FD, Barbee RA. Rhinitis as an independent risk factor for adult-onset asthma. J Allergy Clin Immunol 2002; 109:419–425.

15. Rackemann FM, Edwards RN. Asthma in Children. A Follow-up Study of 688 Patients After An Interval of Twenty Years. N Engl J Med 1952; 246:815–823.

16. Linna O, Kokkonen J, Lukin M. A 10-year prognosis for childhood allergic rhinitis. Acta Paediatr 1992; 81:100–102.

17. Pedersen PA, Weeke ER. Asthma and allergic rhinitis in the same patients. Allergy 1983; 38:25–29.

18. Settipane RJ, Hagy GW, Settipane GA. Long-term risk factors for developing asthma and allergic rhinitis: a 23-year follow-up study of college students. Allergy Proc 1994; 15:21–25.

19. Townley RG, Ryo UY, Kolotkin BM, Kang B. Bronchial sensitivity to methacholine in current and former asthmatic and allergic rhinitis patients and control subjects. J Allergy Clin Immunol 1975; 56:429–442.

20. Ramsdale EH, Morris MM, Roberts RS, Hargreave FE. Asymptomatic bronchial hyperresponsiveness in rhinitis. J Allergy Clin Immunol 1985; 75:573–577.

21. Madonini E, Briatico Vangosa G, Pappacoda A, Maccagni G, Cardani A, Saporiti F. Seasonal increase of bronchial reactivity in allergic rhinitis. J Allergy Clin Immunol 1987; 79:358–363.

22. von Mutius E. Atopy and bronchial hyperresponsiveness in children. ACI 1995; 7:179–182.

23. Ciprandi G, Pronzato C, Passalacqua G, Ricca V, Bagnasco M, Grogen J, Mela GS, Canonica GW. Topical azelastine reduces eosinophil activation and intercellular adhesion molecule-1 expression on nasal epithelial cells: An antiallergic activity. J Allergy Clin Immunol 1996; 98:1088–1096.

24. Braunstahl GJ, Prins JB, Kleinjan A, Overbeek SE, Hoogsteden HC, Fokkens WJ. Nose and lung cross-talk in allergic airways disease. Clin Exp Allergy Rev 2003; 3:38–42.

25. Jacobsen L. Preventive aspects of immunotherapy: Prevention for children at risk of developing asthma. Ann Allergy Asthma Immunol 2001; 87:43–46.

26. Silvestri M, Rossi GA, Cozzani S, Pulvirenti G, Fasce L. Age-dependent tendency to become sensitized to other classes of aeroallergens in atopic asthmatic children. Ann Allergy Asthma Immunol 1999; 83:335–340.

27. Varney VA, Gaga M, Frew AJ, Aber VR, Kay AB, Durham SR. Usefulness of immunotherapy in patients with severe summer hay fever uncontrolled by antiallergic drugs (see comments). Br Med J 1991; 302:265–269.

28. Varney VA, Edwards J, Tabbah K, Brewster H, Mavroleon G, Frew AJ. Clinical efficacy of specific immunotherapy to cat dander: A double-blind placebo-controlled trial. Clin Exp Allergy 1997; 27:860–867.

29. Hedlin G, Graff Lonnevig V, Heilborn H, Lilja G, Norrlind K, Pegelow K, Sundin B, Lowenstein H. Immunotherapy with cat and dog dander extracts. V. Effects of 3 years of treatment. J Allergy Clin Immunol 1991; 87:955–964.

30. Pichler CE, Marquardsen A, Sparholt S, Lowenstein H, Bircher A, Bischof M, Pichler WJ. Specific immunotherapy with *Dermatophagoides pteronyssinus* and *D. farinae* results in decreased bronchial hyperreactivity. Allergy 1997; 52:274–283.

31. Walker SM, Pajno GB, Lima MT, Wilson DR, Durham SR. Grass pollen immunotherapy for seasonal rhinitis and asthma: A randomized, controlled trial. J Allergy Clin Immunol 2001; 107:87–93.

32. Mosbech H, Osterballe O. Does the effect of immunotherapy last after termination of treatment? Follow-up study in patients with grass pollen rhinitis. Allergy 1988; 43:523–529.

33. Jacobsen L, Nuchel PB, Wihl JA, Lowenstein H, Ipsen H. Immunotherapy with partially purified and standardized tree pollen extracts: IV. Results from long-term (6-year) follow-up. Allergy 1997; 52:914–920.

34. Durham SR, Walker SM, Varga EM, Jacobson MR, O'Brien F, Noble W, Till SJ, Hamid QA, Nouri-Aria KT. Long-term clinical efficacy of grass-pollen immunotherapy (see comments). N Engl J Med 1999; 341:468–475.

35. Des RA, Paradis L, Knani J, Hejjaoui A, Dhivert H, Chanez P, Bousquet J. Immunotherapy with a standardized *Dermatophagoides pteronyssinus* extract: V. Duration of the efficacy of immunotherapy after its cessation. Allergy 1996; 51:430–433.

36. Hedlin G, Heilborn H, Lilja G, Norrlind K, Pegelow KO, Schou C, Lowenstein H. Long-term follow-up of patients treated with a three-year course of cat or dog immunotherapy. J Allergy Clin Immunol 1995; 96:879–885.

37. Johnstone DE, Dutton A. The value of hyposensitization therapy for bronchial asthma in children: A 14-year study. Pediatrics 1968; 42:793–802.

38. Bauer CP. Untersuchung zur Asthmaprävention durch die specifische Immuntherapie bei Kindern. Allergologie 1993; 468.

39. Grembiale RD, Camporota L, Naty S, Tranfa CM, Djukanovic R, Marsico SA. Effects of specific immunotherapy in allergic rhinitic individuals with bronchial hyperresponsiveness (in process). Am J Respir Crit Care Med 2000; 162:2048–2052.

40. Moller C, Dreborg S, Ferdousi HA, Halken S, Host A, Jacobsen L, Koivikko A, Koller DY, Niggemann B, Norberg LA, Urbanek R, Valovirta E, Wahn U. Pollen immunotherapy reduces the development of asthma in children with seasonal rhinoconjunctivitis (the PAT-study). J Allergy Clin Immunol 2002; 109:251–256.

41. Jacobsen L, Möller C, Dreborg D, Ferdousi HA, Halken S, Høst A, Norberg LA, Koivikko A, Valovirta E, Niggemann B, Wahn U. Five-year follow-up on the PAT study: A 3-year course of specific immunotherapy (SIT) results in long-term prevention of asthma in children. Allergy 2003; 58(suppl 74):3.

42. Johnstone DE, Crump L. Value of hyposensitization therapy for perennial bronchial asthma in children. Pediatrics 1961; 61:44.

43. Des Roches A, Paradis L, Menardo JL, Bouges S, Daures JP, Bousquet J. Immunotherapy with a standardized *Dermatophagoides pteronyssinus* extract: VI. Specific immunotherapy prevents the onset of new sensitizations in children. J Allergy Clin Immunol 1997; 99:450–453.

44. Pajno GB, Barberio G, De Luca F, Morabito L, Parmiani S. Prevention of new sensitizations in asthmatic children monosensitized to house dust mite by specific immunotherapy: A six-year follow-up study. Clin Exp Allergy 2001; 31:1392–1397.

45. Eng PA, Reinhold M, Gnehm HP. Long-term efficacy of preseasonal grass pollen immunotherapy in children. Allergy 2002; 57:306–312.

46. Purello-D'Ambrosio F, Gangemi S, Merendino RA, Isola S, Puccinelli P, Parmiani S, Ricciardi L. Prevention of new sensitizations in monosensitized subjects submitted to specific immunotherapy or not. A retrospective study. Clin Exp Allergy 2001; 31:1295–1302.

47. Durham SR, Varney VA, Gaga M, Jacobson MR, Varga EM, Frew AJ, Kay AB. Grass pollen immunotherapy decreases the number of mast cells in the skin. Clin Exp Allergy 1999; 29:1490–1496.

48. Bousquet J, Van Cauwenberge P, Khaltaev N. Allergic rhinitis and its impact on asthma. J Allergy Clin Immunol 2001; 108:S147–S334.

29

Immunotherapy for Hymenoptera Venom and Biting Insect Hypersensitivity

ULRICH R. MÜLLER

Spital Bern Ziegler, Bern, Switzerland

DAVID B.K. GOLDEN

Johns Hopkins University, Baltimore, Maryland, U.S.A.

PATRICK J. DEMARCO and RICHARD F. LOCKEY

*University of South Florida College of Medicine and James A. Haley
Veterans' Hospital, Tampa, Florida, U.S.A.*

I. INTRODUCTION

Insect stings, especially by Hymenoptera of the families Apidae (the honeybee and the bumblebee), Vespidae (with the species *Vespula, Dolichovespula, Vespa*, and *Polistes*), and in some regions also Formicidae (the ants), are one of the major causes of severe, generalized, IgE-mediated hypersensitivity reactions, which may be fatal. According to the registered data of the Swiss Statistical Department, 120 individuals died from Hymenoptera stings between 1961 and 1999. Extrapolated to Western and Central Europe, these data correspond to about 160 yearly fatalities from Hymenoptera stings in the region. Government statistics in the United States show at least 40 deaths each year from insect stings, although it is likely that many others are not reported.

The first attempts at immunotherapy for Hymenoptera sting–allergic patients were made at the end of the 1920s. Insect venom or venom sac extracts/vaccines were first used. The high frequency of side effects with these extracts/vaccines and the report of the successful treatment of a beekeeper with whole-body extract/vaccine of bees led to the worldwide use of these better-tolerated whole-body extracts/vaccines of the respective insects. The results of immunotherapy with these extracts/vaccines were favorable in many uncontrolled studies (1). It was only in the late 1960s and 1970s that venoms were shown to be superior to whole-body extracts for diagnosis. Finally, two controlled studies documented the superiority of venoms over whole-body extracts/vaccines for immunotherapy of Hymenoptera sting–allergic individuals (2,3). Venoms obtained by electrostimulation or by venom sac extraction were commercially introduced in 1979 and have since been used successfully worldwide for immunotherapy of patients allergic to stings by Apidae and Vespidae; such preparations are not yet commercially available for Formicidae. Sections II to VI deal with various aspects of immunotherapy in Hymenoptera sting hypersensitivity. Systemic allergic reactions to biting insects, such as mosquitos or horseflies, are much less common, and their treatment is dealt with in Section VII. (See Chapter 19.)

II. INDICATIONS

A. History

The indications for venom immunotherapy (VIT) include only two factors: a history of systemic allergic reaction to a sting and positive diagnostic tests (4,5). The history is especially important because diagnostic tests with venoms are positive in many asymptomatic individuals (6). There is an absolute need to correlate the history with the test results.

Systemic reactions to stings consist of one or more of the signs and symptoms of anaphylaxis or may be limited to cutaneous manifestations, which is more common in children (60%) than in adults (15%) (7). Respiratory symptoms occur with equal frequency, in about 40% of children and adults. Cardiovascular signs and symptoms are common in adults (30%) but uncommon in children (10%). It is sometimes difficult to ascertain whether the symptoms are truly anaphylactic because they may result from anxiety, pain, or toxic effects. It is most helpful when objective signs of anaphylaxis are noted (e.g., widespread urticaria, angioedema, documented hypotension, wheezing, reduced airflow, or oxygen desaturation). The severity of the reaction is one of the most important factors determining the need for and duration of treatment and the chance of adverse reactions to injections (8). Although identification of the stinging insect by patients and physicians is unreliable, the identity of the culprit insect is important because honeybee allergy is associated with greater risks and less reliable treatment efficacy (9). In the absence of history of sting-induced allergic reaction, sensitization by an asymptomatic sting has been reported to be associated with a 17% chance of a systemic reaction to a future sting but is not considered an indication for VIT, especially since asymptomatic sensitivity is transient in many cases (6). For this reason, venom allergy testing and treatment is not recommended when it is requested by an individual out of fear alone, such as a family member of someone who had a fatal reaction to a sting.

B.   Diagnostic Testing: Skin Tests and Serum IgE (RAST)

The decision to begin venom immunotherapy requires confirmation of allergic sensitivity to venom allergens by positive venom-skin tests or detection of venom-specific IgE antibodies in serum by RAST (Table 1).

The standard skin test utilizes the intradermal test technique with commercially available Hymenoptera venom preparations. For Hymenoptera venom testing, prick tests at 0.001 µg/ml may be used initially for patients with a history of very severe reactions. Intradermal tests use venom concentrations beginning at 0.001 to 0.01 µg/ml and increasing, if necessary, to 1.0 µg/ml to find the minimum concentration giving a positive result. Honeybee venom is somewhat more irritating and can induce weak positive reactions in nonallergic individuals. Yellow jacket (*Vespula*) venom causes false-positive reactions primarily at a 10 µg/ml concentration in 10% of nonallergic subjects (10).

Most patients with a convincing history of insect allergy have positive venom tests, but some are skin test negative (11) (Table 2). Negative skin tests can be due to loss of sensitivity after many years and can also occur in up to 50% during the refractory period of 4 to 6 weeks after a sting reaction. When the venom skin test is negative but there is a history of severe anaphylaxis, in vitro tests for venom-specific IgE antibodies should be performed and the patient should continue avoidance precautions. In most such cases, the sensitivity can be detected with in vitro tests. Some cases of apparent sting anaphylaxis are thought to be non–IgE mediated. Possible mechanisms include mast cell hyperreleasability with nonimmune (toxic) release of mast cell mediators and mastocytosis, which has been suspected or proven in more than 1% of patients with insect sting anaphylaxis (12,13).

The detection of allergen-specific IgE antibodies in serum by RAST or similar serologic tests is potentially useful. A high level of venom-specific IgE is diagnostic but must

Table 1   Clinical Recommendations Based on History of Sting Reactions and Results of Venom Skin Test or RAST

Reaction to previous sting	Skin test or RAST	Risk of systemic reaction	Clinical advice
None	Positive	10–15%	Avoidance
Large local	Positive	5–10%	Avoidance
Cutaneous systemic	Positive: child	10%	No VIT
	Positive: adult	15–20%	VIT
Anaphylaxis	Positive	40–60%	VIT
	Negative	2–5%	Repeat skin test/RAST

Table 2   Diagnosis of Insect Allergy in Patients with a Positive History of Systemic Reaction

Skin test positive	68%
Skin test negative/RAST positive	14%
Skin test negative/RAST negative	18%
Sting challenge negative	17%
Sting challenge positive	1%

be correlated with the history. A low level of venom IgE is more difficult to interpret. Even a very low level of venom IgE can be associated with near-fatal anaphylaxis. The venom skin test and RAST correlate imperfectly (14,15). The RAST is negative in approximately 20% of skin test–positive subjects, so skin tests are preferred clinically because of their higher sensitivity. However, the converse is also true: Approximately 10% of skin test–negative patients have a positive RAST. For this reason European allergists recommend estimation of venom-specific IgE in all individuals with a history of systemic allergic reactions.

Most important, neither the degree of skin test sensitivity nor the titer of specific IgE correlates reliably with the degree of clinical sting reaction. Patients who have had only large local reactions may have very high levels of sensitivity on skin test and RAST but have a very low risk of anaphylaxis, whereas some patients who have had abrupt and near-fatal anaphylactic shock have only weak skin test or serologic positivity. In fact, almost 25% of patients presenting for evaluation of systemic allergic reactions to stings are skin test positive only at the 1.0 µg/ml concentration, demonstrating the importance of testing with the full diagnostic range of concentrations. These points emphasize the importance of the history in making the correct diagnosis and prognosis.

Another diagnostic option is a supervised live sting challenge. The history and skin tests select patients at high risk, but even those patients have only about a 50% chance of reacting to a future sting. The sting challenge seems to select those patients who will have another systemic reaction to a sting (15,16). However, even a negative sting challenge does not rule out future reactions, because 20% of patients who did not react to one challenge sting did react to a repeat challenge sting on another occasion (17). Others consider the diagnostic sting challenge to be unethical and recommend it only as a test to evaluate the efficacy of immunotherapy (18).

Some patients with positive venom skin tests have a low risk of anaphylaxis because their systemic reactions had been mild. Subsequent stings in these patients usually cause no systemic reaction or a reaction that tends to be equal to or less severe than previous reactions. However, there are patients who suffer reactions of increasing severity to subsequent stings. In current practice in North America, adults with sting-induced generalized urticaria and angioedema, and patients of all ages with any degree of throat symptoms, dyspnea, dizziness, or hypotension, are advised to undergo immunotherapy. The majority of children who have systemic reactions have cutaneous reactions (generalized urticaria and angioedema) but no involvement of the tongue, throat, or respiratory or circulatory system. These children have a minimal (1%) risk of a more severe reaction. Actually, during 9 years of follow-up, stings caused no systemic reaction at all in 90% of them; the other 10% had some cutaneous symptoms, which were generally even less severe than previously (7). Therefore, VIT is not generally recommended in this situation but is given to highly exposed children with repeated reactions and consequently greatly reduced quality of life. The same restricted recommendation of VIT is also used in Europe in adult individuals with exclusively cutaneous reactions because prospective studies have indicated a low risk (15–20%) of developing a generalized, most often only cutaneous, reaction at reexposure (4).

Some patients with positive venom tests are at a relatively low risk of anaphylaxis because they never had anaphylaxis to previous stings. Those children and adults with large local but no systemic reactions seem to have a 4–10% chance of a subsequent systemic reaction (19). Therapy is not recommended for asymptomatic skin test–positive individuals and large local reactors to avoid the unnecessary treatment of over 90% of such patients. There is limited evidence that venom immunotherapy prevents large local reactions, but it certainly does prevent systemic reactions (20).

C. Selection of Venoms

The selection of venom vaccines for immunotherapy is dependent on the venom skin test reaction and presence of serum-specific IgE antibodies. North American allergists/immunologists recommend that all venoms resulting in positive tests be included for immunotherapy. Therapy includes all venoms that are positive since prevention of future sting reactions is not possible without specific therapy. Some investigators recommend treatment only with the venom of the suspected insect culprit (21). When vespids are involved, the most common therapy is with *Vespula* venom alone or the mixed vespid venom preparation available in North America. It contains equal parts of yellow jacket (*Vespula* spp.), yellow hornet (*Dolichovespula arenaria*), and white-faced hornet (*Dolichovespula maculata*) venoms (22). Mixed vespid venoms are not available in Europe. Although *Dolichovespula* species are by no means rare, they are responsible for only a small minority of vespid stings. These insects are not interested in human food and sting almost exclusively in the proximity of their nests. The same is true for the European hornet, *Vespa crabro*. Moreover, European *Dolichovespula*, in contrast to American *D. maculata*, the white-faced hornet, can be distinguished from *Vespula* only with a magnifying glass by those with special entomological knowledge. Finally, in vitro studies have documented ample cross-reactivity between venoms of *Vespula, Dolichovespula*, and *Vespa*. Therefore, vespid-allergic patients in Europe are treated by *Vespula* venom alone, which is effective in more than 95% (4,18) of treated patients.

The skin test is also positive to wasp (*Polistes*) venoms in at least 50% of vespid-allergic patients. When positive, it is usually included in therapy as a separate injection, at least in areas where *Polistes* is important, such as the gulf states of the United States and the Mediterranean countries in Europe. Therapy with *Vespula* or mixed vespid venoms protects against *Polistes* stings, but this has been established only for patients whose *Polistes*-specific IgE antibodies completely cross-reacted with *Vespula* venom as assessed by RAST inhibition (22).

Double positivity of diagnostic tests with *Vespula* and honeybee venom is occasionally observed. History sometimes helps to identify the culprit insect, since vespids do not usually sting in the spring and do not—in contrast to the honeybee—usually leave the stinger in the skin. The limited cross-reactivity between *Vespula* and honeybee venom is confined largely to hyaluronidase. When skin tests are definitely positive for the two venoms, both venoms should be included for VIT unless complete cross-reactivity can be demonstrated in RAST inhibition (4).

III. EFFICACY, SAFETY, AND MONITORING OF VENOM IMMUNOTHERAPY

The recommended maintenance dose is 100 µg of each venom that elicited a positive venom test result, both in children and in adults. This dose was originally suggested because it was believed to be equivalent to two stings. This is true of honeybee venom, but the dose may be closer to 10 *Vespula* stings. Doses below 100 µg are not reliably effective in adults (23). Venom immunotherapy with honeybee venom gives full protection in 75–85% of cases, whereas therapy with *Vespula* venoms is effective in 95–98% of patients

(18). When treatment with 100 µg is not fully effective, patients may be protected with a higher dose (24).

Venom immunotherapy has proven to be safer than originally thought. Systemic reactions were expected to be more frequent or more severe because of the underlying anaphylactic syndrome, but that did not occur. The incidence of adverse reactions to venom is similar to that reported for inhalant allergen immunotherapy (25). For unexplained reasons, systemic allergic reactions are considerably more frequent during immunotherapy with honeybee venom (9). Systemic symptoms occur in 5–15% of patients on vespid venoms and 20–40% of those on honeybee venom, most often during the first weeks of treatment, regardless of the regimen used. Most reactions are mild. In the unusual case of recurrent systemic reactions to injections, therapy may be streamlined to a single venom and given in divided doses, 30 minutes apart. Large local reactions, which may be larger (8–10 cm) than are generally acceptable during inhalant allergen immunotherapy, occur in up to 50% of patients, especially in the dose range of 20–50 µg. Large local reactions are, however, not predictive of systemic reactions to subsequent injections and will not prevent attainment of the maintenance target dose of venom immunotherapy.

There is minimal need for monitoring the patient with diagnostic tests during maintenance venom immunotherapy. Annual visits with the allergist serve to review the treatment plan and to ensure that the patient does not have a new medication or medical condition that might influence therapy. There is no need for annual skin tests or blood tests, although repeating the skin tests every 2 to 3 years is recommended to identify patients who could stop treatment because skin tests become negative. The venom-specific IgE level and skin test sensitivity usually increase in the first months of therapy, return to baseline after 12 months, and then decline steadily during maintenance treatment. This decline continues even after therapy is stopped or after a sting (26) (Fig. 1). Even after 3 to 5 years of treatment these tests turn negative only in a minority of patients. Less than 20% of patients are skin test negative after 5 years, but 50–60% become negative after 7–10 years (28). Specific IgE may decrease more rapidly than skin sensitivity, but also may persist at very low levels even when venom skin tests become negative (26).

Venom-specific IgG antibodies, especially IgG4, are high in beekepers, and passive immunotherapy with beekeeper gamma globulin has been shown to protect bee venom–allergic individuals (29). Assays for venom-specific IgG correlate with clinical protection but cannot accurately predict the outcome of every sting in every individual. The test may be used to confirm protective levels after initiating therapy and then to verify that the venom IgG level is adequately maintained at the longer intervals used for maintenance treatment. In one study, the IgG level was considered protective with serum levels >3 µg/ml during the first 4 years of maintenance therapy, but protection was independent of the IgG after 4 years of treatment because other mechanisms of action may become more important (30). Profound changes in the T-cell reactivity to allergen stimulation of venom–allergic patients with a shift from a TH2 to a TH1 or TH0 pattern have been described during venom immunotherapy (31,32). Data on the relation of these alterations to the efficacy of the treatment as indicated by a tolerated sting are not available.

IV. IMMUNOTHERAPY PROTOCOLS

The starting dose is between 0.001 and 0.1 µg. The recommended maintenance dose is 100 µg of venom protein, corresponding to one to two bee stings and probably many more *Vespula* stings (33). Higher maintenance doses (200 µg or more) are recommended for

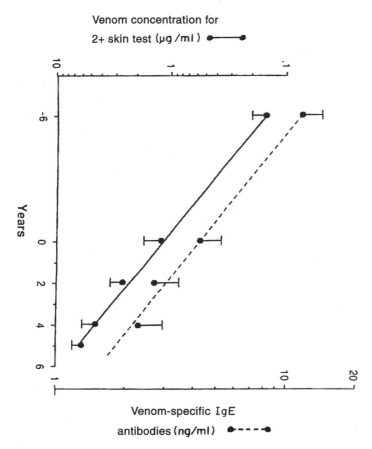

Figure 1 Mean venom skin test sensitivity (concentration in μg/ml for 2+ reaction) and venom-specific IgE antibody level (in ng/ml) shown before venom immunotherapy (time, –6 years); after a mean of 6 years of treatment (time 0); and 2, 4, and 5 years after stopping therapy. (From Golden DBK, Kwiterovich KA, Kagey-Sobotka A, et al. Discontinuing venom immunotherapy: Outcome after five years. J Allergy Clin Immunol 1996; 97:579, with permission.)

beekeepers (34), who may be stung by several insects at the same time, and in treatment failures or incomplete treatment success (4,24). The success rate undoubtedly rises with higher maintenance doses, but so too does the incidence of adverse reactions (34).

A number of protocols have been proposed for the build-up phase, some of which are summarized in Table 3 (conventional, cluster, rush, or ultrarush protocols) (4,35). Many allergists in Europe use aluminium hydroxide–adsorbed venom for conventional protocols, while others use aqueous preparations for the build-up with accelerated protocols and then change to aluminium hydroxide–adsorbed venoms, which are usually somewhat better tolerated, for maintenance immunotherapy. One commercially available preparation is dialyzed to remove small-molecular-weight compounds. In the United States only aqueous preparations are available. Rush and ultrarush protocols (35) have the advantage of inducing a more rapid protection, which is preferred in highly exposed individuals during the flying season of Hymenoptera. Moreover, the number of visits during the build-up phase

Table 3 Treatment Protocols for Venom Immunotherapy

Day	Hour	Dose in µg venom				
		Ultrarush	Rush	Cluster	Conventional	Alhydroxide ads.
1	0	0.1	0.01	0.001	0.01	0.02
	0.5	1	0.1	0.01	0.1	
	1	10	1	0.1		
	1.5	20				
	2.5	30	2			
	3.5	40				
2	0		4			
	1		8			
	2		10			
	3		20			
3	0		40			
	1		60			
	2		80			
4	0		100			
8	0		100	1	1	0.04
	1			5	2	
	2			10		
15	0	50	100	20	4	0.08
	1	50		30	8	
22	0	100		50	10	0.2
	1			50	20	
29			100	100	40	0.4
36				100	60	0.8
43		100	100		80	2
50					100	4
57					100	6
64				100		8
71		100	100		100	10
78						20
85					100	40
92				100		60
99		100	100			80
106					100	100

Further injections of the maintenance dose are 100 mg every 4 weeks during the first year, and every 6 weeks during further years of venom immunotherapy.
Source: Based on Ref. 4.

is greatly reduced. However, the rate of side effects is higher in these rapid build-up protocols, especially in bee venom–allergic individuals (9) and in rush protocols with high cumulative daily doses (35).

Once the maintenance dose has been reached, the interval between injections is extended to 4 weeks in the first year and to 6 to 8 weeks for the second year of immunotherapy and thereafter, provided that the treatment is tolerated. While the build-up phase of venom immunotherapy should be performed by an allergist, injections can be continued by the general practitioner once the maintenance dose is tolerated. Some allergists premedicate with antihistamines during the build-up phase because controlled studies demonstrate that they significantly reduce side effects. One study demonstrated an enhanced efficacy of venom immunotherapy using antihistamine premedication (36).

V. DURATION OF VENOM IMMUNOTHERAPY

After its introduction in 1979, venom immunotherapy was—and by some still is today—continued for life or at least until both skin tests and serum venom-specific IgE become negative. However, after prolonged VIT, only a small proportion of patients developed negative diagnostic tests, and compliance with continuation of VIT for many years often decreased (1,4).

For this reason a number of studies were initiated that addressed the protection rate after stopping VIT of a limited duration (Table 4) (37–42). In one series, the reaction to a sting challenge (CH) 1 to 3 years after stopping VIT of at least 3 years duration was analyzed. All studies, with a relatively short observation period after stopping successful VIT, reported continued protection in the vast majority (83–100%) of patients. Results were somewhat more favorable in *Vespula* than in bee venom–allergic individuals and in children than in adults.

In four studies (27,28,43,44) long-term protection up to 7 years after discontinuing VIT (Table 5) was analyzed. Reisman (43) found relapses following a field sting up to

Table 4 Prospective Studies with Sting Provocation Test After Stopping Venom Immunotherapy

Author	No. of patients	Insect	Sting challenge After years	No. with GR (%)
Urbanek (37)	29	Honeybee	1	1 (3)
	14		2	2 (14)
Golden (38)	29	m *Vespula*	1	0
Müller (39)	86	Honeybee	1	15 (17)
Haugaard (40)	25	*Vespula*	2	0
Keating (41)	51	m *Vespula*	1	2 (4)
van Halteren (42)	75	*Vespula*	1–3	6 (8)

GR = generalized allergic reaction, m *Vespula* = mostly *Vespula*.

Table 5 Long-Term Protection After Discontinuation of Venom Immunotherapy

Author	No. of patients	Insect	Observation yrs. after stop	Reexposure	No. with GR (%)
Reisman (43)	113	mV	1–>5	FS	10 (9)
Golden (26)	74	mV	5	CH	7 (9.5)
Golden (27)	26	mV	3–7	FS	5 (19)
Lerch (44)	120	B	3–7	FS/CH	19 (15.8)
	80	V	3–7	FS/CH	6 (7.5)

GR = generalized allergic reaction, mV = mostly *Vespula*, B = honeybee, V = *Vespula*, FS = field sting, CH = sting challenge.

more than 5 years after stopping in 10 of 113 (9%) mostly *Vespula* venom–allergic patients. Golden (26) followed 74 predominantly *Vespula* venom–allergic patients for 5 years after stopping VIT of at least 5 years duration with a CH every year (29 patients), every second year (25 patients), or only after 2 years (20 patients). Seven (9.5%) developed at least one generalized allergic reaction (GR), which was always mild. The same group (27) observed GR to a field sting in 5 of 26 (19%) patients out of 125 who were followed up to 7 years after VIT, and some of these reactions were severe. Finally, Lerch (44) reported on 358 patients who were controlled up to 7 years after stopping successful VIT. Two hundred were reexposed by either a field sting or a CH, and 25 (12.5%) developed a (mostly mild) GR. Taken together, these studies with a prolonged observation after stopping VIT found relapses somewhat more frequently than the earlier studies with a shorter follow-up. Still, the great majority, 80% or more, remained protected when restung up to 7 years after VIT.

By careful analysis of these prospective studies, a number of risk factors for the recurrence of GR following Hymenoptera stings can be identified:

1. *Age*. Children generally have a more favorable prognosis than adults (7), both without VIT and also after discontinuing VIT. Urbanek (37) saw relapses in only 3% of bee venom (BV)–allergic children, whereas Müller (39) observed a relapse rate of 17% in 86 mostly adult patients after BV immunotherapy. Lerch (44) recorded a 8.3% relapse rate in 24 children compared with 13.1% in 176 adults who were reexposed up to 7 years after stopping VIT.

2. *Insect*. Analysis of the results presented in Table 3 as well as the recurrence rates after VIT reported by Lerch (44) of 7.5% for *Vespula* venom and 15.8% for bee venom–treated patients indicate a higher risk of relapse in bee venom than in *Vespula* venom–allergic patients. The reason for this difference is not entirely clear but has been discussed elsewhere (4,9,18).

3. *Severity of pretreatment reaction*. In four prospective studies involving 386 patients, relapses were observed in 5 (4.1%) of 123 with mild but 38 (14.5%) of 263 with severe pretreatment GR (41,43–45) ($\chi^2 = 9.128$, $p < 0.01$). In addition, there is a higher risk that a recurring reaction after stopping VIT in these patients will be more severe than in those with milder pretreatment reactions.

4. *Safety and efficacy of VIT*. Patients who developed generalized allergic side effects to VIT injections were at a relapse risk of 38%, whereas those who didn't of only 7% according to one study (39). Similarly, incomplete protection when restung during VIT is associated with an increased risk of relapse (26).

5. *Duration of VIT*. With more prolonged VIT the risk of a relapse seems to be reduced. Thus, in one study (44) only 4.8% of 82 patients with a VIT duration of ≥ 50 months as opposed to 17.8% of 118 with a VIT duration of 33–49 months developed GR when restung after discontinuation ($\chi^2 = 7.382$, $p < 0.01$).

6. *Elevated basal serum tryptase, mastocytosis*. Insect venom allergy in patients with urticaria pigmentosa is most often associated with severe shock reactions (13). Two female patients with urticaria pigmentosa and *Vespula* venom sensitivity died from a re-sting 1.3 and 9 years after stopping venom immunotherapy (12). Up to one-quarter of patients with severe shock reactions following Hymenoptera stings have an elevated basal serum tryptase level, indicating the presence of an increased whole-body mast cell load (46). It is assumed that patients in this situation are at an increased risk to develop a severe reaction after stopping VIT.

7. *Repeated reexposure after stopping VIT*. According to Lerch (44), about half of the relapses occur after the first and half after later re-stings. In the presence of repeated

re-stings, the risk of a severe reaction increases significantly. Golden et al. (28) also described an increased frequency of generalized reactions 4 years after stopping VIT compared with the first 1–2 years, as well as in patients who developed such reactions after 7–13 years off VIT despite nonreaction to a previous sting in the first few years after discontinuation.

8. *High sensitivity according to diagnostic tests.* An association of re-sting reactions has been observed after stopping VIT with a persisting high sensitivity with intradermal skin testing (30,31). Others (39,44) were unable to confirm this. Specific serum IgE and IgG antibodies per se have no predictive value with regard to re-sting risk after stopping therapy. Currently used diagnostic tests are of limited predictive value with regard to long-term protection after VIT. Only the combination of a negative intracutaneous skin test at 1 µg/ml with the absence of venom-specific serum IgE antibodies is associated with a strongly diminished risk of relapse (39,44). Sex and a history of atopic disease do not seem to influence the risk of a relapse after stopping VIT.

In conclusion, most patients with Hymenoptera venom sensitivity remain protected for many years following discontinuation of VIT of at least 3 to 5 years duration. In the high-risk situations mentioned above, an even longer treatment duration has to be considered. Because of the small but relevant risk of re-sting reactions, emergency medications for self-administration, including epinephrine for injection, should be considered with patients stopping VIT.

VI. SPECIAL ASPECTS OF ANT HYPERSENSITIVITY

A. Classification

There are nearly 10,000 species of ants (order Hymenoptera, family Formicidae) recognized worldwide. Some of these sting victims, as do other Hymenoptera, and human reactions span the spectrum from a self-limited local reaction to life-threatening anaphylaxis. In the United States, only members of the genera *Solenopsis* (*S.*), the imported fire ant (IFA), and *Pogonomyrmex*, the harvester ant, induce such reactions (47). In Australia 88 species of the genus *Myrmecia* (bull ants) are of clinical relevance (48). The best known, the jack jumper ant (*Myrmecia pilosula*), is responsible for one-quarter of all anaphylaxis treated in some Australian areas. Different species of stinging ants that cause anaphylaxis have also been found in other parts of the world. Details of the taxonomy of stinging ants and their worldwide significance in Hymenoptera venom allergy are given in Chapter 18.

B. Reactions

The IFA attaches to the skin by means of a powerful mandible and stings, releasing venom that produces a characteristic "fire-like" pain. If not removed, the IFA will continue to rotate in a pivotal fashion, repeatedly injecting small amounts of venom and provoking a sharp pain. An initial local reaction begins as a 25–50 mm erythematous flare. This is followed a few minutes later by a larger wheal, and within the next 24 hours an umbilicated pustule forms and usually remains for 3–10 days, later rupturing and leaving a residual macule, nodule, or scar.

Stings of the IFA commonly produce large local reactions that are similar to those induced by stings of the other flying Hymenoptera. Following an initial wheal-and-flare, a large local reaction may develop several hours later. This includes erythema and edema that extends more than 10 cm from the initial sting site. This reaction is thought to occur in up to 30–50% of IFA stings.

Systemic allergic reactions can manifest all the symptoms of anaphylaxis, including generalized erythema, urticaria, angioedema, nausea, vomiting, diarrhea, laryngeal edema, asthma, as well as shock and death. Anaphylaxis to the IFA sting is thought to occur in up to 1% of stings (49). In 1989 a survey of 29,300 physicians reported a total of 32 deaths thought to be secondary to anaphylaxis induced by ant stings (50). Although the species of ant was not identified in most cases, *Solenopsis* and *Pogonomyrmex* species were implicated in these deaths. Postmortem case reports of deaths following IFA stings describe findings of acute pulmonary changes and cerebral vascular congestion compatible with shock due to anaphylaxis. Neurological sequelae due to the IFA are rare but include mononeuropathy, and focal motor and grand mal epileptic seizures (51).

C. Allergens of the Imported Fire Ant

The venoms of the IFA, unlike other Hymenoptera venom, has an extremely low protein content in the aqueous fraction, less than 0.1%, with a prominence of toxic alkaloids. The aqueous component contains the allergenic proteins. Alkaloids compose 95% and the aqueous 5% of the venom. The alkaloids are responsible for the hemolytic, bactericidal, and cytotoxic properties that result in formation of a sterile pustule. This alkaloid portion, however, is nonallergenic (52). The venom of the harvester ant, *Pogonomyrmex*, more closely resembles that of the flying Hymenoptera and consists of 73% protein. *Solenopsis* and *Pogonomyrmex* proteins do not cross-react (52).

IFA whole-body extract (WBE), unlike the WBE of other members of Hymenoptera, contains the clinically important allergens responsible for hypersensitivity (52). Both IFA WBE and venom produce positive skin tests in sensitized individuals. Skin testing with IFA venom is more sensitive and specific than with IFA WBE. The venom is also thought to be 10 times more potent and better tolerated for skin testing, and RAST testing with IFA venom is more sensitive than with WBE. IFA venom, however, is not commercially produced currently, leaving IFA WBE as the only available option for testing and immunotherapy. Similarly, WBE and not venoms are available for *Pogonomyrmex* species.

D. Diagnosis

There is a high rate of false-positive results when skin testing is performed on patients in endemic regions. Therefore, only patients who have experienced a systemic allergic reaction following an ant sting should undergo skin testing with IFA WBE. Skin testing should be done at least 30 days after the systemic reaction. A prick-puncture test with IFA WBE is performed first, and if there is no response, it is followed by serial intradermal testing beginning with a 1:1,000,000 weight/volume (wt/vol) dilution. A great majority of patients who are sensitive react before reaching a 1:500 wt/vol dilution (53). In vitro tests for IFA IgE should be obtained in history-positive, skin test–negative patients.

E. Immunotherapy

With other Hymenoptera (honeybee, wasp, hornet, and yellow jacket), children who have had only a cutaneous systemic reaction (generalized erythema, urticaria, and/or pruritus) are not candidates for immunotherapy. However, with IFA, there are no data to indicate that children who have had only a cutaneous reaction to an IFA sting will not respond to subsequent stings with a more serious systemic reaction. Therefore, patients of all age groups with positive skin or in vitro tests should receive IFA immunotherapy, regardless of the severity of their systemic reaction to IFA.

IFA immunotherapy is begun with 0.05 ml of the highest dilution of WBE that produces a positive skin test (usually 1:10,000 or 1:100,000 wt/vol). The dose is increased with each injection, either weekly or biweekly. Once a maximum tolerated dose or 0.5 ml of a 1:10 wt/vol is achieved, the interval between injections is extended to every 4–6 weeks. A 2-day rush protocol for IFA immunotherapy has been studied in a small population of patients and shown to be safe and efficacious (54).

IFA immunotherapy can be discontinued when the individual becomes negative on repeat skin testing (54). Otherwise, the decision to discontinue such therapy after 5 years is determined by the physician in consultation with the patient, since no data exist on when IFA immunotherapy can be discontinued when skin tests remain positive.

A double-blind placebo-controlled study on venom immunotherapy in patients allergic to the jack jumper ant, *Myremcia pilosula*, was reported from Tasmania, Australia (55). Of 29 patients on placebo, 21 (72%) developed a systemic allergic skin reaction, while all 23 on ant venom were completely protected when purposely stung.

VII. SPECIAL ASPECTS OF BITING INSECT HYPERSENSITIVITY

Local, and very rarely, generalized allergic reactions to insect bites are due to sensitization to insect salivary proteins introduced during the process of blood sucking. Specific IgE antibodies to various salivary proteins have been demonstrated and their clinical relevance documented by passive cutaneous transfer studies. The responsible insects belong to the orders Diptera (mosquitos, flies), Hemiptera (bugs), and Siphonaptera (fleas). The relevant biting insects and their allergens are described in detail in Chapter 19.

A. Clinical Symptoms (56)

Local reactions may be of the immediate, delayed, or combined type. Immediate skin reactions of the wheal-and-flare type are pruritic, usually appear within 10 to 15 minutes after the bite, and disappear within an hour. Delayed reactions develop 12 to 24 hours after the bite and consist of pruritic erythema and papules that may last for days to weeks. They may become vesicular, bullous, or even necrotic. The presence of specific IgE and IgG4 antibodies to salivary proteins in patients with local reactions to mosquito bites (57) indicate that immediate reactions are most likely IgE mediated while the role of IgG antibodies is less clear. They may just reflect exposure or also be involved in the pathogenesis of the local reaction (58). In delayed reactions cell-mediated immunity against salivary secretions could be involved. Systemic anaphylactic reactions to insect bites have been described, especially to horseflies (*Tabanus* spp.) and the kissing bug (*Triatoma*), but are very much rarer than with Hymenoptera stings (56,59).

B. Immunotherapy

Commercially available extracts of biting insects are whole-body extracts. Their diagnostic and therapeutic value is controversial. Case reports have been published on successful treatment with these vaccines for local and systemic reactions (56,60), but controlled trials have not been performed. In one study of five patients with systemic anaphylactic reactions to *Triatoma protracta* (61), a salivary gland vaccine was used for immunotherapy and the patients subjected to a bite challenge during treatment. All five patients had positive skin tests and specific IgE antibodies to the extract and did not react to the challenge. In only local reactions, which are most often due to mosquito bites, avoidance measures such as screens and repellents and prophylactic medication with cetirizine (62) in high-exposure areas are preferable.

In the presence of definite anaphylactic reactions immunotherapy may be discussed but ideally should be performed in the frame of a clinical, preferably controlled trial. The report on the cloning and expression of three major salivary allergens from the mosquito *Aedes aegypti* (63) is promising with regard to both improved diagnostic possibilities and the use of a mixture of these recombinant allergens for immunotherapy.

VIII. NEW APPROACHES TO IMMUNOTHERAPY

Insect venom allergy is often considered as a model for IgE-mediated allergy. Diagnostic tests, skin tests, and RAST are reliable, and specific immunotherapy with venoms is safe and effective. However, at a closer look, the specificity of the main diagnostic tests, skin tests with insect venom extracts and tests for venom-specific serum IgE antibodies, is far from perfect. Up to 20% of individuals with no history of systemic sting reactions have positive tests (1) and only 30–50% of those with positive tests and history will react to a subsequent sting by the incriminated insect (18). According to a sting provocation test during venom immunotherapy, about 95% of patients allergic to vespid stings are completely protected, compared with only 80–90% (9,18) of those allergic to honeybee venom. Systemic allergic side effects to immunotherapy injections may occur in 20–40% of patients during immunotherapy with honeybee and 5–10% during immunotherapy with vespid venoms. There is thus a considerable potential for improvement in both diagnosis and immunotherapy of Hymenoptera venom allergy.

A. Recombinant Venom Allergens

Modern molecular biology technology has made available today a number of major venom allergens in recombinant form from the honeybee, different vespids, and ants (Table 6) (64). The IgE-binding capacity of these recombinant allergens correlates closely with the respective natural purified preparations. Some disparities, however, were revealed by RAST inhibition and Western blot studies, which indicated that all natural preparations were contaminated with trace amounts of other venom allergens. Recombinant allergens should therefore be superior to highly purified natural preparations when the true clinical relevance of the individual allergen is determined. The use of recombinant cocktails is also promising for diagnosis. In a preliminary study, venom-specific IgE antibodies were measured in 85 bee venom–allergic patients with positive and 20 nonallergic controls with negative skin tests to bee venom. None of the negative controls reacted to a recombinant cocktail containing phospholipase A_2, hyaluronidase, and melittin, compared with 15% who reacted to the whole bee venom, indicating superior specificity of the recombinant cocktail. On the other hand, 87% of the patients were positive with the recombinant cocktail versus 95% with the whole bee venom (64). The somewhat lower sensitivity of the cocktail could probably be improved by the addition of further relevant bee venom allergens such as acid phosphatase and protease in recombinant form. Once all relevant allergens of a venom are available in recombinant form, the sensitization pattern of an individual patient can be determined. A patient-tailored cocktail containing all the allergens to

Table 6   Recombinant Hymenoptera Venom Allergens

Species	Allergen	MW (kDa)
Apis mellifera	Api m 1 phospholipase A_2	16–20
	Api m 2 hyaluronidase	43
	Api m 4 acid phosphatase	49
Vespula vulgaris	Ves v 1 phospholipase A_1	35
	Ves v 2 hyaluronidase	45
	Ves v 5 antigen 5	25
Dolichovespula maculata	Dol m 1 phospholipase A_1	35
	Dol m 2 hyaluronidase	45
	Dol m 5 antigen 5	25
Polistes annularis	Pol a 5 antigen 5	25
Solenopsis invicta	Sol i 2	30
	Sol i 3 antigen 5	25
Myrmecia pilosula	Myr p 1	7.5

Source: Ref. 64.

which the patient has IgE antibodies could then be prepared for immunotherapy (65). The mostly conformational B-cell epitopes have been shown to be reduced in unrefolded or point-mutated recombinant allergens. Cocktails of such preparations will have a strongly reduced reactivity to IgE antibodies fixed on effector cells and therefore will induce much less mediator release and be better tolerated. Their capacity to interact with T-cells and thus to induce protective immunological effects will be preserved. So far no clinical trials on immunotherapy with recombinant venom allergens have been performed.

B.   T-Cell Epitope Peptides

T-cell epitope peptides can be prepared synthetically or expressed as recombinant fragments of 11 to 30 amino acids. They have been used for immunotherapy in preliminary studies, including some for bee venom allergy (66,67). Three short linear peptides of 11–18 amino acids of phospholipase A_2 (the major bee venom allergen) were identified that were unable to bind to the respective specific IgE antibodies in sera from bee venom–allergic patients, but induced strong proliferation of their T lymphocytes in vitro (66). Immunotherapy with an equimolar mixture of these major synthesized T-cell epitope peptides was performed in five bee venom–allergic patients. A sting challenge with a live honeybee after 10 weeks of peptide immunotherapy indicated complete protection of three and partial protection of two of the five patients (66). In vitro studies on lymphocyte cultures of the patients suggested the induction of phospholipase A_2–specific tolerance by this form of peptide immunotherapy.

C.   DNA Vaccination (68)

The technique of DNA vaccination consists of the injection of DNA plasmids that encode the allergen. This kind of vaccination induces a TH1 response. Successful DNA vaccination of phospholipase A–sensitized mice with phospholipase A sequence DNA plasmids has been reported (68). Protection from anaphylaxis was complete when vaccination was done before sensitization, but only 65% of the mice survived when it was performed after intraperitoneal sensitization.

D. Antihistamine Premedication (36)

Premedication with antihistamines during the initial phase of venom imunotherapy has resulted in a significant reduction of side effects in a number of placebo-controlled, double-blind studies. A retrospective analysis of one of these double-blind trials suggests that antihistamine premedication during the initial dose-increase phase enhanced the long-term efficacy of venom immunotherapy. Of 52 bee venom–allergic patients, 26 each had been premedicated in a double-blind trial with either terfenadine or placebo during the initial 3 weeks of a rush immunotherapy. After 3 years of maintenance immunotherapy, 41 had been reexposed either by a sting challenge or a field sting, 21 originally on placebo and 20 originally on terfenadine. Six patients developed mostly mild systemic allergic reactions, and all were in the placebo group. This interesting observation needs confirmation in a prospective study.

IX. SALIENT POINTS

1. Venom immunotherapy is a highly effective treatment for Hymenoptera venom allergy.
2. Indication for venom immunotherapy is based on a history of systemic allergic reactions to Hymenoptera stings and positive diagnostic tests to the respective venoms.
3. Rush and ultrarush protocols for starting immunotherapy provide more rapid protection than conventional protocols but may be associated with more side effects.
4. With venom immunotherapy of 3 to 5 years duration, most patients remain protected for many years after stopping this treatment.
5. Immunotherapy with whole-body vaccines of the fire ant (*Solenopsis invicta*) and some other ants appears to be effective, in contrast to the case with other Hymenoptera, where only venoms induce protection.
6. The use of immunotherapy for biting insect hypersensitivity is controversial.
7. The most promising new approaches to venom immunotherapy are based on genetic engineering and include treatment with modified recombinant allergens, T-cell epitope peptides, and DNA vaccination.

REFERENCES

1. Müller UR. Insect Sting Allergy: Clinical Picture, Diagnosis and Treatment. Stuttgart/New York: Gustav Fischer, 1990.
2. Hunt KJ, Valentine MD, Sobotka AK, Benton AW, Amodia FJ, Lichtenstein LM. A controlled trial of immunotherapy in insect hypersensitivity. N Engl J Med 1978; 299:157–161.
3. Müller U, Thurnheer U, Patrizzi R, Spiess J, Hoigne R. Immunotherapy in bee sting hypersensitivity: Bee venom versus wholebody extract. Allergy 1979; 34:369–378.
4. Müller U, Mosbech H. Position paper: Immunotherapy with Hymenoptera venoms. Allergy 1993; 48:37–46.
5. Portnoy JM, Moffitt JE, Golden DBK, Bernstein IL, Berger WE, Dykewicz MS, et al. Stinging insect hypersensitivity: A practice parameter. J Allergy Clin Immunol 1999; 103:963–980.
6. Golden DBK, Marsh DG, Kagey-Sobotka A, Addison BI, Freidhoff L, Szklo M, et al. Epidemiology of insect venom sensitivity. J Am Med Assoc 1989; 262:240–244.

7. Valentine MD, Schuberth KC, Kagey-Sobotka A, Graft DF, Kwiterovich KA, Szklo M, Lichtenstein LM. The value of immunotherapy with venom in children with allergy to insect stings. N Engl J Med 1990; 323:1601–1613.

8. Reisman RE. Natural history of insect sting allergy: Relationship of severity of symptoms of initial sting anaphylaxis to re-sting reactions. J Allergy Clin Immunol 1992; 90:335–339.

9. Müller U, Helbling A, Berchtold E. Immunotherapy with honeybee venom and yellow jacket venom is different regarding efficacy and safety. J Allergy Clin Immunol 1992; 89:529–535.

10. Schwartz HJ, Lockey RF, Sheffer AL, Parrino J, Busse WW, Yuninger JW. A multicenter study on skin test reactivity of human volunteers to venom as compared with whole body Hymenoptera antigens. J Allergy Clin Immunol 1981; 67:81–85.

11. Golden DBK, Kagey-Sobotka A, Hamilton RG, Norman PS, Lichtenstein LM. Insect allergy with negative venom skin tests. J Allergy Clin Immunol 2001; 107:897–901.

12. Oude-Elberink J, deMonchy J, Kors J, vanDoormaal J, Dubois A. Fatal anaphylaxis after a yellow jacket sting despite venom immunotherapy in two patients with mastocytosis. J Allergy Clin Immunol 1997; 99:153–154.

13. Fricker M, Helbling L, Schwartz L, Müller U. Hymenoptera sting anaphylaxis and urticaria pigmentosa: Clinical findings and results of venom immunotherapy in ten patients. J Allergy Clin Immunol 1997; 100:11–15.

14. Hunt KJ, Valentine MD, Sobotka AK, Lichtenstein LM. Diagnosis of allergy to stinging insects by skin testing with Hymenoptera venoms. Ann Intern Med 1976; 85:56–59.

15. Day J, Buckeridge D, Welsh A. Risk assessment in determining systemic reactivity to honeybee stings in sting-threatened individuals. J Allergy Clin Immunol 1994; 93:691–705.

16. van der Linden PG, Hack CE, Struyvenberg A, Zwan JKvd. Insect-sting challenge in 324 subjects with a previous anaphylactic reaction: Current criteria for insect-venom hypersensitivity do not predict the occurrence and the severity of anaphylaxis. J Allergy Clin Immunol 1994; 94:151–159.

17. Franken HH, Dubois AEJ, Minkema HJ, vanderHeide S, deMonchy JGR. Lack of reproducibility of a single negative sting challenge response in the assessment of anaphylactic risk in patients with suspected yellow jacket hypersensitivity. J Allergy Clin Immunol 1994; 93:431–436.

18. Rueff F, Przybilla B, Muller U, Mosbech H. The sting challenge test in Hymenoptera venom allergy. Allergy 1996; 51:216–225.

19. Graft DF, Schuberth KC, Kagey-Sobotka A, Kwiterovich KA, Niv Y, Lichtenstein LM, Valentine MD. A prospective study of the natural history of large local reactions following Hymenoptera stings in children. J Pediatr 1984; 104:664–668.

20. Hamilton RG, Golden DB, Kagey-Sobotka A, Lichtenstein LM. Case report of venom immunotherapy for a patient with large local reactions. Ann Allergy Asthma Immunol 2001; 87:134–137.

21. Reisman RE. Venom hypersensitivity. J Allergy Clin Immunol 1994; 94:651–658.

22. Hamilton RG, Wisenauer JA, Golden DB, Valentine MD, Adkinson NF Jr. Selection of Hymenoptera venoms for immunotherapy based on patients' IgE antibody cross-reactivity. J Allergy Clin Immunol 1993; 92:651–659.

23. Golden DBK, Kagey-Sobotka A, Valentine MD, Lichtenstein LM. Dose dependence of Hymenoptera venom immunotherapy. J Allergy Clin Immunol 1981; 67:370–374.

24. Rueff F, Wenderoth A, Przybilla B. Patients still reacting to a sting challenge while receiving conventional Hymenoptera venom immunotherapy are protected by increased venom doses. J Allergy Clin Immunol 2001; 108:1027–1032.

25. Lockey RF, Turkeltaub PC, Olive ES, Hubbard JM, Baird-Warren IA, Bukantz SC. The Hymenoptera venom study III: Safety of venom immunotherapy. J Allergy Clin Immunol 1990; 86:775–780.

26. Golden DBK, Kagey-Sobotka A, Lichtenstein LM. Survey of patients after discontinuing venom immunotherapy. J Allergy Clin Immunol 2000; 105:385–390.

27. Golden DBK, Kwiterovich KA, Kagey-Sobotka A, Valentine MD, Lichtenstein LM. Discontinuing venom immunotherapy: Outcome after five years. J Allergy Clin Immunol 1996; 97:579–587.

28. Golden DBK, Kwiterovich KA, Addison BA, Kagey-Sobotka A, Lichtenstein LM. Discontinuing venom immunotherapy: Extended observations. J Allergy Clin Immunol 1998; 101:298–305.

29. Müller UR, Morris T, Bischof M, Friedli H, Skarvil F. Combined active and passive immunotherapy in honeybee-sting allergy. J Allergy Clin Immunol 1986;78:115–122.

30. Golden DBK, Lawrence ID, Kagey-Sobotka A, Valentine MD, Lichtenstein LM. Clinical correlation of the venom-specific IgG antibody level during maintenance venom immunotherapy. J Allergy Clin Immunol 1992; 90:386–393.

31. Jutel M, Pichler WJ, Skrbic D, Urwyler A, Dahinden C, Müller UR. Bee venom immunotherapy results in decrease of IL-4 and IL-5 and increase of IFN-γ secretion in specific allergen stimulated T cell cultures. J Immunol 1995; 154:4187–4194.

32. Adkis CA, Blesken T, Adkis M, Wuthrich B, Blazer K. Role of interleukin 10 in specific immunotherapy. J Clin Invest 1998; 102:98–106.

33. Hoffman DR, Jacobson RS. Allergens in Hymenoptera venoms: XII. How much venom is in a sting? Ann Allergy 1984; 52:276–278.

34. Bousquet J, Ménardo JL, Michel FB. Systemic reactions during maintenance immunotherapy with honeybee venom. Ann Allergy 1988; 61:63–68.

35. Birnbaum J, Charpin D. Vervloet D. Rapid Hymenoptera venom immunotherapy: Comparative safety of three protocols. Clin Exp Allergy 1993; 23:226–230.

36. Müller U, Hari Y, Berchtold E. Premedication with antihistamines may enhance efficacy of specific-allergen immunotherapy. J Allergy Clin Immunol 2001; 197:81–86.

37. Urbanek R, Forster J, Kuhn W, Ziupa J. Discontinuation of bee venom immunotherapy in children and adolescents. J Pediatr 1985; 107:367–371.

38. Golden DBK, Addison BI, Gadde J, Kagey-Sobotka A, Valentine MD, Lichtenstein LM. Prospective observations on stopping prolonged venom immunotherapy. J Allergy Clin Immunol 1989; 84:162–167.

39. Müller U, Berchtold E, Helbling A. Honeybee venom allergy: Results of a sting challenge 1 year after stopping successful venom immunotherapy in 86 patients. J Allergy Clin Immunol 1991; 87:702–709.

40. Haugaard L, Nörregaard OF, Dahl R. In-hospital sting challenge in insect venom–allergic patients after stopping venom immunotherapy. J Allergy Clin Immunol 1991; 87:699–702.

41. Keating MU, Kagey-Sobotka A, Hamilton RG, Yunginger JW. Clinical and immunologic follow-up of patients who stop venom immunotherapy. J Allergy Clin Immunol 1991; 88:339–348.

42. van Halteren HK, van der Linden PWG, Burgers JA, Bartelink AKM. Discontinuation of yellow jacket venom immunotherapy: Follow-up of 75 patients by means of deliberate sting challenge. J Allergy Clin Immunol 1997; 100:767–770.

43. Reisman RE. Duration of venom immunotherapy: Relationship to the severity of symptoms of initial insect sting anaphylaxis. J Allergy Clin Immunol 1993; 92:831–836.

44. Lerch E, Müller UR. Long-term protection after stopping venom immunotherapy: Results of re-stings in 200 patients. J Allergy Clin Immunol 1998; 101:606–612.

45. Golden D, Johnson K, Addison BI, Valentine M, Kagey-Sobotka A, Lichtenstein L. Clinical and immunologic observations in patients who stop venom immunotherapy. J Allergy Clin Immunol 1986; 77:435–442.

46. Ludolph-Hauser D, Rueff F, Fries C, Schöpf P, Przybilla B. Constitutively raised serum concentration of mast-cell tryptase and severe anaphylactic reactions to Hymenoptera stings. Lancet 2001; 357:361–362.

47. Lockey RF. Systemic reactions to stinging ants. J Allergy Clin Immunol 1974; 54:132–46.

48. Brown SGA, WO Kelsall RH, Heddle RJ, Baldo DA. Fatal anaphylaxis following jack jumper ant sting in southern Tasmania. Med J Aust 2001; 175:644–647.

49. deShazo RD, Butcher BT, Banks WA. Reactions to the stings of the imported fire ant. N Engl J Med 1990; 323:462–466.

50. Rhoades RB, Stafford CT, James FK Jr. Survey of fatal anaphylactic reactions to imported fire ant stings: Report of the Fire Ant Subcommittee of the American Academy of Allergy and Immunology. J Allergy Clin Immunol 1989; 84:159–162.

51. Candiotti KA, Lamas AM. Adverse neurologic reactions to the sting of the imported fire ant. Int Arch Allergy Immunol 1993; 102:417–420.

52. Hoffman DR. Fire ant venom allergy. Allergy 1995; 50:535–544.

53. Moffitt J, Barker J, Stafford C. Management of imported fire ant allergy: Results of a survey. Ann Allergy Asthma Immunol 1997; 79:125–130.

54. Tankersley MS, Walker RL, Butler WK, Hagan LL, Napoli DC, Freeman TM. Safety and efficacy of an imported fire ant rush immunotherapy protocol with and without prophylactic treatment. J Allergy Clin Immunol 2002; 109:556–562.

55. Brown S, Wiese M, Blackman K, Heddle R. Ant venom immunotherapy: A double-blind placebo-controlled, crossover trial. Lancet 2003; 361:1001–1006.

56. Hoffman DR. Allergic reactions to biting insects. In: Monograph on Insect Allergy, 3rd ed, (Levine MI, Lockey RF, eds.). Milwaukee: American Academy of Allergy, Asthma and Immunology, 1995: 99–108.

57. Palosuo K, Brummer-Korvenkontio H, Mikkola J, Sahi T, Reunala T. Seasonal increase in human IgE and IgG4 antisaliva antibodies to *Aedes* mosquito bites. Int Arch Allergy Immunol 1997; 114:367–372.

58. Peng Z, Simons FE. A prospective study of naturally acquired sensitization and subsequent desensitization to mosquito bites and concurrent antibody responses. J Allergy Clin Immunol 1998; 101:284–286.

59. Hemmer W, Focke M, Vieluf D, Berg-Drevnilok B, Gîtz M, Jarisch R. Anaphylaxis induced by horsefly bites: Identification of a 69 kd IgE-binding salivary gland protein from *Chrysops* spp (Diptera Tabanidae) by western blot analysis. J Allergy Clin Immunol 1998; 101:134–136.

60. McCormack DR, Salata KF, Hershey JN, Carpenter GB, Engler RJ. Mosquito bite anaphylaxis: Immunotherapy with wholebody extracts. Ann Allergy Asthma Immunol 1995; 74:39–44.

61. Rohr AS, Marshall NA, Saxon A. Successful immunotherapy for *Triatoma protracta*–induced anaphlaxis. J Allergy Clin Immunol 1984; 73:369–375.

62. Reunala T, Brummer-Korvenkontio H, Palosuo T. Are we really allergic to mosquito bites? Ann Med 1994; 26:301–306.

63. Simons FE, Peng Z. Mosquito allergy: Recombinant mosquito salivary antigens for new diagnostic tests. Int Arch Allergy Immunol 2001; 124:403–405.

64. Müller U. Recombinant Hymenoptera venom allergens. Allergy 2002; 57:570–576.

65. Valenta R, Lidholm J, Niederberger V, Hajek B, Kraft D, Gronlund H. The recombinant allergen–based concept of component resolved diagnostics and immunotherapy. Clin Exp Allergy 1999; 29:896–904.

66. Carballido J, Carballido M, Kägi M, Meloen T, Wüthrich B, Heusser C, Blaser K. T cell epitope specificity in human allergic and nonallergic subjects to bee venom phospholipase A_2. J Immunol 1993; 150:3582–3591.

67. Müller U, Akdis C, Fricker M, Akdis M, Blesken T, Bettens F, Blaser K. Successful immunotherapy with T-cell epitope peptides of bee venom phospholipase A_2 induces specific T-cell anergy in patients allergic to bee venom. J Allergy Clin Immunol 1998; 101:747–754.

68. Jilek S, Barbey C, Spertini F, Corthésy B. Antigen-independent suppression of the allergic immune response to bee venom phospholipase A_2 by DNA vaccination in CBA/J mice. J Immunol 2001; 166:3612–3621.

30

Immunotherapy Combined with Pharmacotherapy

ANTHONY J. FREW

University of Southampton School of Medicine, Southampton, England

I. INTRODUCTION

Specific allergen immunotherapy (SIT) is a highly effective means of reducing sensitivity to specific allergens, and thereby reducing or abolishing the symptoms of allergic rhinoconjunctivitis and asthma. In most cases SIT is partially rather than fully effective, and patients continue to have some residual allergic symptoms, for which they may continue to take anti-allergic medication. SIT is often given to patients whose allergic conditions have not been well controlled with standard drug therapy, and it is common for these patients to continue their drug therapy during the course of SIT. Immunotherapy is thus combined with drug therapy in many patients. Separately, SIT carries a significant risk of side effects, largely but not exclusively due to allergic reactions to the vaccines. Some allergists have therefore tried to reduce the incidence of side effects by premedicating their patients with antihistamines before each SIT injection. Evidence from some research studies suggests that co-administration of SIT and drug therapy may modify the clinical response to SIT. This chapter reviews the evidence for this phenomenon and the possible mechanisms by which pharmacotherapy may diminish or increase the efficacy of SIT.

II. MECHANISMS OF IMMUNOTHERAPY

Several mechanisms have been proposed to explain the beneficial effects of immunotherapy, but there is an emerging consensus that the main cellular target for SIT is the allergen-specific T-cell. Both in the skin and in the nose, successful SIT is accompanied by a reduction in T-cell and eosinophil recruitment in response to allergen challenge. In parallel, there is a shift in the balance of TH1 and TH2 cytokine expression in the allergen-challenged site. TH2 cytokine expression is not affected, but there is an increased proportion of T-cells expressing the TH1 cytokines IL-2, IFN-γ, and IL-12 (1–3). After venom SIT, there is induction of regulatory T-cells producing IL-10 as well as an increase in TH1 response (4,5). Similar findings have also been reported following SIT with inhalant allergens (1,3,6). IL-10 has a complex series of actions on the immune response, including stimulating production of the IgG4 subclass, which may therefore rise as an indicator of the beneficial effect rather than as a direct player in the mechanism of SIT (7,8). Taken together, these findings suggest that SIT has a modulatory effect on allergen-specific T-cells, which helps to explain why the clinical and late-phase responses are attenuated without a large effect on allergen-specific antibody levels.

III. ANTIHISTAMINE PREMEDICATION FOR SIT

Antihistamines have often been used to pretreat SIT patients who have experienced previous adverse reactions to SIT injections, but it is difficult to draw any useful conclusions from such nonrandomized use in selected patients. Indeed, many clinicians have argued against the use of antihistamine premedication on the grounds that it might mask mild systemic side effects that would have led to a reduction in dosage, perhaps preventing more serious side effects at the next visit. In one of the earliest reported studies, Berchtold et al. used terfenadine premedication in a double-blind, placebo-controlled study of patients receiving rush SIT for bee venom allergy. They found a clear reduction in large local reactions and itching at the site of the injections in the actively treated group (9). Nielsen et al. reported a double-blind, placebo-controlled study of loratadine premedication in patients receiving cluster SIT for birch pollen allergy (10). Although loratadine did not prevent all systemic side effects, it reduced the number of patients affected from 79% to 33% and reduced the severity of adverse reactions by preventing 58% of systemic side effects. Concerns that antihistamine premedication might lead to an increased rate of severe side effects proved unfounded, in that the reduction in adverse events was seen across the spectrum of severity, suggesting that premedication with loratadine did not mask mild side effects that would have warned about impending severe adverse events. Moreover, pretreatment with loratadine did not delay the onset of systemic adverse events. In contrast to the previous study (9) there was no effect on the size of delayed (late-phase) allergic reactions to the SIT injections.

In the largest double-blind, placebo-controlled trial to date, 121 patients were premedicated with either placebo, terfenadine, or terfenadine plus ranitidine before SIT with bee venom. In the two terfenadine-treated groups, fewer patients had to discontinue treatment due to side effects (1/82 versus 6/39 in the placebo group) and fewer patients had local side effects, especially in the first 4 weeks of SIT. No additional benefit was observed among those who received ranitidine as well as terfenadine (11).

In another double-blind, placebo-controlled study of 57 patients, Reimers et al. found a reduction in the size and duration of large local reactions when fexofenadine was given as premedication before SIT with bee venom (12). Although there was no overall reduction in systemic side effects, urticaria, angioedema, and pruritus were all reduced after fexofenadine premedication. Similar results have been reported with cetirizine, which was very effective in reducing local side effects but did not alter the rate of systemic side effects (13).

Taken together, these studies have shown that antihistamine premedication is effective in reducing the incidence of the typical immediate, histamine-associated side effects of SIT, including urticaria, angioedema, and itching, but is less effective against delayed local reactions. However, not all side effects were equally responsive to antihistamines, suggesting that other mechanisms and mediators may underpin these antihistamine-resistant side effects.

Despite previous concerns that premedication might lead to masking of mild side effects and hence to more serious systemic events, which might have been avoided had the previous mild event been noted, premedication was not associated with any excess of serious systemic adverse events.

IV. IMMUNOMODULATORY EFFECTS OF HISTAMINE AND ANTIHISTAMINES

Interest in the possible immunomodulatory role of histamine goes back many years (14) (Fig. 1). In vitro, histamine suppresses mitogen-induced and antigen-driven proliferation of T-cells. This phenomenon appears to be mediated by T-cells with suppressor function and is dependent on H_2 receptors, which can be abrogated in vitro by ranitidine and other H_2-antagonists (15). Histamine, working through its H_2 receptor, also inhibits the ability of bacterial lipopolysaccharide to induce tumor necrosis factor–alpha in monocytes (16). The discovery of H_3 and H_4 histamine receptors has rekindled interest in this area (17), not least because H_4 receptors mediate recruitment of eosinophils and mast cells (18,19) and allow histamine to stimulate the release of several cytokines, including IL-16 (20). In vitro, H_1 antihistamines have been shown to suppress the generation and release of TH2-type cytokines from cultured T-cells (21). This suggests that the release of histamine in allergic responses may upregulate TH2 responses, possibly through inhibition of TH1-type cytokines, whose production has been shown to be inhibited by histamine (22,23). In mice, deletion of the H_1 receptor results in suppression of interferon-gamma and dominant secretion of the TH2-type cytokines IL-4 and IL-13, with associated increases in allergen-specific IgE and IgG antibodies (23).

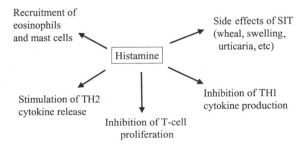

Figure 1 Pro-allergic actions of histamine.

Local release of histamine could influence the immune response as well as have an immunomodulatory effect on T-cell function by increasing tissue permeability, hence affecting the delivery of allergenic proteins to the immune system. This mechanism is thought to be at least partially responsible for the broadening of allergic sensitivities with age in patients with allergic rhinitis. This may underpin the observation that children with allergic rhinitis who receive SIT may have a reduced risk of developing sensitization to allergens to which they are not already sensitized (24).

It follows that antihistamines may have beneficial effects on responses to SIT, through blockade of these immunomodulatory effects of histamine. Support for this hypothesis comes from a retrospective analysis of the use of antihistamines in patients receiving bee venom SIT. In this study, 52 patients were randomized to receive terfenadine or placebo before their initial course of rush immunotherapy in 1988–1989. When 47 of these patients were traced in 1992–1993, 41 had been stung by bees (17 field stings and 21 in hospital). Six (29%) of the 21 subjects who had received placebo premedication reported systemic allergic reactions to the stings, while none of 20 who had received terfenadine had any systemic reaction (25). This study suggests that far from impairing the efficacy of SIT, antihistamine premedication may in fact enhance its efficacy. Further work is needed to determine the mechanisms of this phenomenon, and whether this effect is a general property of antihistamines or specific to terfenadine.

V. COMPARISON OF SIT WITH OTHER TYPES OF TREATMENT FOR ASTHMA

The majority of clinical trials of SIT for asthma have compared SIT either with historical controls or with a matched placebo-treated group. To date, the effectiveness of specific SIT in asthma has rarely been compared with conventional management (with avoidance measures and conventional inhaled or oral drugs). One study assessed SIT in asthmatic children receiving conventional drug therapy and found no additional benefit in patients who were already receiving optimal drug therapy (26). There are some significant criticisms of this study, and further work of this type is needed. Another study compared short-course preseasonal immunotherapy with topical nasal steroids in patients with birch pollen allergy. After one course of therapy, this study found that nasal symptoms were better controlled with topical steroids, but immunotherapy prevented the seasonal rises in blood eosinophils and airway responsiveness to methacholine, while topical nasal steroids were ineffective against these parameters (27). Future comparative trials need to include several measures of clinical effectiveness as well as analysis of cost benefit and cost-effectiveness since purchasers of health care are increasingly demanding this evidence before agreeing to fund therapies.

VI. SALIENT POINTS

1. Until new and improved forms of SIT are designed, it is likely that SIT will be combined with drug therapy to achieve optimal control of allergic symptoms.
2. Adequate literature on combined therapy is lacking, and there is a need for further research to assess the potential for optimal combined therapy.
3. Histamine has an immunomodulatory effect on T-cells, biasing them toward production of TH2 cytokines.

4. Antihistamine premedication may offer a means of enhancing the effectiveness of conventional SIT, possibly through blocking the pro-allergic effects of locally released histamine.

REFERENCES

1. Durham SR, Ying S, Varney VA, Jacobson MR, Sudderick RM, Mackay IS, Kay AB, Hamid QA. Grass pollen immunotherapy inhibits allergen-induced infiltration of CD4+ T-lymphocytes and eosinophils in the nasal mucosa and increases the number of cells expressing mRNA for interferon-gamma. J Allergy Clin Immunol 1996; 97:1356–1365.
2. McHugh SM, Deighton J, Stewart AG, Lachmann PJ, Ewan PW. Bee venom immunotherapy induces a shift in cytokine responses from a Th2 to a Th1 dominant pattern: Comparison of rush and conventional immunotherapy. Clin Exp Allergy 1995; 25:828–838.
3. Ebner C, Siemann U, Bohle B, Willheim M, Wiedermann U, Schenk S, Klotz F, Ebner H, Kraft D, Scheiner O. Immunological changes during specific immunotherapy of grass pollen allergy: Reduced lymphoproliferative responses to allergen and shift from Th2 to Th1 in T-cell clones specific for Phl p 1, a major grass pollen allergen. Clin Exp Allergy 1997; 27:1007–1015.
4. Bellinghausen I, Metz G, Enk AH, Christmann S, Knop J, Saloga J. Insect venom immunotherapy induces IL-10 production and a Th2 to Th1 shift, and changes surface marker expression in venom-allergic subjects. Eur J Immunol 1997; 27:586–596.
5. Nasser SM, Ying S, Meng Q, Kay AB, Ewan PW. IL-10 levels increase in cutaneous biopsies of patients undergoing wasp venom immunotherapy. Eur J Immunol 2001; 31:3704–3713.
6. Akdis CA, Blesken T, Akdis M, Wuthrich B, Blaser K. Role of IL-10 in specific immunotherapy. J Clin Investig 1998; 102:98–106.
7. Akdis CA, Blaser K. IL-10 induced anergy in peripheral T cells and reactivation by microenvironmental cytokines: Two key steps in specific immunotherapy. FASEB J 1999; 13:603–609.
8. Bellinghausen I, Knop J, Saloga J. The role of IL-10 in the regulation of allergic immune responses. Int Arch Allergy Appl Immunol 2001; 126:97–101.
9. Berchtold E, Maibach F, Muller U. Reduction of side-effects from rush immunotherapy with honeybee venom pretreatment with terfenadine. Clin Exp Allergy 1992; 22:59–65.
10. Nielsen L, Johnsen CR, Mosbech H, Poulsen LK, Malling HJ. Antihistamine premedication in specific cluster immunotherapy: A double-blind, placebo-controlled study. J Allergy Clin Immunol 1996; 97:1207–1213.
11. Brockow K, Kiehn M, Riethmuller C, Vieluf D, Berger J, Ring J. Efficacy of antihistamine pretreatment in the prevention of adverse reactions to Hymenoptera immunotherapy: A prospective randomised, placebo-controlled trial. J Allergy Clin Immunol 1997; 100:458–463.
12. Reimers A, Hari Y, Muller U. Reduction of side-effects from ultrarush immunotherapy with honeybee venom by pretreatment with fexofenadine: A double-blind, placebo-controlled trial. Allergy 2000; 55:484–488.
13. Herman D, Melac M. Effect of pretreatment with cetirizine on side-effects from rush immunotherapy with honey bee venom (abstr). Allergy 1996; 51(suppl 31):68.
14. Beer DJ, Rocklin RE. Histamine modulation of lymphocyte biology: Membrane receptors, signal transduction and functions. Crit Rev Immunol 1987; 7:55–97.
15. Hol BE, Krouwels FH, Bruiner B, Lutter R, Bast A, Wieringa EA, Jausen HM, Out TA. Heterogeneous effects of histamine on proliferation of lung and blood derived T-cell clones from healthy and asthmatic patients. Am J Respir Cell Mol Biol 1993; 8:647–654.
16. Morichika T, Takahashi HK, Iwagaki H, Yoshino T, Tamura R, Yokoyama M, Mori S, Akagi T, Nishibori M, Tanaka N. Histamine inhibits lipopolysaccharide-induced tumor necrosis factor–alpha production in an intercellular adhesion molecule-1- and B7.1-dependent manner. J Pharmacol Exp Ther 2003; 304:624–633.

17. Repka-Ramirez MS. New concepts of histamine receptors and actions. Curr Allergy Asthma Rep 2003; 3:227–231.
18. O'Reilly M, Alpert R, Jenkinson S, Gladue RP, Foo S, Trim S, Peter B, Trevethick M, Fidock M. Identification of a histamine H4 receptor on human eosinophils: Role in eosinophil chemotaxis. J Recept Signal Transduct Res 2002; 22:431–448.
19. Hofstra CL, Desai PJ, Thurmond RL, Fung-Leung WP. Histamine h4 receptor mediates chemotaxis and calcium mobilization of mast cells. J Pharmacol Exp Ther 2003; 305:1212–1221.
20. Gantner F, Sakai K, Tusche MW, Cruikshank WW, Center DM, Bacon KB. Histamine h(4) and h(2) receptors control histamine-induced interleukin-16 release from human CD8(+) T cells. J Pharmacol Exp Ther 2002; 303:300–307.
21. Munakata Y, Umezawa Y, Iwata S, Dong RP, Yoshida S, Ishii T, Morimoto C. Specific inhibition of Th2-type cytokine production from human peripheral T cells by terfenadine in vitro. Clin Exp Allergy 1999; 29:1281–1286.
22. Poluektova LY, Huggler GK, Patterson EB, Khan MM. Involvement of protein kinase A in histamine-mediated inhibition of IL-2 mRNA expression in mouse splenocytes. Immunopharmacology 1999; 41:77–87.
23. Jutel M, Watanabe T, Klunker S, Akdis M, Thomet OAR, Malolepszy J, Zak-Nejmark T, Koga R, Kobayashi T, Blaser K, Akdis C. Histamine regulates T-cell and antibody responses by differential expression of H1 and H2 receptors. Nature 2001; 413:420–425.
24. Des Roches A, Paradis L, Menardo JL, Bouges S, Daures JP, Bousquet J. Immunotherapy with a standardized *Dermatophagoides pteronyssinus* extract: VI. Specific immunotherapy prevents the onset of new sensitizations in children. J Allergy Clin Immunol 1997; 99:450–453.
25. Muller U, Hari Y, Bercthold E. Premedication with antihistamines may enhance efficacy of specific allergen immunotherapy. J Allergy Clin Immunol 2001; 107:81–86.
26. Adkinson NF, Eggleston PA, Eney D, Goldstein EO, Schuberth KC, Bacon JR, Hamilton RG, Weiss ME, Arshad H, Meinert CL, Tonascia J, Wheeler B. A controlled trial of immunotherapy for asthma in allergic children. N Engl J Med 1997; 336:324–331.
27. Rak S, Heinrich C, Jacobsen L, Scheynius A, Venge P. A double-blinded, comparative study of the effects of short preseason specific immunotherapy and topical steroids in patients with allergic rhinoconjunctivitis and asthma. J Allergy Clin Immunol 2001; 108:921–928.

31

Immunotherapy in Young Children

**PIERRE SCHEINMANN, CLAUDE PONVERT, PATRICK RUFIN, and
JACQUES DE BLIC**

Hôpital Necker-Enfants Malades, Paris, France

I. INTRODUCTION

Specific allergen immunotherapy (SIT) is based on the progressive administration of increasing quantities of allergen vaccine to an allergic patient to ameliorate symptoms and to reduce the effects of subsequent exposure to causative allergens.

According to the 1998 international consensus (1) SIT is primarily indicated in patients with such allergic diseases of the respiratory tract as rhinoconjunctivitis and/or mild to moderate asthma, provided that asthma symptoms are controlled by bronchodilators and inhaled corticosteroids (ICS). Allergic diseases of the respiratory tract are a major concern for allergists for various reasons:

1. Studies show that allergen-induced IgE-mediated inflammation should be considered a multiorgan disease. Thus, conjunctivitis, rhinitis, and asthma should be considered as a single entity, leading to the designation by some of

"united airways disease"; links between the upper and lower respiratory airways have been reviewed (2,3).

2. Minimal persistent nasal and bronchial inflammation induced by repeated exposure to low and noneliciting concentrations of allergens is also important. This phenomenon may account for the relationship between allergic inflammation; upper respiratory tract infections, perhaps due to increased potency of rhinovirus infections due to ICAM-1 expression on epithelial cells; and symptoms in children (3,4).

Thus, an "integrated" model for respiratory allergy therapy should combine allergen avoidance, anti-allergic and anti-inflammatory medications, and SIT to control factors involved in the allergic inflammatory cascade. Measures, including SIT, should be developed as soon as possible in allergic children to modify the natural course of respiratory allergy. Airway remodeling may start early in life, especially in children with severe asthma (5) , and ongoing airway inflammation and remodeling in adolescents and young adults may increase the risk of asthma later in life (6). Moreover, there is evidence that early SIT significantly reduces the risk of asthma in children with allergic rhinitis (7,8) and diminishes the risk of new sensitizations in monosensitized children (9–11). In addition, children seem to respond more favorably to SIT than do adults.

The development of new perspectives in SIT is highly desirable for children with food allergy. Indeed, foods are a major cause of life-threatening reactions in children with both asthma and food allergy. Accidental ingestion of the causative or cross-reactive foods is a frequent occurrence in children with food allergies. Unfortunately, food allergy may actually be worsened by current forms of SIT, as shown by Pajno et al. (12), and in any case, SIT for food allergy is not yet available for clinical practice (see Chapter 36). The use of immunotherapy in atopic dermatitis requires further investigation, as the data currently available are insufficient to formulate recommendations about efficacy and ability to prevent the onset of allergic rhinitis and/or asthma (13a).

Immunotherapy with Hymenoptera venoms is described in Chapter 29. This chapter will deal primarily with immunotherapy using vaccines of inhaled allergens. In practice, two routes are used in children: subcutaneous immunotherapy (SCIT), where injections of allergen vaccines are administered by injection subcutaneously; and sublingual immunotherapy (SLIT), where the vaccine is given orally, held under the tongue for at least 2 minutes, and then swallowed (SLIT-swallow). The excellent safety profile of SLIT-swallow and the fact that injections are not required with this method may extend the indications for immunotherapy to children below the age of 5 years in an attempt to modify the natural course of allergic diseases. SLIT-swallow is currently under assessment in the United States (13b). SLIT-swallow is widely used in Southern Europe, according to ARIA's data (2) and Cochrane's meta-analysis showing good efficacy and tolerance in allergic rhinitis (13c).

II. SUBCUTANEOUS SIT (SCIT)

A. Efficacy of SCIT

1. Current Knowledge

Controlled studies show that SIT is effective in patients with allergic rhinitis and rhinoconjunctivitis and/or asthma (1,2,14). Cochrane's meta-analysis was restricted to randomized trials conducted with SCIT from 1966 to 1997. SCIT significantly reduces asthma symptoms and the medication scores in patients with asthma. Indeed, one of the principal aims of immunotherapy is to decrease the need for medication. Any method would be welcome that made it possible to decrease ICS therapy, the mainstay of asthma management, while maintaining good asthma control. SCIT also significantly reduces allergen-specific bronchial hyperreactivity (BHR), thereby decreasing the risk of sudden deterioration in patients with brittle allergic asthma exposed to an increase in the levels of an aeroallergen to which they are sensitive. Fairly consistent results have been obtained in studies carried out in children. However, the effects of SCIT on lung function were not consistent, and nonspecific BHR was only moderately reduced (14).

2. What Should Be Determined?

Several questions were raised in Cochrane's meta-analysis and in other reviews (2,15): (1) How do the benefits of SCIT compare with those of other measures, especially ICS? (2) What is the risk/benefit ratio, considering the risk of potentially fatal anaphylaxis associated with SCIT? (3) Should patients with mild to moderate, well-controlled asthma receive SIT because the available drugs are effective and safe at moderate doses? Some pediatric studies have presented strong arguments in favor of SIT.

B. Combination of Anti-inflammatory Drugs and SIT

Interfering with the inflammatory cascade at various levels seems to be one of the best ways to improve clinical outcome and quality of life (2,16). Costa et al. (17) studied children, adolescents, and young adults with asthma caused by allergy to house dust mite (HDM). All patients were treated with ICS for 18 months. The combination of SCIT, with a monthly maintenance dose of 12,000 biological units (BU) for 27 months, and ICS gave a faster, more marked improvement in symptom scores, reducing short-acting bronchodilator needs and BHR and lowering the rate of relapse after ICS withdrawal.

Hedlin et al. (18) studied 27 children with moderate to severe allergic asthma treated with ICS. Children were randomly assigned to groups receiving SCIT for 3 years against cat or *Dermatophagoides pteronyssinus* allergens or placebo, and against birch or timothy pollen or placebo. SCIT was associated with a continuous decrease in bronchial histamine reactivity and a significant reduction in bronchial sensitivity to allergens. Moreover, SCIT induced clinical allergen tolerance in cat-allergic children. However, it was difficult to distinguish between the effects of SIT and ICS in this study. Nevertheless, the decrease in bronchial reactivity was greatest in children treated with a combination of SIT and ICS, suggesting that a combination of these two anti-inflammatory treatments is beneficial to allergic children.

Assessment of direct and indirect airway responsiveness (13b) shows that SLIT decreases BHR. Grüber et al. (19) studied BHR to a cold, dry air challenge in asthmatic children allergic to HDM. A significant decrease in BHR was observed in SCIT-treated children, but not in children receiving only anti-asthma drugs. It has been suggested that adenosine-5′-monophosphate (AMP) provocative concentration reducing the FEV_1 by 20% from baseline (PC_{20}) is useful for detecting early inflammatory changes in asthmatic airways. SIT may prevent the seasonal increase in airway responsiveness to AMP (20,21).

These studies performed in SCIT-treated patients indicate that this therapy decreases BHR in response to various specific and nonspecific stimuli, including methacholine, cold air, and AMP, by directly or indirectly affecting bronchial smooth muscle. Another common finding of these studies is that the beneficial effects of SIT are more pronounced at the end of the second versus the end of the first year of treatment.

C. Long-Term Effects of SIT

The duration of clinical efficacy, when SIT is discontinued, depends on the duration of SIT, as demonstrated by retrospective (22) and prospective (23a) studies. Relapses are reported in most children treated for only 2 years (19). In contrast, several years after the cessation of SIT, there is a significant decrease in symptom scores and a nonsignificant decrease in medication scores observed in young adults treated for allergic asthma during childhood for ~3 years (generally for 5 years) (22). The long-term effects of SIT contrast with the short-term effects of pharmacotherapy (15).

D. SIT as a Preventive Treatment for Allergic Diseases

Other studies suggest that SIT prevents the development of asthma in allergic rhinitis patients and the onset of new sensitizations in monosensitized children.

1. Prevention of Asthma

Grembiale et al. (7) compared disease progression in two groups of children, adolescents and young adults, with allergic rhinitis and BHR. All subjects were monosensitized to *D. pteronyssinus*. A significant increase in methacholine PD_{20} FEV_1 was observed in the SIT group (monthly maintenance dose, 800 BU) after 1 year of treatment. The beneficial effects of SIT on BHR were even greater after 2 years of treatment. The disease severity score was significantly reduced in SIT-treated patients, and none of them developed asthma. In contrast, 9% of the 22 patients in the placebo group developed mild asthma. This study highlights the link between allergic rhinitis and asthma, especially in patients allergic to perennial allergens with BHR. This study also suggests that early SIT may be effective in patients with mild BHR, because airway remodeling is less advanced in such patients.

Asthma was prevented in adults with allergic rhinitis investigated 6 years after the termination of SCIT (23b). Asthma prevention was also observed in children with seasonal rhinoconjunctivitis after 3 years of SIT with birch and/or grass pollen allergen vaccines (8). Asthma symptoms were less frequent and responses in allergen conjunctival provocation and methacholine provocation tests were significantly lessened in the SIT group compared with children receiving only anti-asthma drugs. This study also suggests that early SIT should be considered in allergic rhinitis patients, with the aim of preventing the subsequent development of BHR and/or asthma.

2. Prevention of New Sensitivities

Studies show that a large number of monosensitized children develop sensitizations to new allergens later in life. Results suggest that SCIT, performed with a single allergen, can prevent sensitization to other allergens in monosensitized children. Eng et al. (10) followed children with severe hay fever prospectively, before, during, and after a successful 3-year course of grass pollen SIT. Six years after SCIT was terminated, overall hay fever, eye, nose, and chest symptoms during the pollen season were significantly milder in the SIT-treated children than in children treated only with drugs. Fewer SIT-treated children experienced seasonal pollen asthma, and quality of life (QOL), as assessed by the Visual Analog Scale (VAS), was significantly higher in the SIT-treated group. Finally, 61% of children in the SIT-treated group developed new sensitizations to perennial allergens versus 100% of children in the control group.

The benefits of early SCIT in asthmatic children monosensitized to HDM were studied by Pifferi et al. (24). Fifteen children, including 7 children with asthma and perennial rhinitis, were given SIT over 3 years. Doses of allergen vaccines were gradually increased to the maximal tolerated dose, using a flexible dosing schedule. Outcome was significantly better for the SIT group than for the control group ($n - 10$, pharmacological treatment only) in terms of symptoms, particularly in decreasing asthma exacerbations; drug use, including systemic corticosteroids; and BHR (PD_{20}, methacholine). A decrease in BHR was observed in children treated with SIT but not with ICS. The beneficial effects of SIT increased significantly with increased duration of treatment. Five children in the control group developed new sensitizations to pollen and animal danders, whereas none of the SIT-treated children developed new sensitizations. The authors stressed the value of early SIT in asthmatic children monosensitized to HDM and argued against the use of therapeutic vaccines containing mixtures of up to seven perennial and seasonal allergen sources, including pollen, mites, and molds. The dilution, by using multiple allergens, may result in suboptimal doses, reducing the potency of individual allergen vaccines.

These studies, conducted in small numbers of children (<20), confirm the results of Pajno et al. (11), who prospectively followed the 123 asthmatic children monosensitized to HDM, 40% of whom had rhinitis and asthma, for 6 years. Sixty-nine children received SIT for 3 years and 54 were treated only with drugs. Three years after SIT was terminated, 52 of the 69 children (75.4%) in the SIT group showed no new sensitization, whereas 18 of the 54 (33.3%) children in the control group ($p < 0.0002$) had developed new sensitizations, for which pollens were the allergens most frequently responsible. The authors stressed the importance of the early use of SIT administered by physicians trained in allergy/immunology. They also advocated the early use of SIT combined with inhaled anti-inflammatory drugs to reverse the ongoing allergic inflammation in the respiratory tract.

Pajno's study provides support for the work of Des Roches et al. (9), which shows that early SIT is effective in preventing new sensitizations in young children. Des Roches et al. studied children below the age of 6 years who had asthma and were monosensitized to HDM. Twenty-two children were given SCIT for 3 years and 22 received only anti-allergic drugs. At the end of the study, 12 of the SIT-treated children and all of the control children had developed new sensitizations. Cat and dog danders, *Alternaria*, and grass pollen were the most common allergens.

These results also confirm the retrospective data reported by Purello-d'Ambrosio et al. (25) for patients over the age of 14 years with pollen- or HDM-allergic asthma and/or rhinitis. In the monosensitized patients, 4 years of SIT ($n = 7182$) was associated with a significantly lower number of new sensitizations than observed in patients receiving only anti-asthma drugs ($n = 1214$). The beneficial effects of SIT were significantly greater in asthmatic patients with or without rhinitis, who are more likely to be polysensitized, than in patients only with rhinitis—not only at the end of SIT, but also 3 years after SIT was terminated.

E. Immunological Effects

Studies describe changes in children in total and specific IgE and in specific IgG associated with SIT similar to those observed in adults (see Chapter 5).

The allergic state results from dysregulation of the TH1/TH2 immune response to allergens, with a shift toward a TH2-like response. SIT normalizes immunologicaly reactivity, inducing a shift toward a TH1-like response. Van Bever et al. (26a) showed that blood mononuclear cells (BMCs) from children given SIT with HDM are less reactive than cells from nontreated children and that the level of production of interleukin-4 (IL-4) and interleukin-5 (IL-5) in vitro by allergen-activated BMCs is significantly lower in SIT-treated children. However, changes in the production of TH1-type cytokines by the BMCs of treated children are not significant, except for IL-2. SIT also reduces T lymphocyte reactivity to allergens, as shown by the significant decrease in soluble IL-2 receptor (sIL-2R, sCD25) levels in the sera of house dust mite SIT-treated children (26b). However, SIT induced a significant increase in CD25 expression on the CD4+ and CD8+ T-cells of HDM-treated children (27a). The increase in CD25 expression on CD8+ T-cells is positively and significantly correlated with serum-specific IgG4 levels and with the cumulative dose of allergen vaccine, whereas increased CD25 expression on CD4+ T-cells is similar in both the nonimmunotherapy and immunotherapy groups. These data suggest that SIT induces the activation of specific "suppressor" T-cells, regulating allergen-specific T-cells probably via IL-10 production (15,27b). Finally, SIT induces a significant decrease in serum immuno-enhancing neurohormone levels, melatonin and β-endorphin, in pollen-allergic children (28). These changes were correlated with the clinical efficacy of SIT but not with changes in serum-specific IgE and IgG4 levels.

III. OTHER ROUTES OF IMMUNOTHERAPY

There is increased interest in allergen immunotherapy that does not involve injection therapy. SLIT-swallow may be of particular value for children because it avoids the psychological stress and decreases the risk of severe systemic reaction associated with SCIT. SLIT-swallow is safe for both children and adults (29,30). Moreover, SLIT-swallow can be administered at home, provided appropriate information is given to the patient or to the child's parents.

A. Efficacy of SLIT-Swallow

SLIT has been administered in two different ways: sublingual-spit or sublingual-swallow (2,31). With the SLIT-spit technique, the allergen vaccine is held in the mouth for 2 minutes and then spit out, whereas with sublingual-swallow, the allergen is held in the mouth for 2 minutes and then swallowed (Fig. 1). Most controlled studies have been conducted using the SLIT-swallow method.

Studies have been conducted exclusively in children or in populations including children. Pajno et al. (32) studied children with mild to moderate asthma, monosensitized to *D. pteronyssinus*. Sublingual-spit was initiated after a full year of baseline assessment so that the effects of treatment could be accurately evaluated. Asthma symptoms, including nocturnal symptoms, medication use, and quality of life (QOL), improved significantly in the group treated with sublingual-spit and was also found to be more effective at the end of the second year than at the end of the first year. Shorter therapeutic trials may yield false-negative results.

Bousquet et al. (33) studied children and young adults with HDM-allergic asthma. SLIT-swallow was administered for 2 years, and the cumulative dose of allergen was 200 times higher than that administered by SCIT. Improvements in lung function, BHR, and QOL were more pronounced, although not significantly, in the twenty-fifth month than at the eleventh month.

In children allergic to *Parietaria judaica*, which causes almost year-round symptoms, La Rosa et al. (34) showed that SLIT-swallow significantly diminished symptoms of rhinoconjunctivitis and asthma and decreased reactivity to allergen, as assessed by

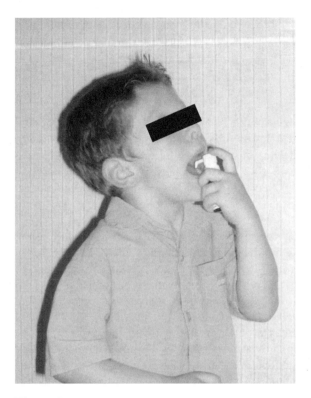

Figure 1   Self-administration of SLIT-swallow by a 5-year-old child (under parental supervision).

conjunctival provocation tests. The cumulative dose of allergen vaccine was 375 times higher than with SCIT. Consistent with other studies, efficacy significantly increased with longer duration of SLIT-swallow. In this study, children in the active group had more severe symptoms than children in the placebo group at the start of the trial. These findings suggest that patients selected for such therapy have more severe symptoms and hence a greater chance for improvement (15).

B. Long-Term Effects of SLIT

Until 2003, only SCIT had been shown to result in long-term benefits. However, results now suggest that SLIT-swallow has long-term beneficial effects in children. Di Rienzo et al. (35) prospectively studied 35 children with HDM-allergic asthma and/or rhinitis. The children received a 4- to 5-year course of SLIT-swallow and were compared with 25 children receiving only drug therapy. Four to 5 years following discontinuation of SLIT-swallow, significant improvements in asthma symptoms, PEFR, and use of asthma medication with respect to baseline were observed in treated children. No change was observed in the control group. However, unlike SCIT, SLIT-swallow did not seem to affect the development of sensitizations to new allergens.

Finally, two reviews suggest that SLIT-swallow is as effective as, or only slightly less effective than, SCIT (3,33); however, this is not endorsed by all investigators (15).

C.   Immunological Effects of SLIT-Swallow

A few studies of the immunological effects of SLIT-swallow have been performed in children. In HDM-allergic children, SLIT-swallow induced a significant decrease in skin test reactivity to *D. pteronyssinus* (Dp) or *Dermatophagoides farinae* (Df) with respect to placebo-treated children (36). However, Hirsch et al. (37) could not confirm these findings. Serum total IgE levels did not change in SLIT-swallow – treated children (38), and there were no significant differences between SLIT-swallow and placebo-treate children for serum-specific IgE, IgG, and IgG4 levels after 1 and 2 years of treatment (32). However, Tari et al. (39) reported a decline in serum-specific IgE antibody levels in the SLIT-swallow group, during the fall, after 12 and 24 months of treatment. In contrast, Hirsch et al. (37) found that specific IgE levels increased in the third and twelfth months of treatment. Serum-specific IgG and IgG4 levels have been found to increase (39) or to remain unchanged during SLIT-swallow (37). Finally, SLIT-swallow induced a significant decrease in ICAM-1 expression on nasal epithelial cells (38), a significant increase in the number of blood CD8+ cells, and a significant decrease in the CD4+/CD8+ ratio (39).

After 2 years of SLIT-swallow treatment, pollen-allergic children were found to have significantly lower levels of skin test reactivity to *P. judaica* and olive pollen than did placebo-treated children (34,40). No within- or between-group differences were found for serum-specific IgE and IgG4 levels (40). In contrast, La Rosa et al. (34) reported significantly higher specific IgG4 levels in pollen-treated children than in the placebo group. Compared with a placebo group, preseasonal oromucosal-swallow immunotherapy (tablets of monomeric allergoid grass pollen allergens to be held in the mouth until they dissolve, 1–2 min) reduced total symptoms significantly and was particularly effective against bronchial symptoms in children with conjunctivitis and/or rhinitis and/or asthma. The EG_2/EG_1 ratio increased significantly during the pollen season only in the placebo group, suggesting that oromucosal swallow may decrease eosinophil activation (the monoclonal antibodies EG_1 and EG_2 detect total and activated ECP, respectively) (41). SLIT-swallow significantly decreased the eosinophilic cation protein (ECP) concentration during the first pollen season (40) but not during the second one. Finally, SLIT-swallow was shown to decrease urinary levels of LTB_4 and LTE_4 significantly in children with grass pollen rhinitis but not in children with seasonal asthma (42).

Four days of SLIT-swallow desensitization resulted in negative allergen-specific provocation tests (conjunctival, oral, and cutaneous) together with clinical tolerance to latex in patients allergic to latex (43).

D.   Nasal, Oral, and Bronchial Immunotherapy

In children, most alternative methods for allergen immunotherapy have focused on SLIT-swallow. However, a pediatric study showed that low-dose local nasal immunotherapy (LNIT) is effective in children with HDM-allergic rhinitis (44). At the end of the second year of LNIT, the medication score, nasal symptoms, and reactivity to allergen provocation were significantly better in the treated than in the placebo group. However, the long-term efficacy, preventive effects, and immunological effects of LNIT in children have not yet been determined.

Bronchial immunotherapy cannot currently be recommended for clinical use in children. More data are required for oral immunotherapy, in which the allergen is immediately swallowed following ingestion and not held in the mouth 2 minutes before it is swallowed, as is done with SLIT-swallow. Positive results for cow milk allergy await confirmation (45).

IV. SAFETY OF SIT

A. SCIT

The major risks associated with SIT (see Chapter 39) are acute asthma and anaphylaxis (1) especially in patients treated by the SC route. Such effects may be prevented by the use of low doses of allergen, but low-dose SIT is not clinically effective. The optimal dose of allergen vaccine should both induce a clinically relevant effect and be safe. Doses of 5–20 µg of major allergens are considered to be optimal for HDM, cat dander, and pollen. Allergists are trained to know how to adjust doses of allergen vaccines in patients with local or systemic reactions. There are no differences in making such adjustments between children and adults.

Nettis et al. (46) observed 34 serious side effects (0.093% of 36,359 injections), including 14 cases of anaphylactic shock, in 29 (5.2%) of the 555 children and adult patients treated with SCIT of absorbed standardized vaccines of HDM, olive, grass, or *P. judaica* pollen. These absorbed vaccines are used in Europe and not in the United States. Most reactions occurred within 30 minutes of the injection. The main risk factors were symptomatic asthma and the injection of increasing doses during the build-up treatment phase of SLIT. Side effects were not associated with sex, age, skin prick test reactivity, or type of allergen. These results are consistent with those of Cantani et al. (47), who showed that severe reactions are rare in children. In other studies, most SCIT-treated children tolerated injections of allergen vaccines, but anaphylactic reactions were reported in up to 6% of children, especially in children treated with molds (1).

Fatal reactions are rare. The main risk factors are errors in SCIT administration, extension beyond recommended intervals between injections, inadequate dose of epinephrine to treat a systemic reaction, and inadequate medical supervision during the 30 minutes following injection of the allergen vaccine.

B. Safety of SLIT-Swallow

The safety of SLIT-swallow administered at home under parental supervision has been demonstrated. Data highlight the absence of urticaria, angioedema, and life-threatening events. Wheezing occurs less frequently in patients receiving SLIT-swallow than in patients receiving placebo. Respiratory symptoms including dyspnea decrease in children receiving SLIT-swallow (40). Mouth burning/itching, lip swelling, and gastrointestinal symptoms (e.g., vomiting, abdominal pain, and diarrhea) are the most common side effects, mostly occurring during the build-up phase. Repeated oral/gastrointestinal symptoms and/or increases in their severity were the main reasons for patients dropping out of SLIT-swallow trials (29,30). Gastrointestinal side effects responded to a reduced allergen dose and to pretreatment with antihistamines (34).

V. NEW THERAPEUTIC APPROACHES

Increasing the understanding of the basic mechanisms responsible for allergic diseases will lead to new therapies. The first drug to be made available for children will probably be the anti-IgE monoclonal antibody omalizumab. Kuehr et al. (48) conducted a double-blind trial to assess the efficacy of omalizumab in more than 200 children with birch and grass pollen-induced seasonal allergic rhinitis. They received preseasonal SCIT with either birch allergen vaccines, mean cumulative dose 48.50 µg of major allergen Bet v 1, or grass pollen, mean cumulative dose 68.83 μg of major allergen. Clinical efficacy was assessed by determining the symptom load score (symptom severity and rescue medication used during the pollen season). Anti-IgE therapy conferred a protective effect independent of the type of allergen used. Treatment with monoclonal anti-IgE antibody and SIT was more effective than SIT alone. This combination therapy facilitated the management of complex cases of seasonal allergic rhinitis. The additive effects of combined SCIT and anti-IgE reduced the requirements for additional rhinitis medication. Whereas worsening of atopic dermatitis was considered a risk of SCIT alone, in fact, eczema was observed only in the placebo group.

The in vitro release of sulfidoleukotrienes (SLT) (LTC$_4$, D$_4$, and E$_4$) in response to allergens was assessed in the peripheral blood leukocyte pellet (49). The combination of SCIT and anti-IgE led to significantly lower levels of SLT release in vitro than did exclusive SCIT with birch or grass pollen allergens. This in vitro response paralleled the clinical results. SCIT alone did not decrease SLT release, perhaps because the duration of SCIT was too short (i.e., 9 months).

Combination therapy with monoclonal anti-IgE antibody and SCIT might prove useful in polysensitized children during the first few years of SIT when the response to SIT is incomplete. Anti-IgE antibody may also reduce the risk of IgE-mediated systemic early and late-phase reactions associated with SCIT and may make it possible to use rush SCIT and/or to achieve higher doses of therapeutic allergens.

VI. INDICATIONS FOR SIT

A. Seasonal or Perennial Rhinitis and/or Asthma

The indications for SIT should be based on allergen sensitization rather than a particular disease (2,50). Moreover, studies suggest that SIT interferes with the "allergic march" and could be indicated very early in children with allergic rhinitis, possibly below 5 years, to prevent the onset of asthma (7,8,51) and in monosensitized children to prevent new sensitizations (9–11).

The indications for SIT are based on the results of studies of efficacy in children with allergic diseases. According to the international consensus (1,2),

1. SIT is primarily indicated for children with proven IgE-dependent sensitization (skin test and/or specific IgE determination), and positive clinical SIT is indicated only in patients with demonstrable evidence of specific IgE directed against clinically relevant allergens where it is impossible to completely avoid those allergens. Nasal provocation tests can be performed in children whose clinical history and allergy tests do not agree (52).

2. SIT is also indicated for children with moderate to severe conjunctivitis, rhinitis, and/or mild to moderate asthma. For children with pollen allergy, immunotherapy is indicated if the pollen season is prolonged and/or the severity of symptoms increases over 2 consecutive years. Subjects with mild symptoms, easily controlled with pharamacotherapy, should not be placed on SIT. Immunotherapy is indicated for children whose symptoms warrant the time and risks necessarily associated with allergen immunotherapy (1,2). However, parents and children may be reluctant to undergo a prolonged course of pharmacological treatment and may prefer immunotherapy. The allergist should inform parents and children that SIT is not immediately effective and provide information about the duration of SIT, usually administered for 3–5 years, and its possible adverse effects.

3. SIT is indicated for children with monosensitization to specific allergens. Some authors argue against the use of therapeutic vaccines containing mixtures of perennial and

seasonal allergens, including pollen, molds, animal danders, and house dust mites, in multisensitized children. Indeed, the mixing of multiple allergens may lead to a decrease in the levels of individual allergens, and the enzymatic activity of some allergens may decrease the allergenic potential of other allergens in the vaccine.

B. SIT with Hymenoptera Venom in Children

The indications for venom immunotherapy (VIT) are based on a history of life-threatening allergic reaction to a Hymenoptera sting and positive venom skin tests and/or specific IgE determinations (see Chapter 8). VIT is also indicated in patients reporting non–life-threatening generalized reactions but with additional risk factors, such as a high risk of exposure (beekeepers and gardeners) (1,2,53). Indications for VIT are more restricted in children than in adults. Severe reactions to Hymenoptera stings are less common in children than in adults, and deaths are rare. Moreover, the re-sting reaction rate is lower in children than in adults, and worsening reactions are rare. Finally, indicators of efficacy such as tolerance to venom injection (54), decreased reactivity to skin tests and/or decreased specific IgE levels, increased serum-specific IgG levels, and tolerance to field re-stings are more common in children than in adults. Thus, the decision to stop VIT, after at least 3 years of treatment, is also easier in children (1,2,53).

During the initial phase of rush (54) and even ultrarush VIT, the frequency of systemic immediate reactions does not differ significantly between adults and children (10.8% versus 11.2%) (55). The incidence of systemic reactions is higher with honeybee venom vaccine (12%) than with yellow jacket venom vaccine (2%) (54). The usual monthly maintenance dose, 100 µg, is reached in the vast majority of children and is usually tolerated. Some authors recommend pretreatment with an antihistamine during rush VIT (54,56). Systemic reactions can occur and the physician should be prepared to immediately administer appropriate treatment (see Chapter 39).

VII. TECHNICAL PRINCIPLES OF IMMUNOTHERAPY

A. SCIT

1. Basic Principles

High-quality and, where possible, standardized allergen vaccines should be used, where available. The vaccines most commonly used in children in Europe are those from house dust mite, *D. pteronyssinus* and *D. farinae*, either alone or combined, and various types of pollen, birch and other members of the Betulaceae, grass, ragweed, and *J. parietaria*. Animal danders and *Alternaria* SIT have not been extensively studied in children (57).

2. Practical Recommendations

The basic treatment principles are similar for adults and children. The optimal maintenance dose in either biological units or micrograms of major allergens should induce clinically relevant benefits without inducing unacceptable side effects. Doses of 5–20 µg of the major allergen constitute the optimal maintenance dose for most common inhalant allergens. The dose of allergen is gradually increased weekly or twice weekly until a maintenance dose is reached, which is then given every 4 weeks (in some cases, every 6 weeks). It should be continued for at least 3–5 years.

It is essential to observe the following recommendations to minimize the risks associated with SCIT. Children should be asymptomatic, with $FEV_1 > 70\%$ of predicted values (1,2), at the time injections are administered. Allergen dosing should be delayed with concurrent or recent infections or exacerbation of allergic symptoms (58). The dose should not be increased if there is a large immediate local reaction, with wheals >3 cm, and should be decreased with wheals >5 cm associated with the preceding dose. Dose adjustments are necessary for delayed local reactions that cause the patient considerable discomfort, and if the planned interval between two injections is exceeded by 2. In cases of a severe systemic reaction, IT is generally stopped. Venom allergy, because of the risk of death from an in-field sting, should be continued, but only after appropriate dose adjustment.

The child should be observed for at least 30 minutes after an injection, and the physician should be present for the time necessary to appropriately treat an acute allergic reaction. It remains controversial whether antihistamines given prophylactically are helpful in preventing systemic reactions (54,56,59).

When the source of the commercial extract used to constitute a vaccine must be changed because a child moves from one physican to another, it is preferable initially to use a lower dose of the new vaccine.

B. SLIT-Swallow

Children may find it difficult to retain the dose of allergen under the tongue for the required 2 minutes before swallowing. The maintenance dose is reached in approximately 2 weeks and is then administered daily or three times per week (Table 1). The dose should be reduced once by half if the planned interval between two doses is lengthened to >1 week. The mean cumulative dose is at least 100 times greater than that for SCIT. Relatively high

Table 1 Proposed Schedule for Grass Pollen SLIT

D1	100 µl	10 IR
D2	200 µl	10 IR
D3	400 µl	10 IR
D4	600 µl	10 IR
D5	100 µl	100 IR
D6	200 µl	100 IR
D7	400 µl	100 IR
D8	600 µl	100 IR
D9	100 µl	300 IR
D10	200 µl	300 IR
D11	400 µl	300 IR
D12	600 µl	300 IR
D13	800 µl	300 IR

Allergen vials are supplied with a micropump, delivering 100 µl.
SLIT-swallow ideally should be initiated two months before beginning of the allergenic season but is also efficacious if initiated just at the beginning of the season.
An allergen extract is attributed a value of 100 IR/ml when it induces a mean 7 mm wheal in a skin prick test using a Stallerpoint needle in 30 subjects sensitized to allergen in question. The reactivity of subjects is also demonstrated by a positive response to a skin prick test with codeine phosphate (9%) or histamine (10 mg/ml). Doses are taken once daily with a rapid increase from 100 µl of a solution of 10 IR/ml to 800 µl of a solution of 300 IR/ml (maintenance dose). The maintenance dose is administered daily or three times per week until the end of the pollen season.

Table 2 Comparison Between SCIT and SLIT-Swallow

Route	SCIT	SLIT-swallow
Indications	Rhinitis, conjunctivitis, and asthma Insect venom allergy	Rhinitis, conjunctivitis, and asthma
Allergens	Aeroallergens (mites, pollen, molds, animal danders) and insect venoms	Aeroallergens (mites, pollen)
Acceptability, ease of administration	Low (administration at the practitioner's office	Good (self-administration at home)
Compliance, adherence	Usually moderate (up to 50% of noncompliant patients)	Unknown
Tolerability, safety	Frequent local reactions Risk of systemic reaction (0.8–46.7%)	Good: no systemic reaction, but oral and gastrointestinal side effects (increasing frequency with increased dosage) (Di Rienzo et al, Allergy 1999)
Efficacy	Good and long-lasting (up to adult age)	Probably lower than efficacy of SCIT. Duration up to 4–5 years after discontinuation of SLIT-swallow.
Optimal cumulative dose of major allergen	5–20 µg	20 to 375 times the dose of SCIT
Prevention of asthma in rhinitis	Yes	Unknown
Prevention of new sensitizations	Yes	No
Mode of action	Known	Largely unknown
Estimated cost (per year)	$534	$460 (formal cost-benefit analysis still lacking)

Based mainly on Canonica and Passalacqua (60).

initial doses are tolerated, and administering SLIT-swallow during the pollen season does not seem to increase the risk of side effects (29). Antihistamines can be used for patients with oral and gastrointestinal side effects.

VIII. SALIENT POINTS

1. SIT is indicated to treat allergic rhinitis, allergic asthma, and Hymenoptera hypersensitivity.
2. SIT may decrease the onset of asthma in children who have only allergic rhinitis and decreases the risk of polysensitization.
3. The most common route for SIT in children is the subcutaneous route.
4. SLIT-swallow may be a viable alternative for such therapy, but few studies have been conducted comparing its efficacy to SCIT (Table 2) (60).

5. Whatever the route of administration, a key element contributing to SIT success is the demonstration that the child's symptoms are related to the clinically relevant allergens.

6. Allergen immunotherapy should be prescribed only by physicians trained in the specialty of allergy and immunology.

7. Therapeutic compliance is essential for SIT because treatment is necessary for at least 3–5 years.

8. SIT is essential to the appropriate management of allergic respiratory deseases. Used together with allergen avoidance and pharmacotherapy, SIT decreases the requirement for drugs and improves the quality of life and long-term prognosis of children with allergic diseases.

REFERENCES

1. Allergen immunotherapy: Therapeutic vaccines for allergic diseases: Geneva, January 27–29, 1997. Allergy 1998; 53:1–42.

2. Bousquet J, Van Cauwenberge P, Khaltaev N. Allergic rhinitis and its impact on asthma. J Allergy Clin Immunol 2001; 108:S147–S334.

3. Passalacqua G, Canonica GW. Treating the allergic patient: Think globally, treat globally. Allergy 2002; 57:876–883.

4. Green RM, Custovic A, Sanderson G, Hunter J, Johnston SL, Woodcock A. Synergism between allergens and viruses and risk of hospital admission with asthma: Case-control study. Br Med J 2002; 324:763.

5. Delacourt C, Benoist MR, Waernessyckle S, et al. Relationship between bronchial responsiveness and clinical evolution in infants who wheeze: A four-year prospective study. Am J Respir Crit Care Med 2001; 164:1382–1386.

6. Van Den Toorn LM, Overbeek SE, Prins JB, Hoogsteden HC, De Jongste JC. Asthma remission: Does it exist? Curr Opin Pulm Med 2003; 9:15–20.

7. Grembiale RD, Camporota L, Naty S, Tranfa CM, Djukanovic R, Marsico SA. Effects of specific immunotherapy in allergic rhinitic individuals with bronchial hyperresponsiveness. Am J Respir Crit Care Med 2000; 162:2048–2052.

8. Moller C, Dreborg S, Ferdousi HA, et al. Pollen immunotherapy reduces the development of asthma in children with seasonal rhinoconjunctivitis (the PAT-study). J Allergy Clin Immunol 2002; 109:251–256.

9. Des Roches A, Paradis L, Menardo JL, Bouges S, Daures JP, Bousquet J. Immunotherapy with a standardized *Dermatophagoides pteronyssinus* extract: VI. Specific immunotherapy prevents the onset of new sensitizations in children. J Allergy Clin Immunol 1997; 99:450–453.

10. Eng PA, Reinhold M, Gnehm HP. Long-term efficacy of preseasonal grass pollen immunotherapy in children. Allergy 2002; 57:306–312.

11. Pajno GB, Barberio G, De Luca F, Morabito L, Parmiani S. Prevention of new sensitizations in asthmatic children monosensitized to house dust mite by specific immunotherapy. A six-year follow-up study. Clin Exp Allergy 2001; 31:1392–7.

12. Pajno GB, La Grutta S, Barberio G, Canonica GW, Passalacqua G. Harmful effect of immunotherapy in children with combined snail and mite allergy. J Allergy Clin Immunol 2002; 109:627–629.

13a. Mastrandrea F. Immunotherapy in atopic dermatitis. Expert Opin Investig Drugs 2001; 10:49–63.

13b. GINA Workshop Report, Global Strategy for Asthma Management and Prevention—updated April 2002. Scientific Information and Recommendations for Asthma Programs. NIH Publication No. 02–3659.

13c. Wilson DR, Torres Lima M, Durham SR. Sublingual immunotherapy for allergic rhinitis (Cochrane review). In: The Cochrane Library, issue 2. Oxford: Update Software, 2003.

14. Abramson MJ, Puy RM, Weiner JM. Allergen immunotherapy for asthma (Cochrane review). Cochrane Database Syst Rev 2003.

15. Frew AJ. Immunotherapy of allergic disease. J Allergy Clin Immunol 2003; 111: 712–719.

16. Yilmaz M, Bingol G, Altintas D, Kendirli SG. Effect of SIT on quality of life. Allergy 2000; 55:302.

17. Costa JC, Placido JL, Silva JP, Delgado L, Vaz M. Effects of immunotherapy on symptoms, PEFR, spirometry, and airway responsiveness in patients with allergic asthma to house-dust mites (*D. pteronyssinus*) on inhaled steroid therapy. Allergy 1996; 51: 238–244.

18. Hedlin G, Wille S, Browaldh L, et al. Immunotherapy in children with allergic asthma: Effect on bronchial hyperreactivity and pharmacotherapy. J Allergy Clin Immunol 1999; 103:609–614.

19. Gruber W, Eber E, Mileder P, Modl M, Weinhandl E, Zach MS. Effect of specific immunotherapy with house dust mite extract on the bronchial responsiveness of pediatric asthma patients. Clin Exp Allergy 1999; 29:176–181.

20. Polosa R. Can immunotherapy prevent progression to asthma in allergic individuals? J Allergy Clin Immunol 2002; 110:672–673.

21. Spicuzza L, Polosa R. The role of adenosine as a novel bronchoprovocant in asthma. Curr Opin Allergy Clin Immunol 2003; 3:65–69.

22. Cools M, Van Bever HP, Weyler JJ, Stevens WJ. Long-term effects of specific immunotherapy, administered during childhood, in asthmatic patients allergic to either house-dust mite or to both house-dust mite and grass pollen. Allergy 2000; 55:69–73.

23a. Durham SR, Walker SM, Varga EM, et al. Long-term clinical efficacy of grass-pollen immunotherapy. N Engl J Med 1999; 341:468–475.

23b. Jacobsen L, Nüchel Petersen B, Wihl JÅ, Løwenstein H, Ipsen H. Immunotherapy with partially purified and standardized tree pollen extracts: IV. Results from long-term (6-year) follow-up. Allergy 1997; 52:914–920.

24. Pifferi M, Baldini G, Marrazzini G, et al. Benefits of immunotherapy with a standardized *Dermatophagoides pteronyssinus* extract in asthmatic children: A three-year prospective study. Allergy 2002; 57:785–790.

25. Purello-D'Ambrosio F, Gangemi S, Merendino RA, et al. Prevention of new sensitizations in monosensitized subjects submitted to specific immunotherapy or not. A retrospective study. Clin Exp Allergy 2001; 31:1295–1302.

26a. Van Bever HP, Vereecke IF, Bridts CH, De Clerck LS, Stevens WJ. Comparison between the in vitro cytokine production of mononuclear cells of young asthmatics with and without immunotherapy (IT). Clin Exp Allergy 1998; 28:943–949.

26b. Hsieh KH. Decreased production of interleukin-2 receptors after immunotherapy to house dust. J Clin Immunol 1988; 8:171–177.

27a. Bonno M, Fujisawa T, Iguchi K, et al. Mite-specific induction of interleukin-2 receptor on T lymphocytes from children with mite-sensitive asthma: Modified immune response with immunotherapy. J Allergy Clin Immunol 1996; 97:680–688.

27b. Francis JN, Till SJ, Durham SR. Induction of IL-10+CD4+CD25+ T cells by grass pollen immunotherapy. J Allergy Clin Immunol 2003; 111:1255–1261.

28. Giron-Caro F, Munoz-Hoyos A, Ruiz-Cosano C, et al. Melatonin and beta-endorphin changes in children sensitized to olive and grass pollen after treatment with specific immunotherapy. Int Arch Allergy Immunol 2001; 126:91–96.

29. Grosclaude M, Bouillot P, Alt R, et al. Safety of various dosage regimens during induction of sublingual immunotherapy: A preliminary study. Int Arch Allergy Immunol 2002; 129:248–253.

30. Andre C, Vatrinet C, Galvain S, Carat F, Sicard H. Safety of sublingual-swallow immunotherapy in children and adults. Int Arch Allergy Immunol 2000; 121:229–234.

31. Kagi MK, Wuthrich B. Different methods of local allergen-specific immunotherapy. Allergy 2002; 57:379–388.

32. Pajno GB, Morabito L, Barberio G, Parmiani S. Clinical and immunologic effects of long-term sublingual immunotherapy in asthmatic children sensitized to mites: A double-blind, placebo-controlled study. Allergy 2000; 55:842–849.

33. Bousquet J, Scheinmann P, Guinnepain MT, et al. Sublingual-swallow immunotherapy (SLIT-swallow) in patients with asthma due to house-dust mites: A double-blind, placebo-controlled study. Allergy 1999; 54:249–260.

34. La Rosa M, Ranno C, Andre C, Carat F, Tosca MA, Canonica GW. Double-blind placebo-controlled evaluation of sublingual-swallow immunotherapy with standardized *Parietaria judaica* extract in children with allergic rhinoconjunctivitis. J Allergy Clin Immunol 1999; 104:425–432.

35. Di Rienzo V, Marcucci F, Puccinelli P, et al. Long-lasting effect of sublingual immunotherapy in children with asthma due to house dust mite: A 10-year prospective study. Clin Exp Allergy 2003; 33:206–210.

36. Bahceciler NN, Isik U, Barlan IB, Basaran MM. Efficacy of sublingual immunotherapy in children with asthma and rhinitis: A double-blind, placebo-controlled study. Pediatr Pulmonol 2001; 32:49–55.

37. Hirsch T, Sahn M, Leupold W. Double-blind placebo-controlled study of sublingual immunotherapy with house dust mite extract (*D. pt.*) in children. Pediatr Allergy Immunol 1997; 8:21–27.

38. Silvestri M, Spallarossa D, Battistini E, et al. Changes in inflammatory and clinical parameters and in bronchial hyperreactivity asthmatic children sensitized to house dust mites following sublingual immunotherapy. J Investig Allergol Clin Immunol 2002; 12:52–59.

39. Tari MG, Mancino M, Madonna F, Buzzoni L, Parmiani S. Immunologic evaluation of 24 month course of sublingual immunotherapy. Allergol Immunopathol 1994; 22:209–216.

40. Vourdas D, Syrigou E, Potamianou P, et al. Double-blind, placebo-controlled evaluation of sublingual immunotherapy with standardized olive pollen extract in pediatric patients with allergic rhinoconjunctivitis and mild asthma due to olive pollen sensitization. Allergy 1998; 53:662–672.

41. Caffarelli C, Sensi LG, Marcucci F, Cavagni G. Preseasonal local allergoid immunotherapy to grass pollen in children: A double-blind, placebo-controlled, randomized trial. Allergy 2000; 55:1142–1147.

42. Yuksel H, Tanac R, Gousseinov A, Demir E. Sublingual immunotherapy and influence on urinary leukotrienes in seasonal pediatric allergy. J Investig Allergol Clin Immunol 1999; 9:305–313.

43. Patriarca G, Nucera E, Pollastrini E, et al. Sublingual desensitization: A new approach to latex allergy problem. Anesth Analg 2002; 95:956–960.

44. Marcucci F, Sensi LG, Caffarelli C, et al. Low-dose local nasal immunotherapy in children with perennial allergic rhinitis due to *Dermatophagoides*. Allergy 2002; 57:23–28.

45. Patriarca G, Buonomo A, Roncallo C, et al. Oral desensitisation in cow milk allergy: Immunological findings. Int J Immunopathol Pharmacol 2002; 15:53–58.

46. Nettis E, Giordano D, Pannofino A, Ferrannini A, Tursi A. Safety of inhalant allergen immunotherapy with mass units–standardized extracts. Clin Exp Allergy 2002; 32:1745–1749.

47. Cantani AD, Gagliesi D. Specific immunotherapy (SIT) in children. Allergy 1996; 51:365–366.

48. Kuehr J, Brauburger J, Zielen S, et al. Efficacy of combination treatment with anti-IgE plus specific immunotherapy in polysensitized children and adolescents with seasonal allergic rhinitis. J Allergy Clin Immunol 2002; 109:274–280.

49. Kopp MV, Brauburger J, Riedinger F, et al. The effect of anti-IgE treatment on in vitro leukotriene release in children with seasonal allergic rhinitis. J Allergy Clin Immunol 2002; 110:728–735.

50. Bousquet J, Lockey R, Malling HJ. Allergen immunotherapy: Therapeutic vaccines for aller-gic diseases. A WHO position paper. J Allergy Clin Immunol 1998; 102:558–562.

51. Jacobsen L, Nuchel Petersen B, Wihl JA, Lowenstein H, Ipsen H. Immunotherapy with partially purified and standardized tree pollen extracts: IV. Results from long-term (6-year) follow-up. Allergy 1997; 52:914–920.

52. Jean R, Rufin P, Pfister A, et al. Diagnostic value of nasal provocation challenge with aller-gens in children. Allergy 1998; 53:990–994.

53. Portnoy JM, Moffitt JE, Golden DB, et al. Stinging insect hypersensitivity: A practice param-eter. J Allergy Clin Immunol 1999; 103:963–980.

54. Sturm G, Kranke B, Rudolph C, Aberer W. Rush Hymenoptera venom immunotherapy: A safe and practical protocol for high-risk patients. J Allergy Clin Immunol 2002; 110:928–933.

55. Birnbaum J, Ramadour M, Magnan A, Vervloet D. Hymenoptera ultra-rush venom immunotherapy (210 min): A safety study and risk factors. Clin Exp Allergy 2003; 33:58–64.

56. Tankersley MS, Walker RL, Butler WK, Hagan LL, Napoli DC, Freeman TM. Safety and effi-cacy of an imported fire ant rush immunotherapy protocol with and without prophylactic treat-ment. J Allergy Clin Immunol 2002; 109:556–562.

57. Tabar AI, Lizaso MT, Garcia BE, Echechipia S, Olaguibel JM, Rodriguez A. Tolerance of immunotherapy with a standardized extract of *Alternaria tenuis* in patients with rhinitis and bronchial asthma. J Investig Allergol Clin Immunol 2000; 10:327–333.

58. Mellerup MT, Hahn GW, Poulsen LK, Malling H. Safety of allergen-specific immunotherapy: Relation between dosage regimen, allergen extract, disease and systemic side-effects during induction treatment. Clin Exp Allergy 2000; 30:1423–1429.

59. Ewbank PA, Murray J, Sanders K, Curran-Everett D, Dreskin S, Nelson HS. A double-blind, placebo-controlled immunotherapy dose-response study with standardized cat extract. J Allergy Clin Immunol 2003; 111:155–161.

60. Canonica GW, Passalacqua G. Noninjection routes for immunotherapy. J Allergy Clin Immunol 2003; 111:437–448.

32

Drug Allergy: Desensitization and Treatment of Reactions to Antibiotics and Aspirin

ROLAND SOLENSKY

The Corvallis Clinic, Corvallis, Oregon, U.S.A.

I. INTRODUCTION

Adverse drug reactions (ADRs) commonly encountered in clinical medicine today are broadly categorized into predictable and unpredictable reactions (Table 1) (1). Predictable reactions are generally dose dependent, are related to the known pharmacological actions of the drug, and occur in otherwise normal individuals. Unpredictable reactions are usually dose independent, are not related to the known pharmacological actions of the drug, and occur only in susceptible individuals.

Allergic drug reactions, constituting 6–10% of all ADRs (2), are also known as hypersensitivity reactions and are distinguished from other unpredictable reactions by being mediated by an immunological mechanism. Allergic drug reactions can be classified according to the Gell and Coombs hypersensitivity reaction scheme (Table 2). Treatment with penicillin has been associated with each of the four types of hypersensitivity

Table 1 Classification of Adverse Drug Reactions

Predictable reactions	Examples
Overdosage	Acetaminophen: hepatic necrosis
Side effect	Albuterol: tremor
Secondary effect	Clindamycin: *C. difficile* pseudomembranous colitis
Drug–drug interaction	Terfenadine/erythromycin: cardiac arrhythmia

Unpredictable reactions	Examples
Intolerance	Aspirin: tinnitus (at usual doses)
Idiosyncratic	Dapsone: hemolytic anemia in G6PD-deficient patient
Allergic	Penicillin: anaphylaxis
Pseudoallergic	Radiologic contrast media: anaphylactoid reaction

Table 2 Gell and Coombs Classification of Allergic Drug Reactions

Reaction type	Mechanism
Type I	Drug-specific IgE leading to mast cell/basophil activation
Type II	Antibody-mediated (IgG, IgM) cytotoxic reaction against cell surface
Type III	Immune complex deposition reaction with activation of complement
Type IV	Drug-specific T lymphocyte–mediated reaction

reactions: anaphylaxis (type I), hemolytic anemia (type II), serum sickness–like reaction (type III), and contact dermatitis when applied topically (type IV). It is not possible to classify all allergic drug reactions because for some the mechanism responsible for elicitation is not known, or the mechanism is known but does not fall into an existing classification (3). Examples of such reactions include Stevens-Johnson syndrome, toxic epidermal necrolysis, interstitial nephritis, hypersensitivity syndrome, fixed drug eruptions, drug fever, immune-mediated hematological disorders, and hepatitis. Patients who have experienced these types of reactions are not candidates for desensitization.

Many patients classified as drug allergic, when properly evaluated are found not to be truly allergic and can tolerate the implicated medication. For example, "penicillin allergy" is reported by up to 10% of the population, yet 80–90% of these patients can be treated safely with penicillins and other β-lactam antibiotics (4,5). Many of these individuals were likely mislabeled as allergic during or soon after their reactions, since patients and physicians commonly refer to all ADRs as allergic. Alternatively, some patients who experienced truly allergic drug reactions lose their sensitivity over time. About 80% of patients with type I allergic reactions to penicillin lose drug-specific IgE antibodies during the 10 years following their reaction (6). Nevertheless, a proportion of patients who undergo a thorough evaluation by allergists/immunologists are proven or suspected to be drug allergic. This chapter focuses on the treatment of these patients when administration of the sensitizing drug, or a cross-reacting drug, is required. The chapter is concerned with commonly encountered clinical situations, including rapid desensitization of patients with IgE-mediated sensitization to antibiotics, treatment of penicillin-allergic patients with other β-lactam antibiotics, graded drug challenges, sulfonamide desensitization of HIV-positive patients, and aspirin desensitization of patients with respiratory-related (aspirin triad) aspirin sensitivity. Because of space limitations, it is impractical to include information on all drugs to which patients become allergic and may need to be desensitized. However, in such cases, the approach is similar to that outlined in this chapter.

II. RAPID ANTIBIOTIC DESENSITIZATION: PENICILLIN

A. Background

Among patients with a history of penicillin allergy, approximately 10% have penicillin-specific IgE antibodies on skin testing with major and minor penicillin antigenic determinants (6). The positive predictive value of penicillin skin testing, based on a limited number of challenges of skin test–positive patients, has been found to be between 40% and 100% (6), which is comparable to the positive predictive value of Hymenoptera or food skin testing. Patients with a positive skin test response to any of the penicillin determinants should be assumed to be at high risk of an IgE-mediated, potentially fatal anaphylactic reaction on administration of any penicillin-class antibiotic (7). Hence, these patients must avoid all penicillins, unless skin testing at a later time shows them to have lost their sensitivity.

If skin test–positive patients require treatment with penicillin, it can be administered via rapid desensitization. The aim of desensitization is to convert a penicillin-allergic individual to a state that will tolerate treatment with penicillin. Penicillin desensitization should be considered only when an alternative antibiotic cannot be used or for patients who have failed treatment with an alternative antibiotic. In such cases, the risk of not properly treating the underlying infection should outweigh the risk of desensitization. Today, the most common clinical scenario in which an absolute need for penicillin arises is treatment of syphilis during pregnancy, since alternative antibiotics such as erythromycin and clindamycin have inferior cure rates and may not cross the placenta in sufficient quantities.

B. Desensitization Procedure

1. Oral

Penicillin desensitization, accomplished by oral administration of gradually increasing doses, was first reported in 1946 (8). In the following 3 decades, additional cases of penicillin desensitization were reported, many of which involved significant allergic reactions during or immediately after the procedure (9). The current form of oral penicillin desensitization, as established by Sullivan, is a relatively safe procedure (Table 3) (9–11). Mild systemic reactions occur in about one-third of patients, but no fatal or life-threatening reactions have been reported (9–11). Only rarely are patients unable to complete the procedure due to the development of allergic symptoms. The starting dose for desensitization is determined by the amount of penicillin G the patient tolerated during skin testing. This dose generally translates to about 1/10,000 of the therapeutic dose. Doubling doses are administered every 15 minutes until the full dose is reached. Once desensitization is completed, the patient can receive the full therapeutic course of penicillin via the desired route. For example, in treating syphilis during pregnancy, intramuscular benzathine penicillin G can be given following successful oral desensitization with penicillin VK (11). To maintain the patient in a desensitized state, penicillin should be continually administered twice daily. If penicillin is discontinued for more than 48 hours, the patient is again at risk of penicillin-induced anaphylaxis, and desensitization needs to be repeated if re-administration is contemplated (10,12,13).

Table 3   Penicillin Oral Desensitization Protocol

Step[a]	Penicillin (mg/ml)	Amount (ml)	Dose given (mg)	Cumulative dose (mg)
1	0.5	0.1	0.05	0.05
2	0.5	0.2	0.1	0.15
3	0.5	0.4	0.2	0.35
4	0.5	0.8	0.4	0.75
5	0.5	1.6	0.8	1.55
6	0.5	3.2	1.6	3.15
7	0.5	6.4	3.2	6.35
8	5	1.2	6	12.35
9	5	2.4	12	24.35
10	5	5	25	49.35
11	50	1	50	100
12	50	2	100	200
13	50	4	200	400
14	50	8	400	800

[a] Interval between doses is 15 minutes.
Observe patient for 30 minutes, then give full therapeutic dose by the desired route.
Source: From Sullivan TJ. Drug allergy. In: Allergy: Principles and Practice, 4th ed. (Middleton E, Reed CE, Ellis EF, Adkinson NF, Yunginger JW, eds.). St. Louis: Mosby, 1993: 1726–1746.

2. Intravenous

Rapid penicillin desensitization can also be accomplished via the intravenous route (Tables 4 and 5) (14,15). Although there is no randomized prospective trial comparing the safety of oral and intravenous penicillin desensitization, the oral route appears to be safer. Sullivan et al. hypothesized that oral desensitization is safer because it is less likely to expose patients to multivalent penicillin conjugates and polymers, which likely play an important role in IgE-mediated allergic reactions (9). Epidemiological evidence also indicates that oral administration of penicillin induces fewer allergic reactions than parental administration (16); only six deaths have been reported secondary to immediate-type allergic reactions to oral penicillin, compared with thousands following parental administration (9). Oral desensitization is also preferred because of its ease of administration and cost savings; at a single medical center, the oral regimen was approximately half as expensive as the intravenous regimen (14).

Acute penicillin desensitization should be performed only by physicians familiar with the procedure, with intravenous access, and with preparedness to treat potential anaphylaxis. Patients should be continuously observed for the appearance of IgE-mediated allergic symptoms or signs, with regular monitoring of vital signs and peak inspiratory flow values. Initially, patients undergoing penicillin desensitization were admitted to an intensive care unit. However, experience has shown the procedure to be relatively safe, when properly performed, in a general ward or in an outpatient setting. Patients with asthma or other pulmonary disorders should be optimally controlled prior to undergoing the procedure. Treatment with β-adrenergic-blocking medications should be discontinued prior to desensitization. Mild allergic reactions should be treated, and if they do not progress, the dose of penicillin can be advanced. Desensitization (to IgE-mediated reactions) does not prevent non–IgE-mediated allergic reactions, as evidenced by reports of

Table 4 Penicillin Intravenous Desensitization Protocol with Drug Added by Piggyback Infusion

Step[a]	Penicillin (mg/ml)	Amount (ml)	Dose given (mg)	Cumulative dose (mg)
1	0.1	0.1	0.01	0.01
2	0.1	0.2	0.02	0.03
3	0.1	0.4	0.04	0.07
4	0.1	0.8	0.08	0.15
5	0.1	1.6	0.16	0.31
6	1	0.32	0.32	0.63
7	1	0.64	0.64	1.27
8	1	1.2	1.2	2.47
9	10	0.24	2.4	4.87
10	10	0.48	4.8	10
11	10	1	10	20
12	10	2	20	40
13	100	0.4	40	80
14	100	0.8	80	160
15	100	1.6	160	320
16	1000	0.32	320	640
17	1000	0.64	640	1280

[a] Interval between doses is 15 minutes.
Observe patient for 30 minutes, then give full therapeutic dose by the desired route.
Source: From Sullivan TJ. Drug allergy. In: Allergy: Principles and Practice. 4th ed. (Middleton E, Reed CE, Ellis EF, Adkinson NF, Yunginger JW, eds.). St. Louis: Mosby, 1993: 1726–1746.

serum sickness–like reactions and hemolytic anemia in patients who were successfully desensitized (15,17).

C. Mechanism

In simplest terms, rapid desensitization "fools" the immune system into accepting a medication to which specific IgE antibodies are present. It is clear that penicillin desensitization somehow renders mast cells unresponsive to the relevant allergic determinants, but the exact immunological mechanism remains elusive. One possible explanation is that cross-linking of penicillin-specific IgE on the surface of mast cells occurs in gradual fashion, thereby keeping the intracellular signal (which would otherwise result in degranulation) below a clinical threshold. Another theory is that univalent penicillin-carrier protein molecules prevent cross-linking of surface IgE and hence the transmission of an intracellular signal.

Although the precise mechanism underlying acute desensitization is not known, the process appears to be antigen specific. A number of investigators have demonstrated that skin test responses to penicillin determinants diminish or become negative in a majority of patients following penicillin desensitization (10,13,17). Sullivan also showed that skin test responses to aeroallergens, histamine, and compound 48/80 (a chemical inducer of mast cell degranulation) were unchanged after penicillin desensitization (17). These findings indicate that mast cells do not become unresponsive to all IgE signals, and that desensitization does not result in a depletion of mast cell mediators or tachyphylaxis to the effects of these mediators.

Table 5　Penicillin Intravenous Desensitization Protocol Using a Continuous Infusion Pump

Step[a]	Penicillin (mg/ml)	Flow rate (ml/h)	Dose given (mg)	Cumulative dose (mg)
1	0.001	4	0.001	0.001
2	0.001	8	0.002	0.003
3	0.001	16	0.004	0.007
4	0.001	32	0.008	0.015
5	0.001	60	0.015	0.03
6	0.001	120	0.03	0.06
7	0.001	240	0.06	0.12
8	0.1	5	0.125	0.245
9	0.1	10	0.25	0.495
10	0.1	20	0.5	1
11	0.1	40	1	2
12	0.1	80	2	4
13	0.1	160	4	8
14	10	3	7.5	15
15	10	6	15	30
16	10	12	30	60
17	10	25	62.5	123
18	10	50	125	250
19	10	100	250	500
20	10	200	500	1000

[a] Interval between doses is 15 minutes.
Observe patient for 30 minutes, then give full therapeutic dose by the desired route.

III.　RAPID ANTIBIOTIC DESENSITIZATION: NON-PENICILLINS

The principles learned from rapid oral or intravenous penicillin desensitization can be applied to any antibiotic to which a patient has an IgE-mediated allergy. In the last 2 decades, a number of investigators have successfully desensitized patients with IgE-mediated allergies to cephalosporins, monobactams, aminoglycosides, sulfonamides, fluoroquinolones, macrolides, and vancomycin (18–22). The desensitization protocol usually parallels penicillin desensitization, with progressively increasing doses of the drug administered every 15 minutes. For example, Lantner administered doubling doses of oral ciprofloxacin every 15 minutes starting at 0.05 mg (1/10,000 of the therapeutic dose) until the full 500 mg dose was reached (22). In some intravenous desensitization protocols, the antibiotic was continuously infused, with a gradual increase in the infusion rate, instead of being given via bolus administration. While there are some differences among the desensitization protocols, these case reports demonstrate that gradually increasing doses of an antibiotic can be given over several hours to individuals with an IgE-mediated allergy to the antibiotic using a wide variety of antimicrobial agents.

As with penicillin, desensitization with other antibiotics should be performed only in a medical setting, with intravenous access and readiness to treat severe allergic reactions. All other practical aspects related to carrying out desensitization that were discussed for penicillin apply to the procedure with other antibiotics. Following desensitization, it is necessary to administer the drug continuously to maintain the desensitized state.

The immunological mechanism responsible for rapid desensitization is presumably identical for penicillin and non-penicillin antibiotics. There are limited data demonstrating a decreased responsiveness of mast cells to the antibiotic following desensitization. For example, both Anne et al. and Lin demonstrated a loss of skin test reactivity to vancomycin following successful desensitization (23,24). Although these investigators did not evaluate the ability of mast cells to react to other allergens, it is likely that desensitization with any antibiotic is antigen specific and does not diminish other hypersensitivities.

The indication for desensitization with other antibiotics is the same as described for penicillin. It should be considered for patients allergic to the medication only as a last resort and where an alternative non–cross-reacting antibiotic cannot be used instead. There are no valid diagnostic tests for drug-specific IgE antibodies directed against non-penicillin antibiotics because of a lack of understanding of the relevant allergenic determinants produced by metabolism or degradation of these medications. As a result, it is more difficult for the clinician to determine the allergy status of patients who present with histories of immediate-type reactions to most antibiotics.

Skin testing with concentrations of antibiotics that are nonirritating in control subjects yields some useful information, since a positive response strongly suggests the presence of drug-specific IgE antibodies. Table 6 lists nonirritating concentrations of commonly used antibiotics, as determined by intradermal skin testing of 25 nonallergic individuals. Hence, patients who test positive to a nonirritating concentration of the antibiotic should undergo desensitization if the clinical condition necessitates its use. The amount of drug tolerated during skin testing can serve as the starting dose for desensitization. Since the negative predictive value of testing with nonirritating concentrations is not perfect, administration of the selected antibiotic to skin test–negative patients must be done cautiously. Depending on the severity and time elapsed since the previous reaction,

Table 6 Nonirritating Intradermal Skin Test Concentrations of Selected Intravenous Antibiotics

Antibiotic	Full-strength concentration (mg/ml)	Nonirritating concentration (dilution from full-strength)
Cefotaxime	100	10-fold
Cefuroxime	100	10-fold
Cefazolin	330	10-fold
Ceftazidime	100	10-fold
Ceftriaxone	100	10-fold
Tobramycin	40	10-fold
Ticarcillin	200	10-fold
Clindamycin	150	10-fold
Trimethoprim-sulfa	80 (sulfa component)	100-fold
Gentamycin	40	100-fold
Aztreonam	50	1000-fold
Levofloxacin	25	1000-fold
Erythromycin	50	1000-fold
Nafcillin	250	10,000-fold
Vancomycin	50	10,000-fold
Azithromycin	100	10,000-fold
Ciprofloxacin	10	10,000,000-fold

Source: Data from Empedrad RB, Earl HS, Gruchalla RS. Determination of non-irritating concentrations of commonly used antimicrobial drugs (abstract). J Allergy Clin. Immunol 2000; 105:S272.

the antibiotic should be reintroduced either via desensitization or graded challenge (which is discussed in more detail later in this chapter). For example, if a patient had developed a pruritic eruption with no other symptoms after the first dose of a sulfonamide 15 years ago and now requires treatment with a sulfonamide, a graded challenge should be performed; if the previous reaction consisted of severe anaphylaxis 2 years ago, acute desensitization should be performed. However, when in doubt about the severity or the type of a reaction, acute desensitization should be carried out.

IV. TREATMENT OF PENICILLIN-ALLERGIC PATIENTS WITH OTHER β-LACTAM ANTIBIOTICS

A. Background

Administration of non-penicillin β-lactams to patients with a history of penicillin allergy warrants further comment because it is frequently encountered in clinical practice. Ideally, penicillin skin testing should be used to guide the approach to these patients. Patients who test negative to penicillin determinants can safely receive all β-lactam antibiotics, and, fortunately, this group includes about 90% of all individuals who present with a history of "penicillin allergy" (6). Penicillin skin test–positive patients, on the other hand, are more difficult to manage since the understanding of the degree of allergic cross-reactivity between penicillin and other β-lactams is incomplete. The following discussion focuses on the treatment of penicillin-allergic patients to whom it is necessary to administer cephalosporins, monobactams, or carbapenems (Fig. 1).

B. Cephalosporins

When cephalosporins were introduced into clinical use in the 1960s, they were found to have in vitro cross-reactivity with penicillin (25), and there were reports of patients with histories of penicillin allergy experiencing anaphylactic reactions to first-generation cephalosporins (26,27). Some retrospective surveys of cephalosporin reaction rates have found them to be higher in patients with a history of penicillin allergy (28,29), whereas

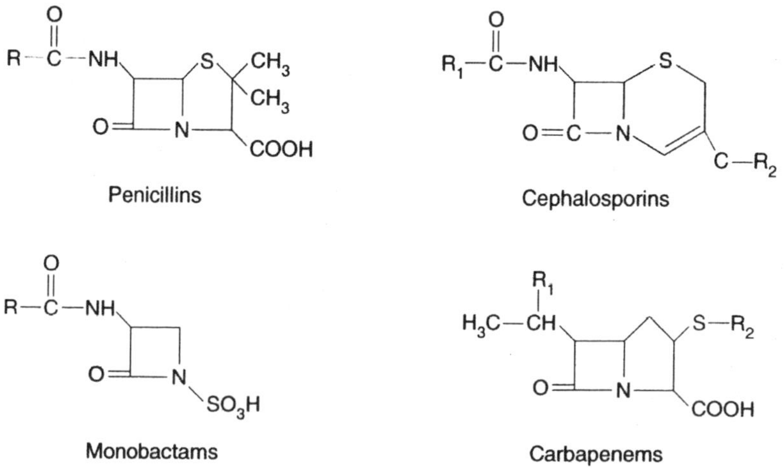

Figure 1   Structures of the major classes of β-lactam antibiotics.

others have not (30,31). The most convincing evidence for a lack of extensive allergic cross-reactivity between penicillin and cephalosporins comes from studies in which patients with positive penicillin skin tests received cephalosporins. A review of the literature revealed that only about 4% of penicillin skin test–positive patients experienced allergic reactions when challenged with cephalosporins (6). Moreover, in nearly all of the cases, the cephalosporin responsible for the reaction shared a similar R-group side chain with benzylpenicillin, suggesting that the immune response may have been directed at the side chain rather than the core β-lactam portion of the molecule. "Disease Management of Drug Hypersensitivity: A Practice Parameter" suggests three options for penicillin skin test–positive patients who are to receive cephalosporins: administration of an alternative non–β-lactam antibiotic, administration of the cephalosporin via graded challenge, or desensitization with the cephalosporin (7). While cephalosporin desensitization is the more conservative approach, based on the data discussed earlier, administration of the medication via graded challenge is appropriate for most patients who require treatment with cephalosporins.

C. Monobactams

Aztreonam is the representative monobactam antibiotic, and its potential immunologic cross-reactivity with penicillin has been studied extensively. There is no in vitro evidence of cross-reactivity between these two β-lactam classes (32). Many penicillin skin test–positive patients have been challenged with aztreonam, and none has experienced allergic reactions (33,34). Hence, administration of monobactams to patients with a history of penicillin allergy is safe and requires no special precautions or prior penicillin skin testing.

D. Carbapenems

Carbapenems appear to cross-react with penicillin, based on limited data. Saxon et al. skin-tested 40 patients with a history of penicillin allergy with penicillin determinants and analogous specially prepared imipenem determinants, that were previously found to be nonirritating in control subjects (35). Twenty of the 40 patients reacted positively to penicillin, and 10 of these also reacted to imipenem determinants. The other 20 patients were penicillin skin test negative and none of them reacted to imipenem reagents. No patients were challenged with imipenem to confirm the suspected cross-reactivity. McConnell et al. retrospectively reviewed the records of 63 patients with histories of penicillin allergy who received imipinem during hospitalization (36). Only 4 of the patients (6%) developed mild, possibly allergic reactions (mostly cutaneous eruptions), but none of the patients underwent penicillin skin testing to confirm whether they were in fact allergic at the time they received imipenem. Pending further research into cross-reactivity between penicillins and carbapenems, patients who demonstrate penicillin-specific IgE antibodies should receive carbapenems only via acute desensitization or possibly cautious graded challenge.

V. GRADED CHALLENGE

Graded challenge (incremental test dosing) is a method of administering a medication to patients who are most likely not allergic to it. This is in contrast to rapid desensitization, where the patient is known or is assumed to be allergic. Graded challenge also differs from desensitization in that there is no attempt to modify the immunological response to the medication. The intention of a graded challenge is to administer a medication in a manner not likely to cause a severe reaction. By giving a medication in frequent incremental doses, any allergic reaction provoked should be minor and easily treatable. Graded challenge should be performed only when another medication cannot be substituted.

A graded challenge is used when available diagnostic testing has inadequate negative predictive value to rule out an allergy to a given medication. For instance, if a practitioner does not have access to all penicillin minor antigenic determinants and performs skin testing only with Pre-Pen and penicillin G, penicillin should be administered via graded test dosing because some allergic patients may have been missed (7). Cephalosporins (and possibly carbapenems) may be given to penicillin skin test–positive patients by graded challenge, since they have a low probability of inducing a reaction (7). Patients who have reacted to a non–β-lactam antibiotic and require treatment with the same or a similar antibiotic may also be treated by a graded challenge. One example is a patient who reports a distant previous immediate-type reaction to ciprofloxacin and now needs a fluoroquinolone. If skin testing with a nonirritating concentration of another fluoroquinolone is negative, it only gives the physician some assurance that there is no IgE-mediated allergy. Furthermore, the extent of allergic cross-reactivity within this antibiotic family is unknown and, in such a case, it would be appropriate to perform a graded challenge with another fluoroquinolone, such as levofloxacin.

Most graded challenges can be carried out in an outpatient setting without intravenous access but with full preparedness to treat severe allergic reactions. The starting dose should be sufficiently small to avoid causing a serious reaction—typically 1/100 of the treatment dose, or lower if the previous reaction was severe. Next, relatively large incremental increases (usually 5- to 10-fold) are administered until the therapeutic dose is reached. The pace of the challenge and degree of caution exercised depends on the likelihood that the patient may react during the procedure. This is determined by the severity of the previous reaction, the length of time elapsed since the reaction, and the probability that the present medication cross-reacts with the previous reactive drug (if the two medications are different). Additional factors include the physician's experience and comfort level with graded challenges and the clinical stability of the patient. The shortest graded challenge involves only two steps, whereas more cautious procedures can include 10 or more doses. For example, the drug allergy "Practice Parameter" recommends that patients who test negative to Pre-Pen and penicillin G (without availability of other minor determinants) initially receive a 1/100 test dose, followed by the full therapeutic dose (assuming no reaction occurs during a brief observation period) (7). Table 7 shows a typical several-step graded challenge with levofloxacin in the hypothetical patient described in the previous paragraph who previously experienced a reaction to ciprofloxacin.

For immediate-type allergic reactions, the doses during a graded challenge may be given at 30-minute intervals. Before each dose, the patient should be examined and questioned for any signs and symptoms of an allergic reaction. If an allergic reaction occurs, the procedure should be abandoned and the patient's reaction treated accordingly. If at a later point re-administration of the medication is required, it should be administered only via desensitization. For delayed, usually dermatological, allergic reactions the doses may be spaced out to a few hours or as much as a full day. In this case, unless the patient is hospitalized, he or she self-administers the doses outside a medical facility and should be instructed to contact the allergist with regular progress reports. Graded challenges should not be performed with drugs known to have caused Stevens-Johnson syndrome, toxic epidermal necrolysis, severe exfoliative dermatitis, hypersensitivity syndrome, hepatitis, or immune-mediated hematologic disorders.

Table 7   Example of Graded Challenge[a] with Oral Levofloxacin

Step[b]	Levofloxacin (mg/ml)	Amount (ml)	Dose (mg)
1	5	0.2	1
2	5	1	5
3	50	0.5	25
4	50	2	100
5	N/A	1 tablet	500

[a] Patient previously experienced an immediate-type reaction to ciprofloxacin and now needs another fluoroquinolone.
[b] Interval between doses is 30 minutes. If an allergic reaction occurs, formal desensitization should be performed. Liquid oral suspension used in first four steps can be prepared by compounding pharmacists.

Patients who have experienced previous allergic drug reactions are usually anxious and fearful during the graded challenge procedure. As a result, some patients (particularly adults) may report psychosomatic-induced subjective symptoms, such as cutaneous pruritus, chest tightness, dyspnea, throat fullness, dysphagia, nausea, and abdominal pain. When these symptomatic individuals have no objective signs of an allergic reaction, the practitioner may need to use his or her "art of medicine" skills to help guide the patient through the procedure. In such situations, utilization of placebos during a graded challenge may be useful.

VI. SULFONAMIDE DESENSITIZATION OF HIV-POSITIVE PATIENTS

A. Background

Sulfonamides have been associated with a variety of allergic reactions. These include anaphylaxis, vasculitis, serum sickness–like reactions, interstitial nephritis, hepatitis, pneumonitis, hypersensitivity syndrome, drug fever, immune-mediated hematologic disorders, and various cutaneous eruptions (37). Skin rashes are by far the most common allergic reactions to sulfonamides, occurring in up to 5% of treated patients (37). They range from benign and self-limited maculopapular and morbilliform rashes to severe and potentially life-threatening exfoliative dermatoses such as Stevens-Johnson syndrome and toxic epidermal necrolysis. Patients infected with human immunodeficiency virus (HIV) appear to be at much increased risk of cutaneous reactions with sulfonamides, as well as many other, unrelated drugs (38). For example, while the incidence of skin rashes to trimethoprim/sulfamethoxazole (TMP/SMX) in normal individuals is 3.3% (39), reaction rates of 40–80% have been reported in patients with HIV (38). The typical reaction to TMP/SMX in HIV-positive patients consists of a generalized maculopapular eruption that occurs during the second week of treatment and is usually accompanied by pruritus and fever (37).

TMP/SMX is a recommended first-line antibacterial for a number of HIV-associated infectious diseases. Most important, it is the drug of choice for both prophylaxis and treatment of *Pneumocystis carinii* pneumonia (PCP) as well as other potentially life-threatening opportunistic infections (40). Hence, it is not uncommon for clinicians to be confronted with patients with HIV who have previously reacted to TMP/SMX and now require treatment with the antimicrobial. As a result, investigators have devised protocols to safely administer TMP/SMX to HIV-positive patients who are allergic to the medication.

B. Desensitization Procedure

Although TMP/SMX desensitization is commonly used to describe procedures of incremental TMP/SMX administration, the term "desensitization" is used loosely since drug-specific IgE antibodies are not implicated in these reactions. "Graded challenge" has also been used to describe the procedures, but this term is also imprecise, since it ideally refers to situations where a patient has a low likelihood of truly being allergic to the medication (as discussed earlier). The lack of an appropriate term for TMP/SMX incremental dose regimens in HIV-positive patients has to do with our lack of understanding of the pathogenesis of these reactions, as well as the responsible mechanisms that allow re-administration of the medication. For the purpose of this discussion, however, the procedure will be referred to as desensitization.

Over the last 20 years, dozens of reports of TMP/SMX desensitization in HIV-positive patients have appeared in the literature (11 are summarized in Table 8). Some of these publications consist of single patient case reports, whereas others are series of as many as 48 patients. The study designs vary greatly in terms of the starting dose, the incremental increase between doses, the time interval between doses, and total duration of the desensitization. Furthermore, some researchers pretreated patients with antihistamines or corticosteroids, chose to treat through minor reactions, or added anti-allergy medications upon the appearance of a reaction. No attempt has been made to standardize the procedures, and there are no comparative studies of different protocols.

In critically analyzing these protocols, another confounding factor is the lack of a diagnostic test for TMP/SMX hypersensitivity to prove that patients undergoing desensitization are truly allergic. It is conceivable that some patients who experienced previous reactions to TMX/SMX had lost their sensitivity by the time they underwent desensitization. In fact, some data indicate that patients with more recent reaction histories are more likely to fail desensitization than patients with distant histories (52). In a multicenter, randomized trial, Bonfanti et al. compared the effectiveness of desensitization (via a 2-day, 40-dose protocol) and re-challenge (single dose) in HIV-positive patients with documented reactions to TMP/SMX who required PCP prophylaxis (50). They found

Table 8 Representative Summary of 11 Published TMP/SMX Desensitization Protocols in HIV Patients (1994–2000)

Study	No. of patients	Initial dose	No. of steps	Total duration	Success rate (%)
Absar (41)	27	2 mg	10	10 days	85
Gluckstein (42)	21	0.02 mg	5	5 hours	71
Nguyen[a] (43)	45	10 ng	40	36 hours	60
Belchi-Hernandez (44)	34	1 mg	21	11 days	79
Kalanadhabhatta (45)	13	20 ng	37	27 hours	100
Caumes (46)	48	4 mg	8	3 days	77
Rich (47)	22	20 ng	24	8 days	86
Ryan (48)	14	2 mg	33	33 days	69
Demoly (49)	44	1 μg	12	6 hours	95
Bonfanti (50)	34	10 ng	40	36 hours	79
Yoshizawa (51)	17	2 mg	10	5 days	88

[a] Indicates identical protocols; dose is expressed as sulfamethoxazole portion of TMP/SMX.

success rates of 79% and 72% in the desensitization and re-challenge groups, respectively, and the difference was not statistically significant. These results place into question the validity of previously reported desensitization success rates in studies that did not include a "control" group of patients who were simply re-challenged with TMP/SMX. In uncontrolled studies, the desensitization success rates ranged from 60% to 100% (Table 8). The widely ranging efficacy values are probably due to different protocols and endpoints that defined success. They are also likely due to inclusion of varying numbers of patients who were not truly TMP/SMX sensitive at the time of desensitization, particularly since most studies consisted of small groups of patients and therefore would be susceptible to such a variable.

A representative sample of published TMP/SMX desensitization protocols is shown in Table 8. The duration of the procedures ranged from several hours to 33 days. Most investigators used the oral route to administer the antibiotic. The starting dose and intervals between doses differed greatly among the studies. Desensitizations were carried out in inpatient or outpatient settings, or completed by patients at home after discharge. In virtually all studies, patients with histories of severe allergic reactions to TMP/SMX, such as anaphylaxis, Stevens-Johnson syndrome, and toxic epidermal necrolysis, were not included. In general, the desensitizations were described as being safe and reactions during or after the procedure were minor and easily treated. However, despite the exclusion of high-risk patients, there were rare occurrences of anaphylaxis, toxic epidermal necrolysis, and hypotension with myocardial infarction.

Selection of HIV-positive patients for TMP/SMX desensitization should be limited to those with a history of the typical delayed maculopapular eruption. Although there is a single case report of successful desensitization in two patients who had previously developed TMP/SMX-induced Stevens-Johnson syndrome (53), most experts recommend that patients with histories of exfoliative dermatitis to TMP/SMX should not receive sulfonamide antibiotics under any circumstance (7). Patients with a suspected history of an IgE-mediated reaction to TMP/SMX should undergo rapid desensitization using a protocol based on penicillin desensitization (as discussed earlier in this chapter), rather than one of the protocols shown in Table 8.

For the clinician faced with an HIV-positive patient with the usual TMP/SMX hypersensitivity, who requires treatment with the sulfonamide, it is impossible to recommend any single published desensitization protocol. There are no comparative trials, and even indirect comparison is difficult due to the large number of variables among the studies. The success rates of many dissimilar protocols are comparable, and there are no apparent differences in safety. It is also not feasible to "tailor" a particular protocol to a specific type of patient, since predictors of success and failure are discordant. Some investigators found low CD4+ counts to be predictive of successful desensitization (46,54), whereas others found no such correlation (43,50). In summary, available data do not permit selection of any single desensitization protocol as most effective, and there is great need for comparative studies of different protocols. Pending further research, it appears that a number of different protocols may be employed with similar hopes for success.

C. Mechanism

Since the pathogenesis of TMP/SMX-induced delayed reactions in HIV-positive patients has not been elucidated, understanding of the mechanism of desensitization is also limited. The vast majority of adverse reactions to TMP/SMX are directed against

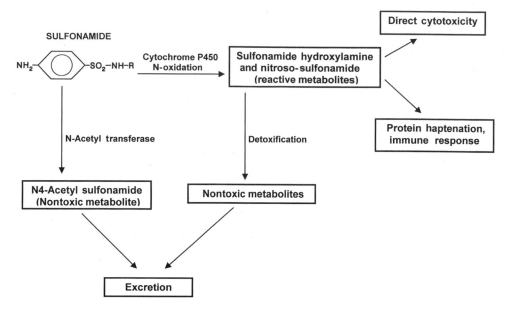

Figure 2 Sulfonamide metabolic pathways. *N*-acetylation yields nontoxic metabolites that are excreted. N-oxidation forms reactive intermediates that can cause direct cytotoxicity or haptenate proteins and lead to an immunological response. Glutathione reduces reactive metabolites to nontoxic products that are excreted.

sulfamethoxazole, although some patients may react to the trimethoprim portion (37). Sulfonamide antimicrobials are metabolized in the liver by *N*-acetylation, yielding nontoxic metabolites that are excreted (Fig. 2). Alternatively, sulfonamides are oxidized and catalyzed by cytochrome P_{450} enzymes to form reactive hydroxylamines, which can be further auto-oxidized to reactive nitroso species. Reactive metabolites can cause direct cytotoxicity or alternatively act as haptens, bind to host proteins, and induce an immunological response. Reactive metabolites can also form in monocytes and neutrophils via the myoloperoxidase pathway. Reactive intermediates are normally detoxified by glutathione or other scavengers, via a reduction reaction.

Although the extent to which immune effects and direct toxicity influence sulfonamide adverse reactions is unknown, there is evidence to suggest that both mechanisms contribute to a variety of sulfonamide-induced reactions (37,52). Regardless of the final pathway of damage, the aromatic amine (i.e., arylamine) group at the N4 position is considered critical for the development of most sulfonamide adverse reactions. Among sulfonamide compounds, only antibacterial sulfonamides contain an arylamine group at the N4 position. Other sulfonamides, such as diuretics, hypoglycemic agents, celecoxib, and sumatriptan, lack an N4 arylamine group and therefore would not be expected to cross-react with sulfonamide antibiotics, although clinical proof for this is limited (37,52,55,56).

There is no evidence that cutaneous eruptions in patients with HIV are caused by TMP/SMX-specific IgE or IgG antibodies (52). Rather, the delayed onset of these rashes is more suggestive of a possible T-cell–mediated mechanism. There are a number of possible explanations of the increased risk of HIV-positive patients reacting to sulfonamides. First, "slow" acetylation may cause more of the parent drug to be shunted toward the oxidative cytochrome P_{450} pathway with subsequent formation of reactive hydroxylamine and nitroso metabolites. Second, a relative deficiency of glutathione or other scavengers would have a similar effect, resulting in an excess of reactive intermediates. Third, viral or other opportunistic infections may stimulate the activity of cytochrome P_{450} enzymes and lead to an increased rate of oxidation and production of reactive metabolites. Finally, viral infections are known to stimulate production of interferon-gamma, which leads to increased expression of major histocompatibility complex (MHC) class I and class II cell surface molecules, including those on keratinocytes. This would favor the presentation of processed drug antigens on MHC molecules to drug-specific CD4+ and CD8+ T-cells, resulting in delayed skin rashes. The pathogenesis of TMP/SMX reactions in HIV-positive patients is probably multifactorial, and there are limited data to suggest that all these elements play some role in the process (3,37,38,52).

VII. ASPIRIN DESENSITIZATION OF ASPIRIN-EXACERBATED RESPIRATORY DISEASE

A. Background

Aspirin (acetylsalicylic acid, ASA) and other nonsteroidal anti-inflammatory drugs (NSAIDs) can cause a number of unpredictable adverse reactions—including urticaria/angioedema, Stevens-Johnson syndrome, toxic epidermal necrolysis, interstitial nephritis, anaphylaxis, aseptic meningitis, and acute worsening of asthma/rhinitis (57). A varied nomenclature has described respiratory reactions to ASA (aspirin triad or Samter syndrome), but this chapter uses the term "ASA-exacerbated respiratory disease" (AERD), which was proposed in a new classification system of allergic and pseudo-allergic reactions to NSAIDs (58). It is estimated that about 5–10% of adult asthmatics have AERD, whereas the prevalence increases to about one-third in adult patients with asthma and nasal polyposis (59). The presence of AERD is rare in prepubescent children. Patients with AERD exhibit cross-reactivity with all NSAIDs, but they can tolerate cyclo-oxygenase-2 enzyme (COX-2) selective inhibitors (60). There are no in vitro tests to detect ASA sensitivity, and oral challenge remains the "gold standard" diagnostic test for AERD (59).

B. Desensitization Procedure

ASA desensitization is the induction of a state of tolerance that permits patients with AERD to take ASA and other NSAIDs without experiencing adverse sequelae. The term "desensitization" is used in a broad sense, since IgE antibodies are not involved in AERD. Furthermore, whereas the goal of desensitization with penicillin and other antibiotics is to safely administer a medication without inducing an allergic reaction, ASA desensitization strives to cause a reaction following which the patient becomes refractory to the deleterious effects of the NSAID. The existence of a refractory period following an ASA respiratory reaction was first reported in a single patient by Widal, et al in 1922 (61), and it became generally recognized with descriptions by Zeiss and Lockey (62) and Stevenson et al. (63). Characterization of the refractory period in 30 patients with AERD showed that it ranged from 2 to 5 days, and ASA sensitivity returned in gradual fashion (64). Desensitization using oral ASA, as opposed to inhaled or intranasal ASA-lysine, is associated with the most experience and broadest use (57). Additionally, ASA-lysine, unlike oral ASA, is unavailable to certain allergists worldwide, including ones practicing in the United States. Hence, this discussion will focus on the oral method of ASA desensitization.

Table 9   ASA Oral Challenge/Desensitization Protocol Used at the Scripps Clinic

Time	Day 1	Day 2	Day 3
8 A.M.	Placebo	15–30 mg	150 mg
11 A.M.	Placebo	45–60 mg	325 mg

Source: From Stevenson DD. Adverse reactions to nonsteroidal anti-inflammatory drugs. Immunol Allergy Clin North Am 1998; 18:773–798.

ASA desensitization is an extension of the ASA oral challenge procedure that is used for diagnosis of AERD. The most commonly used protocol, developed by researchers at the Scripps Clinic, is shown in Table 9. For the practicing allergist, it is reasonable to exclude the placebo portion of the challenge. Additionally, the ASA dosages suggested by this protocol cannot be easily derived from commercially available 81-mg and 325-mg ASA tablets. While ASA in liquid suspension can be prepared by compounding pharmacists, this likewise may not be practical for many clinicians. Therefore, for most patients it is reasonable to modify the Scripps Clinic ASA challenge protocol to allow use of commercially available ASA tablets, as shown in Table 10. During the procedure, most patients with AERD develop a combined lower and upper respiratory reaction with a decrease in forced expiratory volume (FEV_1) and naso-ocular symptoms (59). A minority of patients exhibit purely asthmatic or purely upper respiratory reactions. Once an asthmatic reaction occurs, it should be treated with a rapid-acting inhaled bronchodilator. Other symptoms can be treated with a topical nasal decongestant and an antihistamine, depending on the type of symptoms experienced. After the patient is stabilized and the FEV_1 returns to baseline values, the identical dose of ASA that caused the reaction is re-administered, and if tolerated, progressively higher doses (according to the protocol) are given until the 650-mg dose is reached. Following a respiratory reaction, most patients enter a refractory state and are able to tolerate the remaining doses; but if another reaction occurs, it should be treated. Once the patient is again stabilized, proceed as described above.

Patients who undergo ASA desensitization should be clinically stable with baseline FEV_1 of >70% predicted and >1.5 liters (59). Some patients may require a short course of systemic corticosteroids prior to desensitization in order to achieve clinical stability. Patients should continue to take maintenance asthma medications, with the exception of cromolyn and nedocromil, which delay the onset of ASA-induced respiratory reactions and may allow patients to erroneously receive a higher dose of ASA before they manifest a reaction (57). Concomitant treatment of patients with leukotriene-modifier drugs (LTMDs) during ASA desensitization attenuates lower respiratory tract reactions in some patients, with more experiencing pure naso-ocular reactions (65). Hence, pretreatment with LTMDs appears to make ASA desensitization a safer procedure and should be

Table 10   Modified ASA Oral Challenge/Desensitization Protocol Using Doses Derived from Commercially Available 81-mg and 325-mg ASA Tablets

Time	Day 1	Day 2
8 A.M.	40 mg	162 mg
11 A.M.	81 mg	325 mg
2 P.M.	121 mg	650 mg

strongly considered for patients undergoing the procedure. ASA desensitization should be performed only by clinicians familiar with the procedure, in a controlled clinical setting, with intravenous access and readiness to treat potentially severe bronchospastic reactions.

Selection of patients for ASA desensitization falls into two categories. First, there are patients with AERD whose respiratory disease is well controlled but who require ASA or NSAIDs for other indications, such as cardiac prophylaxis or treatment of arthritis. With the introduction of newer platelet inhibitors (such as clopidogrel) and COX-2 inhibitors, which patients with AERD are able to tolerate, this indication is not encountered as frequently as in the past. Secondly, ASA desensitization should be considered for patients with AERD who have poor control of their disease despite use of appropriate medications, and for patients who require chronic treatment with systemic corticosteroids. Several long-term studies of patients maintained on chronic ASA desensitization demonstrated improved clinical courses (66–68). For upper respiratory disease, long-term ASA desensitization was associated with significant improvements in nasal symptom scores, frequency of sinusitis, need for polypectomies or sinus surgeries, sense of smell, and dose of intranasal corticosteroids (66–68). For lower respiratory disease, improved clinical outcomes included reductions in asthma symptom scores, hospitalizations, emergency room visits, and dose of inhaled corticosteroids (66–68). Importantly, ASA desensitization also resulted in a reduction in the number of bursts of oral corticosteroids and allowed patients on chronic corticosteroids to decrease their dose (66–68).

C. Mechanism

The pathogenesis of AERD is partially understood and involves aberrant arachidonic acid metabolism (Fig. 3). At baseline (prior to the addition of ASA), patients with AERD synthesize higher quantities of both COX and 5-lipoxygenase (5-LO) products, including cysteinyl leukotrienes, phospholipase A_2, and thromboxane B_2, compared with non–ASA-sensitive asthmatics (59). They also have increased respiratory tract expression of the cysteinyl leukotriene-1 receptor ($CysLT_1$) and heightened airway responsiveness to inhaled leukotriene E_4 (LTE_4) (69,70). Patients with AERD appear to be exquisitely susceptible to inhibition of COX by ASA (71). Challenge with ASA/NSAIDs leads to inhibition of COX-1 with a resultant decrease in the synthesis of prostaglandin E_2 (PGE_2) (Fig. 3). PGE_2 normally inhibits 5-LO, but with a loss of this modifying effect, arachidonic acid molecules are preferentially metabolized in the 5-LO pathway, resulting in increased production of cysteinyl leukotrienes. This theory of ASA-induced respiratory reactions is supported by the following observations during ASA challenge: an acute rise of leukotriene C_4 (LTC_4) in nasal and bronchial secretions, a decrease in PGE_2 in nasal and bronchial secretions, and an increase in urinary LTE_4. Additionally, pretreatment of patients with inhaled PGE_2 has been shown to inhibit ASA-lysine–induced bronchospasm (72).

During chronic ASA desensitization, there is continual inhibition of COX-1 and probable direct or indirect inhibition of phospholipase A_2. This leads to diminished synthesis of both prostanoids and leukotrienes. During ASA desensitization, LTC_4 in nasal secretions disappears, urinary LTE_4 decreases to baseline levels, bronchial responsiveness to LTE_4 is greatly abated, and LTB_4 synthesis in monocytes is reduced to the same level found in normal controls (59). Moreover, ASA desensitization is associated with a decrease in the number of respiratory inflammatory cells expressing the $CysLT_1$ receptor (70).

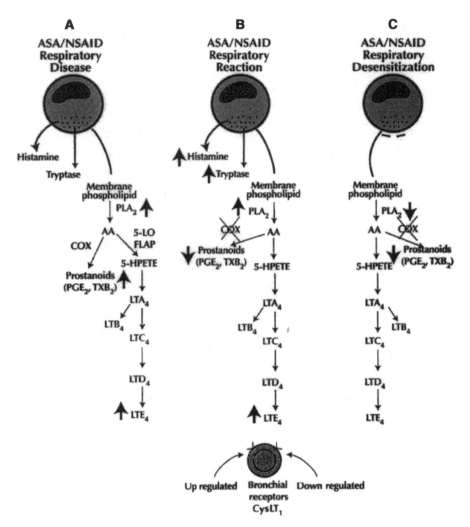

Figure 3   Pathogenesis of aspirin (ASA) respiratory disease, reaction, and desensitization. *A*: At baseline, there is excess production of prostanoids and leukotrienes. Prostaglandin E_2 (PGE_2) partially inhibits 5-lipoxygenase (5-LO). *B*: During an ASA-induced reaction, inhibition of cyclooxygenase (COX) enzymes decreases synthesis of PGE_2, which enhances the activity of 5-LO and leads to increased production of leukotrienes. Upregulated cysteinyl leukotriene-1 ($CysLT_1$) receptors augment the effects of the leukotrienes. *C*: During ASA desensitization, there is continual inhibition of COX and direct or indirect inhibition of phospholipase A_2 (PLA_2), with decreased synthesis of leukotrienes. Downregulation of $CysLT_1$ expression further diminishes the effect of leukotrienes on target organs. NSAID = nonsteroidal anti-inflammatory drug, AA = arachidonic acid, FLAP = 5-lipoxygenase activating protein, 5-HPETE = 5-hydroperoxyeicosatetrenoic acid, TXB_2 = thromboxane B_2, LTA_4–LTE_4 = leukotrienes A_4 to E4. (From Ref. 57.)

VIII. SALIENT POINTS

1. Many patients who present with a history of drug "allergy," after a thorough evaluation turn out not to be allergic and may tolerate treatment with the drug in question.

2. Patients who have penicillin-specific IgE antibodies and require treatment with the medication can receive penicillins via rapid desensitization.

3. Patients with IgE-mediated allergies to non-penicillin antibiotics can receive these antibiotics via rapid desensitization protocols patterned on penicillin desensitization.

4. Patients with confirmed penicillin allergy appear at very low risk of reacting to cephalosporins, but these antibiotics should be administered cautiously via either graded challenge or desensitization. Penicillin-allergic patients may safely receive monobactams, but the clinical cross-reactivity between penicillin and carbapenems is unknown.

5. Graded challenge is a method of cautious administration of a medication in two or more incremental steps. It is used in cases when diagnostic testing cannot sufficiently rule out an allergy and the patient is unlikely to be allergic.

6. A large proportion of HIV-positive patients experience reactions to TMP/SMX, yet this antibiotic is the drug of choice for many HIV-related infections. The majority of these individuals can safely receive TMP/SMX via one of a number of desensitization protocols.

7. Aspirin desensitization induces a state in which patients with AERD are refractory to ASA- and NSAID-induced reactions. It should be considered in patients with AERD who have poor control of their respiratory disease and in patients who require ASA or NSAIDs for other disease states.

REFERENCES

1. Rawlins MD, Thompson W. Mechanisms of adverse drug reactions. In: Textbook of Adverse Drug Reactions (Davies DM, ed.). New York: Oxford University Press, 1991: 18–45.

2. DeSchazo RD, Kemp SF. Allergic reactions to drugs and biologic agents. J Am Med Assoc 1997; 278:1895–1906.

3. Solensky R, Gruchalla RS. Non-anaphylactic drug disorders. In: Inflammatory Mechanisms in Allergic Diseases (Zweiman B, Schwartz LB, eds.). New York: Marcel Dekker, 2001: 411–433.

4. Gadde J, Spence M, Wheeler B, Adkinson NF. Clinical experience with penicillin skin testing in a large inner-city STD Clinic. J Am Med Assoc 1993; 270:2456–2463.

5. Sogn DD, Evans R, Shepherd GM, Casale TB, Condemi J, Greenberger PA, Kohler PF, Saxon A, Summers RJ, Van Arsdel PP, Massicot JG, Blackwelder WC, Levine BB. Results of the National Institute of Allergy and Infectious Diseases collaborative clinical trial to test the predictive value of skin testing with major and minor penicillin derivatives in hospitalized adults. Arch Intern Med 1992; 152:1025–1032.

6. Solensky R. Hypersensitivity reactions to beta-lactam antibiotics. Clin Rev Allergy Immunol 2003; 24:201–219.

7. Bernstein IL, Gruchalla RS, Lee RE, Nicklas RA, Dykewicz MS. Disease management of drug hypersensitivity: A practice parameter. Ann Allergy Asthma Immunol 1999; 83:665–700.

8. O'Donovan WJ, Klorfajn I. Sensitivity to penicillin: Anaphylaxis and desensitization. Lancet 1946; 2:444–446.

9. Sullivan TJ, Yecies LD, Shatz GS, Parker CW, Wedner HJ. Desensitization of patients allergic to penicillin using orally administered beta-lactam antibiotics. J Allergy Clin Immunol 1982; 69:275–282.

10. Stark BJ, Earl HS, Gross GN, Lumry WR, Goodman EL, Sullivan TJ. Acute and chronic desensitization of penicillin-allergic patients using oral penicillin. J Allergy Clin Immunol 1987; 79:523–532.

11. Wendel GD, Stark BJ, Jamison RB, Molina RD, Sullivan TJ. Penicillin allergy and desensitization in serious infections during pregnancy. N Engl J Med 1985; 312:1229–1232.

12. Naclerio RM, Mizrahi EA, Adkinson NJ. Immunologic observations during desensitization and maintenance of clinical tolerance to penicillin. J Allergy Clin Immunol 1983; 71:294–301.

13. Brown LA, Goldberg ND, Shearer WT. Long-term ticarcillin desensitization by the continuous oral administration of penicillin. J Allergy Clin Immunol 1982; 69:51–54.

14. Chisholm CA, Katz VL, McDonald TL, Bowes WA. Penicillin desensitization in the treatment of syphilis during pregnancy. Am J Perinatol 1997; 14:553–554.

15. Borish L, Tamir R, Rosenwasser LJ. Intravenous desensitization to beta-lactam antibiotics. J Allergy Clin Immunol 1987; 80:31–19.

16. Herman R, Jick H. Cutaneous reaction rates to penicillins: Oral versus parental. Cutis 1979; 24:232–234.

17. Sullivan TJ. Antigen-specific desensitization of patients allergic to penicillin. J Allergy Clin Immunol 1982; 69:500–508.

18. Wazny LD, Daghigh B. Desensitization protocols for vancomycin hypersensitivity. Ann Pharmacother 2001; 35:1458–1464.

19. Earl HS, Sullivan TJ. Acute desensitization of a patient with cystic fibrosis allergic to both beta-lactam and aminoglycoside antibiotics. J Allergy Clin Immunol 1987; 79:477–483.

20. Chandler MJ, Ong RC, Grammer LC, Sullivan TJ. Detection, characterization, and desensitization of IgE to streptomycin (abstr). J Allergy Clin Immunol 1992; 89:178.

21. Laurie S, Khan D. Successful clarithromycin desensitization in a macrolide-sensitive patient (abstr). Ann Allergy Asthma Immunol 2000; 84:116.

22. Lantner RR. Ciprofloxacin desensitization in a patient with cystic fibrosis. J Allergy Clin Immunol 1995; 96:1001–1002.

23. Anne S, Middleton E, Reisman RE. Vancomycin anaphylaxis and successful desensitization. Ann Allergy 1994; 73:402–404.

24. Lin RY. Desensitization in the management of vancomycin hypersensitivity. Arch Intern Med 1990; 150:2197–2198.

25. Abraham GN, Petz LD, Fudenberg HH. Immunohaematological cross-allergenicity between penicillin and cephalothin in humans. Clin Exp Immunol 1968; 3:343–357.

26. Scholand JF, Tennenbaum JI, Cerilli GJ. Anaphylaxis to cephalothin in a patient allergic to penicillin. J Am Med Assoc 1968; 206:130–132.

27. Kabins SA, Eisenstein B, Cohen S. Anaphylactoid reaction to an initial dose of sodium cephalothin. J Am Med Assoc 1965; 193:165–166.

28. Petz LD. Immunologic cross-reactivity between penicillins and cephalosporins: A review. J Infect Dis 1978; 137(suppl):S74–S79.

29. Dash CH. Penicillin allergy and the cephalosporins. J Antimicrob Chemother 1975; 1(suppl):107–118.

30. Daulat SB, Solensky R, Earl H, Gruchalla R. Safety of cephalosporin administration to patients with histories of penicillin allergy (abstr). J Allergy Clin Immunol 2002; 109:S268.

31. Goodman EJ, Morgan MJ, Johnson PA, Nichols BA, Denk N, Gold BB. Cephalosporins can be given to penicillin-allergic patients who do not exhibit an anaphylactic response. J Clin Anesth 2001; 13:561–564.

32. Saxon A, Swabb EA, Adkinson NF. Investigation into the immunologic cross-reactivity of aztreonam with other beta-lactam antibiotics. Am J Med 1985; 78(suppl 2A):19–26.

33. Adkinson NF. Immunogenicity and cross-allergenicity of aztreonam. Am J Med 1990; 88(suppl 3C):S3–S14.

34. Vega JM, Blanca M, Garcia JJ, Miranda A, Carmona MJ, Garcia A, Moya MC, Sanchez F, Terrados S. Tolerance to aztreonam in patients allergic to betalactam antibiotics. Allergy 1991; 46:196–202.

35. Saxon A, Adelman DC, Patel A, Hajdu R, Calandra GB. Imipenem cross-reactivity with penicillin in humans. J Allergy Clin Immunol 1988; 82:213–217.

36. McConnell SA, Penzak SR, Warmack TS, Anaissie EJ, Gubbins PO. Incidence of imipenem hypersensitivity reactions in febrile neutropenic marrow transplant patients with a history of penicillin allergy. Clin Infect Dis 2000; 31:1512–1514.

37. Cribb AE, Lee BL, Trepanier LA, Spielberg SP. Adverse reactions to sulphonamide and sulphonamide-trimethoprim antimicrobials: Clinical syndromes and pathogenesis. Adverse Drug React Toxicol Rev 1996; 15:9–50.

38. Koopmans PP, Van der Ven AJ, Vree TB, Van der Meer JW. Pathogenesis of hypersensitivity reactions to drugs in patients with HIV infection: Allergic or toxic? AIDS 1995; 9:217–222.

39. Jick H. Adverse reactions to trimethoprim-sulfamethoxazole in hospitalized patients. Rev Infect Dis 1982; 4:426–428.

40. Center for Disease Control. 1997 USPHS/IDSA guidelines for the prevention of opportunistic infections in persons infected with human immunodeficiency virus. MMWR 1997; 46:4–6.

41. Absar N, Daneshvar H, Beall G. Desensitization to trimethoprim/sulfamethoxazole in HIV-infected patients. J Allergy Clin Immunol 1994; 93:1001–1005.

42. Gluckstein D, Ruskin J. Rapid oral desensitization to trimethoprim-sulfamethoxazole (TMP-SMZ): Use in prophylaxis for *Pneumocystis carinii* pneumonia in patients with AIDS who were previously intolerant to TMP-SMZ. Clin Infect Dis 1995; 20:849–853.

43. Nguyen M, Weiss PJ, Wallace MR. Two-day oral desensitization to trimethoprim-sulfamethoxazole in HIV-infected patients. AIDS 1995; 9:573–575.

44. Belchi-Hernandez J, Espinosa-Parra FJ. Management of adverse reactions to prophylactic trimethoprim-sulfamethoxazole in patients with human immunodeficiency virus infection. Ann Allergy Asthma Immunol 1996; 76:355–358.

45. Kalanadhabhatta V, Muppidi D, Sahni H, Robles A, Kramer M. Successful oral desensitization to trimethoprim-sulfamethoxazole in acquired immune deficiency syndrome. Ann Allergy Asthma Immunol 1996; 77:394–400.

46. Caumes E, Guermonprez G, Lecomte C, Katlama C, Bricaire F. Efficacy and safety of desensitization with sulfamethoxazole and trimethoprim in 48 previously hypersensitive patients infected with human immunodeficiency virus. Arch Dermatol 1997; 133:465–469.

47. Rich JD, Sullivan T, Greineder D, Kazanjian PH. Trimethoprim/sulfamethoxazole incremental dose regimen in human immunodeficiency virus–infected persons. Ann Allergy Asthma Immunol 1997; 79:409–414.

48. Ryan C, Madalon M, Wortham DW, Graziano FM. Sulfa hypersensitivity in patients with HIV infection: Onset, treatment, critical review of the literature. Wis Med J 1998; 97:23–27.

49. Demoly P, Messaad D, Sahla H, Fabre J, Faucherre V, Andre P, Reynes J, Godard P, Bousquet J. Six-hour trimethoprim-sulfamethoxazole–graded challenge in HIV-infected patients. J Allergy Clin Immunol 1998; 102:1033–1036.

50. Bonfanti P, Pusterla L, Parazzini F, Libanore M, Cagni AE, Franzetti M, Faggion I, Landonio S, Quirino T. The effectiveness of desensitization versus rechallenge treatment in HIV-positive patients with previous hypersensitivity to TMP-SMX: A randomized multicentric study. Biomed Pharmacother 2000; 54:45–49.

51. Yoshizawa S, Yasuoka A, Kikuchi Y, Honda M, Gatanaga H, Tachikawa N, Hirabayashi Y, Oka S. A 5-day course of oral desensitization to trimethoprim/sulfamethoxazole (T/S) in patients with human immunodeficiency virus type-1 infection who were previously intolerant to T/S. Ann Allergy Asthma Immunol 2000; 85:241–244.

52. Choquet-Kastylevsky G, Vial T, Descotes J. Allergic adverse reactions to sulfonamides. Curr Allergy Asthma Rep 2002; 2:16–25.

53. Douglas R, Spelman D, Czarny D, O'Hehir RE. Successful desensitization of two patients who previously developed Stevens-Johnson syndrome while receiving trimethoprim-sulfamethoxazole. Clin Infect Dis 1997; 25:1480.

54. Carr A, Penny R, Cooper DA. Efficacy and safety of rechallenge with low-dose trimethoprim-sulphamethoxazole in previously hypersensitive HIV-infected patients. AIDS 1993; 7:65–71.

55. Patterson R, Bello AE, Lefkowith F. Immunologic tolerability profile of celecoxib. Clin Ther 1999; 21:2065–2079.

56. Knowles S, Shapiro L, Shear NH. Should celecoxib be contraindicated in patients who are allergic to sulfonamides? Drug Saf 2001; 24:239–247.

57. Namazy JA, Simon RA. Sensitivity to nonsteroidal anti-inflammatory drugs. Ann Allergy Asthma Immunol 2002; 89:542–550.

58. Stevenson DD, Sanchez-Borges M, Sczeklik A. Classification of allergic and pseudoallergic reactions to drugs that inhibit cyclooxygenase enzymes. Ann Allergy Asthma Immunol 2001; 87:177–180.

59. Stevenson DD. Adverse reactions to nonsteroidal anti-inflammatory drugs. Immunol Allergy Clin North Am 1998; 18:773–798.

60. Stevenson DD, Simon RA. Lack of cross-reactivity between rofecoxib and aspirin in aspirin-sensitive patients with asthma. J Allergy Clin Immunol 2001; 108:47–51.

61. Widal MF, Abrami P, Lermeyez J. Anaphylaxie et idiosyncrasie. Presse Med 1922; 30:189–192.

62. Zeiss CR, Lockey RF. Refractory period to aspirin in a patient with aspirin-induced asthma. J Allergy Clin Immunol 1976; 57:440–448.

63. Stevenson DD, Simon RA, Mathison DA. Aspirin-sensitive asthma: Tolerance to aspirin after positive oral aspirin challenges. J Allergy Clin Immunol 1980; 66:82–88.

64. Pleskow WW, Stevenson DD, Mathison DA, Simon RA, Schatz M, Zeiger RS. Aspirin desensitization in aspirin-sensitive asthmatic patients: Clinical manifestations and characterization of the refractory period. J Allergy Clin Immunol 1982; 69:11–19.

65. Berges-Gimeno MP, Simon RA, Stevenson DD. The effect of leukotriene-modifier drugs on aspirin-induced asthma and rhinitis reactions. Clin Exp Allergy 2002; 32:1491–1496.

66. Berges-Gimeno MP, Simon RA, Stevenson DD. Long-term treatment with aspirin desensitization in asthmatic patients with aspirin-exacerbated respiratory disease. J Allergy Clin Immunol 2003; 111:180–186.

67. Stevenson DD, Hankammer MA, Mathison DA, Christiansen SC, Simon RA. Aspirin desensitization treatment of aspirin-sensitive patients with rhinosinusitis-asthma: Long-term outcomes. J Allergy Clin Immunol 1996; 98:751–758.

68. Sweet JM, Stevenson DD, Simon RA, Mathison DA. Long-term effects of aspirin desensitization-treatment for aspirin-sensitive rhinosinusitis-asthma. J Allergy Clin Immunol 1990; 85:59–65.

69. Arm JP, O'Hickery SP, Spur BW, Lee TH. Airway responsiveness to histamine and leukotriene E4 in aspirin-induced asthma. Am Rev Respir Dis 1989; 140:148–153.

70. Sousa AR, Parikh A, Scadding G, Corrigan C, Lee TH. Leukotriene-receptor expression on nasal mucosal inflammatory cells in aspirin-sensitive rhinosinusitis. N Engl J Med 2002; 347:1493–1499.

71. Juergens UR, Christiansen SC, Stevenson DD, Zuraw BL. Arachidonic acid metabolism in monocytes of aspirin-sensitive asthmatic patients before and after oral aspirin challenge. J Allergy Clin Immunol 1992; 90:636–645.

72. Sestini P, Armetti L, Gambaro G, Pieroni MG, Refini RM, Sala A, Vaghi A, Folco GC, Bianco S, Robuschi M. Inhaled PGE2 prevents aspirin-induced bronchoconstriction and urinary LTE4 excretion in aspirin-sensitive asthma. Am J Respir Crit Care Med 1996; 153:572–575.

33

Non-Injection Routes for Immunotherapy of Allergic Diseases

ERKKA VALOVIRTA

Turku Allergy Center, Turku, Finland

GIOVANNI PASSALACQUA and WALTER G. CANONICA

University of Genoa, Genoa, Italy

I. Introduction
II. Oral Immunotherapy
III. Local Bronchial Immunotherapy (LBIT)
IV. Local Nasal Immunotherapy
V. Sublingual-Swallow Immunotherapy (SLIT-Swallow)
VI. Immunological Aspects
VII. Local Routes: Open Questions, Concerns, and Future Developments
VIII. Salient Points
References

I. INTRODUCTION

The non-subcutaneous routes for immunotherapy have been variously named "alternative," "non-parenteral," "non-injection," and "local," but presently the most appropriate terms are "local" and "non-injection." The word "alternative" has been abandoned. The non-injection routes include

1. Oral (OIT): The allergen vaccine, prepared as drops, capsules or tablets, is immediately swallowed with water.
2. Sublingual (SLIT): The allergen vaccine is kept under the tongue for 1–2 minutes and then swallowed (SLIT-swallow) or spat (SLIT-spit). At present, only the sublingual-swallow route is used.
3. Local nasal (LNIT): The allergen vaccine, prepared as on aqueous solution or dry powder, is sprayed into a nostril.
4. Local bronchial (LBIT): The allergen is inhaled as an aerosolized preparation.

At present, SLIT-swallow is the most commonly used route of administration, and its use is supported by an increasing number of controlled trials.

In terms of a historical perspective, 1911 is regarded as the official birth date of allergen immunotherapy (1), and since that date allergens have been administered largely via the subcutaneous route (Fig. 1). Attempts to "immunize" against hay fever by the oral route had already been tried by 1900 (2). During the last century, routes differing from the subcutaneous one were investigated—such as oral (3), nasal (4), and bronchial (5)—but the studies remained anecdotal until the 1970s, when systematic studies on the oral and nasal routes were undertaken.

In 1986, the British Committee for the Safety of Medicines (6) and the American Academy of Allergy, Asthma and Immunology study by Lockey et al. (7) reported deaths caused by SCIT, raising serious concerns about the safety and the risk/benefit ratio of immunotherapy. Retrospective studies showed that life-threatening events were sometimes, but not always, due to human error (8). Interest in non-injection routes rapidly increased, and in addition to studies on LNIT, published during the 1970s, OIT was extensively investigated. The sublingual route was introduced in 1986 (9). Non-injection routes were mentioned for the first time in the European Academy of Allergology and Clinical Immunology (EAACI) position paper published in 1993 (10). In that document there was a request for more studies and research in this area. After a number of clinical studies were published, the 1998 World Health Organization (WHO) position paper (11) stated that

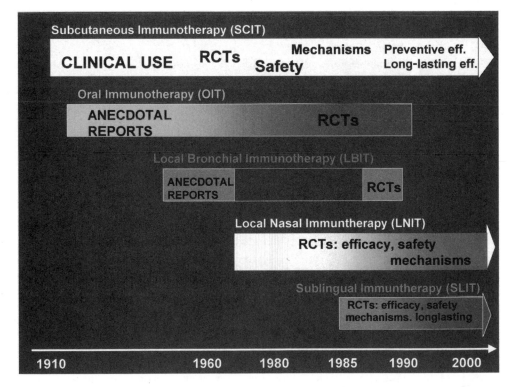

Figure 1 The historical evolution of the different routes for allergen immunotherapy. RCTs = randomized controlled trials.

SLIT and LNIT are viable alternatives to subcutaneous allergen immunotherapy (SCIT), at least in adults. OIT and LBIT were not recommended for clinical use. These conclusions were confirmed in a position paper of the EAACI and ESPACI (European Society of Pediatric Allergology and Clinical Immunology) dedicated entirely to local routes of immunotherapy (12). Finally, in 2001, the publication of "Allergic Rhinitis and Its Impact on Asthma" (ARIA) extended the indication of SLIT-swallow to children with allergic rhinitis (13) (Fig. 2).

II. ORAL IMMUNOTHERAPY

The oral route was the first alternative used for administering immunotherapy. It was hypothesized, in the first years of the twentieth century, that administration of the allergen via the gastrointestinal tract would achieve immunization. The value of giving the allergen orally was supported when it was later shown that the gastrointestinal tract has an abundant mucosal immune system, making effective antigen presentation possible. The results of the earliest controlled studies with OIT, performed at the beginning of the 1980s, were controversial or negative (14,15). New trials carried out by Scandinavian investigators using high amounts of allergen yielded some positive results.

There have been nine double-blind, placebo-controlled (DBPC) trials of OIT, performed with various allergens, in patients with allergic rhinitis; four of these were conducted in pediatric patients (Table 1). Three out of the nine studies (16–18) yielded evidence of a statistically significant improvement of rhinitis symptoms and a decrease in

NON INJECTION ROUTES IN GUIDELINES				
	EAACI 1993	**BSACI 1993**	**WHO 1998**	**ARIA 2001**
Oral route (OIT)	Good clinical results Further studies required How does it work? Not a practical option	Not considered	No demonstration of efficacy Not recommended for clinical use	Not recommended for clinical use
Sublingual route (SLIT)	Benefical effects More conclusive data required before routine employment	Not considered	Viable alternative to SCIT in adults Studies needed in children	Can be administered in adults and children
Nasal route (LNIT)	Clinical efficacy Risk of rapid absorption No comparison with SIT Further studies needed	Not considered	Viable alternative to SCIT for rhinitis in adults One single study in children	Viable alternative to SCIT for rhinitis in adults One single study in children
Bronchial route	There is evidence but is still questionable	Not considered	Not recommended for clinical use	Not recommended for clinical use

Figure 2 Recommendations about non-injection routes in the different guidelines.

Table 1 Double-Blind, Placebo-Controlled Trials of OIT[a]

Author, year (reference)	Age range (years)	Allergen	Duration	Patients, A/P	Extract	Disease
Cooper, 1984 (60)	5–15	Grass	4 months	22/22	Aqueous drops	R
Taudorf, 1985 (61)	11–44	Grass	6 months	25/27	Enteric-coated tabs	R
Moller, 1986 (16)	9–17	Birch	10 months	14/16	Enteric-coated tabs	R
Mosbech, 1987 (62)	15–38	Grass	12 months	24/27	Enteric-coated tabs	R
Taudorf, 1987 (63)	16–47	Birch	18 months	18/21	Enteric-coated tabs	R
Oppenheimer, 1994 (18)	3–13	Mite	3 years	10/8	Aqueous drops	R/A
Giovane, 1994 (17)	7–15	Mite	6 months	8/7	Aqueous drops	R/A
Van Deusen, 1997 (64)	19–49	Ragweed	14 weeks	12/11	Capsules	R
Litwin, 1997 (65)	21–50	Ragweed	4 months	20/21	Capsules	R

[a] Reviewed in Refs. 11 and 14.
A = active, P = placebo, R = rhinitis, R/A = rhinitus and asthma.

medication intake. In one study performed with dust mite vaccine (17), the clinical effect became measurable after 2 years of therapy for rhinitis and after 3 years for asthma. The pharmaceutical preparation, drops or capsules, seemed not to affect the outcome. Some studies observe systemic and local immunological changes, e.g., increases of IgG subclasses and a reduction of specific reactivity at the target organs, resembling those induced by SCIT. Thus, it is possible that the oral administration of allergens really interacts with the immune system.

It is also noteworthy that in almost all studies, many non–life-threatening adverse effects occurred, including nausea, vomiting, abdominal pain, diarrhea, and urticaria.

It was concluded that when evaluated through a rigorous experimental design, the clinical efficacy of OIT is marginal and can be achieved only with very high doses of allergen, and that side effects are frequent, although not severe. For these reasons, OIT is not recommended for clinical use, and OIT with allergens was abandoned in the early 1990s (11,13).

III. LOCAL BRONCHIAL IMMUNOTHERAPY (LBIT)

Local bronchial immunotherapy was proposed as early as 1951 (5), but there have been only two DBPC trials, both with dust mite vaccines (19,20). In the first study, of 22 adults treated for about 3 months, no significant clinical improvement was found, although there was a significant decrease of bronchial specific reactivity during the early and late-phase reactions with allergen bronchial challenge. The majority of patients had a significant fall in their FEV_1 after LBIT administration, and one experienced bronchospasm. In the other study, of 24 adult patients treated for 2 years, there was significant clinical improvement and a decrease of medication intake. The authors reported that some patients (numbers not provided) experienced bronchospasm and needed bronchodilator therapy. The results of the controlled trials indicate that clinical efficacy was not sufficient and the risk/benefit ratio is unfavorable. For these reasons LBIT has been abandoned.

Table 2 LNIT Studies

Author, year (reference)	Age range (years)	Patients, A/P	Allergen	Duration	Type of vaccine
Johansson, 1979 (66)	Ad	12/11	Grass mix	14 weeks	Aqueous, modified
Nickelsen, 1981 (67)	16–66	38/34	Ragweed	3 months	Aqueous, modified
Welsh, 1981 (68)	13–58	18/15	Ragweed	20 weeks	Aqueous
Schumacher, 1981 (69)	20–53	8/7	Grass mix	10 weeks	Powder, modified
Georgitis, 1983 (70)	16–67	31/13	Grass mix	10 weeks	Aqueous, modified
Georgitis, 1984 (71)	Ad	29/16	Grass mix	10 weeks	Aqueous, modified
Andri, 1992 (72)	14–54	8/8	Wall pellitory	18 weeks	Powder, modified
Andri, 1993 (73)	15–54	11/10	Mite	12 months	Powder
Passalacqua, 1995 (74)	20–56	9/9	Wall pellitory	5 months	Powder
D'Amato, 1995 (23)	13–37	10/10	Wall pellitory	8 months	Powder
Andri, 1995 (75)	17–56	14/14	Birch	22 weeks	Powder
Andri, 1996 (76)	14–52	13/15	Grass mix	4 months	Powder
Cirla, 1996 (77)	17–44	11/11	Birch/alder	4 months	Powder
Bardare, 1996 (78)	5–15	19/20	Grass mix	3 months	Powder
Bertoni, 1999 (79)	18–43	10/10	Grass mix	3 months	Aqueous
Motta, 2000 (80)	13–55	55/47	Grass mix/mite	8 months	Aqueous
Pocobelli, 2001 (81)	16–45	22/21	Grass mix	4 months	Powder, modified
Marcucci, 2002 (82)	4–15	16/16	Mite	18 months	Powder, modified

A = active, P = placebo.

IV. LOCAL NASAL IMMUNOTHERAPY

A. Experimental Evidence: Efficacy and Safety

The first attempts to selectively desensitize the nose were made in the 1970s. Nasal administration is supported by the observation that hyporesponsiveness of the nasal mucosa occurs after repeated intranasal administration of low doses of allergen. To date, there have been 18 DBPC studies of LNIT (Table 2). All but one of these studies documented a significant reduction of symptom scores and/or drug intake. The magnitude of clinical efficacy for rhinitis symptoms was comparable to SCIT, and in several trials a reduction of specific nasal reactivity was demonstrated. Classical systemic immunological changes induced by LNIT (e.g., reduction of IgE with an increase of IgG subclasses) were reported only rarely in the mentioned trials, suggesting that the beneficial effect of LNIT was local, not systemic. Nevertheless, one open study with grass vaccine (21) demonstrated that LNIT decreased the proliferation of allergen-specific T lymphocyte clones in the peripheral blood. Also in this case, only SCIT, but not LNIT, induced an increase of circulating IgG4. LNIT was clinically effective with the relevant pollen, birch, ragweed, grasses, *Parietaria judaica*, and *Parietaria officinalis* in adults, but only two studies in adults were performed with a house dust mite vaccine. One mite and one grass study were carried out in children; therefore, LNIT use in mite- or grass-induced rhinitis in the pediatric age group is not yet sufficiently evidence based. A long-term follow-up study suggested that LNIT does not sustain clinical efficacy once it is discontinued, and that with pollen a preseasonal course must be given every year (22).

Aqueous vaccines of unmodified allergens were effective but often caused rhinitis symptoms, whereas allergoids, chemically modified allergens, were devoid of local side effects but were less potent. These facts suggest that LNIT is of little use in clinical practice, since symptoms are reduced during environmental allergen exposure but are present, although mild, at each LNIT administration. The new vaccines, prepared as dry powders, appear to have solved this problem. The vaccine granules, with diameters of 40–50 µm, are uniformly deposited on the nasal mucosa and do not provoke clinical symptoms. In fact, in all studies with dry powders, negligible or no side effects were reported. In one study (23), three patients withdrew because of bronchospasm after administration, but this was ascribed to accidental inhalation of an excess of the vaccine.

B. Practical Aspects

LNIT vaccines were originally prepared as aqueous solutions to be sprayed into the nares. Newer vaccines are usually prepared as dry powders contained in predosed capsules. At each administration, a capsule with the selected dosage is put into an appropriate device, which breaks it; it is then sprayed into the nostril.

In order to avoid bronchial inhalation, the subject must be instructed to vocalize while actuating the spray. Premedication with nasal cromolyn before each dose is recommended by some authors, but there are no data to support this.

LNIT can be administered either preseasonally, for pollen allergens, or continuously, for dust mites. Usually, LNIT consists of a build-up phase with increasing doses, followed by a maintenance phase with a constant dose administered two or three times a week continuously, depending on the manufacturer's recommendations. A simplified schedule also has been proposed. The dose of allergen to be administered is titrated for each patient by skin test reactivity, and once the dose has been established, it is used from the beginning to the end of treatment. This steady-dose schedule is simple, patient friendly, and virtually error free (24).

Despite its optimal safety profile and its efficacy, the use of LNIT is progressively declining. This is primarily because SLIT-swallow is easier to manage and can be used in patients with concomitant asthma. LNIT remains a viable alternative to SCIT for adults with pollen-induced rhinitis and for adult patients who refuse SCIT or do not tolerate injections.

V. SUBLINGUAL-SWALLOW IMMUNOTHERAPY (SLIT-SWALLOW)

The original rationale for SLIT-swallow was to achieve a prompt and rapid absorption of the vaccine to avoid its possible gastrointestinal degradation (Fig. 3). Although it was demonstrated that there is no direct absorption through the sublingual mucosa, SLIT-swallow proved to be the most effective non-injection route, and therefore, it is presently the most widely used form of local immunotherapy.

A. Experimental Evidence: Efficacy and Safety

The first controlled study with SLIT-swallow was published in 1986 (9). To date, 25 DBPC trials have been conducted and published in peer-reviewed journals (25) (Table 3). A Cochrane Review (26) from the year 2003 concludes that SLIT is a safe treatment and significantly reduces symptoms and medication requirements in allergic rhinitis.

Nineteen of the studies confirmed statistically the clinical efficacy of SLIT-swallow with the most common allergens: grass, house dust mites, birch, and *P. judaica* and *officinalis*. There were also single positive studies with olive, cypress, and mixed tree vaccines. The magnitude of the clinical efficacy ranged between a 20% and a 50% reduction of

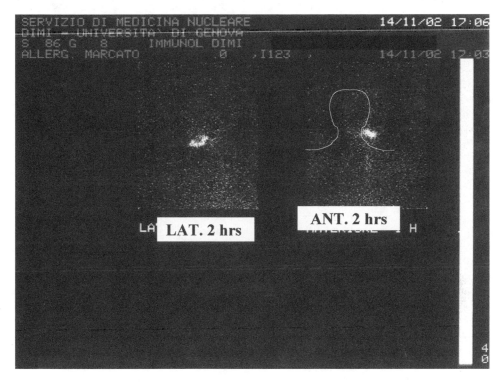

Figure 3 Scintiscan of the head and neck, 2 hours after sublingual administration of a radiolabeled Der p 1 allergoid. The persistence of the allergen in the mouth is apparent.

symptom and/or medication scores, which is superior to the placebo effect and similar to the effects reported with SCIT.

A study published in 2002 (27) failed to demonstrate a significant clinical effect on either the symptom scores or medication intake of SLIT-swallow for allergic rhinitis due to grass, even though the self-evaluation by patients largely favored active treatment. A systemic immunological effect was shown (27). In studies conducted using mite vaccines, SLIT-swallow performed poorly. A trend toward clinical improvement was seen in the active groups, but it did not reach statistical significance (28,29). SCIT is less effective in mite-allergic than in pollen-sensitive patients.

The earliest studies with SLIT-swallow were performed in allergic rhinitis patients, but such treatment also improves asthma symptoms. It decreases asthma symptoms, reduced the use of β_2 agonists, and decreased the need for systemic glucocorticosteroids. One study also demonstrated a measurable effect of SLIT-swallow on the quality of life of patients (30). SLIT-swallow was found to maintain its clinical efficacy for at least 5 years after discontinuation in a study published in 2003 (31). Of 60 children suffering from mite-induced allergic asthma, 35 underwent a 4- to 5-year course of SLIT-swallow and 25 received only drug therapy. The patients were evaluated at baseline, at the end of SLIT-swallow, and 4 to 5 years later. A significant difference versus baseline for the presence of asthma ($p < 0.001$) was found in the SLIT-swallow–treated group.

The original objective for SLIT-swallow and other non-injection routes was to minimize adverse events. SLIT-swallow, based on over 15 years of clinical studies, has an

Table 3 SLIT-Swallow Studies

Author, year (reference)	Age range (years)	Patients, A/P	Allergen	Duration	Disease
Tari, 1990 (83)	5–12	30/28	Mites	18 months	R/A
Sabbah, 1994 (84)	13–51	19/29	Grasses	17 weeks	R
Feliziani, 1995 (85)	14–48	18/16	Grasses	3.5 months	R
Troise, 1995 (86)	17–60	15/16	Wall pellitory	10 months	R
Hirsch, 1997 (28)	6–16	15/15	Mites	1 years	R/A
Passalacqua, 1998 (49)	15–46	10/9	Mites (monomeric allergoid)	2 years	R
Vourdas, 1998 (87)	7–17	33/31	Olive	2 years	R/A
Clavel, 1998 (88)	8–55	62/28	Grasses	6 months	R/A
Horak, 1998 (89)	16–48	18/16	Birch	4 months	R
Hordijk 1998 (90)	18–45	30/27	Grasses	6 months	R/A
Bousquet, 1999 (30)	15–37	15/15	Mites	2 years	A
Passalacqua, 1999 (50)	15–42	15/15	Wall pellitory	8 months	R/A
Pradalier, 1999 (91)	6–25	59/61	Grasses	4 months	R/A
La Rosa, 1999 (32)	6–14	20/21	Wall pellitory	6 months	R/A
Purello, 1999 (92)	14–50	14/16	Wall pellitory	8 months	R/A
Pajno, 2000 (93)	8–15	12/12	Mites	2 years	A
Guez, 2000 (29)	6–51	24/18	Mites	2 years	R
Caffarelli, 2000 (94)	4–14	24/20	Grasses	3 months	R/A
Ariano, 2001 (95)	19–50	10/10	Cypress	8 months	R/A
Bahcecilier, 2001 (96)	7–15	8/7	Mites	6 months	R/A
Voltolini, 2001 (97)	15–52	24/13	Trees	24 months	R
Torres Lima, 2002 (27)	16–48	24/22	Grasses	18 months	R
Mortemousque 2003 (98)	6–60	26/19	Mites	24 months	C
Andre 2003 (99)	6–55	48/51	Ragweed	7 months	R
Ippoliti 2003 (100)	5–12	47/39	Mites	6 months	R/A

A/P = active/placebo, R = rhinitis, A = Asthma.

excellent safety profile (Fig. 4). The most frequently reported side effect in the published literature is onset of oral/sublingual itching following the dose. This side effect is mild and self-resolving, and in pediatric studies side effects are negligible. The rate of gastrointestinal side effects was particularly high in one study where very high doses of allergen vaccines were used, 375 times the amount of a standard SCIT course (32). Systemic side effects, such as headache, rhinorrhea, asthma, and urticaria, were reported only sporadically and their incidence did not differ from the placebo groups. No severe systemic adverse event has been reported over these same years. André et al. reviewed the safety of controlled trials performed with the vaccines of a single manufacturer (33). Six hundred and ninety subjects were enrolled, 347 active and 343 placebo, with 218 children, 103 active and 115 placebo. There was no significant difference in systemic side effects between active and placebo-treated patients, whereas oral and gastrointestinal side effects were more frequent in SLIT patients. Two pharmacosurveillance studies reported side effects of SLIT observed in everyday clinical practice. There are two postmarketing studies. Of these two studies, the first (34) was performed on 268 children between 2 and 15 years of age. The overall incidence of systemic side effects was 3% of the patients in 1/12,000 doses. Of eight reported side effects, only one was moderate in severity, and no

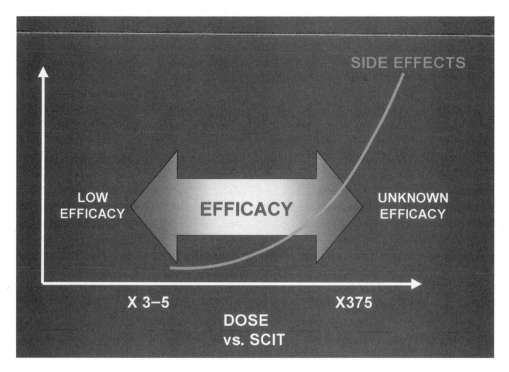

Figure 4 The wide dose interval of efficacy of SLIT, in relation to the occurrence of side effects.

patient discontinued therapy. The second study (35) followed up 198 patients and reported that side effects occurred in 7.5% of the patients and at a rate of 5.2 of every 10,000 doses administered. A temporary dose adjustment resulted in no major recurrence, and in no case was treatment discontinued. The sublingual-swallow administration of allergens did not affect the levels of sublingual tryptase and eosinophilic cationic protein (ECP), even in the one patient who had oral itching after sublingual intake (36). In conclusion, the data from randomized controlled trials and pharmacosurveillance studies confirm the safety of SLIT-swallow in adults and children.

B. Practical Aspects

SLIT-swallow involves a build-up phase of vaccine administered at increasing doses (daily or on alternate days, depending on the manufacturer), followed by a maintenance phase, where the maximum dose is administered two or three times a week. In some experimental studies, a once-a-day maintenance schedule was proposed. SLIT-swallow can be administered either preseasonally and pre-coseasonally or continuously. In the pre-coseasonal modality, the SLIT-swallow begins 2 or 3 months before the expected pollen season, and the doses are reduced by one-third or halved, as a precautionary measure, during the pollen season. For perennial allergens, the treatment is continuous, as with traditional SCIT. SLIT-swallow can be administered as drops or soluble tablets depending on the patient's preference. Accelerated build-up schedules, over 20 days, have been used with no safety problems. Also, a one-day ultrarush build-up with a cypress vaccine was used without side effects (37).

C. Studies Comparing SLIT and SCIT

The double-blind, double-dummy study is the gold standard for comparing two different routes of administration, such as SLIT-swallow and SCIT. Only one such study has been published (38). It shows that the clinical efficacy of SLIT-swallow in grass pollen–allergic patients is equivalent to SCIT. Another double-blind, double-dummy trial with birch pollen vaccine is to be published (39), showing that SLIT and SCIT are equally effective, although safety was superior with the non-injection route.

There have been other comparative but uncontrolled studies. Ongari et al. (40) demonstrated that SLIT-swallow and SCIT were equally efficacious in 20 patients with grass allergy, and both treatments were significantly more effective than pharmacotherapy. Another open study (41) compared SLIT and SCIT for efficacy and safety in 23 *Alternaria tenuis*–allergic patients and showed that both routes provided a clinical improvement versus pretreatment conditions, with no difference between SLIT and SCIT. In another study (42), SLIT-swallow, SCIT, and LNIT were compared in 43 patients with house dust mite–induced rhinitis; in this study, only the immunological changes were measured. The authors highlighted the tolerability of SLIT-swallow, but SCIT was more effective in inducing immunological changes. Finally, a comparative study (43), again in house dust mite–allergic patients, showed that clinical improvement was more prompt with SCIT, especially for relieving asthma symptoms, although SLIT-swallow controlled rhinitis symptoms.

VI. IMMUNOLOGICAL ASPECTS

SCIT regulates cytokine and mediator release, inhibits activation and recruitment of effector cells, and downregulates the TH2 while upregulating the TH1 response. Altering the TH1/TH2 response probably accounts for the prolonged efficacy after discontinuing SCIT and also may account for its preventive effect. Local IT has primarily been studied clinically.

The immunological rationale for the local administration of allergen vaccines is supported by several experimental observations in animal models. The oral route is "tolerogenic" and can redirect the TH1/TH2 paradigm (44–46). Also, the dendritic cells of oral mucosa are efficient antigen-presenting cells and produce IL-12 (47); in mice, the intranasal administration of an antigen was demonstrated to be capable of inducing tolerance by selecting out a functionally inactive subset of CD4+ cells (48).

The immunological effects of local immunotherapy differ from those of SCIT. In fact, OIT and SLIT-swallow affected serum immunoglobulins only in a minority of studies (27). In general, local routes do not induce a decrease of IgE and an increase of IgG1 and IgG4.

SLIT-swallow can decrease the mucosal expression of the ICAM-1 adhesion molecule and, as a consequence, inflammatory infiltration in humans. (49,50). An open study in 10 children confirmed that SLIT-swallow reduced ICAM-1 expression on nasal epithelial cells and decreased methacholine responsiveness (51).

Some interesting suggestions about the possible mechanism of action of SLIT comes from two pharmacokinetics studies (52,53). Radiolabeled purified allergen (Par j 1) is not directly absorbed through the sublingual mucosa in humans, but the allergen is retained in the mouth for up to 40 hours. The allergen seems to be absorbed as peptides, and not as native protein, in the gut, even though trace amounts of the chemically modified allergen, monomeric allergoid, could be detected in plasma. These data suggest that contact of the allergen with the oral mucosa is critical and that the allergen is not directly absorbed through the mucosa in the mouth. This may be the reason why OIT does not work.

VII. LOCAL ROUTES: OPEN QUESTIONS, CONCERNS, AND FUTURE DEVELOPMENTS

Randomized clinical trials and postmarketing surveys done during the last 15 years provide data on the clinical efficacy and general safety of some local routes for SLIT and the general use of SLIT-swallow and LNIT for clinical use in many parts of the world. LNIT has limited indications, since its efficacy is primarily for allergic rhinitis and not asthma and its use is progressively declining. SLIT-swallow is more attractive because of its efficacy and lack of side effects. However, SCIT remains better understood than SLIT-swallow, and more studies are necessary comparing the two modes of therapy.

A. The Optimal Dose of Allergen

The optimal dose for SLIT-swallow has yet to be determined. The available studies indicate that doses of allergen ranging between 3 to 5 and 375 times the dose of a corresponding SCIT dose are effective in most patients (54). This range is wide and imprecise, and there is no formal proof that one particular dose is better than another. Moreover, there is no clear evidence that the efficacy is dose dependent within the mentioned range; in particular, it is unknown if there is still a dose response at doses higher than 375 times that used for SCIT, although it is clear that higher amounts of allergen are associated with more gastrointestinal symptoms whereas too-low doses are ineffective.

Dose-ranging studies have not been performed with SLIT-swallow, in contrast to SCIT. Second, the methods used for standardization often do not allow for a comparison of vaccines from different manufacturers. Some studies with SLIT-swallow were performed using vaccines with defined content of major allergen(s). Additional studies of this type should permit a better idea about this form of therapy. The term "high-dose SLIT-swallow" simply means that the dose of allergen used should be, on average, considerably greater than that used for SCIT.

B. Preventive Effect and Long-Lasting Efficacy

SCIT treatment for 3 to 5 years maintains clinical efficacy, with a continual reduction of symptoms and medication intake for 3 to 5 years after it is discontinued (55). The same effect has been demonstrated for SLIT-swallow in pediatric patients with asthma treated with house dust mite vaccine (31). SCIT also modifies the natural history of the disease, i.e., the onset of asthma in rhinitis patients (54). This has not yet been demonstrated for SLIT-swallow; however lack of such data can be explained by the fact that this form of therapy has been used only for the last decade.

C. Compliance and Costs

It is impossible to assess compliance with a self-administered treatment modality such as SLIT-swallow. Assessment of compliance with SCIT is better since it is prescribed and administered by physicians and can be monitored on an ongoing basis. The studies show that between 10% and 34% of individuals discontinue SCIT (56) and up to 50% of patients who have side effects become noncompliant (57). Better compliance would be expected with SLIT-swallow administration because of its better safety profile compared with SCIT, but to date, no compliance studies have been completed.

The cumulative dose of allergen given via SLIT-swallow is 3–5 to 375 times the usual dose of SCIT, and therefore, the cost of the vaccine is higher than with SCIT. This higher cost is balanced by the reduced need for medical and nursing time (25), so that the total cost of SLIT-swallow should be less than that of SCIT. Again, formal cost-benefit analyses are lacking.

D. Future Developments

Accelerated build-up schedules have been studied for SLIT-swallow based on its safety profile. A 1-day ultrarush build-up with cypress vaccine produced no increase in side effects (37). A four-parallel-group study using different build-up regimens showed that starting with higher doses, 100-fold with respect to a traditional schedule, did not modify the safety profile of SLIT-swallow (58). An accelerated or ultrarush build-up phase, taking advantage of the safety profile of treatment, should result in time saving and probably in an easy-to-use therapy.

VIII. SALIENT POINTS

1. OIT and LBIT are not indicated for clinical practice.
2. LNIT remains an alternative to SCIT for adult patients with pollen-induced allergic rhinitis, especially if the patient does not want or does not tolerate SCIT.
3. SLIT-swallow is effecive for common allergens such as grass, birch, house dust mites, and *P. judaica* and *officinalis*.
4. The safety of SLIT is satisfactory and has been documented in both clinical trials and postmarketing surveillance study. No severe or life-threatening adverse event has been described so far (59).
5. Further studies are needed to document the preventive effect, especially in children, and to better define the optimal maintenance dose.

REFERENCES

1. Noon L. Prophylactic inoculation against hay fever. Lancet 1911; (i)1:1572–1573.
2. Curtis HH. The immunizing cure of hayfever. Med News (NY) 1900; 77:16–18.
3. Black JH. The oral administration of pollen. J Lab Clin Med 1927; 12:1156.
4. Taylor G, Shivalkar PR. Local nasal desensitization in allergic rhinitis. Clin Allergy 1972; 2:125–126.
5. Herxeimer H. Bronchial hypersensitization and hyposensitization in man. Int Arch Allergy Appl Immunol 1951; 40:40–57.
6. Committee on the Safety of Medicines. CSM update: Desensitizing vaccines. Br Med J 1986; 293:948.
7. Lockey RF, Benedict LM, Turkeltaub PC, Bukantz SC. Fatalities from immunotherapy and skin testing. J Allergy Clin Immunol 1987; 79:660–677.
8. Reid MJ, Lockey RF, Turkeltaub PC, Platt-Mills TAE. Survey of fatalities from skin testing and immunotherapy. J Allergy Clin Immunol 1993; 92:6–15.
9. Scadding K, Brostoff J. Low dose sublingual therapy in patients with allergic rhinitis due to dust mite. Clin Allergy 1986; 16:483–491.
10. Malling HJ, Weeke B, eds. EAACI immunotherapy position paper. Allergy 1993; 48:9–35.

11. Bousquet J, Lockey R, Malling HJ, eds. World Health Organization position paper. Allergen immunotherapy. Therapeutical vaccines for allergic diseases. Allergy 1998, 53(suppl).1–42.

12. Malling HJ, ed. EAACI/ESPACI position paper on local immunotherapy. Allergy 1998; 53:933.

13. Bousquet J, Van Cauwenberge P, eds. ARIA: Allergic rhinitis and its impact on asthma. J Allergy Clin Immunol 2001; S147–S336.

14. Rebien W, Wahn U, Puttonen E, Maasch HG. Comparative study of immunological and clinical efficacy of oral and subcutaneous hyposensitization. Allergologie 1980; 3:101–109.

15. Taudorf E, Weeke B. Orally administered grass pollen. Allergy 1983; 38:561–564.

16. Moller C, Dreborg S, Lanner A, Bjorksten B. Oral immunotherapy of children with rhinoconjunctivitis due to birch pollen allergy. Allergy 1986; 41:271–279.

17. Giovane A, Bardare M, Passalacqua G, Ruffoni S, Scordamaglia A, Ghezzi E, Canonica GW. A three year double blind placebo-controlled study with specific oral immunotherapy to *Dermatophagoides*: Evidence of safety and efficacy in pediatric patients. Clin Exp Allergy 1994; 24:53–59.

18. Oppenheimer J, Areson JG, Nelson HS. Safety and efficacy of oral immunotherapy with standardized cat extract. J Allergy Clin Immunol 1994; 93:61–67.

19. Crimi E, Voltolini S, Troise C, Gianiorio P, Crimi P, Brusasco V, Negrini AC. Local immunotherapy with *Dermatophagoides* extract in asthma. J Allergy Clin Immunol 1991; 87:721–728.

20. Tari MG, Mancino M, Monti G. Immunotherapy by inhalation of allergen in powder in house dust allergic asthma: A double blind study. J Investig Allergol Clin Immunol 1992; 2:59–67.

21. Giannarini L, Maggi E. Decrease of allergen specific T cell response induced by nasal immunotherapy. Clin Exp Allergy 1998; 28:404–412.

22. Passalacqua G, Albano M, Pronzato C, Riccio A, Falagiani P, Canonica GW. Nasal immunotherapy to *Parietaria*: Long term follow up of a double blind study. Clin Exp Allergy 1997; 27:904–908.

23. D'Amato G, Lobefalo G, Liccardi G, Cazzola M. A double blind placebo controlled trial of local nasal immunotherapy in allergic rhinitis to *Parietaria* pollen. Clin Exp Allergy 1995; 25:141–148.

24. Pocobelli D, Del Bono A, Venuti L, Falagiani P, Venuti A. Nasal immunotherapy at constant dosage: A double blind placebo controlled study in grass allergic rhinoconjunctivitis. J Invest, Allergol Clin Immunol 2001; 11:79–88.

25. Canonica GW, Passalacqua G. Noninjection routes for immunotherapy. J Allergy Clin Immunol 2003; 111:437–48.

26. Wilson DR, Torres Lima M, Dirham SR. Sublingual immunotherapy for allergic rhinitis (Cochrane review). In: The Cochrane Library, issue 2. Oxford: Update Software, 2003.

27. Lima MT, Wilson D, Pitkin L, Roberts A, Nouri-Aria K, Jacobson M, Walker S, Durham S. Grass pollen sublingual immunotherapy for seasonal rhinoconjunctivitis: A randomized controlled trial. Clin Exp Allergy 2002; 32:507–514.

28. Hirsch T, Sahn M, Leupold W. Double blind controlled study of sublingual immunotherapy with house dust mite extracts in children. Pediatr Allergy Immunol 1997; 8:21–27.

29. Guez S, Vatrinet C, Fadel R, André C. House dust mite sublingual swallow immunotherapy in perennial rhinitis: A double blind placebo controlled study. Allergy 2000; 55:369–375.

30. Bousquet J, Scheinmann P, Guinnepain MT, Perrin-Fayolle M, Sauvaget J, Tonnel AB, Pauli G, Caillaud D, Dubost R, Leynadier F, Vervloet D, Herman D, Galvain S, Andre C. Sublingual swallow immunotherapy (SLIT) in patients with asthma due to house dust mites: A double blind placebo controlled study. Allergy 1999; 54:249–260.

31. Di Rienzo V, Marcucci F, Puccinelli P, Parmiani S, Frati F, Sensi I, Canonica GW, Passalacqua G. Long lasting effect of sublingual immunotherapy in children with asthma due to house dust mites: A ten-year prospective study. Clin Exp Allergy 2003; 33:206–210.

32. La Rosa M, Ranno C, André C, Carat F, Tosca MA, Canonica GW. Double blind placebo controlled evaluation of sublingual swallow immunotherapy with standardized *Parietaria judaica* extract in children with allergic rhinoconjunctivitis. J Allergy Clin Immunol 1999; 104:425–432.

33. André C, Vatrinet C, Galvain S, Carat F, Sicard H. Safety of sublingual swallow immunotherapy in children and adults. Int Arch Allergy Immunol 2000; 121:229–234.

34. Di Rienzo V, Pagani A, Parmiani S, Passalacqua G, Canonica GW. Post-marketing surveillance study on the safety of sublingual immunotherapy in children. Allergy 1999; 54:1110–1113.

35. Lombardi C, Gargioni S, Melchiorre A, Canonica GW, Passalacqua G. Safety of sublingual immunotherapy in adults: A post marketing surveillance study. Allergy 2001; 56:889–892.

36. Marcucci F, Sensi L, Frati F, Senna GE, Canonica GW, Parmiani S, Passalacqua G. Sublingual tryptase and ECP in children treated with grass pollen sublingual immunotherapy (SLIT): Safety and immunologic implications. Allergy 2001; 56:1091–1095.

37. Vervloet D, Birnbaum J, Laurent P, et al. Safety and clinical efficacy of rush sublingual cypress immunotherapy: preliminary results (abstr). Allergy 2002; 57(suppl 73):70.

38. Quirino T, Iemoli E, Siciliani E, Parmiani S. Sublingual vs. injective immunotherapy in grass pollen allergic patients: A double blind double dummy study. Clin Exp Allergy 1996; 26:1253–1261.

39. Khinchi S, Poulsen LK, Carat F, André C, Hansen AB, Malling HJ. Clinical efficacy of sublingual and subcutaneous birch pollen allergen specific immunotherapy: A randomized placebo controlled double blind dummy study. Allergy 2004, in press.

40. Ongari S, Domeneghetti P, Parmiani S. Comparison among drugs, injective IT and sublingual IT in grass allergic patients. Allergy 1995; 50(26):358.

41. Bernardis P, Agnoletto M, Puccinelli P, Parmiani S, Pozzan M. Injective VS sublingual immunotherapy in *Alternaria tenuis* allergic patients. J Investig Allergol Clin Immunol 1996; 6:55–62.

42. Piazza I, Bizzarro N. Humoral response to subcutaneous, oral and nasal immunotherapy for allergic rhinitis due to *Dermatophagoides pteronyssinus*. Ann Allergy 1993; 71:461–469.

43. Mungan D, Misirligil Z, Gurbuz L. Comparison of the efficacy of subcutaneous and sublingual immunotherapy in mite sensitive patients with rhinitis and asthma: A placebo controlled study. Ann Allergy Asthma Immunol 1999; 82:485–490.

44. Chen Y, Kuchroo VK, Inobe J, Hafler DA, Weiner HL. Regulatory T cell clones induced by oral tolerance: Suppression of autoimmune enkephalomyelitis. Science 1994; 265: 1237–1240.

45. Holt PG, Vines J, Britten D. Sublingual allergen administration: I. Selective suppression of IgE production in rats with high allergen doses. Clin Allergy 1988; 18:229–234.

46. Miller A, Lider O, Roberts AB, Sporn MB. Suppressor T cells generated by oral tolerization to myelin basic protein suppress both in vitro and in vivo immune response by the release of TGFbeta following antigen specific triggering. Proc Natl Acad Sci USA 1992; 89:421–425.

47. Macatonia SE, Hosken NA. Dendritic cells produce IL-12 and direct the development of TH1 cells from naive CD4+ T cells. J Immunol 1995; 154:5071–5079.

48. Tsitoure DC, DeKruyff RH, Lamb JR, Umetsu DT. Intranasal exposure to antigen induces immunological tolerance mediated by functionally disabled CD4+ T cells. J Immunol 1999; 163:2592–2600.

49. Passalacqua G, Albano M, Fregonese L, Riccio A, Pronzato C, Mela GS, Canonica GW. Randomised controlled trial of local allergoid immunotherapy on allergic inflammation in mite induced rhinoconjunctivitis. Lancet 1998; 351:629–632.

50. Passalacqua G, Albano M, Riccio A, Fregonese L, Puccinelli P, Parmiani S, Canonica GW. Clinical and immunological effects of a rush sublingual immunotherapy to *Parietaria* species: A double blind placebo controlled trial. J Allergy Clin Immunol 1999; 104:964–968.

51. Silvestri M, Spallarossa D, Battistini E, Sabatini F, Pecora S, Parmiani S, Rossi GA. Changes in inflammatory and clinical parameters and in bronchial hyperreactivity asthmatic children

sensitized to house dust mites following sublingual immunotherapy. J Investig Allergol Clin Immunol 2002; 12:52–59.

52. Bagnasco M, Mariani G, Passalacqua G, Motta C, Bartolomei M, Falagiani P, Mistrello G, Canonica GW. Absorption and distribution kinetics of the mayor *Parietaria* allergen administered by noninjectable routes to healthy human beings. J Allergy Clin Immunol 1997; 100:121–129.

53. Bagnasco M, Passalacqua G, Villa G, Augeri C, Flamigni G, Borini E, Falagiani P, Mistrello G, Canonica GW, Mariani G. Pharmacokinetics of an allergen and a monomeric allergoid for oromucosal immunotherapy in allergic volunteers. Clin Exp Allergy 2001; 31:54–60.

54. Moller C, Dreborg S, Ferdousi HA, Halken S, Host A, Jacobsen L, Koivikko A, Koller DY, Niggemann B, Norberg LA, Urbanek R, Valovirta E, Wahn U. Pollen immunotherapy reduces the development of asthma in children with seasonal rhinoconjunctivitis (the PAT-study.) J Allergy Clin Immunol 2002; 109:251–256.

55. Passalacqua G, Canonica GW. Long lasting efficacy of specific immunotherapy. Allergy 2002; 57:275–276.

56. Lower T, Hensy J, Mandik L, Janosky J, Friday GA Jr. Compliance with allergen immunotherapy. Ann Allergy 1993; 70:480–482.

57. Cohn JR, Pizzi A. Determinants of patient compliance with allergen immunotherapy. J Allergy Clin Immunol 1993; 91:734–737.

58. Grosclaude M, Bouillot P, Alt R, Leynadier F, Scheinmann P, Basset D, Fadel R, Andrè C. Safety of various dosage regimens during induction of sublingual immunotherapy. Int Arch Allergy Immunol 2002; 129:248–253.

59. Passalacqua G, Baena Cagnani C, Berardi M, Canonica GW. Oral and sublingual immunotherapy in pediatric patients. Curr Opin Allergy Clin Immunol 2003; 3:139–145.

60. Cooper PJ, Darbyshire J, Nunn AJ, Warner JO. A controlled trial of oral hyposensitization in pollen asthma and rhinitis in children. Clin Allergy 1984; 14:541–550.

61. Taudorf E, Laursen LC Djurup, et al. Oral administration of grass pollen to hay fever patients: An efficacy study in oral hyposensitization. Allergy 1985; 40:321–335.

62. Mosbech H, Dreborg S, Madsenn F, et al High dose grass pollen tablets used for hyposensitization in hay fever patients: A one year double blind placebo controlled study. Allergy 1987; 42:415–455.

63. Taudorf E, Laursen CL, Lanner A, et al. Oral immunotherapy to birch pollen hay fever. J Allergy Clin Immunol 1987; 80:153–161.

64. Van Deusen MA, Angelini BL, Gordoro KM, et al. Efficacy and safety of oral immunotherapy with short ragweed extract. Ann Allergy Asthma Immunol 1997; 78:573–580.

65. Litwin A, Flanagan M, Entis G, et al. Oral immunotherapy with short ragweed in a novel encapsulated preparation: A double blind study. J Allergy Clin Immunol 1997; 100:30–38.

66. Johansson SGO, Deuschl H, Zetterström O. Use of glutaraldehyde-modified timothy grass pollen extract in nasal hyposensitization of hay fever. Int Arch Allergy Appl Immunol 1979; 60:447–460.

67. Nickelsen JA, Goldstein S, Mueller U, et al. Local intranasal immunotherapy for ragweed allergic rhinitis: Clinical response. J Allergy Clin Immunol 1981; 68:33–40.

68. Welsh PW, Zimmermann EM, Yunginger JW, et al. Preseasonal intranasal immunotherapy with nebulized short ragweed extract. J Allergy Clin Immunol 1981; 67:237–242.

69. Schumacher MJ, Pain MCF. Intranasal immunotherapy with polymerized grass pollen allergens. Allergy 1981; 37:241–245.

70. Georgitis JW, Reisman RE, Clayton WF, et al. Local nasal immunotherapy for grass allergic rhinitis. J Allergy Clin Immunol 1983; 71:71–76.

71. Georgitis JW, Clayton WF, Wypych JI, et al. Further evaluation of local nasal immunotherapy with aqueous and allergoid grass extract. J Allergy Clin Immunol 1984; 74:694–700.

72. Andri L, Senna GE, Betteli C, et al. Local nasal immunotherapy in allergic rhinitis to *Parietaria*. Allergy 1992; 47:318–323.

73. Andri L, Senna GE, Betteli C. Local nasal immunotherapy for *Dermatophagoides*-induced rhinitis: Efficay of a powder extract. J Allergy Clin Immunol 1993; 91:587–596.

74. Passalaqua G, Albano M, Ruffoni S, et al. Local nasal immunotherapy to *Parietaria*: Evidence of reduction of allergic inflammation. Am J Respir Crit Care Med 1995; 152:461–466.

75. Andri L, Senna GE, Andri G, et al. Local nasal imuunotherapy for birch allergic rhnitis with extract in powder form. Clin Exp Allergy 1995; 25:1092–1099.

76. Andri L, Senna GE, Betteli C, et al. Local nasal immunotherapy with extract in powder form is effective and safe in grass pollen rhinitis: A double blind study on 32 patients. J Allergy Clin Immunol 1996; 97:37–41.

77. Cirla A, Sforza N, Roffi GP, et al. Preseasonal intranasal immunotherapy in birch-alder rhinitis: A double blind study. Allergy 1996; 51:299–305.

78. Bardare M, Zaini C, Novembre E , Vierucci A. Local nasal immunotherapy with a powder extract for grass pollen rhinitis in pedaitric ages: A controlled study. J Investig Allergol Clin Immunol 1996; 97:34–41.

79. Bertoni M, Cosmi F, Bianchi I, Di Berardino L. Clinical efficacy and tolerability of a steady dosage schedule of local immunotherapy: Results of preseasonal treatment in grass pollen rhinitis. Ann Allergy Asthma Immunol 1999; 82:47–51.

80. Motta G, Passali D, De Vincentis I, et al. A multicenter trial of specific local nasal immunotherapy. Laryngoscope 2000; 110:132–139.

81. Pocobelli D, Del Bono A, Venuti L, et al. Nasal immunotherapy at constant dose: A double blind placebo controlled study in grass allerg rhinoconjunctivitis. J Investig Allergol Clin Immunol 2001; 11:79–88.

82. Marcucci F, Sensi LG, Caffarelli, et al. Low-dose local nasal immunotherapy in children with perennial allergic rhinitis due to *Dermatophagoides*. Allergy 2002; 57:23–28.

83. Tari M G, Mancino M, Monti G. Efficacy of sublingual immunotherapy in patients with rhinitis and asthma due to house dust mite: A double blind study. Allergol Immunopathol 1990; 18:277–284.

84. Sabbah A, Hassoun S, Le Sellin J, et al. A double blind placebo controlled trial by the sublingual route of immunotherapy with a standardized grass pollen extract. Allergy 1994; 49:309–313.

85. Feliziani V, Lattuada G, Parmiani S, Dall'Aglio PP. Safety and efficacy of sublingual rush immunotherapy with grass allergen extracts: A double blind study. Allergol Immunopathol 1995; 23:173–178.

86. Troise C, Voltolini S, Canessa A, et al. Sublingual immunotherapy in *Parietaria* pollen induced rhinitis: A double blind study. J Investig Allergol Clin Immunol 1995; 5:25–30.

87. Vourdas D, Syrigou E, Potamianou P, et al. Double blind placebo controlled evaluation of sublingual immunotherapy with a standardized olive tree pollen extract in pediatric patients with allergic rhinoconjunctivitis and mild asthma due to olive tree pollen sensitization. Allergy 1998; 53:662–671.

88. Clavel R, Bousquet J, Andre C. Clinical efficacy of sublingual swallow immunotherapy: A double blind placebo controlled trial of a standardized five grass pollen extract in rhinitis. Allergy 1998; 53:493–498.

89. Horak F, Stubner UE, Berger U, ct al. Immunotherapy with sunlingual birch pollen extract: A short term double blind study. J Investig Allergol Clin Immunol 1998; 8:165–171.

90. Hordijk GJ, Antwelink JB, Luwema RA. Sublingual immunotherapy with a standardized grass pollen extract: A double blind placebo controlled study. Allergol Immunopathol 1998; 26:234–240.

91. Pradalier A, Basset D, Claudel A, et al. Sublingual swallow immunotherapy (SLIT) with a standardized five grass pollen extract (drops and sublingual tablets) versus placebo in seasonal rhinitis. Allergy 1999; 54:819–828.

92. Purello D'Ambrosio F, Gangemi S, Isola S, et al. Sublingual immunotherapy: A double blind placebo controlled trial with *Parietaria judaica* extract standardized in mass units in patients with rhinoconjunctivitis, asthma or both. Allergy 1999; 54:968–973.

93. Pajno GB, Morabito L, BarberioG, Parmiani S. Clinical and immunological effects of longterm sublingual immunotherapy in asthmatic children sensitized to mite: A double blind study. Allergy 2000; 55:842–849.

94. Caffarelli C, Sensi LG, Marcucci F, Cavagni C. Preseasonal local allergoid immunotherapy to grass pollen in children: A double-blind, placebo-controlled, randomized trial. Allergy 2000; 55:1142–1147.

95. Ariano R, Spadolini I, Panzani RC. Efficacy of sublingual specific immunotherapy in Cupressaceae allergy using an extract of *Cupressus arizonica*: A double blind study. Allergol Immunopathol (Madr) 2001; 29:238–244.

96. Bahcecilier NN, Isik U, Barlan IB, Basaran N. Efficay of sublingual immunotherapy in children with asthma and rhinitis: A double-blind, placebo-controlled study. Pediatr Pulmonol 2001; 32:49–55.

97. Voltolini S, Modena P, Minale P, et al. Sublingual immunotherapy in tree pollen allergy: Double blind, placebo controlled study with a biologically standardized extract of tree pollen (alder, birch and hazel) administered by a rush schedule. Allergol Immunopathol 2001; 29:103–110.

98. Mortemousque B, Bertel F, De Casamayor J, Verin P, Colin J. House-dust mite sublingual-swallow immunotherapy in perennial conjunctivitis: a double-blind, placebo-controlled study. Clin Exp Allergy. 2003; 33:464–9.

99. Andrè C, Perrin-Fayolle M, Grosclaude M, et al. A double blind placebo controlled evaluation of SLIT with a standardized ragweed extract in patients with seasonal rhinitis. Int Arch Allergy Immunol 2003; 131:111–118.

100. Ippoliti F, De Sanctis W, Volterrani A, et al. Immunomodulation during sublingual therapy in allergic children. Pediatr Allergy Immunol 2003; 14:216–21.

34

Anti-IgE Therapy

ULRICH WAHN and ECKARD HAMELMANN

University Hospital Charité-Virchow, Berlin, Germany

I. INTRODUCTION

The first implication of a transferable/soluble factor as the mediator of an allergic reaction was published in 1919. In that case report, Ramirez describes a man who experienced an acute asthmatic episode while entering a horse-drawn coach in New York's Central Park 2 weeks after having received a 600-ml blood transfusion from a man with a known horse allergy (1). The first scientific description of the mechanism of the allergic reaction was provided 1921 by Prausnitz and Küstner, who showed that a serum factor ("reagin") passively transferred hypersensitive reactivity from the serum of an allergic patient to the skin of a nonallergic patient (2). Ishizaka and colleagues (3,4) and Johannson and colleagues (5) independently showed 45 years later that this "reagin" was a novel class of serum antibodies—immunoglobulin E: IgE (6). Now, 35 years later, we stand on the brink of a novel therapeutic option for the treatment of allergic diseases, by directly targeting increased serum IgE with neutralizing antibodies: anti-IgE antibodies.

II. ROLE OF IgE IN ALLERGIC DISEASES

IgE, similar to other immunoglobulins, is composed of two heavy and two light chains (Fig. 1). It is produced by allergen-specific plasma cells after isotype switch to the ε-chain. IgE production is mainly under the control of T-cells and T-cell cytokines (Fig. 2) (7,8). In the case of allergic immune reactions, naive T-cells develop toward the so-called TH2 type, defined by the predominant production of TH2 cytokines, especially IL-4, IL-5, and IL-13 (9). Differentiation of B-cells to IgE-producing plasma cells requires two distinct signals, the first provided by IL-4 and IL-13 (10,11) and the second by interaction between the costimulatory antigen CD40 on the surface of B-cells with CD40 ligand on T-cell surfaces (12,13).

Biological activities of IgE are mediated through specific receptors. The high-affinity receptor (FcεRI) is expressed mainly on mast cells and basophils (14,15), and the low-affinity receptor (FcεRII, CD23) is expressed on B-cells (16,17). Whereas free serum IgE has a very short half-life of about $2\frac{1}{2}$ days, mast cells remain sensitized for up to 12 weeks following binding of IgE to high-affinity receptors.

Reexposure of sensitized patients to allergens leads to binding of specific allergen to IgE-FcεRI complexes on mast cells. This activates the allergic cascade characteristic of the early IgE-mediated reaction (18,19) (Fig. 2). The cross-linking of receptors immediately triggers the release and production of preformed and newly synthesized mediators, such as leukotrienes, prostaglandins, cytokines, and chemokines. These pro-inflammatory mediators cause, depending on the site of allergen exposure, immediate reactions such as airway smooth muscle contraction, mucus hypersecretion, mucosal edema of upper or lower airways, or conjunctivitis. The finding that human mast cells, after IgE-mediated activation, produce a wide range of cytokines (20,21) suggests that IgE may contribute to subse-

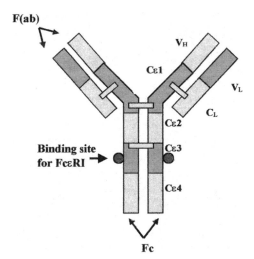

Figure 1 Structure of IgE and position of binding site for FcεRI, which is recognized by the recombinant humanized anti-IgE. Variable (V) and constant (C) regions of the heavy (H) and light (L) chains are linked by disulfide bridges. Allergen is recognized by the F(ab) part, binding to the IgE receptor, indicated by the Fc part. Indicated is the binding site of the high-affinity IgE receptor (FcεRI) within the third domain of the constant region of the heavy chain (Cε3).

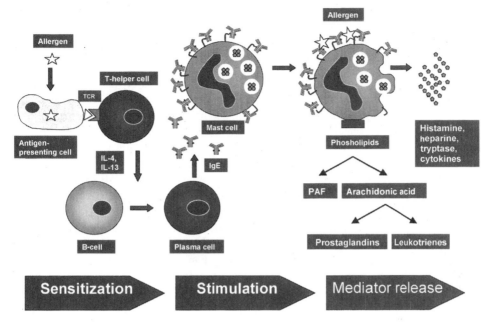

Figure 2 The allergic cascade: IgE production, mast cell activation, and degranulation. Allergen is processed by antigen-presenting cells and recognized by the specific T-cell receptor (TCR) on the T-cells. T-helper cell type II cytokines interleukin-4 (IL-4) and -13 (IL-13) induce isotype switch and differentiation of IgE-producing B-cells. IgE binds to specific IgE receptors on mast cells, recognizes specific allergen, and activates mast cell degranulation and de-novo synthesis of pro-inflammatory mediators, inducing the immediate type of hypersensitivity reaction.

quent inflammatory reaction, such as airway eosinophilia and airway remodeling associated with the late allergic response.

III.   ANTI-IgE FOR THE TREATMENT OF ALLERGIC DISEASES

A.   Mechanism of Anti-IgE

The binding site of IgE for the high-affinity receptor FcεRI is located within the third domain of the heavy chain, Cε3 (22). A murine antibody, MAE1, was generated that recognizes the same residues in the Cε3 domain of IgE that are responsible for binding to FcεRI (23). To avoid sensitization with foreign proteins, a humanized version, containing 95% of a human IgG1 antibody and only 5% of the murine IgE-specific epitope, was constructed and named recombined humanized monoclonal antibody (rhuMAb)-E25, or omalizumab (24).

The main features of anti-IgE are that it

1.   Recognizes and binds IgE, but not IgG or IgA
2.   Inhibits the binding of IgE to FcεRI
3.   Does not bind to IgE bound to mast cells or basophils and thus does not cause degranulation ("non-anaphylactic antibody")
4.   Blocks mast cell degranulation following passive sensitization in vitro or challenge with allergen in vivo

5. Is nonspecific for the allergen specificity of the IgE antibody, meaning that it binds to any IgE molecule

B. Safety, Tolerability, and Route of Administration

A series of preclinical and phase I studies were conducted to test safety and efficacy of anti-IgE. Studies in cynomolgus monkeys showed that anti-IgE binds IgE, resulting in the formation of small (~1000 kDa), nonprecipitating and non–complement-activating immune complexes that are no longer able to bind IgE receptors. When E25 was at its highest concentration in the serum compartment, no specific organ deposition was observed, and immune complexes were eliminated by urinary excretion (25).

In addition to the effect on circulating IgE, treatment with anti-IgE suppresses IgE-receptor expression on basophils in vitro (26) as well as in vivo (27), supporting the concept that IgE receptor expression is regulated by and associated with IgE serum levels.

Single- and multi-dose trials in adults with and without allergic disease showed that anti-IgE was tolerated and decreased IgE serum levels in a dose-dependent manner as soon as 5 min after intravenous and within 24 h after subcutaneous administration (28,29). The decrease of IgE lasted, depending on the antibody dose, for about 4–6 weeks after a single dose.

A large phase II study in adults with seasonal allergic rhinitis (SAR) compared subcutaneous (SC) versus intravenous (IV) treatment at different dosages (0.15 mg/kg body weight SC; 0.15 mg/kg IV; or 0.5 mg/kg IV, seven injections within 84 days) (30). The pharmacodynamics of the SC and IV routes of administration did not differ. Anti-IgE decreased serum IgE levels in a dose- and baseline IgE–dependent fashion (Fig. 3).

Not all routes of administration of anti-IgE are similarly effective. Fahy et al. found that aerosolized anti-IgE in patients with mild allergic asthma did not significantly suppress serum IgE levels and did not, despite detectable levels of omalizumab, affect the early asthmatic response to allergen (31).

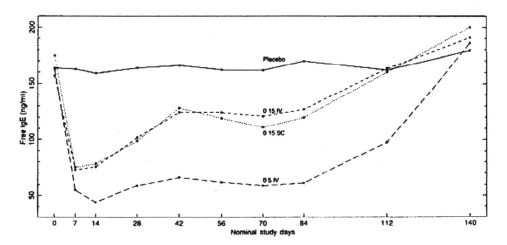

Figure 3   Anti-IgE reduces free IgE antibody serum levels (53). IV or SC injection of anti-IgE antibodies resulted in rapid and sustained reduction of free IgE serum levels for up to 12 weeks in a dose-dependent manner (30).

In summary, the data show that anti-IgE is a safe and well-tolerated drug that can effectively reduce serum IgE levels.

IV. ANTI-IgE AND ASTHMA

A. Effects of Anti-IgE on Early- and Late-Phase Allergic Responses (Phase I/II Studies)

Two studies were performed in patients with mild asthma to test the ability of anti-IgE to inhibit early and late-phase allergic responses after bronchial challenge with allergen (32,33). Anti-IgE treatment was found to significantly decrease IgE serum levels and reduce the early allergic response, as demonstrated by a significant smaller reduction in Forced expiratory volume in 1 second (FEV_1) and a significant increase in median allergen PC15 after allergen challenge on days 27, 55, and 77 (32). A similar effect was observed for the late-phase response to allergen, assessed 2 to 7 hours after allergen provocation (33). Anti-IgE treatment significantly reduced the rise in sputum eosinophils following allergen challenge, an inflammatory reaction linked to the development of the late asthmatic response. No improvement of nospecific hyperresponsiveness, asthma symptom score, or overall lung function was shown after treatment with anti-IgE, compared with placebo. Still, the studies demonstrated that intravenous or subcutaneous administration of anti-IgE is able to reduce early and late-phase allergic responses in patients with asthma.

B. Effects of Anti-IgE on Asthma Symptom Scores (Phase II Study)

The promising results of the early studies had to be confirmed in a large-scale study investigating the efficacy of anti-IgE in the treatment of asthma. Dosing was adapted to individual body weight and serum IgE levels to ensure a constant ratio of IgE to anti-IgE antibody. Administration was by IV route (34).

Treatment with anti-IgE led to a fast decrease in serum IgE levels, which remained stable and below 5% of mean baseline values for 20 weeks. Following treatment with the low or high dose of anti-IgE, the proportion of patients at 12 weeks with at least a 50% reduction in asthma symptom scores was significantly higher than in the placebo group (49% and 47% vs. 24%, $p < 0.001$). The mean reduction of symptom scores from mean baseline score 4.0 for all patients was significantly higher in both the low- (2.8) and the high-dose (2.8) anti-IgE group, compared with placebo (3.1), although patients in the placebo also improved during the course of the study (34).

The requirements for inhaled or oral steroids were reduced in patients treated with anti-IgE: 78% of patients receiving the high dose ($p = 0.04$) and 57% of the low-dose group ($p = 0.23$, n.s.) had at least a 50% reduction in overall steroids after 20 weeks, compared with 33% of patients receiving placebo. The decrease in oral or inhaled steroid medications was associated with a decrease of β_2 agonist use by 1.8 puffs/day in the high-dose anti-IgE group ($p = 0.02$) and by 1.2 puffs/day in the low-dose anti-IgE group ($p = 0.24$), compared with 0.8 puff/day in the placebo group (34).

Treatment with anti-IgE increased morning peak expiratory flow (PEF) at 12 weeks, compared with placebo (low dose, 18.6 l/min, $p = 0.10$; high dose, 30.7 l/min, $p = 0.001$; placebo, 11.3 l/min). Similarly, PEF was improved at the end of the study after 20 weeks (low dose 20.8 l/min, $p = 0.046$; high dose, 29.9 l/min, $p = 0.02$; placebo, 10.2 l/min). FEV_1 improvements were statistically not significant (low dose, +2.1%, $p = 0.49$; high dose, +1.9%, $p = 0.81$; placebo, +1.0%) (34).

During the 20-week study period, 28% of patients in the low-dose anti-IgE group ($p = 0.01$) and 30% of patients in the high-dose anti-IgE group ($p = 0.03$) reported asthma exacerbation, compared with 45% of patients receiving placebo, even though steroid use was reduced to a higher degree in the anti-IgE groups.

In summary, this study showed that anti-IgE improved asthma symptoms, reduced exacerbation rates, and reduced oral or inhaled steroid medications without requirement for increased rescue medication. Improvements by anti-IgE therapy were modest but significantly better than in the placebo group, and occurred despite reductions in steroid and β_2 agonist therapy. There were no complaints concerning the safety and tolerability of anti-IgE antibodies. These promising results inspired succeeding studies with anti-IgE at a larger scale and with modified settings.

C. Effects of Anti-IgE on Asthma Exacerbation (Phase III Studies)

Three identically designed large-scale phase III studies were performed to evaluate the efficacy of anti-IgE in the treatment of asthma: protocol 008 in the United States (35); protocol 009 in the EU, United States, South Africa and Australia (36); and protocol 010 in asthmatic children in the United States (37). In contrast to the phase II study (34), anti-IgE was administered SC rather than IV and only once every 4 weeks for patients with low and intermediate IgE baseline serum levels. The duration of the trial was extended, and the age range of the adult patients increased; the primary endpoints now were frequency of asthma exacerbations. In contrast to the studies in adults, asthma was controlled (not symptomatic) on entry in the children study (37). Differences between anti-IgE– and placebo-treated patients therefore were obvious only during the steroid withdrawal phase in this particular trial.

The main findings of the phase III trials were similar and confirmed the results of the phase II trial (34). Treatment with anti-IgE was significantly more effective than placebo in reducing the number of exacerbations, the primary endpoint of the trials, in both the stable-steroid and the steroid withdrawal phases (Fig. 4). The mean number of exacerbations in the anti-IgE treatment group during the stable-steroid and the steroid withdrawal phases were 58% and 52% lower, respectively ($p < 0.001$ for both) (35). This reduction in asthma exacerbations in the anti-IgE treatment group was obvious despite significantly

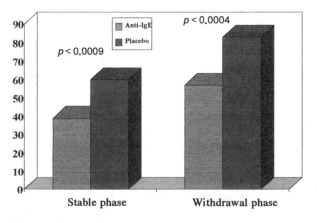

Figure 4 Percentage of patients with asthma exacerbations during stable-steroid and steroid withdrawal phases of a double-blind, placebo-controlled study with anti-IgE (36).

lower use of Inhaled corticosteroids (ICS) (126 µg/d beclamethasone diproprionate (BDP) in the anti-IgE vs. 210 µg/d in the placebo group) or complete withdrawal of BDP (43% anti-IgE vs 19% placebo, $p < 0.001$) during the steroid withdrawal phase.

Symptom scores improved in both the placebo-treated and the anti-IgE–treated patients, but the improvement was significantly higher in the latter group, despite the lower use of corticosteroids. Similar, β_2 agonist use was significantly lower in the anti-IgE group than in the placebo group during the stable-steroid phase (Fig. 5). Lung function improved significantly in patients receiving anti-IgE compared with placebo, as indicated by increases in PEF (18.5 l/min vs. 6.9 l/min, $p < 0.05$) and a small but significant improvement in FEV$_1$ (4.3% vs 1.4%, $p < 0.02$). Most important, anti-IgE treatment was associated with clinically significant improvement in all aspects of asthma-related quality of life (QOL) (38).

Similarly, treatment of asthmatic children with anti-IgE showed significantly better results than placebo during the steroid withdrawal phase for frequency and incidence of exacerbation (number of episodes per patient: 0.42 vs. 2.72, $p < 0.001$), median reduction of BDP doses (100% vs. 67%, $p = 0.001$), complete discontinuation of steroids (55% vs. 39% of patients, $p = 0.004$), and requirements for rescue medication (daily number of puffs 0 vs. 0.46, $p = 0.004$). No statistical differences were found for symptom scores or spirom-

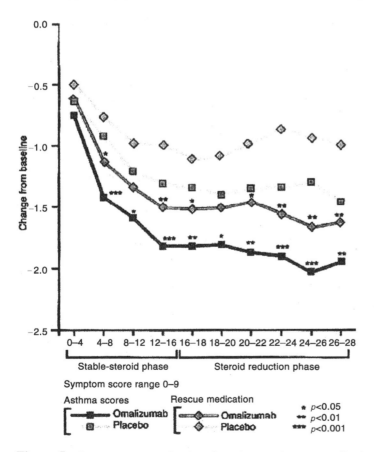

Figure 5 Symptom scores of asthmatic patients and rescue medication use during stable-steroid and steroid withdrawal phases of a double-blind, placebo-controlled study with anti-IgE (35).

etry measurements (PEF) between the two groups in either the stable-steroid or the steroid withdrawal phase (37).

Taken together, the phase III studies show that treatment of adults and children with moderate to severe asthma with anti-IgE is safe, statistically lowering the number of disease exacerbations and reducing ICS use. A pooled analysis of all phase-III studies also demonstrated a reduced need for unscheduled outpatient visits, emergency room treatment, and hospitalization (39).

V. ANTI-IgE AND ALLERGIC RHINITIS

Seasonal allergic rhinitis (SAR) is a frequently underestimated disease with impairment of patients' QOL. Allergen avoidance as a method of secondary intervention is difficult to achieve for these patients, who may be sensitized to multiple outdoor allergens. So far, specific immunotherapy (SIT) is the only available approach (40,41), but its application is restricted somewhat with polysensitized and very young patients. The polysensitized group of patients require therapy for several months of the year and suffer most from decreased QOL (42,43) and reduced productivity at school or the work place (44). Despite optimized treatment regimens, including antihistamines, corticosteroids, and mast cell stabilizers, a subgroup of patients with SAR have insufficient symptom control (45). Therefore, new treatment options are desirable that target more specifically and earlier in the allergic cascade.

A. Efficacy of Anti-IgE in Treatment of SAR in Adults (Phase II Study)

A large-scale trial was performed to assess optimal dosing regimens (30). Anti-IgE decreased serum IgE levels in a dose- and baseline IgE–dependent fashion (Fig. 3), and the specific IgE levels achieved correlated significantly with symptom scores. In none of the treatment groups were IgE levels consistently decreased to less than 25 IU/ml. Patients with IgE levels below detection level (<25 IU/ml) experienced a marked reduction of symptoms, a group of patients too small ($n = 11$) to show significance. Moreover, the averaged symptom score before and during the peak of the season was low (before season 0.6, during season 0.91 in placebo and 0.7 to 0.8 in anti-IgE groups, n.s.), and use of rescue medication was similar for both groups. The QOL scores did not differ between the groups, nor was specific skin test reactivity altered over the course of the study, with the exception of the high-dose anti-IgE group, which developed a marginally significant increase in average endpoint concentration.

These data showed that (1) clinical efficacy is achieved only in patients with significantly reduced IgE levels, and (2) significant suppression of IgE levels requires higher doses of anti-IgE. This necessitated a dosing regimen taking individual body weight and basic IgE levels into account: 0.005 mg anti-IgE/kg body weight/week for each IU baseline IgE /ml serum, doses between 150 and 375 mg per application period of 2 or 4 weeks. Because equivalent results were seen with IV and SC dosing regimens, the latter was preferred in consecutive trials for practical reasons.

B. Effects of Anti-IgE on Symptom Scores in SAR in Adults (Phase III Study)

The results of the previous study (30) warranted further evaluations of the efficacy of anti-IgE therapy in SAR, utilizing higher anti-IgE doses in a randomized, double-blind, placebo-controlled study (46). Serum IgE levels at weeks 3–4 were decreased to less than 25 IU/ml in 113 (69%) of subjects treated with anti-IgE, and exceeded 50 IU/ml only in 3 of these patients. In the placebo group, free IgE levels at weeks 3–4 exceeded 50 ng/ml in all but one subject. A better clinical outcome was significantly correlated with IgE levels below 25 IU/ml. Average daily nasal symptom severity did not change during the course of the study in the anti-IgE group (0.71 at baseline vs. 0.70 total average during study) but increased in the placebo group (0.78 vs. 0.98, $p < 0.001$). Ocular symptom severity scores decreased from 0.47 to 0.43 in anti-IgE–treated patients, but increased from 0.43 to 0.54 in the placebo group ($p = 0.031$). The average use of rescue medication was significantly lower in the anti-IgE group compared with the placebo group (0.59 vs. 1.37 tablets per day, $p < 0.001$), and the proportion of days on which no SAR medication was required was almost twice as high (49% vs. 28%, $p < 0.001$). Statistically significant differences in favor of anti-IgE were similarly observed for estimation of QOL (activities, nasal symptoms, non–nose-eye symptoms, and practical problems). Patients' evaluation of efficacy of treatment favored anti-IgE treatment ($p = 0.001$). Twenty-one percent of serum-treated patients reported complete control of symptoms (vs. 2% of placebo treated), 59% estimated improvement (vs. 35%), and only 2% experienced worsening (vs. 13%) (46).

In conclusion, anti-IgE was safe and effective in controlling birch pollen–induced SAR compared with placebo, with less use of rescue medication and improved QOL. The rather shallow effect of anti-IgE treatment may be explained by an unexpected early pollen season during that specific year of the trial in Scandinavia, which resulted in the beginning of anti-IgE treatment less than 1 week in advance of the first pollen exposure in more than 50% of all patients.

C. Anti-IgE in Combination with SIT in Children with SAR (Phase III Study)

SIT is considered the only curative treatment for SAR and allergic asthma, as long as its prerequisites are fulfilled: small scale of sensitizations and administration of adequate doses of standardized allergens (47,48). Beneficial effects of SIT can be observed even years after discontinuation (49,50). Especially in children, administration of SIT may prevent the extension of upper airway disease to the lower airways. However, SIT carries the risk of side effects. Since anti-IgE reduces the serum concentration of IgE and thereby reduces IgE-mediated reactions, it was hypothesized that concomitant treatment with anti-IgE and SIT would improve the risk/benefit ratio of SIT in polysensitized patients during the consecutive pollen seasons and thereby prove clinically superior to treatment with SIT alone. Therefore, a randomized, double-blind, placebo-controlled study in children with SAR was initiated to investigate whether combined therapy with SIT and anti-IgE is superior to single treatment (51).

Two hundred and twenty-one patients (6–17 years) with moderate to severe SAR and sensitization to birch *and* grass pollen (history ≥2 years, IgE specific to birch and grass CAP class ≥2, total serum IgE levels 30–1300 IU/ml) were included in the study. There were four treatment arms: Each subject was started on SIT-birch (2 groups) *or* SIT-grass (two groups) for ≥14 weeks prior to the start of birch pollen season (build-up phase: 12 injections, 1-week intervals; maintenance phase: 5 injections, 4-week intervals). After SIT titration (12 weeks), placebo *or* anti-IgE was added for 24 weeks to either of the two groups of the respective SIT arms. When analyzed separately by season, the two groups receiving unrelated SIT were considered placebo controls. Anti-IgE was administered SC

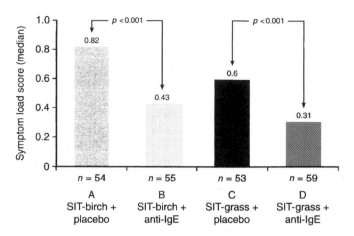

Figure 6   Symptom load (syptom score + rescue medication score) of children with seasonal allergic rhinoconjunctivitis and allergy to grass and birch pollens during the entire pollen season (birch and grass) after preseasonal specific immunotherapy (SIT) with either pollen extract ± anti-IgE (51).

at 2- or 4-week intervals at a dose equivalent to a minimum of 0.016 mg/kg/IU IgE/ml serum in 4 weeks. As primary outcome, the "symptom load" (mean daily symptom severity score plus mean daily rescue medication use) was chosen.

As a result, combination therapy of anti-IgE and SIT was found to reduce the symptom load over the entire pollen seasons (birch and grass) by 48% compared with SIT alone ($p < 0.001$). Reduction was highly significant for both analyses, SIT-birch + anti-IgE vs. SIT-birch + placebo, and SIT-grass + anti-IgE vs. SIT-grass + placebo (Fig. 6).

In the birch pollen season, the addition of anti-IgE to the relevant SIT-birch reduced symptom load by 50% compared with SIT alone (median symptom score 0.46 vs. 0.23, $p = 0.003$). Anti-IgE reduced symptom load in comparison with the irrelevant SIT-grass alone by 39% (0.44 vs. 0.27, $p = 0.1$). Unexpectedly, the patients treated with SIT-birch (+placebo) alone showed a comparable symptom load of 0.46 versus 0.44 ($p = 0.43$) compared with the group treated with SIT-grass (+placebo). This may have been caused by pollen exposure before adequate cumulative SIT doses were administered and may also reflect the very modest symptom load scores in this group.

In the grass pollen season, the relevant SIT-grass reduced symptom load by 32% compared with the irrelevant SIT-birch + placebo (0.61 vs. 0.89, $p = 0.1$). The addition of anti-IgE to the relevant SIT-grass had a highly significant effect, with a 57% decrease in mean symptom load compared with SIT-grass alone (0.26 vs. 0.61, $p = 0.001$). The addition of anti-IgE to the unrelated SIT-birch (considered as treatment with anti-IgE alone) reduced the symptom load by 45% compared with unrelated SIT-birch alone (0.49 vs. 0.89, $p < 0.001$) (51).

Over both pollen seasons, the addition of omalizumab resulted in reduction of the median rescue medication score by 78% compared with the SIT-birch groups (0.06 vs. 0.27; $p < 0.001$) and by as much as 81% compared with the SIT-grass groups (0.03 vs. 0.16; $p = 0.001$).

The results of the study strongly support the primary hypothesis that the combined treatment of SIT and anti-IgE is more effective than SIT alone. Patients receiving anti-IgE required almost no additional rhinitis medication.

In conclusion, the three studies of patients with SAR, together with a published Japanese study of efficacy of omalizumab on SAR associated with cedar pollen allergy (52), suggest the following requirements for successful anti-IgE therapy:

1. The dose regimen must be adapted to personal body weight and IgE base levels.
2. IgE serum levels have to be reduced substantially.
3. Initiation of the anti-IgE treatment has to be far enough in advance of the pollen season/allergen exposure.

VI. ANTI-IgE AND PEANUT ALLERGY

IgE-mediated allergic reactions to peanut may occur early in childhood and are potentially life threatening, especially since allergen avoidance is difficult due to unintended ingestion. Anti-IgE therapy was used in a double-blind, randomized dose-ranging trial in 84 adult patients with a history of immediate hypersensitivity reactions to peanut confirmed by challenge tests with peanut flour. A 450-mg dose of anti-IgE injected subcutaneously every 4 weeks increased the threshold of allergic reactions to peanut upon oral food challenge from a level equal to half a peanut (178 mg) to one equal to almost nine peanuts (2805 mg), an effect that should translate into protection against most unintended ingestions of peanuts (Fig. 7) (53). This study is the first proof of the concept that anti-IgE therapy is a novel and effective approach in the treatment of food allergies.

VII. CONCLUSION

The most advanced of a variety of novel therapeutic approaches to allergic diseases is treatment with recombinant humanized anti-IgE antibodies. Targeting IgE aims at the common and most distinct phenotype in all patients suffering from allergic diseases: increased IgE production. There are extensive evidential data demonstrating a pivotal role for IgE in the development of bronchial asthma. These include increased IgE serum levels associated with prevalence rates and disease severity (54,55), asthma in children almost

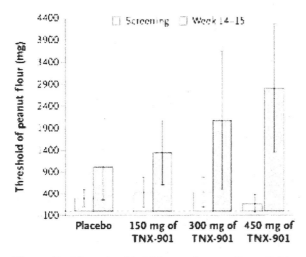

Figure 7 Mean threshhold doses of peanut flour eliciting symptoms in patients receiving placebo or anti-IgE (53).

always associated with production of allergen-specific IgE and positive skin test reactivity against environmental allergens (54), and even in patients with nonallergic asthma with normal IgE serum levels, extensive production of IgE in large areas of the airways (56). On the other hand, experimental data from murine models demonstrate that development of airway inflammation and hyperreactivity, two main features of the disease, may occur independently of B-cells (57), IgE production (58) or IgE-mediated mast cell activation (59). Concordantly, in animals with a robust allergen-mediated inflammatory response in the airways, treatment with anti-IgE antibodies does not inhibit development of airway inflammation or hyperreactivity (60).

The findings of clinical phase II and III trials with anti-IgE antibody treatment in asthmatic patients show that anti-IgE is an effective therapy for moderate to severe allergic asthma. It reduces the frequency of exacerbations, improves symptom scores, and reduces the requirements for steroid medication, important especially in consideration of future treatment strategies for childhood asthma. Similarly important, it is safe and tolerated. Some improvements in symptom scores, exacerbation rates, and lung function during the course of the trials were also seen in the placebo-treated group, presumably demonstrating the benefits of continuous physician monitoring; but the differences between the anti-IgE– and the placebo-treated groups reached significance for almost all important endpoints in favor of anti-IgE. The results show that anti-IgE is efficacious and safe for treatment of asthma.

The situation for SAR appears to be less complicated. SAR clearly is a mainly IgE-mediated disease, in which chronic inflammation and remodeling of anatomical structures are not as important as in asthma. The immediate hypersensitivity reaction to environmental allergens, triggered by allergen-specific IgE and IgE-mediated mast cell activation, is the basic pathophysiological correlate to the symptoms apparent in patients with SAR. Thus, targeting IgE is a plausible way of preventive therapy for SAR.

Clinical phase II and III trials investigating the safety and efficacy of anti-IgE for treatment of SAR demonstrated that anti-IgE effectively reduces serum IgE levels and allergen-related symptoms and increases QOL. Moreover, anti-IgE is not allergen specific and thus adds to the beneficial effects of SIT—a very significant improvement for the often multisensitized SAR patients, who suffer from long pollen seasons and frequent comorbidity of the lower airways. In contrast to SIT, anti-IgE has the drawback that its effect may be transient, but the advantage that it is not allergen specific. Even more important, treatment with anti-IgE antibodies may help to prevent the "allergic march," the development of allergen-mediated airway diseases such as bronchial asthma in patients with predisposing SAR. Effective control of SAR thus may provide preventive and/or therapeutic treatment of concomitant respiratory diseases.

In patients with peanut allergy, there is currently no adequate treatment of or protection against the accidental ingestion of peanuts other than avoidance. The first clinical trial demonstrates that anti-IgE is able to increase the threshold of sensitivity to peanuts.

Future trials should examine the efficacy of anti-IgE in comparison with standard medication for treatment of allergic diseases, and perform cost-related analysis of the advantages of anti-IgE treatment. New areas of potential indications for anti-IgE should be investigated, especially those where IgE plays a major role in development of the disease. Food allergies in infancy require expensive diets, insect venom–allergic patients are at risk of anaphylactic reactions, side effects during (rush) SIT are a major safety issue, and severe atopic dermatitis is often associated with high IgE serum levels. Here, anti-IgE may be a very valuable and even cost-reducing addition to standard therapies. Finally, future trials must identify and/or predict "responders" versus "nonresponders." This will help to outline the optimal target group of patients that may ideally benefit from anti-IgE therapy.

VIII. SALIENT POINTS

1. Anti-IgE therapy is effective for seasonal allergic rhinitis, allergic bronchial asthma and food allergy.
2. The efficacy of anti-IgE therapy is dose dependent.
3. For optimal efficacy, anti-IgE must be adjusted to personal body weight and baseline total IgE serum levels: 0.016 mg anti-IgE mAb per kg body weight and IU of IgE per ml serum.
4. Anti-IgE may be administered IV or SC, and injections have to be repeated every 4 to 6 weeks to maintain reduction of IgE serum levels.
5. For optimal efficacy, anti-IgE therapy has to be started far in advance of the pollen season/allergen exposure.
6. The optimal duration of anti-IgE therapy is unknown, but it is likely that anti-IgE has to be administered continuously (for food and perennial allergies) or every season (for seasonal allergic rhinitis and/or asthma).
7. Anti-IgE therapy is effective in all age groups that have been studied so far: greater than 6 and less than 60 years of age.
8. The combination of anti-IgE therapy with specific immune therapy (SIT) is superior to both treatment strategies alone in terms of symptom severity and concomitant medication use. Combination therapy may permit a broader use of SIT by reducing the risk of anaphylactic side effects after SIT injections.

REFERENCES

1. Ramirez M. Horse asthma following blood transfusion: Report on a case. J AM Med Assoc 1919;1 73:984.
2. Prausnitz C, Küstner H. Studienüber die Überempfindlichkeit Zbl Bakt 1921; 86:160–160.
3. Ishizaka K, Ishizaka T, Hornbrook MM. Physico-chemical properties of human reaginic antibody: IV. Presence of a unique immunoglobulin as a carrier of reaginic activity. J Immunol 1966; 97:75–85.
4. Ishizaka K, Ishizaka T. Identification of gamma-E-antibodies as a carrier of reaginic activity. J Immunol 1967; 99:1187–1198.
5. Johansson SG. Raised levels of a new immunoglobulin class (IgND) in asthma. Lancet 1967; 2:951–953.
6. Bennich HH, Ishizaka K, Johansson SG, Rowe DS, Stanworth DR, Terry WD. Immunoglobulin E: A new class of human immunoglobulin. Immunology 1968; 15:323–324.
7. Coffman RL, Seymour BW, Lebman DA, Hiraki DD, Christiansen JA, Shrader B, Cherwinski HM, Savelkoul HF, Finkelman FD, Bond MW. The role of helper T cell products in mouse B cell differentiation and isotype regulation. Immunol Rev 1988; 102:5–28.
8. Coffman RL, Carty J. A T cell activity that enhances polyclonal IgE production and its inhibition by interferon-gamma. J Immunol 1986; 136:949–954.
9. Mosmann TR, Cherwinski H, Bond MW, Giedlin MA, Coffman RL. Two types of murine helper T cell clone: I. Definition according to profiles of lymphokine activities and secreted proteins. J Immunol 1986; 136:2348–2357.
10. Lebman DA, Coffman RL. Interleukin 4 causes isotype switching to IgE in T cell–stimulated clonal B cell cultures. J Exp Med 1988; 168:853–862.

11. Jabara HH, Schneider LC, Shapira SK, et al. Induction of germline and mature Ce transcripts in human B cells stimulated with rIL-4 and EBV. J Immunol 1990; 145:3468–3473.

12. Vercelli D, Jabara HH, Arai K, Geha RS. Induction of human IgE synthesis requires interleukin 4 and T-B cell interaction involving the T cell receptor/CD3 complex and MHC-class II antigens. J Exp Med 1989; 169:1295–1307.

13. Jabara HH, Fu SM, Geha RS, Vercelli D. Synergism between anti-CD40 mAb and IL-4 in the induction of IgE synthesis by highly purified human B cells. J Exp Med 1990; 172:1861–1864.

14. Blank U, Ra C, Miller L, White K, Metzger H, Kinet JP. Complete structure and expression in transfected cells of high affinity IgE receptor. Nature 1989; 337:187–189.

15. Gounni AS, Lamkhioued B, Delaporte E, Dubost A, Kinet JP, Capron A, Capron M. The high-affinity IgE receptor on eosinophils: From allergy to parasites or from parasites to allergy?. J Allergy Clin Immunol 1994; 94:1214–1216.

16. Kehry MR, Yamashita LC. Low-affinity IgE receptor (CD23) function on mouse B cells: Role in IgE-dependent antigen focusing. Proc Natl Acad Sci U S A 1989; 86:7556–7560.

17. Conrad DH. Fc epsilon RII/CD23: The low affinity receptor for IgE. Annu Rev Immunol 1990; 8:623–645.

18. Holgate ST, Robinson C, Church MK, Howarth PH. The release and role of inflammatory mediators in asthma. Clin Immunol Rev 1985; 4:241–288.

19. Holgate ST. Contribution of inflammatory mediators to the immediate asthmatic reaction. Am Rev Respir Dis 1987; 135:S57–S62.

20. Bradding P, Roberts JA, Britten KM, et al. Interleukin-4, -5, and -6 and tumor necrosis factor–alpha in normal and asthmatic airways: Evidence for the human mast cell as a source of these cytokines. Am J Respir Cell Mol Biol 1994; 10:471–480.

21. Galli SJ, Wershil BK, Gordon JR, Martin TR. Mast cells: Immunologically specific effectors and potential sources of multiple cytokines during IgE-dependent responses. Ciba Found Symp 1989; 147:53–65, discussion 65–73.

22. Presta L, Shields R, O'Connell L, et al. The binding site on human immunoglobulin E for its high affinity receptor. J Biol Chem 1994; 269:26368–26373.

23. Saban R, Haak-Frendscho M, Zine M, et al. Human FcɛRI-IgG and humanized anti-IgE monoclonal antibody MaE11 block passive sensitization of human and rhesus monkey lung. J Allergy Clin Immunol 1994; 94:836–843.

24. Presta LG, Lahr SJ, Shields RL, et al. Humanization of an antibody directed against IgE. J Immunol 1993; 151:2623–2632.

25. Fox JA, Hotaling TE, Struble C, Ruppel J, Bates DJ, Schoenhoff MB. Tissue distribution and complex formation with IgE of an anti-IgE antibody after intravenous administration in cynomolgus monkeys. J Pharmacol Exp Ther 1996; 279:1000–1008.

26. MacGlashan D Jr, Bochner BS, Adelman DC, Jardieu PM, Togias A, McKenzie-White J, Sterbinsky SA, Hamilton RG, Lichtenstein LM. Down-regulation of FcɛRI-expression on human basophils during in vivo treatment with anti-IgE antibody. J Immunol 1997; 158:1438–1445.

27. Boesel KM, Griffith DT, Prussin C, Foster B, Liu H, Casale TB. Rapid reduction of basophil FcɛRI expression by omalizumab. J Allergy Clin Immunol 2003; III:264.

28. Fick RBJ. Anti-IgE as novel therapy for the treatment of asthma. Curr Opin Pulm Med 1999; 5:76–80.

29. Jardieu PM, Fick RBJ. IgE inhibition as a therapy for allergic disease. Int Arch Allergy Immunol 1999; 118:112–115.

30. Casale TB, Bernstein IL, Busse WW, et al. Use of an anti-IgE humanized monoclonal antibody in ragweed-induced allergic rhinitis. J Allergy Clin Immunol 1997; 100:110–121.

31. Fahy JV, Cockcroft DW, Boulet LP, et al. Effect of aerosolized anti-IgE (E25) on airway responses to inhaled allergen in asthmatic subjects. Am J Respir Crit Care Med 1999; 160:1023–1027.

32. Boulet LP, Chapman KR, Cote J, et al. Inhibitory effects of an anti-IgE antibody E25 on allergen-induced early asthmatic response. Am J Respir Crit Care Med 1997; 155: 1835–1840.

33. Fahy JV, Fleming HE, Wong HH, et al. The effect of an anti-IgE monoclonal antibody on the early- and late-phase responses to allergen inhalation in asthmatic subjects. Am J Respir Crit Care Med 1997; 155:1828–1834.

34. Milgrom H, Fick RBJ, Su JQ, et al. Treatment of allergic asthma with monoclonal anti-IgE antibody: rhuMAb-E25 Study Group. N Engl J Med 1999; 341:1966–1973.

35. Busse W, Corren J, Lanier BQ, et al. Omalizumab, anti-IgE recombinant humanized monoclonal antibody, for the treatment of severe allergic asthma. J Allergy Clin Immunol 2001; 108:184–190.

36. Soler M, Matz J, Townley R, et al. The anti-IgE antibody omalizumab reduces exacerbations and steroid requirement in allergic asthmatics. Eur Respir J 2001; 18:254–261.

37. Milgrom H, Berger W, Nayak A, et al. Treatment of childhood asthma with anti–immunoglobulin E antibody (omalizumab). Pediatrics 2001; 108:E36.

38. Buhl R, Hanf G, Solèr M, Bensch G, Wolfe J, Everhard F, Champain K, Fox H, Thirlwell J. The anti-IgE antibody omalizumab improves asthma-related quality of life in patients with allergic asthma. ERS 2002; 20:1088–1094.

39. Corren J, Casale T, Deniz Y, Ashby M. Omalizumab, a recombinant humanized anti-IgE antibody, reduces asthma-related emergency room visits and hospitalizations in patients with allergic asthma. J Allergy Clin Immunol 2003; 111:87–90.

40. Norman PS. Modern concepts of immunotherapy. Curr Opin Immunol 1993; 5:968–973.

41. Lieberman P, Patterson R. Immunotherapy for atopic disease. Adv Intern Med 1974; 19:391–411.

42. Juniper EF, Guyatt GH, Dolovich J. Assessment of quality of life in adolescents with allergic rhinoconjunctivitis: Development and testing of a questionnaire for clinical trials. J Allergy Clin Immunol 1994; 93:413–423.

43. Juniper EF, Guyatt GH, Griffith LE, Ferrie PJ. Interpretation of rhinoconjunctivitis quality of life questionnaire data. J Allergy Clin Immunol 1996; 98:843–845.

44. Malone DC, Lawson KA, Smith DH, Arrighi HM, Battista C. A cost of illness study of allergic rhinitis in the United States. J Allergy Clin Immunol 1997; 99:22–27.

45. White P, Smith H, Baker N, Davis W, Frew A. Symptom control in patients with hay fever in UK general practice: How well are we doing and is there a need for allergen immunotherapy? Clin Exp Allergy 1998; 28:266–270.

46. Adelroth E, Rak S, Haahtela T, Assand G, Rosenhall L, Zetterstrom O, Byrne A, Champain K, Thirlwell J, Cioppa GD, Sandstrom T. Recombinant humanized mAb-E25, an anti-IgE mAb, in birch pollen–induced seasonal allergic rhinitis. J Allergy Clin Immunol 2000; 106:253–259.

47. Practice parameters for allergen immunotherapy. Joint Task Force on Practice Parameters, representing the American Academy of Allergy, Asthma and Immunology, the American College of Allergy, Asthma and Immunology, and the Joint Council of Allergy, Asthma and Immunology. J Allergy Clin Immunol 1996; 98:1001–1011.

48. Bousquet J, Lockey RF, Malling H (eds.). Allergen immunotherapy: Therapeutic vaccines for allergic diseases. Geneva: January 27–29, 1997. Allergy 1998; 53:1–42.

49. Durham SR, Walker SM, Varga EM, Jacobson MR, O'Brien F, Noble W, Till SJ, Hamid QA, Nouri-Aria KT. Long-term clinical efficacy of grass-pollen immunotherapy. N Engl J Med 1999; 341:468–475.

50. Walker SM, Varney VA, Gaga M, Jacobson MR, Durham SR. Grass pollen immunotherapy: Efficacy and safety during a 4-year follow-up study. Allergy 1995; 50:405–413.

51. Kuehr J, Brauburger J, Zielen S, Schauer U, Kamin W, Von Berg A, Leupold W, Bergmann KC, Rolinck-Werninghaus C, Gräve M, Hultsch T, Wahn U. Efficacy of combination treatment with anti-IgE plus specific immunotherapy in polysensitized children and adolescents with seasonal allergic rhinitis. J Allergy Clin Immunol 2001 (in press).

52. Ishikawa T. Clinical Efficacy of omalizumab on seasonal allergic rhinitis associated with Japanese cedar pollen. J Allergy Clin Immunol 2003; 111:84.

53. Leung DYM, Sampson HA, Yunginger JW, Burks AW Jr, Schneider LC, Wortel CH, Dabis FM, Hyun JD, Shanahan WR Jr. TNX-901Peanut Allergy Study Group: Effect of Anti-IgE therapy in patients with peanut allergy. N Engl J Med 2003; 348:986–993.

54. Sears MR, Burrows B, Flannery EM, Herbison GP, Hewitt CJ, Holdaway MD. Relation between airway responsiveness and serum IgE in children with asthma and in apparently normal children. N Engl J Med 1991; 325:1067–1071.

55. Burrows B, Martinez FD, Halonen M, Barbee RA, Cline MG. Association of asthma with serum IgE levels and skin-test reactivity to allergens. N Engl J Med 1989; 320:271–277.

56. Humbert M, Grant JA, Taborda-Barata L, Durham SR, Pfister R, Menz G, Barkans J, Ying S, Kay AB. High-affinity IgE receptor (FcεRI)-bearing cells in bronchial biopsies from atopic and nonatopic asthma. Am J Respir Crit Care Med 1996; 153:1931–1937.

57. Hamelmann E, Takeda K, Schwarze J, Vella AT, Irvin CG, Gelfand EW. Development of eosinophilic airway inflammation and airway hyperresponsiveness requires interleukin-5 but not immunoglobulin E or B lymphocytes (see comments). Am J Respir Cell Mol Biol 1999; 21:480–489.

58. Oettgen HC, Martin TR, Wynshaw BA, Deng C, Drazen JM, Leder P. Active anaphylaxis in IgE-deficient mice. Nature 1994; 370:367–370.

59. Takeda K, Hamelmann E, Joetham A, et al. Development of eosinophilic airway inflammation and airway hyperresponsiveness in mast cell-deficient mice. J Exp Med 1997; 186:449–454.

60. Hamelmann E, Cieslewicz G, Schwarze J, et al. Anti-interleukin 5 but not anti-IgE prevents airway inflammation and airway hyperresponsiveness. Am J Respir Crit Care Med 1999; 160:934–941.

35

Modifying Allergens and Using Adjuvants for Specific Immunotherapy

MARK LARCHÉ

*Imperial College London Faculty of Medicine,
London, England*

FATIMA FERREIRA

University of Salzburg, Salzburg, Austria

SHYAM S. MOHAPATRA

*University of South Florida College of Medicine and James A. Haley
Veterans' Hospital, Tampa, Florida, U.S.A.*

I. INTRODUCTION

Allergen specific immunotherapy (SIT) is an effective form of treatment for allergic diseases caused by inhalant allergens (e.g., pollen, mites, animal dander) and insect venom. Despite being initially described at the turn of the twentieth century, SIT remains the only "curative" approach to atopic allergic disease. In addition to the ability to modulate existing disease, SIT is capable of modifying the natural course by preventing the worsening of symptoms (from rhinitis to asthma) and the onset of sensitization against new allergens (1,2). SIT consists of administering increasing doses of natural allergen preparations on a regular basis; the beneficial effects for the patient depend on the amount of allergen given. Typically, between 5 and 20 µg of the major allergen is required in each monthly maintenance injection to achieve optimal clinical efficacy. Because SIT involves injecting allergens into a sensitized individual, the occurrence of typical allergic symptoms is frequent, with risks increasing with higher concentration of the allergen injected. Several immunological pathways are involved in the clinical improvement achieved by the usual SIT schedules (3,4): a rise in allergen-specific IgG antibodies, in particular IgG4, which exerts its effect by neutralizing allergen and blocking IgE-facilitated allergen presentation to T-cells (5); generation of antigen-specific CD8+ suppressor T-cells (6); a reduction in the number of mast cells and eosinophils, and diminished release of mediators (7,8); modulation of allergen-specific T-cells—a shift from the TH2 to the TH1 cytokine pattern with a decrease of IL-4 and IL-5 production accompanied by an increase of IFN-γ (immune deviation) (9,10). Moreover, the induction of an anergic state in peripheral T-cells (immunological tolerance) has been reported. The latter may be mediated by IL-10 and has been characterized by suppressed proliferative and cytokine responses against major allergens (11).

Although this type of therapy is widely established, three major problems are still associated with SIT:

1. SIT is performed with allergen vaccines that contain mixtures of extracts of allergens, nonallergenic and/or toxic proteins including bacterial endotoxin, and other macromolecules that are difficult to standardize. Indeed, it has been shown that SIT administration of allergen vaccines can lead to the development of new specific IgE reactivities to allergenic components in the vaccines (12).
2. Severe IgE-mediated side effects can occur during the treatment due to systemic administration of fully active allergens.
3. Therapeutically effective doses often cannot be achieved because of adverse events or poor standardization of extracts.

II. RECOMBINANT AND ENGINEERED ALLERGENS

Many of the problems associated with SIT could be overcome by the use of genetically engineered allergens (13,14). Cocktails of pure and standardized recombinant allergens can be formulated to replace natural extracts, and the selected recombinant allergens can be engineered to reduce the risk of IgE-mediated side effects. Genetic engineering of allergens for SIT aims at the production of modified molecules with reduced IgE-binding epitopes (hypoallergens) while preserving structural motifs necessary for T-cell receptor recognition and for induction of IgG antibodies (blocking antibodies) reactive with the natural allergen. The uptake of allergens by antigen-presenting cells (APCs) is mediated and facilitated by the interaction of the allergen with specific IgE (15,16) and leads to enhanced production of TH2 cytokines and IgE production. Engineered allergens lacking IgE binding are designed to avoid these pathways and preferentially target APCs (e.g., monocytes, macrophages, and dendritic cells) that utilize phagocytosis or pinocytosis for antigen uptake. This in turn induces a balanced TH0- or TH1-like cytokine production by T-cells, and low IgE and high IgG production by B-cells. The presence of intact T-cell epitopes in hypoallergens enables targeting of T-cells, allowing administration of higher doses to induce tolerance of allergen-specific T-cells and alteration of cytokine production toward a TH1-like pattern. In this way, vaccines containing recombinant allergens could replace natural extracts and increase the efficacy and safety of SIT.

A. Low IgE-Binding Natural Isoforms

cDNA cloning of allergens has demonstrated that many major allergens are encoded by gene families. Within individual allergen sequences, polymorphisms have been described such as those found in ragweed Amb a 1 (17), hazel Cor a 1 (18), birch Bet v 1 (19), Group 1 and Group 5 grass allergens (20,21), apple Mal d 1 (22), celery Api g 1 (23), *Parietaria* Par j 1 (24), olive Ole e 1 (25), Group 2 dust mite allergens (26), latex Hev b 7 (27), and cow dander Bos d 2 (28). Due to sequence variations, it was proposed that isoallergens might have different antigenic and/or allergenic activities. Differences in T-cell reactivity of isoforms has previously been reported for Cor a 1 (29), Bet v 1 (30), Phl p 5 (31), and Der p 2 (32).

Investigation of the IgE-binding activity of isoallergens led to the identification of naturally occurring Bet v 1 hypoallergens (33). Isoforms Bet v 1d, Bet v 1g, and Bet v 1l were found to be highly antigenic in T-cell proliferation assays and poorly allergenic in vitro and in vivo. The crystal structure of the hypoallergenic isoform Bet v 1l was determined (34) and shown not to differ significantly from the high IgE-binding isoform Bet v 1a. Thus, the low IgE-binding activity of certain isoforms is not due to problems in the recombinant production. Such well-characterized low IgE-binding molecules would be excellent candidates for specific immunotherapy. However, naturally occurring hypoallergens have not been identified for other allergen families and, instead, genetic engineering has been widely used to generate low-IgE binding variants.

B. Engineered Allergens

Genetic engineering involves the modification of a targeted protein in order to alter its function or properties in a predictable manner. This requires the complete understanding of the relationship between structure and function/properties for precise and effective manipulation. Alteration of the encoding gene includes changing specific basepairs (mutated gene), introduction of a new piece of DNA into the existing gene DNA molecule (chimeric or hybrid gene), and deletions (truncated gene or fragments) (Fig. 1). With the exception of the DNA shuffling approach (described later), which bypasses the need to identify amino acid residues or motifs that are important to structure and function, engineering of allergens usually requires knowledge of B- and T-cell epitopes and, in some cases, also of the three-dimensional structure of the allergen. No matter how allergen genes have been altered, putative hypoallergens must be subjected to a series of in vitro and in vivo evaluation procedures before being considered for therapeutic purposes (Fig. 1). To date, cDNA sequences of approximately 345 allergens (60 pollens, 39 mites, 17 mammalian, 74 fungi, 63 insects, 79 foods, and 13 latex) have been deposited in the allergen databank (http://www.allergen.org). Some examples of engineered inhalant allergens and their evaluation are discussed later. The use of engineered allergens for the treatment of food allergies has also generated interest (35).

1. Site-Directed Mutants

After identification of crucial amino acid residues or motifs involved in IgE recognition, dominant epitopes can be targeted using site-directed mutagenesis. The observation that Bet v 1 and other, closely related tree pollen allergens consist of a mixture of closely related isoforms displaying striking differences in their ability to bind IgE (36) constituted the basis for engineering a Bet v 1 hypoallergen (37). The patterns of amino acid substitutions in tree pollen isoallergens and their IgE-binding activities were analyzed using a

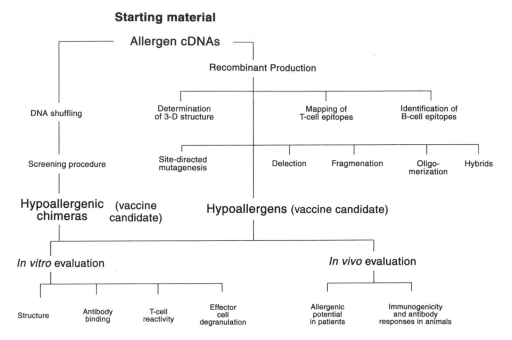

Figure 1 Task tree for genetic engineering and evaluation of hypoallergens for specific immunotherapy.

computer algorithm developed to predict functional residues in protein sequences (38). Using in vitro site-directed mutagenesis, the amino acid residues occurring in positions 113, 57, 125, 112, 30, and 10 of Bet v 1a were substituted with those present in the same positions of low IgE-binding isoforms. Thus, a Bet v 1 mutant was produced carrying six point mutations that displayed extremely low IgE-binding activity for all patients tested. In vivo (skin prick) tests indicated that the potency of the six-point mutant to induce typical wheal-and-flare skin reactions in allergic individuals was dramatically reduced (100- to 1000-fold) compared with Bet v 1a. T-cell clones (TCC) established from the peripheral blood of birch pollen–allergic patients and reactive with Bet v 1a were also activated by the six-point mutant.

B- and T-cell epitope mapping and sequence comparison of Group 5 allergens from different grasses provided the basic information for introducing point mutations in highly conserved sequence domains of rye grass pollen Lol p 5. Hypoallergenic forms of Lol p 5 were produced that contained all relevant T-cell epitopes (39). Similarly, hypoallergenic variants of latex Hev b 5 (40), apple Mal d 1 (22), egg Gal d 1 (41), and peanut Ara h 1, Ara h 2, and Ara h 3 (35,42) were also generated by site-directed mutagenesis. Peanut hypoallergens have been tested in a murine model of peanut anaphylaxis (43).

2. Conformational Variants

Bee venom phospholipase A_2 (PLA) preparations, lacking native conformation and antibody-binding activity, were exclusively presented by monocytes and induced a TH1-biased cytokine profile leading to IgG4 production by B-cells (44). In contrast, folded PLA with full antibody-binding activity, processed and presented by B-cells, stimulated TH2-like cytokines and induced IgE antibodies. Thus, the three dimensional structure of an antigen and its recognition by different APCs has a crucial influence on the development of distinct T-cell cytokine patterns. These findings further support the use of hypoallergens in aeroallergen immunotherapy. This led to production of hypoallergenic variants of the major allergen of Par j 1 (45). Par j 1 is a member of the nonspecific lipid transfer proteins (nsLTPs) with a characteristic α-α-α-α-β structure, which is stabilized by four disulfide bonds. Targeting these disulfide bonds by site-directed mutagenesis produced molecules with altered conformation and decreased IgE-binding activity that retained their ability to stimulate T-cell proliferation. Disruption of native conformation by targeting disulfide bonds could be a generally applicable approach for engineering allergenic nsLTPs, including food-derived members. Disulfide bonds stabilizing the antigenic structure of major allergens of dust mites have also been targeted by site-directed mutagenesis. Hypoallergenic variants of Der p 2 (46), Der f 2 (47), and Lep d 2 (48) were produced and evaluated for their IgE-mediated reactions and cellular responses. However, caution is required in targeting the conformation of allergens, as this may reduce the solubility of the final product, since denatured or unfolded proteins tend to form aggregates.

3. Deletion Mutants

Knowledge of IgE-reactive regions of allergens can be used to engineer hypoallergenic variants by deleting the corresponding DNA segment in the gene. This approach was successfully used for the timothy grass pollen allergen Phl p 5b (49). Epitope mapping was performed using overlapping recombinant fragments, and at least four continuous IgE-binding epitopes were identified. Deletions avoiding identified T-cell epitopes were then performed within these IgE-binding regions. Some of these deletion mutants showed reduced IgE-binding properties, no histamine-releasing activity, reduced skin reactivity, and no significant changes in T-cell reactivity. A similar approach was used to engineer hypoallergens of the American cockroach Per a 1 allergen (50). Based on the results obtained by proteolytic fingerprinting, a deletion mutant of ryegrass Lol p 1 was produced, which displayed decreased IgE-binding activity and did not trigger histamine release up to a concentration of 10 mg/ml (51). The mutant was not tested in T-cell proliferation assays or for skin reactivity.

4. Allergen Oligomers

Vrtala et al. (52) constructed a Bet v 1 oligomeric form consisting of three copies of full-length Bet v 1 cDNA linked by short oligonucleotide spacers in one open reading frame. Recombinant Bet v 1 monomer and trimer produced in *Escherichia coli* showed comparable in vitro IgE-binding activity and strongly stimulated Bet v 1–specific TCC and PBMC from birch pollen-allergic patients. The Bet v 1 trimer exhibited extremely low histamine release from patients' basophils, and its skin reactivity compared to the monomer. When injected in mice and rabbits, the trimer induced IgG antibodies that inhibited human IgE binding to Bet v 1 monomer. Several explanations were proposed to explain why the IgE-binding Bet v 1 trimer showed reduced anaphylactic potential: lower affinity for IgE binding; reorientation of IgE epitopes preventing efficient cross-linking of FcεRI-bound IgE antibodies; and microaggregation, steric hindrance, and/or unfavorable charge interactions causing concealment of IgE epitopes required for efficient cross-linking.

5. Allergen Chimeras

King et al. (53) genetically modified allergens by preparing hybrids consisting of a small portion of the "guest" allergen of interest and a large portion of a homologous but weakly cross-reacting host protein. The homologous host protein serves as a scaffold to maintain the native structure of the guest allergen of interest in order to preserve conformation-dependent B-cell epitopes, but at a reduced density. The homologous allergens from yellow jacket venom Ves v 5 and from paper wasp Pol a 5 (59% sequence identity) show very limited cross-reactivity of antibodies from sensitized patients. Hybrids of these two molecules containing 10–49 residues of Ves v 5 showed 100- to 3000-fold reduction in allergenicity in histamine release assay with basophils from yellow jacket–sensitized patients.

Hybrids consisting of head-to-tail fusions of Phl p 5 and Phl p 1 and of Phl p 6 and Phl p 2 allergens were engineered by PCR with the aim of producing combination vaccines for grass pollen immunotherapy (54). These hybrids were not hypoallergens and contained most of the IgE and T-cell epitopes of natural grass pollen extract. However, these hybrids showed higher immunogenic activity than the individual allergens when injected in mice, and thus may be useful for vaccine development.

As discussed previously, directed mutagenesis has been used widely to generate hypoallergens. As with other rational design methods, understanding of the relationship between structure and function/properties is required. The approach has the limitation that substitutions of amino acids or segments must be appropriate for the specific position in which they are found in the protein. The effects of substitutions, even chemically conserved ones, are practically impossible to predict with the current knowledge-based system. DNA shuffling or molecular breeding is a novel approach that mimics natural evolution and can be performed without prior knowledge of structural or functional characteristics of the target molecules (55). It allows the generation of large and complex libraries of novel chimeric genes, from which variants with desired properties can be selected using appropriate screening methods. The features of the DNA family shuffling method would allow the generation of allergen chimeras having T-cell epitopes derived from several family members, but at the same time with reduced anaphylatic potential and increased immunogenicity (56). This could prove to be an extremely efficient approach for the production of optimal molecules for more efficient and safer forms of allergen vaccines.

6. Allergen DNA Vaccines

An attractive alternative for immunotherapy using allergen proteins is the use of allergen genes in genetic immunization approaches. Intramuscular or intradermal injection of plasmid DNA encoding clinically relevant allergens can induce long-lasting immune responses with a TH1 bias and promote the formation of IFN-γ–producing CD4+ T-cells (57–59). After subcutaneous administration of plasmid DNA encoding an allergen, transcripts have been simultaneously detected in several tissues. Furthermore, immunization of mice with an allergen cDNA cloned in a plasmid vehicle resulted in an allergen-specific IgG2a and TH1-like response, with no detectable IgE response. This was in contrast to immunization with allergen, which induced an IgE antibody response. However, despite the potential of this approach, no studies have been performed in humans to date, largely due to concerns over the introduction of "active" genetic material into humans.

III. ALLERGEN FRAGMENTS

A. Large Allergen Fragments

IgE epitopes can be formed by linear sequences of amino acids (continuous epitopes) or by nonadjacent sequence elements brought together by folding (discontinuous or contormation-dependent epitopes). IgE recognition of continuous epitopes may also depend on their conformation, which might occur only in the context of the folded allergen molecule. Thus, disruption of the three-dimensional structure by fragmentation could be a useful approach to reduce the anaphylactic potential of allergens. The three-dimensional structure of Bet v 1 was disrupted by expressing in *E. coli* two fragments of the cDNA, which corresponded to amino acids 1–74 and 75–160 (60). The fragments exhibited random coil conformation and almost no allergenicity. Together, the fragments harbored all relevant T-cell epitopes. Skin reactivity and histamine release greatly reduced compared with the native intact Bet v 1 allergen (61). Moreover, immunization of mice and rabbits with Bet v 1 fragments induced IgG antibodies that inhibited binding of IgE from allergic patients to wild-type Bet v 1 (62). Clinical trials are currently being performed to determine the efficacy of vaccines based on Bet v 1 fragments for immunotherapy of birch pollen–allergic patients.

Non-anaphylactic fragments of the major house dust mite allergen Der f 2 were produced by C- and N-terminal deletions and mixed after separate refolding of the denatured fragments (63). Fragments of the calcium-binding allergens Bet v 4 (64) and Aln g 4 (65), and an N-terminal fragment of Lol p 1 from ryegrass (51) also showed decreased IgE-binding activities. However, these fragments have yet to be studied with respect to T-cell reactivity and immunogenicity.

B. T-Cell Peptide Epitopes

Peptide immunotherapy is an approach that targets CD4+ T-cells by using allergen-derived peptides containing short linear T-cell epitopes to induce tolerance. This approach is similar in many ways to the use of allergen fragments but employs smaller sequences specifically selected for activity as T-cell epitopes. The principle has been established in animal models, and the reduced ability of short peptide epitopes to cross-link surface-bound IgE may provide an attractive alternative to SIT in humans.

In vitro experiments have demonstrated that different concentrations of peptides can induce activation or hyporesponsiveness depending on the dose. Lamb and colleagues (66) employed high doses (50 μg) of peptide to render human T-cells nonresponsive in vitro. Influenza virus hemagglutinin-specific human TH0 T-cell clones were exposed to supraoptimal doses of peptide in the absence of antigen-presenting cells. Subsequent whole antigen challenge was characterized by antigen-specific T-cell hyporesponsiveness (anergy), which could be prevented or reversed by the addition of IL-2 (67). Further studies using supraoptimal doses of peptides in human CD4+ T-cell clones reactive to house dust mite reproduced clonal anergy and showed that this state was accompanied by downregulation of IL-2 and IL-4 and maintenance of IFN-γ secretion (68).

The principle that T-cell peptide epitopes may be employed to induce antigen-specific hyporesponsiveness has been extensively investigated in rodent models of autoimmune disease and, more recently, in models of allergic sensitization. Translation of the approach to human subjects was first attempted in individuals allergic to cats.

1. Allervax CAT

Approximately 95% of individuals with a clinical history of cat allergy are sensitive to one protein, Fel d 1 (*Felis domesticus*), found in cat dander and saliva. The allergen is ubiquitous in the environment, present not only in the homes of cat owners but also in public places, and is transported on clothing (69). Cloning, sequencing, epitope mapping, and preclinical studies resulted in the selection of two 27-amino-acid sequences, IPC-1 and IPC-2, for evaluation in clinical trials (70).

The efficacy of Allervax CAT (IPC-1/IPC-2) was evaluated by Norman and colleagues in a double-blind, placebo-controlled trial (71). Four weekly subcutaneous injections of placebo or peptides at doses of 7.5 µg, 75 µg, or 750 µg were administered. Modest improvements in symptom and medication scores were observed in the highest dose group, 6 weeks after treatment. Clinical outcomes included nasal and lung symptoms during a 60-minute exposure in a "cat room." Treatment was associated with a significant number of early and late adverse events, including chest tightness, nasal congestion, and flushing. These occurred a few minutes to several hours after administration of the peptides. In an associated study, a decrease in IL-4 production by IPC-1/IPC-2–specific T-cell lines from subjects in the high group was demonstrated. However, proliferative responses to either peptide or whole allergen remained unchanged (72).

Immunotherapy with Allervax CAT was also evaluated in cat-allergic asthmatic subjects using inhaled allergen challenge (73). The investigators performed allergen PD_{20} before and after a variable cumulative dose of peptides. Six weeks after ending therapy, posttreatment PD_{20} FEV_1 was not significantly different between the treated and placebo groups. However, in the middle- and high-dose groups, there was a significant increase in allergen tolerance between baseline and posttreatment days. In addition, IL-4 release was significantly reduced in the high-dose group. No change was observed in IFN-γ production.

In a randomized, double-blind, parallel-group study (74), 40 cat-allergic subjects received SC injections of 250 µg of the same peptide preparation as used in the two studies described previously, weekly for 4 consecutive weeks. No change was seen in either early or late-phase skin reactivity to whole cat extract up to 24 weeks after the last injection. No significant change in cat antigen–specific cytokine production was observed. Frequent adverse events, including symptoms of asthma, rhinitis, and pruritus, were reported.

In a further multicenter, randomized, double-blind, placebo-controlled study of 133 cat-allergic patients, Maguire and co-workers demonstrated modest improvements in some clinical outcome measures (75). Subjects received SC injections of either 75 µg or 750 µg peptides or placebo twice weekly for 2 weeks in two treatment phases, 4 months apart (a total of eight injections). Pulmonary function was improved in the 750 µg group, but only in those subjects with reduced baseline FEV_1, at a single time-point 3 weeks post–initial treatment phase. A large number of adverse events were recorded, including the requirement for systemic epinephrine in 3 peptide-treated patients. The majority of adverse events were associated with respiratory symptoms, occurred a few hours after injection, and declined with successive doses.

2. MHC-Based Peptide Vaccines

Haselden and colleagues (76) administered a mixture of three short (16/17 mers compared with to 27 mers in Allervax CAT) peptides from the cat allergen Fel d 1, intradermally, to cat-allergic asthmatics. In a proportion of individuals, an isolated late asthmatic reaction (LAR) was observed characterized by a decline in FEV_1 2–4 hours after peptide administration. Induction of bronchoconstriction was demonstrated to be IgE independent and MHC restricted, implying a T-cell–mediated reaction. Interestingly, subjects receiving Fel d 1 peptides and experiencing isolated LAR subsequently displayed markedly reduced reactivity to injected peptides. In later studies, 12 overlapping peptides (16/17 residues long each) spanning the majority of chains 1 and 2 of Fel d 1 were synthesized. Encompassing the majority of the molecule increased the number of HLA haplotypes able to bind and present peptide (77). Using this preparation of peptides, it was demonstrated that the magnitude, as well as the frequency, of isolated LARs in cat-allergic asthmatic subjects was dose dependent, with 50% of individuals developing a LAR when challenged with a single dose of 5 µg of peptides. A second injection of peptides was associated with a marked reduction or absence of the LAR with a return to baseline values of responsiveness over a period of up to 40 weeks. Thus, peptide-induced hyporesponsiveness was long lived.

An open study employing an up-dosing protocol with peptides (0.1, 1.0, 5, 10, 25 µg) injected at biweekly intervals demonstrated the ability to induce T-cell hyporesponsiveness in the absence of LAR. These results indicate that incremental dosing protocols, starting at a dose that is too low to induce LAR, may allow peptide immunotherapy to be used safely in the treatment of asthma, without undesirable bronchoconstriction (78).

Following a single peptide injection, cutaneous late-phase reactions (LPR) to intradermal challenge with whole cat dander extract were significantly reduced (77). To confirm these observations, a small, double-blind, placebo-controlled study was initiated. Subjects received either placebo or peptides via an incremental dosing protocol, to a total dose of 90 µg (79). Following peptide treatment a significant reduction in both the early and late cutaneous reactions to allergen challenge were observed, indicating peptide-induced modulation of both B-cell (early-phase reaction) and T-cell function (late phase reaction), respectively. Changes in late cutaneous reactions were observed within weeks of completing treatment and persisted for several months (Fig. 2). Changes in early cutaneous reactions were apparent only at long-term follow-up (3–9 months). No significant differences were demonstrated in bronchial responsiveness to either methacholine or whole cat dander. However, the study was not designed to detect such outcomes in the group of subjects studied. Importantly, peptide treated subjects were better able to tolerate subsequent exposure to cats.

In vitro T-cell responses measured before and after peptide treatment demonstrated a significant decrease in peptide- and whole allergen–induced proliferation of PBMCs and the production of IL-4, IL-13, and IFN-γ in cultures. Furthermore, peptide treatment was associated not only with decreases in whole cat dander–induced pro-inflammatory cytokines by PBMCs, but also with increased IL-10 production. Thus, induction of T-cell hyporesponsiveness in humans may be associated with the induction/expansion of a population of regulatory T-cells.

IV. ADJUVANTS

Approaches that have been exploited to enhance the immunogenicity of the vaccine antigens include strategies based on adjuvants, epitopes, and particulate antigens. An emerging area of vaccinology of allergic diseases involves the use of various adjuvants to direct and redirect protective immune responses. Substantial progress has been made in some of these approaches, leading to clinical trials and licensure however, safety concerns and economic considerations have limited their commercialization. The experimental research on improving immunotherapy has involved a combination of standardized allergens or purified/cloned allergens with an appropriate adjuvant. The latter may consist of a live or killed microorganism as a vaccine vector, or molecular immunostimuants such as those carrying CpG sequences or plasmids (pDNA) encoding protective cytokines (80).

A

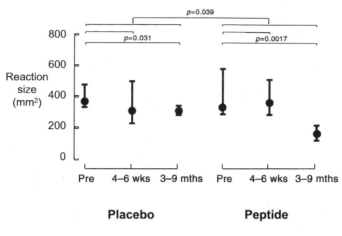

Placebo   Peptide

B

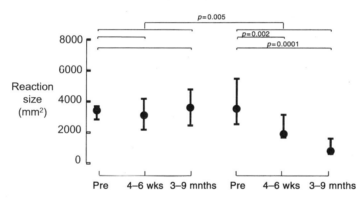

Figure 2 Peptide immunotherapy reduced both the early-phase cutaneous reaction to allergen challenge (*A*) and the late-phase cutaneous response to allergen challenge (*B*). A randomized, double-blind, placebo-controlled study of peptide immunotherapy with a mixture of 12 synthetic overlapping peptides derived from the primary sequence of the major cat allergen Fel d 1 was performed in cat-allergic asthmatic volunteers. A total of 90 µg of each peptide was administered. Measurements of early-phase (15 minutes) and late-phase (6 hours) skin reactions to intradermal challenge with purified Fel d 1 protein were recorded before therapy, 4–6 weeks after therapy, and 3–9 months after therapy. Statistically significant reductions in the magnitude of both early and late reactions were observed in the peptide-treated group.

A.   Microbial Adjuvants

To date, a large repertoire of live vaccine vectors, either avirulent or nonpathogenic organisms capable of expressing important immunomodulatory molecules, have been investigated. These include vectors with small genome sizes, such as vaccinia virus, avipoxviruses, adenoviruses, polioviruses, and salmonella, and vectors with large genomes, such as the herpes viruses and the mycobacterium BCG (81–83). cDNAs encoding major allergens are available that can be cloned in these nonpathogenic organisms to generate the effective reagents for prophylaxis and treatment of allergies. Such organisms are expected to provide more effective and longer-lasting adjuvant effect compared with the pDNA immunostimulants (84), presumably because of their persistence within cells of the body.

1. Live BCG

BCG is considered an excellent vaccine vector because it offers the following unique advantages (85,86). (1) It lends itself to the development of a multi-antigen vaccine, as would be required for downregulation of specific allergies. (2) Live attenuated BCG has been used for immunization of more than 2.5 billion people worldwide since 1948, with a low incidence of serious complications (case fatality rates of $0.19/10^6$). (3) BCG has been shown to be a potent adjuvant in experimental animals and humans particularly in relation to induction of TH1 cells. (4) BCG is heat stable and inexpensive to produce. (5) It can be administered by the oral route. (6) It can be given at birth or at any time afterward and is unaffected by maternal antibodies. (7) BCG given as single inoculum sensitizes to tuberculoproteins for 5–50 years. (8) Various in vitro studies of human and murine systems show that BCG-reactive CD4+ T-cells are potent producers of IFN-γ (87), the principal mediator of anti-tuberculous resistance. (9) The evidence that BCG can be a resident within the phagosome of the long-lived macrophage for years suggest that BCG-based vaccine may induce a potentially persistent or long-lasting allergen-specific immune response (88). Controversial evidence in support of a role for BCG vaccination in the determination of allergic phenotype has come from the observation that Japanese children displaying a positive delayed-type hypersensitivity skin test reaction, following prior BCG immunization, exhibited lower prevalence of atopic allergic disease (89).

Previously, Erb et al. demonstrated that infection of mice with BCG suppressed allergen-induced airway eosinophilia (90). In order to establish if live BCG would provide an adjuvant effect similar to that of complete Freund's adjuvant, mice were vaccinated with BCG, then immunized with recombinant allergen in alum. This protocol induced a decrease in total IgE and specific IgE by 5- and 10-fold, respectively. Concomitantly, IgG2a increased by 10-fold (Mohapatra, unpublished data). Furthermore, in vitro stimulation (with Kentucky bluegrass allergen) of cells from mice vaccinated with BCG followed by immunization with recombinant allergen in alum, led to an increase in the synthesis of IFN-γ, resulting in an increase in the IFN-γ:IL-4 ratio. These results demonstrated that live BCG as an adjuvant is capable of inducing a protective TH1 type of response.

In an effort to provide specificity in the effects of BCG, centers have developed recombinant BCG-producing foreign antigens within the macrophage. Oral immunization with recombinant BCG (rBCG) was shown to induce both cellular and humoral responses against foreign antigen (91). Experiments to examine the effects of rBCG vaccination on allergic responses in a murine model (88) have been conducted. A BCG–*E. coli* shuttle vector was developed with the promoter and signal sequence of the a-antigen of *Mycobacterium bovis*, and the vector was tested using *E. coli* β-galactosidase as the model antigen and allergen (88). This vector enabled the expression of the *E. coli* β-galactosidase (GAL) gene in BCG, which was detected in its protein extract by immunoblotting analysis. Vaccination of mice with a single dose of 10^6 rBCG generated a β-galactosidase–specific antibody response. The splenocytes of vaccinated mice, compared with controls, produced significantly higher levels of IFN-γ ($p < 0.01$) and interleukin-2 (IL-2) ($p < 0.05$) and lower levels of IL-5 ($p < 0.01$). Mice vaccinated with rBCG had significantly less ($p < 0.01$) serum IgE compared with controls. These results together demonstrate that rBCG-secreting antigens or allergens may be utilized for the induction of a TH1-like response and the downregulation of IgE antibody response.

2.   Mycobacterium vaccae

M. vaccae has been examined for its therapeutic effect for allergy and asthma. Wang and Rook showed that *M. vaccae* injected twice after mice were sensitized with ovalbumin led to a reduction in IgE and allergen-specific IL-5 synthesis, suggesting a potential clinical application of this organism in the immunotherapy of allergic diseases (87). Like BCG, *M. vaccae* also evokes a strong IFN-γ response and has been suggested to be effective in enhancing anti-allergic response in clinical trials. In a murine model of asthma, *M. vaccae* inhibited airway inflammation via regulation of TH1/TH2 balance, suggesting that it may be beneficial in the treatment of asthma (92,93). Further studies have demonstrated that immunization of newborn mice with *M. vaccae* would prevent some of the chronic airway changes in asthma. Furthermore, treatment of mice with SRP299 (a killed *M. vaccae* suspension) gave rise to allergen-specific CD4+CD45RB$_{(Lo)}$ regulatory T-cells that conferred protection against airway inflammation (94). This specific inhibition was mediated through interleukin-10 (IL-10) and transforming growth factor–beta (TGF-β), as antibodies against IL-10 and TGF-β completely reversed the inhibitory effect. Thus, regulatory T-cells generated by mycobacterial treatment may have an essential role in restoring the balance of the immune system to prevent and treat allergic diseases.

A double-blind, randomized study was conducted to investigate whether heat-killed *M. vaccae* (SRL172), a potent downregulator of TH2 cytokines, could reduce allergen-induced airway responses in patients with atopic asthma (95). A total of 24 male asthmatics participated in this study. Bronchial allergen challenge was performed along with measurement of early (EAR) and late asthmatic responses (LAR) 2 weeks before and 3 weeks after a single intradermal injection of SRL172 or placebo. SRL172 caused a mean 34% reduction of the area under the curve of the FEV changes during the LAR; however, this was not statistically different from placebo. SRL172 caused a trend for a reduction in serum IgE and IL-5 synthesis in vitro 3 weeks posttreatment ($p = 0.07$). These results suggest that multiple dosing of *M. vaccae* may be required to achieve significant benefit in asthma.

These studies have identified the potential of live BCG or other microorganisms, either by themselves or in the form of recombinant organisms expressing desirable allergens, as adjuvants for the potentiation of treatments for allergic diseases. However, these preliminary studies need to be extended at the clinical and epidemiological levels to determine if such compounds offer real advantages to the management of allergic diseases.

3.   Adjuvant Effects of CpG Motifs

Bacterial toxins are commonly used as adjuvants in animal models, but they are too toxic for use in humans. In contrast to eukaryotic DNA, the genetic material of prokaryotes is rich in sequences containing unmethylated cytosine-phosphoguanosine (CpG) dinucleotide motifs. CpG DNA is most often co-administered with antigen in the form of synthetic oligodeoxynucleotides (CpG ODN), which are made with a nuclease-resistant phosphorothioate backbone. Synthetic oligonucleotides (ODNs) containing CpG motifs are able to activate both innate and acquired immune responses through a signaling pathway involving Toll-like receptor 9 (TLR9) (Fig. 3). Depending on the sequence, length, and number and positions of CpG motifs in an ODN, distinct immunostimulatory profiles can be observed. These immunostimulatory profiles can be further modified and fine-tuned by appropriate chemical modifications, leading to preclinical and clinical development of

CpG ODNs in cancer, allergy, asthma, and infectious diseases. CpG ODN sequences tend to induce TH1-like cytokine response (81,96). The adjuvant may be injected with natural allergens or may be genetically linked with allergen cDNA.

CpG ODN, administered in conjunction with antigen, has been shown to be effective in downregulation of established TH2 responses. Protection is neither murine strain dependent nor model dependent. Although the effects of CpG ODN are associated with the induction of the TH1 cytokines IFN-γ and IL-12, neither cytokine is absolutely required for protection (97). The majority of studies evaluating CpG DNA as an adjuvant have been designed with parenteral delivery. However, mucosal immunization with CpG DNA has also been shown to induce both systemic (humoral and cellular) and mucosal antigen-specific immune responses (98).

Allergen-ISS Conjugates.   Specific immunostimulatory sequences (ISS) containing CpG motifs have been evaluated in allergen immunotherapy (99,100). The allergen-ISS conjugates (AICs) were found to be not only less allergenic, but more effective (than allergen alone) in inducing protective anti-allergic responses (TH1 cytokines and IgG antibody response) in preclinical studies in a mouse model and in human PBMC. Preliminary (unpublished; oral presentation by P.S. Creticos, American Academy of Allergy, Asthma and Immunology, Denver 2003) results from an initial clinical trial of ragweed AIC therapy for allergic rhinitis indicated that AIC treatment was well tolerated and resulted in statistically significant improvements in symptom and medication scores. Furthermore, the effect of treatment prior to one ragweed season was maintained through the next season, in the absence of additional therapy suggesting a long-lasting effect of treatment. AIC treatment was associated with an increase in allergen-specific IgG and antibodies and the absence of the normal seasonal rise in allergen-specific IgE. At present the mechanism of action of AIC remains unclear but may involve the induction of both TH1 and regulatory responses to allergen (101). Phase III clinical studies are currently being designed.

B. Cytokines as Adjuvants

Advances in gene transfer technology now make it possible to deliver cytokine genes to the target organ, either alone or in combination with allergens/allergen genes (Fig. 3). This approach will allow the evaluation of cytokines as adjuvants in immunotherapy formulation. IL-12 and IFN-γ have been considered potentially important adjuvants for the induction of TH1 cell-mediated protective immunity (102). The functional effects of IL-12 in many systems are likely to be mediated through secondary production of IFN-γ. However, the TH1-inducing effect of IL-12 in vivo may not be accompanied by a long-lasting suppression of TH2 development, and IL-12 has been demonstrated to be toxic in some systems. IFN-τ, a type I interferon that lacks the toxicity associated with other type I interferons, inhibited IgE production in a murine model allergy and also in an IgE-producing human myeloma cell line (103).

Administration of recombinant allergen (ovalbumin) with an IL-12 (subunit p40) fusion protein vaccine downregulated ovalbumin-specific IgE responses in vivo (82). In another model, IL-12 was delivered intranasally during allergen immunotherapy (104). In a typical protocol, DBA/2 mice were immunized intraperitoneally with grass pollen allergen and then immunized parenterally with grass allergen with or without IL-12. Treatment of sensitized mice with a combination of allergen plus IL-12 showed the highest IFN-γ production and decreased the TH2-like response in GAL-stimulated splenocyte culture. IL-12 also inhibited GAL-induced IgE production and enhanced GAL-specific IgG2a in

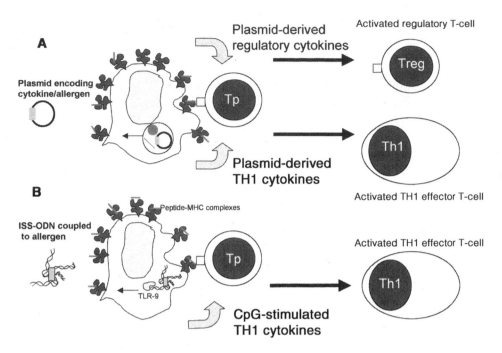

Figure 3 DNA-based approaches for the treatment of allergic diseases. *A*: Plasmid DNA vectors encoding allergens and cytokine genes may be used to generate allergen-specific responses in an environment rich in pro-inflammatory TH1 cytokines such as IL-12 and IFN-γ, or regulatory cytokines such as IL-10 and TGF-β. Presentation of allergen-derived peptides to precursor T-cells (Tp) leads to the generation of robust TH1 or T regulatory allergen-specific responses. *B*: Allergens covalently coupled to immunostimulatory oligodeoxynucleotides (ISS-ODN) may be used to deliver allergen molecules to antigen-presenting cells together with Toll-like receptor-9 (TLR-9) activation, leading to the production of TH1-stimulating cytokines such as IL-12. Presentation of allergen-derived peptides to precursor T-cells (Tp) leads to the generation of robust TH1 allergen-specific responses.

GAL-presensitized mice. Intranasal delivery of IL-12 attenuated airway hyperresponsiveness and BAL eosinophilia in sensitized mice. Analysis of IL-12 receptor expression suggested a shift in the expression profile of IL-12Rβ1 and β2 in the lung tissue, consistent with the observed shift in the cytokine profile from a TH2- to a TH1-like response. These results suggest that intranasal delivery of IL-12 inhibits allergic airway inflammation in asthma via a IFN-γ–independent pathway, involving regulation of the expression of IL-12 receptor.

The immunomodulatory role of plasmid DNA–expressing cytokines IFN-γ (pIFN-γ) and/or IL-12 (pIL-12) as adjuvants was assessed in a murine model of Kentucky bluegrass (KBG) allergy (104). Mice vaccinated with the cytokine plasmid adjuvants had relatively less total serum IgE and higher levels of grass allergen–specific IgG2a than did control mice injected with the empty vector plasmid. The lowest IgE and the highest IgG2a levels were found in mice vaccinated with combined pIFN-γ and pIL-12 as adjuvant. The IgG1 titers of all mice remained unchanged. The greatest decrease in airway hyperresponsiveness and pulmonary inflammation occurred in mice receiving both pIFN-γ and pIL-12 as adjuvants. These studies provide evidence that a combination of pIFN-γ and pIL-12 provides a more effective adjuvant to the grass allergen vaccine than either one of these plasmids alone and may enhance the effectiveness of allergen immunotherapy in humans.

V. CONCLUSIONS

Rapid progress is being made in the development of novel immunotherapies for the treatment of allergic diseases. Recombinant DNA technology has enabled the cloning and sequencing of genes encoding several hundred important aeroallergens. Knowledge of nucleotide and amino acid sequences has allowed the standardized production of recombinant molecules, fragments, and peptides to high degrees of purity for development as vaccine candidates. Furthermore, detailed evaluation of structural features of allergens and their isoforms has led to strategies aimed at decreasing the allergenicity of proteins while retaining the ability to induce protective immunity.

Parallel development of adjuvant technology, including the use of bacteria or their products to activate the innate immune response and also the use of TH1-stimulating plasmid-encoded cytokines, offers the potential to redirect allergic responses effectively and safely. Many of these approaches are currently being evaluated in clinical trials and hold considerable promise for future therapeutic interventions in allergic diseases.

VI. SALIENT POINTS

1. Specific immunotherapy may be improved for safety and efficacy using recombinant and engineered allergens, which may include low IgE-binding natural isoforms, conformational variants, deletion mutants, allergen oligomers, and allergen chimeras. These may be administered either as recombinant proteins or as DNA vaccines.
2. Large allergen fragments composed of either T-cell peptides such as Allervax CAT or MHC-based peptide vaccines may also be used for specific immunotherapy.
3. Adjuvants may augment safety and efficacy of allergen specific immunotherapy. These may include microbial adjuvants such as BCG or *M. vaccae*, immunostimulatory sequences containing CpG motif, or cytokines suh as IFN-γ and/or IL-12.

REFERENCES

1. Bousquet J, Lockey R, Malling HJ, Alvarez-Cuesta E, Canonica GW, Chapman MD, Creticos PJ, Dayer JM, Durham SR, Demoly P, Goldstein RJ, Ishikawa T, Ito K, Kraft D, Lambert PH, Lowenstein H, Muller U, Norman PS, Reisman RE, Valenta R, Valovirta E, Yssel H. Allergen immunotherapy: Therapeutic vaccines for allergic diseases. World Health Organization. American Academy of Allergy, Asthma and Immunology. Ann Allergy Asthma Immunol 1998; 81(5 pt 1):401–405.
2. Durham SR, Walker SM, Varga EM, Jacobson MR, O'Brien F, Noble W, Till SJ, Hamid QA, Nouri-Aria KT. Long-term clinical efficacy of grass-pollen immunotherapy. N Engl J Med 1999; 341(7):468–475.
3. Durham SR, Till SJ. Immunologic changes associated with allergen immunotherapy. J Allergy Clin Immunol 1998; 102(2):157–164.
4. Akdis CA, Blaser K. Immunologic mechanisms of allergen-specific immunotherapy. Adv Exp Med Biol 2001; 495:247–259.
5. van Neerven RJ, Wikborg T, Lund G, Jacobsen B, Brinch-Nielsen A, Arnved J, Ipsen H. Blocking antibodies induced by specific allergy vaccination prevent the activation of CD4+

T cells by inhibiting serum-IgE-facilitated allergen presentation. J Immunol 1999; 163(5):2944–2952.

6. Rocklin RE, Sheffer AL, Greineder DK, Melmon KL. Generation of antigen-specific suppressor cells during allergy desensitization. N Engl J Med 1980; 302(22):1213–1219.

7. Otsuka H, Mezawa A, Ohnishi M, Okubo K, Seki H, Okuda M. Changes in nasal metachromatic cells during allergen immunotherapy. Clin Exp Allergy 1991; 21(1):115–119.

8. Durham SR, Varney VA, Gaga M, Jacobson MR, Varga EM, Frew AJ, et al. Grass pollen immunotherapy decreases the number of mast cells in the skin. Clin Exp Allergy 1999; 29(11):1490–1496.

9. Secrist H, Chelen CJ, Wen Y, Marshall JD, Umetsu DT. Allergen immunotherapy decreases interleukin 4 production in CD4+ T cells from allergic individuals. J Exp Med 1993; 178(6):2123–2130.

10. Ebner C, Siemann U, Bohle B, Willheim M, Wiedermann U, Schenk S et al. Immunological changes during specific immunotherapy of grass pollen allergy: Reduced lymphoproliferative responses to allergen and shift from TH2 to TH1 in T-cell clones specific for Phl p 1, a major grass pollen allergen. Clin Exp Allergy 1997; 27(9):1007–1015.

11. Akdis CA, Blesken T, Akdis M, Wuthrich B, Blaser K. Role of interleukin 10 in specific immunotherapy. J Clin Investig 1998; 102(1):98–106.

12. Moverare R, Elfman L, Vesterinen E, Metso T, Haahtela T. Development of new IgE specificities to allergenic components in birch pollen extract during specific immunotherapy studied with immunoblotting and Pharmacia CAP System. Allergy 2002; 57(5):423–430.

13. Chapman MD, Smith AM, Vailes LD, Arruda LK, Dhanaraj V, Pomes A. Recombinant allergens for diagnosis and therapy of allergic disease. J Allergy Clin Immunol 2000; 106(3):409–418.

14. Valenta R. The future of antigen-specific immunotherapy of allergy. Nat Rev Immunol 2002; 2(6):446–453.

15. van der Heijden FL, Joost van Neerven RJ, van Katwijk M, Bos JD, Kapsenberg ML. Serum-IgE–facilitated allergen presentation in atopic disease. J Immunol 1993; 150(8 pt 1):3643–3650.

16. Maurer D, Ebner C, Reininger B, Fiebiger E, Kraft D, Kinet JP, Stingl G. The high affinity IgE receptor (Fc epsilon RI) mediates IgE-dependent allergen presentation. J Immunol 1995; 154(12):6285–6290.

17. Griffith IJ, Pollock J, Klapper DG, Rogers BL, Nault AK. Sequence polymorphism of Amb a I and Amb a II, the major allergens in *Ambrosia artemisiifolia* (short ragweed). Int Arch Allergy Appl Immunol 1991; 96(4):296–304.

18. Breiteneder H, Ferreira F, Hoffmann-Sommergruber K, Ebner C, Breitenbach M, Rumpold H, et al. Four recombinant isoforms of Cor a I, the major allergen of hazel pollen, show different IgE-binding properties. Eur J Biochem 1993; 212(2):355–362.

19. Swoboda I, Jilek A, Ferreira F, Engel E, Hoffmann-Sommergruber K, Scheiner O, et al. Isoforms of Bet v 1, the major birch pollen allergen, analyzed by liquid chromatography, mass spectrometry, and cDNA cloning. J Biol Chem 1995; 270(6):2607–2613.

20. Chang ZN, Peng HJ, Lee WC, Chen TS, Chua KY, Tsai LC, et al. Sequence polymorphism of the group 1 allergen of Bermuda grass pollen. Clin Exp Allergy 1999; 29(4):488–496.

21. Muller WD, Karamfilov T, Kahlert H, Stuwe HT, Fahlbusch B, Cromwell O, Fiebig H, Jager L. Mapping of T-cell epitopes of Phl p 5: Evidence for crossreacting and non-crossreacting T-cell epitopes within Phl p 5 isoallergens. Clin Exp Allergy 1998; 28(12):1538–1548.

22. Son DY, Scheurer S, Hoffmann A, Haustein D, Vieths S. Pollen-related food allergy: Cloning and immunological analysis of isoforms and mutants of Mal d 1, the major apple allergen, and Bet v 1, the major birch pollen allergen. Eur J Nutr 1999; 38(4):201–215.

23. Hoffmann-Sommergruber K, Ferris R, Pec M, Radauer C, O'Riordain G, Laimer Da Camara MM, et al. Characterization of api g 1.0201, a new member of the Api g 1 family of celery allergens. Int Arch Allergy Immunol 2000; 122(2):115–123.

24. Duro G, Colombo P, Assunta CM, Izzo V, Porcasi R, Di Fiore R, Locorotondo G, Cocchiara R, Geraci D. Isolation and characterization of two cDNA clones coding for isoforms of the *Parietaria judaica* major allergen Par j 1.0101. Int Arch Allergy Immunol 1997; 112(4):348–355.

25. Gonzalez EM, Villalba M, Lombardero M, Aalbers M, van Ree R, Rodriguez R. Influence of the 3D-conformation, glycan component and microheterogeneity on the epitope structure of Ole e 1, the major olive allergen: Use of recombinant isoforms and specific monoclonal antibodies as immunological tools. Mol Immunol 2002; 39(1–2):93–101.

26. Smith AM, Benjamin DC, Derewenda U, Smith WA, Thomas WR, Chapman MD. Sequence polymorphisms and antibody binding to the group 2 dust mite allergens. Int Arch Allergy Immunol 2001; 124(1–3):61–63.

27. Sowka S, Hafner C, Radauer C, Focke M, Brehler R, Astwood JD, Arif SA, Kanani A, Sussman GL, Scheiner O, Beezhold DH, Breiteneder H. Molecular and immunologic characterization of new isoforms of the *Hevea brasiliensis* latex allergen hev b 7: Evidence of no cross-reactivity between hev b 7 isoforms and potato patatin and proteins from avocado and banana. J Allergy Clin Immunol 1999; 104(6):1302–1310.

28. Rautiainen J, Auriola S, Konttinen A, Virtanen T, Rytkonen-Nissinen M, Zeiler T, et al. Two new variants of the lipocalin allergen Bos d 2. J Chromatogr B Biomed Sci Appl 2001; 763(1–2):91–98.

29. Schenk S, Hoffmann-Sommergruber K, Breiteneder H, Ferreira F, Fischer G, Scheiner O, Kraft D, Ebner C. Four recombinant isoforms of Cor a 1, the major allergen of hazel pollen, show different reactivities with allergen-specific T-lymphocyte clones. Eur J Biochem 1994; 224(2):717–722.

30. Ferreira F, Hirtenlehner K, Jilek A, Godnik-Cvar J, Breiteneder H, Grimm R, et al. Dissection of immunoglobulin E and T lymphocyte reactivity of isoforms of the major birch pollen allergen Bet v 1: Potential use of hypoallergenic isoforms for immunotherapy. J Exp Med 1996; 183(2):599–609.

31. Wurtzen PA, Bufe A, Wissenbach M, Madsen HO, Ipsen H, Arnved J, et al. Identification of isoform-specific T-cell epitopes in the major timothy grass pollen allergen, Phl p 5. Clin Exp Allergy 1999; 29(12):1614–1625.

32. Hales BJ, Hazell LA, Smith W, Thomas WR. Genetic variation of Der p 2 allergens: Effects on T cell responses and immunoglobulin E binding. Clin Exp Allergy 2002; 32(10):1461–1467.

33. Arquint O, Helbling A, Crameri R, Ferreira F, Breitenbach M, Pichler WJ. Reduced in vivo allergenicity of Bet v 1d isoform, a natural component of birch pollen. J Allergy Clin Immunol 1999; 104(6):1239–1243.

34. Markovic-Housley Z, Degano M, Lamba D, Roepenack-Lahaye E, Clemens S, Susani M, Ferreira F, Scheiner O, Breiteneder H. Crystal structure of a hypoallergenic isoform of the major birch pollen allergen Bet v 1 and its likely biological function as a plant steroid carrier. J Mol Biol 2003; 325(1):123–133.

35. Bannon GA, Cockrell G, Connaughton C, West CM, Helm R, Stanley JS, et al. Engineering, characterization and in vitro efficacy of the major peanut allergens for use in immunotherapy. Int Arch Allergy Immunol 2001; 124(1–3):70–72.

36. Ferreira F, Hirtenlehner K, Jilek A, Godnik-Cvar J, Breiteneder H, Grimm R, et al. Dissection of immunoglobulin E and T lymphocyte reactivity of isoforms of the major birch pollen allergen Bet v 1: Potential use of hypoallergenic isoforms for immunotherapy. J Exp Med 1996; 183(2):599–609.

37. Ferreira F, Ebner C, Kramer B, Casari G, Briza P, Kungl AJ, et al. Modulation of IgE reactivity of allergens by site-directed mutagenesis: Potential use of hypoallergenic variants for immunotherapy. FASEB J 1998; 12(2):231–242.

38. Casari G, Sander C, Valencia A. A method to predict functional residues in proteins. Nat Struct Biol 1995; 2(2):171–178.

39. Swoboda I, De Weerd N, Bhalla PL, Niederberger V, Sperr WR, Valent P, et al. Mutants of the major ryegrass pollen allergen, Lol p 5, with reduced IgE-binding capacity: Candidates for grass pollen-specific immunotherapy. Eur J Immunol 2002; 32(1):270–280.

40. Beezhold DH, Hickey VL, Sussman GL. Mutational analysis of the IgE epitopes in the latex allergen Hev b 5. J Allergy Clin Immunol 2001; 107(6):1069–1076.

41. Mine Y, Sasaki E, Zhang JW. Reduction of antigenicity and allergenicity of genetically modified egg white allergen, ovomucoid third domain. Biochem Biophys Res Commun 2003; 302(1):133–137.

42. Li XM, Srivastava K, Huleatt JW, Bottomly K, Burks AW, Sampson HA. Engineered recombinant peanut protein and heat-killed *Listeria* monocytogenes coadministration protects against peanut-induced anaphylaxis in a murine model. J Immunol 2003; 170(6):3289–3295.

43. Li X-M, Srivastava K, Grishin A, Huang C-K, Schofield B, Burks W, Sampson H. Persistent protective effect of heat-killed *Escherichia coli* producing "engineered," recombinant peanut proteins in a murine model of peanut allergy. J Allergy Clin Immunol 2003; 112:159–167.

44. Akdis CA, Blesken T, Wymann D, Akdis M, Blaser K. Differential regulation of human T cell cytokine patterns and IgE and IgG4 responses by conformational antigen variants. Eur J Immunol 1998; 28(3):914–925.

45. Bonura A, Amoroso S, Locorotondo G, Di Felice G, Tinghino R, Geraci D, Colombo P. Hypoallergenic variants of the *Parietaria judaica* major allergen Par j 1: A member of the non-specific lipid transfer protein plant family. Int Arch Allergy Immunol 2001; 126(1):32–40.

46. Smith AM, Chapman MD. Reduction in IgE binding to allergen variants generated by site-directed mutagenesis: Contribution of disulfide bonds to the antigenic structure of the major house dust mite allergen Der p 2. Mol Immunol 1996; 33(4–5):399–405.

47. Takai T, Yokota T, Yasue M, Nishiyama C, Yuuki T, Mori A, et al. Engineering of the major house dust mite allergen Der f 2 for allergen-specific immunotherapy. Nat Biotechnol 1997; 15(8):754–758.

48. Kronqvist M, Johansson E, Whitley P, Olsson S, Gafvelin G, Scheynius A, van Hage-Hamsten M. A hypoallergenic derivative of the major allergen of the dust mite *Lepidoglyphus destructor*, Lep d 2.6Cys, induces less IgE reactivity and cellular response in the skin than recombinant Lep d 2. Int Arch Allergy Immunol 2001; 126(1):41–49.

49. Schramm G, Kahlert H, Suck R, Weber B, Stuwe HT, Muller WD, et al. "Allergen engineering": Variants of the timothy grass pollen allergen Phl p 5b with reduced IgE-binding capacity but conserved T cell reactivity. J Immunol 1999; 162(4):2406–2414.

50. Wu CH, Lee MF, Yang JS, Tseng CY. IgE-binding epitopes of the American cockroach Per a 1 allergen. Mol Immunol 2002; 39(7–8):459–464.

51. Tamborini E, Faccini S, Lidholm J, Svensson M, Brandazza A, Longhi R, Groenlund H, Sidoli A, Arosio P. Biochemical and immunological characterization of recombinant allergen Lol p 1. Eur J Biochem 1997; 249(3):886–894.

52. Vrtala S, Hirtenlehner K, Susani M, Hufnagl P, Binder BR, Vangelista L, et al. Genetic engineering of recombinant hypoallergenic oligomers of the major birch pollen allergen, Bet v 1: Candidates for specific immunotherapy. Int Arch Allergy Immunol 1999; 118(2–4):218–219.

53. King TP, Jim SY, Monsalve RI, Kagey-Sobotka A, Lichtenstein LM, Spangfort MD. Recombinant allergens with reduced allergenicity but retaining immunogenicity of the natural allergens: Hybrids of yellow jacket and paper wasp venom allergen antigen 5s. J Immunol 2001; 166(10):6057–6065.

54. Linhart B, Jahn-Schmid B, Verdino P, Keller W, Ebner C, Kraft D, Valenta R. Combination vaccines for the treatment of grass pollen allergy consisting of genetically engineered hybrid molecules with increased immunogenicity. FASEB J 2002; 16(10):1301–1303.

55. Crameri A, Raillard SA, Bermudez E, Stemmer WP. DNA shuffling of a family of genes from diverse species accelerates directed evolution. Nature 1998; 391(6664):288–291.

56. Punnonen J. Molecular breeding of allergy vaccines and antiallergic cytokines. Int Arch Allergy Immunol 2000; 121(3):173–182.

57. Hsu CH, Chua KY, Tao MH, Huang SK, Hsieh KH. Inhibition of specific IgE response in vivo by allergen-gene transfer. Int Immunol 1996; 8(9):1405–1411.

58. Raz E, Tighe H, Sato Y, Corr M, Dudler JA, Roman M, et al. Preferential induction of a Th1 immune response and inhibition of specific IgE antibody formation by plasmid DNA immunization. Proc Natl Acad Sci U S A 1996; 93(10):5141–5145.

59. Hartl A, Kiesslich J, Weiss R, Bernhaupt A, Mostbock S, Scheiblhofer S, Ebner C, Ferreira F, Thalhamer J. Immune responses after immunization with plasmid DNA encoding Bet v 1, the major allergen of birch pollen. J Allergy Clin Immunol 1999; 103(1 pt 1):107–113.

60. Vrtala S, Hirtenlehner K, Vangelista L, Pastore A, Eichler HG, Sperr WR, et al. Conversion of the major birch pollen allergen, Bet v 1, into two nonanaphylactic T cell epitope-containing fragments: Candidates for a novel form of specific immunotherapy. J Clin Investig 1997; 99(7):1673–1681.

61. Hage-Hamsten M, Kronqvist M, Zetterstrom O, Johansson E, Niederberger V, Vrtala S, et al. Skin test evaluation of genetically engineered hypoallergenic derivatives of the major birch pollen allergen, Bet v 1: Results obtained with a mix of two recombinant Bet v 1 fragments and recombinant Bet v 1 trimer in a Swedish population before the birch pollen season. J Allergy Clin Immunol 1999; 104(5):969–977.

62. Vrtala S, Akdis CA, Budak F, Akdis M, Blaser K, Kraft D, et al. T cell epitope-containing hypoallergenic recombinant fragments of the major birch pollen allergen, Bet v 1, induce blocking antibodies. J Immunol 2000; 165(11):6653–6659.

63. Takai T, Mori A, Yuuki T, Okudaira H, Okumura Y. Non-anaphylactic combination of partially deleted fragments of the major house dust mite allergen Der f 2 for allergen-specific immunotherapy. Mol Immunol 1999; 36(15–16):1055–1065.

64. Twardosz A, Hayek B, Seiberler S, Vangelista L, Elfman L, Gronlund H, Kraft D, Valenta R. Molecular characterization, expression in *Escherichia coli*, and epitope analysis of a two EF-hand calcium-binding birch pollen allergen, Bet v 4. Biochem Biophys Res Commun 1997; 239(1):197–204.

65. Hayek B, Vangelista L, Pastore A, Sperr WR, Valent P, Vrtala S, Niederberger V. Twardosz A, Kraft D, Valenta R. Molecular and immunologic characterization of a highly cross-reactive two EF-hand calcium-binding alder pollen allergen, Aln g 4: Structural basis for calcium-modulated IgE recognition. J Immunol 1998; 161(12):7031–7039.

66. Lamb JR, Skidmore BJ, Green N, Chiller JM, Feldmann M. Induction of tolerance in influenza virus-immune T lymphocyte clones with synthetic peptides of influenza hemagglutinin. J Exp Med 1983; 157(5):1434–1447.

67. Essery G, Feldmann M, Lamb JR. Interleukin-2 can prevent and reverse antigen-induced unresponsiveness in cloned human T lymphocytes. Immunology 1988; 64(3):413–417.

68. O'Hehir RE, Yssel H, Verma S, de Vries JE, Spits H, Lamb JR. Clonal analysis of differential lymphokine production in peptide and superantigen induced T cell anergy. Int Immunol 1991; 3(8):819–826.

69. Custovic A, Green R, Taggart SC, Smith A, Pickering CA, Chapman MD, Woodcock A. Domestic allergens in public places: II. Dog (Can f 1) and cockroach (Bla g 2) allergens in dust and mite, cat, dog and cockroach allergens in the air in public buildings. Clin Exp Allergy 1996; 26(11):1246–1252.

70. Counsell CM, Bond JF, Ohman JL, Greenstein JL, Garman RD. Definition of the human T-cell epitopes of Fel d 1, the major allergen of the domestic cat. J Allergy Clin Immunol 1996; 98(5 pt 1):884–894.

71. Norman PS, Ohman JL, Long AA, Creticos PS, Gefter MA, Shaked Z, et al. Treatment of cat allergy with T-cell reactive peptides. Am J Respir Crit Care Med 1996; 154(6 pt 1):1623–1628.

72. Marcotte GV, Braun CM, Norman PS, Nicodemus CF, Kagey-Sobotka A, Lichtenstein LM, et al. Effects of peptide therapy on ex vivo T-cell responses. J Allergy Clin Immunol 1998; 101(4 pt 1):506–513.

73. Pene J, Desroches A, Paradis L, Lebel B, Farce M, Nicodemus CF, Yssel H, Bousquet J. Immunotherapy with Fel d 1 peptides decreases IL-4 release by peripheral blood T cells of patients allergic to cats. J Allergy Clin Immunol 1998; 102(4 pt 1):571–578.

74. Simons FE, Imada M, Li Y, Watson WT, HayGlass KT. Fel d 1 peptides: Effect on skin tests and cytokine synthesis in cat-allergic human subjects. Int Immunol 1996; 8(12): 1937–1945.

75. Maguire P, Nicodemus C, Robinson D, Aaronson D, Umetsu DT. The safety and efficacy of Allervax CAT in cat allergic patients. Clin Immunol 1999; 93(3):222–231.

76. Haselden BM, Kay AB, Larche M. Immunoglobulin E–independent major histocompatibility complex–restricted T cell peptide epitope-induced late asthmatic reactions. J Exp Med 1999; 189(12):1885–1894.

77. Oldfield WL, Kay AB, Larche M. Allergen-derived T cell peptide-induced late asthmatic reactions precede the induction of antigen-specific hyporesponsiveness in atopic allergic asthmatic subjects. J Immunol 2001; 167(3):1734–1739.

78. Alexander C, Oldfield WL, Shirley K, Larche M, Kay AB. A dosing protocol of allergen-derived T cell peptide epitopes for the treatment of allergic disease (abstr). J Allergy Clin Immunol 2001; 107:716.

79. Oldfield WL, Larche M, Kay AB. Effect of T-cell peptides derived from Fel d 1 on allergic reactions and cytokine production in patients sensitive to cats: A randomised controlled trial. Lancet 2002; 360(9326):47–53.

80. Hedley ML. Gene therapy of chronic inflammatory disease. Adv Drug Deliv Rev 2000; 44(2–3):195–207.

81. van Ginkel FW, Nguyen HH, McGhee JR. Vaccines for mucosal immunity to combat emerging infectious diseases. Emerg Infect Dis 2000; 6(2):123–132.

82. Bumann D, Hueck C, Aebischer T, Meyer TF. Recombinant live *Salmonella* spp. for human vaccination against heterologous pathogens. FEMS Immunol Med Microbiol 2000; 27(4):357–364.

83. Broder CC, Earl PL. Recombinant vaccinia viruses: Design, generation, and isolation. Mol Biotechnol 1999; 13(3):223–245.

84. Yew NS, Zhao H, Wu IH, Song A, Tousignant JD, Przybylska M, et al. Reduced inflammatory response to plasmid DNA vectors by elimination and inhibition of immunostimulatory CpG motifs. Mol Ther 2000; 1(3):255–262.

85. Husson RN, James BE, Young RA. Gene replacement and expression of foreign DNA in mycobacteria. J Bacteriol 1990; 172(2):519–524.

86. Stover CK, de la Cruz, VF, Fuerst TR, Burlein JE, Benson LA, Bennett LT, Bansal GP, Young JF, Lee MH, Hatfull GF, Snapper SB, Barletta RG, Jacobs WR & Bloom BR. New use of BCG for recombinant vaccines. Nature 1991; 351(6326):456–460.

87. Wang CC, Rook GA. Inhibition of an established allergic response to ovalbumin in BALB/c mice by killed *Mycobacterium vaccae*. Immunology 1998; 93(3):307–313.

88. Kumar M, Behera AK, Matsuse H, Lockey RF, Mohapatra SS. A recombinant BCG vaccine generates a Th1-like response and inhibits IgE synthesis in BALB/c mice. Immunology 1999; 97(3):515–521.

89. Shirakawa T, Enomoto T, Shimazu S, Hopkin JM. The inverse association between tuberculin responses and atopic disorder. Science 1997; 275(5296):77–79.

90. Erb KJ, Holloway JW, Sobeck A, Moll H, Le Gros G. Infection of mice with *Mycobacterium bovis-Bacillus* Calmette-Guerin (BCG) suppresses allergen-induced airway eosinophilia. J Exp Med 1998; 187(4):561–569.

91. Lagranderie M, Murray A, Gicquel B, Leclerc C, Gheorghiu M. Oral immunization with recombinant BCG induces cellular and humoral immune responses against the foreign antigen. Vaccine 1993; 11(13):1283–1290.

92. Ozdemir C, Akkoc T, Bahceciler NN, Kucukercan D, Barlan IB, Basaran MM. Impact of *Mycobacterium vaccae* immunization on lung histopathology in a murine model of chronic asthma. Clin Exp Allergy 2003; 33(2):266–270.

93. Hopfenspirger MT, Parr SK, Hopp RJ, Townley RG, Agrawal DK. Mycobacterial antigens attenuate late phase response, airway hyperresponsiveness, and bronchoalveolar lavage eosinophilia in a mouse model of bronchial asthma. Int Immunopharmacol 2001; 1(9–10):1743–1751.

94. Zuany-Amorim C, Sawicka E, Manlius C, Le Moine A, Brunet LR, Kemeny DM, Bowen G, Rook G, Walker C. Suppression of airway eosinophilia by killed *Mycobacterium vaccae*–induced allergen-specific regulatory T-cells. Nat Med 2002; 8(6):625–629.

95. Camporota L, Corkhill A, Long H, Lordan J, Stanciu L, Tuckwell N, et al. The effects of *Mycobacterium vaccae* on allergen-induced airway responses in atopic asthma. Eur Respir J 2003; 21(2):287–293.

96. Roman M, Martin-Orozco E, Goodman JS, Nguyen MD, Sato Y, Ronaghy A, Kornbluth RS, Richman DD, Carson DA, Raz E. Immunostimulatory DNA sequences function as T helper-1-promoting adjuvants. Nat Med 1997; 3(8):849–854.

97. Bohle B, Jahn-Schmid B, Maurer D, Kraft D, Ebner C. Oligodeoxynucleotides containing CpG motifs induce IL-12, IL-18 and IFN-gamma production in cells from allergic individuals and inhibit IgE synthesis in vitro. Eur J Immunol 1999; 29(7):2344–2353.

98. McCluskie MJ, Weeratna RD, Payette PJ, Davis HL. The potential of CpG oligodeoxynucleotides as mucosal adjuvants. Crit Rev Immunol 2001; 21:103–120.

99. Creticos PS, Eiden JJ, Balcer S, Van Nest G, Kagey-Sobotka A, Tuck S, Norman PS, and Lichtenstein LM. Immunostimulatory oligonucleotides conjugated to Amb a 1: Safety, skin test reactivity and basophil histamine release (abstr). J Allergy Clin Immunol 2000; 105(1):S70.

100. Creticos PS, Balcer S, Schroeder JT, Hamilton RG, Chung B, Norman PS, Lichtenstein LM, and Eiden JJ. Initial immunotherapy trial to explore the safety, tolerability and immunogenicity of subcutaneous injections of an Amb a 1 immunostimulatory oligonucleotide conjugate (Aic) in ragweed allergic adults (abstr). J Allergy Clin Immunol 2001; 107:S216.

101. Creticos PS, Lighvani SS, Bieneman AP, Balcer-Whaley SL, Norman PS, Lichtenstein LM, Schroeder JT. Enhanced IL-10 secretion by PBMC during the ragweed season: Effect of AIC immunotherapy versus placebo (abstr). J Allergy Clin Immunol 2003; III:S201.

102. Bliss J, Van C, V, Murray K, Wiencis A, Ketchum M, Maylor R, et al. IL-12, as an adjuvant, promotes a T helper 1 cell, but does not suppress a T helper 2 cell recall response. J Immunol 1996; 156(3):887–894.

103. Mujtaba MG, Villarete L, Johnson HM. IFN-tau inhibits IgE production in a murine model of allergy and in an IgE-producing human myeloma cell line. J Allergy Clin Immunol 1999; 104:1037–1044.

104. Matsuse H, Kong X, Hu J, Wolf SF, Lockey RF, Mohapatra SS. Intranasal IL-12 produces discreet pulmonary and systemic effects on allergic inflammation and airway reactivity. Int Immunopharmacol 2003; 3(4):457–468.

36

Novel Approaches to Immunotherapy for Food Allergy

XIU-MIN LI and HUGH A. SAMPSON

Mount Sinai School of Medicine, New York, New York, U.S.A.

I. INTRODUCTION

Food allergy affects up to 6% of children less than 4 years of age and about 2% of the U.S. population beyond the first decade of life (1). It is the single leading cause of anaphylaxis treated in hospital emergency departments in the United States and many "Westernized" countries. Extrapolating from a survey in Olmstead County, Minnesota, it is estimated that food allergy accounts for about 30,000 anaphylactic reactions, 2000 hospitalizations, and 150 deaths each year in the United States (2). Peanut (PN) and tree nut allergies account for the vast majority of fatal and near-fatal anaphylactic reactions (3,4). Food allergy research is receiving increased attention due to the apparently increasing prevalence of food allergy and the frequency and severe consequences of food-induced anaphylactic reactions. However, there is still no treatment for this disorder (5), and the number of severe and fatal food-allergic reactions indicate that allergen avoidance is not adequate for dealing with this disorder. Monthly injections of humanized recombinant anti-IgE antibodies, which reduce mast cell– and basophil-bound IgE, appears to be effective in preventing allergic responses in peanut-sensitive subjects, at least to small amounts of peanut protein (6). However, this treatment cannot cure allergy, and continued protection would depend on monthly injections for an indefinite period of time. Additional therapeutic approaches for the treatment of food allergy are needed.

Peanut allergy (PNA) is an IgE-mediated type I hypersensitivity reaction in which allergen-specific IgE antibodies that bind to high-affinity receptors (FcεRI) on the surface of mast cells and basophils are central to the immunopathology of food allergy. In patients with food allergy, reexposure to the relevant foods triggers degranulation of mast cells/basophils, resulting in the release of histamine and other mediators, provoking symptoms of anaphylaxis. Early symptoms of food-induced anaphylaxis often include oral pruritus, colicky abdominal pain, nausea, vomiting, diarrhea, cutaneous flushing, urticaria, and angioedema. Progressive respiratory symptoms, hypotension, and dysrhythmias typically develop in fatal and near-fatal cases (7). Numerous studies have shown that TH2 cytokines are central to the pathogenesis of allergic disorders (8). A TH2-skewed response has been observed in food allergy. PN-specific TH2 clones have also been generated from patients with PNA (9,10). It has been suggested that tolerance to food antigen induced via the gut is dependent on an IFN-γ–involved immune mechanism (11,12). Another study suggested that peanut allergic status is characterized by a TH2 response, whereas TH1-skewed responses underlie oral tolerance (13). According to the hygiene hypotheses, the increasing incidence of allergy in Westernized societies over the last decades (14) may be explained, to some extent, by a reduced microbial load early in infancy, which results in too little TH1 cell activity and therefore insufficient IFN-γ to optimally cross-regulate TH2 responses (11,15–17).

Advances in the understanding of the immunological mechanisms of food allergy, in characterization of allergens (18), and in novel vaccination approaches make possible the development of new immunotherapeutic approaches for treatment of food allergy. However, the probability of a life-threatening reaction following exposure to even minute amounts of peanut reinforces the need for a suitable animal model.

We generated the first murine models of IgE-mediated cow milk hypersensitivity (19) and peanut anaphylaxis (20) using C3H/HeJ mice. In the peanut anaphylaxis model, peanut-specific IgE levels were induced by intragastric (ig) peanut sensitization, and systemic anaphylactic symptoms were provoked by peanut ingestion. It was also found that T- and B-cell responses to the major peanut allergens resemble those of human peanut allergy. This model physiologically and immunologically mimics human PNA and is a suitable tool to investigate the efficacy of novel treatments for peanut anaphylaxis. Over the past several years, this model has been used to test several novel approaches, including "engineered" (modified) recombinant protein immunotherapy (21), DNA based immunotherapy (22), bacterial adjuvant therapy (23), cytokine-modulated immunotherapy (24), and Chinese herbal medicine (25) to the treatment of PNA. In those studies, treatment efficacy was evaluated by determining anaphylactic symptom scores, plasma histamine levels, and percent mast cell degranulation. The effects on B-cell antibody synthesis (IgE/IgG2a) and T-cell cytokine patterns were also determined. In some cases, core body temperature and peak expiratory flow (PEF) measurements were performed. This chapter highlights the results of these antigen-specific and non–antigen–specific immunotherapies.

II. ANTIGEN-SPECIFIC IMMUNOTHERAPY

A. Purified "Engineered" (Modified) Recombinant Protein Immunotherapy

Antigen-specific immunotherapy is used to generate tolerance to specific allergens, but unlike traditional immunotherapy for inhalant and Hymenoptera sting allergy, the benefit-

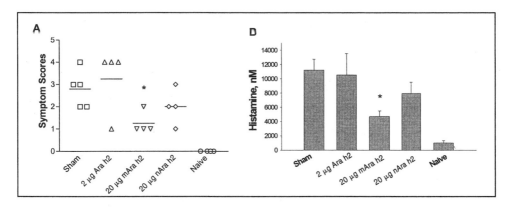

Figure 1 mAra h2 protection against peanut-induced anaphylactic reactions. *A: Anaphylactic symptom scores.* Mice were sensitized intragastrically (ig) with PN and then subjected to a 4-week desensitization protocol and challenged 4 weeks after the last desensitization. Symptoms were scored 30 min following oral peanut challenge as follows: 0—no reaction; 1—scratching and rubbing around the nose and head; 2—puffiness around eyes and snout, pilar erecti, diarrhea, reduced activity, or standing still with an increasing respiratory rate; 3—wheezing, labored respiration, cyanosis around the mouth and tail; 4—no activity after prodding, or tremor and convulsion; 5—death. Symbols indicate individual mice (*n* = 4–5 in each group) *B: Plasma histamine levels.* Blood was collected 30 min post-challenge, and plasma histamine levels were determined using an enzyme immunoassay kit (ImmunoTECH Inc.). Data are mean ± SEM. **p* < 0.05 vs. sham. (Source: King et al., manuscript submitted.)

to-risk ratio for traditional injections of peanut allergen was found to be unacceptable (26). To investigate safe and effective immunotherapeutic approaches for treating peanut allergy, engineered (modified) peanut proteins mAra h1, mAra h2, and mAra h3 (mAra-h123) have been developed; i.e., IgE-binding epitopes have been altered by a critical amino acid within the IgE binding site (epitope) to eliminate or drastically reduce IgE binding to the protein (27,28) and therefore carry less risk of eliciting allergic reactions. The efficacy of immunotherapy with modified peanut allergen to wild type (WT) peanut allergen protein was first compared using our murine model of peanut allergy. Peanut-allergic mice were desensitized by intranasal administration of mAra h2 (2 μg and 20 μg) or wild type Ara h2 (20 μg) given to them, three doses per week for 4 weeks. Treatment with mAra h2, but not wild type Ara h2, significantly reduced peanut-specific IgE (data not shown), symptom scores, and histamine levels (Fig. 1) compared with sham-treated mice. These results indicate that modified, but not wild type, peanut protein immunization provided some protection against peanut hypersensitivity. However, desensitization required frequent administrations (King et al., manuscript submitted). In a separate experiment, subcutaneous (SC) desensitization, the standard route for immunotherapy, produced modest protection, even with a higher dose (30 μg) (Li et al., unpublished data). These results suggest that engineered peanut protein alone may not be an adequate approach to treating peanut allergy.

B. Co-administration of Engineered Recombinant Peanut Protein and Heat-Killed *Listeria monocytogenes* Protects Against Peanut-Induced Anaphylaxis in a Murine Model

Heat-killed *Listeria monocytogenes* (HKLM), a potent activator of the innate immune system, has been employed as an adjuvant in immunotherapeutic desensitization of mice. For example, Yeung et al. showed that co-administration of HKLM and keyhole limpet hemocyanin (KLH) to KLH-sensitized mice reduced TH2 cytokines and IgE production and increased IFN-γ production (29). Hansen et al. showed that co-administration of HKLM and OVA prevented and reversed established airway hyperreactivity (AHR) in a murine model of allergic asthma (30). The findings that HKLM is a strong TH1 adjuvant suggest that HKLM might enhance the efficacy of modified peanut protein–based immunotherapy.

Therefore, the effect of co-administration of modified peanut proteins (mAra h123) and HKLM as an adjuvant (mAra h123 + HKLM) on a murine model of peanut hypersensitivity was investigated (31). In this study, peanut-allergic mice were treated SC with mAra h123 + HKLM (30 μg each) three times at weekly intervals or with mAra h123 alone (30 μg each) three times a week for 4 weeks. All mice in the sham and HKLM-alone–treated groups developed anaphylactic reactions (median symptom scores 3 and 2.7, respectively), whereas only 31% of mice in the mAra h123 + HKLM–treated group developed anaphylactic symptoms (median score 0.5) following peanut challenge. Rectal temperature and PEF, 20 and 30 min following challenge, respectively, were also determined, since a drop in body temperature and peak expiratory flow (PEF) in mice are correlated with the severity of anaphylaxis. Temperatures and PEF levels were significantly higher in the mAra h123 + HKLM–treated group compared with the sham-treated group (Fig. 2). Plasma histamine levels were markedly reduced (31). Furthermore, IgE levels were significantly reduced and IgG2a levels were significantly increased in the mAra h123 + HKLM–treated group compared with the sham-treated group (Fig. 3). Treatment with mAra h123 alone had significantly less effect on hypersensitivity reactions and histamine release and no effect on IgE synthesis despite increased numbers of treatments. Furthermore, splenocyte IL-4, IL-5, and IL-13 production were significantly reduced and IFN-γ production was significantly increased only in cultured lymphocytes from mAra h123 + HKLM–treated mice (31). These results suggest that immunotherapy with modified PN protein and HKLM, as an adjuvant, is superior to purified modified protein alone and may be a potential approach to treating PN hypersensitivity.

C. Potency and Persistency of Heat-Killed *E. coli*–Producing mAra h123 Effects on PN Hypersensitivity

Since engineered PN proteins are generated in *Escherichia coli*, which itself may serve as an adjuvant promoting a TH1 response, subsequent studies investigated the efficacy of a mixture of heat-killed *E. coli*–producing mAra h123 (HKE-MP123). Administering this mixture subcutaneously or rectally, but not intragastrically, suppressed PNA (Li et al., manuscript in preparation). The subcutaneous route of HKE-MP123 was abandoned because it induced skin inflammation (Li et al., unpublished data) and is unlikely to be acceptable for human use. Since the rectal mucosa is heavily colonized with *E. coli* and other organisms, it was felt that the rectal route of administering HKE-MP123 could provide an acceptable alternative.

The efficacy of rectal administration of HKE-MP123 to a mixture of the same purified modified PN allergenic proteins alone (MP-123) were also compared in a separate

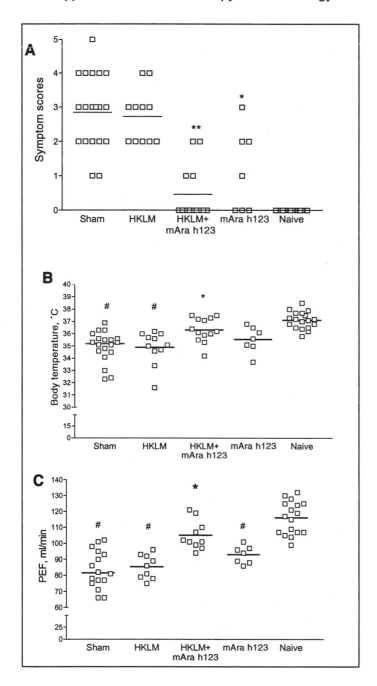

Figure 2 Protection against peanut-induced anaphylactic reactions by mArah123 + HKLM. *A: Anaphylactic symptom scores*. Anaphylactic symptoms were scored as described in Fig. 1. *B: Core temperatures*. Core temperatures were measured 20 min after ig peanut challenge. *C: Immediate airway responses (PEF)*. PEF measurements were performed immediately after evaluation of anaphylactic symptoms. Symbols indicate individual mice from three separate experiments (sham, $n = 19$; HKLM, $n = 11$; mAra h123 + HKLM, $n = 13$; mAra h123, $n = 7$; naive, $n = 18$). Bars indicate the medians. $*p < 0.05$ vs. sham; $**p < 0.01$ vs. sham; $\#p < 0.05$ vs. naive. (From Ref. 31.)

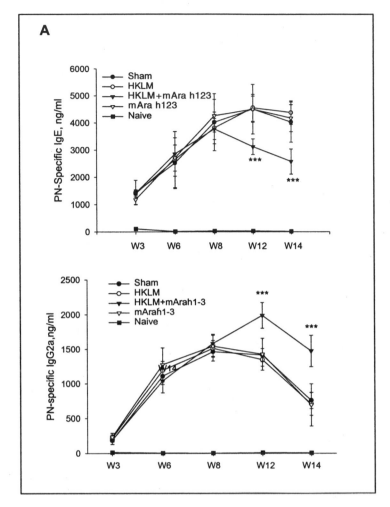

Figure 3 Reduction of IgE and increase in IgG2a by mAra h123 + HKLM treatment. Sera from all groups of mice were obtained during desensitization (3, 6, and 8 weeks), after 2 weeks treatment, and at the time of challenge (weeks 12 and 14). PN-specific IgE levels and IgG2a levels were determined by ELISA. Data are mean ± SEM for each group from three separate experiments as in Fig. 2. ***$p < 0.001$ vs. sham. (From Ref. 31.)

study. The therapeutic efficacy of low (9 μg, or 3 μg each of mAra h123 proteins) and high doses (90 μg or 30 μg each of mAra h123 proteins) of HKE-MP123 on PNA compared with MP-123 (a mixture of mAra h1, mAra h2, and mAra h3) treatment in PN-allergic mice were tested. HKE-MP123 treatment, even at low dose, significantly reduced anaphylactic symptom scores, plasma histamine levels, and serum IgE levels, and increased IgG2a levels compared with the sham-treated group. MP-123 did not produce significant protection of PN-induced anaphylactic reactions regardless of the dose and nine additional administrations. HKE-MP123 increased TH1 and decreased TH2 cytokine production. These results demonstrate that HKE-MP123 significantly protects against PN-induced anaphylaxis in this model and also exhibits beneficial immunoregulatory effects on T-cells (Li et al., manuscript in preparation).

Next, the persistence of pr HKE-MP123 effects (32) were evaluated. In this study, PN-allergic C3H/HeJ mice received 0.9 μg (low dose, or 0.3 μg each of mAra h123 proteins), 9 μg (medium dose, or 3 μg each of mAra h123 proteins) or 90 μg (high dose, or 30 μg each of mAra h123 proteins) HKE-MP123, HKE-containing vector (HKE-V) alone, or vehicle alone (sham) weekly for 3 weeks. Mice were challenged 2 weeks later. A second and third challenge were performed at 4-week intervals. Following the first challenge, all HKE-MP123– and HKE-V–treated groups exhibited reduced symptom scores ($p < 0.01, 0.01, 0.05, 0.05$, respectively, Fig. 4A) compared with the sham-treated group. Only the medium- and high-dose HKE-MP123–treated mice remained protected for up to 10 weeks following treatment (Fig. 4B and C). These mice also showed a significant reduction of plasma histamine levels compared with sham-treated mice ($p < 0.05$ and 0.01, respectively) (32). IgE levels were significantly lower in all HKE-MP123–treated groups ($p < 0.001$), being the lowest in the high-dose HKE-MP123–treated group at the time of challenges. IgG2a levels were significantly increased in all HKE-MP123–treated groups ($p < 0.001$), being the highest in the high-dose HKE-MP123–treated group (32). Furthermore, IL-4, IL-5, IL-13, and IL-10 production by splenocytes of high-dose HKE-MP123–treated mice was significantly lower (Fig. 5A, B, C, and F; $p < 0.01$, $p < 0.001$, $p < 0.001$, and $p < 0.001$, respectively). IFN-γ and TGF-β production was significantly higher (Fig. 5D and E, $p < 0.001$ and $p < 0.01$, respectively) compared with sham-treated mice at the time of the last challenge, showing a beneficial immunoregulatory effect. These results demonstrate that treatment with rectally administered HKE-MP123 can induce long-term "downregulation" of PN hypersensitivity.

In addition to HKE's probable adjuvant activity, HKE-MP123 treatment has several other benefits as a novel immunotherapeutic approach to PNA treatment. First, because the engineered recombinant PN proteins are generated in *E. coli*, using HKE-producing engineered PN protein does not require purifying the recombinant PN proteins from *E. coli* and is therefore less time-consuming and costly. Second, *E. coli* cells are still intact after heat killing, preventing the proteins from activating mast cells and resulting in an additional level of safety. Finally, since the HKE-MP123 is administered into an environment replete with *E. coli* and other bacteria, there is little concern about safety of such vaccine administration. Therefore, this approach appears to be superior to co-administration of HKL and purified engineered PN proteins. Although rigorous investigation is required to confirm the safety of this approach, no signs of anaphylaxis or local inflammation have occurred during desensitization. These studies suggest that HKE-MP123 may be a potential therapeutic approach for PNA.

D. Plasmid DNA–Based Immunotherapy

Plasmid DNA–based immunotherapy (DNA vaccine) is a novel method of generating immune responses by immunizing with bacterial plasmid DNA (pDNA), encoding specific antigens. DNA vaccination can induce prolonged humoral and cellular immune responses and is of particular interest for treatment of allergy because it induces a TH1 response (33). Since treatment of peanut-allergic mice with modified peanut allergen protein produced some protection, it was hypothesized that plasmid DNA encoding mutated peanut allergens may provide a more effective immunotherapy for peanut allergy. Therefore, a plasmid DNA construct encoding mAra h2 (pST2mAra h2) was generated and Ara h2–sensitized C3H/HeJ mice treated. pST2mAra h2 attenuated peanut hypersensitivity reactions following oral Ara h2 challenge.

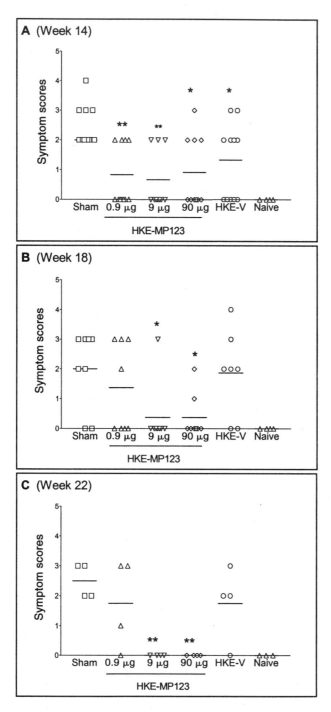

Figure 4   Persistent HKE-MP123 protection against peanut-induced anaphylactic reactions. Mice were challenged at weeks 2 (*A*), 6 (*B*), and 10 (*C*) following the last HKE-MP123 treatment. Anaphylactic symptom scores were determined 30 min following challenge. Each point indicates an individual mouse. Bars indicate the median scores of 12 mice (*A*), 8 mice (*B*), and 4 mice (*C*) in each group. *$p < 0.05$, **$p < 0.01$ vs. sham. (From Ref. 32.)

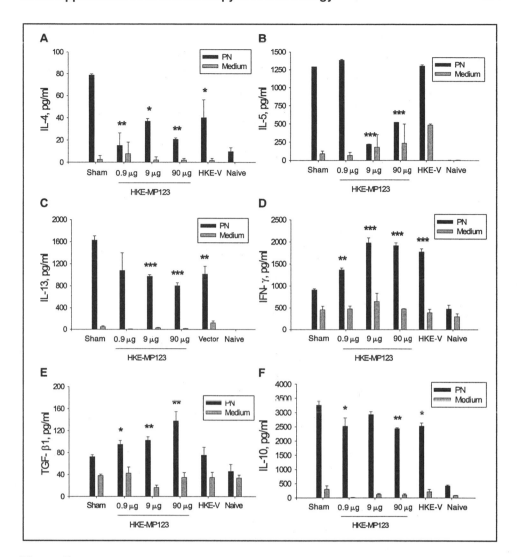

Figure 5 Effect of HKE-MP123 therapy on cytokine production. Splenocytes were collected immediately following anaphylaxis evaluation from four mice in each group at week 10 following the last HKE-MP123 treatment. Cell suspensions were cultured in complete culture medium in the presence of CPE, or medium alone or Con A (data not shown). Supernatants were collected 72 hours later, and cytokine levels were determined by ELISA. Results are expressed as mean ± SEM of two duplicate cultures of four mice. *$p < 0.05$, **$p < 0.01$, ***$p < 0.001$ vs. sham. (From Ref. 32.)

In addition, both intranasal and rectal administration of pST2mAra h (100 μg/mouse, three times at weekly intervals) suppressed peanut hypersensitivity reactions induced by whole peanut sensitization and challenge. As shown in Fig. 6, anaphylactic symptom scores and peanut-specific IgE were markedly reduced in pST2mAra h–treated groups compared with the sham and mock DNA treated–groups (Fig. 2A and B, $p < 0.05$ and 0.01, respectively). This protection was associated with suppression of T-cell proliferative responses, reduction of IL-4, and induction of IFN-γ (Zhang et al., unpublished

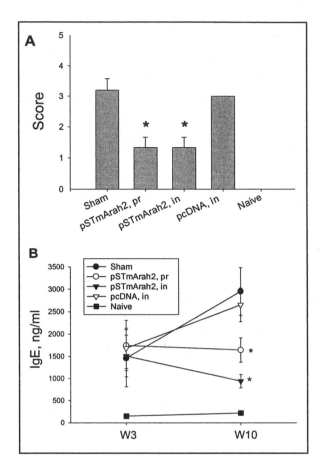

Figure 6 pST2mAra h2 suppresses peanut hypersensitivity. *A*: PN-specific IgE levels. Blood was collected 1 day prior to initiating treatment at week 3 and 1 day prior to challenge at week 10. PN-specific IgE levels were measured by ELISA. *B*: Anaphylactic symptom scores. Anaphylactic symptom scores were evaluated as described in Fig. 1. Data are mean ± SEM ($n = 4,5$), *$p < 0.05$ vs. sham in = intranasal, pr = per rectum. (Source: Zhang et al., manuscript in preparation.)

data). That this approach required only three administrations suggests that plasmid DNA encoding of mutated major peanut allergens is more potent than purified recombinant mutated protein alone. This might be a potential immunotherapeutic approach for peanut allergy. However, the protection was only partial against peanut anaphylaxis mediated by pSTmAra h2 in this study. Whether efficacy might be improved by increasing the dose of pSTmAra h2 has not yet been determined. Administration of a mixture of the three constructs encoding mutated peanut allergens (pST2mAra h123) may also further increase efficacy. Since the advantage of plasmid DNA–based vaccination is its long-lasting effect, we are also interested in investigating whether pST2mAra h2 or pST2mAra h123 has long-lasting protection against peanut allergy.

III. NON–ANTIGEN-SPECIFIC APPROACHES TO PEANUT ALLERGY

A. Cytokine Therapy: Effect of IL-12 on Peanut Allergy

IL-12, a heterodimeric cytokine produced by antigen-presenting cells, promotes differentiation of TH1 cells and IFN-γ production and inhibits the differentiation of TH0 cells into IL-4–secreting TH2 cells, thereby suppressing IgE production (34–38). Intraperitoneal IL-12 treatment of mice has been shown to inhibit antigen-induced eosinophilic inflammation, airway hyperresponsiveness, and IgE production (39–41) and to switch a TH2 to a TH1-type response in established *Leishmania* major infections (42). Lee et al. used a mouse model of peanut anaphylaxis to evaluate the possible prophylactic and therapeutic effects of orally administered IL-12 on peanut allergy. They found that oral IL-12 administration initiated 3 weeks after sensitization as well as at the time of sensitization attenuated anaphylactic reactions triggered by peanut challenge of allergic mice (43). Symptom reduction was accompanied by reduction in peanut-specific IgE and reversal or reduction of the IgG1/IgG2a ratio. Furthermore, oral IL-12 treatment increased the IFN-γ/IL-4 and IFN-γ/IL-5 ratios (43). These results suggest some potential for the use of IL-12, either alone or in combination with other immunomodulatory agents, as a treatment for peanut allergy. Further studies are required to evaluate dose-related and long-term effects of IL-12 therapy on peanut hypersensitivity.

Other cytokines such as IFN-γ and transforming growth factor–β (TGF-β) have been suggested as important in the induction of oral tolerance to food (44). As discussed earlier, persistence of heat-killed *E. coli*–producing mAra h123 effects on peanut hypersensitivity was associated with induction of IFN-γ and TGF-β. However, there are no studies on the effects of administering IFN-γ and/or TGF-β on food allergy.

B. CpG Oligonucleotides Protect Against Anaphylaxis

Bacterial DNA and synthetic oligodeoxynucleotides (ODN) containing CpG motifs are potent inducers of TH1-like responses characterized by production of IL-12, IFN-γ, and IgG2a (45,46). Consequently, immunomodulatory protocols employing CpG-ODN have been applied to murine models of allergic asthma. CpG-ODN treatment, at the time of Ag sensitization or before Ag challenge, have a prophylactic effect on Ag-induced airway eosinophilia and AHR (47–50). In addition to its known preventive effects, CpG-ODN administration following Ag challenge also significantly reduces Ag-specific IgE production, eosinophilic inflammation, and AHR, which are associated with upregulation of IFN-γ and downregulation of IL-4, IL-5, and IL-13 (51). The use of CpG for the treatment of peanut allergy in a murine model of peanut-induced anaphylaxis was investigated (52). C3H/HeJ mice were orally sensitized with peanut and cholera toxin over 7 weeks. Mice were subsequently treated with CpG intranasally weekly for 3 weeks or left untreated. One week following the final treatment, mice were orally challenged with PN. CpG-treated mice were completely protected from anaphylactic reactions in response to PN challenge, whereas 67% of untreated mice displayed symptoms of anaphylaxis. Core body temperatures following challenge of CpG-treated mice ($35.15 \pm 0.6°C$) were higher than in the untreated group ($32.3 \pm 2.0°C$). A slight reduction in peanut-specific IgE levels was seen in CpG-treated mice (1553 ± 156 ng/ml) compared with the untreated mice (1738 ± 290 ng/ml). PN-specific IgG2a levels in CpG-treated mice (234.5 ± 90.3 μg/ml) were more than threefold higher than in untreated mice (68.4 ± 4.1 μg/ml). Intranasal CpG treatment was shown to protect PN-allergic mice from anaphylactic reactions to oral PN challenge, suggesting that CpG may be a potential therapeutic approach for peanut allergy in humans. As seen in the asthma model, CpG-ODN alone was also partially effective in suppression of anaphylactic reactions. This approach may have potential for all TH-2 mediated food-allergic reactions regardless of the specific food allergen (Srivastava et al., manuscript in preparation).

C. Chinese Herbal Medicine Therapy for Food Allergy

Traditional Chinese medicine (TCM), one of the oldest medical systems in the world, has been used for thousands of years in China and is attracting interest in Western countries as a source of potential therapies for a variety of diseases. There is some scientific evidence to support the use of TCM-derived treatments for allergy and asthma (53–55). Food Allergy Herbal Formula–1 (FAHF-1), developed from a TCM herbal formula, completely protected against peanut anaphylaxis in a murine model of peanut hypersensitivity (25) (Fig. 7). FAHF-1 also markedly reduced mast cell degranulation (Fig. 8) and histamine release. FAHF-1 protection against peanut allergy is associated with significantly reduced peanut-specific IgE, lymphocyte proliferation to peanut allergen stimulation, and IL-4, IL-5, and IL-13 production (25). No toxic effects on liver or kidney functions and no overall immune suppression was observed (25). Although animal models of disease do not translate to human disease, this study suggests that FAHF-1 and possible other herbal formulas may prove useful for the treatment of peanut allergy and other IgE-mediated food allergy. Although the mechanisms are not fully understood, it is possible that FAHF-1 may target multiple parts of food-allergic reaction cascade such as suppressing antigen-specific B-cell, TH2 cell, and mast cell activation. It is also conceivable that FAHF-1 may reduce intestinal permeability, thereby reducing the amount of peanut allergens available to interact with mast cells. These features may prove to be particularly advantageous compared with other immunotherapies that target only antigen, TH2 cytokines, or IgE antibodies. However, pharmacological level standardization of this formula would be a major undertaking.

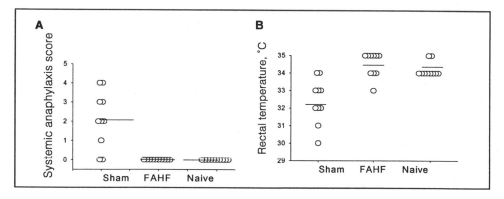

Figure 7 Complete protection against symptoms of peanut anaphylaxis by FAHF-1. *A*: Anaphylactic symptom scores. Anaphylactic symptoms were scored as described in Fig. 1. *B*: Core body temperatures. Core temperatures were measured 20 min after intragastric gavage peanut challenge. Symbols in *A* and *B* (open circles) indicate individual mice from two sets of experiments (*n* = 10). Bars are medians of scores. **$p < 0.01$ vs. sham. (From Ref. 25.)

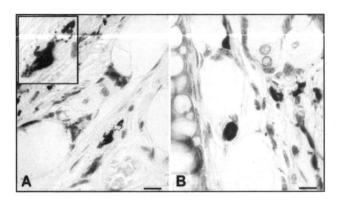

Figure 8   FAHF-1 suppression of mast cell degranulation. Paraffin sections of ear samples (5 μm) collected 40 min after challenge were stained with toluidine blue and examined by light microscopy. *A*: Degranulated mast cells in dermis of sham-treated mice following challenge (bar = 10 μm). Inset is high magnification showing granules outside degranulating mast cells. *B*: Normal mast cells in an ear sample of FAHF-1-treated mice. (From Ref. 25.)

IV.   CONCLUSION

Although there is no effective and safe therapy for food allergy, many novel approaches are under investigation. Some of these approaches may provide allergists with effective treatments in the near future.

V.   SALIENT POINTS

1.   The incidence of food allergy is increasing. Peanut allergy is one of the major causes of food-induced fatal and near-fatal anaphylactic reactions in both adults and children.
2.   PNA is an IgE-mediated type I hypersensitivity. Peanut allergic status is characterized by a TH2 response whereas TH1-skewed responses underlie oral tolerance.
3.   Antigen-specific immunotherapy is used to generate tolerance to specific allergens, but unlike traditional immunotherapy for inhalant and bee sting allergy, the benefit-to-risk ratio for traditional injections of peanut allergen is unacceptable.
4.   Animal models of food hypersensitivity that mimic human food allergy have facilitated the investigation of novel therapies for food allergy.
5.   Engineered (mutated) peanut proteins carry less risk of eliciting allergic reactions. However, engineered peanut proteins are inadequate for treating peanut allergy. Treatment with a mixture of mutated peanut proteins and HKLM, or with HKE containing mutated peanut proteins, produced protection against peanut anaphylaxis. The effect was associated with upregulation of TH1 cytokines and downregulation of TH2 cytokines. Induction of TGF-β, the T-regulatory cytokine, may also play an important role in mediating desensitization of peanut allergy.

6. Other immunomodulators such as IL-12 and CpG oligonucleotides showed partial protection against peanut anaphylaxis. This type of therapy does not require specific allergen administration.

7. Chinese herbal medicine formulas, including FAHF-1, appear to have potential for treating peanut allergy and perhaps other food allergies. However, it will be challenging to determine the effective components in the formula and to purify the active constituents responsible for its therapeutic effect.

ACKNOWLEDGEMENTS

The authors thank Kamala Srivastava, Teng-Fei Zhang, Chih-Kang Huang, Soo-Young Lee, Jacob Kattan, Brian Schofield, Gary Bannon, and Wesley Burks for their contributions to this work. This work was supported by the Clarissa Sosin Allergy Foundation, the Dugan Family Foundation, and by National Institutes of Health grant #AI 43668.

REFERENCES

1. Sampson HA. Food allergy. Part 1: Immunopathogenesis and clinical disorders. J Allergy Clin Immunol 1999; 103:717–728.

2. Sampson HA. Clinical practice: Peanut allergy. N Engl J Med 2002; 346:1294–1299.

3. Sampson HA, Mendelson L, Rosen JP. Fatal and near-fatal anaphylactic reactions to food in children and adolescents. N Engl J Med 1992; 327:380–384.

4. Bock SA, Munoz-Furlong A, Sampson HA. Fatalities due to anaphylactic reactions to foods. J Allergy Clin Immunol 2001; 107:191–193.

5. Bock SA. The natural history of food sensitivity. J Allergy Clin Immunol 1982; 69:173–177.

6. Leung DY, Sampson HA, Yunginger JW, Burks AWJ, Schneider LC, Wortel CH, Davis FM, Hyun JD, Shanahan WRJ. Effect of anti-IgE therapy in patients with peanut allergy. N Engl J Med 2003; 348:986–993.

7. Yocum MW, Butterfield JH, Klein JS, Volcheck GW, Schroeder DR, Silverstein MD. Epidemiology of anaphylaxis in Olmsted County: A population-based study. J Allergy Clin Immunol 1999; 104:452–456.

8. Romagnani S. The role of lymphocytes in allergic disease. J Allergy Clin Immunol 2000; 105:399–408.

9. de Jong EC, Van Zijverden M, Spanhaak S, Koppelman SJ, Pellegrom H, Penninks AH. Identification and partial characterization of multiple major allergens in peanut proteins. Clin Exp Allergy 1998; 28:743–751.

10. Dorion BJ, Burks AW, Harbeck R, Williams LW, Trumble A, Helm RM, Leung DY. The production of interferon-gamma in response to a major peanut allergy, Ara h II, correlates with serum levels of IgE anti–Ara h II. J Allergy Clin Immunol 1994; 93:93–99.

11. Brandtzaeg P. Current understanding of gastrointestinal immunoregulation and its relation to food allergy. Ann N Y Acad Sci 2002; 964:13–45.

12. Strobel S, Mowat AM. Immune responses to dietary antigens: Oral tolerance. Immunol Today 1998; 19:173–181.

13. Turcanu V, Maleki SJ, Lack G. Characterization of lymphocyte responses to peanuts in normal children, peanut-allergic children, and allergic children who acquired tolerance to peanuts. J Clin Investig 2003; 111:1065–1072.

14. von Mutius E. The environmental predictors of allergic disease. J Allergy Clin Immunol 2000; 105:9–19.

15. Erb KJ. Atopic disorders: A default pathway in the absence of infection? Immunol Today 1999; 20:317–322.

16. International Study of Asthma and Allergies in Childhood Steering Committee. Worldwide variation in the prevalence of symptoms of asthma, allergic rhinoconjunctivitis and atopic eczema: ISAAC. Lancet 1998; 351:1225–1232.

17. Rook GA, Stanford JL. Give us this day our daily germs. Immunol Today 1998; 19:113–116.

18. Burks W, Helm R, Stanley S, Bannon GA. Food allergens. Curr Opin Allergy Clin Immunol 2001; 1:243–248.

19. Li XM, Schofield BH, Huang CK, Kleiner GA, Sampson HA. A murine model of IgE mediated cow milk hypersensitivity. J Allergy Clin Immunol 1999; 103:206–214.

20. Li XM, Serebrisky D, Lee SY, Huang CK, Bardina L, Schofield BH, Stanley JS, Burks AW, Bannon GA, Sampson HA. A murine model of peanut anaphylaxis: T- and B-cell responses to a major peanut allergen mimic human responses. J Allergy Clin Immunol 2000; 106:150–158.

21. Srivastava K, Li XM, King N, Stanley S, Bannon GA, Burks W, Sampson HA. Immunotherapy with modified peanut allergens in a murine model of peanut allergy (abstr). J Allergy Clin Immunol 2002; 109:S287–S287.

22. Li X, Huang CK, Schofield BH, Burks AW, Bannon GA, Kim KH, Huang SK, Sampson HA. Strain-dependent induction of allergic sensitization caused by peanut allergen DNA immunization in mice. J Immunol 1999; 162:3045–3052.

23. Li JH, Srivastava K, Huleatt J, Bottomly K, Burks W, Li XM, Sampson HA. Investigation of efficacy of co-administration of heat killed *Listeria* with modified peanut protein for the treatment of peanut-induced hypersensitivity in a murine model (abstr). J Allergy Clin Immunol 2002; 109:S93–S93.

24. Lee SY, Huang CK, Zhang TF, Schofield BH, Burks AW, Bannon GA, Sampson HA, Li XM. Oral administration of IL-12 suppresses anaphylactic reactions in a murine model of peanut hypersensitivity. Clin Immunol 2001; 101:220–228.

25. Li XM, Zhang TF, Huang CK, Srivastava K, Teper AA, Zhang L, Schofield BH, Sampson HA. Food Allergy Herbal Formula–1 (FAHF-1) blocks peanut-induced anaphylaxis in a murine model. J Allergy Clin Immunol 2001; 108:639–646.

26. Oppenheimer JJ, Nelson HS, Bock SA, Christensen F, Leung DY. Treatment of peanut allergy with rush immunotherapy. J Allergy Clin Immunol 1992; 90:256–262.

27. Stanley JS, King N, Burks AW, Huang SK, Sampson H, Cockrell G, Helm RM, West CM, Bannon GA. Identification and mutational analysis of the immunodominant IgE binding epitopes of the major peanut allergen Ara h 2. Arch Biochem Biophys 1997; 342:244–253.

28. Schramm G, Kahlert H, Suck R, Weber B, Stuwe HT, Muller WD, Bufe A, Becker WM, Schlaak MW, Jager L, Cromwell O, Fiebig H. "Allergen engineering": Variants of the timothy grass pollen allergen Phl p 5b with reduced IgE-binding capacity but conserved T cell reactivity. J Immunol 1999; 162:2406–2414.

29. Yeung VP, Gieni RS, Umetsu DT, DeKruyff RH. Heat-killed *Listeria monocytogenes* as an adjuvant converts established murine Th2-dominated immune responses into Th1-dominated responses. J Immunol 1998; 161:4146–4152.

30. Hansen G, Yeung VP, Berry G, Umetsu DT, DeKruyff RH. Vaccination with heat-killed *Listeria* as adjuvant reverses established allergen-induced airway hyperreactivity and inflammation: Role of CD8+ T cells and IL-18. J Immunol 2000; 164:223–230.

31. Li XM, Srivastava K, Huleatt JW, Bottomly K, Burks AW, Sampson HA. Engineered recombinant peanut protein and heat-killed *Listeria monocytogenes* coadministration protects against peanut-induced anaphylaxis in a murine model. J Immunol 2003; 170:3289–3295.

32. Li XM, Srivastava K, Grishin A, Huang CK, Schofield BH, Burks AW, Sampson HA. Persistent protective effect of heat killed *E. coli* producing "engineered," recombinant peanut proteins in a murine model of peanut allergy. J Allergy Clin Immunol 2003 (in press).

33. Raz E, Tighe H, Sato Y, Corr M, Dudler JA, Roman M, Swain SL, Spiegelberg HL, Carson DA. Preferential induction of a Th1 immune response and inhibition of specific IgE antibody formation by plasmid DNA immunization. Proc Natl Acad Sci USA 1996; 93:5141–5145.

34. Seder RA, Gazzinelli R, Sher A, Paul WE. Interleukin 12 acts directly on CD4+ T cells to enhance priming for interferon gamma production and diminishes interleukin 4 inhibition of such priming. Proc Natl Acad Sci USA 1993; 90:10188–10192.

35. Wills-Karp M. IL-12/IL-13 axis in allergic asthma. J Allergy Clin Immunol 2001; 107:9–18.

36. Hsieh CS, Macatonia SE, Tripp CS, Wolf SF, O'Garra A, Murphy KM. Development of TH1 CD4+ T cells through IL-12 produced by *Listeria*-induced macrophages. Science 1993; 260:547–549.

37. Trinchieri G. Interleukin-12 and its role in the generation of TH1 cells. Immunol Today 1993; 14:335–338.

38. Manetti R, Parronchi P, Giudizi MG, Piccinni MP, Maggi E, Trinchieri G, Romagnani S. Natural killer cell stimulatory factor (interleukin 12 [IL-12]) induces T helper type 1 (Th1)–specific immune responses and inhibits the development of IL-4-producing Th cells. J Exp Med 1993; 177:1199–1204.

39. Gavett SH, O'Hearn DJ, Li X, Huang SK, Finkelman FD, Wills-Karp M. Interleukin 12 inhibits antigen-induced airway hyperresponsiveness, inflammation, and Th2 cytokine expression in mice. J Exp Med 1995; 182:1527–1536.

40. Stampfli MR, Scott NG, Wiley RE, Cwiartka M, Ritz SA, Hitt MM, Xing Z, Jordana M. Regulation of allergic mucosal sensitization by interleukin-12 gene transfer to the airway. Am J Respir Cell Mol Biol 1999; 21:317–326.

41. Kim TS, DeKruyff RH, Rupper R, Maecker HT, Levy S, Umetsu DT. An ovalbumin-IL-12 fusion protein is more effective than ovalbumin plus free recombinant IL-12 in inducing a T helper cell type 1–dominated immune response and inhibiting antigen-specific IgE production. J Immunol 1997; 158:4137–4144.

42. Nabors GS, Afonso LC, Farrell JP, Scott P. Switch from a type 2 to a type 1 T helper cell response and cure of established *Leishmania* major infection in mice is induced by combined therapy with interleukin 12 and Pentostam. Proc Natl Acad Sci USA 1995; 92:3142–3146.

43. Lee SS, Lee KY, Noh G. The necessity of diet therapy for successful interferon-gamma therapy in atopic dermatitis. Yonsei Med J 2001; 42:161–171.

44. Husby S. Sensitization and tolerance. Curr Opin Allergy Clin Immunol 2001; 1:237–241.

45. Krieg AM, Yi AK, Matson S, Waldschmidt TJ, Bishop GA, Teasdale R, Koretzky GA, Klinman DM. CpG motifs in bacterial DNA trigger direct B-cell activation. Nature 1995; 374:546–549.

46. Klinman DM, Yi AK, Beaucage SL, Conover J, Krieg AM. CpG motifs present in bacteria DNA rapidly induce lymphocytes to secrete interleukin 6, interleukin 12, and interferon gamma. Proc Natl Acad Sci USA 1996; 93:2879–2883.

47. Kline JN, Waldschmidt TJ, Businga TR, Lemish JE, Weinstock JV, Thorne PS, Krieg AM. Modulation of airway inflammation by CpG oligodeoxynucleotides in a murine model of asthma. J Immunol 1998; 160:2555–2559.

48. Broide D, Schwarze J, Tighe H, Gifford T, Nguyen MD, Malek S, Van UJ, Martin-Orozco E, Gelfand EW, Raz E. Immunostimulatory DNA sequences inhibit IL-5, eosinophilic inflammation, and airway hyperresponsiveness in mice. J Immunol 1998; 161:7054–7062.

49. Sur S, Wild JS, Choudhury BK, Sur N, Alam R, Klinman DM. Long term prevention of allergic lung inflammation in a mouse model of asthma by CpG oligodeoxynucleotides. J Immunol 1999; 162:6284–6293.

50. Jahn-Schmid B, Wiedermann U, Bohle B, Repa A, Kraft D, Ebner C. Oligodeoxynucleotides containing CpG motifs modulate the allergic TH2 response of BALB/c mice to Bet v 1, the major birch pollen allergen. J Allergy Clin Immunol 1999; 104:1015–1023.

51. Serebrisky D, Teper A, Huang CK, Lee SY, Zhang TF, Schofield BH, Kattan M, Sampson HA, Li XM. CpG Oligodeoxynucleotides can reverse Th2-associated allergic airway respones and alter the B7, 1/B7, 2 expression in a murine model of asthma. J Immunol 2000; 165:5906–5912.

52. Kattan JD, Srivastava KD, Sampson HA, Li XM. Intranasal treatment with CpG oligonucleotides provides protection from anaphylaxis in a murine model of peanut allergy (abstr). J Allergy Clin Immunol 2003; 111:S206.

53. Bielory L, Lupoli K. Herbal interventions in asthma and allergy. J Asthma 1999; 36:1–65.

54. Ziment I, Tashkin DP. Alternative medicine for allergy and asthma. J Allergy Clin Immunol 2000; 106:603–614.

55. Li XM, Huang CK, Zhang TF, Teper AA, Srivastava K, Schofield BH, Sampson HA. The Chinese herbal medicine formula MSSM-002 suppresses allergic airway hyperreactivity and modulates TH1/TH2 responses in a murine model of allergic asthma. J Allergy Clin Immunol 2000; 106:660–668.

37

Tolerance Induced by Allergen Immunotherapy

MARSHALL PLAUT and DANIEL ROTROSEN

National Institute of Allergy and Infectious Diseases, National Institutes of Health, Bethesda, Maryland, U.S.A.

I. INTRODUCTION

"Immunologic tolerance" describes the inhibition or absence of an immune response and, when used in the therapeutic sense, inhibition or elimination of only pathogenic immune responses, leaving the beneficial functions, such as protective immunity, intact (1). Although tolerance is often used to refer to responses to self-antigens, tolerant T- and B-cell responses can occur to both self and non-self antigens. In contrast to immunosuppressive and/or anti-inflammatory drugs, tolerizing agents induce an altered immune response that persists after the agent has been stopped. Tolerance in this chapter denotes a clinical state in which the allergen, after the discontinuation of allergen immunotherapy, no longer induces allergic symptoms. Studies to demonstrate that allergen immunotherapy induces long-term changes in the natural history of allergy have only recently become convincing because they included critical controls. The most detailed studies of immunotherapy have focused on 1 year or less of allergen injections, and such short duration of therapy does not generally induce tolerance. Several studies have demonstrated that, following prolonged insect venom immunotherapy, patients are protected from systemic reactions to stings for at least several years after therapy is stopped. In addition, a carefully controlled study of immunotherapy with grass pollen allergen provides strong evidence that allergen immunotherapy induces a clinical effect which persists at least 3 years after therapy is stopped (2).

There is strong clinical evidence for tolerance induction during allergen immunotherapy. However, investigators have not yet carried out the sophisticated immunological studies that are required to understand the basis of tolerance induction or to identify biomarkers of tolerance induction. Indeed, there are no known biomarkers of immunotherapy that predict whether symptom relief will persist after immunotherapy is discontinued. There are only two published papers, both using aeroallergen immunotherapy, that describe immune parameters that persist after immunotherapy is discontinued: blockade of postseasonal increases in IgE antibody (3), and blockade of allergen-induced late-phase skin reactions and of cellular components of the reaction, including reduction in the number of IL-4–expressing cells (2). With insect venom immunotherapy, there are no comparable parameters.

II. TOLERANCE INDUCTION*

A. General Principles

A major goal of modern clinical immunology is the development of new strategies and treatments that induce a state of immune tolerance by selectively blocking or eliminating pathogenic immune responses while maintaining protective immunity. Enthusiasm for the development of tolerizing therapies has been fueled by many anecdotal cases in which transplant recipients have discontinued immunsuppressive medications and maintained functioning grafts without evidence of rejection (4–6). The prospects for tolerizing therapies are now quite promising, as research into basic immunology has helped to unravel the fundamental processes responsible for self-tolerance and immune regulation. A variety of agents and approaches to induce immune tolerance are now entering clinical trials and, if successful, will find applications in a range of clinical scenarios, spanning allergy and autoimmunity, in addition to transplantation.

During immune development, the thymus molds the developing T-cell repertoire centrally by deletion of self-reactive clones. Small numbers of autoreactive T-cells escape to the periphery, either through incomplete negative selection or because not all peripheral antigens are displayed within the thymus. These self-reactive T-cells are inactivated at extrathymic sites, primarily lymph nodes and spleen, when mature T-cells encounter self-antigens. The processes that regulate peripheral tolerance—clonal inactivation, clonal deletion, and cytokine-dependent suppression and immune deviation—operate to varying degrees in the generation and maintenance of tolerance, although their relative contribu-

---

*Section II of this manuscript is reproduced almost verbatim from: Rotrosen D, Matthews JB, Bluestone JA. The immune tolerance network: A new paradigm for developing tolerance-inducing therapies. J Allergy Clin Immunol 2002; 110:17–23. (The U.S. government holds the copyright to this material.)

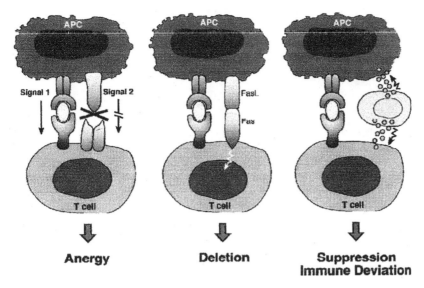

Figure 1 Molecular basis of immune tolerance. Schematic diagram of molecular pathways of tolerance induction. *Anergy*, left panel. T-cells that receive signal 1 in the absence of signal 2 (costimulatory blockade) become nonresponsive or anergic, and remain anergic upon subsequent antigen-specific stimulation, even in the presence of signal 2. A number of other approaches that interrupt signaling through the TCR may also lead to anergy (see text). *Deletion*, center panel. Activated T-cells upregulate the expression of Fas; subsequent binding of Fas ligand (FasL) induces T-cells to undergo apoptotic cell death. FasL may be expressed on APCs, activated T-cells, and stromal cells of immunologically privileged sites. *Suppression* and *immune deviation*, right panel. Stimulated T-cells may be tolerized via direct cell-cell contact (suppression) or soluble factors derived from regulatory T-cells (immune deviation). (Appeared in: Rose SM, Turka L, Kerr L, Rotrosen D. Advances in immune-based therapies to improve solid organ graft survival. In: Advances in Internal Medicine, volume 47 (Schrier RW, Dzau VJ, Baxter JD, Fauci AS, eds.). St. Louis, MO: Mosby, 2001:293–331.) (The U.S. government holds the copyright to this material.)

tions may vary depending upon the nature of the antigen and the location in which tolerization occurs (Fig. 1) (7). The existence of multiple pathways presents a wide range of potential targets for intervention. Indeed, dozens of ligands, receptors, and signaling intermediates provide the structural underpinnings for a host of candidate drugs. This complexity also introduces many practical challenges, due to the potential for functional redundancies in the targeted pathways, and heterogeneity in their expression among different diseases and affected individuals.

B. Targets for Intervention

1. Signal 1 and Signal 2

Naive T-cells require two distinct signals to become fully activated (Fig. 2). Signal 1 is propagated on presentation of antigen to the T-cell, initiating a signaling cascade involving a number of molecules including the CD4 or CD8 co-receptors and their associated kinases. Professional antigen-presenting cells (APC) deliver additional costimulatory signals, termed signal 2, that elicit robust and durable T-cell responses. Costimulation is

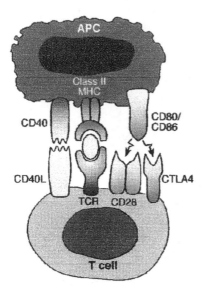

Costimulation

Figure 2 Molecular interactions leading to T-cell activation. Schematic diagram of the antigen-specific (signal 1) and costimulatory (signal 2) interactions between an APC and the T-cell. Signal 1 depends on interactions of the MHC-peptide complex with the T-cell receptor. Signal 2 is illustrated here by interactions of CD80 or CD86 with CD28. In contrast, CTLA4 acts as a competitive inhibitor of CD28, blocking CD28-mediated events. *Abbreviations. APC*, antigen-presenting cell; *MHC*, major histocompatibility complex; *TCR*, T-cell receptor. (Appeared in: Rose SM, Turka L, Kerr L, Rotrosen D. Advances in immune-based therapies to improve solid organ graft survival. In: Advances in Internal Medicine, volume 47 (Schrier RW, Dzau VJ, Baxter JD, Fauci AS, eds.). St. Louis, MO: Mosby, 2001:293–331.) (The U.S. government holds the copyright to this material.)

required for complete T-cell activation, whereas propagation of signal 1 in the absence of signal 2 leads to aborted T-cell responses, anergy, or death (8).

The most extensively studied of the costimulatory pathways involves the APC proteins, CD80 (B7-1) and CD86 (B7-2), and their T-cell receptor, CD28 (9,10). Other APC proteins including CD40, 4-1BB ligand, and a molecule called LIGHT provide costimulation through their T-cell receptors, CD40L, 4-1BB, and HVEM (for *herpes virus entry molecule*), respectively (11–13). These receptors act either directly in a costimulatory fashion or by upregulating other receptors and ligands needed for generation of signal 2, including CD28 itself. A major effect of costimulation is production of IL-2 and other cytokines required for T-cell proliferation and for arming differentiated T-cells to take on effector functions. Once fully differentiated and armed for effector functions, neither CD4+ nor CD8+ T-cells require costimulatory signals to respond; signal 1 is sufficient to stimulate secondary responses.

Interrupting signal 1 at a number of points may lead to tolerance, which may be antigen-specific depending on the approach—e.g., by monoclonal antibodies directed at the TCR and co-receptor molecules, by MHC-derived peptides, through presentation of altered TCR ligands, or through alloantigen pretreatment when donor-specific transfusion is combined with solid organ transplantation (14). Several of these have been, or are ready to be, applied clinically. Promising candidates include nonmitogenic anti-CD3 mAb, CD4 mAbs, anti-CD52 mAb (Campath-1), and systemic and oral peptide therapies (Copaxone and MHC peptides). It is possible that peptide-based immunotherapies for asthma and allergy induce clinical effects by allowing signal 1 in the absence of signal 2.

Costimulatory blockade with anti-CD40 ligand greatly prolongs renal allograft survival in nonhuman primates without the need for other immunosuppressives. For example, monkeys infused monthly with anti-CD40 ligand remained rejection-free and maintained functioning allografts for up to 2 years (15). Similarly encouraging results were achieved in pancreatectomized rhesus monkeys that received islet transplants under cover of anti-CD40 ligand alone (16). However, in neither of these experimental systems did the animals become fully tolerant. Future studies targeting both signal 1 and signal 2 (e.g., with nonmitogenic anti-CD3 plus anti-CD 80/86 or anti-CD40 ligand) may result in synergistic effects on tolerance induction. Such therapies represent some of the most promising approaches in transplantation and autoimmune diseases.

2. Clonal Deletion

Multiple approaches are being pursued to promote clonal deletion, either centrally within the thymus or in the periphery. T-cell–depleting antibodies and immunotoxin conjugates have been given at the time of transplantation, establishing a "window" for regeneration of the T-cell repertoire in the presence of alloantigen. This approach leads to long-term graft survival—and perhaps true tolerance—in rodent and nonhuman primate models (17–20).

Another approach that is being applied in large animal models clinically involves combining renal transplantation with myeloablation and allogeneic bone marrow transplantation (21,22). The resulting bone marrow chimerism leads to immune reconstitution characterized by central deletion of graft-reactive cells, with robust tolerance in rodent and some large animal models. Other approaches take advantage of the Fas, TNF, and Trance pathways to promote activation-induced cell death (AICD). T-cells become susceptible to AICD on repetitive stimulation, due to upregulation of IL-2 and cell surface death receptors, primarily Fas (23). Another form of T-cell apoptosis, termed "death by neglect," occurs when activated T-cells are deprived of growth factors such as IL-2 and other cytokines. One well-studied pathway involves the CD28 homologue, CTLA4, which also binds CD80/86, but with a higher affinity than that of CD28. CTLA4 acts as a competitive inhibitor of CD28, blocking CD28-mediated clonal expansion and triggering cell cycle arrest through downregulation of IL-2. Gene knockout experiments highlight the importance of these mechanisms in immune homeostasis, as Fas- and CTLA4-deficient mice develop fatal lymphoproliferative syndromes and autoimmunity (24).

3. Immune Deviation and Suppression

These forms of peripheral tolerance are characterized by downregulation of stimulated T-cells by soluble factors (immune deviation or suppression) or by direct cell-to-cell contact (suppression). Cytokines such as TGF-β, IL-10, and others may broadly suppress pathogenic T-cells, while IL-4 and IFNγ can alter the balance or character of Th1 and Th2 responses. Certain indirect means to alter the cytokine environment during antigen presentation appear promising in animal models, e.g., by delivering allergen in the presence of immunostimulatory DNA, driving allergen-specific responses in a Th1 direction (25).

III. ALLERGEN IMMUNOTHERAPY AND TOLERANCE: OVERVIEW

A. Effects of Allergen Immunotherapy

The preceding section has provided an overview on the T-cell mechanisms that induce tolerance. While the tolerogenic pathways induced by allergen immunotherapy are not known, the remainder of the chapter will review the clinical and laboratory changes induced by allergen immunotherapy and relate these changes to the mechanisms that have been discussed.

As described both here and in other chapters in this book, allergen immunotherapy induces at least three long-lasting changes: (1) induction of tolerance to the allergen, (2) prevention of sensitization to new allergens, and (3) prevention of asthma. Of these three effects, only the first has been shown convincingly to persist after immunotherapy is stopped. This chapter will also mention prevention of sensitization to new allergens, because, based on limited data, this effect also persists after immunotherapy is stopped (26).

Two distinct patient groups have been studied for tolerance induction in allergen immunotherapy trials. These two groups are considered separately in this chapter. Patients undergo immunotherapy (1) with aeroallergens such as ragweed and grass pollen allergens for rhinitis and/or asthma, and (2) with allergens derived from insect venom for systemic reactions to stinging insects. Natural aeroallergen exposure by low-dose inhalation occurs over many years, either seasonally or perennially. Individuals allergic to aeroallergens are atopic with dysregulated immunity and an enhanced Th2 response. Their symptoms and IgE antibodies to one or more aeroallergens generally persist for years. In contrast, insect venom allergy occurs independently of the atopic state of the patient, and exposure to venom allergen is sporadic, generally subcutaneous, by insect stings. In untreated patients over a period of years, both the risk of systemic reactions and IgE antibody levels decline substantially.

B. Clinical Trial Design for Studying Tolerance Induction

Tolerance is best studied by a blinded clinical trial analogous to the design published by Durham (2). Group 1 receives placebo throughout the course of the trial. Group 2 receives immunotherapy throughout the course of the trial. Group 3 receives immunotherapy for the first part of the trial, and then immunotherapy is discontinued for the second part. If immunotherapy is effective, then symptoms should be reduced in group 2 compared with group 1. If tolerance is induced, then symptoms in group 3 should not be different from group 2 and should be reduced compared with group 1. Figure 3 illustrates this trial design and also portrays a hypothetical result of a clinical trial, with tolerance during the allergy season persisting for 2 years after therapy is discontinued and partial reversal of the tolerogenic effect with recurrence of symptoms in the third year.

C. Limitations in Design of Trials to Induce Tolerance

There are several issues that limit interpretation of the majority of published trials in allergen immunotherapy. First, in contrast to the hypothetical study in Fig. 3, many published studies of discontinuation of immunotherapy have not included both a placebo group and an uninterrupted immunotherapy group, so the magnitude of the tolerance effect is difficult to estimate. Second, until recently there were no data on the safety of discontinuation of venom immunotherapy. Thus, most published studies evaluated individuals who stopped because of a personal choice rather than a defined protocol. Third, the study

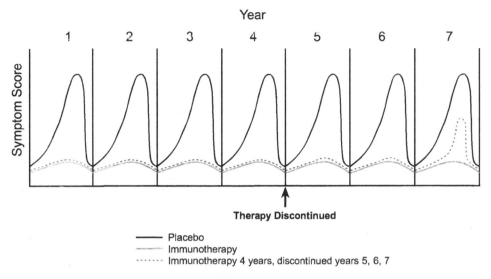

Figure 3 Idealized graph of a 7-year clinical trial to determine allergen immunotherapy-mediated induction and duration of tolerance. One group of participants was treated with placebo immunotherapy only. A second group was treated with allergen immunotherapy continuously for 7 years. A third group was treated with allergen immunotherapy for 4 years, and then immunotherapy was discontinued and placebo therapy was used for years 5, 6, and 7. The graph shows symptom scores, from just before the allergen season to just after the season, for each of the 7 years of the study.

design of immunotherapy trials has not been optimized for tolerance induction. Thus, the maintenance dose for aeroallergens of approximately 5–20 μg of the major allergen (e.g., *Amb a* 1 for ragweed) is said to be optimal, based on either short-term (i.e., weeks to months) clinical benefit and/or stimulating the highest levels of IgG or IgG4 antibody to allergen and/or reducing responses to nasal allergen challenge (27,28). In aeroallergen immunotherapy, IgG antibody level does not correlate with clinical benefit. In insect venom immunotherapy, while the IgG antibody level appears to be a marker for successful short-term protection against systemic reactions, the level does not correlate with tolerance induction. It is only within the past few years that it has been demonstrated that allergen immunotherapy induces tolerance. Although the optimal doses, as described above, induce both tolerance and also T-cell changes (27) that may be relevant to tolerance, such as reductions in IL-4–expressing T-cells, there are no published data on optimal conditions for inducing tolerance with allergen immunotherapy. Indeed, there are no proven biomarkers of tolerance induction, so additional lengthy clinical trials are required to measure tolerance.

IV. CLINICAL TOLERANCE INDUCED BY ALLERGEN IMMUNOTHERAPY

A. Subcutaneous Aeroallergen (Standard Immunotherapy) and Immunotherapy with Allergoid

One year of standard allergen immunotherapy is not sufficient to induce tolerance to aeroallergens. A single year of immunotherapy reduces allergy symptoms during treatment, but symptoms recur in the succeeding year (29). A longer duration of immunotherapy (more than 3 years) is more likely to result in persistent symptom improvement after therapy is stopped than a shorter course (30). Indeed, several years of immunotherapy do induce tolerance, as demonstrated by two published controlled studies. Naclerio (3) investigated discontinuation after ragweed allergen immunotherapy. Participants received immunotherapy for at least 3 years with a maintenance dose of 12 µg of *Amb a* 1 and then were randomized to either continuation or discontinuation of immunotherapy. For the first year after therapy was discontinued, the symptom scores of the discontinued group were not different from the group continuing immunotherapy, indicating that ragweed immunotherapy does induce tolerance. However, the study was not extended to examine the duration of the tolerance effect.

Durham (2) performed a 6-year controlled study of immunotherapy with aluminum hydroxide–adsorbed depot grass pollen allergen. After 3 years of immunotherapy, symptoms were markedly suppressed. After the first 3 years of the trial, one group had therapy discontinued for 3 years. In the discontinued group, the reduction of symptoms persisted throughout the 3-year discontinuation period, and symptoms were nearly as low as in the group that received immunotherapy for the entire 6 years. This 3-year persistence of symptom relief after discontinuing immunotherapy is impressive and strongly supports the concept of tolerance induction.

More recent data (31) indicate that when patients receive 2 years of grass pollen immunotherapy, discontinuation results in marked symptom relief for at least 2 additional years, including reduction in nonspecific bronchial hyperreactivity. The symptoms in the discontinued group were not significantly different from the group that had continuous immunotherapy for 4 years.

At least four other studies indicate that tolerance is induced following standard immunotherapy with tree, cat, dog, and house dust mite aeroallergens, although these studies all lack control groups (30,32–34). Similar results were obtained with immunotherapy with allergoids, which are allergens that are chemically modified, typically by formaldehyde (26,35). These studies were carried out with up to 3 years of immunotherapy and a 5- to 6-year follow-up after immunotherapy was discontinued. In one of the studies, in addition to persistent reduction of symptoms, asthma development may have been inhibited as no patients with rhinitis developed asthma (33).

B. Novel Approaches to Immunotherapy

1. Rush Immunotherapy

Rush immunotherapy utilizes a dose escalation regimen resembling, but more rapid than, standard subcutaneous immunotherapy. With conventional immunotherapy, maintenance doses are achieved after approximately 3 months, but with rush immunotherapy, maintenance doses are typically achieved in days or a few weeks. There is currently no information on tolerance induction following rush immunotherapy with aeroallergens. However, venom immunotherapy (discussed below), which induces tolerance, is typically administered via a modified rush regimen, which suggests that rush immunotherapy will mimic conventional immunotherapy in inducing tolerance.

2. Sublingual Immunotherapy

Sublingual immunotherapy (SLIT) with conventional allergen preparations has been shown to be a safe therapeutic approach; there is apparently a very low risk of systemic reactions. An unblinded study (36) compared untreated children to mite-allergic children with allergic asthma and rhinitis treated with SLIT with mite, for 4–5 years. After discontinuation of

SLIT for 4–5 years, there was a significant reduction in asthma and in use of asthma medication, and the peak expiratory flow rate (PEFR) was significantly higher than in untreated individuals. Surprisingly, although the PEFR was higher in the treated group at the end of SLIT, this difference was not statistically significant.

3. Allergen Peptides

Several investigators have proposed that cat allergy can be treated by a modified form of immunotherapy with peptides derived from the major cat allergen. Kay and colleagues have studied the effect of peptide injections, which induce isolated late-phase (no immediate phase) asthmatic reactions in a subset of patients. A second injection of peptide attenuates these late-phase responses. In one placebo-controlled study (37), patients were injected intradermally with peptides for 2 weeks. Three to nine months after therapy was stopped, the ability of treated individuals to tolerate cat exposure was enhanced, but the differences from placebo were not statistically significant. Further data are needed to evaluate the capacity of this approach to induce long-term symptom improvement.

4. Immunostimulatory Oligonucleotides

One interesting new approach to immunotherapy is the use of a chemical conjugate of allergen and immunostimulatory oligonucleotide sequences of (unmethylated) DNA (38). In mice, a conjugate of *Amb a* 1 (the major allergen in ragweed) with immunostimulatory oligonucleotides (AIC) induces a marked shift in cytokine production, to Th1-predominant, and a blockade of IgE antibody production. In ragweed-allergic humans, compared with unconjugated allergen, 30-fold higher levels of AIC are necessary to induce basophil histamine release (39). In vitro studies with peripheral blood indicate that AIC induces a shift from Th2 to Th1 cytokines (40). A placebo-controlled study tested the effect of six injections, prior to the 2001 ragweed season, of AIC (38). AIC induced a reduction in symptoms during the 2001 season and also during the 2002 season, indicating that tolerance was achieved. The statistical significance of these reduced symptoms is currently being evaluated. If the significance is confirmed, the results indicate that a tolerogenic effect may not require years of therapy but may be induced with a limited course of an allergen–oligonucleotide conjugate.

5. Anti-IgE and Allergen

Two distinct preparations of humanized monoclonal anti-IgE antibodies, omalizumab and TNX-901, have been used immunotherapeutically. The first (omalizumab) significantly improved symptoms of allergic rhinitis and allergic asthma (41), and the second (TNX-901) significantly improved the ability of peanut-allergic individuals to ingest peanuts (41,42). One trial demonstrated that anti-IgE and allergen act synergistically in improving seasonal allergic rhinitis symptoms (43). It is possible that anti-IgE will increase the dose of allergen that can be tolerated during immunotherapy and that higher doses of allergen will increase the likelihood of inducing tolerance as a result of immunotherapy. Anti-IgE may have other immune effects that facilitate tolerance induction. The Immune Tolerance Network is currently conducting a trial to evaluate the potential tolerizing effects of omalizumab in combination with ragweed allergen immunotherapy.

C. Venom Immunotherapy

The balance of currently available data indicates that there is substantial protection from systemic reactions after insect venom therapy is discontinued, strongly suggesting that venom immunotherapy induces tolerance. However, the scientific design of such studies has not been well controlled. First, discontinuation of therapy has generally been a personal decision rather than by randomization. Second, stings are not fully controlled, as the estimated frequency of accidental insect stings among venom-allergic patients is 10% per year, and the results of such stings (where the insect may not be identified accurately) have been used for analyzing the clinical outcomes.

When patients with venom allergy are placed on immunotherapy and reach a maintenance dose, the risk of sting-induced systemic reactions falls to 5%, and even those systemic reactions are mild. When immunotherapy is stopped after 5 years, the risk of systemic reactions remains substantially reduced compared with untreated patients.

The persistence of tolerance following immunotherapy with vespid venom (yellow jacket, yellow hornet, polistes) appears to be superior to persistence following honeybee (44), although the basis for this difference is not understood.

As discussed in Section IV A, tolerance induction with aeroallergen immunotherapy depends on the duration of therapy. More extensive data with immunotherapy to stinging insect venoms provide strong evidence that a long duration of immunotherapy is needed to induce tolerance.

Short-term immunotherapy with venom is associated with minimal tolerance induction after immunotherapy is stopped. Thus, when immunotherapy is stopped after 1–2 years, the systemic reaction rate to stings, the reaction rate within 1–2 years after discontinuation, is as high as 30% (Fig. 4) (45,46). In contrast, a longer course of venom immunotherapy induces a more prolonged effect on symptoms after therapy is discontinued. Only 5% of venom-allergic individuals who had been treated for more than 50 months had a systemic reaction, compared to 18% of those treated 50 months or less (47). Golden found that for individuals discontinuing immunotherapy following a long (average 6 years)

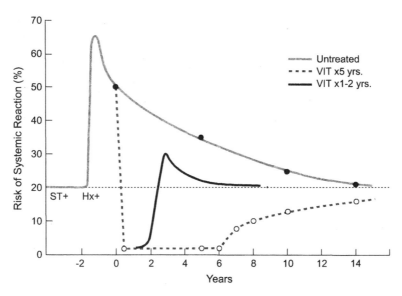

Figure 4   Natural history of insect sting allergy showing the risk of systemic reaction to a sting in untreated patients (gray line) and in patients who received venom immunotherapy for a duration of either 1 to 2 years (solid black line) or for a mean of 6 years (dashed line). (Reprinted from Golden DB, Kagey-Sobotka A, Lichtenstein, LM. Survey of patients after discontinuing venom immunotherapy. J Allergy Clin Immunol 2000; 105:385–90. It is reprinted with permission from Elsevier.)

course of immunotherapy with insect venom, the sting-induced systemic reaction rate was approximately 0% in 1 year off therapy and then increased each year to a plateau of 15% in 10 years off therapy (Fig. 4) (48). Lerch and Muller reported similar data (47).

Because of these results, the American Academy of Allergy, Asthma and Immunology has suggested that immunotherapy to venom should be discontinued after 5 or 6 years, since the resultant risk of systemic reactions is 5–10%, and these reactions are generally mild (49). Now that discontinuation of therapy after 5 years has become a clinical recommendation, data from future studies may provide better controls to analyze the magnitude of the tolerance effect.

V. IMMUNOLOGICAL CHANGES ASSOCIATED WITH ALLERGEN IMMUNOTHERAPY AND WITH TOLERANCE

Many immunological changes are associated with standard aeroallergen immunotherapy, including blockade of the postseasonal increase in IgE antibody to allergen, increases in IgG (including IgG4) antibodies to allergen, and increases in secretory IgA and IgG antibodies. In some patients, mostly children, basophil responsiveness to allergen is reduced. Nasal mediator release in response to nasal allergen challenge is diminished. Immediate skin test responses to intradermal allergen are modestly reduced. Late-phase skin reactions to intradermal allergen are markedly reduced. In addition, as discussed in detail in Section VI, there is evidence of reduced production of Th2 cytokines and/or increased production of regulatory cytokines and/or anergy. However, there are limited data on the utility of any of these measurements for either predicting, or serving as a biomarker of, the tolerant state.

Allergen-specific IgE and IgG antibody levels are commonly assessed in immunotherapy trials, and the relevance of such measurements to tolerance induction is discussed below. Total IgE and total IgG do not change as a consequence of immunotherapy.

A. IgE Antibody Response

1. Subcutaneous Aeroallergen (Standard Immunotherapy)
Since tolerance is targeted to eliminating the pathogenic immune response, and the IgE antibody response is the immune response that is most clearly associated with the expression of allergic diseases, an obvious candidate marker of tolerance induction is inhibition of the production of allergen-specific IgE antibody.

Two different measures of changes in allergen-specific IgE antibody levels have been used in evaluating immunotherapy trials. The first, which is used to compare IgE antibody levels from year to year, is called the "average IgE antibody." This is the average of multiple measurements over the course of a year, although in many studies only a single preseasonal measurement is taken. However, results from several immunotherapy trials suggest that the variation in IgE antibody over the course of 1 year is greater than the change in average IgE antibody from one year to the next. The pattern of IgE antibody within a year is consistent. Seasonal aeroallergen exposure induces a twofold increase in IgE antibody, which then falls during the remainder of the year. The twofold increase in IgE antibody to ragweed pollen typically represents, in the eastern and Midwestern United States, the change from early August (about 1–2 weeks before the start of the pollen season) to mid-October (about 1–2 weeks after the end of the pollen season) and has been a useful parameter for immunotherapy studies.

Immunotherapy to aeroallergens blocks the postseasonal increases in IgE antibody. In contrast, immunotherapy induces either no reduction or only small reductions in the average IgE antibody levels (32–35,50).

There is only one analysis of pre- versus postseasonal IgE antibody responses during controlled discontinuation of conventional aeroallergen immunotherapy (3). One year after discontinuation of ragweed immunotherapy, postseasonal increases in IgE antibody were blocked to the same degree as in those who continued immunotherapy, suggesting that this blockade was a useful marker of tolerance. However, further work is needed to analyze the reproducibility of this effect and its causal relationship, if any, to tolerance induction.

Other studies have measured only the average IgE antibody levels. Even though at least one study shows that discontinuation of immunotherapy maintains up to a twofold reduction of average IgE antibody compared with pre-immunotherapy (34), in general there is no change in the average IgE antibody level with either immunotherapy itself or when immunotherapy is discontinued (32), and thus the value of average IgE antibody levels as a biomarker of tolerance is doubtful.

2. Sublingual Immunotherapy

Although Di Rienzo demonstrated a tolerogenic effect of SLIT with house dust mite, the only laboratory data mentioned is the average IgE antibody level (36). After 4–5 years of SLIT followed by 4–5 years without immunotherapy, the IgE antibody level was unchanged in the SLIT treated group, with a trend ($p = 0.06$) for an increase in the untreated individuals.

3. Immunostimulatory Oligonucleotides

Preliminary data indicate that AIC therapy was associated with very modest changes in IgE antibody. The capacity of AIC to block postseasonal increases in IgE has not been analyzed (38). The results of additional mechanistic studies are in progress.

4. Venom Immunotherapy

Venom immunotherapy results in a marked reduction of both immediate skin test responses and IgE responses, and both reductions persist after therapy is stopped. However, the natural history of untreated insect venom allergy differs substantially from that of aeroallergen allergy, in that IgE antibody levels to insect venom apparently fall in untreated individuals, even if the individual is stung. This fall in IgE levels is associated with a drop in the systemic reaction rate of untreated subjects, to 20%. The fall in IgE anti-venom appears to be greater in untreated patients than in immunotherapy-treated patients (51).

It has been suggested that the most effective protection against systemic reactions after therapy is stopped occurs in those individuals (up to 25% of venom immunotherapy–treated patients) who have developed negative immediate skin tests and/or undetectable (i.e., <1 ng/ml) or nearly undetectable IgE anti-venom antibodies (47,52,53). IgE anti-venom antibody levels do not generally increase after therapy is stopped. However, more recent data suggest that there is a risk for systemic reactions after therapy is stopped even in those individuals who have a loss of skin test sensitivity and a marked reduction of IgE levels (48,54).

B. IgG Antibody Responses

Both aeroallergen immunotherapy and venom immunotherapy induce increases in allergen-specific IgG (predominantly IgG4) antibody. When therapy is discontinued, within

9 months the IgG antibody levels fall to the level of untreated patients (55), suggesting that the IgG antibody level is not a useful marker for tolerance induction. Indeed, as discussed below, venom immunotherapy demonstrates both an IgG-dependent and an IgG-independent phase, and tolerance induction probably occurs during the IgG-independent phase.

1. Subcutaneous Aeroallergen (Standard Immunotherapy)

Immunotherapy induces substantial increases in IgG antibody, and these levels fall when immunotherapy is discontinued. Similar effects are seen when the IgG antibodies of the relevant subclass (i.e., IgG4) are measured (34). Results from a controlled trial confirm that IgG antibody levels fall within the first year of discontinuation of immunotherapy (3).

2. Venom Immunotherapy

IgG anti-venom antibodies increase during immunotherapy so that the majority of patients have high levels of specific IgG antibodies (i.e., 3–10 µg/ml). After therapy is stopped, IgG antibodies fall to baseline within 6 to 12 months (55). Laboratory parameters, such as high IgG antibody when therapy is stopped, have no predictive value in estimating the likelihood of systemic reactions after stopping immunotherapy (47).

C. Immediate Skin Test Responses

1. Subcutaneous Aeroallergen (Standard Immunotherapy)

In untreated individuals, immediate skin test responses to allergen typically correlate with circulating IgE antibody levels. Several studies have demonstrated that immediate skin test reactivity is reduced by immunotherapy (27), but a detailed analysis suggests that this reduction is more clearly seen 1–3 hours after allergen administration, time points which are later than the typical 15-minute immediate skin reaction (56). The reduction in skin test reactivity appears not to be accompanied by a change in IgE antibody responses (56), suggesting that immunotherapy acts by reducing cutaneous mast cell responsiveness to allergen.

Persistence of symptom improvement correlated with decreased immediate skin test reactivity (30). Two studies confirm for grass pollen allergen that immunotherapy reduces the magnitude of skin test responses (2,26). In both of these studies, discontinuation of immunotherapy resulted in persistent reduction of immediate skin test response, although Durham's study suggests that 3 years after discontinuation, the immediate skin test response had begun to increase toward the pre-immunotherapy level. Neither of these studies measured IgE antibody levels, but other studies suggest that IgE antibody responses to grass are not reduced by immunotherapy. A study of tree pollen immunotherapy demonstrates that IgE antibody did not fall, but immediate skin test responses were reduced. After immunotherapy was discontinued, the IgE antibody levels did not change and the immediate skin test responses were the same as at the end of immunotherapy and did not increase to the pre-immunotherapy level (33). The results suggest that immunotherapy may reduce skin mast cell mediator release or other components of the immediate response, and that the reduced wheal and flare is a marker of tolerance.

2. Allergen Peptides

In a placebo-controlled study, peptides derived from *Fel d* 1, the major cat allergen, were injected subcutaneously, and patients were followed for 3 to 9 months after therapy was discontinued. The treatment resulted in a significant reduction in both early- and late-phase skin reactions to *Fel d* 1 and a reduction in early- and late-phase skin reactions to cat dander, although the skin reaction to cat dander did not differ significantly from placebo. Cytokine production by peripheral blood mononuclear cells did not differ between placebo- and peptide-treated subjects (37).

3. Venom Immunotherapy

In individuals treated with venom immunotherapy, IgE antibody levels and immediate skin test responses fall in parallel, and both remain reduced after immunotherapy is stopped (51).

D. Late-Phase Skin Reactions

Immunotherapy leads to inhibition of late-phase skin reactions much more than inhibition of immediate-phase skin reactions (56–58). One study evaluated late-phase skin reactions when tolerance is induced and demonstrated that inhibition of the late-phase reaction correlated with persistent symptom relief after immunotherapy was discontinued (2) (see Section VI also). These late-phase parameters were virtually identical between those on maintenance immunotherapy and those who discontinued immunotherapy. A second study (31) found that after 2 years of immunotherapy, the late-phase skin test response was equally suppressed in those remaining on immunotherapy for 2 additional years and those given placebo. These data suggest that inhibition of late-phase skin responses may be a marker of tolerance.

E. Nasal Allergen Challenge

Immunotherapy results in inhibition of allergen nasal challenge–induced symptoms and mediators, but 1 year after immunotherapy was stopped, immediate symptoms and mediator release in response to nasal allergen challenge return toward pretreatment levels (3). Late-phase responses were not evaluated. In the same study, symptoms during seasonal allergen exposure remain reduced during the discontinuation period. Thus, the nasal allergen challenge appears to be more resistant to inhibition than symptom scores, perhaps because the dose of allergen for nasal challenge is much larger than allergen levels deposited in the respiratory tract during the pollen season. Data from bronchial challenge, in a study that was not optimally controlled (34), were similar in that immunotherapy with cat allergen reduced bronchial reactivity to allergen challenge, and 5 years after discontinuing, the bronchial reactivity had returned to pretreatment levels.

F. Venom Immunotherapy: IgG Antibody–Dependent Early Protection, IgG Antibody–Independent Late Protection, and Late Tolerance Induction

A study of venom immunotherapy provides important information about the role of IgG antibody (59). It indicates that the mechanisms underlying the clinical improvement within the first year of immunotherapy are distinct from those underlying clinical improvement after several years of immunotherapy. In individuals treated with vespid venoms for less than 4 years, effective protection from systemic reactions to sting challenge occurs in only those individuals whose IgG anti-vespid venom is >3 μg/ml. After 4 year of immunotherapy, the reaction rate in all individuals was low, regardless of the IgG antibody levels.

These data must be considered in the context of other results that have been discussed. That is, tolerance induction, or long-term protection from systemic reactions after therapy is stopped, requires a long period of immunotherapy (44,48). Thus, the early IgG antibody–dependent protective effects of venom immunotherapy are probably unrelated to the induction of tolerance.

G.   Allergen Specificity of Allergen Immunotherapy-Induced Tolerance

Because tolerance is induced by immunotherapy with a specific allergen, it might be expected to induce allergen-specific effects. On the other hand, potent immune stimuli may induce more global effects. Currently available data are too limited to provide definitive conclusions about the immunological specificity of immunotherapy-induced tolerance. One long-term study evaluated the allergen specificity of immunotherapy itself and demonstrated that symptom relief was allergen-specific over 3 years (60).

Only one study has examined the allergen specificity of immunotherapy-induced tolerance. It was not optimally controlled and measured not symptoms but immediate skin test responses. Participants received 3 years of immunotherapy with grass allergoid and then were followed for 6 years after stopping therapy and compared to controls who did not receive immunotherapy (26). Some results demonstrate allergen specificity: Compared with the controls, the skin prick response to grass was diminished but that to three tree pollens (birch, alder, and hazel) was not diminished. Other data are not consistent with allergen specificity: The prick test to rye was reduced, but the reduction was not statistically significant, which is unexplained since the immunotherapy mix contained mixed grass and rye and also because mixed grass and rye (grass) would be expected to be antigenically related. Other results indicate a strong allergen-nonspecific effect; e.g., 39% of the treated group (versus 0% of the control group) developed no new allergen sensitivity over the course of the study. The results suggest that immediate skin test "tolerance" induced by grass pollen allergoid is both allergen-specific and allergen-nonspecific.

H.   Immunological Changes Induced by Natural Allergen Exposure That May Be Relevant to Immunotherapy and to Tolerance Induction

Natural but high-dose exposure to certain aeroallergens, especially cat and dog, induces long-lasting immunological and clinical effects. While medium-dose exposure to cats is associated with the production of IgE antibodies to cat allergen and asthma, high-dose exposure is associated with less IgE antibody, high levels of IgG4 antibody, and a low rate of asthma (61). These results raise the possibility that there may be parallels between "tolerance" induced by natural aeroallergen exposure and that induced by allergen immunotherapy.

A second study demonstrated that early-life exposure to two or more dogs or cats causes a long-lasting reduction of IgE antibody production to a large number of antigenically unrelated allergens (62). This effect is not allergen-specific: The development of IgE responses to dog, cat, and other indoor and outdoor allergens is inhibited.

The mechanisms underlying these long-lasting effects of natural aeroallergen exposure are uncertain. Exposure to cats and dogs is associated with exposure not only to allergens but also to other potentially immunomodulatory molecules derived from microbial agents, such as endotoxin. Further research is needed to confirm these results; to determine whether these effects are, at least partially, allergen-specific; to measure the levels of aeroallergens that interact with the host immune system following natural exposure; and to evaluate whether the mechanisms of "tolerance" are similar to the mechanisms by which allergen immunotherapy induces tolerance. Nevertheless, the magnitude of effects is striking, suggesting that allergen inhalation induces long-term immunological changes even though the doses of allergen inhaled are thought to be considerably less than those injected in immunotherapy.

I.   What Is in Allergen Vaccines?

Many commercial allergen extracts contain a mixture of allergenic and nonallergenic proteins plus variable amounts of endotoxin (63). In contrast, grass and ragweed extracts contain only low levels of endotoxin, suggesting that at least some of the effects of allergen immunotherapy might be independent of endotoxin. However, further studies of the role of endotoxin are necessary.

VI.   SINCE AEROALLERGEN IMMUNOTHERAPY INDUCES REGULATORY AND/OR TH1 CYTOKINE–PREDOMINANT RESPONSE, WHY ARE IgE ANTIBODY RESPONSES NOT INHIBITED?

As discussed in Section VII, allergen immunotherapy induces IL-10, TGF-β, IL-12, and increased IFN-γ/IL-4 ratios, yet appears to induce minimal changes in average IgE levels. Durham clearly demonstrated that the elevated IFN-γ/IL-4 ratio in allergen-induced late-phase skin reactions persists when therapy is stopped (2). An explanation for the lack of effect on average IgE antibody levels will require additional research. It is possible that blockade of the postseasonal increase in IgE antibody, which persists when immunotherapy is discontinued, is the proper measure of IgE blockade (3). It is also possible that the IgE antibody response resists control by regulatory and TH1 cytokines. For example, IgE secreted by long-lived antibody-producing plasma cells may be an important contributor to IgE levels (64,65), and IgE formation by these cells may be difficult to inhibit.

VII.   TOLEROGENIC MECHANISMS UNDERLYING ALLERGEN IMMUNOTHERAPY

The potential mechanisms for central and peripheral T-cell tolerance are described in Section II. In addition, B-cell tolerance (not shown in Fig. 1) may also contribute to maintenance of tolerance. All of these mechanisms may operate to induce tolerance to exogenous allergens and may explain the effects of immunotherapy.

Immunotherapy has been reported to induce at least four distinct cytokine patterns, any one of which could account for the tolerogenic effects of allergen immunotherapy. These four patterns are (1) a shift from TH2 cytokines to TH1 cytokines, (2) the production of IL-10, (3) the production of TGF-β, and (4) anergy or the absence of cytokine production. Most likely, immunotherapy induces a spectrum of cytokine shifts. However, most of the studies have been carried out with short-term (1 year or less) allergen immunotherapy. The relevance to tolerance of short-term immunotherapy changes is uncertain, since tolerance appears to require more than 1 year of standard immunotherapy. From published data as of May 2003, of these cytokine patterns, only the shift from TH2 to TH1 cytokines has been shown to persist after therapy is stopped (2).

A.   Immunotherapy and TH2 to TH1 Shift

Four weeks of cluster cat allergen immunotherapy induced a reduction in the percent of IL-4+ cells from peripheral blood CD4+ T-cells (27). Other studies also suggest that immunotherapy increases the IFN-γ/IL-4 ratio in peripheral blood CD4+ T-cells (66). Still other studies have demonstrated increases in cells containing IL-12 mRNA in late-phase skin reactions (67). Furthermore, immunotherapy to grass pollen increases the nasal mucosal IFN-γ/IL-5 mRNA (68) and blocks seasonal increases in IL-5 mRNA (69).

B. Immunotherapy and IL-10 and TGF-β

Akdis et al. (70) demonstrated that a 28-day rush immunotherapy regimen with phospholipase A2 (PLA2) (the major allergen in bee venom) not only induced anergy (see below) but also stimulated the production of IL-10. The IL-10 was produced initially by CD4+CD25+ allergen-specific T-cells, and later by B-cells and monocytes. Since anti–IL-10 antibody reversed the anergy, the data indicate that IL-10 is responsible for anergy induced by short-term allergen immunotherapy. Other results from this group (71) indicate that over 70 days of immunotherapy with the aeroallergens house dust mite or birch pollen, T-cells produce both IL-10 and TGF-β, and that both cytokines are responsible for peripheral T-cell anergy. Furthermore, immunotherapy for 70 days with peptides from PLA2 decreased T-cell proliferation and stimulated secretion of IL-10 and IFN-γ from short-term T-cell lines (72). Durham has demonstrated that 1 year of immunotherapy with grass pollen induces local nasal mucosal IL-10 (68), and he has also shown that 2 years of immunotherapy induces IgG4 antibody, which is associated with IL-10 production. Indeed, allergen immunotherapy to either aeroallergens or insect venom is known to stimulate consistently the production of IgG4 antibodies to allergen, and IgG4 production is thought to be IL-10 dependent. However, since IgG (including IgG4) antibody production falls rapidly when immunotherapy is discontinued, the relevance of IgG4 to tolerance induction is uncertain.

C. Immunotherapy and T-Cell Anergy

Akdis et al. demonstrated that 28-day modified rush immunotherapy with bee venom induces peripheral blood T-cells to become anergic to PLA2, in that the cells did not make either TH1 or TH2 cytokines (73). The T-cell anergy could be reversed, to producing TH1 cytokines, by IL-2 or IL-15, and IL-4 partially reversed anergy and stimulated TH2 cytokines. Further studies, as discussed in Section VII B, indicate that anergy is associated with the production of IL-10 and TGF-β.

D. T-Cell Cytokine Patterns During Tolerance Induction

A single published study identified persistent changes in allergen challenge–induced T-cell function (TH2 to TH1 cytokine shifts) associated with immunotherapy-induced tolerance (2). Immunotherapy almost completely inhibited both the 24-hour skin reaction and the number of IL-4–producing cells, and reduced by more than threefold the number of CD3+ cells. These late-phase parameters were virtually identical between those on maintenance immunotherapy and those who discontinued immunotherapy for 3 years. Data from another Durham study indicate that 2 years of grass pollen immunotherapy induced a significant increase in the local (nasal mucosal) expression of IFN-γ/IL-5 mRNA. Since this 2-year immunotherapy trial apparently induced tolerance (31,68), these cytokine data may support the TH2 to TH1 cytokine shift reported in Durham's earlier study.

VIII. SUMMARY

This chapter has reviewed the large number of studies demonstrating that allergen immunotherapy, after it is discontinued, results in long-term clinical improvement. These studies strongly suggest that tolerance is induced by allergen immunotherapy. Additional research is needed so that the mechanisms underlying tolerance induction can be understood. Because the number of allergen-specific T-cells, particularly in blood, is quite small, analysis of these mechanisms will not be easy.

A number of key questions should guide future studies of tolerance induced by allergen immunotherapy: (1) What biomarkers are associated with tolerance induction? Although some data suggest that allergen immunotherapy leads to blockade of postseasonal increases in IgE antibody, diminution in the size of immediate skin tests to allergen, and diminution in the size of late skin tests to allergen (associated with reduction in IL-4–producing cells), only limited data support these as biomarkers of the tolerant state. (2) What T-cell (and/or B-cell) tolerogenic mechanism(s) are associated with the clinical and biomarker evidence of tolerance? (3) What explains the prolonged (for years) duration of tolerance? (4) Why is tolerance eventually broken? (5) Is tolerance antigen-specific? (6) What therapeutic agents, other than allergen immunotherapy, induce or contribute to tolerance? (7) With the possible exception of AIC therapy, allergen immunotherapy apparently requires at least 2 years to induce tolerance. Are there protocols that will allow tolerance to be induced rapidly? (8) Does early-life "natural" exposure to certain allergens induce tolerance by a mechanism analogous to that induced by allergen immunotherapy?

IX. SALIENT POINTS

1.   In the setting of allergen immunotherapy, tolerance is characterized by a reduction in symptoms that persists for several years after therapy is stopped.
2.   With allergen immunotherapy as currently practiced, the tolerant state develops only after at least 2 years of treatment.
3.   Immunotherapy targeted against both aeroallergens (e.g., ragweed pollen, grass pollen) and stinging-insect venom allergens induces tolerance.
4.   There are no known biomarkers during immunotherapy that predict whether tolerance will be induced.
5.   There are two biomarkers that appear to correlate with a tolerant clinical state after discontinuing aeroallergen immunotherapy: (1) blockade of postseasonal increases in IgE antibody, and (2) blockade of allergen-induced late-phase skin reactions. Levels of IgG antibody do not correlate with a tolerant state.
6.   There are no known biomarkers that correlate with tolerance after stinging-insect venom allergen immunotherapy.

REFERENCES

1.   Bluestone JA, Matthews JB, Krensky AM. The immune tolerance network: The "Holy Grail" comes to the clinic. J Am Soc Nephrol 2000; 11:2141–2146.
2.   Durham SR, Walker SM, Varga EM, Jacobson MR, O'Brien F, Noble W, Till SJ, Hamid QA Nouri-Aria KT. Long-term clinical efficacy of grass pollen immunotherapy. N Engl J Med 1999; 341:468–475.
3.   Naclerio RM, Proud D, Moylan B, Balcer S, Freidhoff L, Kagey-Sobotka A, Lichtenstein LM, Creticos PS, Hamilton RG, Norman PS. A double-blind study of the discontinuation of ragweed immunotherapy. J Allergy Clin Immunol 1997; 100:293–300.
4.   Starzl TE, Demetris AJ, Trucco M, Murase N, Ricordi C, Ildstad S, Ramos H, Todo S, Tzakis A, Fung JJ, et al. Cell migration and chimerism after whole-organ transplantation: The basis of graft acceptance. Hepatology 1993; 17:1127–1152.

5. Mazariegos GV, Reyes J, Marino IR, Demetris AJ, Flynn B, Irish W, McMichael J, Fung JJ Starz TE. Weaning of immunosuppression in liver transplant recipients. Transplantation 1997; 63:243–249.

6. Devlin J, Doherty D, Thomson L, Wong T, Donaldson P, Portmann B, Williams R. Defining the outcome of immunosuppression withdrawal after liver transplantation. Hepatology 1998; 27:926–933.

7. Gudmundsdottir H, Turka LA. Transplantation tolerance: Mechanisms and strategies? Semin Nephrol 2000; 20:209–216.

8. Weaver CT, Hawrylowicz CM, Unanue ER. T helper cell subsets require the expression of distinct costimulatory signals by antigen-presenting cells. Proc Natl Acad Sci U S A 1988; 85:8181–8185.

9. Jenkins MK, Schwartz RH. Antigen presentation by chemically modified splenocytes induces antigen-specific T cell unresponsiveness in vitro and in vivo. J Exp Med 1987; 165:302–319.

10. Jenkins MK, Ashwell JD, Schwartz RH. Allogeneic non-T spleen cells restore the responsiveness of normal T cell clones stimulated with antigen and chemically modified antigen-presenting cells. J Immunol 1988; 140:3324–3330.

11. DeBenedette MA, Shahinian A, Mak TW, Watts TH. Costimulation of CD28- T lymphocytes by 4-1BB ligand. J Immunol 1997; 158:551–559.

12. Tamada K, Shimozaki K, Chapoval AI, Zhu G, Sica G, Flies D, Boone T, Hsu H, Fu YX, Nagata S, Ni J, Chen L. Modulation of T-cell-mediated immunity in tumor and graft-versus-host disease models through the LIGHT co-stimulatory pathway. Nat Med 2000; 6:283–289.

13. Tamada K, Shimozaki K, Chapoval AI, Zhai Y, Su J, Chen SF, Hsieh SL, Nagata S, Ni J, Chen L. LIGHT, a TNF-like molecule, costimulates T cell proliferation and is required for dendritic cell-mediated allogeneic T cell response. J Immunol 2000; 164:4105–4110.

14. Brennan DC, Mohanakumar T, Flye MW. Donor-specific transfusion and donor bone marrow infusion in renal transplantation tolerance: A review of efficacy and mechanisms. Am J Kidney Dis 1995; 26:701–715.

15. Kirk AD, Harlan DM, Armstrong NN, Davis TA, Dong Y, Gray GS, Hong X, Thomas D, Fechner JH Jr, Knechtle SJ. CTLA4-Ig and anti-CD40 ligand prevent renal allograft rejection in primates. Proc Natl Acad Sci U S A 1997; 94:8789–8794.

16. Kenyon NS, Fernandez LA, Lehmann R, Masetti M, Ranuncoli A, Chatzipetrou M, Iaria G, Han D, Wagner JL, Ruiz P, Berho M, Inverardi L, Alejandro R, Mintz DH, Kirk AD, Harlan DM, Burkly LC, Ricordi C. Long-term survival and function of intrahepatic islet allografts in baboons treated with humanized anti-CD154. Diabetes 1999; 48:1473–1481.

17. Woodle ES, Xu D, Zivin RA, Auger J, Charette J, O'Laughlin R, Peace D, Jollife LK, Haverty T, Bluestone JA, Thistlethwaite JR Jr. Phase I trial of a humanized, Fc receptor nonbinding OKT3 antibody, huOKT3gamma1(Ala-Ala) in the treatment of acute renal allograft rejection. Transplantation 1999; 68:608–616.

18. Friend PJ, Hale G, Chatenoud L, Rebello P, Bradley J, Thiru S, Phillips JM, Waldmann H. Phase I study of an engineered aglycosylated humanized CD3 antibody in renal transplant rejection. Transplantation 1999; 68:1632–1637.

19. Calne R, Moffatt SD, Friend PJ, Jamieson NV, Bradley JA, Hale G, Firth J, Bradley J, Smith KG, Waldmann H. Prope tolerance with induction using Campath 1H and low-dose cyclosporin monotherapy in 31 cadaveric renal allograft recipients. Nippon Geka Gakkai Zasshi 2000; 101:301–306.

20. Thomas JM, Neville DM, Contreras JL, Eckhoff DE, Meng G, Lobashevsky AL, Wang PX, Huang ZQ, Verbanac KM, Haisch CE, Thomas FT. Preclinical studies of allograft tolerance in rhesus monkeys: A novel anti-CD3-immunotoxin given peritransplant with donor bone marrow induces operational tolerance to kidney allografts. Transplantation 1997; 64:124–135.

21. Kimikawa M, Sachs DH, Colvin RB, Bartholomew A, Kawai T, Cosimi AB. Modifications of the conditioning regimen for achieving mixed chimerism and donor-specific tolerance in cynomolgus monkeys. Transplantation 1997; 64:709–716.

22. Spitzer TR, Delmonico F, Tolkoff-Rubin N, McAfee S, Sackstein R, Saidman S, Colby C, Sykes M, Sachs DH, Cosimi AB. Combined histocompatibility leukocyte antigen-matched donor bone marrow and renal transplantation for multiple myeloma with end stage renal disease: The induction of allograft tolerance through mixed lymphohematopoietic chimerism. Transplantation 1999; 68:480–484.

23. Van Parijs L, Refaeli Y, Lord JD, Nelson BH, Abbas AK, Baltimore D. Uncoupling IL-2 signals that regulate T cell proliferation, survival, and Fas-mediated activation-induced cell death. Immunity 1999; 11:281–288.

24. Straus SE, Sneller M, Lenardo MJ, Puck JM, Strober W. An inherited disorder of lymphocyte apoptosis: The autoimmune lymphoproliferative syndrome. Ann Intern Med 1999; 130:591–601.

25. Broide DH, Stachnick G, Castaneda D, Nayar J, Miller M, Cho JY, Roman M, Zubeldia J, Hayashi T, Raz E, Hyashi T. Systemic administration of immunostimulatory DNA sequences mediates reversible inhibition of Th2 responses in a mouse model of asthma. J Clin Immunol 2001; 21:175–182.

26. Eng PA, Reinhold M, Gnehm HP. Long-term efficacy of preseasonal grass pollen immunotherapy in children. Allergy 2002; 57:306–312.

27. Ewbank PA, Murray J, Sanders K, Curran-Everett D, Dreskin S, Nelson HS. A double-blind, placebo-controlled immunotherapy dose-response study with standardized cat extract. J Allergy Clin Immunol 2003; 111:155–161.

28. Creticos PS, Marsh DG, Proud D, Kagey-Sobotka A, Adkinson NF Jr, Friedhoff L, Naclerio RM, Lichtenstein LM, Norman PS. Responses to ragweed-pollen nasal challenge before and after immunotherapy. J Allergy Clin Immunol 1989; 84:197–205.

29. Lowell FC, Franklin W. A double-blind study of the effectiveness and specificity of injecton therapy in ragweed hay fever. N Engl J Med 1965; 273:675–679.

30. Des Roches A, Paradis L, Knani J, Hejjaoui A, Dhivert H, Chanez P, Bousquet J. Immunotherapy with a standardized *Dermatophagoides pteronyssinus* extract. V. Duration of the efficacy of immunotherapy after its cessation. Allergy 1996; 51:430–433.

31. Walker SM, Jacobson M, Durham SR. Grass pollen immunotherapy for two years has sustained effects during two years double-blind placebo-controlled withdrawal of treatment. J Allergy Clin Immunol 2003; 111:S267, abst. 799.

32. Mosbech H, Osterballe O. Does the effect of immunotherapy last after termination of treatment? Follow-up study in patients with grass pollen rhinitis. Allergy 1988; 43: 523–529.

33. Jacobsen L, Nuchel Petersen B, Wihl JA, Lowenstein H, Ipsen H. Immunotherapy with partially purified and standardized tree pollen extracts. IV. Results from long-term (6-year) follow-up. Allergy 1997; 52:914–920.

34. Hedlin G, Heilborn H, Lilja G, Norrlind K, Pegelow KO, Schou C, Lowenstein H. Long-term follow-up of patients treated with a three-year course of cat or dog immunotherapy. J Allergy Clin Immunol 1995; 96:879–885.

35. Ariano R, Kroon AM, Augeri G, Canonica GW, Passalacqua G. Long-term treatment with allergoid immunotherapy with Parietaria. Clinical and immunologic effects in a randomized, controlled trial. Allergy 1999; 54:313–319.

36. Di Rienzo V, Marcucci F, Puccinelli P, Parmiani S, Frati F, Sensi L, Canonica GW, Passalacqua G. Long-lasting effect of sublingual immunotherapy in children with asthma due to house dust mite: A 10-year prospective study. Clin Exp Allergy 2003; 33:206–210.

37. Oldfield WL, Larche M, Kay AB. Effect of T-cell peptides derived from Fel d 1 on allergic reactions and cytokine production in patients sensitive to cats: A randomised controlled trial. Lancet 2002; 360:47–53.

38. Creticos PS. Clinical trials of oligonucleotide coupled allergen vaccines. 60th anniversary meeting American Academy of Allergy, Asthma, and Immunology, Denver, CO, March 7–12, 2003.

39. Tighe H, Takabayashi K, Schwartz D, Van Nest G, Tuck S, Eiden JJ, Kagey-Sobotka A, Creticos PS, Lichtenstein LM, Spiegelberg HL, Raz E. Conjugation of immunostimulatory

DNA to the short ragweed allergen amb a 1 enhances its immunogenicity and reduces its allergenicity. J Allergy Clin Immunol 2000; 106:124–134.

40. Marshall JD, Abtahi S, Eiden JJ, Tuck S, Milley R, Haycock F, Reid MJ, Kagey-Sobotka A, Creticos PS, Lichtenstein LM, Van Nest G. Immunostimulatory sequence DNA linked to the Amb a 1 allergen promotes T(H)1 cytokine expression while downregulating T(H)2 cytokine expression in PBMCs from human patients with ragweed allergy. J Allergy Clin Immunol 2001; 108:191–197.

41. Casale TB, Condemi J, LaForce C, Nayak A, Rowe M, Watrous M, McAlary M, Fowler-Taylor A, Racine A, Gupta N, Fick R, Della Cioppa G. Effect of omalizumab on symptoms of seasonal allergic rhinitis: A randomized controlled trial. JAMA 2001; 286:2956–2967.

42. Leung DY, Sampson HA, Yunginger JW, Burks AW Jr, Schneider LC, Wortel CH, Davis FM, Hyun JD, Shanahan WR Jr. Effect of anti-IgE therapy in patients with peanut allergy. N Engl J Med 2003; 348:986–993.

43. Kuehr J, Brauburger J, Zielen S, Schauer U, Kamin W, Von Berg A, Leupold W, Bergmann KC, Rolinck-Werninghaus C, Grave M, Hultsch T, Wahn U. Efficacy of combination treatment with anti-IgE plus specific immunotherapy in polysensitized children and adolescents with seasonal allergic rhinitis. J Allergy Clin Immunol 2002; 109:274–280.

44. Muller U, Berchtold E, Helbling A. Honeybee venom allergy: Results of a sting challenge 1 year after stopping successful venom immunotherapy in 86 patients. J Allergy Clin Immunol 1991; 87:702–709.

45. Reisman RE, Dvorin DJ, Randolph CC, Georgitis JW. Stinging insect allergy: Natural history and modification with venom immunotherapy. J Allergy Clin Immunol 1985; 75:735–740.

46. Golden DB, Johnson K, Addison BI, Valentine MD, Kagey-Sobotka A, Lichtenstein LM. Clinical and immunologic observations in patients who stop venom immunotherapy. J Allergy Clin Immunol 1986; 77:435–442.

47. Lerch E, Muller UR. Long-term protection after stopping venom immunotherapy: Results of re-stings in 200 patients. J Allergy Clin Immunol 1998; 101:606–612.

48. Golden DB, Kagey-Sobotka A, Lichtenstein LM. Survey of patients after discontinuing venom immunotherapy. J Allergy Clin Immunol 2000; 105:385–390.

49. The discontinuation of Hymenoptera venom immunotherapy. Report from the Committee on Insects. J Allergy Clin Immunol 1998; 101:573–575.

50. Gleich GJ, Zimmermann EM, Henderson LL, Yunginger JW. Effect of immunotherapy on immunoglobulin E and immunoglobulin G antibodies to ragweed antigens: A six-year prospective study. J Allergy Clin Immunol 1982; 70:261–271.

51. Golden DB, Marsh DG, Freidhoff LR, Kwiterovich KA, Addison B, Kagey-Sobotka A, Lichtenstein LM. Natural history of Hymenoptera venom sensitivity in adults. J Allergy Clin Immunol 1997; 100:760–766.

52. Reisman RE. Duration of venom immunotherapy: Relationship to the severity of symptoms of initial insect sting anaphylaxis. J Allergy Clin Immunol 1993; 92:831–836.

53. Haugaard L, Norregaard OF, Dahl R. In-hospital sting challenge in insect venom-allergic patients after stopping venom immunotherapy. J Allergy Clin Immunol 1991; 87:699–702.

54. Golden DB, Kwiterovich KA, Kagey-Sobotka A, Lichtenstein LM. Discontinuing venom immunotherapy: Extended observations. J Allergy Clin Immunol 1998; 101:298–305.

55. Golden DB, Addison BI, Gadde J, Kagey-Sobotka A, Valentine MD, Lichtenstein LM. Prospective observations on stopping prolonged venom immunotherapy. J Allergy Clin Immunol 1989; 84:162–167.

56. Nish WA, Charlesworth EN, Davis TL, Whisman BA, Valtier S, Charlesworth MG, Leiferman KM. The effect of immunotherapy on the cutaneous late phase response to antigen. J Allergy Clin Immunol 1994; 93:484–493.

57. Pienkowski MM, Norman PS, Lichtenstein LM. Suppression of late-phase skin reactions by immunotherapy with ragweed extract. J Allergy Clin Immunol 1985; 76:729–734.

58. Iliopoulos O, Proud D, Adkinson NF Jr, Creticos PS, Norman PS, Kagey-Sobotka A, Lichtenstein LM, Naclerio RM. Effects of immunotherapy on the early, late, and rechallenge nasal reaction to provocation with allergen: Changes in inflammatory mediators and cells. J Allergy Clin Immunol 1991; 87:855–866.

59. Golden DB, Lawrence ID, Hamilton RH, Kagey-Sobotka A, Valentine MD, Lichtenstein LM. Clinical correlation of the venom-specific IgG antibody level during maintenance venom immunotherapy. J Allergy Clin Immunol 1992; 90:386–393.

60. Norman PS, Lichtenstein LM. The clinical and immunologic specificity of immunotherapy. J Allergy Clin Immunol 1978; 61:370–377.

61. Platts-Mills T, Vaughan J, Squillace S, Woodfolk J, Sporik R. Sensitisation, asthma, and a modified Th2 response in children exposed to cat allergen: A population-based cross-sectional study. Lancet 2001; 357:752–756.

62. Ownby DR, Johnson CC, Peterson EL. Exposure to dogs and cats in the first year of life and risk of allergic sensitization at 6 to 7 years of age. JAMA 2002; 288:963–972.

63. Trivedi B, Valerio C, Slater JE. Endotoxin content of standardized allergen vaccines. J Allergy Clin Immunol 2003; 111:777–783.

64. Han S, Yang K, Ozen Z, Peng W, Marinova E, Kelsoe G, Zheng B. Enhanced differentiation of splenic plasma cells but diminished long-lived high-affinity bone marrow plasma cells in aged mice. J Immunol 2003; 170:1267–1273.

65. Okudaira H, Ishizaka K. Reaginic antibody formation in the mouse. XI. Participation of long-lived antibody-forming cells in persistent antibody formation. Cell Immunol 1981; 58:188–201.

66. Majori M, Caminati A, Corradi M, Brianti E, Scarpa S, Pesci A. T-cell cytokine pattern at three time points during specific immunotherapy for mite-sensitive asthma. Clin Exp Allergy 2000; 30:341–347.

67. Hamid QA, Schotman E, Jacobson MR, Walker SM, Durham SR. Increases in IL-12 messenger RNA+ cells accompany inhibition of allergen-induced late skin responses after successful grass pollen immunotherapy. J Allergy Clin Immunol 1997; 99:254–260.

68. Durham SR. Clinical efficacy of immunotherapy. 60th anniversary meeting American Academy of Allergy, Asthma, and Immunology, Denver, CO, March 7–12, 2003.

69. Wilson DR, Nouri-Aria KT, Walker SM, Pajno GB, O'Brien F, Jacobson MR, Mackay IS, Durham SR. Grass pollen immunotherapy: Symptomatic improvement correlates with reductions in eosinophils and IL-5 mRNA expression in the nasal mucosa during the pollen season. J Allergy Clin Immunol 2001; 107:971–976.

70. Akdis CA, Blesken T, Akdis M, Wuthrich B, Blaser K. Role of interleukin 10 in specific immunotherapy. J Clin Invest 1998; 102:98–106.

71. Jutel M, Akdis M, Budak F, Aebischer-Casaulta C, Wrzyszcz M, Blaser K, Akdis CA. IL-10 and TGF-beta cooperate in the regulatory T cell response to mucosal allergens in normal immunity and specific immunotherapy. Eur J Immunol 2003; 33:1205–1214.

72. Fellrath JM, Kettner A, Dufour N, Frigerio C, Schneeberger D, Leimgruber A, Corradin G, Spertini F. Allergen-specific T-cell tolerance induction with allergen-derived long synthetic peptides: Results of a phase I trial. J Allergy Clin Immunol 2003; 111:854–861.

73. Akdis CA, Akdis M, Blesken T, Wymann D, Alkan SS, Muller U, Blaser K. Epitope-specific T cell tolerance to phospholipase A2 in bee venom immunotherapy and recovery by IL-2 and IL-15 in vitro. J Clin Invest 1996; 98:1676–1683.

38

Unproven and Controversial Forms of Immunotherapy

ABBA I. TERR

University of California, San Francisco, School of Medicine, San Francisco, California, U.S.A.

I. INTRODUCTION

Specific allergen immunotherapy is currently an accepted practice among allergy specialists throughout the world for the treatment of selected patients with respiratory atopic allergy or Hymenoptera venom anaphylaxis. The vast majority of placebo-controlled clinical trials support its use. Standardized protocols are of limited value because the specific allergens and the dosage necessary to optimize efficacy and safety must be tailored to each patient. Nevertheless, the basic procedures used in this form of therapy include a perennial subcutaneous injection schedule, beginning with progressively increasing quantities of allergen, that culminate in a program of stable high doses of allergen maintained for a period of several years.

Such a program differs little from that recommended empirically by Noon and Freeman in 1910. Numerous efforts have been made over the past century to improve

Table 1 Unconventional Forms of Immunotherapy

Serial endpoint titration
Neutralization or symptom-relieving therapy
Enzyme-potentiated desensitization
Autogenous urine injections

allergen immunotherapy because it is time-consuming, costly, and has potentially serious adverse effects, including death. These efforts at improvement have been mostly empirical, because the precise mechanism by which allergen immunotherapy makes the patient clinically tolerant to ambient allergen exposure remains elusive. Such efforts include changes in the structure of the administered allergen, the use of immunological adjuvants, and different routes of administration.

The purpose of this chapter is to describe certain alternative and unconventional methods of allergen immunotherapy (Table 1) that have been tried but cannot be recommended because they (1) are unproven, based on the results of clinical trials; (2) are controversial in concept; or (3) entail potential risk to the patient without sufficient evidence of efficacy.

II. IMMUNOTHERAPY BASED ON SERIAL ENDPOINT TITRATION

Serial endpoint titration refers to a method that links semi-quantitative skin testing to specific doses of allergen for initiating and optimizing injection treatment of allergic disease. It was devised by Rinkel, whose name is usually associated with this method and its modifications by others. The method was recommended first for treatment of respiratory diseases caused by the common inhalant allergens but was later adopted for use with food allergens (1–4). It is currently favored particularly by some otolarygologists in the United States who include allergy practice in their specialty.

Rinkel's method of testing uses serial fivefold decreasing dilutions (i.e., increasing concentrations) of allergen injected intradermally in a volume of 0.01 ml to establish an "endpoint." Skin testing to each allergen is repeated, using as many as nine serial intradermal injections. The initial test dose could therefore be as dilute as 1:1,953,125 of the concentrated allergen. The wheal diameter is recorded 10 min after injection (5,6). The "endpoint" of the test for each allergen is the dilution that initiates a serial 2-mm incremental increase in wheal diameter with decreasing fivefold dilutions.

Certain features of this testing protocol must be considered in assessing its relationship to treatment. The presence or absence of erythema accompanying the wheal is ignored (7), which could be responsible for false-positive results. The use of a latent period of only 10 minutes for an IgE-mediated allergic skin test reaction could lead to a false-negative interprctation. In somc cascs this tcsting mcthod docs not produce the expected progres sive increase in wheal diameter. These variations are referred to as bizarre, hourglass, plateau, and flash responses (7), which proponents of the Rinkel method attribute to extraneous factors such as concurrent infection, airborne allergen exposure, or incidental food allergy, although there is no proof of such associations.

The "endpoint," as it is defined above, is considered to be a safe dose to initiate immunotherapy for that particular allergen and patient. In fact, this procedure has been shown to be a safe method for preventing a systemic reaction to the first intracutaneous treatment dose, although it is almost always too conservative (i.e., excessively dilute). It underestimates the initial dose and unnecessarily prolongs the course of treatment (8–11).

In addition to establishing the initial dose of immunotherapy, an "optimal" dose is calculated at certain arbitrary multiples of the endpoint, usually between 25 and 50 times the quantity of allergen producing the endpoint. Practitioners of this procedure may vary these multiples in an empirical fashion, depending on the allergen.

The "optimal dose," as determined in this way, is believed to be the dose at which symptoms will be controlled during immunotherapy. Clinical trials, however, have shown that such a calculated "optimal" immunotherapy dose is almost always too low, so that treatment based on the endpoint procedure leads to therapy that is ultimately no more effective than placebo (12).

Proponents of the Rinkel method recommend retesting during the course of immunotherapy to establish a new "endpoint" if the patient fails to improve as expected. There are no studies to assess the clinical validity of this recommendation.

III. PROVOCATION-NEUTRALIZATION

"Neutralization" (also called "symptom-relieving" or "tolerance") therapy is also based on a procedure in which the technique for testing is related to the method of treatment. The testing procedure is known as provocation-neutralization, which evolved from serial endpoint titration, described in the previous section. It is based on the concept that an extremely small quantity of allergen can cause the immediate appearance of a symptomatic allergic reaction or the prompt disappearance ("neutralization") of ongoing allergic symptoms. In actual practice, the symptoms that are provoked and cleared in this way are subjective, nonspecific, and not consistent with the symptoms that are widely recognized in allergic disease (13–18).

Provocation-neutralization testing is performed in a manner similar to that of skin endpoint titration, using increasing or decreasing fivefold serial dilutions of the allergen (4). Many practitioners of this procedure use skin test allergen extracts that include not only the usual inhalant and food allergens, but also solutions of environmental chemicals, drugs, hormones, and many other items that are unlikely to cause atopic disease.

The testing is performed by exposing the patient to the allergen for testing via the intracutaneous, subcutaneous, or sublingual route. There is no rational explanation for these three choices. Intracutaneous testing is done with injected volumes of 0.01, 0.02, or 0.05 ml. Injections are given in the arm. Regardless of the route of administration, the patient keeps a written record of all "sensations" (i.e., any symptom) that is experienced over a 10-min period following each injection or application of the sublingual drop. There is no standardized protocol for grading the subjective response, so any symptom or sensation reported by the patient constitutes a positive test result. If the patient reports no symptoms, higher doses are administered in a serial fashion until symptoms are reported. Once a test result is considered positive, further testing proceeds by the administration of a progressive series of lower concentrations until a dose is reached at which the patient reports no sensations. This particular dose of the test substance is considered to be the "neutralizing dose," which is then used for subsequent treatment.

To accomplish this form of testing, each allergen or other test substance must be given separately in a serial fashion, so that the entire testing procedure can require many days, weeks, or months to complete. This method of testing does include negative controls, and there is no provision for accounting for spontaneous symptoms.

There are variations on this basic protocol. Wheal diameter may be used in addition to subjective symptoms in determining a positive response, but there are no published criteria for wheal sizes to indicate whether the test is positive or negative (14). Some practitioners of provocation-neutralization use the *absence* of symptoms as an indication of a positive test (14,16). In this scheme, a negative test result is followed by serially lowering the subsequent doses; following a positive test doses are serially raised until a negative ("neutralizing") dose is reached.

The sublingual route for provocation-neutralization is used especially—although not exclusively—to diagnose food allergy.

After testing, the "neutralizing" doses of one or more tested substances are self-administered by the patient as treatment. Where multiple substances are required for treatment, they can be combined or used separately. Treatment can be carried out by the intracutaneous, subcutaneous, or sublingual route. The choice is arbitrary, because there are no established protocols. The patient is advised to administer the neutralizing solution either after symptoms appear or before anticipated exposure to a substance that the patient believes is the cause of the illness. Treatment can also be given on a regular maintenance schedule, usually daily or twice weekly.

Historically, this procedure evolved from the serial intradermal endpoint technique, and certain theories have been offered to justify the results. It has been claimed that allergen is present in the wheal and is released into the systemic circulation, from which it elicits symptoms (13), but the minute amount of allergen and the nonallergic nature of induced symptoms make this theory unlikely. Another hypothesis states that allergen introduced into the skin or under the tongue induces antibody formation with the development of circulating immune complexes, but the kinetics and time required for these events make this an untenable scenario. Other theories postulate antigen stimulation or suppression of lymphocyte function, and the induction of immunological tolerance. Sublingual "desensitization" of lymphocytes has also been postulated as a consequence of antigen absorption from the sublingual route, which bypasses its gastrointestinal metabolism. There have been no published results of experiments to test any of these theories.

Neutralizing therapy has been recommended for treating a wide variety of conditions, including atopic allergy, rheumatic diseases, premenstrual syndrome, viral infections, headache, musculoskeletal complaints, attention deficit disorder in children, and others. Neutralizing "antigens" have consisted of extracts of atopic allergens, environmental chemicals, hormones, viral vaccines, foods, histamine, serotonin, saline, and even distilled water.

Published clinical trials of "neutralization" therapy are few in number (17–25). One preliminary report of a double-blind, placebo-controlled crossover study of subcutaneous injections of foods administered daily to 8 patients revealed improvement with both placebo and active vaccines, but the results from the latter were said to be superior (21). Another report claimed both subjective and objective improvement in 20 patients with perennial rhinitis treated with sublingual dust vaccine, but the results are of questionable significance since the duration of the study period was only 2 weeks, and 5 of the subjects were, in fact, not allergic to the house dust mite as determined by the investigators reporting the study (25).

IV.   ENZYME-POTENTIATED DESENSITIZATION

In 1973, McEwen reported that the enzyme β-glucuronidase acts as an adjuvant or promoter of an immune response when added to the antigen immediately before injection

(26). Since then, a small number of allergists have recommended a procedure known as enzyme-potentiated desensitization (EPD) as an improvement over conventional immunotherapy, claiming that it requires many fewer injections compared with conventional immunotherapy and has 80% effectiveness.

A very low dose of allergen (1–2.5 Noon units), which is approximately the amount delivered into the skin in a standard prick test, is mixed with partially purified enzyme, β-glucuronidase, in a dose (100 Fishman units, <40 μg) equivalent to the amount of enzyme normally present in 4 ml of human blood. The mixture is immediately injected intradermally in a volume of approximately 0.125 ml. This is considered sufficient immunization as a single dose preseasonally to produce a therapeutic effect for an entire pollen season. For perennial allergy, the intradermal injections are given every 2 to 6 months. Both inhalant and food allergens have been used in this fashion. A single intradermal injection may contain as many as 150 allergens, typically including inhalants, foods, and certain food additives.

Proponents of this form of treatment have claimed success in treating not only allergic rhinitis, asthma, and eczema, but also sinusitis, nasal polyposis, urticaria, migraine headaches, ulcerative colitis, irritable bowel syndrome, chronic fatigue syndrome, "immune dysfuntion," hyperactivity anxiety, rheumatoid arthritis, grand mal and petit mal seizures, and anaphylaxis from food allergy.

To date, there have been no published research findings in patients treated by this method to substantiate this theory. The effectiveness of enzyme-potentiated desensitization and the presumed pharmacological property of β-glucuronidase on the immune system are based on anecdotal evidence only. Several published double-blind reports claim symptomatic improvements in adults or children with allergic rhinitis or asthma along with conflicting results of immunological changes (27–31). These studies have been done on 10 to 20 subjects only in the active and placebo groups, have been of short duration, and generally lacked objective measurements of disease activity.

The proponents of enzyme-potentiated desensitization hypothesize that the enzyme recruits and activates a new population of CD8 lymphocytes that suppress or downregulate the response to the injected antigens, thereby suppressing the immune response. The claim that this method of treatment requires infrequent injections of allergen is based on the supposition that specific "suppressor" CD8 T-cells persist for up to 2 years. When prescribed for perennial allergies, the first few injections are given every 2 months, after which the frequency may decrease to as little as once or twice yearly. For treatment of seasonal pollen allergy, a single dose is given not more than 4 months before the expected arrival of the season. Boosting doses are given "as required." The effectiveness for house dust allergy is said to be evident almost immediately, for hay fever after 3 to 4 weeks, and for food allergy after 6 to 9 months.

Advocates of this treatment require their patients to follow certain rules to avoid treatment failure. The patients must not be exposed to allergens for which they are being treated for a period of 24 hours before and 48 hours after the injection. They must consume a special "EPD diet" of lamb, sweet potatoes, carrots, celery, lettuce, sago, tapioca, rhubarb, sea salt, and bottled water for 24 hours before and 48 hours after the injection. They are prescribed specific vitamins and minerals. The injection is given only during the first 2 weeks of the menstrual cycle, and a number of specified medications must be avoided. It is not to be used during pregnancy or within 5 days of an upper respiratory infection. The patient must not use scented products or ointments on the skin near the injection site. Exposure to heat, stress, environmental chemicals, smoke, air conditioning, newsprint, and photocopiers must be avoided. Efficacy also is believed to be enhanced by taking zinc, folic acid, vitamins A and B$_6$, and magnesium orally or intravenously for several days before the injection.

Delayed reactions, described as a temporary return of the allergic symptoms for which the patient is being treated, are considered a favorable sign that the treatment will be effective.

V. AUTOGENOUS URINE IMMUNOTHERAPY

In the early 1930s, several medical publications appeared claiming that a specific substance, called "proteose," is present in the urine during the course of allergic disease (32,33). Urinary proteose refers to a mixture of partially to completely hydrolyzed protein from the glomerular filtrate. It is therefore postulated to contain allergen peptide fragments, and in particular those peptides that are "specific" or most allergenic for each individual allergic person. This substance was believed to be a source of allergen for therapy superior to the usual allergen vaccines used in immunotherapy.

Several chemical extraction procedures were recommended for obtaining "proteose" from the urine of allergic patients. The extract was suspended in a buffered solution and then used for intradermal testing and for subcutaneous therapeutic injections. This practice seems to have thrived briefly about 50 years ago, subsided after several years, and has resurfaced recently.

The published reports consist of uncontrolled anecdotal histories of apparently successful treatment of a variety of allergic conditions, including asthma, rhinitis, anaphylaxis, urticaria, angioedema, and serum sickness (34–36). None of these studies used proper controls and therefore cannot be used to show efficacy.

There has been no investigation of long-term safety. This is a critical issue, since small quantities of glomerular basement membrane antigens are found in normal urine. It is not unreasonable to assume that alteration by chemical treatment during the extraction process could lead to the production of altered renal proteins that might prove to be antigenic for the induction of autoantibodies.

VI. SCOPE OF THE PROBLEM

Some of the unproven treatment methods discussed here, such as urine therapy, are rarely encountered today. Others, however, persist. In particular, neutralization therapy using either the injection or sublingual route and enzyme-potentiated desensitization form an important part of the practice of those who subscribe to the theory of "multiple chemical sensitivities," whereby certain people are believed to react to ordinary or even exceedingly minute exposures to common environmental items that can be detected by odor, such as perfumes, organic solvents, and other ubiquitous chemicals. The clinical manifestations of this condition are numerous but entirely subjective. Extracts of chemicals and foods are typically included in the "neutralizing" or "enzyme-potentiating" treatment. The current preferred name for multiple chemical sensitivities is idiopathic environmental intolerances, which reflects the fact that the condition has never been shown to be caused by chemicals or to involve a physical sensitivity (37).

VII. COSTS TO THE HEALTH CARE SYSTEM

There is no reliable method to assess or even estimate the cost of these unproven immunotherapy methods in either absolute amounts or as a percentage of the total health care expenditure. Since they are controversial and not considered standard forms of medical practice, they are not listed or codified in the Common Procedural Terminology publication (38). It is likely that in most instances payment for these services in the United States is made by the patient directly to the practitioner and not by third-party payers.

VIII. SALIENT POINTS

1. The same controversial treatment is often claimed to be efficacious for a variety of unrelated illnesses.
2. Theories in support of controversial allergy procedures freqently change.
3. Controversial allergy treatments are often linked to unproven forms of allergy diagnostic testing.
4. Clinicians should be familiar with unproven and controversial treatments and their pitfalls to properly advise their patients.
5. Unproven treatments flourish in part because of the placebo effect inherent in every form of treatment.

REFERENCES

1. Rinkel HJ. The management of clinical allergy. Part II: Etiologic factors and skin titration. Arch Otolaryngol 1963; 77:42–89.
2. Rinkel HJ. The management of clinical allergy. Part III: Inhalation allergy therapy. Arch Otolaryngol 1963; 77:205.
3. Rinkel HJ. The management of clinical allergy. Part IV: Food and mold allergy. Arch Otolaryngol 1963; 77:302.
4. Rinkel HJ, Lee CH, Brown DW Jr, et al. The diagnosis of food allergy. Arch Otolaryngol 1964; 79:71–80.
5. Williams RI. Skin titration: Testing and treatment. Otolaryngol Clin North Am 1971; 3:507–521.
6. Richardson AS. Titration: Evaluation of an office system of allergy diagnosis and treatment. Its use in otolaryngology. Ann Otol Rhinol Laryngol 1961; 70:344.
7. Willoughby JW. Serial dilution titration skin tests in inhalant allergy: A clinical quantitative assessment of biologic skin reactivity to allergenic extracts. Otolaryngol Clin North Am 1974; 7:579.
8. Hirsch S, Kalbfleisch JH, Golbert TM, et al. Rinkel method: A controlled study. Second report. J Allergy Clin Immunol 1980; 65:192.
9. Hirsch S, Kalbfleisch JH, Golbert TM, Josephson BM, McConnell LG, Scanlon R, Kniker WT, Fink JN, Murphree JJ, Cohen SH. Rinkel injection therapy: A multicenter controlled study. J Allergy Clin Immunol 1981; 68:133–155.
10. Van Metre TE, Adkinson NF, Amodio FJ, Lichtenstein LM, Mardiney MR, Norman PS, Rosenberg GL, Sobotka AK, Valentine MD. A comparative study of the effectiveness of the Rinkel method and the current standard method of immunotherapy for ragweed pollen hay fever. J Allergy Clin Immunol 1980; 66:500–513.
11. Van Metre TE, Adkinson NF, Lichtenstein LM, Mardiney MR, Norman PS, Rosenberg GL, Sobotka AR, Valentine MD. A controlled study of the effectiveness of the Rinkel method of immunotherapy for ragweed pollen hay fever. J Allergy Clin Immunol 1980; 65:288–297.
12. Van Metre TE. Critique of controversial and unproven procedures for diagnosis and therapy of allergy disorders. Ped Clin North Am 1983; 30:807–817.
13. Morris DL. Use of sublingual antigen in diagnosis and treatment of food allergy. Ann Allergy 1971; 27:289.
14. Lee CH, Williams RT, Binkley EL, Jr. Provocative testing and treatment for foods. Arch Otolaryngol 1969; 90:87–94.

15. Breneman JC, Crook WC, Deamer W, et al. Report of the Food Allergy Committee on the sublingual method of provocation testing for food allergy. Ann Allergy 1973; 31:382.

16. Willoughby JW. Provocative food test technique. Ann Allergy 1965; 23:543.

17. Lee CH, Williams RT, Binkley EL, Jr. Provocative inhalation testing and treatment. Arch Otolaryngol 1969; 90:173–177.

18. Kailin EW, Collier R. "Relieving" therapy for antigen exposure. J Am Med Assoc 1971; 217:78.

19. Dickey LD, Pfeiffer G. Sublingual therapy in allergy. Trans Am Soc Ophthal Otolaryngol Allergy 1964; 5:37.

20. Warren CM. Inhalant allergy: Diagnosis and treatment by provocation intracutaneous method. Med Dig 1978; 33.

21. Miller JB. A double-blind study of food extract injection therapy: A preliminary report. Ann Allergy 1977; 38:185–191.

22. Morris DL. Use of sublingual antigen in diagnosis and treatment of food allergy. Ann Allergy 1969; 27:289–294.

23. Morris DL. Treatment of respiratory disease with ultra-small doses of antigen. Ann Allergy 1970; 28:494–500.

24. Morris DL. Treatment of atopic dermatitis with tolerogenic doses of antigen. Acta Dermatovenerol 1980; 92(suppl):97.

25. Scadding GK, Brostoff J. Low dose sublingual therapy in patients with allergic rhinitis due to house dust mite. Clin Allergy 1986; 16:483–491.

26. McEwen LM, Nicholson M, Kitchen I, White S. Enzyme potentiated desensitization: III. Control by sugars and diols of the immunological effect of glucuronidase in mice and patients with hay fever. Ann Allergy 1973; 31:543–550.

27. Fell P, Brostoff J. A single dose desensitization for summer hay fever: Results of a double blind study—1988. Eur J Clin Pharmacol 1990; 38:77–79.

28. Cantani A, Ragno V, Monteleone MA, Lucenti P, Businco L. Enzyme-potentiated desensitization in children with asthma and mite allergy: A double-blind study. J Invest, Allergol Clin Immunol 1996; 6:270–276.

29. Astarita C, Scala G, Sproviero S, Franzese A. Effects of enzyme-potentiated desensitization in the treatment of pollinosis: A double-blind placebo-controlled trial. J Invest Allergol Immunol 1996; 6:248–255.

30. Di Stanisloa C, Di Berardino L, Bianchi I, Bologna G. A double-blind, placebo controlled study of preventive immunotherapy with E.P.D., in the treatment of seasonal allergic disease. Allerg Immunol (Paris) 1997; 29:39–42.

31. Caramia G, Franceschini F, Cimarelli ZA, Ciucchi MS, Gagliardini R, Ruffini E. The efficacy of E.P.D., a new immunotherapy, in the treatment of allergic diseases in children. Allerg Immunol (Paris) 1996; 28:308–310.

32. Steel RS. The specificity of urinary proteose. Med J Aust 1932; 2:800.

33. Oriel OH, Barber HW. Proteose in urine excreted in anaphylactic and allergic conditions. Lancet 1930; 2:1304.

34. Whitehead RW, Darley W, Dickman PA. Therapeutic use of urinary proteose. Colorado Med 1934; 56.

35. Liberman I, Bigland AD. Autogenous urinary proteose in asthma and other allergic conditions. Br Med J 1937; 1:62.

36. Plesch J. Urine therapy. Med Press 1947; 218:128.

37. United Nations Environment Program—International Labor Office—World Health Organization. Conclusions and recommendations of a workshop on multiple chemical sensitivities (MCS). Reg Toxicol Pharmacol 1996; 24:S188–S189.

38. International Classification of Diseases, 9th rev. Clinical modification, Chicago, AMAPress, 2003.

39

Adverse Effects and Fatalities Associated with Subcutaneous Allergen Immunotherapy

SAMUEL C. BUKANTZ and RICHARD F. LOCKEY

University of South Florida College of Medicine and James A. Haley Veterans' Hospital, Tampa, Florida, U.S.A.

I. INTRODUCTION

Most local and systemic reactions that develop during allergen immunotherapy occur within 20 to 30 min of injection but can occur later than 30 min afterward. Subcutaneous nodules at the site of injection are more common with aluminum-adsorbed vaccines, may persist but usually disappear, and do not necessitate an adjustment in the immunotherapy dose. Patients who develop nodules that persist should be injected with aqueous preparations.

Van Arsdel and Sherman's (1) comprehensive review in 1957 analyzed retrospectively the incidence of constitutional reactions in a population of 8706 patients who had received a total of 1,250,000 allergen injections during the 21 years between 1935 and

1955. Their patients experienced a total of 1774 constitutional reactions, corresponding to about 1 in 700 of the 1,250,000 injections given. The reactions occurred in 663 patients, an incidence of 1.9% [vs. the 3.5% reported in 1916 by Cooke and Vanderveer (2)]. Of the 663 reacting patients, 635 were pollen sensitive, representing about 15% of the 4215 pollen-sensitive patients, contrasted with an 0.6% incidence in the remaining 4491 patients. Most of the studies on adverse reactions to allergen immunotherapy have been concerned with reactions resulting from the injection itself.

Reports of adverse effects from prick puncture skin tests prompted an analysis of data derived from the Second National Health and Nutrition Examination Survey (NHANES II) (3). This study revealed that the risk of prick puncture allergy skin testing was low when carried out with eight vaccines licensed by the U.S. Food and Drug Administration on a randomly selected population.

The incidence of adverse reactions during immunotherapy reported in retrospective and prospective studies has varied considerably depending on several factors, including the type of antigen vaccine preparation, the patients selected, route of administration, and treatment schedule used, with or without pretreatment and/or preventive procedures (4–12). All of these studies carried out between 1980 and 1989 established the safety of immunotherapy when performed on selected patients by experienced physicians who exercised caution and provided adequate monitoring and appropriate treatment, when anaphylaxis does occur. The nonfatal adverse reaction rate ran from less than 1% of patients on immunotherapy to 36.2% on rush immunotherapy, without pretherapy.

These data have been obtained in studies utilizing the subcutaneous route of injection of allergen vaccines obtained by aqueous extraction of allergens. An "Immunotherapy Coalition" consisting of the American College of Allergy, Asthma and Immunology (ACAAI), the American Academy of Allergy, Asthma and Immunology (AAAAI), and allergy extract manufacturers supported the benefits of immunotherapy and pretreatment to reduce adverse effects associated with the therapy (13–24).

Other allergen molecules and techniques of immunotherapy have been explored to decrease the potential for adverse reactions and to increase efficacy (25–33). These have included oral administration (34,35), nasal administration (36,37), and sublingual-swallow immunotherapy (SLIT), a method used primarily by some Europeans and South American allergists (38–42). A review of the available literature by WHO in 1998 concluded that oral immunotherapy was ineffective, whereas SLIT is a viable alternative to the subcutaneous injection route. These conclusions were also made in a position paper of the European Academy of Allergy and Clinical Immunology. This is reviewed in the paper by Passalacqua et al. (40). However, in the United States such therapy is not routinely used because it has not been approved by the U.S. FDA.

The traditionally protein-based immunotherapy (IT) has a limited scope of efficacy. A number of reagents, however, termed DNA-based immunotherapeutics, have been effective in the prevention and reversal of TH2-mediated hypersensitivity states in mouse models of allergic disease (43). The four basic DNA-based IT modalities used include immunization with gene vaccines, allergen mixed with immunostimulating oligodeoxynucleotides (ISS-ODN), and physical allergen–ISS-ODN conjugates, as well as immunomodulation with ISS-ODN alone. As the review by Horner et al. review concluded, "If these reagents prove as effective in humans, as they have proven to be in rodents and nonhuman primates, then DNA-based immunotherapeutics are likely to revolutionize the standard of care for the treatment of allergic disease." However, for the time being, subcutaneous allergen immunotherapy will remain the standard of care throughout most of the world.

II.   FREQUENCY OF IgE SYSTEMIC REACTIONS

The risk of death after the injection of a foreign substance has been known since Lamson's report in 1924 (44). No other cited studies had reported fatalities; however, in 1942 Vance and Strassman (45) reported seven cases of sudden death following injection of foreign protein, and James and Austen (46) published an analysis of six instances of fatal anaphylaxis in humans following parenteral administration of antigen (penicillin, guinea pig hemoglobin, bee venom, and ragweed vaccine), citing several single case reports by Sheppe (47) and Blanton and Sutphin (48), as well as the seven cases of Vance and Strassman cited by Rosenthal (49) following penicillin injection.

Rands, a general practitioner in the United Kingdom, published a report of a single fatality of a 19-year-old female due to nonresponsive bronchoconstriction developing within 5 min following the injection of her usual maintenance dose of Pollinex (a pollen vaccine) given 5 weeks after the same dose had been administered without effect (50). This was followed by a report of 26 fatalities due to immunotherapy and the recommendations of the Committee on Safety of Medicine in the United Kingdom (51), which established preconditions for immunotherapy that temporarily resulted in the virtual abandonment of immunotherapy in the United Kingdom.

A major objective of this chapter is to compare the retrospective reviews of fatalities occurring during skin testing and immunotherapy made by the Committee on Allergen Standardization of the American Academy of Allergy, Asthma and Immunology and by the Paul Ehrlich Institute, German Federal Agency for Sera and Vaccines (52). These studies analyzed the factors contributing to fatalities occurring during skin tests or immunotherapy with a view to diminishing and, hopefully, eliminating them.

III.   NON–IgE-MEDIATED ADVERSE REACTIONS

It is appropriate to review reports of some aspects of adverse reactions to immunotherapy that are controversial. The possible role of precipitins as responsible for adverse reactions was addressed by Busse et al. in a study correlating *Alternaria* IgG precipitins and adverse reactions (53). Their prospective study revealed that 5 of 23 *Alternaria*-sensitive persons had IgG precipitins before immunotherapy and another 6 developed precipitins during therapy. Only 1 of the 23 experienced a reaction to *Alternaria* 4 to 6 h after an injection of *Alternaria* vaccine. They concluded that precipitins to *Alternaria* are common and do not seem to be the basis for late reactions, and their presence is not a contraindication to immunotherapy. A contrasting report by Kaad and Ostergaard suggested that immunotherapy of asthmatic children with mold vaccines might be hazardous by provoking immune complex reactions (54). Of 38 children with bronchial asthma who were immunized with mold vaccines, 7 (19%) were withdrawn from immunotherapy due to "serious" side effects that were considered clinically consistent with an immune complex reaction. These 7 children exhibited a two- to fourfold increase in circulating precipitating antibodies to the injected vaccines. Of the remaining 31 patients also treated with mold vaccines, 14, who were without side effects, did not develop precipitating antibodies. The sera of these patients were not examined for immune complexes, and the authors quote the contradictory findings of the Kemler and Stein (55,56) groups as well as apparently supportive reports by Stendardi et al., Cano et al., El-Hefny et al., Moore and Fink, and Kuuliala et al. (57–61).

Relevant to these studies is the report by Clausen and Yanari that immune complex–mediated disease is not a factor in patients on maintenance venom immunotherapy (62). They evaluated the problem in 30 adults and 15 pediatric patients receiving regular monthly doses of venom (100 µg of antigen), all for between 9 and 12 months. A serum sickness–like presentation had been reported as a sequel of Hymenoptera stings, but the possible role of immune complexes had not been addressed.

No patients developed clinical manifestations suggestive of immune complex pathology: All urinalyses were negative for gross and microscopic hematuria, no sera showed an elevation of Clq, and only 4 of the 45 patients had significantly elevated Raji cell assays. Prospective reevaluation showed the presence of immune complexes before venom administration with no change in acute-phase reactants or Raji cell titers 12 h later. The authors concluded that monthly administration of Hymenoptera venom does not appear to be associated with immune complex disease by either clinical or immunological parameters. A further relevant article was contributed by Umetsu et al., who described an 8-year-old male child with rhinitis and asthma who developed serum sickness triggered by anaphylaxis complicating immunotherapy with multiple inhalant allergens (ragweed, grass, and tree pollens; mold spores; and dust) (63). This child developed puffy eyelids 1 h following a half dose of his vaccine and progressed thereafter to an impressive serum sickness syndrome characterized by severe generalized raised annular urticaria, severe asthma, angioedema, severe arthralgias, fever, and episodes of confusion and disorientation. The authors hypothesized that the enhanced vascular permeability that accompanied the anaphylaxis allowed immune complexes, which may have persisted in the circulation, to deposit in the blood vessels of the patient. The immune complexes may or may not have been related to the immunotherapy itself. Tests for these complexes, however, were negative. Clemmensen and Knudsen reported a patient with eczema who apparently developed contact sensitivity to aluminum while receiving immunotherapy for hay fever with an aluminum-precipitated allergen (64). Standard patch testing was positive to the aluminum discs used for testing and negative in 53 controls; the eczema disappeared when therapy was discontinued.

An association between brachial plexus neuropathy and allergen immunotherapy was reported by Wolpow (65). Two patients were described who developed acute, self-limiting, unilateral brachial plexus neuropathy in association with subcutaneous injections of dust and molds. Previous reports of this neurological illness had "in many cases followed injection of foreign substances, but usually of animal rather than vegetable origin."

Schatz et al. call attention to what they termed nonorganic adverse reactions to allergen immunotherapy (66). They described 10 patients who presented adverse reactions to immunotherapy that mimicked immunologically mediated reactions but were believed to be "nonorganic in etiology—with a high incidence of coexisting or contributory psychiatric problems."

IV. LONG-TERM SEQUELAE

The possibility that chronic injection of foreign proteins might induce long-term sequelae had been addressed by both experimental animal studies and anecdotal reports in humans. Rabbits hyperimmunized with various vaccines make cryoprecipitating proteins, monoclonal antibodies, rheumatoid factor, and anti-DNA antibodies (67–69), and such hyperimmunized animals may develop amyloidosis and myeloma (70,71). There have been anecdotal reports of multiple myeloma and Waldenström's macroglobulinemia in patients on long-term immunotherapy (72) and a report of a striking incidence of positive rheumatoid factors in atopic children on such therapy (73).

Levinson et al. undertook to determine if long-term allergen immunotherapy caused late sequelae, particularly those reflecting abnormal immunological responses (74). Their study, the first systematic investigation of potential adverse effects of long-term immunotherapy, examined 41 patients between 18 and 50 years of age who had received regular immunotherapy with three or more allergen vaccines for 5 or more years at the Walter Reed Army Medical Center Allergy Clinic. Twenty-one age- and gender-matched atopic individuals served as controls prior to initiating such therapy. The treated individuals showed no increased autoimmune, collagen, vascular, or lymphoproliferative disease. Furthermore, long-term allergen immunotherapy had no adverse effects on immunological reactivity as assessed by a number of immunological parameters—with a particularly noteworthy absence of immune complexes in the serum of patients undergoing long-term immunotherapy. The patients in this study were mostly Caucasian females, of an average age of 30, treated for allergic rhinitis and asthma.

Phanuphak and Kohler (75) described in 6 of 20 consecutive patients the onset of polyarteritis nodosa, vasculitic symptoms that coincided with allergen immunotherapy for presumptive atopic (IgE-mediated) respiratory disease. Compared with 14 other patients with polyarteritis nodosa, the 6 on immunotherapy had significantly greater skin involvement and peripheral blood eosinophils. There was evidence of circulatory complexes with decreased hemolytic complement, increased cryoglobulins, or increased Clq binding in both groups but no allergen-precipitating antibodies.

A possible association between pemphigus vulgaris and allergen injections with cat pelt vaccine was raised by McCombs et al. (76). Although intriguing, it seems irrelevant since such therapy today is performed with purified cat allergens.

The conflicting results of studies in patients receiving long-term immunotherapy might be explained by the nonuniformity of detection methods used. This prompted a group of Australian investigators to examine a population of older patients with documented prolonged immunotherapy extending over many years. They examined 35 older patients (mean age 62, range 53 to 85 years) who received injections of allergen vaccines for between 2 and 30 years (mean of 13 years) and compared them with an age-matched control group (mean age 64.7, range 42–87 years). Treated patients had significantly higher IgG and lower total IgE than controls, but no increased incidence of paraproteins or evidence of immune complex disease such as urinary abnormalities, increased Clq binding levels, cryoglobulins, or rheumatoid (*sic*) fever (77).

V. FATALITIES

Fatalities, carefully documented, constitute a less controversial measure of adverse effects related to either skin testing or allergen immunotherapy. Since Lamson's first description of death from anaphylaxis associated with immunotherapy (44), six fatalities have been reported related to or associated with immunotherapy (45,46,50,78–80). More than 70 deaths (between 1895 and 1964) have been reported after skin testing, the majority of these associated with antigens such as horse serum–derived tetanus or diphtheria antitoxins and pneumococcus antiserum, none of which is currently in use. Nine of these 70 deaths from skin testing were associated with allergens similar to allergens used today. No articles on fatalities associated with immunotherapy or skin testing were published in the United States between 1980 and 1987.

A project defining risk factors for fatalities from skin testing and immunotherapy was instituted as a retrospective study by the Committee on Allergen Standardization of the American Academy of Allergy and Immunology in 1983. For this project, Lockey and his co-workers composed a 64-item questionnaire designed to obtain data on fatalities from skin testing and immunotherapy. The questionnaire was mailed to the then 3400 members and fellows of the American Academy of Allergy and Immunology, and its analysis was published in the *Journal of Allergy and Clinical Immunology* in April 1987 (81). Although 46 fatalities had been reported from 1945 to 1984, only 30 (6 fatalities from skin testing and 24 from immunotherapy) had sufficient data for analysis. Tables 1 and 2 summarize the data on fatalities associated with skin testing and immunotherapy, respectively.

Although all ages were affected (range 7–70), the mean ages of the fatalities following skin testing and immunotherapy were 30 and 34 years, respectively. There was no gender predilection. Errors of administration appeared to be responsible for three fatalities and were questionable for an additional three. Ten patients had died after skin tests or immunotherapy during a seasonal exacerbation of the patients' allergic disease—four in patients who had been symptomatic at the time of injection, two of whom had been receiving β-adrenergic blockers. Of the 24 fatalities associated with immunotherapy, 4 had experienced previous reactions, 11 had a high degree of sensitivity, and 4 had been injected with newly prepared vaccines. Fifteen of the total of 30 fatalities had received a pollen vaccine as part of the fatal injection. Five of the six fatalities associated with skin testing had occurred without prior prick puncture testing. Signs and symptoms of systemic reactions were not reliable predictors of death. The onset of systemic reactions was 30 min or less after injection in 23 of 30 patients, was more than 30 min after injection in 2, and had not been reported in 5. The cause of death in 14 of 16 patients with asthma was respiratory. Epinephrine had been administered to 18 patients, was not given to 3, and was either not recorded or unknown in 9 patients.

A later supplemental survey conducted by Reid, Lockey, Turkeltaub, and Platts-Mills on deaths in the United States from immunotherapy between 1985 and 1989 was reported at the 1990 American Academy of Allergy, Asthma and Immunology meeting in Baltimore, Maryland (82). There were no deaths from skin testing reported; however, 16 deaths were reported from immunotherapy. These deaths were reported in the *Journal of Allergy and Clinical Immunology* and included 1 additional death, for a total of 17 (83). The mean age was 36 years (range 10–77), and there were 5 males and 11 females (gender of one subject not reported) versus 11 males and 13 females in the earlier study. Eighty-seven percent of the subjects had asthma, 1 was on beta-blocker therapy, and 10 of 17 were "highly sensitive" by skin testing or the radioallergosorbent test (RAST). Fourteen of 17 were on aqueous vaccines, 10 of 17 were on increasing doses, and 9 of 17 received epinephrine. The results obtained in this study are very similar to those reported previously.

Reid and Gurka presented at the 1996 American Academy of Allergy, Asthma and Immunology meeting an abstract of a continuation of the above-mentioned study that covered events from January 1990 to June 1995 (84). They reported 28 deaths during this time, an average of 5 deaths per year, with incomplete data for 19 of the 28 reports. One of the 28 deaths was associated with intradermal skin testing and 27 with immunotherapy. Four of the immunotherapy deaths occurred following home injections or injections given with no physician present, 3 were associated with an incorrect dose, 19 occurred in individuals with atopic asthma, and 5 deaths occurred despite postreaction intervention. The age range at the time of death was 12 to 73 years and there was no gender predilection. Data in this study are similar to previous reports of fatalities.

Table 1 Case Reports from the Literature: Fatalities from Skin Test

Author/year	Age/medical disease	Injected vaccine	Onset of symptoms	Initial symptoms	Cause of death
Baagoe, 1928	Unknown	Egg white, 0.1 cc	Sudden	Dyspnea	Unknown
Lamson, 1929	5 mo, eczema	Ovomucoid, 0.05 cc	2 min	Cyanosis	Respiratory arrest
Lamson, 1929	34 yr, asthma	Buckwheat 1:500, ID	2–3 min	Lacrimation, cyanosis, respiratory difficulty	Anaphylactic shock
Vance and, Strassman, 1942	4 yr	Silkworm, sheep's wool, kapok extracts, IC	5 min	Shock/unconsciousness	Anaphylactic shock[a]
Wiseman and McCarthy-Brough, 1945	78 yr, asthma	17 environmental allergens, 0.01 cc, IC	5 min	Cough, asthma	Anaphylactic arrest
Swineford, 1946	49 yr, asthma	56 food extracts, 8–9 inhalant extracts, IC	3 min	"Not feeling well," dyspnea	Cardiovascular collapse
Blantin and Sutphin, 1949	57 yr, asthma	56 skin tests, scratch and IC	Sudden	Air hunger	Anaphylactic shock[a]
Harris and Shure, 1950	25 yr, asthma	Environmental substances, ID	1 min	Dyspnea	Respiratory arrest[a]
Dogliotti, 1968	35 yr	Penicillin scratch	4–5 min	Flush, abdominal pain	Anaphylactic shock
Lockey et al., 1987	6 subjects, 10–50 yrs	Variable	3–20 min	Variable	Asthma, anaphylactic shock, others
Reid et al., 1995	1 subject	Unknown	Unknown	Unknown	Unknown

[a] Autopsy confirmed anaphylactic shock.
Source: Adapted from Ref. 81.

Table 2 Case Reports from the Literature: Fatalities from Immunotherapy

Author	Gender	Age (yr)	Medical disease	Allergen	Status of IT	Onset of symptoms	Symptoms	Cause of death
Lamson, 1929	M	34	Asthma	Bermuda grass pollen, 0.05 cc, 1:100	Because of "nervousness" with preceding reaction	<3 min	Flushing, athetoid movements, dyspnea	Anaphylactic shock[a]
Waldbott, 1932	F	40		Ragweed vaccine, 1400 units	Unknown	<3 min	Dyspnea, urticaria	Anaphylactic shock
Vaughn, Black, 1939	Unknown	Unknown	Unknown	Unknown	Unknown	Unknown	Unknown	Unknown
Vance, Strassman, 1964	M	35	Asthma	Ragweed vaccine	Unknown	1 hr	Unknown	Anaphylactic shock[a]
James, Austen, 1964	M	56		Hay fever desensitization	Unknown (11 of 21)	<45 min	Dyspnea	Anaphylactic shock[a]
Rends, 1980	F	19	Asthma	Pollinex, Migen[b]	Maintenance	3–10 min	Rushing, tachycardia	Anaphylactic shock[a]
Pellard, 1980	M	24	Asthma	Bencard product[c]	Unknown (15th injection)	25 min	Unknown	Status asthmaticus
CSM Update, 1986	F, 13 M, 12 Unknown, 1	11–57 x,31	Asthma, hay fever, Unknown	Varied, mite	Normal course, 16[d] Maintenance, 4 Unknown, 6	<10 min, 14 <30 min, 4 <90 min, 2 Unknown, 6	Asthma and anaphylaxis	Asthma and anaphylaxis
Lockey et al., 1987	F, 13 M, 11	7–70 x,34	Unknown[e]	Varied pollens, molds	Maintenance, 7 Increasing, 9 Decreasing, 1 1st injection, 1 NA, 6	<20 min, 15 20–30 min, 3 >30 min, 2 Unknown, 4	Pruritus, 3 Angioedema, 0 Airway obstruction and/or asthma, 12	Airway obstruction and/or asthma, 13 Cardiovascular, 6 Anaphylactic shock, 13

(Continued)

Table 2 Continued

Author	Gender	Age (yr)	Medical disease	Allergen	Status of IT	Onset of symptoms	Symptoms	Cause of death
							Shock, 4 Coma, 9 Hypotension, 6 Myocardial infarction, 1 NA or Unknown, 6	Others, 4 NA or Unknown, 3
Reid, Lockey, et al., 1989	F, 11 M, 5 Unknown, 1	10–77 x,36	Asthma, 13 AR, 7 CV, 3 DM, 1 HtD, 1 Unknown, 1	Aqueous, 14 Unknown, 2	Maintenance, 3 Increasing, 9 Decreasing, 1 Unknown, 3	<20 min, 8 20–30 min, 3 >30 min, 1[f] Unknown, 4	Urticaria and angioedema, 1 L airway ob, 5 U&L airway ob, 4 U airway ob, 1 Shock, 4 Unknown, 5	Resp, 8 Shock, 0 Both, 4 Other, 1 Unknown, 3
Reid et al., 1995	Unknown	12–73	Asthma, 19	Unknown	Unknown	Unknown	Unknown	Unknown
Lüderitz-Puchel et al., 1996	Unknown, 40 28 analyzed	Unknown	Aqueous, 6 Semidepot, 22	Unknown	Unknown	Unknown	Anaphylactic shock, 7 Unknown, 21	Unknown

[a] Autopsy confirmed.
[b] Not in article. Listed only as Pollinex, pollen vaccine; Migen, house dust-mite vaccine.
[c] Bencard Allergy Unit, Brentford, Middlesex, United Kingdom.
[d] ? meaning of normal course.
[e] Not requested.
[f] Not witnessed.

AR, allergic rhinitis; CV, cardiovasular; DM, diabetes mellitus; HtD, heart disease; NA, not available.
Source: Adapted from Ref. 81.

The Committee on the Safety of Medicine of the United Kingdom reported in 1986 that 26 deaths from anaphylaxis due to allergen immunotherapy had occurred in the United Kingdom since 1957. All died from immunotherapy-induced bronchospasm and/or anaphylaxis, 11 of these since 1980 and 5 during the preceding 18 months. In most of the cases, adequate facilities for cardiorespiratory resuscitation were not available. Asthma was the indication for treatment in 16 of the 26, allergic rhinitis in 1, and the indicator was unknown in 9. In 2 patients, the ultimately fatal systemic reaction allegedly began more than 30 min after injection, resulting in a recommendation that patients remain in a medical facility for 2 h after injection (51).

In Sweden, introduction of potent mite, mold, and animal dander vaccines was accompanied by some anaphylactic deaths that prompted the regulatory agency to restrict the use of these vaccines to physicians and clinics specializing in this area (85).

The Paul Ehrlich Institute in Germany reported 40 fatalities between 1977 and 1994, with complete data available for 20 reports in Germany and 8 reports elsewhere in Europe. For 23 of the 28 reports analyzed, it was not possible to rule out error on the part of the physician and/or inadequate information given to the patient as factors contributory to the fatal outcome (52). Three cases with permanent hypoxic brain damage as a result of anaphylactic shock were also reported. Semidepot preparations, which are not used in the United States, were involved in most of the adverse and fatal reactions. Mite allergen vaccines were used in 18 of the cases reported.

VI. FATALITIES ASSOCIATED WITH SKIN TESTING AND IMMUNOTHERAPY IN THE 1980S AND 1990S

The study by Van Arsdel and Sherman (1) supports the general safety of immunotherapy for the control of IgE-mediated allergic diseases in that over 1 million allergen vaccine injections given to 8700 patients from 1935 to 1955 had been administered without a fatality. The prospective study by Hepner et al. on immunotherapy reported in 1987 that 25 out of 2989 patients, over a 7-month period, experienced systemic reactions and there were no fatalities (11). Based on annual studies from a panel of 2000 physicians in the United States, the National Disease and Therapeutic Index indicated that in each of the 5 previous years, 7 to 10 million allergen injections had been given (86). Since so many injections are administered yearly, the risk of a fatal reaction is low. Lockey et al. reported that 45 (1.4%) of 3236 patients who had a clinical history of Hymenoptera hypersensitivity and were skin tested had systemic hypersensitivity reactions during skin testing, and 8 of these (0.25% of the subjects tested) were severe (87). Of 1410 patients placed on immunotherapy, 171 experienced 327 systemic reactions, of which 28 reactions (9%) were severe but not fatal (88). These studies illustrate that immunotherapy with a standardized vaccine, used as indicated in individuals with an allergic disease that may be life threatening, induces a low incidence of adverse reactions, most of which are mild to moderate.

A review by Stewart and Lockey (89) in 1992, which examined the incidence of systemic reactions to immunotherapy, concluded that the percentage of subjects experiencing a systemic reaction from immunotherapy is small but will probably increase as the immunotherapy schedule is accelerated and when or if high-dose regimens are required in highly sensitive subjects. In addition, maintenance immunotherapy is associated with fewer systemic reactions than the build-up period of rush and accelerated schedules of immunotherapy.

Premedication with a combination of methylprednisolone, ketotifen (a mast cell stabilizer not available in the United States), and long-acting theophylline may decrease the incidence of systemic reactions associated with rush protocols, although such studies have not been done with conventional protocols. Concern was voiced over masking a mild reaction by using premedication, which might therefore be followed by a later, more serious reaction or delay the onset of a reaction beyond the waiting period. In other studies, however, premedication with antihistamines significantly reduced the incidence of systemic reactions during rush immunotherapy or specific cluster immunotherapy (90–92). There was no evidence that antihistamines masked the early warning signs or delayed the onset of systemic reactions. Further studies involving larger groups of patients and different dosage regimens are necessary to define the future role of antihistamine and other pharmacological pretreatment in immunotherapy. Finally, a 20–30-min waiting period, as recommended by the AAAAI and ACAAI's "Allergen Immunotherapy: A Practice Parameter," was deemed appropriate, with a longer waiting period for high-risk patients (22).

VII.   RISK FACTORS FOR SKIN TESTING AND IMMUNOTHERAPY

It is essential that strict attention be paid to risk factors for systemic reactions and that techniques of management be initiated both before and after skin testing or immunotherapy to minimize these risks. Several guidelines have been suggested that emphasize thorough training of all personnel involved in these procedures as well as the prompt treatment of systemic reactions (81,85). These have encouraged the development and use of standardized vaccines and emphasize certain risk factors, including

1. Patients, particularly asthmatics, suffering a seasonal exacerbation of their symptoms
2. Patients who demonstrate exquisite sensitivity to particular allergen(s)
3. Patients on beta-blockers (93)
4. Patients with asthma, especially when their asthma is unstable
5. Patients in whom rush immunotherapy is used (both venoms and inhalant allergens) (89,90,92)
6. Patients in whom high doses of potent standardized allergen vaccines are utilized

VIII.   PRECAUTIONS FOR SKIN TESTING AND IMMUNOTHERAPY

The following guidelines are suggested:

1. Always begin with a percutaneous procedure for skin testing (i.e., prick puncture).
2. When possible, do not use β-adrenergic blocking agents concomitantly during skin testing or immunotherapy.
3. Keep patients under observation for 20 to 30 minutes, or even longer for those at greatest risk, since most fatal systemic reactions begin within that time (22).
4. When immunotherapy is prescribed, give the patient written and/or verbal guidelines outlining methods of immunotherapy and the importance of adherence to these guidelines to prevent an adverse reaction (see Chapter 41).

5. Inform patients receiving immunotherapy of its potential risk and obtain informed consent.
6. Administer immunotherapy in an office or clinical setting with a physician present and with optimal care available for the treatment of a systemic reaction.
7. Monitor patients to ensure that they are waiting the proper time in the facility where they receive their immunotherapy.
8. Provide adequate instructions to another physician who may give the injections elsewhere from vials of vaccine taken from the prescribing physician's office or clinic (see Chapter 25).

The safety of allergen immunotherapy has been reviewed in detail by Norman and Van Metre (94).

IX. EQUIPMENT RECOMMENDED FOR SETTINGS WHERE ALLERGEN IMMUNOTHERAPY IS ADMINISTERED

The following equipment is recommended by the Joint Task Force on Practice Parameters (22):

1. Stethoscope and sphygmomanometer
2. Tourniquets, syringes, hypodermic needles, large-bore needles (14 gauge)
3. Aqueous epinephrine HCl 1:1000
4. Equipment for administering oxygen
5. Equipment for administering intravenous fluids
6. Oral airway
7. Antihistamines for injection
8. Corticosteroids for intravenous injection
9. Vasopressor (dopamine hydrochloride)

The prompt recognition of systemic reactions and the immediate use of epinephrine are the mainstays of therapy (95–97).

X. SALIENT POINTS

1. Physicians who administer allergen immunotherapy should have the appropriate equipment and personnel to treat a systemic reaction.
2. No allergen vaccine can be considered completely safe for a given patient allergic to that vaccine.
3. The risk of a fatal reaction can be reduced and even eliminated by the careful selection and monitoring of allergic patients on immunotherapy, by using improved, biologically standardized vaccines, and by skilled and timely treatment of systemic reactions.
4. A wait period of 20 to 30 minutes is adequate for most patients, but should be extended for high-risk patients.
5. Patients at highest risk for allergen immunotherapy are those with asthma, especially unstable asthma.
6. Other high-risk patients include those with a seasonal exacerbation and exquisite sensitivity, and those on beta-blockers and rush schedules.

REFERENCES

1. Van Arsdel PP, Sherman W. The risk of inducing constitutional reactions in allergic patients. J Allergy 1957; 28:251.
2. Cooke RA, Vanderveer A Jr. Human sensitization. J Immunol 1916; 1:201.
3. Turkeltaub PC, Gergen PJ. The risk of adverse reactions from percutaneous prick puncture allergen skin testing, venipuncture, and body measurements: Data from the second National Health and Nutrition Examination Survey 1976–80 (NHANES II). J Allergy Clin Immunol 1989; 84:886.
4. Levine MI. Systemic reactions to immunotherapy. J Allergy Clin Immunol 1979; 63:209.
5. Rawlins MD, Wood S. Hazards with desensitizing vaccines. In: Arbeiten aus dem Paul-Ehrlich-Institut (Bulzdcsamt fur Scra uizd Impfstoffe). Stuttgart: Band 82 Gustav Fischer Verlag, 1988: 147.
6. Rieckenberg MR, Khan RH, Day IH. Physician reported patient response to immunotherapy: A retrospective study of factors affecting the response. Ann Allergy 1990; 64:364.
7. Vervloet D, Khairallah E, Amaud A, Charpin J. A prospective national study of the safety of immunotherapy. Clin Allergy 1980; 10:59.
8. Osterballe O. Side effects during immunotherapy with purified grass pollen extracts. Allergy 1982; 37:553.
9. Nelson BL, Dupont LA, Reid MJ. Prospective survey of local and systemic reactions to immunotherapy with pollen extracts. Ann Allergy 1986; 56:331.
10. Greenberg MA, Gonzalez GE, Rosenblatt CD, Sununers RJ. Late and immediate systemic-allergic reactions to inhalant allergen immunotherapy. J Allergy Clin Immunol 1986; 77:865.
11. Hepner M, Ownby D, MacKechnie H, Rowe M, Anderson J. The safety of immunotherapy: A prospective study. J Allergy Clin Immunol 1987; 79:133.
12. Hejjaoui A, Dhivert H, Michel FB, Bousquet J. Immunotherapy with a standardized *Dermatophagoides pteronyssinus* extract. J Allergy Clin Immunol 1990; 85:473.
13. Tankersley MS, Butler KK, Butler WK, Goetz DW. Local reactions during allergen immunotherapy do not require dose adjustment. J Allergy Clin Immunol 2000; 106:840–843.
14. Mellerup MT, Hahn GW, Poulsen LK, and Malling H. Safety of allergen-specific immunotherapy: Relation between dosage regimen, allergen extract, disease and systemic side-effects during induction treatment. Clin Exp Allergy 2000; 30:1423–1429.
15. Malling HJ. Minimizing the risks of allergen-specific injection immunotherapy. Drug Saf 2000; 23:323–332.
16. Akcakaya N, Hassanzadeh A, Camcioglu Y, Cokugras H. Local and systemic reactions during immunotherapy with adsorbed extracts of house dust mite in children. Ann Allergy Asthma Immunol 2000; 85:317–321.
17. Karaayvaz M, Erel F, Caliskaner Z, Ozanguc N. Systemic reactions due to allergen immunotherapy. J Investig Allergol Clin Immunol 1999; 9:39–44.
18. Lockey RF, Nicoara-Kasti GL, Theodoropoulos DS, Bukantz SC. Systemic reactions and fatalities associated with allergen immunotherapy. Ann Allergy Asthma Immunol 2001; 87:47–55.
19. Brockow K, Kiehn M, Riethmuller C, Vieluf D, Berger J, Ring J. Efficacy of antihistamine pretreatment in the prevention of adverse reactions to Hymenoptera immunotherapy: A prospective, randomized, placebo-controlled trial. J Allergy Clin Immunol 1997; 100:458–463.
20. Machin IS, Robaina JCG, Bonnet C, de Blas C, Fernandez-Caldas E, Trivino MS, de la Morin FT. Immunotherapy units: A follow-up study. J Investig Allergol Clin Immunol 2001; 11:167–171, 2001.
21. Nettis E, Giordano D, Pannofino A, Ferrannini A, Tursi A. Safety of inhalant allergen immunotherapy with mass units–standardized extracts. Clin Exp Allergy 2002; 32(12):1745–1749.
22. Li JT, Lockey RF, Bernstein IL, et al. (eds.). Joint Task Force on Practice Parameters. Allergen immunotherapy: A practice parameter. American Academy of Allergy, Asthma and

Immunology. American College of Allergy, Asthma and Immunology. Ann Allergy Asthma Immunol 2003; 90(suppl 1):1–40.

23. Wuthrich B, Gumowski PL, Fah J, Hurlimann A, Deluze C, Andre C, Fadel R, Carat F. Safety and efficacy of specific immunotherapy with standardized allergenic extracts adsorbed on aluminium hydroxide. J Investig Allergol Clin Immunol 2001; 11:149–156.

24. Winther L, Malling HJ, Mosbech H. Allergen-specific immunotherapy in birch- and grass-pollen-allergic rhinitis: II. Side-effects. Allergy 2000; 55:827–835.

25. Bhalla PL. Genetic engineering of pollen allergens for hayfever immunotherapy. Expert Rev Vaccines 2003; 2(1):75–84.

26. Chen D, Maa YF, Haynes JR. Needle-free epidermal powder immunization. Expert Rev Vaccines 2002; 1(3):265–276.

27. Spiegelberg HL, Takabayashi K, Beck L, Raz E. DNA-based vaccines for allergic disease. Expert Rev Vaccines 2002; 1(2):169–177.

28. Tella R, Bartra J, San Miguel M, Olona M, Bosque M, Gaig P, Garcia-Ortega P. Effects of specific immunotherapy on the development of new sensitizations in monosensitized patients. Allergol Immunopathol (Madr) 2003; 31(4):221–225.

29. Holt PG, Rowe J, Loh R, Sly PD. Developmental factors associated with risk for atopic disease: Implications for vaccine strategies in early childhood. Vaccine 2003; 21(24):3432–3435.

30. Koh YY, Kim CK. The development of asthma in patients with allergic rhinitis. Curr Opin Allergy Clin Immunol 2003; 3(3):159–164.

31. Tarzi M, Larche M. Peptide immunotherapy for allergic disease. Expert Opin Biiol Ther 2003; 3(4):617–626.

32. Reyes Moreno A, Castrejon Vazquez MI, Miranda Feria AJ. [Failure of allergen-based immunotherapy in adults with allergic asthma]. Rev Alerg Mex 2003; 50(1):8–12.

33. Di Gioacchino M, Cavallucci E, Di Sciascio MB, Di Stefano F, Verna N, Raimondo S, Lobefalo L, Conti P, Cuccurullo F. Allergen immunotherapy: An effective immune-modifier. Int J Immunopathol Pharmacol 1999; 12(1):1–5.

34. Litwin A, Flanagan M, Entis G, Gottschlich G, Esch R, Gartside P, Michael JG. Oral immunotherapy with short ragweed extract in a novel encapsulated preparation: A double-blind study. J Allergy Clin Immunol 1997; 100:30–38.

35. Molina AC, Pasadas, FG, Munoz JC, Munoz DJC, Aguilar CM, Llamas AE, Gomariz EM, Ugalde EF, Diaz AC, Cardenas GM, Guigo SP. Immunotherapy with an oral *Alternaria* extract in childhood asthma: Clinical safety and efficacy and effects on in vivo and in vitro parameters. Allergol Immunopathol 2002; 30:319–330.

36. Passali D, Bellussi L, Passali GC, and Passali FM. Nasal immunotherapy is effective in the treatment of rhinitis due to mite allergy: A double-blind, placebo-controlled study with rhinological evaluation. Int J Immunopathol Pharmacol 2002; 15:141–147.

37. Liu YH, Kao MC, Lai YL, Tsai JJ. Efficacy of local nasal immunotherapy for Dp2-induced airway inflammation in mice: Using Dp2 peptide and fungal immunomodulatory peptide. J Allergy Clin Immunol 2003; 112(2):301–310.

38. Andre C, Perrin-Fayolle M, Grosclaude M, Couturier P, Basset D, Cornillon J, Piperno D, Girodet B, Sanchez R, Vallon C, Bellier P, Nasr M. A double-blind placebo-controlled evaluation of sublingual immunotherapy with a standardized ragweed extract in patients with seasonal rhinitis: Evidence for a dose-response relationship. Int Arch Allergy Immunol 2003; 131:111–118.

39. Cirla AM, Cirla PE, Parmiani S, Pecora S. A pre-seasonal birch/hazel sublingual immunotherapy can improve the outcome of grass pollen injective treatment in bisensitized individuals: A case-referent, two-year controlled study. Allergol Immunopathol 2002; 30: 319–330.

40. Passalacqua G, Baena-Cagnani CE, Berardi M, Canonica GW. Oral and sublingual immunotherapy in paediatric patients. Curr Opin Allergy Clin Immunol 2003; 3:139–145.

41. Grosclaude M, Bouillot P, Alt R, Leynadier F, Scheinmann P, Rufin P, Basset D, Fadel R, Andre C. Safety of various dosage regimens during induction of sublingual immunotherapy: A preliminary study. Int Arch Allergy Immunol 2002; 129:248–253.

42. Di Rienzo V, Marcucci F, Puccinelli P, Parmiani S, Frati F, Sensi L, Canonica GW, Passalacqua G. Long-lasting effect of sublingual immunotherapy in children with asthma due to house dust mite: A 10-year prospective study. Clin Exp Allergy 2003; 33:206–210.

43. Horner AA, Van Uden JH, Zubeldia JM, Broide D, Raz E. DNA-based immunotherapeutics for the treatment of allergic disease. Immunol Rev 2001; 179:102–118.

44. Lamson RW. Sudden death associated with injection of foreign substances. J Am Med Assoc 1924; 82:1090.

45. Vance BM, Strassman G. Sudden death following injection of foreign protein. Arch Pathol 1942; 34:849.

46. James LP, Austen KF. Fatal systemic anaphylaxis in man. N Engl J Med 1964; 270:597.

47. Sheppe WM. Fatal anaphylaxis in man. J Lab Clin Med 1930; 16:372.

48. Blanton WV, Sutphin AK. Death during skin testing. Am J Med Sci 1949; 217:169.

49. Rosenthal A. Fatal anaphylactic reactions to penicillin. NY State J Med 1954; 54:1485.

50. Rands DA. Anaphylactic reaction to desensitization for allergic rhinitis and asthma. Br Med J 1980; 281:854.

51. Committee on Safety of Medicines. CSM Update: Desensitization vaccines. Br Med J 1986; 293:948.

52. Lüderitz-Puchel U, May S, Haustein D. Incidents following hyposensitization. Münch Med Wschr 1996; 138:1–7.

53. Busse WW, Storms WW, Flaherty DK, Crandall M, Reed CE. *Alternaria* IgG precipitins and adverse reactions. J Allergy Clin Immunol 1976; 57:367.

54. Kaad PH, Ostergaard PA. The hazard of mould hyposensitization in children with asthma. Clin Allergy 1982; 12:317.

55. Kemler BJ, Franklin WD, Alpert E, Bloch KJ. Failure to detect circulating immune complexes in allergic patients on injection therapy. Clin Allergy 1979; 9:473.

56. Stein MR, Brown GL, Lima JE, Carr RI. A laboratory evaluation of immune complexes in patients on inhalant immunotherapy. J Allergy Clin Immunol 1978; 62:211.

57. Stendardi L, Delespesse G, Debisschop MJ. Circulating immune-complexes in bronchial asthma. Clin Allergy 1980; 10:405.

58. Cano PO, Chow M, Jerry LM, Sladowski JP. Circulating immune-complexes in patients with atopic allergy. Clin Allergy 1977; 7:167.

59. El-Hefny A, Ekladious EM, El-Sharkawy S, El-Ghadban H, El-Heneidy F, Franklin AW. Extrinsic allergic bronchiole-alveolitis in children. Clin Allergy 1980; 10:651.

60. Moore VL, Fink IN. Immunologic studies in hypersensitivity pneumonitis-quantitative precipitins and complement-fixing antibodies in symptomatic and asymptomatic pigeon-breeders. J Lab Clin Med 1975; 85:540.

61. Kuuliala O, Palosuo T, Aho K, Jarvinen AJ. Haemagglutinating antibodies to cat dander in relation to exposure and respiratory allergy. Clin Allergy 1979; 9:391.

62. Clausen RW, Yanari SS, Immune complex–mediated disease not a factor in patients on maintenance venom immunotherapy. J Allergy Clin Immunol 1983; 72:199–203.

63. Umetsu DT, Hahn JS, Perez-Atayde AR, Geha RS. Serum sickness triggered by anaphylaxis: A complication of immunotherapy. J Allergy Clin Immunol 1985; 76:713.

64. Clemmensen O, Knudsen HE. Contact sensitivity to aluminum in a patient hyposensitized with aluminum precipitated grass pollen. Contact Derm 1979; 6:305.

65. Wolpow ER. Brachial plexus neuropathy. J Am Med Assoc 1975; 234:620.

66. Schatz M, Patterson R, DeSwarte R. Nonorganic adverse reactions to aeroallergen immunotherapy. J Allergy Clin Immunol 1976; 58:198.

67. Bokisch VA, Bernstein D, Krause RM. Occurrence of 19S and 7S anti-IgG's during hyperimmunization of rabbit with streptococci. J Exp Med 1972; 136:799.

68. Eichmann K, Braun DG, Krause RM. Influence of genetic factors on the magnitude and the heterogeneity of the immune response in the rabbit. J Exp Med 1971; 134:48.

69. Christian CI, DeSimone AR, Abruzzo JL. Anti-DNA antibodies in hyperimmunized rabbits. J Exp Med 1965; 121:309.

70. Abruzzo n, Gross AF, Christian CL. Studies on experimental amyloidosis. Br J Exp Pathol 966; 47:52.

71. Potter M. Myeloma proteins (M-components) with antibody-like activity. N Engl J Med 1971; 284:8831.

72. Penny R, Hughes S. Repeated stimulation of the reticuloendothelial system and the development of plasma-cell dyscrasias. Lancet 1970; 1:77.

73. Raphael SA, Nell PA, Hymchuk IM, Lischner HW. Positive late antiglobulin test in atopic pediatric subjects receiving hyposensitization therapy. J Allergy Clin Immunol 1976; 57:103.

74. Levinson AI, Summers RJ, Lawley TJ, Evans R, Frank MM. Evaluation of the adverse effects of long-term hyposensitization. J Allergy Clin Immunol 1978; 62:109.

75. Phanuphak P, Kohler PF. Onset of polyarteritis nodosa during allergic hyposensitization treatment. Am J Med 1980; 68:479.

76. McCombs CC, Michalski JP, Jerome DC. Case 26-1980: Pemphigus vulgaris after hyposensitization injections. N Engl J Med 1980; 303:1179.

77. Katelaris CH, Walls RS. A study of possible ill effects from prolonged immunotherapy in treatment of allergic diseases. Ann Allergy 1984; 53:257.

78. Waldbott GL. The prevention of anaphylactic shock. J Am Med Assoc 1932; 98:446.

79. Vaughan VA, Black JR. Practice of Allergy. St. Louis: C.V. Mosby, 1939.

80. Pollard RCH. Anaphylactic reaction to desensitization. Br Med J 1980; 281:1429.

81. Lockey RF, Benedict LM, Turkeltaub PC, Bukantz SC. Fatalities from immunotherapy (IT) and skin testing (ST). J Allergy Clin Immunol 1987; 79:660.

82. Reid MJ, Lockey RF, Turkeltaub PC, Platts-Mills TAB. Fatalities (F) from immunotherapy (IT) and skin testing (ST). J Allergy Clin Immunol 1990; 85:180.

83. Reid M, Lockey RF, Turkeltaub PC, Platts-Mills TAE. Survey of fatalities from skin testing and immunotherapy 1985–1989. J Allergy Clin Immunol 1993; 92:6–15.

84. Reid M, Gurka G. Deaths associated with skin testing and immunotherapy. J Allergy Clin Immunol 1996; 97:231.

85. Norman PS. Fatal misadventures. J Allergy Clin Immunol 1987; 79:572.

86. National Disease and Therapeutic Index. Ambler: IMS America, Ltd.

87. Lockey RF, Turkeltaub PC, Olive CA, Baird-Warren LA, Olive ES, Bukantz SC. The Hymenoptera venom study II: Skin test results and safety of venom skin testing. J Allergy Clin Immunol 1989; 84:967.

88. Lockey RF, Turkeltaub PC, Olive ES, Hubbard JM, Baird-Warren IA, Bukantz SC. The Hymenoptera venom study III: Safety of venom immunotherapy. J Allergy Clin Immunol 1990; 86:775.

89. Stewart E, Lockey FR. Systemic reactions from allergen immunotherapy. J Allergy Clin Immunol 1992:567–578.

90. Portnoy J, Bagstad K, Kanarek H, Pacheco F, Hall B, Barnes C. Premedication reduces the incidence of systemic reactions during inhalant rush immunotherapy with mixtures of allergenic extracts. Ann Allergy 1994; 73:409–418.

91. Nielsen L, Johnsen CR, Mosbech H, Poulsen LK, Malling HJ. Antihistamine premedication in specific cluster immunotherapy: A double-blind, placebo-controlled study. J Allergy Clin Immunol 1996; 97:1207–1213.

92. Berchtold E, Maibach R, Muller U. Reduction of side effects from rush-immunotherapy with honey bee venom by pretreatment with terfenadine. Clin Exp Allergy 1992; 22:59–65.

93. Kaplan AP, Anderson JA, Valentine MD, Lockey RF, Pierson WE, Zweiman B, Kaliner MA, Lichtenstein LM, Settipane GA, Sheffer AL, Yunginger JW. Position statement: Beta-adrenergic blockers, immunotherapy, and skin testing. J Allergy Clin Immunol 1989; 55:129.

94. Norman PS, Van Metre TE. The safety of allergenic immunotherapy. J Allergy Clin Immunol 1990; 85:522.

95. Executive Committee, American Academy of Allergy, Asthma and Immunology. Position statement: Personnel and equipment to treat systemic reactions caused by immunotherapy with allergenic extracts. J Allergy Clin Immunol 1986; 77:271–273.

96. Bousquet J, Lockey RF, Malling H-J. WHO position paper. Allergen immunotherapy: Therapeutic vaccines for allergic disease. Allergy 1998; 53S:1–42.

97. Kemp SF, Lockey RF. Anaphylaxis: A review of causes and mechanisms. J Allergy Clin Immunol 2002; 110:341–348.

40

Prevention and Treatment of Anaphylaxis

STEPHEN F. KEMP and RICHARD D. DESHAZO

University of Mississippi Medical Center, Jackson, Mississippi, U.S.A.

I. INTRODUCTION

Anaphylaxis is not a reportable disease, and both its morbidity and its mortality are probably underestimated. A variety of statistics on the epidemiology of anaphylaxis have been published (1–10) (Table 1). There is no universally accepted clinical definition of anaphylaxis (11,12). In this discussion, anaphylaxis is defined as an acute life-threatening reaction, usually, but not always, mediated by an immunological mechanism (*anaphylactoid* reactions are thought to be IgE independent), that results from the sudden systemic release of mediators from mast cells and basophils. It has varied clinical presentations that consist of some or all of the following signs and symptoms: pruritus, flushing, urticaria and/or angioedema, bronchospasm, dysphonia, laryngeal edema, hyperperistalsis, hypotension, and/or cardiac arrhythmias. Other symptoms can occur, such as dysphagia, nausea, vomiting, rhinitis, lightheadedness, headache, feeling of impending doom, and unconsciousness.

Generalized urticaria and angioedema are the most common manifestations of anaphylaxis [772 of 835 (92%) subjects in retrospective series] (13–15) and occur as the initial signs and symptoms or are associated with severe anaphylaxis (16). However,

Table 1 Epidemiology of Anaphylaxis

Statistic	Value	Reference
Incidence	30/100,000 person-years	1
Risk/person in U.S.	1–3%/person	1,2
	1.24–16.74%	3
Risk in hospitalized patients	1/2700	4
Hospital fatalities	$154/10^6$ patients	5
Mortality rate	1%	2
Food anaphylaxis fatalities	150/yr	6
Peanuts or tree nuts	94% fatalities in registry	7
Fatal reactions to β-lactam antibiotics	400–800/yr	4
Fatalities from allergen immunotherapy	1/2,000,000 injections	8
Systemic reactions to Hymenoptera stings	0.4–4%	9
Prevalence of idiopathic anaphylaxis	34,000 subjects	10

cutaneous manifestations may be delayed or absent in rapidly progressive anaphylaxis. Respiratory symptoms are the next most common manifestations, followed by dizziness, unconsciousness, and gastrointestinal symptoms. The more rapid the onset of the signs and symptoms of anaphylaxis, the more likely the reaction is to be severe and life threatening (17,18). Anaphylaxis often produces signs and symptoms within 5 to 30 minutes, but reactions may not develop for several hours.

A. Immunotherapy and Anaphylaxis

Three surveys reported that fatalities from allergen immunotherapy occur at a rate of approximately 1 per 2,000,000 injections administered by allergists (surveys included only members of the American Academy of Allergy, Asthma and Immunology) (18–20). The rate of fatalities resulting from immunotherapy by physicians who are not specially trained to practice allergy and immunology remains unknown. The three studies evaluated 63 fatalities from immunotherapy or skin testing between 1945 and 1995. Most of the fatalities occurred when reactions took place within 20 minutes of the injection. Subjects with symptomatic asthma or with high levels of allergen-specific IgE (as indicated by skin testing or RAST) were more likely to die from anaphylaxis. Subjects who were symptomatic, especially with asthma, at the time of the injection or who were in their "allergy season" were also at increased risk. Occasional errors in vial selection, especially in advancing to a higher concentration of allergen, and mistakes in dosage or administration were important causes of preventable anaphylaxis and subsequent fatality in both surveys.

Lüderitz-Püchel, May, and Haustein analyzed 28 of 48 immunotherapy-related fatalities reported from Germany and other countries between 1977 and 1994 (21) and 3 additional subjects who experienced hypoxic brain injury following anaphylaxis. In 23 of the 28 fatalities, the authors could not exclude medical error and/or inadequate information provided to the subjects as contributory factors to fatal anaphylaxis. Common errors included mistakes in dosage and administration of allergen vaccines and failure to adhere to the recommended 30-minute period of observation following injection.

Stewart and Lockey (22) reviewed 38 studies in which systemic reactions were associated with immunotherapy. One or more systemic reactions occurred in 0.8% to 46.7% of subjects on conventional dose schedules (mean 12.92%, SD 10.8%). Systemic reactions per injection during build-up occurred in 0.05% to 3.2% of subjects (mean 0.5%, SD 0.87%). All but one study reported rates per injection of 0.6% or less. The 23 studies in which rush or accelerated schedules were used were also reviewed. The percentage of subjects experiencing one or more systemic reactions during the maintenance phase of immunotherapy ranged from 0% to 21.1% (mean 4.77%, SD 6.47%). However, the number of systemic reactions was higher during build-up when the interval between injections was reduced ("rush" or "semi-rush" protocols). Subjects experiencing one or more systemic reactions ranged from 0% to 66.7% with these accelerated schedules (mean 21.33%, SD 17.86%). These protocols were associated with rates of systemic reactions per injection ranging from 0% to 6.4% (mean 2.36%, SD 1.7%).

B. Chemical Mediators of Anaphylaxis

The chemical mediators that are associated with anaphylaxis are preformed and released from granules (histamine, tryptase, glycosidases, and granulocyte chemotactic factors) or are generated from membrane lipids (prostaglandin D_2, leukotrienes, and platelet activating factor) by the activated mast cell or basophil (23). The immunologically induced ("anaphylactic") release of mediators results from the interaction of specific IgE antibody with the responsible allergen. Nonimmunological triggers, such as radiocontrast media, directly activate the mast cell and/or basophil via IgE-independent ("anaphylactoid") mechanisms.

Histamine is only one of the mast cell mediators released in anaphylaxis, but its systemic effects have been studied more than those of any other mediator. Kaliner et al. infused histamine into normal volunteers at doses ranging from 0.05 to 1.0 µg/kg/min over 30 minutes to determine the plasma levels required to elicit symptoms of anaphylaxis (24). A mean plasma level of 1.61 ± 0.30 ng/ml induced a 30% increase in heart rate, a level of 2.39 ± 0.52 ng/ml induced flushing and headaches, and a level of 2.45 ± 0.13 ng/ml induced a 30% increase in pulse pressure. Pretreatment with an H_2 antagonist (cimetidine) did not alter these reactions. However, pretreatment with the H_1 antagonist hydroxyzine increased the level of histamine necessary to increase the heart rate by 30%. Combining the two antihistamines significantly raised the level at which histamine elicited all responses. On the basis of these results, the authors concluded that flushing, hypotension, and headache associated with histamine infusion are mediated by both H_1 and H_2 receptors, whereas tachycardia, pruritus, rhinorrhea, and bronchospasm are associated only with H_1 receptors.

H_3 receptors have been implicated in a canine model of anaphylaxis (25). These inhibitory presynaptic receptors modulate endogenous release of norepinephrine from sympathetic fibers that innervate the cardiovascular system. Pretreatment of study animals with thioperamide maleate, an H_3 receptor antagonist, was associated with higher heart rate and greater left ventricular systolic function compared to a non-treatment group or the other treatment arms involving receptor blockade for H_1, H_2, cyclooxygenase, and leukotriene pathways (25). Potential implications for human subjects have not been studied.

Histamine levels correlate with the severity and persistence of cardiopulmonary manifestations, but they do not correlate with the development of urticaria during anaphylaxis (26,27). Gastrointestinal signs and symptoms in anaphylaxis also have a greater association with histamine than with tryptase elevations (26).

Tryptase is the only protein known to be concentrated selectively in the secretory granules of all human mast cells and is released when these cells degranulate. Its plasma levels during mast cell degranulation correlate with the clinical severity of anaphylaxis (28). Since β-tryptase is stored in the secretory granules, its release may be more specific for mast cell activation than α-protryptase, which appears to be secreted constitutively (29).

Postmortem measurements of serum tryptase may be useful in establishing anaphylaxis as the cause of death in subjects experiencing sudden death of uncertain cause (30–33), and serum for postmortem tryptase levels should be obtained within 15 hours of death to exclude nonspecific elevations (31). Elevated postmortem tryptase levels have been reported in 12% of otherwise healthy adults who died suddenly and in at least 40% of victims of sudden infant death syndrome (32,34,35). Causation, however, is challenged by one report that found 40% of infants with SIDS had tryptase elevations, but only those in the prone position at death (36). Buckley et al. observed that 5 of 32 cases (16%) had abnormally high tryptase levels, reflecting elevated β-tryptase (anaphylaxis specific) but no elevated α-tryptase levels (37).

Histamine can stimulate endothelial cells to produce nitric oxide (NO), an autacoid formerly known as endothelium-derived relaxing factor (38). NO is synthesized from the amino acid L-arginine by a family of enzymes known as nitric oxide synthetases. NO is a potent vasodilator when it is released from vascular endothelial cells and it relaxes all kinds of smooth muscle. Physiologically, NO participates in the homeostatic control of vascular tone and regional blood pressure. NO is also involved in the regulation of various gastrointestinal, respiratory, and genitourinary tract functions that are beyond the scope of this review (39).

NO appears to be involved in a complex interaction of regulatory and counter-regulatory mediators in mast cell activation, including anaphylaxis (40). L-arginine is converted to NO as histamine binds to H_1 receptors during phospholipase-C–dependent calcium mobilization. NO activates guanylate cyclase, leading to the production of cyclic GMP and vasodilation. Enhanced formation of NO due to activation of endothelial cell NO synthase decreases venous return, contributing to the vasodilation that occurs with anaphylaxis. However, in vivo studies with mice, rabbits, and dogs have demonstrated that NO inhibitors cause myocardial depression by facilitating histamine release, production of cysteinyl leukotrienes, and coronary vasoconstriction. NO inhibitors also promote bronchospasm during anaphylaxis. These findings suggest that NO may decrease the signs and symptoms of anaphylaxis, except those associated with vasodilation (39).

Metabolites of arachidonic acid include products of lipoxygenase and cyclooxygenase pathways. Of note, leukotriene B_4 is a chemotactic agent and thus can solicit other cells to participate in an anaphylactic or anaphylactoid event. These cells theoretically may contribute to the late phase of anaphylaxis and to protracted reactions. Other effects of arachidonic acid metabolites may reflect mast cell degranulation since elevations in tryptase and histamine occur. These effects include bronchospasm, hypotension, and erythema (41).

Inflammatory mediators activate the contact (kallikrein-kinin) system. Release of kininogenase, kallikrein, and tryptase may induce formation of bradykinin as well as the activation of factor XII. This, in turn, may produce clotting, clot lysis, and subsequent activation of complement. In contrast, some mediators may have a salubrious affect that limits the anaphylactic or anaphylactoid episode. For example, chymase may activate angiotensin II, which can modulate hypotension. Heparin inhibits clotting, kallikrein, and plasmin. It also opposes complement formation and modulates tryptase activity (41).

There are other inflammatory pathways that participate in anaphylactic episodes. These may be extremely important in the prolongation and amplification of anaphylaxis. Much of the supporting evidence derives from data obtained during experimental insect sting challenges. During severe episodes of anaphylaxis, there is concomitant activation of complement, coagulation pathways, and the contact (kallikrein kinin) system. Decreases in C4 and C3, as well as the formation of C3a, have been observed in anaphylaxis. Coagulation pathway activation may decrease factor V, factor VIII, and fibrinogen levels. Contact system recruitment is indicated by decreased high-molecular-weight kininogen and the formation of kallikrein-C1 inhibitor complexes and factor XIIa–C1 inhibitor complexes. Kallikrein activation not only results in the formation of bradykinin but also activates factor XII. Factor XII in itself can lead to clotting and clot lysis via plasmin formation. Plasmin can also activate complement (41).

C. The Heart in Anaphylaxis

Reports have focused on the effects of anaphylaxis on cardiac function, as refractory shock associated with anaphylaxis suggests that the mediators of anaphylaxis directly affect the myocardium (27,42) Histamine exerts its pathophysiological effects via both H_1 and H_2 receptors. H_1 receptors mediate coronary artery vasoconstriction and increased vascular permeability. H_2 receptors mediate atrial and ventricular inotropy, atrial chronotropy, and coronary artery vasodilation. The interaction of H_1 and H_2 receptor stimulation appears to mediate increased pulse pressure and decreased diastolic pressure (43). Platelet activating factor (PAF) also produces negative inotropic effects on the heart, decreases coronary blood flow, and delays atrioventricular conduction (44). As discussed earlier, the role of H_3 receptors in anaphylaxis is unknown.

Anaphylaxis has been associated with myocardial ischemia and a variety of electro-cardiographic changes, including atrial and ventricular arrhythmias, conduction defects, and T wave changes (44). However, it is not clear whether such changes are related to direct mediator effects on the myocardium or to preexisting myocardial insufficiency exacerbated by the hemodynamic events that occur with anaphylaxis. This issue was clarified somewhat by a report describing two previously healthy subjects who developed profound anaphylactic shock (42). Hemodynamic measurements, echocardiography, and nuclear imaging techniques established the presence of myocardial dysfunction. Their anaphylaxis was treated medically and with intra-aortic balloon counter-pulsation. Although other clinical signs of anaphylaxis resolved, myocardial dysfunction persisted and balloon counter-pulsation was required for up to 72 hours. Both subjects recovered and subsequently demonstrated no evidence of myocardial dysfunction or underlying heart disease.

Thus, the heart may be the primary target organ in anaphylaxis, even in subjects without preexisting cardiac disease. It is therefore important that the cardiac status of subjects with anaphylaxis and persistent shock be evaluated so that appropriate therapy may be initiated when necessary.

Increased vascular permeability during anaphylaxis can produce a shift of 50% of intravascular fluid to the extravascular space within 10 minutes (45,46). This dramatic shift of effective blood volume causes compensatory catecholamine release and activates the renin-angiotensin-aldosterone system (47–49). These internal compensatory responses produce variable effects during anaphylaxis. Some subjects experience increased peripheral vascular resistance, indicating maximal vasoconstriction (50), while others have depressed systemic vascular resistance, despite elevated catecholamine levels (51).

Mast cells accumulate at sites of coronary plaque erosion and rupture, and they may play a part in thrombotic coronary occlusion (52). Since antibodies attached to mast cells can trigger mast cell degranulation and the release of chemical mediators, it has been suggested that allergic reactions may promote the disruption of plaques (53). Histamine released from mast cells may also facilitate plaque disruption by inducing vasospasm, by increasing arterial pressure and the hemodynamic stress on the plaque, or both (54).

Hemodynamic collapse may occur immediately with no cutaneous or respiratory symptoms (55,56). Of 27 subjects with anaphylaxis in Scandinavia who received prehospital treatment, there were 2 fatalities and 23 hospitalizations. Only 70% of subjects with cardiovascular collapse and/or respiratory failure had cutaneous symptoms, whereas 30% had gastrointestinal manifestations and, interestingly, 85% had neurological deficits (55).

D. Agents That Cause Anaphylaxis or Anaphylactoid Reactions

No evaluation can prove causation of anaphylaxis without directly challenging the subject with the suspected agent. Direct challenge is generally contraindicated due to safety concerns in subjects who have experienced potentially life-threatening anaphylaxis. Cause and effect may often be identified historically in subjects who experience recurrent, objective findings of anaphylaxis upon inadvertent reexposure to the offending agent. Specific diagnostic testing, where appropriate, may confirm the presence of specific IgE and/or mediators produced by the degranulation of mast cells and basophils.

Virtually any agent capable of activating mast cells or basophils may potentially precipitate anaphylactic or anaphylactoid reactions. Table 2 lists common causes of anaphylaxis classified by pathophysiological mechanism. Idiopathic anaphylaxis arguably is the most common cause since this diagnosis accounts for approximately one-third of cases in retrospective studies of anaphylaxis (1,14,57,58). It remains a diagnosis of exclusion, however. Serial histories diagnostic tests for foods, spices, and vegetable gums have occasionally identified the culprit agent in subjects previously presumed to have idiopathic anaphylaxis (41). The most common identifiable causes of anaphylaxis are foods, medications, insect stings, and immunotherapy injections (1,22,41,57) (Figs. 1 and 2). Anaphylaxis to peanuts and/or tree nuts causes the greatest concern because of its life-threatening severity, especially in subjects with asthma, and because of the propensity for life-long allergic sensitivity to these foods. Of added importance, it has been reported that the majority (52%) of peanut-allergic children will experience life-threatening symptoms with subsequent exposure, even if atopic dermatitis has previously been the only adverse clinical manifestation (59). A radioallergosorbent test to quantify the level of food-specific IgE antibodies can be essentially diagnostic; subjects with peanut-specific IgE levels of at least 15 kU/liter have at least a 95% chance of peanut anaphylaxis if they eat peanuts (60).

E. Exercise-Induced Anaphylaxis

Anaphylaxis associated with exercise occurs as two syndromes of physical allergy: exercise-induced anaphylaxis (EIA) and cholinergic urticaria (61). EIA occurs with prolonged strenuous exercise, frequently in conditioned athletes such as marathon runners, and is usually accompanied by a short prodrome of cutaneous warmth and generalized pruritus. It may occur only after certain foods (such as lettuce or celery) or medications (such as aspirin) are ingested prior to exercise. Clinical manifestations may progress to generalized erythema and urticaria, nausea or diarrhea, upper or lower airway obstruction, hypotension, and possibly syncope if exercise continues (15,61). Administration of antihistamines, corticosteroids, or cromolyn prior to exercise does not consistently prevent EIA. Episodes occur sporadically, which distinguishes EIA from other forms of physical urticaria in which exercise provocation invariably produces symptoms (61). Some individuals may demonstrate symptoms

Table 2 Representative Agents That Cause Anaphylaxis

Anaphylactic (IgE-dependent)
    Foods (such as peanut, tree nuts, and crustaceans)
    Medications (such as antibiotics)
    Venoms (fire ants, jumper ants, yellow jackets, others)
    Allergen vaccines
    Latex
    Exercise (possibly, in food- and medication-dependent events)
    Hormones
    Animal or human proteins
    Colorants (insect-derived, such as carmine)
    Polysaccharides
    Enzymes
Anaphylactoid (IgE-independent)
    Nonspecific degranulation of mast cells and basophils
        Opioids
        Muscle relaxants
        Idiopathic
        Physical factors
            Exercise
            Temperature (cold, heat)
    Disturbance of arachidonic acid metabolism
        Aspirin and other nonsteroidal anti-inflammatory drugs (NSAIDs)[a]
    Immune aggregates
        Intravenous immunoglobulin
        Dextran (possibly)
        Possibly antihaptoglobin in anhaptoglobinemia (in Asians)
    Cytotoxic
        Transfusion reactions to cellular elements (IgM, IgG)
    Multimediator complement activation/activation of contact system
        Radiocontrast media
        ACE-inhibitor administered during renal dialysis with sulfonated polyacrylonitrile, cuprophane, or polymethylmethacrylate dialysis membranes
        Ethylene oxide gas on dialysis tubing
        Protamine (possibly)
Psychogenic
    Factitious
    Munchausen syndrome by proxy
    Undifferentiated somatoform idiopathic anaphylaxis

[a] Some authors suggest that reactions to NSAIDs should be classified as anaphylactic, even though there is no reliable or consistent detection of agent-specific IgE. These reactions almost always are drug specific [unlike the cross-reactivity observed in aspirin-sensitive respiratory disease (also known as Samter syndrome or aspirin triad)], they require two or more previous specific drug exposures, and the subject group characteristically has no underlying asthma or nasal polyps. (Stevenson DD. Anaphylactic and anaphylactoid reactions to aspirin and other non-steroidal anti-inflammatory drugs. Immunol Allergy Clin N Am 2001; 21:745–768.)
Source: Modified from Kemp SF, Lockey RF. Anaphylaxis: A review of causes and mechanisms. J Allergy Clin Immunol 2002; 110:341–348.

during a controlled exercise challenge, but the test is often negative despite a classical clinical history (61). Subjects with EIA should learn how to self-administer epinephrine and preferably should exercise with a partner educated about EIA and how to treat it.

A

B

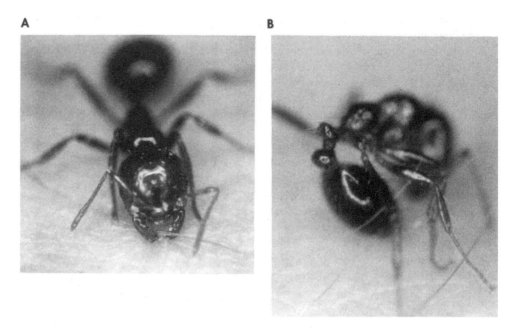

Figure 1 Imported fire ant attaches itself with its mandibles (A) and then stings about this anchor point in a circular pattern (B).

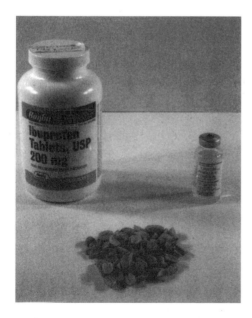

Figure 2 Nonsteroidal anti-inflammatory drugs, penicillin, and peanuts are examples of agents that cause anaphylaxis and anaphylactoid reactions.

Exercise avoidance remains the best treatment since the natural history of the syndrome is not fully understood. Shadick et al. surveyed 365 subjects with EIA for an average of 10.6 years. Of survey respondents, 47% had fewer episodes and 46% had stabilized since diagnosis. Forty one percent reported no episodes in the year preceding the survey. Successful respondents apparently had moderated their exercise programs and avoided provocative factors (62).

F. Cholinergic Urticaria

Cholinergic urticaria, also called "heat urticaria," is caused by increased core body temperature due to fever, stress, environmental factors, or exercise. Skin lesions frequently appear as 2–4-mm pruritic wheals ("microhives") surrounded by marked erythema. Systemic manifestations like those described for EIA may also occur but are unusual. Subjects with this syndrome may develop wheals at the site where methacholine is injected or generalized urticaria when the body is warmed, as with a plastic occlusive suit (61).

G. Idiopathic Anaphylaxis

Idiopathic anaphylaxis is a syndrome of repeated anaphylactic episodes for which no cause can be determined despite extensive evaluation (63). It may occur in children as well as adults (13,64). Three large retrospective series suggest that 20% to 33% of all anaphylactic episodes are idiopathic (1,14,58). Fatalities are rare (64). Within one year, almost all subjects enter a period of prolonged remission or have infrequent and less severe episodes (13). Failure to respond to prednisone should prompt consideration of another diagnosis (13). (See Section II for management of idiopathic anaphylaxis.)

The usefulness of prick skin testing for reactions to food allergens was tested in 102 subjects with idiopathic anaphylaxis (65). One-third had positive tests to one or more foods from a battery of 79 food allergens. Five subjects experienced anaphylaxis after eating a food implicated by a positive skin test. Two subjects stopped having reactions after they eliminated the implicated food from their diet, but they refused subsequent confirmatory oral food challenge. The 10 allergens that provoked anaphylaxis in these 7 subjects were aniseed, cashew, celery, flaxseed, hops, mustard, mushroom, shrimp, sunflower, and walnut. The authors concluded that skin testing with selected foods may be useful in identifying food allergens that cause anaphylaxis since 7% of subjects in the reference group previously presumed to have idiopathic anaphylaxis instead had food-induced anaphylaxis.

H. Anaphylaxis Attributed to Endogenous Progesterone

A syndrome of recurrent anaphylaxis apparently triggered or exacerbated by progesterone has been described in five female subjects (66,67). Four of these subjects reported attacks that exacerbated during pregnancy, lessened during lactation, and increased when lactation ceased. Three of the five subjects experienced remission when treated with a luteinizing hormone–releasing hormone (LHRH) analogue, which apparently antagonized LHRH and inhibited progesterone. Immediate skin test reactions to intradermal injection of 40–2000 μg of medroxyprogesterone were present in responders to LHRH analogue therapy. Systemic reactions characterized by urticaria and hypotension developed in two subjects after 100 μg of LHRH was administered intravenously during the luteal phase of their menstrual cycles. The authors postulated that progesterone, in some undefined way, facilitates mast cell mediator release. The three subjects whose anaphylactic symptoms were dramatically reduced by LHRH analogue therapy subsequently underwent oophorectomy with long-lasting reduction in their symptoms. One subject, however, continued to require combined H_1 and H_2 antihistamine therapy to control attacks.

I. Recurrent and Persistent Anaphylaxis

Depending on the report, recurrent or biphasic anaphylaxis occurs in up to 20% of subjects who experience anaphylaxis (14,68–71). Stark and Sullivan reported biphasic anaphylaxis in 5 of 25 subjects (20%) (71). Another study comprising 44 outpatient and 59 inpatient cases of anaphylaxis, however, observed incidences of 5% and 7%, respectively, over a 4-year period (69). Brazil and MacNamara retrospectively reviewed 34 subjects admitted for observation after anaphylaxis who required epinephrine treatment (68). Six (18%) had biphasic episodes. The investigators observed that subjects who had experienced biphasic episodes did not differ clinically at initial presentation but required significantly more epinephrine to ameliorate their initial symptoms (1.2 mg) than did those with uniphasic reactions, who required only 0.6 mg ($p = 0.03$).

Persistent anaphylaxis, anaphylaxis that may last from 5 to 32 h, occurred in 7 of 25 subjects (28%) in the Stark and Sullivan report (71). Of 13 subjects analyzed in a report on fatal or near-fatal anaphylaxis to foods, 3 (23%) similarly experienced persistent anaphylaxis (70). Data from other investigators, however, suggest that persistent anaphylaxis is uncommon. Kemp et al. retrospectively analyzed 266 consecutive subjects with nonfatal anaphylaxis, none of whom had biphasic or persistent anaphylaxis (14).

Neither biphasic nor persistent anaphylaxis can be predicted from the severity of the initial phase of an anaphylactic reaction. Since life-threatening manifestations of anaphylaxis may recur, it may be necessary to monitor subjects up to 24 h after their apparent recovery from the initial phase.

J. Clinical Manifestations of Anaphylaxis

The broad spectrum of clinical presentations may complicate the diagnosis of anaphylaxis. Special attention should be directed toward assessment of both upper and lower airways, respiratory and pulse rates, blood pressure, tissue perfusion, and appearance of the skin. Measurements of peak expiratory flow rate and pulse oximetry are also useful. Anaphylaxis consists of the following signs and symptoms, alone or in combination: diffuse erythema, pruritus, urticaria, angioedema, bronchospasm, laryngeal edema, hyperperistalsis, hypotension, or cardiac arrhythmias. Urticaria and angioedema were the most common manifestations [772 (92%) of 835 subjects in retrospective series] (13–15). However, cutaneous findings may be delayed or absent in rapidly progressive anaphylaxis. The next most frequent manifestations of anaphylaxis in order of occurrence are respiratory symptoms, dizziness, syncope, and gastrointestinal symptoms. The more rapidly anaphylaxis occurs after exposure to its stimulus, the more likely the reaction is to be severe and potentially life threatening (17,18).

K. Differential Diagnosis of Anaphylaxis

Several systemic disorders share clinical features with anaphylaxis. The vasodepressor (vaso-vagal) reaction probably is the condition most commonly confused with anaphylactic and anaphylactoid reactions. In vasodepressor reactions, however, urticaria is absent, the heart rate is typically slow, bronchospasm or other breathing difficulty is absent, the blood pressure is usually normal or elevated, and the skin is typically cool and pale. Tachycardia is the rule in anaphylaxis, but it may be absent in subjects with conduction defects, increased vagal tone due to a cardioinhibitory (Bezold-Jarisch) reflex, activated by ischemic effects on sensory receptors in the inferoposterior wall of the left ventricle, or in those who take sympatholytic medications. Myocardial dysfunction may cause sudden hemodynamic collapse with or without arrhythmia. A pulmonary embolism may produce tachycardia, dyspnea, tachypnea, and chest discomfort that is often pleuritic. Systemic mastocytosis, a disease characterized by mast cell proliferation in multiple organs, usually features urticaria pigmentosa (brownish macules that transform into wheals upon stroking) and recurrent episodes of pruritus, flushing, tachycardia, abdominal pain, diarrhea, syncope, or headache. Other diagnostic considerations for children, in particular, include foreign body aspiration, acute poisoning, and seizure disorder.

Signs and symptoms frequently observed in anaphylaxis may occur by themselves in other disorders. Subjects with hereditary angioedema, for example, experience episodes of nonpruritic, typically painless edema of the extremities that may be associated with laryngeal edema or abdominal discomfort due to visceral angioedema. Factitious anaphylaxis is a psychiatric disorder characterized by repeated, self-induced episodes of anaphylaxis. Anaphylaxis alternatively may be inflicted surreptitiously upon a susceptible subject (an example of Munchausen syndrome by proxy). Undifferentiated somatoform idiopathic anaphylaxis likewise is a psychiatric disorder in which subjects report symptoms identical to those encountered in idiopathic anaphylaxis, but objective findings are absent and the subjects meet established diagnostic criteria for undifferentiated somatoform disorder (64).

II. MANAGEMENT OF ANAPHYLAXIS

A. General

Practice parameters (72) and consensus emergency management guidelines (11,73) concerning anaphylaxis and its management have been published. As in asthma and other diseases for which there are published guidelines, however, physicians and other health care professionals may not apply them. In a standardized clinical setting of anaphylaxis as defined by UK Resuscitation Council guidelines, only 5% of 78 senior house officers beginning emergency department responsibilities would, in the judgment of investigators, administer epinephrine appropriately and with the proper dose and route of administration as recommended by the published guidelines (74).

A sequential approach to management is outlined in Table 3. Anaphylactic and anaphylactoid reactions differ mechanistically, but the management of acute episodes is the same. Assessment and maintenance of airway, breathing, and circulation (the ABCs of basic life support) are necessary before proceeding to other management steps. Subjects are monitored continuously to facilitate the prompt detection of any complications resulting from subsequent therapeutic intervention. Judicious use of epinephrine and the maintenance of adequate oxygenation and effective circulatory volume are paramount. Systemic absorption of an agent causing anaphylaxis must be minimized. This includes stopping intravenous infusions of offending medications. Vasoconstrictor properties of epinephrine may also limit systemic absorption if injected into the site of an insect sting or needle stick. Severe laryngospasm may develop within 30 min to 3 h of the onset of anaphylaxis (11). An endotracheal tube should be inserted as soon as possible if laryngospasm does not reverse promptly after parenteral administration of epinephrine. Epinephrine and atropine may be administered endotracheally if establishing intravenous access is difficult. H_1 and H_2 antagonists, corticosteroids, and volume expanders can be infused once intravenous access is established.

Table 3 Physician-Supervised Sequential Management of Anaphylaxis

I. Immediate intervention
    a. Assessment of airway, breathing, circulation, and adequacy of mentation.
    b. Administer aqueous epinephrine 1:1000 dilution, 0.2–0.5 ml (0.01 mg/kg in children, max 0.3 mg dosage) *intramuscularly* into the arm (deltoid) every 5 min, as necessary, to control symptoms and blood pressure. The arm permits easy access for administration of epinephrine, although intramuscular injection into the anterolateral thigh (vastus medialis) produces higher and more rapid peak plasma levels than injections intramuscularly in the arm. Subjects with moderate, severe, or progressive anaphylaxis should receive epinephrine injections in the anterolateral thigh. Alternatively, an epinephrine autoinjector [e.g., EpiPen (0.3 mg) or EpiPen Jr. (0.15 mg)] may be administered, through clothing if necessary, into the lateral thigh. Repeat every 5 min as necessary (avoid toxicity).[a]
    c. *For moribund subjects* not responding to epinephrine injections and volume replacement, an intravenous infusion may be prepared by adding 1.0 mg (1.0 ml) of 1:1000 dilution of epinephrine to 500 ml of 5% dextrose to yield a concentration of 2.0 µg/ml. This 1:10,000 solution is infused at a rate of 1.0 µg/min (15 drops/min) using a micro-drop apparatus), increasing to a maximum of 10.0 µg/min for adults and adolescents. A dosage of 0.01 mg/kg (0.1 ml/kg of a 1:10,000 solution) is recommended for children. CONTINUOUS HEMODYNAMIC MONITORING IS ESSENTIAL WHEN INTRAVENOUS EPINEPHRINE IS ADMINISTERED.[a] (See also IV below.)
II. General measures
    a. Place subject in recumbent position and elevate lower extremities.
    b. Establish and maintain airway (endotracheal tube or cricothyrotomy may be required).
    c. Administer oxygen at 6–8 liters/min.
    d. Establish venous access.
    e. Normal saline IV for fluid replacement. May require large volumes of crystalloid (1–2 liters normal saline to adults can be given at 5–10 ml/kg in first 5 min; children can receive up to 30 ml/kg in first hour). If severe hypotension exists, rapid infusion of volume expanders (colloid-containing solutions) may be necessary.
III. Specific measures that depend on the clinical condition
    a. Aqueous epinephrine 1:1,000, 1/2 dose (0.1–0.2 mg) at the reaction site following sting or injection may delay allergen absorption via local vasoconstriction.
    b. Diphenhydramine, 1–2 mg/kg or 25–50 mg/dose parenterally.
    c. Consider ranitidine (administer only *after* diphenhydramine), 50 mg in adults and 12.5–50 mg (1 mg/kg) in children, which may be diluted in 5% dextrose (D5W) to a total volume of 20 ml and injected IV over 5 min. Cimetidine (4 mg/kg) alternatively may be administered IV to adults, but no pediatric dosage in anaphylaxis has been established. *Note:* In the management of anaphylaxis, a combination of diphenhydramine and ranitidine is superior to diphenhydramine alone.
    d. For bronchospasm resistant to epinephrine, nebulized albuterol 2.5–5 mg in 3 ml saline, and repeat as necessary.
    e. For hypotension refractory to volume replacement and epinephrine injections, dopamine, 400 mg in 500 ml D5W, may be administered IV at 2–20 µg/kg/min with the rate titrated to maintain adequate blood pressure. Continuous hemodynamic monitoring is essential.
    f. Glucagon, 1–5 mg [20–30 µg/kg (max. 1 mg) in children], administered IV over 5 min followed by an infusion, 5–15 µg/min, may be utilized in patients receiving chronic beta-blocker therapy who do not respond to epinephrine. Aspiration precautions should be observed because glucagon usually causes nausea and emesis.
    g. Systemic glucocorticosteroids, such as methylprednisolone 1–2 mg/kg per 24 h, may prevent prolonged reactions or relapses.

(Continued)

Table 3   Continued

IV. Key additional interventions for cardiopulmonary arrest occurring during anaphylaxis
   a. Cardiopulmonary resuscitation and advanced cardiac life support measures.
   b. High-dose epinephrine IV (i.e., rapid progression to high dose). A commonly used sequence is 1 to 3 mg (1:10,000 dilution) IV slowly administered over 3 min, 3 to 5 mg IV over 3 min, and then 4–10 µg/min infusion. The recommended initial resuscitation dosage in children is 0.01 mg/kg (0.1 ml/kg of a 1:10,000 solution), repeated every 3 to 5 min for ongoing arrest. Higher subsequent dosages (0.1–0.2 mg/kg; 0.1 ml/kg of a 1:1,000 solution) may be considered for unresponsive asystole or pulseless electrical activity (PEA). These arrhythmias are often observed during cardiopulmonary arrest that occurs in anaphylaxis.
   c. Rapid volume expansion is mandatory.
   d. Atropine and transcutaneous pacing if asystole/PEA are present.
   e. Prolonged resuscitation efforts are encouraged, if necessary, since efforts are more likely to be successful in anaphylaxis where the subject is young and has a healthy cardiovascular system.
V. Observation
Follow-up after reactions: (1) at home if the reaction is mild or (2) in a medical setting for more severe reactions characterized by (a) a slow onset, (b) occurrence in a severe asthmatic or in association with a severe asthma component, (c) a possibility of continuing absorption of allergen, or (4) subjects with a previous history of recurrent or protracted anaphylaxis.

---

[a] There is no absolute contraindication to epinephrine administration in anaphylaxis. However, several anaphylaxis fatalities have been attributed to the overuse of intravenous epinephrine (12).
Source: Modified from Kemp SF, Lockey RF. Anaphylaxis: A review of causes and mechanisms. J Allergy Clin Immunol 2002; 110:341–348.

B.   How to Use Epinephrine

Epinephrine is generally acknowledged to be the most important drug for use in severe anaphylaxis (13,72,73). It is used in all cases of anaphylaxis to restore vasomotor tone, and all subsequent therapeutic interventions depend on the severity of the reaction and the initial response to epinephrine.

The α-adrenergic effect causes peripheral vasoconstriction, which alleviates hypotension and also reduces angioedema and urticaria. It may also minimize further absorption of antigen from a sting or injection. The β-adrenergic properties of epinephrine cause bronchodilation, increase myocardial output and contractility, and suppress further mediator release from mast cells and basophils (75).

Overzealous treatment with epinephrine can potentially be as hazardous as the reaction itself. Excessive α-adrenergic activity may cause hypertension and excessive β-adrenergic stimulation will increase myocardial oxygen consumption, possibly leading to myocardial ischemia or arrhythmias (75). Pulmonary edema may result from large doses, especially if epinephrine is administered intravenously (76,77). Pathophysiological mechanisms include peripheral vasoconstriction with effective transfer of blood volume to the pulmonary vasculature, increased pulmonary vascular pressure due to elevated left atrial pressure and/or pulmonary vasoconstriction, ventricular dysfunction resulting from increased peripheral resistance and concomitantly decreased diastolic filling time imposed by tachycardia, and autonomic sensory input (78). Pumphrey reviewed data from 164 cases of fatal anaphylaxis that occurred in the UK from 1992 to 1998 and reports that *intravenous* epinephrine overdoses caused at least 3 of these fatalities (79).

Fatalities during witnessed anaphylaxis usually result from delayed administration of epinephrine and from severe respiratory and/or cardiovascular complications. In a retrospective review of 6 fatal and 7 nonfatal episodes of food-induced anaphylaxis in children and adolescents, all subjects who survived had received epinephrine before or within 5 min of developing severe respiratory symptoms. None of the subjects with fatal attacks had received epinephrine prior to the onset of severe respiratory symptoms (70). Analysis of data from a national case registry of fatal food anaphylaxis in the United States indicates that very few individuals (3 of 32) had epinephrine syringes available at the time of fatal reaction (7). Similarly, Pumphrey determined that epinephrine was administered in 62% of the fatal anaphylactic reactions that he reviewed, only 14% prior to cardiac arrest (79).

The most commonly recommended dosage of epinephrine for the treatment of anaphylaxis in adults or adolescents without cardiovascular compromise is 0.2 to 0.5 mg of a 1:1000 dilution administered intramuscularly every 5 min, as clinically needed in both adults and children (11,12,72,73). Age alone does not contraindicate epinephrine administration (80). However, epinephrine should be used more cautiously in subjects over 55 years of age because of the risk for coexisting atherosclerotic cardiovascular disease in this population. Test doses of 0.1 mg may be appropriate and sufficient in some circumstances. The dosage of epinephrine generally recommended for children is 0.01 mg/kg (maximum 0.5 mg) of a 1:1000 dilution administered intramuscularly every 5 min for 2 doses and then every 4 h as needed (11,12,72,73). Absorption is more rapid and plasma levels are higher in children who receive epinephrine intramuscularly in the thigh with an autoinjector (81). Intramuscular injection into the thigh (vastus lateralis) in adults is also superior to intramuscular or subcutaneous injection into the arm (deltoid), neither of which achieves elevated plasma epinephrine levels compared with endogenous levels associated with saline injection. Spring-loaded, automatic epinephrine devices (e.g., EpiPen) administered intramuscularly and intramuscular epinephrine injections through a syringe into the thigh in adults provide dose-equivalent plasma levels (82).

A subject with persistent hypotension rarely requires intravenous administration of epinephrine. No established dosage or regimen for intravenous epinephrine is recognized. Because of the risk for potentially lethal arrhythmias, epinephrine should be administered intravenously only during cardiac arrest or to profoundly hypotensive subjects who have failed to respond to intravenous volume replacement and several injected doses of epinephrine. Adults or adolescents should receive an initial dose of 0.1 mg (0.1 ml) of a 1:1000 dilution of epinephrine in 10 ml of normal saline, administered over 5 min (72). Additional dosage increments of 0.1 mg of this 1:10,000 dilution may be administered every 5 to 15 min depending upon the clinical response, but a continuous infusion may also be prepared in more critical situations. An infusion may be prepared by adding 1.0 mg (1.0 ml) of 1:1000 dilution of epinephrine to 500 ml of D5W to yield a concentration of 2.0 µg/ml. This 1:10,000 solution is infused at a rate of 1.0 µg/min (15 drops/minute using a micro-drop apparatus), increasing to a maximum of 10.0 µg/min for adults and adolescents. A dosage of 0.01 mg/kg (0.1 ml/kg of a 1:10,000 solution) is recommended for children (72). Continuous hemodynamic monitoring is essential.

High-dose intravenous epinephrine (i.e., rapid progression to high dose) should be used without delay for subjects in cardiopulmonary arrest. A commonly used sequence is 1 to 3 mg (1:10,000 dilution) IV slowly administered over 3 min, 3 to 5 mg IV over 3 min, and then 4–10 µg/min infusion (73). The recommended initial resuscitation dosage in children is 0.01 mg/kg (0.1 ml/kg of a 1:10,000 solution), repeated every 3 to 5 min for ongoing arrest. Higher subsequent dosages (0.1–0.2 mg/kg, 0.1 ml/kg of a 1:1000 solution) may be considered for nonresponsive asystole or pulseless electrical activity (PEA). These arrhythmias are often observed during cardiopulmonary arrest that occurs in anaphylaxis. Administration of atropine and transcutaneous pacing in accordance with asystole/PEA algorithms may also be appropriate. Additionally, prolonged resuscitation efforts are encouraged, if necessary, since such efforts are more likely to be successful in anaphylaxis, where the subject is often a young individual with a healthy cardiovascular system (73).

C. How to Use Ancillary Medications

1. H_1 and H_2 Antagonists

The standard treatment of anaphylactic episodes should include antihistamines and corticosteroids in addition to epinephrine. Even at maximum dosages, however, antihistamines (H_1 antagonists) cannot abort anaphylaxis if histamine already occupies its receptor. Thus, antihistamines should never be administered alone as treatment for anaphylaxis. These agents, however, may attenuate cutaneous symptoms, such as urticaria or generalized pruritus, and they may prevent relapse. Diphenhydramine, 25–50 mg for adults and 12.5–25 mg for children, may be administered intravenously once the cardiovascular and respiratory conditions are stabilized. The role of H_2 antagonists, such as cimetidine and ranitidine, is more controversial but their use is recommended (41). H_2 receptors mediate coronary vasodilation and some case reports suggest that intravenously administered H_2 antagonists may help to relieve persistent hypotension during anaphylaxis. Because cimetidine may inhibit the metabolism of β-adrenergic antagonists in vitro and may also inhibit theophylline metabolism in vivo, ranitidine, 50 mg (1 mg/kg) in adults and 12.5–50 mg in children, infused over 10 to 15 min is recommended (83). When bolus intravenous administration is desired, ranitidine may be diluted in 5% dextrose to a total volume of 20 ml and injected over 5 min. Cimetidine, 4 mg/kg in adults, should be administered slowly since rapid intravenous administration may produce hypotension (84). There are no established dosages for cimetidine in children with anaphylaxis. Since H_2 blockade without concomitant H_1 blockade could increase available histamine and increase H_1 receptor stimulation, H_2 antagonists should not be administered prior to administration of H_1 antagonists.

2. Corticosteroids

Systemic corticosteroids may have no effect for 4 to 6 hours, but they potentially may prevent persistent or biphasic reactions. Subjects with asthma or other conditions recently treated with corticosteroids are at increased risk for severe or fatal anaphylaxis (because of possible adrenal suppression) and may receive additional benefit if corticosteroids are administered to them during anaphylaxis. We recommend corticosteroid treatment for all subjects with anaphylaxis. Corticosteroids should be given intravenously early in the treatment of anaphylaxis at a dosage equivalent to 1.0 mg/kg of methylprednisolone every 6 hours. Oral administration of prednisone, 0.5 mg/kg, may suffice for milder attacks.

3. Oxygen and $β_2$ Agonists

Oxygen should be administered to subjects with anaphylaxis who require multiple doses of epinephrine, have protracted anaphylaxis, or have preexisting hypoxemia or myocardial dysfunction. Oxygen therapy should be regulated by arterial blood gas determination or continuous pulse oximetry.

Inhaled $β_2$ agonists (e.g., albuterol, 0.5 ml or 2.5 mg of a 5% solution) may be administered for bronchospasm refractory to epinephrine.

4. Persistent Hypotension: Appropriate Roles of Volume Replacement and Glucagon

Usual doses of epinephrine administered during anaphylaxis to subjects taking β-adrenergic antagonists may not produce the desired clinical response and may instead cause predominantly α-adrenergic effects. In such situations, both isotonic volume expansion (in some circumstances, up to 7 liters of crystalloid are necessary) and glucagon administration are recommended (41). Glucagon may potentially reverse refractory hypotension and bronchospasm during anaphylaxis (85–87). Glucagon directly activates adenyl cyclase and completely bypasses the β-adrenergic receptor. The recommended dosage for glucagon is 1 to 5 mg [20–30 μg/kg (max. 1 kg) in children] administered intravenously over 5 min and followed by an infusion, 5–15 μg/min, titrated to clinical response. Protection of the airway is particularly important in severely drowsy or obtunded subjects since glucagon uses causes emesis with the attendant risk of aspiration.

Some investigators have reported elevated endogenous levels of norepinephrine, epinephrine, and angiotensin II in individuals who experience hypotension during anaphylaxis due to insect stings (48). These findings may explain why epinephrine injections fail to help some subjects with anaphylaxis. The subject whose hypotension persists despite epinephrine injections should receive intravenous crystalloid solutions, and volume expanders, such as hydroxyethyl starch (Hespan), should be ordered for use as necessary. Large volumes are often required. A volume of 1 to 2 liters of normal saline is administered to adults at a rate of 5–10 ml/kg in the first 5 min. Children should receive up to 30 ml/kg in the first hour. Adults receiving colloid solution should receive 500 ml rapidly, followed by slow infusion (41).

Vasopressors, such as dopamine or norepinephrine, should be administered if epinephrine injections with or without antihistamines and volume expansion fail to alleviate hypotension. The vasopressor of choice is probably dopamine (400 mg in 500 ml of 5% dextrose), administered at 2–20 μg/kg/min and titrated to systolic blood pressure. Central venous access should be attempted to facilitate both rapid administration of fluids and continuous assessment of intravascular volume status. As mentioned previously, oxygen should be administered to subjects with protracted anaphylaxis since subjects with prolonged hypoxemia and/or hypotension may experience myocardial dysfunction, possibly resulting in refractory hypotension and/or end organ damage. A critical care specialist may need to be consulted for a subject with intractable hypotension.

D. Management of Persistent Airway Obstruction

1. Persistent Upper Airway Obstruction

Severe laryngospasm may occur so quickly during anaphylaxis that endotracheal intubation is impossible. Therefore, an endotracheal tube should be inserted as soon as possible if laryngospasm does not reverse promptly after parenteral administration of epinephrine. An endotracheal tube measuring at least 7.5 mm in diameter is preferable in adults since larger sizes reduce resistance to airflow. Aerosolized epinephrine, along with supplemental oxygen and extension of the neck, may be helpful if endotracheal intubation proves difficult. A cricothyrotomy likely is the next step since it is accomplished more easily than an emergency tracheostomy. Briefly, the subject's neck is hyperextended, and the area of the cricothyroid membrane is palpated below the thyroid cartilage and above the cricoid cartilage. A small incision is made, the membrane is punctured, and the opening is enlarged with a blunt instrument such as a scalpel handle. Finally, a small-diameter

(4–5 mm) endotracheal tube is inserted. Alternatively, high-flow oxygen delivery through an 11-gauge needle or polyethylene catheter may suffice for the short term if an endotracheal tube is not available. Potential complications of cricothyrotomy include vocal cord injury, bleeding, and subcutaneous emphysema (73).

2. Persistent Lower Airway Obstruction

Attention should be directed toward treating any bronchospasm once the subject's upper airway has been secured. Epinephrine generally reduces the bronchospasm associated with anaphylaxis, but ventilation and oxygenation may remain a problem despite an adequate airway. This persistent airway obstruction should be treated similarly to status asthmaticus. Arterial blood gas determinations and continuous pulse oximetry help to guide therapy. Subjects often respond to inhaled β-agonists, such as albuterol (0.5 ml or 2.5 mg of a 5% solution) delivered with oxygen by nebulization.

Mechanical ventilation itself may present a danger for subjects requiring ventilator support during anaphylaxis. Common complications include pulmonary barotrauma (stretch injury) and hemodynamic compromise, which may result if extremely high inspiratory pressures are needed to overcome airway obstruction. Mechanical ventilation may have serious consequences for subjects with persistent hypotension despite adequate ventilation. High inspiratory pressure and an inadequate internal diameter of the endotracheal tube may decrease venous return and increase right ventricular afterload, which leads to inadequate oxygen delivery, arrhythmias, and possible cardiac arrest.

E. Problems Posed by β-Adrenergic Antagonists During Anaphylaxis

β-adrenergic antagonists (beta-blockers) are used to treat cardiovascular disease, arrhythmias, hypertension, migraine headaches, anxiety, glaucoma, or thyrotoxicosis. Ophthalmic administration of β-antagonists may induce significant systemic effects, and subjects may neglect to report usage of eyedrops unless they are questioned specifically. Subjects taking β-adrenergic antagonists may be more likely to experience severe anaphylactic reactions characterized by paradoxical bradycardia, profound hypotension, and severe bronchospasm. These agents may also impede treatment with epinephrine. Dosage increases of isoproterenol (a β-adrenergic agonist) up to 80-fold are necessary experimentally to overcome β-receptor blockade (88). Use of selective β_1-antagonists does not reduce the risk of anaphylaxis since both β_1- and β_2-antagonists may inhibit the β-adrenergic receptor (89). Nonetheless, data from a meta-analysis of subjects with reactive airway disease suggest that they can tolerate β_1-selective beta-blockers without bronchospasm (90). No similar analysis has been conducted for selective beta-blockers in anaphylaxis.

F. Management of Anaphylaxis in Pregnancy

Anaphylaxis rarely occurs during pregnancy, and data are insufficient for firm treatment recommendations. The uteroplacental arteries are very responsive to α-adrenergic stimulation, and great care is necessary when epinephrine or other agents with α-adrenergic effects are contemplated (91). Obstetric anesthesiologists commonly use ephedrine, 10 to 25 mg intravenously, to support the blood pressure of pregnant subjects, primarily by its β-adrenergic effects, which increase cardiac output (83). Ephedrine will also stimulate α-adrenergic receptors at high doses. Therefore, this medication should be used with caution to avoid jeopardizing the fetal circulation in pregnant subjects.

Table 4 Specific Measures for Idiopathic Anaphylaxis[a]

Reaction	Treatment
Acute	Epinephrine, 0.3 cc of 1:1000 solution IM
	Prednisone, 60 mg orally
	Antihistamine, such as hydroxyzine, 25 mg orally
	Proceed to the nearest emergency room or contact physician for further instructions
Infrequent	Treat as for acute reactions
Frequent and severe	Prednisone, 60–100 mg orally for 1 week or until signs and symptoms are controlled
	Continuous antihistamine (such as hydroxyzine, 25 mg three times daily)
	Continuous sympathomimetic agent (such as albuterol, 2 mg three times daily)
	When all signs and symptoms are controlled, convert to alternate-day prednisone, 60 to 100 mg, cautiously tapering by no more than 5–10 mg/month

[a] Adult/adolescent management and dosages for idiopathic anaphylaxis are listed. Dosages should be adjusted appropriately for children.
Source: Modified from Kemp SF. Anaphylaxis: Current concepts in pathophysiology, diagnosis, and management. Immunol Allergy Clin N Am 2001; 21:611–634.

G. Management of Idiopathic Anaphylaxis

Treatment for subjects with idiopathic anaphylaxis depends on the frequency of episodes. Subjects with single or infrequent episodes may be treated with a combination of epinephrine, an antihistamine, and a single dose of prednisone. Subjects with frequent attacks should receive a combination of prednisone, antihistamines, and a sympathomimetic agent (Table 4). When signs and symptoms are controlled, prednisone may be tapered cautiously by no more than 5 mg/month prior to discontinuing the other two medications (13,64).

H. Self-Treatment by Subject

All subjects at high risk for recurrent anaphylaxis should carry epinephrine syringes and know how to administer them (92). Data from Vander Leek et al. suggest that epinephrine should be provided for use in any child or adult with confirmed peanut allergy, regardless of the nature of the initial reaction (59). A survey determined that more than 80% of subjects who died from food anaphylaxis were not given appropriate information to avoid inadvertent food-induced reactions or epinephrine kits to manage them (7).

Demonstration of proper technique with a placebo trainer is recommended since two studies have reported that many subjects receive improper or no instructions (93,94). Only one device is commercially available in the United States but others are in development. An EpiPen (Dey Laboratories, Napa, CA) is a spring-loaded, pressure-activated syringe that contains a single 0.3-mg dose (1:1000 dilution) of epinephrine (Fig. 3). It is easy to use and will inject through clothing (Fig. 4). An EpiPen Jr., which delivers 0.15 mg (1:2000 dilution) epinephrine, is appropriate for children weighing less than 30 kg or for subjects with a comorbid condition, such as coronary artery disease, that might be affected adversely by higher dosages of epinephrine. Compliance with instructions to carry

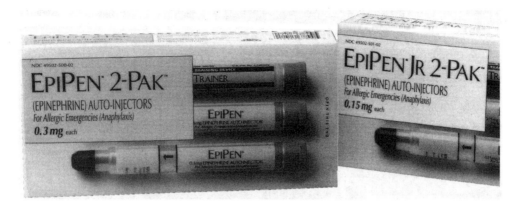

Figure 3 Currently available epinephrine syringes. Single devices are also available. (Photo courtesy of Dey Laboratories, Napa, CA, www.anaphylaxis.com.)

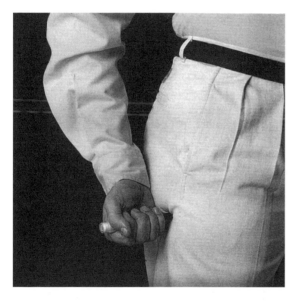

Figure 4 EpiPen Auto-injector. (Photo courtesy of Dey Laboratories, Napa, CA, www.anaphylaxis.com.)

epinephrine syringes must be assessed periodically since many subjects will forget to carry them (93–96) or will prefer to seek emergency medical assistance (79).

Inhalation of high-dose epinephrine from a metered dose aerosol has been studied as a potential alternative to epinephrine injections during anaphylaxis (97,98). High doses are required because 90% of an epinephrine dose administered by metered dose inhaler is swallowed and inactivated in the gastrointestinal tract by monoamine oxidase and catechol *O*-methyltransferase (99). Simons et al. observed in an observer-blinded, placebo-controlled, parallel-group study of 19 asymptomatic children that most (17) children were unable to inhale sufficient epinephrine, despite expert coaching, to increase their plasma epinephrine concentrations significantly (98).

III. PREVENTION OF ANAPHYLAXIS

Some anaphylactic reactions are so severe that treatment will be unsuccessful. This underscores the critical importance of education, avoidance, and prevention. Table 5 outlines basic principles for the prevention of future anaphylactic or anaphylactoid reactions. An allergist-immunologist can provide comprehensive professional advice on these matters.

Agents that cause anaphylaxis must be identified whenever possible, and subjects should be instructed how to minimize future exposure to these agents. β-adrenergic antagonists should be discontinued where substitutions are feasible. Alternatives to angiotensin-converting enzyme (ACE)–inhibitors may also potentially be helpful since ACE-inhibitors may prevent compensatory angiotensin II mobilization during anaphylaxis. However, more clinical data are needed on ACE-inhibitor effects in anaphylaxis (100). Monoamine oxidase inhibitors and some tricyclic antidepressants render epinephrine usage more hazardous by interfering with its degradation.

Meals may have unsavory surprises for highly allergic individuals. A case report illustrates that anaphylaxis may occur in latex-allergic subjects whose food handlers wear latex gloves. Baked goods commonly contain peanuts and nuts, and accidental ingestion of these foods is common. Approximately 35% to 50% of subjects allergic to peanuts will have an inadvertent peanut ingestion within 3 to 4 years (101). Pumphrey observed that commercial catering caused 76% of food-related anaphylactic reactions (79). Education is of paramount importance, and the Food Allergy and Anaphylaxis Network (phone 800-929-4040, www.foodallergy.org) is a helpful nonprofit resource for many food-allergic individuals.

The potential for anaphylaxis may be determined by skin tests in some circumstances (e.g., allergy to β-lactam antibiotics). However, the immunochemistry of most

Table 5 Preventive Measures for Subjects with Anaphylaxis

I. General measures
- Obtain thorough history to diagnose life-threatening food or drug allergy.
- Identify cause of anaphylaxis and those individuals at risk for future attacks.
- Provide instruction on proper reading of food and medication labels, where appropriate.
- Avoid exposure to antigens and cross-reactive substances.
- Practice optimal management of asthma and coronary artery disease.

II. Specific measures for high-risk subjects
- Individuals at high risk for anaphylaxis should carry self-injectable syringes of epinephrine at all times and receive instruction in proper use with placebo trainer.
- Wear a MedicAlert bracelet or chain.
- Substitute other agents for β-adrenergic antagonists, ACE-inhibitors, tricyclic antidepressants, and monoamine oxidase inhibitors whenever possible.
- Employ slow, supervised administration of agents suspected of causing anaphylaxis, orally if possible.
- Where appropriate, utilize specific preventive strategies, including pharmacological prophylaxis, short-term challenge and desensitization, and long-term desensitization.

Source: Modified from Kemp SF. Anaphylaxis: Current concepts in pathophysiology, diagnosis, and management. Immunol Allergy Clin N Am 2001; 21:611–634.

drugs and biologic agents is not well defined, and reliable in vivo or in vitro testing for most agents is unavailable (102). Use of a radioallergosorbent test to quantify the level of food-specific IgE antibodies can be diagnostic in some circumstances. For example, subjects with peanut-specific IgE levels of at least 15 kU/liter have at least a 95% chance of peanut anaphylaxis if they eat peanuts (60).

Situations may arise in which it is medically necessary to administer an agent to an individual in whom it has previously caused an anaphylactic episode. Numerous protocols enable prevention or reduction of the severity of anaphylaxis. All protocols should be conducted only in clinical settings where anaphylaxis, if it occurs, can be managed properly. Examples of these protocols are antihistamine and corticosteroid prophylaxis to prevent or reduce the severity of IgE-independent reactions (e.g., radiocontrast media); administration of gradually increasing incremental doses of medication over several hours (e.g., short-term penicillin desensitization); or the highly effective, long-term desensitization with venom immunotherapy for stinging insect anaphylaxis.

IV. POTENTIAL FUTURE OPTIONS FOR REDUCING THE RISK OF ANAPHYLAXIS

Potential future therapeutic options may feature modification of allergens to reduce allergenicity. Options being explored include novel vaccine delivery systems; DNA-based vaccination; conjugation of immunostimulatory DNA motifs to specific allergens; plasmid vectors containing DNA; vaccines with highly purified and defined allergens; non-anaphylactic allergens/allergen fragments/peptides for active immunotherapy; IgE-binding haptens of major allergens for passive saturation of effector cells and induction of blocking antibodies; allergen-specific antibodies and antibody fragments for passive immunotherapy in the allergic effector organs; and immunotherapy with humanized anti-IgE monoclonal antibodies or IgE-mimotopes (103,104).

V. SALIENT POINTS

1. Fatal anaphylaxis from allergen immunotherapy occurs at a rate of approximately 1 per 2,000,000 injections.
2. Anaphylaxis associated with allergen immunotherapy occurs more frequently with accelerated dosage schedules than with traditional, more leisurely schedules.
3. β-adrenergic antagonists may increase the risk for refractory anaphylaxis in subjects taking immunotherapy injections.
4. Mast cell tryptase levels correlate with the severity of anaphylaxis.
5. Some subjects with anaphylaxis have atypical findings such as bradycardia, vasomotor collapse without urticaria, or isolated gastrointestinal symptoms.
6. Myocardial dysfunction and arrhythmias may be prominent features of anaphylaxis.
7. The peanut allergen causes the greatest concern in food-associated anaphylaxis because of (1) the life-threatening severity of anaphylaxis to peanuts, especially in subjects with concomitant asthma; and (2) the propensity for subjects to remain allergic to peanuts throughout life.
8. Exercise avoidance remains the best treatment for exercise-induced anaphylaxis since medical prophylaxis is not consistently effective.

9. Epinephrine and oxygen are the most important therapeutic agents used in the treatment of anaphylaxis. Epinephrine must be used in appropriate doses. Intravenous doses of epinephrine should be reserved for cardiac arrest or profound hypotension unresponsive to intravenous fluids and multiple injected doses of epinephrine.

10. Glucagon administration may be life saving for subjects on β-blockers who experience anaphylaxis.

REFERENCES

1. Yocum MW, Butterfield JH, Klein JS, Volcheck GW, Schroeder DR, Silverstein MD. Epidemiology of anaphylaxis in Olmsted County: A population-based study. J Allergy Clin Immunol 1999; 104:452–456.

2. Valentine M, Frank M, Friedland L, et al. Allergic emergencies. In: Asthma and Other Allergic Diseases. (Drause RM, ed.). NIAID Task Force Report. Bethesda, MD: National Institutes of Health, 1979: 467–507.

3. Neugat AI, Ghatak AT, Miller RL. Anaphylaxis in the United States: An investigation into its epidemiology. Arch Intern Med 2001; 161:15–21.

4. Porter J, Jick H. Drug-induced anaphylaxis, convulsion, deafness, and extrapyramidal symptoms. Lancet 1977; 1:587–588.

5. International Collaborative Study of Severe Anaphylaxis. An epidemiologic study of severe anaphylactic and anaphylactoid reactions among hospital patients: Methods and overall risks. Epidemiology 1998; 9:141–146.

6. Burks W, Bannon GA, Sicherer S, Sampson HA. Peanut induced anaphylactic reactions. Int Arch Allergy Immunol 1999; 119:165–172.

7. Bock SA, Muñoz-Furlong A, Sampson HA. Fatalities due to anaphylactic reactions to foods. J Allergy Clin Immunol 2001; 107:191–193.

8. Kemp SF. Adverse effects of allergen immunotherapy: Assessment and treatment. Immunol Allergy Clin N Am 2000; 20:571–591.

9. Graft DF, Schuberth KC, Kagey-Sobotka A, Kwiterovich KA, Niv Y, Lichtenstein LM, Valentine MD. A prospective study of the natural history of large local reactions after Hymenoptera stings in children. J Pediatr 1984; 104:664–668.

10. Patterson R, Hogan MB, Yarnold PR, Harris KE. Idiopathic anaphylaxis: An attempt to estimate the incidence in the United States. Arch Intern Med 1995; 155:869–871.

11. Project Team of the Resuscitation Council (UK). Emergency medical treatment of anaphylactic reactions. J Accid Emerg Med 1999; 16:243–247.

12. Kemp SF, Lockey RF. Anaphylaxis: A review of causes and mechanisms. J Allergy Clin Immunol 2002; 110:341–348.

13. Ditto AM, Harris KE, Krasnick J, Miller MA, Patterson R. Idiopathic anaphylaxis: A series of 335 cases. Ann Allergy Asthma Immunol 1996; 77:285–291.

14. Kemp SF, Lockey RF, Wolf BL, Lieberman P. Anaphylaxis: A review of 266 cases. Arch Intern Med 1995; 155:1749–1754.

15. Wade JP, Liang MH, Sheffer AL. Exercise-induced anaphylaxis. Epidemiologic observations. Proc Clin Biol Res 1989; 297:175–182.

16. Lockey RF, Turkeltaub PC, Olive ES, Hubbard JM, Baird-Warren IA, Bukantz SC. The Hymenoptera venom study III: Safety of venom immunotherapy. J Allergy Clin Immunol 1990; 86:775–780.

17. James LP Jr, Austen KF. Fatal and systemic anaphylaxis in man. N Engl J Med 1964; 270:597–603.

18. Lockey RF, Benedict LM, Turkeltaub PC, Bukantz SC. Fatalities from immunotherapy (IT) and skin testing (ST). J Allergy Clin Immunol 1987; 79:660–677.

19. Reid MJ, Lockey RF, Turkeltaub PC, Platts-Mills TAE. Survey of fatalities from skin testing and immunotherapy 1985–1989. J Allergy Clin Immunol 1993; 92:6–15.

20. Reid M, Gurka G. Deaths associated with skin testing and immunotherapy (abstr) J Allergy Clin Immunol 1996; 97:231.

21. Lüderitz-Püchel U, May S, Haustein D. Zwischenfälle nach hyposensibilisierung [Incidents following hyposensitization]. Münch Med Wscher 1996; 138(8):45–48.

22. Stewart GE, Lockey RF. Systemic reactions from allergen immunotherapy. J Allergy Clin Immunology 1992; 90:567–578.

23. Lieberman PL. Specific and idiopathic anaphylaxis: Pathophysiology and treatment. In: Allergy, Asthma, and Immunology from Infancy to Adulthood, 3rd ed. (Bierman CW, Pearlman DS, Shapiro GG, Busse WH, eds.). Philadelphia: W.B. Saunders, 1996: 297–319.

24. Kaliner M, Sigler R, Summers R, Shelhamer JH. Effects of infused histamine: Analysis of the effects of H-1 and H-2 receptor antagonists on cardiovascular and pulmonary responses. J Allergy Clin Immunol 1981; 68:365–371.

25. Chrusch C, Sharma S, Unruh H, Bautista E, Duke E, Becker A, Kepron W, Mink SN. Histamine H3 receptor blockade improves cardiac function in canine anaphylaxis. Am J Respir Crit Care Med 1999; 160:142–149.

26. Lin RY, Schwartz LB, Curry A, Pesola GR, Knight RJ, Lee HS, Bakalchuk L, Tenenbaum C, Westfal RE. Histamine and tryptase levels in patients with acute allergic reactions: An emergency department–based study. J Allergy Clin Immunol 2000; 106:65–71.

27. Smith PL, Kagey-Sobotka A, Bleecker ER, Traystman R, Kaplan AP, Gralnick H, Valentine MD, Permutt S, Lichtenstein LM. Physiologic manifestations of human anaphylaxis. J Clin Invest 1980; 66:1072–1080.

28. Schwartz LB, Bradford TR, Rouse C, Irani A-M, Rasp G, van der Zwan JK, van der Linden PW. Development of a new, more sensitive immunoassay for human tryptase: Use in systemic anaphylaxis. J Clin Immunol 1994; 14:190–204.

29. Kanthawatana S, Carias K, Arnaout R, Hu J, Irani A-MA, Schwartz LB. The potential clinical utility of serum alpha-protryptase levels. J Allergy Clin Immunol 1999; 103:1092–1099.

30. Ansari MQ, Zamora JL, Lipscomb MF. Postmortem diagnosis of acute anaphylaxis by serum tryptase analysis: A case report. Am J Clin Pathol 1993; 99:101–103.

31. Becker AB, Mactavish G, Frith E, Desjardins PRE. Post-mortem stability of serum tryptase and immunoglobulin E (abstr). J Allergy Clin Immunol 1995; 95:369.

32. Schwartz HJ, Yuninger JW, Schwartz LB. Is unrecognized anaphylaxis a cause of sudden unexpected death? Clin Exp Allergy 1995; 25:866–870.

33. Yuninger JW, Nelson DR, Squillace DL, Jones RT, Holley KE, Hyma BA, Biedryzycki L, Sweeney KG, Sturner WQ, Schwartz LB. Laboratory investigations of death due to anaphylaxis. J Forensic Sci 1991; 36:857–865.

34. Holgate ST, Walters C, Walls AF, Lawrence S, Shell DJ, Variend S, Fleming PJ, Berry PJ, Gilbert RE, Robinson C. The anaphylaxis hypothesis of sudden infant death syndrome (SIDS): Mast cell degranulation in cot death revealed by elevated concentrations of tryptase in serum. Clin Exp Allergy 1994; 24:1115–1122.

35. Platt MS, Yuninger JW, Sekula-Perlman A, Irani A-MA, Smialek J, Mirchandani HG, Schwartz LB. Involvement of mast cells in sudden infant death syndrome. J Allergy Clin Immunol 1994; 94:250–256.

36. Edston E, Gidlund E, Wickman M, Ribbing H, Van Hage-Hamsten M. Increased mast cell tryptase in sudden infant death: Anaphylaxis, hypoxemia or artifact? Clin Exp Allergy 1999; 29:1648–1654.

37. Buckley MG, Variend S, Walls AF. Elevated serum concentrations of β-tryptase, but not α-tryptase, in Sudden Infant Death Syndrome (SIDS): An investigation of anaphylactic mechanisms. Clin Exp Allergy 2001; 31:1696–1704.

38. Palmer RMJ, Ferrige AG, Moncada S. Nitric oxide release accounts for the biological activity of endothelium derived relaxing factor. Nature 1987; 327:524–526.

39. Mitsuhata H, Shimizu R, Yokoyama MM. Role of nitric oxide in anaphylactic shock. J Clin Immunol 1995; 15:277–283.

40. Coleman JW. Nitric oxide: A regulator of mast cell activation and mast cell–mediated inflammation. Clin Exp Immunol 2002; 129:4–10.

41. Lieberman P. Anaphylaxis and anaphylactoid reactions. In: Allergy: Principles and Practice, 5th ed. (Middleton E Jr, Reed CE, Ellis EF, Adkinson NF Jr., Yunginger JW, Busse WW, eds.). St. Louis: Mosby–Year Book, 1998: 1079–1092.

42. Raper RF, Fisher MM. Profound reversible myocardial depression after anaphylaxis. Lancet 1988; 1:386–388.

43. Bristow MR, Ginsburg R, Harrison DC. Histamine and the human heart: The other receptor system. Am J Cardiol 1982; 49:249–251.

44. Wasserman SI. The heart in anaphylaxis. J Allergy Clin Immunol 1986; 77:663–666.

45. Fisher M. Clinical observations on the pathophysiology and implications for treatment. In: Update in Intensive Care and Emergency Medicine (Vincent JL, ed.). New York: Springer-Verlag, 1989: 309–316.

46. Fisher MM. Clinical observations on the pathophysiology and treatment of anaphylactic cardiovascular collapse. Anaesth Intensive Care 1986; 14:17–21.

47. Hermann K, Rittweger R, Ring J. Urinary excretion of angiotensin I, II, arginine vasopressin and oxytocin in patients with anaphylactoid reactions. Clin Exp Allergy 1992; 22:845–853.

48. van der Linden P-WG, Struyvenberg A, Kraaijenhagen RJ, Hack CE, van der Zwan JK. Anaphylactic shock after insect-sting challenge in 138 persons with a previous insect-sting reaction. Ann Intern Med 1993; 118:161–168.

49. von Tschirschnitz M, von Eschenbach CE, Hermann K, Ring J. Plasma angiotensin II in patients with Hymenoptera venom allergy during hyposensitization (abstr). J Allergy Clin Immunol 1993; 91.283.

50. Hanashiro PK, Weil MH. Anaphylactic shock in man: Report of two cases with detailed hemodynamics and metabolic studies. Arch Intern Med 1967; 119:129–140.

51. Fahmy NR. Hemodynamics, plasma histamine and catecholamine concentrations during an anaphylactoid reaction to morphine. Anesthesiology 1981; 55:329–331.

52. Kovanen PT, Kaartinen M, Paavonen T. Infiltrates of activated mast cells at the site of coronary atheromatous erosion or rupture in myocardial infarction. Circulation 1995; 92:1084–1088.

53. Constantinides P. Infiltrates of activated mast cells at the site of coronary atheromatous erosion or rupture in myocardial infarction. Circulation 1995; 92:1083.

54. Abela GS, Picon PD, Friedl SE, Gebara OC, Miyamoto A, Federman M, Tofler GH, Muller JE. Triggering of plaque disruption and arterial thrombosis in an atherosclerotic rabbit model. Circulation 1995; 91:776–784.

55. Soreide E, Harboe S. Severe anaphylactic reactions outside hospital: Etiology, symptoms and treatment. Acta Anaesthesiol Scand 1988; 32:339–342.

56. Viner NA, Rhamy RK. Anaphylaxis manifested by hypotension alone. J Urol 1975; 113:108–110.

57. Brown AFT, McKinnon D, Chu K. Emergency department anaphylaxis: A review of 142 patients in a single year. J Allergy Clin Immunol 2001; 108:861–866.

58. Coghlan-Johnston M, Lieberman P. Demographic and clinical characteristics of anaphylaxis (abstr). J Allergy Clin Immunol 2001; 107:S57.

59. Vander Leek TK, Liu AH, Stefanski K, Blacker B, Bock SA. The natural history of peanut allergy in young children and its association with serum peanut-specific IgE. J Pediatr 2000; 137:749–755.

60. Sampson HA. Utility of food-specific IgE concentrations in predicting symptomatic food allergy. J Allergy Clin Immunol 2001; 107:891–896

61. Horan RF, DuBuske LM, Sheffer AL. Exercise-induced anaphylaxis. Immunol Allergy Clin N Am 2001; 21:769–782.

62. Shadick NA, Liang MH, Partridge AJ, et al. The natural history of exercise-induced anaphylaxis: Survey results from a ten year follow-up study. J Allergy Clin Immunol 1999; 104:123–127.

63. Bacale E, Patterson R, Zeiss CR. Evaluation of severe (anaphylactic) reactions. Clin Allergy 1978; 8:295–304.

64. Abraham D, Grammer L. Idiopathic anaphylaxis. Immunol Allergy Clin N Am 2001; 21:783–794.

65. Stricker WE, Anorve-Lopez E, Reed CE. Food skin testing in patients with idiopathic anaphylaxis. J Allergy Clin Immunol 1986; 77:516–519.

66. Slater JE, Raphael G, Cutler GB, Loriaux DL, Meggs WJ, Kaliner M. Recurrent anaphylaxis in menstruating women: Treatment with a luteinizing hormone-releasing hormone agonist—a preliminary report. Obstet Gyn 1987; 70:542–546.

67. Meggs WJ, Pesconitz OH, Metcalfe D, Loriaux DL, Cutler G Jr, Kaliner M. Progesterone sensitivity as a cause of recurrent anaphylaxis. N Engl J Med 1984; 311:1236–1238.

68. Brazil E, MacNamara AF. Not so immediate hypersensitivity: The danger of biphasic allergic reactions. J Accid Emerg Med 1998; 15:252–253.

69. Douglas DM, Sukenick E, Andrade WP, Brown JS. Biphasic systemic anaphylaxis: An inpatient and outpatient study. J Allergy Clin Immunol 1994; 93:977–985.

70. Sampson HA, Mendelson L, Rosen JP. Fatal and near-fatal anaphylactic reactions to food in children and adolescents. N Engl J Med 1992; 327:380–384.

71. Stark BJ, Sullivan TJ. Biphasic and protracted anaphylaxis. J Allergy Clin Immunol 1986; 78:76–83.

72. Lieberman P, Kemp SF, Nicklas R (contr. eds). Joint Task Force on Practice Parameters. The diagnosis and management of anaphylaxis. J Allergy Clin Immunol 2004 (in press).

73. Cummins RO, Hazinski MR (eds). Guidelines 2000 for cardiopulmonary resuscitation and emergency cardiovascular care: An international consensus on science. American Heart Association in collaboration with the International Liaison Committee on Resuscitation (ILCOR). Part 8: Advanced challenges in resuscitation. Section 3: Special challenges in ECC, Anaphylaxis. Circulation 2000; 102(suppl I):I241–I243.

74. Gompels LL, Bethune C, Johnston SL, Gompels MM. Proposed use of adrenaline (epinephrine) in anaphylaxis and related conditions: A study of senior house officers starting accident and emergency posts. Postgrad Med J 2002; 78:416–418.

75. Barach EM, Nowak RM, Lee TG, Tomanovich MC. Epinephrine for treatment of anaphylactic shock. J Am Med Assoc 1984; 251:2118–2122.

76. Ersoz N, Firestone SC. Adrenaline-induced pulmonary edema and its treatment: A report of two cases. Br J Anesth 1971; 43:709–712.

77. Freedman BJ. Accidental adrenaline overdosage and its treatment with piperoxan. Lancet 1955; 2:575–578.

78. Patterson R, Dykewicz MS, Perry JM. Iatrogenic pseudoanaphylaxis. J Allergy Clin Immunol 1987; 79:24–26.

79. Pumphrey RSH. Lessons for management of anaphylaxis from a study of fatal reactions. Clin Exp Allergy 2000; 30:1144–1150.

80. Cydulka R, Davison R, Grammer L. The use of epinephrine in the treatment of older adult asthmatics. Ann Emerg Med 1988; 17:322–326.

81. Simons FER, Roberts JR, Gu X, Simons KJ. Epinephrine absorption in children with a history of anaphylaxis. J Allergy Clin Immunol 1998; 101:33–37.

82. Simons FER, Gu X, Simons KJ. Epinephrine absorption in adults: Intramuscular versus subcutaneous injection. J Allergy Clin Immunol 2001; 108:871–873.

83. Worobec AS, Metcalfe DD. Systemic anaphylaxis. In: Current Therapy in Allergy, Immunology, and Rheumatology, 5th ed. (Lichtenstein LM, Fauci AS, eds.). St. Louis: Mosby–Year Book, 1996: 170–177.

84. Kiowski W, Frei A. Bolus injection of cimetidine and hypotension in patients in the intensive care unit. Arch Intern Med 1987; 147:153–156.

85. Pollack CV. Utility of glucagon in the emergency department. J Emerg Med 1993; 11:195–205.
86. Sherman MS, Lazar EJ, Eichacker P. A bronchodilator action of glucagon. J Allergy Clin Immunol 1988; 81:908–911.
87. Zaloga GP, Delacey W, Holmboe E, Chemow B. Glucagon reversal of hypertension in a case of anaphylactoid shock. Ann Intern Med 1986; 105:65–66.
88. Toogood JH. Beta-blocker therapy and the risk of anaphylaxis. Can Med Assoc J 1987; 136:929–933.
89. Toogood JH. Risks of anaphylaxis in patients receiving beta-blocker drugs (editorial). J Allergy Clin Immunol 1988; 81:1–5.
90. Salpeter SR, Ormiston TM, Salpeter EE. Cardioselective β-blockers in patients with reactive airway disease: A meta-analysis. Ann Intern Med 2002; 137:715–725.
91. Entman SS, Moise KJ. Anaphylaxis in pregnancy. South Med J 1984; 77:402.
92. Board of Directors, American Academy of Allergy and Immunology. The use of epinephrine in the treatment of anaphylaxis (position statement). J Allergy Clin Immunol 1994; 94:666–668.
93. Grouhi M, Alshehri M, Hummel D, Roifman CM. Anaphylaxis and epinephrine auto-injector training: Who will teach the teachers? J Allergy Clin Immunol 1999; 103:190–193.
94. Sicherer SH, Forman JA, Noone SA. Use assessment of self-administered epinephrine among food-allergic children and pediatricians. Pediatrics 2000; 105:359–362.
95. Gold MS, Sainsbury R. First aid anaphylaxis management in children who were prescribed an epinephrine autoinjector device (EpiPen). J Allergy Clin Immunol 2000; 106:171–176.
96. Goldberg A, Confino-Cohen R. Insect sting-inflicted systemic reactions: Attitudes of patients with insect venom allergy regarding after-sting behavior and proper administration of epinephrine. J Allergy Clin Immunol 2000; 106:1184–1189.
97. Heilborn H, Hjemdahl P, Daleskog M, Adamsson U. Comparison of subcutaneous injection and high-dose inhalation of epinephrine: Implications for self treatment to prevent anaphylaxis. J Allergy Clin Immunol 1986; 78:1174–1179.
98. Simons FER, Gu X, Johnston LM, Simons KJ. Can epinephrine inhalations be substituted for epinephrine injections in children at risk for systemic anaphylaxis? Pediatrics 2000; 106:1040–1044.
99. Hoffman BB, Lefkowitz RJ. Catecholamines, sympathomimetic drugs, and adrenergic receptor antagonists. In: Goodman and Gilman's The Pharmacologic Basis of Therapeutics (Hardman JD, Limbird LE, Molinoff PB, Ruddon RW, Gilman AG, eds.). New York: McGraw-Hill, 1996: 204–209.
100. Kemp SF, Lieberman P. Inhibitors of angiotensin II: Potential hazards for patients at risk for anaphylaxis? Ann Allergy Asthma Immunol 1997; 78:527–529.
101. Sampson HA. Food allergy. Part 2: Diagnosis and management. J Allergy Clin Immunol 1999; 103:981–989.
102. deShazo RD, Kemp SF. Allergic reactions to drugs and biologic agents. J Am Med Assoc 1997; 278:1895–1906.
103. Kemp SF. Anaphylaxis: Current concepts in pathophysiology, diagnosis, and management. Immunol Allergy Clin N Am 2001; 21:611–634.
104. Leung DYM, Sampson IIA, Yunginger JW, Burks AW Jr, Schneider LC, Wortel CH, Davis FM, Hynn JD, Shanahan WR. Effect of anti-IgE in patients with peanut allergy. New Engl J Med 2003; 348:986–993.

41

Instructions and Consent Forms for Allergen Immunotherapy

LINDA COX

*Nova Southeastern University College of Osteopathic Medicine,
Ft. Lauderdale, Florida, U.S.A.*

RICHARD F. LOCKEY

*University of South Florida College of Medicine and James A. Haley
Veterans' Hospital, Tampa, Florida, U.S.A.*

I. INTRODUCTION

The primary objective of allergy skin test and immunotherapy forms is to provide sufficient information about the procedures to allow them to be accurately interpreted by physicians and other health care professionals even when they are in an office other than that of the prescribing physician. The immunotherapy and allergy skin test forms also should be sufficiently detailed to allow all physicians to base treatment decisions on their content.

The recommended information to be included on the forms is outlined in "Guidelines for Reporting Immediate Allergy Skin Test Results" by the American Academy of Allergy, Asthma and Immunology's Immunotherapy Committee (AAAAI ICOM) (1) and in the Joint Task Force on Practice Parameters "Allergen Immunotherapy: A Practice Parameter" (JAIPP) (2). The purpose of these guidelines is to promote objective, scientific, and reproducible documentation of skin testing and immunotherapy and to standardize skin testing and immunotherapy procedures. This chapter reviews these guidelines and recommendations and includes examples of the standard immunotherapy and allergy skin test forms developed by the AAAAI ICOM. The immunotherapy forms are also included in "Allergen Immunotherapy: A Practice Parameter" and are provided as a courtesy of the Joint Task Force on Practice Parameter. The forms integrate the guidelines into editable documents. Also included are examples of consent and instruction forms.

Physicians should obtain these forms and customize them for their practice, maintaining the basic information recommended in the published guidelines. Utilization of these forms will lead to uniformity of allergy skin testing and immunotherapy procedures and will maintain the safe and accurate care of the allergic patient.

II. ALLERGY SKIN TEST FORMS

The use of immediate hypersensitivity (allergy) skin testing as a diagnostic tool in clinical allergy dates back to the late 1800s with the work of Charles Blakely (1820–1900), an English physician who proved, through experiments on himself, that hay fever was due to pollen. During these experiments he discovered that he would elicit a response if he rubbed the pollen into his skin scratches (3). Throughout the one hundred–plus years since its inception, allergy skin testing has continued to be the primary diagnostic tool in patients with allergic diseases and clinical trials of allergen immunotherapy. Until recently there has been very little effort made to ensure that the clinical practice of allergy skin testing is uniform and consistent. As a result there is considerable variability in how allergy skin test results are performed and recorded. This variability can adversely impact care of patients, particularly individuals who may require a transfer of their allergy care. Physicians may have difficulty interpreting allergy skin test results performed in an outside office and recommend that the transferring patient repeat the allergy evaluation. The AAAAI ICOM developed guidelines to provide parameters for allergy skin reporting to help the allergy community move toward a more uniform practice. The goal of these guidelines is to improve the quality of allergy skin testing and reduce undesirable variation by documenting the results in an objective, scientific, and reproducible manner.

The completed allergy skin test form should provide enough information to allow other physicians to understand the type of test and how it was performed. Many variables that can potentially affect allergy skin test results and are included in the skin test form developed by the AAAAI ICOM. These variables include location of the testing site, skin test device, testing technician, patient age, sun damage of the skin, and medications.

These variables can influence interpretation of the allergy skin test results. Therefore, it is important to include details about them on the allergy skin test form.

The key purpose of the allergy skin test report is to convey information about the test results. The skin test results should be recorded in a manner permitting other physicians to readily interpret the patient's positive and negative allergy skin test profile. The two most commonly used methods of reporting allergy skin test results are

> *Quantitative:* Results are reported as measurement in millimeters of the longest diameter of wheal and erythema/flare or the longest plus the widest perpendicular diagonal diameter (orthogonal).
> *Semi-quantitative:* Scoring is 0 to 4+. If this method is utilized, the key to scoring must be included and must be based on measurement of wheal and flare.

One of the limitations of the semi-quantitative scoring method is that it fails to provide specific information about degree of skin test reactivity (i.e., a 4 + could represent a wide range of wheal sizes in many of the currently used scoring systems). There are clinical implications associated with the degree of skin test reactivity that are pertinent to patients on allergen immunotherapy:

1. A high degree is associated with greater risk during immunotherapy (4).
2. The starting dose of immunotherapy may be based on skin test reactivity (4).
3. A change in skin test reactivity with immunotherapy may predict who will not relapse after immunotherapy is discontinued (5).

Recording the allergy skin test results as a measurement of the wheal and erythema in millimeters will provide any physician with precise, reproducible information about the patient's degree of allergen sensitivity.

The skin testing form should contain the following information:

A. Patient and prescribing physician information
   1. Patient name, date of birth, and identifying number (if applicable)
   2. Ordering physician's name, address, and telephone number
   3. Testing date
   4. Last administration of medications, which can interfere with interpretation or increase the risk of skin testing (e.g., antihistamine and beta-blocker)
B. Allergy skin test methods
   1. Skin test technician (ideally, the clinic should have some documented evaluation of the technician's skin test performance)
   2. Location of test (e.g., back or arm)
   3. Type of test (e.g., percutaneous and/or intradermal)
   4. Instrument used (e.g., testing device, needle size, and commercial kit)
   5. Elapsed time between application of tests and reading of tests
   6. Amount injected with intradermal technique
C. Testing materials
   1. Positive and negative controls
   2. Manufacturing company or source of reagent
   3. Common name (scientific name optional)
   4. Concentration used in testing
   5. Dilution and diluent where applicable
   6. Contents, concentrations, and diluents of any mixtures
D. Recording of results
   1. *Quantitative:* The preferred method is to record results as the longest diameter of wheal and erythema/flare in millimeters *or* to record both the longest diameter of wheal and erythema/flare and the widest perpendicular diagonal diameter (orthogonal) (Fig. 1).
   2. *Semi-quantitative:* Results are recorded using a numerical scale from 0 through 4+. This method is *not preferred* because it is variable and lacks precision. If this method is used, each score must include a measure of wheal and flare/erythema in millimeters.

The forms in Figs. 2 and 3 were developed by the AAAAI ICOM and include the information recommended in its earlier published guidelines. Figure 2 is an example of an allergy skin test form, and Fig. 3 represents an example of a completed allergy skin test form. It includes the 30 allergens that have been designated by a subcommittee of the AAAAI ICOM assigned to identify key allergens in North America to be prioritized for

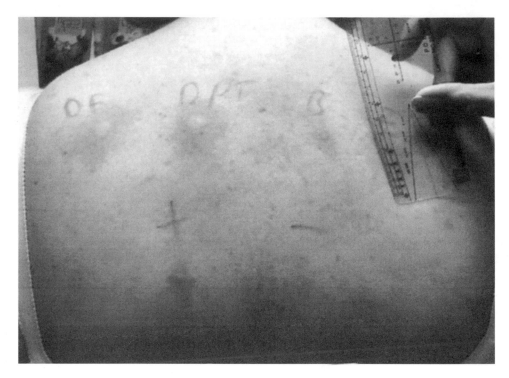

Figure 1 Reporting allergy skin test results as a measurement in millimeters of the longest diameter of the wheal and flare/erythema. (Provided with permission from Dr. Linda Cox.)

standardization. It also contains additional allergens, previously standardized, which are likely to be included in all skin test forms regardless of geographic location.

III. ALLERGY VACCINE PRESCRIPTION FORMS

The immunotherapy prescription form should provide specific information about the contents of the allergy vaccine. Precise details are necessary for any other physician or health care professional to replicate the prescription without significant variation from the previous vaccine aside from known differences of lots and manufacturers. The allergy vaccines differ when there are changes in the constituents of the vaccines, including the diluent, manufacturer, and extract type (aqueous vs. glycerinated) (2). The allergy vaccine label is important and should contain sufficient details to allow physicians, other health care professionals, and the patient to recognize for whom the vaccine is indicated as well as pertinent information about its content. The JAIPP has proposed a nomenclature system for allergy vaccine dilutions. Uniform adoption of this system should reduce errors in administration of allergy vaccines, particularly outside of the prescribing physician's office.

Immunotherapy prescription forms should contain the following information:

A. Patient information
    1   Patient name, patient number (if applicable), birth date, telephone number, and photo (optional but helpful)

Practice name Ordering physician:		
Street address	City	State	Zip
Telephone	Fax	

Patient name: _____ Date of birth: __/__/__ Patient number: _____

Testing Technician: _____

Last use of antihistamine (or other med affecting response to histamine): ___ days

Testing Date (s) and Time: Percutaneous __/__/__   AM PM Intradermal __/__/__   AM PM

1) General information about skin test protocol

    1. **Percutaneous** reported as: **Allergen: Testing concentration: Extract company** (*see below)

        Location: back___ arm___ **Device:** _____

    2. **Intradermal:** 0.___ml injected, **Location:** arm **Testing concentration:** 1:____ w/v or BAU or AU/ml, PNU

    3. **Results** Longest diameter **or** longest diameter and orthogonal diameter (perpendicular diameters) of wheal (W) and erythema (flare) (F) measured in millimeters at 15 minutes

        Blank in results column indicates test was not performed, 0=negative

* Extract manufacturer abbreviations: G=Greer, AL=Allergy Labs, Ohio, LO Allergy Labs, Oklahoma, AK=ALK, HS=Hollister–Stier, C=Center, NE=Nelco, AM=Allermed

Allergen: Concentration: Extract Manufacturer. *	Percutaneous W (mm) F	Intradermal W (mm) F	Allergen: Concentration: Extract Manufacturer. *	Percutaneous W (mm) F	Intradermal W (mm) F
			Controls		
			Percutaneous		
			Negative:		
			Positive:		
			Intradermal		
			Negative		
			Positive:		

Comments:

Figure 2 Allergy skin test form. (Provided with permission of the AAAAI.)

    B. Preparation information
        1. Name and signature of person preparing the vaccine
        2. Date of preparation
        3. Vial name (e.g., trees, grasses). If abbreviations are used, a legend should be included to describe meaning of the abbreviations.
    C. Vaccine content information. The following information for each allergen should be included on the form in a separate column:
        1. Content of the vaccine, including common name or genus and species of individual allergens and detail of all mixes

Dr. Ah Choo, M.D.
Address: 665 Rosebud Lane
Hollywood, Fl. 33424
Telephone: 645-123-4444 Fax: 645-123-4567

Patient name: Jerry Cleanex   Date of birth: 05/05/90   Patient number: 23456
Testing Technician: Mary Lancet
Last use of antihistamine (or other med affecting response to histamine): 10 days ago   medication _____
Testing Date (s) and Time: Percutaneous 5/30/02__10:30_AM   Intradermal 6/2/02 11:15 AM

General information about skin test protocol
1. **Percutaneous** reported as: **Allergen: Testing concentration: Extract company** (*see below)
   Location: back_X__arm___   Device: HS Quintip_____
2. **Intradermal**: 0.02ml injected, **Location**: arm **Testing concentration**: 1:500 w/v, 100 BAU or AU/ml, 400 PNU
3. **Results** Longest diameter (*Left in this example*) **or** longest diameter and orthogonal diameter (*Right in this example*) of wheal (W) and erythema (flare) (F) measured in millimeters at 15 minutes
   Blank in results column indicates test was not performed, O=negative
   * Extract manufacturer abbreviations: G=Greer, AL= Allergy Labs (Oklahoma), AK=ALK Abello, AD=ALK (Denmark), H=Hollister–Stier, AG=Antigen, N=Nelco, AM=Allermed

Allergen: Concentration: Extract Manufacturer. *	Percutaneous W (mm) F		Intradermal W (mm) F		Allergen: Concentration: Extract Manufacturer. *	Percutaneous W (mm) F		Intradermal W (mm) F	
Trees					**Weeds**				
Ulmaceae					*Composite family*				
1. American Elm 1:20 G	0	0			21. Mugwort 10,000 PNU AD	4/6	18/15		
Cupressaceae					22. Short Ragweed 1:10 H	10/6	20/20		
2. Mountain Cedar 1:10 AL	0	0			*Chenopod*				
Betulaceae					23. Russian Thistle 1:20 AG	3/7	10/15		
3. Paper Birch 1:20 AK	3	15			24. Burning Bush 20,000 PNU N	4/6	15/20		
4. Red Alder 1:20 AD	3	10			25. Lamb's Quarter 1:40 AM	6/10	15/20		
Fagaceae					*Amaranth*				
5. White Oak 1:10 H	0	0	10	20	26. Red Root Pigweed G	8/10	20/30		
6. Red Oak 1:10 AG	5	15			*Plantaginaceae*				
Aceraceae					27. English Plantain AK	10/9	20/18		
7. Box Elder 1:20 N	0	0			**Molds/Fungi**				
Oleaceae					28. Alternaria alternata AD	10/9	20/18		
8. White Ash 1:20 AM	0	0			29. Cladosporium herbarum H	0	0	15/18	25/20
9. Olive 1:20 G	5	20			30. Cladosporium cladosporioides AG	0	0	18/22	30/35
Salicaciae					31. Penicillium chrysogenum N	4/5	15/10		
10. Cottonwood Eastern 1.40 AL	6	25			32. Aspergillus fumigatus AM	5/7	20/16		
Moraceae					33. Epicoccum nigrum G	0	0		
11. Mulberry 1:20 AK	7	30			34. Helminthosporium solani AL	0	0		
Juglandaceae									
12. Pecan 1:20 AD	0	0			**Animals/Mites /Cockroach/Others**				
13. Black Walnut 1:20 H	0	0			35. D. Pteronyssinus AK	20/30	40/30		
Plantaceae					36. D. Farinae AD	15/9	32/40		
14. Sycamore 1:40 AG	0	0			37. American Cockroach H	5/6	12/10		
					38. German Cockroach AG	7	18		
Grasses					39. Cat Epithelium N	15	30		
15. Bahia 1:20 N	20	40			40. Dog Epithelium 1:20 AM	0	0	15	25
16. Bermuda 10,000 BAU/ml AM	15	35			**Controls**				
17. Sweet Vernal 1:20 G	25	40			**Percutaneous**				
18. Timothy 100,000BAU/ml AL	30	45			**Negative:** 50% glycerine-saline G	0	0		
19. Johnson 1:10 AK	15	30			**Positive:** Histamine 1mg/ml AL	5/7	20/15		
Weeds					**Intradermal**				
Polygonaceae					**Negative:** 0.05 % glycerine-saline AK			0	7/8
20. Sheep sorrel 1:10 H	4/9	15/12			**Positive:** Histamine 1mg/ml AD			15/20	25/15

Comments:

Figure 3 Example of a completed allergy skin test form. (Provided with permission of Linda Cox, M.D.)

2. Concentration of available manufacturer's extract
3. Volume of manufacturer's extract to add to achieve a selected volume of the projected effective concentration. This can be calculated by dividing the projected effective concentration by the concentration of available manufacturer's extract and multiplying the result by the selected volume. [*Example:* Cat: The recommended maintenance dose for cat is 2000–3000 BAU. To deliver 2000 BAU in a 0.5-ml maintenance injection: 4000 BAU/ml (projected effective concentration) ÷ 10,000 BAU/ml (available

manufacturer's extract concentration) $\times$ 5 cc (selected volume) = 2.00 ml (amount needed to be added to 5-ml vial).]

4. The type of diluent (if used)
5. Extract/vaccine manufacturer
6. Lot number
7. Expiration date, which should not exceed the expiration date of any of the individual components

The AAAAI ICOM developed three forms for immunotherapy prescription writing. These forms can also be found in "Allergen Immunotherapy: A Practice Parameter." One form (Fig. 4) is utilized primarily for the build-up phase of immunotherapy because it includes a section to document subsequent dilutions from the maintenance concentration. The second form (Fig. 5) does not include this section and can be used for the maintenance phase of immunotherapy treatment. The third form (Fig. 6) can be used to document the components of any mixes used in the immunotherapy vaccine and would accompany the primary immunotherapy prescription. Figure 7 is an example of a completed immunotherapy prescription form.

Table 1 presents proposed methods for labeling allergy vaccine dilutions, based on the system proposed by the JAIPP, "Allergen Immunotherapy: A Practice Parameter" (2). Figures 8 and 9 show examples utilizing the proposed labeling system.

IV. IMMUNOTHERAPY ADMINISTRATION FORMS

The fundamental purpose of the immunotherapy administration form is to provide enough information to enable physicians and other health care personal to understand exactly what was administered previously and to furnish a detailed representation of the patient's immunotherapy history, including

1. A record of any systemic reactions and treatment administered
2. Other adverse reactions encountered during immunotherapy (such as large local reactions, bruises, or sore arm)

Several risk factors for immunotherapy have been identified, including presence of symptomatic asthma, high degree of hypersensitivity, use of beta-blockers, dosing errors, and injections giving during periods of exacerbation of symptoms (4). With the exception of dosing errors and high degree of hypersensitivity, these risk factors can be minimized by performing a pre-injection health screen prior the administration of the allergy vaccine. This pre-injection evaluation may include a peak flow measurement for asthmatic patients and a health inquiry administered verbally or as a written questionnaire directed to determine if there were any recent health changes that may require modifying that patient's immunotherapy treatment (e.g., the addition of a beta-blocker medication to treat hypertension). The immunotherapy administration form is used to document an evaluation of the patient's health status prior to administering the allergy vaccine. The form was created by the AAAAI ICOM and is based on the recommendations of the JAIPP. The information recommended on an immunotherapy administration form is summarized below.

    A. Patient information

        1. Patient name, date of birth, telephone number, patient photo (optional but helpful).

Patient Name:	Prescribing Physician:
Patient Number:	Address:
Birth Date:	
Telephone:	Telephone:
	Fax:

Vaccine Name:

Bottle Name Abbreviations

Tree: T	Mold: M
Grass: G	Cat: C
Weed: W	Dog: D
Ragweed: R	Cockroach: Cr
Mixture: Mx	Dust Mite: Dm

Maintenance Concentrate Prescription Form

Prepared by: _____ **Date Prepared:**__/__/__

Dates of subsequent dilutions from maintenance concentration with expiration dates

Vial _____ from Vial _____ on __/__/__ Expiration date: __/__/__
Vial _____ from Vial _____ on __/__/__ Expiration date: __/__/__
Vial _____ from Vial _____ on __/__/__ Expiration date: __/__/__
Vial _____ from Vial _____ on __/__/__ Expiration date: __/__/__

Antigen Number	Extract Name Allergen or Diluent (Common name or Genus/species)*	Concentration and Type Manufacturer's Extract (AU, BAU, W/V, PNU)/ (50% G, Aq, Ly, AP)	Volume of Manufacturer's Extract to Add	Extract Manufacturer	Lot Number	Expiration Date
1						
2						
3						
4						
5						
6						
7						
8						
9						
10						
Diluent						
Total Volume						

* Components of mixes listed on a separate sheet

Specific Instructions:

$$\text{Volume to add} = \frac{\text{Maintenance Concentration}}{\text{Conc. Of Manufacturer's Extract}} \times \text{Total volume}$$

_____

_____

_____

_____

Maintenance concentration and subsequent dilutions reported as volume/volume (v/v) dilutions with maintenance concentration=1:1 v/v

_____ ___/___/___
Prescribing Physician Signature   Date
Patient Consent Form Signed   ___/___/___
                                                       Date

BAU = Bioeqivalent Allergy Unit, AU =Allergy Unit
PNU=Protein Nitrogen Unit
W/V=Weight per Volume Ratio
G= 50 % Glycerinated
Aq=Aqueous, Ly=Lyophilized
AP= Alum precipitated

Figure 4   Immunotherapy prescription form for build-up phase. (Provided with permission of the AAAAI.)

B.   Vaccine information
1.   Vaccine name and dilution from maintenance concentrate in volume per volume (Table 1), vial letter (e.g., A, B), and color or number if used.
2.   Expiration date of all dilutions.

Patient Name:		Prescribing Physician:
Patient Number:		Address:
Birth Date:		
Telephone:		Telephone:
		Fax:

Vaccine Name:	**Maintenance Concentrate Prescription Form**

Bottle Name Abbreviations

Tree: T	Mold: M
Grass: G	Cat: C
Weed: W	Dog: D
Ragweed: R	Cockroach: Cr
Mixture: Mx	Dust Mite: Dm

Prepared by: _____ **Date Prepared:** __/__/__

Antigen Number	Extract Name Allergen or Diluent (*Genus,species* or Common name)*	Concentration and Type Manufacturer's Extract (AU, BAU, W/V, PNU)/ (50% G, Aq, Ly, AP)	Volume of Manufacturer's Extract to Add	Extract Manufacturer	Lot Number	Expiration Date
1						
2						
3						
4						
5						
6						
7						
8						
9						
10						
Diluent						
Total Volume						

* Components of mixes listed on a separate sheet

Specific Instructions:

$$\text{Volume to add} = \frac{\text{Maintenance Concentration}}{\text{Conc. Of Manufacturer's Extract}} \times \text{Total volume}$$

Maintenance concentration and subsequent dilutions reported as volume/volume (v/v) dilutions with maintenance concentration=1:1 v/v

_____

_____

_____

_____

_____ __/__/__
Prescribing Physician Signature Date
Patient Consent Form Signed __/__/__
 Date

BAU = Bioeqivalent Allergy Unit, AU =Allergy Unit
PNU=Protein Nitrogen Unit
W/V=Weight per Volume Ratio
50%G= 50 % Glycerinated
Aq=Aqueous, Ly=Lyophilized
AP= Alum precipitated

Figure 5 Maintenance immunotherapy prescription form. (Provided with permission of the AAAAI.)

 C. Administration information in separate columns
  1. Date of injection.
  2. Patient's health prior to injection. This is obtained via a verbal or written interview of the patient prior to administering the immunotherapy injection. The patient is questioned about increased asthma or allergy symptoms, beta-blocker use, change in health status (including pregnancy), or an

| Practice name |
| Address: |
| Telephone Number   Fax Number |

Immunotherapy Mix Components

Patient Name:_____

Name of Mix:

Extract Name Allergen or Diluent (Common name or *Genus/species*)*	Concentration and Type Manufacturer's Extract (AU, BAU, W/V, PNU)/ (50% G, Aq, Ly, AP)	Volume of Manufacturer's Extract Added	Extract Manufacturer	Lot Number	Expiration Date
			Total:			

| Date Mix Prepared (if mix prepared in the office): __/__/__ |
| Prepared by:_____ |

| BAU = Bioeqivalent Allergy Unit, AU =Allergy Unit |
| PNU=Protein Nitrogen Unit |
| W/V=Weight per Volume Ratio |
| 50%G= 50 % Glycerinated |
| Aq=Aqueous, Ly=Lyophilized |
| AP= Alum precipitated |

Figure 6   Immunotherapy mix components form. (Provided with permission of the AAAAI.)

adverse reaction to previous injection (including delayed large local reactions). Patients with a significant systemic illness usually should not receive an allergy injection.

3. Antihistamine use. It is unclear if an antihistamine prior to an immunotherapy injection decreases the systemic reaction rate. The JAIPP suggests noting if the patient is taking an antihistamine in order to consistently interpret reactions. It may also be desirable for a patient to either take or not

Patient Name: Jerry Cleanex
Patient Number: 23456
Birth Date: 05/05/90
Telephone: 645-345-0987

Prescribing Physician: Dr. Ah Choo
Address: 665 Rosebud Lane
Hollywood, Fl. 33424
Telephone: 645-123-4444
Fax: 645-123-4567

Vaccine Name: C, R, G, T, W

Bottle Name Abbreviations	
Tree: T	Mold: M
Grass: G	Cat: C
Weed: W	Dog: D
Ragweed: R	Cockroach: Cr
Mixture: Mx	Dust Mite: Dm

Maintenance Concentrate Prescription Form

Prepared by: Mary Lancet   Date Prepared: 6/10/02

Dates of subsequent dilutions from maintenance concentration with expiration dates
Vial **4** from Vial **1** on **8/30/02** Expiration date: **10/15/02**
Vial ____ from Vial ____ on _/_/_ Expiration date: _/_/_
Vial ____ from Vial ____ on _/_/_ Expiration date: _/_/_
Vial ____ from Vial ____ on / / Expiration date: / /

Antigen Number	Extract Name Allergen or Diluent (Common name or Genus/species)*	Concentration and Type Manufacturer's Extract (AU, BAU, W/V, PNU)/ (50% G, Aq, Ly, AP)	Volume of Manufacturer's Extract to Add**	Extract Manufacturer	Lot Number	Expiration Date
1	Short ragweed	1:20 w/v G (150 Amb a1)	0.5ml	Greer	12345	1/01/03
2	Amaranthus Retroflexus	1:10 w/v G	0.5ml	H-S	6789	2/07/03
3	Ash	1:10 w/v G	0.5ml	Center	3333	3/17/03
4	Cat	10,000 BAU/ml G	2.00ml	ALO	9898	2/27/03
5	Timothy grass	100,000 BAU/ml G	0.4ml	ALK	56789	7/09/03
6	Johnson grass	1:10 w/v G	0.5ml	Greer	2434	7/20/03
7						
8						
9						
10						
Diluent	HSA		0.6ml	ALK	68597	12/03
Total Volume			5.00 ml			1/01/03

* Components of mixes listed on a separate sheet
** Assumes 0.5 ml injection as target maintenance dose

$$\text{Volume to add} = \frac{\text{Maintenance Concentration}}{\text{Conc. Of Manufacturer's Extract}} \times \text{Total volume}$$

Specific Instructions:

Ah Choo M.D   6/8/02
Prescribing Physician Signature Date
Patient Consent Form Signed   x   5/24/02
                                       Date

Maintenance concentration and subsequent dilutions reported as volume/volume (v/v) dilutions with maintenance concentration=1:1 v/v

BAU = Bioeqivalent Allergy Unit, AU =Allergy Unit
PNU=Protein Nitrogen Unit
W/V=Weight per Volume Ratio
G= 50 % Glycerinated
Aq=Aqueous, Ly=Lyophilized
AP= Alum precipitated

Figure 7 Example of a completed immunotherapy prescription. (Provided with permission of the AAAAI.)

take an antihistamine *consistently* on the day of the injection. The immunotherapy administration form is a means by which antihistamine use is documented and reflects specific instructions from the treating physician about an antihistamine on injections days.

4. Peak flow reading: Symptomatic asthma is a risk factor for immunotherapy (4). Obtaining a peak flow measurement prior to the immunotherapy injection may help screen patients with active asthma who should not receive their

Table 1   Proposed Labeling of Dilutions of Vaccine

Dilution from maintenance concentrate	V/V label[a]	Number[b]	Color
Maintenance concentrate	1:1	1	Red
10-fold	1:10	2	Yellow
100-fold	1:100	3	Blue
1000-fold	1:1000	4	Green
10,000-fold	1:10,000	5	Silver

[a] V/V refers to volume per volume dilution, with 1:1 being the maintenance concentrate and subsequent dilutions based on the maintenance concentrate.
[b] It is recommended that the numbering system begin with the highest concentration, the maintenance concentrate. This will provide consistency in labeling in the event further dilutions are needed.
Provided with permission from the JAIPP.

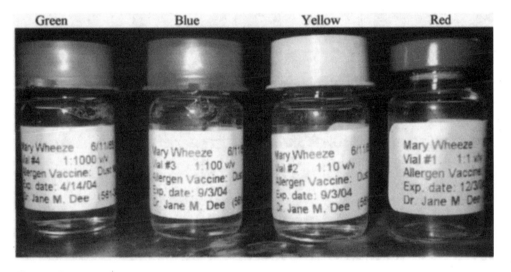

Figure 8   Color-coded labeled allergy vaccine with dilutions from maintenance concentrate. (Provided with permission from Linda Cox, M.D.)

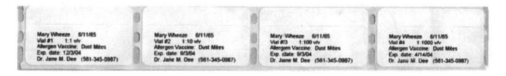

Figure 9   Examples of completed allergy vaccine labels utilizing the Joint Task Force on Practice Parameters' "Allergen Immunotherapy: A Practice Parameter" proposed nomenclature system for vaccine dilutions. (Provided with permission from Linda Cox, M.D.)

immunotherapy injection on that day. The form should provide the patient's best peak flow baseline as a reference, and the health care professional giving the injection should be provided with specific guidelines about the degree of diminished peak flow for which an injection should be withheld.

5. Baseline blood pressure. It is desirable to record the patient's baseline blood pressure for future reference.
6. Arm administered. Noting into which arm each vaccine is injected facilitates identification of the cause of a large local reaction and thus which vaccine should be modified.
7. Projected build-up schedule.
8. Delivered volume reported in milliliters.
9. Injection reaction. The details of any treatment given in response to either a systemic or large reaction should be documented on the health screen (second page of the administration form) or elsewhere in medical record and referenced on the administration form.

The initials of the individual who gives the injection should be included. The immunotherapy administration form was developed as a two-part form (Figs. 10 and 11) and are included in the JAIPP. Figure 10 is used to document the pre-injection screening and allergy immunotherapy injection administration for up to two vaccines. A modification of this form with columns for three vaccines is available but not included here. The second page is used to note the results of the pre-injection screen, including any delayed immunotherapy reactions or immediate systemic reactions. Figures 12 and 13 are the pre-immunotherapy injection questionnaire and the systemic reaction reporting forms (developed by the AAAAI Immunotherapy and Anaphylaxis Committee).

V. IMMUNOTHERAPY INSTRUCTION AND CONSENT FORMS

There are two types of instruction forms pertinent to immunotherapy treatment. One form is designed to instruct physicians and other health care professionals from offices outside the prescribing allergist's office if the patient transfers his or her immunotherapy treatment. The other is directed at the patient or patient's guardian. If a patient's immunotherapy treatment is transferred from one physician to another, there is an added risk of a systemic reaction because of the multiple variables that change because of this transfer. Changes in the vaccine components, such as the extract manufacturer, may be one reason for the added risk following transfer of immunotherapy treatment. Additional risk may come from staff unfamiliar with the prescribing allergist's immunotherapy schedule, the allergy vaccine vial color coding, and the nomenclature system. Therefore, it is important that immunotherapy transfer forms provide clear, specific instructions and information. When such documentation is provided and there is no change in the allergy vaccine components or immunotherapy schedule, the risk of a systemic reaction from transfer of care is minimized (2).

It is important to provide patients with information about immunotherapy prior to starting it. Compliance with immunotherapy treatment is historically poor, but should improve by enhancing the patient's understanding of the immunotherapy process (6,7). A study of patients receiving allergen immunotherapy ($n = 134$ patients, mean age 30 ± 13 with male to female ratio of 1:2 and mean duration of immunotherapy 30 ± 60 months) demonstrates that a substantial number of patients have poor knowledge, many misconceptions, and unfounded expectations concerning various important aspects of immunotherapy (8). Immunotherapy patients should be familiar with the potential risks involved and the time commitment necessary to receive such therapy. They should also have an understanding of the time necessary before they will begin to improve.

Immunotherapy Vaccine Administration Form

Patient Name: Patient Number: Telephone Number:	Date of Birth: Diagnosis:	Prescribing Physician: Address: Telephone:		Fax:

Dilution Color	1:10,000 (v/v) Silver	1:1000 (v/v) Green	1:100 (v/v) Blue	1:10 (v/v) Yellow	Maintenance 1:1 (v/v) Red	Vaccine Name Abbreviations*
Vial number	5	4	3	2	1	Tree: T Mold: M
Expiration date(s)	__/__/__	__/__/__	__/__/__	__/__/__	__/__/__	Grass: G Cat: C Weed: W Dog: D Ragweed: R Cockroach: Cr Mixture: Mx Dust Mite: Dm

Best Baseline Peak Flow: _____
Baseline Blood pressure: _____

Vaccine A: *vaccine contents*＊   Vaccine B: _____

	Date	Time	Health screen abnormal[1]	Anti-histamine taken?[2]	Peak Flow	Arm	Vial Number or Dilution	Delivered Volume	Reaction[3]	Arm	Vial Number or Dilution	Delivered Volume	Reaction	Injector Initials
1.	__/__/__		Y N	Y N	_____	R L				R L				
2.	__/__/__		Y N	Y N	_____	R L				R L				
3.	__/__/__		Y N	Y N	_____	R L				R L				
4.	__/__/__		Y N	Y N	_____	R L				R L				
5.	__/__/__		Y N	Y N	_____	R L				R L				
6.	__/__/__		Y N	Y N	_____	R L				R L				
7.	__/__/__		Y N	Y N	_____	R L				R L				
8.	__/__/__		Y N	Y N	_____	R L				R L				
9.	__/__/__		Y N	Y N	_____	R L				R L				
10.	__/__/__		Y N	Y N	_____	R L				R L				
11.	__/__/__		Y N	Y N	_____	R L				R L				
12.	__/__/__		Y N	Y N	_____	R L				R L				
13.	__/__/__		Y N	Y N	_____	R L				R L				
14.	__/__/__		Y N	Y N	_____	R L				R L				
15.	__/__/__		Y N	Y N	_____	R L				R L				
16.	__/__/__		Y N	Y N	_____	R L				R L				
17.	__/__/__		Y N	Y N	_____	R L				R L				
18.	__/__/__		Y N	Y N	_____	R L				R L				
19.	__/__/__		Y N	Y N	_____	R L				R L				
20.	__/__/__		Y N	Y N	_____	R L				R L				
21.	__/__/__		Y N	Y N	_____	R L				R L				
22.	__/__/__		Y N	Y N	_____	R L				R L				
23.	__/__/__		Y N	Y N	_____	R L				R L				
24.	__/__/__		Y N	Y N	_____	R L				R L				

1. **Health screen** *refers to either a written or verbal interview of the patient prior to the administration of the allergy injection regarding: the presence of increased allergy or asthma symptoms or symptoms of respiratory tract infection, beta-blocker use, change in health status (including pregnancy) or adverse reaction to previous injection. A* **yes** *answer to this health screen may require further evaluation (see health screen record on back page).*

2. **Antihistamine use:** *to improve consistency in interpretation of reactions it should be noted if the patient has taken an antihistamine on injection days. Physician may also request that an* **antihistamine be taken consistently on injection days: recommended: Y N**

3. **Reaction**: *refers to either immediate or delayed systemic or local reactions. Local reactions (noted as LR) can be reported in millimeters as the longest diameter of wheal and erythema.. The details of the symptoms and treatment of a* **systemic reaction** *(noted as SR) would be recorded elsewhere in the medical record. Guidelines for dose reduction after a systemic reaction on a separate instruction sheet.*

Injector signature	Initials	Projected Build-up Schedule				
		Vial 5	Vial 4	Vial 3	Vial 2	Vial 1

Figure 10   Immunotherapy administration form. (Provided with permission of the AAAAI.)

Instruction forms for physicians supervising immunotherapy prescribed by another physician should contain the following information:

1. Detailed documentation of the patient's previous immunotherapy treatment, including specific information about the components of the immunotherapy vaccine, details of any adverse reaction to immunotherapy, schedule, and allergy skin test results

Patient name:_____ Date of birth:_____ Patient number_____

Health Screen Record

1. Date of immunotherapy injection visit: __/__/__
Patient's response to pre-injection screening questions: _____
_____
Staff action taken (if any): _____

2. Date of immunotherapy injection visit: __/__/__
Patient's response to pre-injection screening questions: _____
_____
Staff action taken (if any): _____

3. Date of immunotherapy injection visit: __/__/__
Patient's response to pre-injection screening questions: _____
_____
Staff action taken (if any): _____

4. Date of immunotherapy injection visit: __/__/__
Patient's response to pre-injection screening questions: _____
_____
Staff action taken (if any): _____

5. Date of immunotherapy injection visit: __/__/__
Patient's response to pre-injection screening questions: _____
_____
Staff action taken (if any): _____

6. Date of immunotherapy injection visit: __/__/__
Patient's response to pre-injection screening questions: _____
_____
Staff action taken (if any): _____

7.Date of immunotherapy injection visit: __/__/__
Patient's response to pre-injection screening questions: _____
_____
Staff action taken (if any): _____

8.Date of immunotherapy injection visit: __/__/__
Patient's response to pre-injection screening questions: _____
_____
Staff action taken (if any): _____

9.Date of immunotherapy injection visit: __/__/__
Patient's response to pre-injection screening questions: _____
_____
Staff action taken (if any) : _____

10. Date of immunotherapy injection visit: __/__/__
Patient's response to pre-injection screening questions: _____
_____
Staff action taken (if any): _____

11. Date of immunotherapy injection visit: __/__/__
Patient's response to pre-injection screening questions: _____
_____
Staff action taken (if any): _____

12. Date of immunotherapy injection visit: __/__/__
Patient's response to pre-injection screening questions: _____
_____
Staff action taken (if any): _____

Figure 11   Health screen record. (Provided with permission of the AAAAI.)

2.   Specific instructions for administering immunotherapy and treatment of large local and systemic reactions

3.   Guidelines for dosage adjustments for unexpected gaps in immunotherapy injections and systemic reactions

Instructions for patients beginning immunotherapy should provide the following information:

Immunotherapy Pre-Injection Questionnaire

Patient Name:_____ Date:_____

This questionnaire is designed to optimize safety precautions already in place for your allergen immunotherapy injection (s) (allergy shot). Please review and answer the following questions. The nursing staff will review your responses and notify your physician if they have any questions or concerns whether you should receive your injection(s) today. **If you are pregnant or have been diagnosed with a new medical condition, please notify the staff.** (Please circle the appropriate answer.)

1. Have you had increased asthma symptoms (chest tightness, increased cough, wheezing, or

   felt short of breath) in the past week?   **Yes   No**

2. Have you had a marked increase in allergy symptoms (itching eyes or nose, sneezing, runny

   nose, post-nasal drip, or throat-clearing) in the past week?   **Yes   No**

3. Do you have a cold, respiratory tract infection, or flu-like symptoms?   **Yes   No**

4. Did you have any problems such as increased allergy or asthma symptoms, hives, or

   generalized itching within 12 hours of receiving your last injection or swelling that persisted

   into the next day?   **Yes   No**

5. Are you on any new medications? Any new eye drops? Please specify._____

Staff intervention/office visit:

_____

_____

_____

Figure 12   Pre-immunotherapy health screen form. (Provided with permission of the AAAAI.)

1.   Description of what immunotherapy treatment involves and what alternative treatments are available
2.   Potential benefits to be expected from the treatment and the expecting timing of these benefits
3.   Potential risks of immunotherapy, including the remote possibility of death
4.   Costs associated with immunotherapy and who pays for it
5.   The anticipated duration of treatment
6.   Any specific office policies regarding immunotherapy, such as acute illnesses and deferment of immunotherapy injections

VI.   TRANSFER OF ALLERGY IMMUNOTHERAPY INSTRUCTION FORMS

Figure 14 represents a letter to the physician who will be supervising immunotherapy outside of the prescribing allergist's office. Figure 15 represents a letter to a patient who will receive immunotherapy in an outside office. Figure 16 is a consent form for the patient to sign if he or she is receiving immunotherapy outside of the prescribing allergist's office. Figure 17 represents a patient allergy skin test consent and information sheet with a list of medications to avoid prior to testing. Figure 18 is a patient immunotherapy information sheet. Figure 19 is a patient immunotherapy consent form. Figure 20 presents guidelines for administration of immunotherapy.

Allergen Immunotherapy Systemic Reation/Anaphylaxis Treatment Record

Name:_____ Date_____
Date of Birth_____ Prescribing Physician_____
Allergens: Tree-Grass-Weed-Mites-Cockroach-Animal Dander-Mold-Hymenoptera
Prior systemic rxn:_____ Hx of asthma?_____
Date/time of injection:_____ Date/time of rxn:_____
Dilution (Vial #): _____ New? Yes No
History of the systemic reaction (SR):
Immediate measures:
__Assess airway, breathing, circulation, and orientation
__Epinephrine IM into arm, thigh, or IV
__Activate EMS (call 911 or local rescue squad) Y/N Time called:_____AM/PM
__Management algorithm reviewed (as needed)

Signs & Symptoms:

Respiratory:	Skin :	Eye/Nasal:	Vascular	Other:
Shortness of breath	Hives	Runny nose	Hypotension	Difficulty swallowing
Wheezing	Angioedema	Red eyes	Chest discomfort	Abdominal pain, nausea, diarrhea
Cough	Generalized itch	Congestion	Dizziness	Diaphoresis
Stridor	Flushing	Sneezing	Headache	

Time	Resp. rate/ PEFR	Pulse/ O2 Saturation	BP	Intervention, Medications. Exam Comments

Time (AM/PM)/ Condition upon release:_____
Patient instructions:_____
Follow-up call to patient: Time_____ Comments:_____
Clinical impression: True SR   Questionable SR   No SR
Comments:_____
_____
_____

Dosage adjustment?: _____
Signatures_____ RN _____MD/DO

Figure 13   Systemic reation reporting form. (Provided with permission of the AAAAI.)

Figure 14 Letter to physician supervising immunotherapy from an outside office.

Dr. Ah Choo
Address: 665 Rosebud Lane
Hollywood, Fl. 33424
Telephone: 645-123-4444
Fax: 645-123-4567
Certified by the American Board of Allergy and Immunology

Re: Jerry Cleanex's Allergen Immunotherapy

Dear Supervising Physician:

Jerry Cleanex will receive his allergen immunotherapy injections in your office/clinic.   We are requesting that a physician sign the attached form and return it to our office so that we know that you are aware that this patient is receiving her immunotherapy under your supervision.

We appreciate your assistance and cooperation in this matter and look forward to hearing from you in the near future.

Sincerely,

Ah Choo, M.D.

I have reviewed the attached allergen immunotherapy instruction form and hereby give permission for _____ to receive his allergy immunotherapy injections in my office under my supervision.

Name and Address of physician:
_____   _____
                                      Physician's signature   Date:

_____

_____   _____
                                      Patient's signature   Date

Enclosure: Position Statement on: Administration of immunotherapy outside of the prescribing allergist facility *Drug and Anaphylaxis Committee of ACAAI. Ann Allergy Asthma and Immunol 1998;81: 101-102*
The readers can obtain copies of this document through the American College of Allergy, Asthma and Immunology website www. ACAAI.org and click on the link to the practice resource center or go to the direct address at: http://www.acaai.org/position_statement.html
Modified with permission of Dr. Richard Lockey, M.D.

Figure 14   Letter to physician supervising immunotherapy from an outside office. (Provided with permission from Division of Allergy and Immunology, Department of Internal Medicine, University of South Florida College of Medicine, Tampa, Florida.)

Dr. Ah Choo
Address: 665 Rosebud Lane
Hollywood, Fl. 33424
Telephone: 645-123-4444 Fax: 645-123-4567
Certified by the American Board of Allergy and Immunology

RE: Receiving allergy injections outside of Dr. Ah Choo's office

Dear

We understand that you will receive your allergy injections outside of this office at another health care facility. For your continued safety and well-being, we want to make sure that you are fully aware of several important issues about allergy shots. To do so, I have enclosed a copy of the American College of Allergy Asthma and Immunology 's position statement on this issue for your information.

Allergy injections, when appropriately administered, effectively alleviate symptoms caused by allergic diseases, such as hay fever, eye symptoms, allergic asthma, and insect allergy. However, as is true with any form of treatment, there are potential side effects. By injecting allergic patients with the very things to which they are allergic, it is possible to cause an allergic reaction. Some of the symptoms of such a reaction can include shortness of breath, hives, drop in blood pressure, and even loss of consciousness. Very rarely, these reactions can be life-threatening and result in death.

It is for these reasons that patients are not permitted to receive their allergy injections at home. Also; the physician supervising your allergy injections should be prepared to treat an adverse reaction and have available various medications and equipment (please see the enclosed American College of Allergy, Asthma and Immunology's Position Statement).

It is also important that you remain in the office where you receive your injection for 30 minutes following your injection and that a physician be present during that time Adjustments in your dosage sometimes are necessary when you have worsening of your nasal symptoms or asthma from a cold or allergen exposure. Similarly, dosage adjustments are sometimes necessary if you have large bumps at your injection site or have hay fever symptoms, asthma, or other symptoms following your injection. You should inform the nurse or physician monitoring your injections if you are having increased symptoms or problems before or after your injections. The instructions accompanying your allergen vaccine contain information about adjusting your dose when such changes in your symptoms are present or have occurred.

Together, we can control your allergic problems. Help us help you by receiving your shots on a regular basis. Please feel free to call on us if you have any questions about your injections or injection schedule. We look forward to seeing you at your next office visit.

Sincerely ,

Ah Choo, M.D., F.A.A.A.A.I.

Enclosure: Position Statement on: Administration of immunotherapy outside of the prescribing allergist facility *Drug and Anaphylaxis Committee of ACAAI. Ann Allergy Asthma and Immunol 1998;81: 101-102.* The readers can obtain copies of this document through the American College of Allergy, Asthma and Immunology website www.ACAAI.org and click on the link to the practice resource center or go to the direct address at: http://www.acaai.org/position_statement.html

Modified with permission of Dr. Richard Lockey, M.D.

Figure 15   Letter to patient who will receive immunotherapy in an outside office. (Provided with permission from Division of Allergy and Immunology, Department of Internal Medicine, University of South Florida College of Medicine, Tampa, Florida.)

Dr. Ah Choo
Address: 665 Rosebud Lane
Hollywood, Fl. 33424
Telephone: 645-123-4444 Fax: 645-123-4567
Certified by the American Board of Allergy and Immunology

INJECTIONS ADMINISTERED AT AN OUTSIDE MEDICAL FACILITY

Please complete the following if the allergen vaccine will be administered at an outside medical facility.

I have read (if new patient) or re-read (if established patient) all the information about allergy injections, and I agree that I will not attempt to administer my vaccines to myself nor will I permit anyone who is not a licensed physician or under the supervision of a licensed physician to administer these vaccines. Released with American College of Allergy, Asthma and Immunology Position Statement and the patient's allergy injection form attached.

Patient (or parent if minor)_____Date:_____

Witness_____

FACILITY WHERE IMMUNOTHERAPY INJECTIONS WILL BE ADMINISTERED:
_____

Enclosure: Position Statement on: Administration of immunotherapy outside of the prescribing allergist facility *Drug and Anaphylaxis Committee of ACAAI. Ann Allergy Asthma and Immunol 1998;81: 101-102.* The readers can obtain copies of this document through the American College of Allergy, Asthma and Immunology website www.ACAAI.org and click on the link to the practice resource center or go to the direct address at: http://www.acaai.org/position_statement.html

Modified with permission of Richard Lockey, MD

Figure 16   Consent form for patient to sign if receiving immunotherapy outside of the prescribing allergist's office. (Provided with permission from Division of Allergy and Immunology, Department of Internal Medicine, University of South Florida College of Medicine, Tampa, Florida.)

Richard F. Lockey, M.D.   Roger W. Fox, M.D.   Dennis K. Ledford, N1.D.

13801 Bruce B. Downs Boulevard, Suite 502 Tampa, Florida 33613 - (813) 971-9743

PATIENT INSTRUCTIONS / CONSENT FORM FOR ALLERGY SKIN TESTING

Skin testing is a method to test for allergic antibodies. A test consists of introducing small amounts of the suspected substance, allergen, into the skin and recording the response 20 minutes after application. A positive reaction consists of a wheal (swelling) and flare (surrounding area of redness.) Interpreting the clinical significance of the skin tests requires correlation of the test results with the patient's clinical history.

The skin test methods used

> **Prick-Puncture Method**: The skin is prick-punctured with an applicator coated with allergen.
> **Intradermal Method:** This method consists of injecting small amounts of an allergen into the superficial layers of the skin.
> **Multi-Test Method (optional):** Allergen solutions are placed on individual prongs of a multi-prong plastic device which is placed firmly on the back for 5 to 10 seconds, then removed.

You will be skin tested to important Tampa Bay airborne allergens and possibly some of the major foods. These include trees, grasses, weeds, molds, dust mites, danders, and if necessary, milk, egg, pecan, peanut, and a few other foods. The skin testing appointment takes approximately 2-3 hours. Prick-puncture tests will be performed on your back and intradermal tests on your upper arms. If you have a specific allergic sensitivity to an allergen, a red, raised, itchy hive (caused by histamine release into the skin) appears on your skin within 15-20 minutes. These positive reactions, which will itch, will gradually disappear over 30-60 minutes, and typically, no treatment is necessary. Occasionally local swelling at a test site will begin 4 to 8 hours after the skin tests, particularly at the sites of the intradermal tests. These reactions are not serious and will gradually disappear over the next week or so. You may be scheduled for skin testing to antibiotics, caines, venoms, or other biological agents and the same guidelines apply.

MEDICATIONS YOU NEED TO STOP BEFORE TESTING: Antihistamines block the histamine response making the tests inaccurate.

- No prescription or over-the-counter antihistamines should be used 4-5 days prior to the scheduled skin testing. These include cold tablets, sinus tablets, hay fever medications, or oral treatments for itchy skin. Some of the names of these drugs include Actifed, Allegra, Allerx, Benadryl, Dimetapp, Dristan, Drixoral, Rondec, Trinalin, Zyrtec, and many others. Do not take Allerx-D on the day of the test. If you have any questions whether or not you are using an antihistamine, please ask the nurse or doctor. Astelin nasal spray, Clarinex, Claritin, Phenergan. and Histussin HC need to be stopped 7 days prior to the skin test.

- Medications, such as over-the-counter sleeping medicines (e.g., Nytol and Tylenol PM) should be stopped 4-5 days before skin tests. Prescribed drugs, such as amitriptyline hydrochloride (Elavil), hydroxyzine (Atarax), doxepin (Sinequan), imipramine (Tofranil), Remeron, and meclizine (Antivert), and others have antihistaminic activity and should be discontinued at least 2 weeks prior to skin tests. Please make the doctor and nurse aware of the fact that you are taking these medications so that you may be advised as to how long prior to testing you should stop taking them.

Figure 17 Allergy skin testing information and consent sheet. (Provided with permission from Division of Allergy and Immunology, Department of Internal Medicine, University of South Florida College of Medicine, Tampa, Florida.)—Continued

<u>MEDICATIONS YOU MAY CONTINUE</u>

- Continue on your intranasal allergy sprays such as (Beconase/ Vancenase. Flonase, Nasacort. Nasalide, Nasonex, Rhinocort, or TriNasal.) Afrin or Sudafed may be used temporarily but not the day of the testing.
- Continue asthma inhalers (albuterol [Proventil. Ventolin], beclomethasone (Beclovent, Vanceril). Advair. Aerobid. Alupent, Atrovent, Azmacort, Brethaire, Flovent. Foradil, Intal, Pulmicort. Serevent. Tilade), and oral theophylline (Theo-Dur, T-Phyl, Uniphyl. Theo-24, etc.) They do not interfere with skin testing and should be used as prescribed.
- Please let the nurse know if you are taking a beta-blocker. such as Inderal, Lopressor, Tenormin, and others, and do not take a beta-blocker the morning of your skin test. Also, let the nurse know if you are taking an antidepressant or a monoamine oxidase inhibitor.
➢ Fasting is not necessary, and please avoid sunburns.

Please let the physician and the nurse know:
a) If you are pregnant.
b) If you have a fever or are wheezing.
c) All medications you are taking (bring a list).

PROCEED TO SECOND FLOOR, SUITE 203. Skin testing will be done at this facility. A physician is present since occasional reactions may require therapy. These reactions may consist of any of the following symptoms: itchy eyes, nose, or throat; nasal congestion; runny nose; tightness in the throat or chest; increased wheezing; lightheadedness; faintness; nausea and vomiting; hives; generalized itching; and shock, the latter under extreme circumstances. A severe reaction to skin testing has never occurred in this office, however, if one would occur, the staff is trained to treat you. A separate follow-up appointment will be scheduled and your physician will make further recommendations regarding your treatment.

- **WE REQUEST THAT YOU DO NOT BRING SMALL CHILDREN WITH YOU WHEN YOU ARE SCHEDULED FOR SKIN TESTING UNLESS THEY ARE ACCOMPANIED BY ANOTHER ADULT WHO CAN SIT WITH THEM IN THE RECEPTION ROOM.**

- **ANYONE 17 YEARS OF AGE OR YOUNGER, MUST BE ACCOMPANIED BY A PARENT OR LEGAL GUARDIAN DURING THE ENTIRE PROCEDURE AND VISIT WITH THE PHYSICIAN. IF A PATIENT UNDER 17 YEARS OF AGE IS NOT ACCOMPANIED BY A PARENT OR LEGAL GUARDIAN, A WRITTEN CONSENT MUST BE SIGNED BY THE PARENT OR LEGAL GUARDIAN.**

- **IT IS IMPERATIVE THAT YOU ARE ON TIME FOR THIS APPOINTMENT.**

- **PLEASE DO NOT CANCEL YOUR APPOINTMENT SINCE THE TIME SET ASIDE FOR YOUR SKIN TESTING IS YOURS FOR WHICH SPECIAL ALLERGENS ARE PREPARED.**

- **IF FOR ANY REASON YOU MUST CHANGE YOUR SKIN TEST APPOINTMENT, PLEASE GIVE US AT LEAST 72 HOURS NOTICE. A LAST MINUTE CHANGE RESULTS IN LOSS OF VALUABLE TIME THAT ANOTHER PATIENT COULD HAVE UTILIZED.**

- **IF YOU ARE ON A MANAGED CARE HEALTH PLAN, PLEASE CONTACT YOUR PRIMARY CARE PHYSICIAN TO INITIATE THIS <u>REFERRAL</u>.**

Figure 17 Continued

PATIENT'S NAME:

You will be tested to selected foods. Have you had any reactions /allergies to egg, wheat, milk, fish, soy, peanut, pecan, shellfish, or others?   YES_____NO_____

PHYSICIAN_____ DATE SIGNED_____

I have read the patient information form on allergy skin testing and understand it. The opportunity has been provided for me to ask questions regarding the potential side effects of allergy skin testing and these questions have been answered to my satisfaction. I understand that every precaution consistent with the best medical practice will be carried out to protect me against any reaction to skin testing.

PATIENT_____   DATE SIGNED_____

*Testing takes 2-3 hours

PARENT or LEGAL GUARDIAN_____   DATE SIGNED_____

As parent or legal guardian, I understand that I must accompany my child throughout the entire procedure and visit.

WITNESS_____   DATE SIGNED_____

Richard F. Lockey, M.D.   Roger W. Fox, M.D.   Dennis K Ledford, M.D.

TO BE COMPLETED BY NURSE (circle)

TYPE OF SKIN TEST:_____

SKIN TEST II   MULTI - I II III   VENOM   PCN   FOOD   OTHER_____

Rev. 5/02

Figure 17   Continued

Richard F. Lockey, M.D.   Roger W. Fox, M.D.   Dennis K. Ledford, M.D.
ALLERGY, ASTHMA & IMMUNOLOGY ASSOCIATES OF TAMPA BAY

Antihistamines block the histamine response making the skin test results inaccurate.

Please STOP these medications prior to your skin testing procedure:		
MEDICATION	5 DAYS PRIOR	7 DAYS PRIOR
ACTIFED	X	
ALLEGRA	X	
ALLERX	X	
ASTELIN		X
BENADRYL	X	
CLARINEX		X
CLARITIN		X
DIMETAPP	X	
DRISTAN	X	
HISTUSSIN HC		X
PHENERGAN		X
ZYRTEC	X	
NYTOL AND TYLENOL PM	X	
ALL OTHER DRUGS CONTAINING ANTI-HISTAMINE, SUCH AS ALLEREST, CONTAC, DRIXORAL, FEDAHIST, NOVAFED, ETC.	X	

ALLERX-D - DO NOT TAKE ON THE DAY OF THE TESTING.

The following list of medications should be STOPPED 14 days before your skin test, but only with the approval of your prescribing physician

ANTIVERT (MECLIZINE)   REMERON (MIRTAZAPINE)

ATARAX (HYDROXYZINE)   SINEQUAN (DOXEPIN)

ELAVIL (ANITRIPTYLINE HCL)   TOFRANIL (IMIPRAMINE)
LET THE NURSE KNOW IF YOU ARE TAKING BETA BLOCKERS OR MAO INHIBITORS.

Rev. 8/02

Figure 17   Continued

Richard F. Lockey, M.D. Roger W. Fox, M.D.
Dennis K. Ledford, M.D. 13801 Bruce B. Downs
Boulevard, Suite 502 Tampa, Florida 33613 -
(813) 971-9743

BACKGROUND INFORMATION ABOUT IMMUNOTHERAPY
(ALLERGY SHOTS) FOR PATIENTS

The history and physical examination is the most important part of an allergy evaluation; skin tests are informative and help to make a diagnosis of specific allergy. Treatment must take into account your symptoms, allergic exposure, previous treatments, and other medical problems.

Allergy shots

Allergen immunotherapy or "allergy shots" are prescribed for allergic patients who have symptoms not adequately controlled by environmental control measures or medications, which persist and require medications, or who do not wish to be on continuous medications to treat their allergy.

Effectiveness

Allergen immunotherapy (allergy shots) "turn down" allergic reactions to common pollens, molds, and dusts. The initial 6 to 12 month course of allergy shots gradually decreases your sensitivity and continuation of injections leads to further improvement. The injections do not cure patients but diminish sensitivities, resulting in fewer symptoms and use of fewer medications. It is important to maintain shots at the proper time interval; missing shots for a short time or for some other problem is acceptable but an appropriate adjustment in the dose of vaccine is necessary thereafter. Please see us if you miss receiving your injections for longer than a month.

Figure 18 Immunotherapy information sheet. (Provided with permission from Division of Allergy and Immunology, Department of Internal Medicine, University of South Florida College of Medicine, Tampa, Florida.)—Continued

How long are shots given?

The goal of the maintenance schedule is to increase the interval between shots to 2 to 4 weeks depending upon your allergy sensitivities. Upon obtaining acceptable results for several years, the shots may be discontinued. Some patients will continue to do well and some will have a slight increase in symptoms which are usually controllable with medications; others require resumption of allergy injections in time. You will be re-evaluated periodically while on injections: changes in the allergen vaccine or injection schedule may be necessary to obtain optimal results.

Reactions to allergy infections

It is possible to have an allergic reaction to the allergy injection itself. Reactions can be local (swelling at the injection site) or systemic (affecting the rest of the body). Systemic reactions include hay fever type symptoms, hives, flushing, lightheadedness, and/or asthma, and rarely, life threatening reactions. Some conditions can make allergic reactions to the injections more likely: heavy natural exposure to pollen during a pollen season and exercise after an injection. Reactions to injections can occur, however, even in the absence of these conditions. If any symptoms occur immediately or within hours of your injection, please inform the nurse before you receive your next injection.

PATIENTS MUST WAIT IN THE DOCTOR'S OFFICE FOR 30 MINUTES AFTER RECEIVING AN ALLERGY INJECTION(S). A PHYSICIAN SHOULD BE PRESENT DURING THIS TIME.

....

IF YOU ARE ON A MANAGED HEALTH CARE PLAN, YOU WILL NEED TO OBTAIN A REFERRAL FOR THE VISIT WHEN YOU OBTAIN YOUR ALLERGEN VACCINE VIAL AND/OR IF YOU WISH TO RECEIVE YOUR INJECTIONS IN OUR OFFICE. PLEASE CONTACT YOUR PRIMARY CARE PHYSICIAN TO OBTAIN REFERRALS FOR VIALS AND/OR INJECTIONS. A CO-PAYMENT IS DUE EVERY TIME YOU ARE GIVEN AN ALLERGY INJECTION. PROCEED TO SUITE 504 FOR NEW VIAL APPOINTMENTS.

....

Figure 18   Continued

Richard F. Lockey, M.D. Roger W. Fox, M.D.
Dennis K. Ledford, M.D. 13801 Bruce B.
Downs Boulevard, Suite 502 Tampa, Florida
33613 - (813) 971-9743

IMMUNOTHERAPY PATIENT CONSENT FORM

Immunotherapy, hyposensitization, or allergy injections should be administered at a medical facility with a medical physician present since occasional reactions may require immediate therapy. These reactions may consist of any or all the following symptoms: itchy eyes, nose, or throat; nasal congestion; runny nose; tightness in the throat or chest; coughing; increased wheezing; lightheadedness; faintness; nausea and vomiting; hives; generalized itching; and shock, the last under extreme conditions. Reactions, even though unusual, can be serious and rarely, fatal. You are required to wait in the medical facility in which you receive the injections for 30 minutes after each injection. If the patient is 17 years of age or younger, a parent or legal guardian must be present during the waiting period. I verify that I (or patient) am not taking beta blocker medications or that if I am, I have discussed the risks/benefits of doing so with my physician (see information sheet).

I have read (if new patient) or re-read (if established patient) the patient information sheet on immunotherapy and understand it. The opportunity has been provided for me to ask questions regarding the potential side effects of immunotherapy and these questions have been answered to my satisfaction. I understand that every precaution consistent with the best medical practice will be carried out to protect me against such reactions. I also agree that if I have an allergic reaction to the injections that the physician-in-charge has permission to treat said reaction.

I acknowledge the fact with my signature that I am authorizing the office to bill for allergen vaccines, even if, for any reason, I decide not to initiate the allergen immunotherapy program after the vaccine has been made. Vaccines may be prepared up to 1½ weeks prior to my appointment. I agree to obtain prior authorization, if needed, from my insurance plan.

PATIENT_____ **DATE SIGNED**_____

PARENT OR LEGAL GUARDIAN_____**DATE SIGNED**_____

As parent or legal guardian, I understand that I must accompany my child throughout the entire 30-minute wait.

WITNESS_____**DATE SIGNED**_____

Figure 19 Immunotherapy consent form. (Provided with permission from Division of Allergy and Immunology, Department of Internal Medicine, University of South Florida College of Medicine, Tampa, Florida.)

Richard F. Lockey, M.D. Roger W. Fox,
M.D. Dennis IC Ledford, M.D. 13801 Bruce
B. Downs Boulevard, Suite 502 Tampa,
Florida 33613 - (813) 971-9743

NAME_____ DATE_____

GUIDELINES FOR ADMINSTRAION OF ALLERGY INJECTIONS

TECHNIQUE: Use a 1 ml disposable syringe, graduated to 0.01 cc and a 26 to 27 gauge, ^{1}/2-inch needle. Carefully withdraw the proper amount from the appropriate vial. Check to make sure that it is the correct patient, dilution dose and that the patient did not have any problems with the previous injection. Cleanse the skin area with an alcohol swab before injecting. Give the injection SUBCUTANEOUSLY in the posterior aspect of the middle third of the arm. Gently draw back the plunger before injecting and if blood appears, withdraw the needle and select a new site. Slowly inject the vaccine, withdraw the needle, and apply pressure over the injection site for 15 to 20 seconds. Do not massage the area. Either arm may be used or the arms may be alternated. Allergy vaccines should be refrigerated. Avoid exposure to sunlight, extreme heat of freezing. Do not administer expired vaccines. If the patient is receiving injections twice a week, he or she will need to wait 72 hour between injections.

A 30 MINUTE WAIT: Each patient is required to wait 30 minutes in a medical facility after receiving allergy infection treatment so that he or she can be checked for local and systemic reactions.
NOTE: DO NOT give allergy injection unless a medical doctor is present during the 30 minute waiting period.

MANAGEMENT OF LOCAL REACTIONS:

a.   Negative: Swelling to 15 mm (dime size) - progress according to schedule.

b.   Swelling (as in a welt) 15-20 mm (not redness) (dime to nickel size) - repeat same dosage.

c.   Swelling 20-25 mm (quarter size) - return to the last dosage, which caused no reaction.

d.   Swelling persisting more than 12 hours or over 25 mm (quarter size or larger) - decrease dosage by 50%*

*If reduced dose is tolerated, increase dose by 0.05 to 0.1 cc weekly and resume schedule. If local reaction occurs again, patient should be seen in our office with dosage sheet.

SYSTEMIC REACTIONS: Systemic reactions resulting from injections can occur in the course of treating allergic patients. Most reactions occur within 30 minutes after an injection. Symptoms may include itching of the palms of the hands or other parts of the body, sneezing, coughing, hives (welts), swelling of the lips or other areas, and shortness of breath. With severe reactions, acute asthma or a drop in blood pressure (anaphylaxis) may occur. Fatalities can occur with allergy injections. At the first sign of a systemic reaction epinephrine 1: 1.000 should be administered intramuscularly (about 0.3 cc in adults and 0.01 mg/kg in children under 30 kg). Epinephrine should be repeated if improvement does not occur within minutes, almost immediately. A venous tourniquet applied above the injection site may decrease absorption of the allergen. Any hypotension or loss of consciousness should be treated first with epinephrine, followed by rapid intravenous infusion of normal saline solution. Epinephrine, 1:10,000 w/v,

Figure 20   Immunotherapy administration guidelines. (Provided with permission from Division of Allergy and Immunology, Department of Internal Medicine, University of South Florida College of Medicine, Tampa, Florida.)—Continued

can be given, as needed, intravenously, with severe anaphylaxis. Oxygen by mask or cannula should be administered if respiratory or circulatory compromise occurs. Antihistamines. glucocorticosteroids, vasopressors, and other medications may be necessary for a severe reaction. After a systemic reaction additional allergy injections should not be given. The patient must return to our office with all records for re-evaluation before injections are resumed.

MISSED INJECTIONS:

SERIES- before reaching maintenance or build-up

Up to 7 days, continue as scheduled.
8 to 13 days, repeat previous dose.
14 to 21 days, reduce pervious dose by 25%.' 21 to 28 days reduce previous dose by 50%*
*Increase dose per week one injection (each vial if more than one vial) as directed on the immunotherapy schedule until maintenance reached.

MAINTENANCE

Up to 10 days, repeat last dose.
11 to 20 days, reduce dose by 25%. *
21 to 28 days, reduce dose by 50%. *
Over 28 days, contact physician for orders.
*Increase dose by 0.05 cc one injection per week (each vial, if more than one vial) until maintenance is reached, and then resume maintenance schedule.

NOTE: If patient has a history of previous systemic reactions or severe asthma from injection therapy, discuss with the attending physician if any additional reduction is necessary. If you have any questions, please call our office at: _____

ADDITIONAL CONSIDERATIONS:

a. **REFRIGERATION:** If vaccine is exposed to extreme heat or cold or if serum becomes cloudy, do not administer and notify the office.
b. **EXPIRATION DATE:** Allergen vaccines have an expiration date and should be replaced after this date.
c. **BETA-BLOCKERS:** Oral and eye drop beta-blockers used concomitantly with allergen immunotherapy are a potential problem because the medications can potentate anaphylaxis. **ADVISE THE PHYSICIAN IF PATIENT IS TAKING ANY OF THESE OR OTHER BETA BLOCKERS.**
    a. Blocadren, Brevibloc, Corgard, Inderal, Inderal-LA, Lopressor, Normozide, Sectral Tenoretoz, Tenormin Visken and Inderide.
d. **PREGNANT:** If the patient becomes pregnant, do not administer any further injections. Have her schedule an appointment with our office and bring vials and all dosage sheets for this visit.
e. **WHEEZING:** DO NOT GIVE ALLERGY SHOTS IF THE PATIENT IS HAVING ASTHMA SYMPTOMS.
f. **ASTHMATICS:** PEAK FLOW MEASUREMENT SHOULD IDEALLY BE DONE WHEN THE PATIENT IS SYMPTOMATIC. IF THE MEASUREMENT IS LESS THAN 70% OF PREDICTED, THE ALLERGY INJECTION SHOULD NOT BE GIVEN.
g. **EXERCISE:** NO EXERCISE FOR AT LEAST 2 HOURS AFTER RECEIVING INJECTION.
h. Always send the dosage sheet(s) and remaining vials with the patient when he or she is returning to the office for new vials and/or dosage adjustments.

Rev. 7/00

Figure 20 Continued

REFERENCES

1. American Academy of Allergy, Asthma and Immunology's Immunotherapy Committee's Guidelines for Reporting Immediate Allergy Skin Test Results. Academy News 1999.
2. Li JT, Lockey RF, Bernstein IL, Portnor JM Nicklas RA. Allergen immunotherapy: A practice parameter. Ann Allergy Asthma Immunol 2003; 90(suppl).
3. Simons EF. Ancestors of Allergy. New York: Global Medical Communications, 1994.
4. Bousquet J, Lockey R, Malling HJ. WHO position paper. Allergen immunotherapy: Therapeutic vaccines for allergic diseases. Allergy 1998; 53(suppl 54).

5. Des Roches A, Paradis L, Knani J et al. Immunotherapy with a standardized *Dermatophagogoides pteronyssinus* extract: V. Duration of the efficacy of immunotherapy after cessation. Allergy 1996; 51:430–434.
6. Lower T, Henry J, Mandik L, Janosky J, Friday G. Compliance with allergen immunotherapy. Ann Allergy 1993; 70:480–482.
7. Cohn JR, Pizzi A. Determinants of patients compliance with immunotherapy. J Allergy Clin Immunol 1993; 91:734–737.
8. Sade K, Berkun Y, Kivity S, Shalit M. Knowledge and expectations of patients receiving aeroallergen immunotherapy. Ann Allergy Asthma Immunol 2003; 91:444–449.

Index

About the Editors

RICHARD F. LOCKEY is Professor of Medicine, Pediatrics, and Public Health; the Joy McCann Culverhouse Chair in Allergy and Immunology; and Director of the Division of Allergy and Immunology, University of South Florida College of Medicine, Tampa. Additionally, he is Chief of the Section of Allergy and Immunology, James A. Haley Veterans' Hospital, Tampa, Florida. He is the editor or coeditor of 10 books and the author or coauthor of more than 500 professional publications. A past president and Fellow of the American Academy of Allergy, Asthma and Immunology, and a Fellow of the American College of Physicians American Society of Internal Medicine, Dr. Lockey is a member of several societies, including the American Thoracic Society, the Clinical Immunology Society, and the American Medical Association, and is on the board of the World Allergy Organization. He received the B.S. degree (1961) from Haverford College, Pennsylvania, the M.S. degree (1972) from the University of Michigan, Ann Arbor, and the M.D. degree (1965) from Temple University School of Medicine, Philadelphia, Pennsylvania.

SAMUEL C. BUKANTZ is Professor of Medicine, Professor of Medical Microbiology and Immunology (Research), and Emeritus Director of the Division of Allergy and Immunology, University of South Florida College of Medicine, Tampa. Additionally, he is a Consultant at James A. Haley Veterans' Hospital, Tampa, Florida. He is the author, coauthor, editor, or coeditor of over 110 professional publications and is emeritus editor of the journal *Hospital Practice*. A Fellow and past vice president of the American Academy of Allergy, Asthma, and Immunology, he is also a Fellow of the American College of Physicians, the American College of Allergy, Asthma, and Immunology, the American Society for Clinical Investigation (Emeritus), and the Central Society for Clinical Research (Emeritus), as well as a member of the Society for Experimental Biology and Medicine, the American Medical Association, and the Florida Medical Association. He received the B.S. degree (1930) from Washington Square College, New York University, and the M.D. degree (1934) from New York University College of Medicine.

JEAN BOUSQUET is Professor of Pulmonary Medicine, Montpellier University, France; Head of the Allergy and Clinical Immunology Department of the Chest Clinic at the Montpellier University Hospital; Head of the Laboratory on Asthma Inflammation,

INSERM U454, Montpellier, France; and Director of the Allergy Programme of the Institut Pasteur, Paris, France. The author, editor, or coeditor of numerous professional publications including *Immunotherapy in Asthma,* and *Airway Remodeling,* and *Upper and Lower Respiratory Disease* (Marcel Dekker, Inc.), he is an associate editor of *Allergy,* a Fellow of the American College of Allergy and Immunology, and a Corresponding Fellow of the American Academy of Allergy and Immunology. Dr. Bousquet received the M.D. and Ph.D. degrees (both 1979) from Montpellier University Hospital, Montpellier, France.

ISBN 0-8247-5650-9

90000